OTOLARYNGOLOGY
HEAD AND NECK
SURGERY

OTOLARYNGOLOGY—HEAD AND NECK SURGERY

VOLUME ONE
Part One: General Considerations in Head and Neck
Charles W. Cummings, editor
Paul W. Flint, associate editor
Part Two: Face
Charles J. Krause, editor
J. Regan Thomas, associate editor

VOLUME TWO
Part Three: Nose
Charles J. Krause, editor
J. Regan Thomas, associate editor
Part Four: Paranasal Sinuses
Charles J. Krause, editor
J. Regan Thomas, associate editor
Part Five: Salivary Glands
David E. Schuller, editor
K. Thomas Robbins, associate editor
Part Six: Oral Cavity/Oropharynx/Nasopharynx
David E. Schuller, editor
K. Thomas Robbins, associate editor

VOLUME THREE
Part Seven: Neck
David E. Schuller, editor
K. Thomas Robbins, associate editor
Part Eight: Larynx/Hypopharynx, Trachea/Bronchus and Esophagus
John M. Fredrickson, editor
Bruce H. Haughey, associate editor
Part Nine: Thyroid/Parathyroid
John M. Fredrickson, editor
Bruce H. Haughey, associate editor

VOLUME FOUR
Part Ten: Ear and Cranial Base
Lee A. Harker, editor
Part Eleven: Vestibular System
Lee A. Harker, editor
Part Twelve: Facial Nerve
Lee A. Harker, editor
Part Thirteen: Auditory System
Lee A. Harker, editor
Part Fourteen: External Ear
Lee A. Harker, editor
Part Fifteen: Eustachian Tube, Middle Ear, and Mastoid
Lee A. Harker, editor
Part Sixteen: Inner Ear
Lee A. Harker, editor
Part Seventeen: Skull Base
Lee A. Harker, editor

VOLUME FIVE
Pediatric Otolaryngology
Mark A. Richardson, editor

VOLUME TWO

OTOLARYNGOLOGY HEAD & NECK SURGERY

THIRD EDITION

EDITED BY

Charles W. Cummings, M.D.
Andelot Professor and Chairman
Department of Otolaryngology-Head and Neck Surgery
Johns Hopkins University School of Medicine
Baltimore, Maryland

John M. Fredrickson, M.D.
Lindburg Professor and Head
Department of Otolaryngology
Washington University School of Medicine
St. Louis, Missouri

Lee A. Harker, M.D.
Deputy Director
Boys Town National Research Hospital
Vice Chairman
Department of Otolaryngology and Human Communication
Creighton University School of Medicine
Omaha, Nebraska

Charles J. Krause, M.D.
Professor
Department of Otolaryngology-Head and Neck Surgery
University of Michigan Medical School
Ann Arbor, Michigan

David E. Schuller, M.D.
Professor and Chairman
Department of Otolaryngology
Director, Arthur G. James Cancer Hospital and Research Institute
Co-Director, Comprehensive Cancer Center
The Ohio State University
Columbus, Ohio

Mark A. Richardson
Vice Chairman
Department of Otolaryngology-Head and Neck Surgery
Johns Hopkins University School of Medicine
Baltimore, Maryland

with 333 contributors
with 4061 illustrations, including 18 color plates

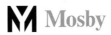

St. Louis Baltimore Boston Carlsbad Chicago Minneapolis New York Philadelphia Portland
London Milan Sydney Tokyo Toronto

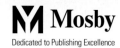

Publisher: Geoff Greenwood
Editor: Robert Hurley
Developmental Editor: Lauranne Billus
Associate Developmental Editor: Marla Sussman
Editorial Assistant: Jori Matison

Project Managers: Christopher Baumle, David Orzechowski
Senior Production Editor: Stacy M. Loonstyn
Production Editor: Susie Coladonato
Designer: Carolyn O'Brien
Manufacturing Manager: William A. Winneberger, Jr.

Third Edition
Copyright © 1998 by Mosby–Year Book, Inc.
Previous editions copyrighted 1986, 1993

Printed in the United States of America
Composition by Maryland Composition
Printing/binding by Maple Vail Book Manufacturing Group

Mosby–Year Book, Inc.
11830 Westline Industrial Drive
St. Louis, Missouri 63146

Library of Congress Cataloging-in-Publication Data

Otolaryngology—head and neck surgery / edited by Charles W. Cummings.
— 3rd ed.
    p.   cm.
    Includes bibliographical references and index.
    Contents: v. 1. General considerations in head and neck, face /
[edited by] Charles W. Cummings, Charles J. Krause — v. 2. Nose,
paranasal sinuses, salivary glands, oral
cavity/oropharynx/nasopharynx / [edited by] Charles J. Krause, David
E. Schuller — v. 3. Neck, larynx/hypopharynx, trachea/bronchus and
esophagus, thyroid/parathyroid / [edited by] David E. Schuller, John
M. Fredrickson — v. 4. General (ear and cranial base), vestibular
system, facial nerve, auditory system, external ear, eustachian
tube, middle ear, and mastoid, inner ear, skull base / [edited by]
Lee A. Harker — v. 5. Pediatric otolaryngology / [edited by] Mark
A. Richardson.
    ISBN 0-8151-2136-9 (set)
    1. Otolaryngology, Operative. 2. Head—Surgery. 3. Neck—
Surgery. I. Cummings, Charles W. (Charles William), 1935– .
    [DNLM: 1. Otorhinolaryngologic Diseases—surgery. WV 168 088
1998]
RF51.086   1998
617.5′ 1059—DC21
DNLM/DLC
for Library of Congress   98-2986
                                                              CIP

Figures 1, 2A, 2C, 3, 5 through 20, 22 through 26, 28, 29, and 31 in Chapter 56 are used with permission from Som PM, Curtin HD: *Head and neck imaging*, ed 3, St Louis, 1996, Mosby.

97 98 99 00 01 / 9 8 7 6 5 4 3 2 1

Associate Editors

Paul W. Flint, M.D.
Associate Professor
Department of Otolaryngology-Head and Neck Surgery
Johns Hopkins University School of Medicine
Baltimore, Maryland

Bruce H. Haughey, M.B., Ch.B.
Associate Professor
Department of Otolaryngology-Head and Neck Surgery
Washington University School of Medicine
Director
Division of Head and Neck Surgical Oncology
Barnes-Jewish Hospital
St. Louis Children's Hospital
St. Louis, Missouri

K. Thomas Robbins, M.D.
Professor and Chairman
Department of Otolaryngology-Head and Neck Surgery
University of Tennessee College of Medicine
Director
Head and Neck Oncology Program
Memphis, Tennessee

J. Regan Thomas, M.D.
Professor and Chairman
Department of Otolaryngology-Head and Neck Surgery
St. Louis University School of Medicine
Director
The Facial Plastic Surgery Center
St. Louis, Missouri

Contributors

Paul J. Abbas, Ph.D.
Professor
University of Iowa
Iowa City, Iowa

George L. Adams, M.D., F.A.C.S.
Professor and Head
Department of Otolaryngology
University of Minnesota
Minneapolis, Minnesota

David Albert, M.B., B.S., F.R.C.S.
Pediatric Otolaryngologist
Hospital for Sick Children
London, United Kingdom

James Alex, M.D.
Assistant Professor
Section of Otolaryngology
Director
Division of Facial Plastic and Reconstructive Surgery
Yale University School of Medicine
New Haven, Connecticut

Eugene L. Alford, M.D., F.A.C.S.
Assistant Professor
Department of Otorhinolaryngology
Baylor College of Medicine
Department of Dermatology and Division of Plastic Surgery
The Methodist Hospital and St. Luke's Hospital
Houston, Texas

Carl M. Allen, D.D.S., M.S.D.
Professor
Oral and Maxillofacial Pathology
Ohio State University
College of Dentistry
Columbus, Ohio

Mário Andrea, M.D., Ph.D.
Head and Chairman
Department of Otolaryngology
Faculty of Medicine
Lisbon, Portugal

Edward L. Applebaum, M.D.
Professor and Department Head
Department of Otolaryngology-Head and Neck Surgery
University of Illinois at Chicago
Chief of Service
Department of Otolaryngology-Head and Neck Surgery
University of Illinois Eye and Infirmary
Chicago, Illinois

Richard L. Arden, M.D., F.A.C.S.
Assistant Professor
Department of Otolaryngology-Head and Neck Surgery
Wayne State University
Detroit, Michigan

William B. Armstrong, M.D.
Adjunct Associate Professor
Department of Otolaryngology-Head and Neck Surgery
University of California, Irvine, College of Medicine
Orange, California

Moisés A. Arriaga, M.D., F.A.C.S.
Adjunct Associate Professor of Surgery
Otorhinolaryngology and Neurosurgery
Director
Hearing and Balance Center
Allegheny University of the Health Sciences
Associate Clinical Professor of Otolaryngology
University of Pittsburgh School of Medicine
Pittsburgh, Pennsylvania

H. Alexander Arts, M.D.
Assistant Professor
Division of Otology/Neurotology
Department of Otolaryngology-Head and Neck Surgery
University of Michigan
Ann Arbor, Michigan

Douglas Backous, M.D.
Otology, Neurotology and Skull Base Surgery
Virginia Mason Medical Center
Seattle, Washington

Shan R. Baker, M.D.
Professor of Otolaryngology
Chief, Division of Facial Plastic Surgery
University of Michigan Medical School
Ann Arbor, Michigan

Thomas Balkany, M.D., F.A.C.S., F.A.A.P.
Hotchkiss Professor and Vice-Chair
Department of Otolaryngology
Professor
Department of Neurological Surgery and Pediatrics
University of Miami School of Medicine
Director
University of Miami Ear Institute
Miami, Florida

Robert W. Baloh, M.D.
Professor of Neurology and Surgery (Head and Neck)
UCLA School of Medicine
Los Angeles, California

Fuad M. Baroody, M.D.
Assistant Professor of Otolaryngology-Head and Neck
    Surgery and Pediatrics
University of Chicago, Pritzker School Of Medicine
Chicago, Illinois

Robert W. Bastian, M.D.
Associate Professor of Otolaryngology
Loyola University of Chicago Stritch School of Medicine
Chicago, Illinois

John G. Batsakis, M.D.
Professor and Chairman
Department of Pathology
University of Texas M.D. Anderson Cancer Center
Houston, Texas

Carol A. Bauer, M.D.
Assistant Professor
Division of Otolaryngology-Head and Neck Surgery
Southern Illinois University School of Medicine
Springfield, Illinois

Daniel G. Becker, M.D.
Instructor
Department of Otolaryngology
University of Pennsylvania
Philadelphia, Pennsylvania

Ferdinand F. Becker, M.D.
Clinical Assistant Professor
University of Florida College of Medicine
Medical Director
Facial Plastic Surgery Center, Inc.
Vero Beach, Florida

G. Jan Beekhuis, M.D.
Clinical Professor
Department of Otolaryngology
Wayne State University School of Medicine
Detroit, Michigan

Bruce Benjamin, F.R.A.C.S., D.L.O., F.A.A.P.
Clinical Professor
Department of Otolaryngology
University of Sydney
Royal Alexandra Hospital for Children
Royal North Shore Hospital
Sydney, Australia

Joseph E. Berg, M.D.
Fellow
Division of Plastic and Reconstructive Surgery
University of Missouri
Kansas City, Missouri

Carol M. Bier-Laning, M.D.
Assistant Professor
Department of Otorhinolaryngology
University of Texas Southwestern Medical Center
Dallas, Texas

James Blaugrund, M.D.
Instructor
Department of Otolaryngology-Head and Neck Surgery
Johns Hopkins University School of Medicine
Baltimore, Maryland

Andrew Blitzer, M.D., D.D.S.
Professor of Clinical Otolaryngology
Columbia University College of Physicians and Surgeons
Director
New York Center for Voice and Swallowing Disorders
New York, New York

George Gordon Blozis, D.D.S., M.S.
Professor Emeritus
Ohio State University College of Dentistry
Consultant
Dayton Virginia Medical Center
Columbus Children's Hospital
Columbus, Ohio

Charles D. Bluestone, M.D.
Eberly Professor of Pediatric Otolaryngology
University of Pittsburgh School of Medicine
Director of Pediatric Otolaryngology
Children's Hospital of Pittsburgh
Pittsburgh, Pennsylvania

Derald E. Brackmann, M.D.
Clinical Professor
Otolaryngology/Head and Neck Surgery and Neurosurgery
University of Southern California School of Medicine
President
House Ear Clinic, Inc.
Los Angeles, California

Gregory H. Branham, M.D., F.A.C.S.
Associate Professor
Department of Otolaryngology-Head and Neck Surgery
St. Louis University School of Medicine
St. Louis, Missouri

Mitchell F. Brin, M.D.
Associate Professor
Department of Neurology
Director
Division of Movement Disorders
Mt. Sinai Medical Center
New York, New York

Kenneth B. Briskin, M.D.
Attending Surgeon
Crozer-Chester Memorial Hospital
Riddle Memorial Hospital
Chester, Pennsylvania

Patrick E. Brookhouser, M.D.
Father Flanagan Professor and Chairman
Department of Otolaryngology and Human
    Communication
Creighton University School of Medicine
Director
Boys Town National Research Hospital
Omaha, Nebraska

Allan C. D. Brown, M.B., Ch.B., F.R.C.A.
Associate Professor
Departments of Anesthesiology and Otorhinolaryngology-
    Head and Neck Surgery
University of Michigan Medical School
Director
The Difficult Airway Clinic
University of Michigan Medical Center
Ann Arbor, Michigan

Karla Brown, M.D.
Fellow
Boston Children's Hospital
Harvard Medical Center
Boston, Massachusetts

Mark T. Brown, M.D.
Assistant Professor
Department of Otolaryngology-Head and Neck Surgery
Johns Hopkins University School of Medicine
Baltimore, Maryland

Orval E. Brown M.D.
Associate Professor
University of Texas Southwestern Medical Center at Dallas
Children's Medical Center of Dallas
Dallas, Texas

J. Dale Browne, M.D., F.A.C.S
Assistant Professor Of Otolaryngology
Bowman Gary School of Medicine of Wake Forest
   University
Winston-Salem, North Carolina

Daniel Buchbinder, M.D.
Associate Professor
Department of Oral, Maxillo-Facial Surgery and
   Otolaryngology
Mt. Sinai School of Medicine
Chief of Oral Maxillo-Facial Surgery
Mt. Sinai Medical Center
New York, New York

Robert M. Bumsted, M.D.
Professor
Department of Otolaryngology and Bronchoesophagology
Rush Medical College
Chicago, Illinois

Michael Cannito, Ph.D., CCC-SLP
Associate Professor
School of Audiology and Speech-Language Pathology
University of Memphis
Adjunct Associate Professor
Department of Otolaryngology-Head and Neck Surgery
University of Tennessee College of Medicine
Memphis, Tennessee

Roy D. Carlson, M.D.
Senior Clinical Instructor
Department of Otolaryngology
Temple University School of Medicine
Philadelphia, Pennsylvania
Memorial Hospital of Burlington County
Mt. Holly, New Jersey

Alan B. Carr, D.M.D., M.S.
Associate Professor
Director
Department of Maxillofacial Prosthetics
Ohio State University College of Dentistry
A.G. James Cancer Hospital and Research Institute
Columbus, Ohio

Roy R. Casiano, M.D.
Associate Professor
Department of Otolaryngology
University of Miami School of Medicine
Director
Center for Sinus and Voice Disorders
Sylvester Comprehensive Cancer Center
Miami, Florida

Sujana S. Chandrasekhar, M.D.
Assistant Professor of Clinical Surgery
University of Medicine and Dentistry of New Jersey-
   New Jersey Medical School
Director of Otology/Neurotology
University of Medicine and Dentistry of New Jersey-
   University Hospital
Newark, New Jersey

Mack L. Cheney, M.D.
Assistant Professor
Harvard Medical School
Director
Facial Plastic and Reconstructive Surgery
Massachusetts Eye and Ear Infirmary
Boston, Massachusetts

Sukgi S. Choi, M.D.
Assistant Professor
Department of Otolaryngology and Pediatrics
George Washington University
Children's National Medical Center
Washington, D.C.

Richard A. Chole, M.D., Ph.D.
Lindburg Professor and Head
Department of Otolaryngology-Head and Neck Surgery
Washington University School of Medicine
St. Louis, Missouri

Moo-Jin Choo, M.D.
Fellow
Department of Otolaryngology
University of California, Davis, Medical Center
Sacramento, California

James M. Chow, M.D.
Associate Professor
Loyola University
Loyola University Medical Center
Maywood, Illinois

John E. Clemons, M.D.
Clinic Instructor
University of Wisconsin
Madison, Wisconsin
Gundersen Lutheran Medical Center
LaCrosse, Wisconsin

Ross A. Clevens, M.D.
Director
The Center for Facial Cosmetic Surgery
Melbourne and Palm Bay, Florida

Lanny Garth Close, M.D.
Howard W. Smith Professor and Chairman
Department of Otolaryngology-Head and Neck Surgery
Columbia University College of Physicians and Surgeons
Director
Department of Otolaryngology-Head and Neck Surgery
Columbia Presbyterian Medical Center
New York, New York

D. Thane Cody, II, M.D.
Fellow in Head and Neck Oncologic and Microvascular
    Surgery
Department of Otolaryngology-Head and Neck Surgery
University of Iowa
Iowa City, Iowa

Noel L. Cohen, M.D.
Professor and Chairman
Department of Otolaryngology
New York University Hospital and Bellevue Hospital
New York, New York

Newton Coker, M.D.
Clinical Professor
Bobby R. Alford Department of Otorhinolaryngology and
    Communicative Sciences
Baylor College of Medicine
Director
Texas Center for Hearing and Balance
Houston, Texas

Jeffrey J. Colton, M.D.
Clinical Assistant Professor
Department of Otolaryngology
University of Michigan, Ann Arbor
Henry Ford Hospital
Detroit, Michigan

Philippe Contencin, M.D.
University of Paris
Hopital St. Vincent-De-Paul
Paris, France

Cheryl S. Cotter, M.D.
Fellow
Department of Pediatric Otolaryngology
Harvard Medical School
Boston Children's Hospital
Boston, Massachusetts

Robin T. Cotton, M.D.
Professor
Department of Otolaryngology and Maxillofacial Surgery
University of Cincinnati College of Medicine
Director
Department of Otolaryngology and Maxillofacial Surgery
Children's Hospital Medical Center
Cincinnati, Ohio

Marion E. Couch, M.D., Ph.D.
Assistant Professor
Johns Hopkins Hospital
Baltimore, Maryland

Mark S. Courey, M.D.
Assistant Professor
Department of Otolaryngology
Vanderbilt University
Medical Director
Vanderbilt Voice Center
St. Thomas Medical Center
Nashville, Tennessee

Roger L. Crumley, M.D.
Professor and Chairman
Department of Otolaryngology
University of California, Irvine, Medical Center
Orange, California

Bernard J. Cummings, M.B., Ch.B
Professor and Chair
Department of Radiation Oncology
University of Toronto
Chief
Department of Radiation Oncology
Princess Margaret Hospital
Toronto, Ontario, Canada

Charles W. Cummings, M.D.
Andelot Professor and Chairman
Department of Otolaryngology-Head and Neck Surgery
Johns Hopkins University School of Medicine
Baltimore, Maryland

Robert W. Dalley, M.D.
Associate Professor
Department of Radiology
University of Washington Medical Center
Seattle, Washington

Terence M. Davidson, M.D.
Professor
Department of Head and Neck Surgery
Associate Dean for Continuing Medical Education
University of California, San Diego, School of Medicine
San Diego, California

Larry E. Davis, M.D.
Professor of Neurology and Microbiology
University of New Mexico School of Medicine
Chief
Neurology Service
Albuquerque Veterans Administration Medical Center
Albuquerque, New Mexico

Antonio De La Cruz, M.D.
Clinical Professor
Department of Otolaryngology-Head and Neck Surgery
University of Southern California
Director of Education
House Ear Institute
Los Angeles, California

Steven R. DeMeester, M.D.
Assistant Professor
Department of Cardiothoracic Surgery
University of Southern California University Hospital
Los Angeles, California

Lawrence W. DeSanto, M.D.
Professor and Chairman Emeritus
Department of Otolaryngology-Head and Neck Surgery
Mayo Clinic
Scottsdale, Arizona

Leigh Anne Dew, M.D.
Resident Physician
University of Utah
Salt Lake City, Utah

Oscar Dias, M.D., Ph.D.
Assistant Professor
Department of Otolaryngology
Faculty of Medicine
Lisbon, Portugal

Robert A. Dobie, M.D.
Chairman and Thomas Walthall Folbre Professor
Department of Otolaryngology-Head and Neck Surgery
University of Texas Health Science Center
San Antonio, Texas

Timothy D. Doerr, M.D.
Department of Otolaryngology-Head and Neck Surgery
Wayne State University School of Medicine
Detroit, Michigan

Larry G. Duckert, M.D., Ph.D.
Professor
Department of Otolaryngology-Head and Neck Surgery
University of Washington School of Medicine
University of Washington Medical Center
Seattle, Washington

Newton O. Duncan, III, M.D.
Clinical Assistant Professor
Departments of Otorhinolaryngology and Pediatrics
Baylor College of Medicine
Co-Director
Texas Pediatric Otolaryngology Center
Houston, Texas

David W. Eisele, M.D.
Associate Professor
Department of Otolaryngology-Head and Neck Surgery
Johns Hopkins University School of Medicine
Director
Division of Head and Neck Surgery
Johns Hopkins Hospital
Baltimore, Maryland

Charles N. Ellis, M.D.
Professor and Associate Chair
Department of Dermatology
University of Michigan Medical School
Chief
Dermatology Service
Veterans Affairs Medical Center
Ann Arbor, Michigan

Jane M. Emanuel, M.D., F.A.C.S.
Assistant Professor
Department of Otolaryngology and Human Communication
Creighton University School of Medicine
Staff Otolaryngologist
Boys Town National Research Hospital
Omaha, Nebraska

Emily J. Erbelding, M.D., M.P.H.
Assistant Professor
Johns Hopkins University School of Medicine
Baltimore, Maryland

Ramon M. Esclamado, M.D.
Associate Professor
Department of Otolaryngology
Director
Division of Head and Neck Surgery
The Cleveland Clinic
Cleveland, Ohio

David N.F. Fairbanks, M.D.
Clinical Professor
Department of Otolaryngology
George Washington University School of Medicine
Sibley Memorial Hospital
Washington, D.C.

Michael L. Farrell, M.B.B.S., F.R.A.C.S.
Visiting Medical Officer
St. George Hospital
Liverpool Hospital
Sydney, New South Wales, Australia

Edward H. Farrior, M.D.
Clinical Associate Professor
University of South Florida
Tampa, Florida

Richard T. Farrior, M.D., F.A.C.S.
Clinical Professor
University of South Florida School of Medicine
Tampa, Florida
Clinical Professor
University of Florida School of Medicine
Gainesville, Florida

Willard E. Fee, Jr., M.D.
Edward C. and Amy H. Sewall Professor and Chairman
Stanford University Medical Center
Stanford, California

Berrylin J. Ferguson, M.D.
Assistant Professor
Department of Otolaryngology
University of Pittsburgh School of Medicine
Director
Sino-Nasal Disorders and Allergies
University of Pittsburgh Medical Center
Pittsburgh, Pennsylvania

Paul W. Flint, M.D.
Associate Professor
Department of Otolaryngology-Head and Neck Surgery
Johns Hopkins University School of Medicine
Baltimore, Maryland

Arlene A. Forastiere, M.D.
Associate Professor
Department of Medical Oncology
Johns Hopkins University
Baltimore, Maryland

L. Arick Forrest, M.D.
Assistant Professor
Department of Otolaryngology
Ohio State University
University Hospital Clinic
Columbus, Ohio

James W. Forsen, Jr., M.D.
Instructor
Pediatric Otolaryngology
Washington University School of Medicine
St. Louis, Missouri

Howard W. Francis, M.D.
Assistant Professor
Johns Hopkins University
Assistant Chief of Service
Johns Hopkins Hospital
Baltimore, Maryland

John M. Fredrickson, M.D.
Lindburg Professor and Head
Department of Otolaryngology
Washington University School of Medicine
Director
Implantable Hearing Aid Development Program
St. Louis, Missouri

John L. Frodel, M.D.
Associate Professor and Director
Division of Facial Plastic Surgery
Department of Otolaryngology-Head and Neck Surgery
John Hopkins University School of Medicine
Baltimore, Maryland

Nabil S. Fuleihan, M.D.
Chairman
Department of Otolaryngology-Head and Neck Surgery
Boston University Medical Center
Boston, Massachusetts

Ruth Gaare, J.D., M.P.H.
Academic Program Director
The Bioethics Institute
Johns Hopkins University
Baltimore, Maryland

Bruce J. Gantz, M.D.
Professor and Head
Department of Otolaryngology-Head and Neck Surgery
University of Iowa College of Medicine
Iowa City, Iowa

C. Gaelyn Garrett, M.D.
Assistant Professor
Department of Otolaryngology
Vanderbilt University Medical Center
Nashville, Tennessee

George A. Gates, M.D.
Professor
Department of Otolaryngology-Head and Neck Surgery
University of Washington School of Medicine
Director
Virginia Merrill Bloedel Hearing Research Center
Seattle, Washington

Scott M. Gayner, M.D.
Instructor in Otorhinolaryngology
Mayo Clinic
Rochester, Minnesota

Eric M. Genden, M.D.
St. Louis, Missouri

Douglas A. Girod, M.D.
Assistant Professor and Vice Chairman
Chief
Department of Otolaryngology
Veteran's Administration Medical Center
Kansas City, Missouri

Harvey S. Glazer, M.D.
Professor of Radiology
Washington University School of Medicine
St. Louis, Missouri

Jack L. Gluckman, M.D.
Professor and Chairman
Department of Otolaryngology-Head and Neck Surgery
University of Cincinnati
Cincinnati, Ohio

George S. Goding, Jr., M.D.
Associate Professor
University of Minnesota
Minneapolis Veterans Administration Medical Center
Minneapolis, Minnesota

W. Jarrard Goodwin, Jr., M.D., F.A.C.S.
Sylvester Professor and Chairman
Department of Otolaryngology
University of Miami School of Medicine
Director
Sylvester Comprehensive Cancer Center
University of Miami Hospitals and Clinics
Jackson Memorial Hospital
Miami, Florida

Michael P. Gorga, Ph.D.
Professor
Department of Otolaryngology and Human Communication
Creighton University School of Medicine
Director
Clinical Sensory Physiology Laboratory
Boys Town National Research Hospital
Omaha, Nebraska

H. Devon Graham, III, M.D., F.A.C.S.
Clinical Assistant Professor
Department of Otolaryngology-Head and Neck Surgery
Tulane University School of Medicine
New Orleans, Louisiana

Daniel O. Graney, M.D.
Associate Professor
Department of Biological Structure
University of Washington School of Medicine
Seattle, Washington

Steven D. Gray, M.D.
Associate Professor
University of Utah School Of Medicine
Primary Children's Medical Center
Alta View Hospital
Salt Lake City, Utah

William C. Gray, M.D.
Associate Professor
Department of Otolaryngology-Head and Neck Surgery
University of Maryland School of Medicine
Baltimore, Maryland

Roy C. Grekin, M.D.
Assistant Professor
Department of Dermatology
University of Michigan Medical School
Ann Arbor, Michigan

Andrew J. Griffith, M.D., Ph.D.
Chief Resident
Department of Otolaryngology-Head and Neck Surgery
University of Michigan Hospitals
Ann Arbor, Michigan

Kenneth M. Grundfast, M.D.
Professor of Otolaryngology and Pediatrics
Georgetown University School of Medicine
Washington, D.C.

Jerry Thomas Guy, M.D.
Clinical Professor of Medicine
Ohio State University
Director of Oncology
Park Medical Center
Regional Oncology Center at Park
Columbus, Ohio

Joseph Haddad, Jr., M.D.
Associate Professor and Vice Chairman
Department of Otolaryngology-Head and Neck Surgery
Columbia University College of Physicians and Surgeons
Director
Pediatric Otolaryngology-Head and Neck Surgery
Babies and Children's Hospital
New York, New York

Jeffrey R. Haller, M.D.
Assistant Professor
Division of Otolaryngology
University of Utah School of Medicine
Salt Lake City, Utah

Ronald C. Hamaker, M.D.
Physician
Head and Neck Surgery Associates
Indianapolis, Indiana

Ehab Y. Hanna, M.D.
Assistant Professor
Department of Otolaryngology-Head and Neck Surgery
University of Arkansas for Medical Science
Little Rock, Arkansas

Lee A. Harker, M.D.
Deputy Director
Boys Town National Research Hospital
Vice Chairman
Department of Otolaryngology and Human
  Communication
Creigton University School of Medicine
Omaha, Nebraska

Stephen G. Harner, M.D.
Professor of Otolaryngology
Mayo Medical School
Consultant, Department of Otolaryngology
Mayo Clinic
Rochester, Minnesota

Jeffrey P. Harris, M.D., Ph.D.
Chief of the Division of Head and Neck Surgery
University of California
San Diego, California

Donald F.N. Harrison, M.D., M.S., Ph.D., F.R.C.S.
Emeritus Professor
Departments of Laryngology and Otology
University of London
Royal National ENT Hospital
London, England

Bruce H. Haughey, M.B., Ch.B.
Associate Professor
Department of Otolaryngology
Washington University School of Medicine
Director
Division of Head and Neck Surgical Oncology
Barnes-Jewish Hospital
St. Louis Children's Hospital
St. Louis, Missouri

Gerald B. Healy, M.D.
Professor of Otology and Laryngology
Harvard Medical School
Otolaryngologist-in-Chief, Surgeon-in-Chief
Children's Hospital
Boston, Massachusetts

Arden K. Hegtvedt, D.D.S.
Assistant Professor
Department of Oral and Maxillofacial Surgery
Ohio State University
Columbus, Ohio

Jay P. Heiken, M.D.
Professor
Department of Radiology
Director
Abdominal Imaging
Co-Director
Body Computed Tomography
Mallinckrodt Institute of Radiology
Washington University School of Medicine
St. Louis, Missouri

David A. Hendrick, M.D.
Clinical Instructor
Veterans Administration Hospital
Denver, Colorado
Private Practice
Vail, Colorado

Hajime Hirose, M.D., D.M.Sc.
Professor
Department of Otolaryngology
School of Allied Health Sciences
Kitasato University and Univeristy Hospital
Sagamihara, Japan

William E. Hitselberger, M.D.
Neurosurgeon
St. Vincent's Hospital
Los Angeles, California

Henry T. Hoffman, M.D.
Associate Professor
Department of Otolaryngology
University of Iowa College of Medicine
Iowa City, Iowa

Lauren D. Holinger, M.D., F.A.C.S, F.A.A.P.
Professor
Department of Otolaryngology
Northwestern University School of Medicine
Head
Pediatric Otolaryngology
Children's Memorial Hospital
Chicago, Illinois

David B. Hom, M.D., F.A.C.S
Assistant Professor
Division of Facial Plastic and Reconstructive Surgery
Department of Otolaryngology-Head and Neck Surgery
University of Minnesota School of Medicine
Associate Physician
Department of Otoalryngology-Head and Neck Surgery
Facial Plastic Surgery
Hennepin County Medical Center
Minneapolis, Minnesota

Vicente Honrubia, M.D.
Professor and Director of Research
Division of Head and Neck Surgery
The Center of the Health Sciences
University of California
Los Angeles, California

John W. House, M.D.
Clinical Professor
Department of Otolaryngology
University of Southern California School of Medicine
House Ear Clinic
Los Angeles, California

Andrew F. Inglis, Jr., M.D.
Associate Professor
Department of Otolaryngology
University of Washington
Children's Hospital and Medical Center
Seattle, Washington

Robert K. Jackler, M.D.
Professor of Otolaryngology and Neurological Surgery
University of California Medical Center
San Francisco, California

John R. Jacobs, M.D.
Professor
Department of Otolaryngology and Radiation Therapy
Wayne State University School of Medicine
Director
Head and Neck Cancer Program
Karmanos Cancer Center
Detroit, Michigan

Ivo P. Janecka, M.D., F.A.C.S.
Director, Longwood Skull Base Program
Departments of Otolaryngology, Neurosurgery and Plastic
  Surgery
Harvard Medical School
Boston, Massachusetts

Pawel J. Jastreboff, M.D.
Professor
Department of Surgery and Physiology
University of Maryland School of Medicine
Director
University of Maryland Tinnitus and Hyperacusis Center
Baltimore, Maryland

Virginia W. Jenison, M.A.
Clinical Instructor
Department of Otolaryngology-Head and Neck Surgery
Washington University School of Medicine
St. Louis, Missouri

Herman Jenkins, M.D.
Professor
Baylor College of Medicine
Houston, Texas

Calvin M. Johnson, Jr., M.D.
Director
Hedgewood Surgical Center
New Orleans, Louisiana

Jonas T. Johnson, M.D.
Professor and Vice Chairman
Department of Otolaryngology
Director
Division of Head and Neck Oncology and Immunology
University of Pittsburgh School of Medicine
Pittsburgh, Pennsylvania

Timothy M. Johnson, M.D.
Assistant Professor
Department of Dermatology, Otolaryngology, Surgery
University of Michigan
Director
Cutaneous Surgery and Oncology Unit
Ann Arbor, Michigan

Kim Richard Jones, M.D., Ph.D.
Assistant Professor
Division of Otolaryngology-Head and Neck Surgery
University of North Carolina School of Medicine
University of North Carolina Hospitals
Chapel Hill, North Carolina

Sheldon S. Kabaker, M.D., F.A.C.S.
Associate Clinical Professor
Division of Facial Plastic Surgery
Department of Otolaryngology
University of California
San Francisco, California

Joel C. Kahane, M.D.
Professor
Director
Anatomical Sciences Laboratory
School of Audiology and Speech-Language Pathology
University of Memphis
Memphis, Tennessee

Michael Kaliner, M.D.
Clinical Professor
George Washington University School of Medicine
Medical Director
Institute of Asthma and Allergy
Washington Hospital/George Washington University
Washington, D.C.

William J. Kane, M.D.
Assistant Professor
Department of Plastic and Reconstructive Surgery
Mayo Clinic
Rochester, Minnesota

Dan H. Kelly, Ph.D.
Associate Professor
Department of Otolaryngology-Head and Neck Surgery
University of Cincinnati College of Medicine
Voice Pathologist
Barrett Cancer Center
ENT Voice Center
Cincinnati, Ohio

Eugene B. Kern, M.D.
Professor
Department of Otorhinolaryngologic Surgery
Endicott Professor of Medicine
Mayo Medical School
Mayo Clinic
Rochester, Minnesota

Robert C. Kern, M.D.
Assistant Professor
Northwestern Medical School
Northwestern Memorial Hospital
Chicago, Illinois

Maurice Morad Khosh, M.D.
Assistant Clinical Professor
Department of Otolaryngology-Head and Neck Surgery
Columbia University School of Medicine
St. Luke's/Roosevelt Hospital Center
New York, New York

S. Khosla, M.D.
Resident
Department of Otolaryngology
Washington University School of Medicine
St. Louis, Missouri

Paul R. Kileny, Ph.D.
Professor
Department of Otolaryngology
University of Michigan Medical School
Director
Audiology and Electrophysiology
University of Michigan Health Systems
Ann Arbor, Michigan

Sam E. Kinney, M.D.
Clinical Associate Professor
Department of Otolaryngology-Head and Neck Surgery
Case Western Reserve University
Head
Section of Otology and Neurotology
Cleveland Clinic Foundation
Cleveland, Ohio

Wayne Martin Koch, M.D.
Associate Professor
Department of Otolaryngology-Head and Neck Surgery
Johns Hopkins University and Hospital
Baltimore, Maryland

James A. Koufman, M.D.
Director
Center for Voice Disorders
Professor
Department of Otolaryngology
Bowman Gray School of Medicine
Wake Forest University Medical Center
Winston-Salem, North Carolina

Frederick K. Kozak, M.D., F.R.C.S.C.
Assistant Professor
University of British Columbia
Pediatric Otolaryngologist
B.C. Children's Hospital
Vancouver, British Columbia, Canada

Eric H. Kraut, M.D.
Professor of Medicine
Ohio State University
Arthur James Cancer Hospital Research Institute
Columbus, Ohio

Dario Kunar, M.D.
Instructor
Department of Otolaryngology-Head and Neck Surgery
Johns Hopkins University School of Medicine
Baltimore, Maryland

Ollivier Laccourreye, M.D.
Department of Otolaryngology-Head and Neck Surgery
Laennec Hospital
University of Rene-Descartes
Paris, France

Paul R. Lambert, M.D.
Professor, Director
Division of Otolaryngology-Neurology
Department Otolaryngology-Head and Neck Surgery
University of Virginia Medical Center
Richmond, Virginia

George E. Laramore, M.D., Ph.D.
Professor
Department of Radiation Oncology
University of Washington
Vice Chairman
Department of Radiation Oncology
University Medical Center
Seattle, Washington

Peter E. Larsen, D.D.S.
Associate Professor
Oral and Maxillofacial Surgery
Ohio State University
College of Dentistry
Columbus, Ohio

Daniel M. Laskin, D.D.S., M.S.
Professor and Chairman
Department Oral and Maxillofacial Surgery
Medical College of Virginia
Virginia Commonwealth University
Director
Temporomandibular Joint and Facial Pain Research Center
Richmond, Virginia

Richard E. Latchaw, M.D.
Professor
Department of Radiology and Neurosurgery
Chief, Interventional Neuroradiology Section
University of Miami School of Medicine
Miami, Florida

Susanna Leighton, B.Sc., F.R.C.S. (Orl)
Pediatric Otolaryngologist
Hospital for Sick Children
London, England

Donald Leopold, M.D.
Associate Professor
Johns Hopkins University
Department of Otolaryngology-Head and Neck Surgery
Baltimore, Maryland

Greg R. Licameli, M.D.
Assistant Professor
Director of Pediatric Otolaryngology
Department of Otolaryngology-Head and Neck Surgery
University of Illinois at Chicago
Chicago, Illinois

William H. Liggett, Jr., M.D., D.M.D., D.M.S.C.
Senior Clinical Fellow in Medical Oncology
Johns Hopkins School of Medicine
Baltimore, Maryland

Raleigh E. Lingeman, M.D.
Betty Morgan Professor
Department of Otolaryngology-Head and Neck Surgery
Indiana University School of Medicine
Indianapolis, Indiana

Neal M. Lofchy M.D., F.R.C.S.C.
Clinical Instructor
Rush Medical College
Rush-Presbyterian-St. Luke's Medical Center
Chicago, Illinois

Jeri Logemann, Ph.D.
Ralph and Jean Sundin Professor
Department of Communication Sciences and Disorders
Professor
Departments of Head and Neck Surgery and
    Neurology and Dental Prosthetics
Northwestern University Medical School
Director
Speech, Voice and Swallowing Service
Northwestern Memorial Hospital
Chicago, Illinois

Brenda L. Lonsbury-Martin, Ph.D.
Chandler Professor
Director of Research
Department of Otolaryngology Research Laboratories
University of Miami Ear Institute
University of Miami School of Medicine
Miami, Florida

Rodney P. Lusk, M.D.
Associate Professor
Department of Otolaryngology
Washington University School of Medicine
Otolaryngologist-in-Chief
St. Louis Children's Hospital
St. Louis, Missouri

Joseph P. Lynch, III, M.D.
Professor
Department of Internal Medicine
Division of Pulmonary and Critical Care Medicine
University of Michigan Medical Center
Ann Arbor, Michigan

Anna Lysakowski, Ph.D.
Assistant Professor
Department of Anatomy and Cell Biology
University of Illinois
Chicago, Illinois

Richard L. Mabry, M.D.
Professor
Department of Otorhinolaryngology
University of Texas Southwestern Medical Center
Dallas, Texas

Michael R. Macdonald, M.D., F.R.C.S.C.
Chief
Division of Head and Neck Surgery
Alameda County Hospital
Oakland, California
Director
Aesthetic Surgery Center
San Francisco, California

Eileen M. Mahoney, M.C., U.S.A., M.D.
Pediatric Staff
Otolaryngology Section
Brook Army Medical Center
Fort Sam
Houston, Texas

Robert H. Maisel, M.D.
Professor
Department of Otolaryngology
University of Minnesota
Chief
Department of Otolaryngology-Head and Neck Surgery
Facial Plastic Surgery
Hennepin County Medical Center
Minneapolis, Minnesota

Patrizia Mancini, M.D.
Policlinico Umberto
Ear Nose and Throat Department
University "La Sapienza"
Rome, Italy

Lee M. Mandel, M.D.
Co-Director
Head and Neck-Facial Plastic Surgery Associates of South
    Florida
Plantation, Florida

Scott C. Manning, M.D.
Associate Professor
Department of Otolaryngology-Head and Neck Surgery
University of Washington School of Medicine
Chief, Pediatric Otolaryngology-Head and Neck Surgery
Children's Hospital and Medical Center
Seattle, Washington

Lawrence J. Marentette, M.D.
Associate Professor
Director
Cranial Base Program
Department of Otolaryngology
University of Michigan
Ann Arbor, Michigan

James E. Marks, M.D.
Radiation Oncologist
Missouri Baptist Medical Center
St. Louis, Missouri

Bernard R. Marsh, M.D.
Professor
Department of Otolaryngology-Head and Neck Surgery
Johns Hopkins University
Johns Hopkins Hospital
Baltimore, Maryland

Michael Marsh, M.D.
The Holt-Krock Clinic
Ear, Nose and Throat
Fort Smith, Arkansas

Glen K. Martin, Ph.D.
Professor
Department of Otolaryngology
University of Miami Ear Institute
Miami, Florida

Robert H. Mathog, M.D.
Professor and Chairman
Wayne State University
Harper Hospital
Detroit, Michigan

Douglas E. Mattox, M.D.
Professor and Head
Department of Otolaryngology-Head and Neck Surgery
Emory University
Atlanta, Georgia

Ernest L. Mazzaferri, M.D., F.A.C.P.
Professor and Chairman
Ohio State University
Columbus, Ohio

Thomas V. McCaffrey, M.D., Ph.D.
Professor
Mayo Medical School
Consultant
Department of Otorhinolaryngology
Mayo Clinic
Rochester, Minnesota

Robert A. McCrea, Ph.D.
Associate Professor
Department of Pharmacological and Physiological Sciences
University of Chicago
Chicago, Illinois

Timothy M. McCulloch, M.D.
Associate Professor
Department of Otolaryngology-Head and Neck Surgery
University of Iowa College of Medicine
Iowa City, Iowa

Thomas J. McDonald, M.D., M.S., F.A.C.S., F.R.C.S. Irel.
Professor
Department of Otolaryngology
Mayo Medical School
Chairman
Department of Otorhinolaryngology
Mayo Clinic and Foundation
Rochester, Minnesota

John T. McElveen, Jr., M.D.
Head
Otology-Neurotology
Carolina Ear and Hearing Clinic
Director
Carolina Ear Research Institute
Raleigh Community Hospital
Rex Hospital
Wake Medical Center
Raleigh, North Carolina

Trevor J.I. McGill, M.D.
Associate Professor
Department of Otolaryngology
Harvard Medical School
Clinical Director of Otolaryngology
The Children's Hospital
Boston, Massachusetts

W. Frederick McGuirt, Sr., M.D.
Professor
Department of Otolaryngology
Bowman Gray School of Medicine
Wake Forest University
Winston-Salem, North Carolina

Christine M. Menapace, M.A.
U.S. Clinical Manager
Symphonix Devices, Inc.
San Jose, California

Saumil N. Merchant, M.D.
Assistant Professor
Department of Otology and Laryngology
Harvard Medical School
Massachusetts Eye and Ear Infirmary
Boston, Massachusetts

Charles A. Miller, Ph.D.
Assistant Research Scientist
Department of Otolaryngology-Head and Neck Surgery
University of Iowa
Iowa City, Iowa

Lloyd B. Minor, M.D.
Associate Professor
Department of Otolaryngology-Head and Neck Surgery
Johns Hopkins University
School of Medicine
Baltimore, Maryland

Mahmood Moosa, M.D.
Clinical Fellow In Endocrinology
Ohio State University, College of Medicine
Ohio State University Medical Center
Columbus, Ohio

Jeffrey Morray, M.D.
Professor
Department of Anesthesiology and Pediatrics
University of Washington School of Medicine
Director
Department of Anesthesia and Critical Care
Children's Hospital and Medical Center
Seattle, Washington

Michael R. Morris, M.D., F.A.C.S.
Staff Otolaryngologist
Moore Regional Hospital
Pinehurst Surgical Clinic
Pinehurst, North Carolina

John B. Mulliken, M.D.
Associate Professor of Surgery
Harvard Medical School
Director
Craniofacial Center
Division of Plastic Surgery
The Children's Hospital
Boston, Massachusetts

Craig S. Murakami, M.D.
Associate Professor
Department of Otolaryngology/Head and Neck Surgery
University of Washington School of Medicine
Seattle, Washington

Alan D. Murray, M.D.
Assistant Professor
Department of Otorhinolaryngology
University of Texas Southwestern Medical Center
Attending Physician
Children's Medical Center of Dallas
Dallas, Texas

Charles M. Myer, III, M.D.
Professor
Department of Otolaryngology and Maxillofacial Surgery
University of Cincinnati College of Medicine
Professor
Department of Otolaryngology and Maxillofacial Surgery
Children's Hospital Medical Center
Cincinnati, Ohio

Eugene N. Myers, M.D.
Professor and Chairman
Department of Otolaryngology
University of Pittsburgh School of Medicine
University of Pittsburgh Medical Center
Pittsburgh, Pennsylvania

Robert M. Naclerio, M.D.
Professor and Chief
Otolaryngology-Head and Neck Surgery
University of Chicago Pritzker School of Medicine
Chicago, Illinois

Joseph B. Nadol, Jr., M.D.
Walter Augustus Lecompte Professor and Chairman
Department of Otology and Laryngology
Harvard Medical School
Chief of Otolaryngology
Massachusetts Eye and Ear Infirmary
Boston, Massachusetts

Philippe Narcy, M.D.
Professeur of Otorhinology
Universite Paris VII
Chief
Department of Pediatric Otorhinolaryngology
Hopital Robert Debre
Paris, France

Julian Nedzelski, M.D., F.A.C.S. (C)
Otolaryngologist in Chief
Sunnybrook Health Science Centre
Professor and Chairman
Department of Otolaryngology
University of Toronto
Toronto, Ontario, Canada

H. Bryan Neel, III, M.D., Ph.D.
Professor and Past Chairman
Mayo Medical School
Consultant
Mayo Clinic
Rochester, Minnesota

John Niparko, M.D.
Professor
Department of Otolaryngology-Head and Neck Surgery
Director of Otology/ Neurotology
Johns Hopkins University School of Medicine
Baltimore, Maryland

Daniel W. Nuss, M.D., F.A.C.S.
Professor and Chairman
Department of Otolaryngology-Head and Neck Surgery
Louisiana State University School of Medicine
New Orleans, Louisiana

Rick M. Odland, M.D, Ph.D., F.A.C.S.
Assistant Professor
Division of Facial, Plastic and Reconstructive Surgery
Department of Otolaryngology-Head and Neck Surgery
University of Minnesota School of Medicine
Hennepin County Medical Center
Minneapolis, Minnesota

Michael J. O'Leary, M.D.
Assistant Clinical Professor of Surgery
Uniformed Services University of the Health Sciences
Chief
Neurotology/Skull Base Surgery Division
Department of Otolaryngology
Navy Medical Center
San Diego, California

Patrick J. Oliverio, M.D.
Instructor
Department of Diagnostic Radiology and Neuroradiology
Johns Hopkins Medical Institution
Staff Neuroradiologist
Radiological Consultants Association
Fairmount, Wisconsin

Bert W. O'Malley, Jr., M.D.
Associate Professor
Department of Otolaryngology-Head and Neck Surgery
Department of Oncology
Johns Hopkins University School of Medicine
Baltimore, Maryland

Lisa A. Orloff, M.D.
Associate Professor of Surgery
University of California, San Diego, Medical Center
San Diego, California

Rosemary J. Orr, M.D.
Clinical Associate Professor
University of Washington
Associate Clinical Director of Operating Room
Children's Hospital Medical Center
Seattle, Washington

Robert H. Ossoff, D.M.D., M.D.
Guy M. Maness Professor and Chairman
Associate Vice Chancellor for Health Affairs
Chief of Staff
Vanderbilt University Hospital
Executive Medical Director
Vanderbilt Voice Center
Nashville, Tennessee

Steven Otto, M.A.
Audiologist and Coordinator
Brain Stem Implant Project
House Ear Institute
Los Angeles, California

John F. Pallanch, M.D., M.S.
The Midlands Clinic
Sioux City, Iowa

William R. Panje, M.D.
Professor and Director
Head and Neck Reconstruction and Skull Base Surgery
Rush-Presbyterian-St. Luke's Medical Center
Chicago, Illinois

Stephen S. Park, M.D., F.A.C.S.
Director
Division of Facial, Plastic and Reconstructive Surgery
Department of Otolaryngology-Head and Neck Surgery
University of Virginia
Charlottesville, Virginia

Carl Patow, M.D., M.P.H., F.A.C.S.
Associate Professor
Johns Hopkins School of Medicine
Baltimore, Maryland

G. Alexander Patterson, M.D.
Joseph C. Bancroft Professor of Surgery
Washington University School of Medicine
Barnes-Jewish Hospital
St. Louis, Missouri

Larry J. Peterson, D.D.S.
Professor
Department of Oral-Maxillofacial Surgery
Ohio State University
Ohio State University Hospitals
Columbus, Ohio

Guy I. Petruzzelli, M.D., Ph.D.
Assistant Professor
Department of Otolaryngology-Head and Neck Surgery
Loyola University Hospital/Medical Center
Maywood, Illinois

Jay F. Piccirillo, M.D.
Assistant Professor
Department of Otolaryngology
Washington University School of Medicine
Barnes-Jewish Hospital
St. Louis, Missouri

Catherine A. Picken, M.D., F.A.C.S.
Assistant Professor
Department of Otolaryngology-Head and Neck Surgery
Georgetown University Medical Center
Washington Hospital Center
Washington, D.C.

Judy Pinborough-Zimmerman, Ph.D.
Adjunct Faculty
Department of Communicative Disorders
University of Utah
Program Director
Child Development Clinic
Utah Department of Health
Salt Lake City, Utah

Jennifer Parker Porter, M.D.
Resident
Department of Otorhinolaryngology
Baylor College of Medicine
Houston, Texas

Gregory N. Postma, M.D.
Assistant Professor
Department of Otolaryngology
Center for Voice Disorders of Wake Forest University
North Carolina Baptist Hospital
Winston-Salem, North Carolina

William P. Potsic, M.D.
Professor of Otorhinolaryngology Head and Neck Surgery
University of Pennsylvania School of Medicine
Director
Pediatric Otolaryngology and Human Communication
Children's Hospital of Philadelphia
Philadelphia, Pennsylvania

Frederic A. Pugliano, M.D.
Resident Physician
Washington University
Resident Physician
Barnes Hospital
St. Louis, Missouri

Vito C. Quatela, M.D.
Associate Professor
University of Rochester School of Medicine and Dentistry
Clinical Instructor
Strong Memorial Hospital Medical Center
Rochester, New York

Leslie E. Quint, M.D.
Department of Radiology
University of Michigan Medical Center
Ann Arbor, Michigan

C. Rose Rabinov, M.D.
Fellow
Department of Facial Plastic and Reconstructive Surgery
University of California, Irvine
Orange, California

Gordon D. Raphael, M.D.
Associate Clinical Professor
George Washington University School of Medicine
Washington, D.C.

Christopher Rassekh, M.D.
Assistant Professor
Department of Otolaryngology-Head and Neck Surgery
University of Texas Medical School at Galveston
Galveston, Texas

Elie E. Rebeiz, M.D.
Associate Professor
Tufts University School of Medicine
Director
Head and Neck Surgery
Tufts-New England Medical Center
Boston, Massachusetts

Lou Reinisch, Ph.D.
Assistant Professor and Director of Laser Research
Department of Otolaryngology
Vanderbilt University Medical Center
Nashville, Tennessee

Bradford D. Ress, M.D.
Chief Resident
Department of Otolaryngology
University of Miami School of Medicine
Miami, Florida

Dale H. Rice, M.D.
Tiber/Alpert Professor and Chair
Department of Otolaryngology-Head and Neck Surgery,
University of Southern California School of Medicine
Los Angeles, California

Brock D. Ridenour, M.D.
Assistant Professor and Director
Facial Plastic Surgery Division
Washington University School of Medicine
Barnes-Jewish Hospital
St. Louis, Missouri

K. Thomas Robbins, M.D., F.R.C.S.C., F.A.C.S.
Professor and Chairman
Department of Otolaryngology-Head and Neck Surgery
University of Tennessee, Memphis College of Medicine
Director
Head and Neck Oncology Program
Memphis, Tennessee

William D. Robertson, M.D.
Professor
Department of Radiology
University of Washington Medical Center
Seattle, Washington

Robert A. Robinson, M.D., Ph.D.
Professor
Department of Pathology
University of Iowa College of Medicine
Iowa City, Iowa

J. Thomas Roland, Jr., M.D.
Assistant Professor
Department of Otolaryngology
New York University School of Medicine
Bellevue Hospital
Manhattan VA Medical Center
New York, New York

Anne M. Rompalo, M.D.
Associate Professor
Johns Hopkins University School of Medicine
Johns Hopkins Hospital
Baltimore, Maryland

Richard M. Rosenfeld, M.D., M.P.H.
Associate Professor
Department of Otolaryngology
SUNY Health Science Center at Brooklyn
Director of Pediatric Otolaryngology
University Hospital Brooklyn and The Long Island College
   Hospital
Brooklyn, New York

Jay T. Rubinstein, M.D., Ph.D.
Assistant Professor
Department of Otolaryngology-Head and Neck Surgery
   and Physiology and Biophysics
University of Iowa
Iowa City, Iowa

Stephen J. Salzer, M.D.
Clinical Instructor in Surgery
Department of Otolaryngology
Yale University School of Medicine
New Haven, Connecticut

Peter A. Santi, Ph.D.
Professor
Departments of Otolaryngology and Neuroscience
University of Minnesota
Minneapolis, Minnesota

Clarence T. Sasaki, M.D.
Charles W. Ohse Professor
Yale School of Medicine
New Haven, Connecticut

Gordon H. Sasaki, M.D.
Chief, Plastic Surgery Section
St. Luke Medical Center
Pasadena, California

Steven D. Schaefer, M.D.
Professor and Chair
Department of Otolaryngology
New York Medical College
Chair
Department of Otolaryngology
New York Eye and Ear Infirmary and Affiliated Hospitals
Valhalla, New York

David Arthur Schessel, M.D., Ph.D.
Assistant Professor
Department of Otolaryngology and Neurosurgery
George Washington University
Assistant Professor
George Washington University Hospital
Washington, D.C.

David E. Schuller, M.D.
Professor and Chairman
Department of Otolaryngology
The Ohio State University
Director
Arthur G. James Cancer Hospital and Research Institute
Columbus, Ohio

Timothy A. Scott, M.D.
Private Practice
John Muir Hospital
Walnut Creek, California

Roy B. Sessions, M.D.
Professor and Chairman,
Department Otolaryngology-Head and Neck Surgery
Georgetown University
Washington, D.C.

Larry R. Severeid, M.D.
Clinical Assistant Professor
University of Wisconsin-Madison Medical School
Gunderson Clinic
LaCrosse, Wisconsin

Robert V. Shannon, Ph.D.
Head
Department of Auditory Implants and Perception
House Ear Institute
Los Angeles, California

Stanley M. Shapshay M.D., F.A.C.S.
Professor
Department Otolaryngology-Head and Neck Surgery
Tufts University School of Medicine
Otolaryngologist-in-Chief (Chairman)
Tufts-New England Medical Center
Boston, Massachusetts

Pramod K. Sharma, M.D.
Oncologic Surgery Fellow
Department of Otolaryngology
Ohio State University Medical Center
Columbus, Ohio

Clough Shelton, M.D., F.A.C.S.
Associate Professor
University of Utah, School of Medicine
Salt Lake City, Utah

Neil T. Shepard, Ph.D.
Associate Professor
Department of Otolaryngology
University of Michigan Medical School
Director
Vestibular Testing Center
University of Michigan Hospital and Clinics
Ann Arbor, Michigan

David A. Sherris, M.D.
Assistant Professor
Mayo Medical School
Senior Associate Consultant
Mayo Clinic
Rochester, Minnesota

Kevin A. Shumrick, M.D.
Associate Professor
Department of Clinical Otolaryngology
University of Cincinnati College of Medicine
Director
Division of Facial Plastic and Maxillofacial Trauma
University Hospital
Cincinnati, Ohio

Kathleen C.Y. Sie, M.D.
Assistant Professor
Department of Otolaryngology-Head and Neck Surgery
University of Washington School of Medicine
Children's Hospital and Medical Center
Seattle, Washington

Robert W. Seibert, M.D.
Professor
Department of Otolaryngology-Head and Neck Surgery
University of Arkansas for Medical Sciences
Chief, Pediatric Otolaryngology
Arkansas Children's Hospital
Little Rock, Arkansas

Marilyn J. Siegel, M.D.
Professor
Department of Radiology and Pediatrics
Washington University School of Medicine
St. Louis, Missouri

Patricia Silva, M.D.
Clinical Assistant Professor
Department of Radiology
University of Miami School of Medicine
Miami, Florida

Jonas Singer, M.D.
Visiting Professor
Mallinckrudt Institute of Radiology, St. Louis Program
Alton Memorial Hospital
Alton, Illinois

Margaret W. Skinner, Ph.D.
Professor
Director of Adult Cochlear Implant Program
Department of Otolaryngology-Head and Neck Surgery
Washington University School of Medicine
St. Louis, Missouri

Richard J.H. Smith, M.D.
Professor and Vice-Chairman
Department of Otolaryngology-Head and Neck Surgery
University of Iowa College of Medicine
Head
Division of Pediatric Otolaryngology
Director
Molecular Otolaryngology Research Laboratories
Iowa City, Iowa

Gordon B. Snow, M.D.
Professor and Chairman
Department of Otolaryngology-Head and Neck Surgery
Free University Hospital
Amsterdam, Netherlands

Robert C. Sprecher, M.D.
Assistant Professor
Departments of Otolaryngology and Pediatrics
Rainbow Babies and Children's Hospital
Case Western Reserve University
Cleveland, Ohio

Steven J. Staller, Ph.D.
Clinical Studies Manager
Cochlear Corporation
Englewood, Colorado

Robert B. Stanley, Jr., M.D., D.D.S.
Professor
Department of Otolaryngology-Head and Neck Surgery
University of Washington School of Medicine
Chief
Department of Otolaryngology-Head and Neck Surgery
Harborview Medical Center
Seattle, Washington

Patricia G. Stelmachowicz, Ph.D.
Professor
Department of Otolaryngology and Human Communication
Creighton University School of Medicine
Director, Audiological Services
Boys Town National Research Hospital
Omaha, Nebraska

Laura M. Sterni, M.D.
Fellow
Division of Pediatric Pulmonary
Johns Hopkins Children's Center
Baltimore, Maryland

Susan Strauss, M.D.
Assistant Professor
University of Washington
Children's Regional Hospital and Medical Center
Seattle, Washington

Barbara S. Stroer, M.A.
Assistant Professor
Department of Communication Disorders
Fontbonne College
St. Louis, Missouri
Coordinator of Audiology Services
St. Joseph Institute for the Deaf
Chesterfield, Missouri

James Y. Suen, M.D.
Professor and Chairman
Department of Otolaryngology-Head and Neck Surgery
University of Arkansas for Medical Sciences
University Hospital of Arkansas
Little, Arkansas

Gordon W. Summers, D.M.D, M.D.
Department of Otolaryngology-Head and Neck Surgery
Providence Medical Center
Portland, Oregon

Neil A. Swanson, M.D.
Professor and Chair
Department of Dermatology
Professor
Department of Otolaryngology-Head and Neck Surgery
Oregon Health Sciences University
Portland VA Medical Center
Lagacy Emmanuel Medical Center
St. Vincent's Hospital
Portland, Oregon

Jonathan M. Sykes, M.D.
Associate Professor
Facial Plastic Surgery
Department of Otolaryngology/Head and Neck Surgery
University of California, Davis, Medical Center
Sacramento, California

M. Eugene Tardy, Jr., M.D.
Professor
Department of Clinical Otolaryngology
Director, Division of Facial Plastic Surgery
University of Illinois College of Medicine
Chicago, Illinois

Steven A. Telian, M.D.
Associate Professor
University of Michigan Medical Center
Ann Arbor, Michigan

Fred F. Telischi, M.D.
Assistant Professor
Department of Otolaryngology
University of Miami Ear Institute
Miami, Florida

Jeffrey E. Terrell, M.D.
Assistant Professor
University of Michigan Medical Center
Ann Arbor, Michigan

Stanley E. Thawley, M.D.
Associate Professor
Department of Otolaryngology
Washington University School of Medicine
Chief Adult Division Department of Otolaryngology
Barnes-Jewish Hospital
St. Louis, Missouri

J. Regan Thomas, M.D.
Professor and Chairman
Department of Otolaryngology-Head and Neck Surgery
St. Louis University School of Medicine
Director
The Facial Plastic Surgery Center
St. Louis, Missouri

James N. Thompson, M.D.
Dean
Wake Forest University
Bowman Gray School of Medicine
North Carolina Baptist Hospital
Winston-Salem, North Carolina

R. David Tomlinson, Ph.D.
Associate Professor
Departments of Otolaryngology, Physiology, and Medicine
University of Toronto
Toronto, Ontario, Canada

Dean M. Toriumi, M.D.
Associate Professor
Division of Facial Plastic and Reconstructive Surgery
Department of Otolaryngology-Head and Neck Surgery
University of Illinois College of Medicine
Chicago, Illinois

Joseph B. Travers, Ph.D.
Associate Professor
Department of Oral Biology
Ohio State University College of Dentistry
Columbus, Ohio

David E. Tunkel, M.D.
Associate Professor
Department of Otolaryngology-Head and Neck Surgery
    and Pediatrics
Johns Hopkins University School of Medicine
Director
Division of Pediatric Otolaryngology
Johns Hopkins Hospital and Outpatient Center
Baltimore, Maryland

Mark L. Urken, M.D., F.A.C.S.
Professor and Chairman
Mt. Sinai School of Medicine
Mt. Sinai Medical Center
New York, New York

Thierry Van Den Abbeele, M.D.
Chef de Clinique
Faculte de Medecine Bichat
Assistant
Service D'or Pediatrique
Hopital Robert Debre
Paris, France

Isaäc van der Waal, D.D.S., Ph.D.
Head
Department of Oral Maxillofacial Surgery Pathology
Professor
Department of Oral Pathology
Hospital of the Free University
Amsterdam, Netherlands

Mark A. Varvares, M.D.
Instructor
Department of Otolaryngology and Laryngology
Harvard Medical School
Massachusetts Eye and Ear Infirmary
Boston, Massachusetts

David L. Walner, M.D.
Assistant Professor
Rush-Presbyterian St. Luke's Medical Center
Chicago, Illinois

Harrison G. Weed, M.D.
Assistant Professor
Department of Internal Medicine
Ohio State University College of Medicine
Arthur G. James Cancer Hospital and Research Institute
Columbus, Ohio

Mark S. Weinberger, M.D.
Clinical Instructor
University of Illinois at Chicago
Fellow
Facial Plastic and Reconstructive Surgery
University of Illinois Eye and Ear Infirmary
Chicago, Illinois

Gregory S. Weinstein, M.D.
Assistant Professor
Department of Otorhinolaryngology-Head and Neck
    Surgery
University of Pennsylvania
Philadelphia, Pennsylvania

Ralph F. Wetmore, M.D.
Associate Professor
Department of Otorhinolaryngology-Head and Neck Surgery
University of Pennsylvania School of Medicine
Children's Hospital Of Philadelphia
Philadelphia, Pennsylvania

Ernest A. Weymuller, Jr., M.D.
Professor and Chairman
Department Otolaryngology-Head and Neck Surgery
University of Washington School of Medicine
Seattle, Washington

Brian J. Wiatrak, M.D.
Associate Professor
Department of Surgery and Pediatrics
University of Alabama School of Medicine
Chief of Pediatric Otolaryngology
Children's Hospital of Alabama
Birmingham, Alabama

Gregory J. Wiet, M.S., M.D.
Fellow
Department of Pediatric Otolaryngology
University of Arkansas for Medical Sciences
Arkansas Children's Hospital
Little Rock, Arkansas

Ewain P. Wilson, M.B., B.Ch.
Assistant Professor
Director, Head and Neck Surgical Oncology
West Virginia University School of Medicine
Morgantown, West Virginia

Franz J. Wippold, II, M.D.
Associate Professor
Mallinckrodt Institute of Radiology
Washington University School of Medicine
Barnes-Jewish Hospital
St. Louis Children's Hospital
St. Louis, Missouri

Gregory T. Wolf, M.D.
Professor and Chair
Department of Otolaryngology
University of Michigan Medical School
Ann Arbor, Michigan

Gayle Ellen Woodson, M.D., F.A.C.S., F.R.C.S.C.
Professor
Department of Otolaryngology-Head and Neck Surgery
Director
Voice Disorder Clinic
University of Tennessee
Memphis, Tennessee

Audie L. Woolley, M.D.
Assistant Professor
Division of Otolaryngology-Head and Neck Surgery
University of Alabama School of Medicine
Birmingham, Alabama

Eiji Yanagisawa, M.D.
Clinical Professor
Department of Otolaryngology
Yale University School of Medicine
New Haven, Connecticut

Charles D. Yingling, Ph.D.
Director
Neurophysiologic Monitoring Service
University of California San Francisco Medical Center
San Francisco, California

Christine Yoshinaga-Itano, Ph.D.
Associate Professor
Department of Speech, Language, and Hearing Sciences
University of Colorado, Boulder
Boulder, Colorado

George H. Zalzal, M.D.
Associate Professor
Department of Otolaryngology and Pediatrics
George Washington University
Chairman
Department of Otolaryngology
Children's National Medical Center
Washington, D.C.

David S. Zee, M.D.
Departments of Neurology, Otolaryngology-Head and Neck
Surgery and Ophthalmology
Johns Hopkins University School of Medicine
Baltimore, Maryland

S. James Zinreich, M.D.
Associate Professor
Johns Hopkins Medical Institution
Baltimore, Maryland

Teresa A. Zwolan, Ph.D.
Director and Assistant
Cochlear Implant Program
Research Scientist
University of Michigan Medical Center
Ann Arbor, Michigan

Preface

Otolaryngology—Head and Neck Surgery was created to fill the needs for a contemporary, definitive textbook on the specialty of otolaryngology-head and neck surgery. The scope of the third edition is a testimonial to the tremendous expansion of knowledge in this specialty. Our desire is to record this expansion in a retrievable fashion so that these volumes become indispensable reference works. The third edition builds on the success of the past two editions. The reader will note new algorithms and boxed lists which serve to enhance learning.

The field of otolaryngology-head and neck surgery is represented in all of its diversity; the extensive interrelationship of its various components provided the skeleton for the table of contents. These volumes are intended as a detailed reference text and not as a surgical atlas: a definitive work, not an introductory overview. It is designed for residents and practitioners alike. We hope that our quest to document significant and up-to-date information in the specialty has been successful.

Another of our goals throughout the pages of this textbook is to acknowledge all those who have contributed to the specialty. Since significant medical expertise has no geographic boundaries, there are contributors from countries all over the world. Recognizing the unique aspects of pediatric otolaryngology-head and neck surgery, the editors have created an additional volume edited by Mark A. Richardson. This freestanding resource meets the global criteria of the comprehensive textbook.

To ensure continuity at the editorship level, Drs. Paul Flint, Bruce Haughey, K. Thomas Robbins, and J. Regan Thomas have assumed associate editorship roles in this expanded effort. It is hoped that the ecumenicism which combines the effort of all the contributors will further the excellence of those now associated with otolaryngology-head and neck surgery and provide the foundation for continued progress by the generations to follow. This third edition builds on the success of the first two. It is more comprehensive, is of broader scope, and continues the tradition established 11 years ago.

Table of Contents

PART THREE

NOSE

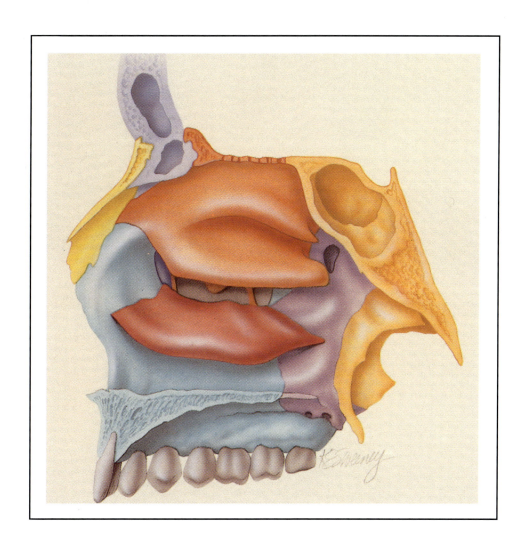

Chapter 40

Anatomy

Daniel O. Graney
Shan R. Baker

NASAL PYRAMID

The nose is a pyramidal structure with its apex projecting anteriorly and its base attached to the facial skeleton. The superior part of the base, consisting of the nasal bones, is raised and projects more anteriorly than the inferior part, creating the *bony vault* of the nose. In contrast, the more anterior part of the apex is formed by cartilage and is called the *cartilaginous vault*. The analogy to a pyramid can be misleading because it implies a quadrilateral base: the base of the nose is actually pear shaped and is named the *piriform aperture*. Furthermore, in the usual concept of a pyramid the base is at the bottom and, until one mentally rotates the image sideways, some confusion may occur. Nevertheless, the concept is useful and has been used extensively for a number of years, especially in the clinical literature. Hinderer[3] has described the nasal pyramid as consisting of four parts: the bony pyramid, the cartilaginous vault, the lobule, and the nasal septum.

Bony pyramid

If one traces the outline of the piriform aperture on a dried skull specimen, all of the parts distal to this outline are clearly the mobile parts of the nose. Beginning at the anterior nasal spine in the midline, the outline of the piriform aperture follows posterolaterally along the floor of the nasal cavity and then ascends the edge of the nasal notch on the anterior surface of the maxilla. Up to that point the plane of the maxillary bone is coronal, but there, the medial edge of the maxillary bone begins to rotate anteriorly until it projects into the sagittal plane that forms the frontal process of the maxilla. Rotation of the frontal process brings it into alignment with the surface of the nasal bone and completes the

outline of the piriform aperture. The projecting frontal processes of the maxillae and the paired nasal bones thus form the bony vault. An important clinical corollary of this is useful to the otolaryngologist when placing the lateral osteotomy to mobilize the bony pyramid. The osteotomy must be placed on the projecting frontal process, rather than on the flat coronal plane on the maxilla, to keep from entering the nasolacrimal canal.

The superior border of the nasal bones forms a suture with the frontal bone and is also an important point of support for the bony vault because of the buttress formed by the underlying nasal spine of the frontal bone. Also buttressing the nasal bones in the midsagittal plane is the perpendicular plate of the ethmoid bone. The midline point at which the nasal bones meet the frontal bone is termed the *nasion*. The inferior point of the midline suture between the nasal bones where they meet the upper lateral cartilages is the *rhinion*.

Cartilaginous vault

The cartilaginous vault consists of the upper lateral cartilages and the adjacent portion of the cartilaginous nasal septum. The details of the septum are discussed in the later section on nasal cavities.

The upper lateral nasal cartilages attach to the undersurface (deep surface) of the nasal bones and extend inferiorly (caudally) to form the cartilaginous portion of the dorsum of the nose (Fig. 40-1). Straatsma and Straatsma[6] describe the amount of overlap as varying between a minimum of 2 mm and a maximum of 15 mm. Laterally the cartilages have a modest attachment to the frontal process of the maxilla. In the midline, the upper lateral cartilages fuse or adhere to the cartilaginous portion of the nasal septum. The articulation between the caudal edge of the upper lateral cartilage and the lower lateral cartilage is of interest both anatomically and clinically. Anatomically, considerable debate exists regarding the precise arrangement of the articulation. Clinically the articulation is the site of the intercartilaginous incision during rhinoplasty.

Two studies of this region are particularly worthwhile because they employed histologic as well as dissection techniques. Drumheller[2] and Dion and others[1] all confirm the variability of the anatomy from specimen to specimen as well as from side to side (see Fig. 40-1). In 52% of 46 sides examined, Dion and others[1] found the articulation between the edges of the upper and lower lateral cartilages to be of an interlocked-scroll type. In this classification the edge of the upper lateral cartilage turns laterally and superiorly and appears concave when viewed from the lateral aspect. In contrast, the convex surface of the lower lateral cartilage turns medially and caudally to interlock with the upper lateral cartilage. The authors point out that in patients with this form of articulation, an intercartilaginous incision is actually intracartilaginous. Other variations noted by these authors (see Fig. 40-1) were classified as: 17% end to end; 20% over-lapping (similar to interlocking but with less curling of the edges); and 11% opposed (edge of the lower lateral cartilage is deep to the edge of the upper lateral cartilage).

Lobule

The nasal lobule includes the tip, lower lateral cartilages, alae, vestibular regions, and columella. Each lower lateral cartilage is shaped approximately in the form of an inverted U and consists of a medial and lateral crus. The crura under-

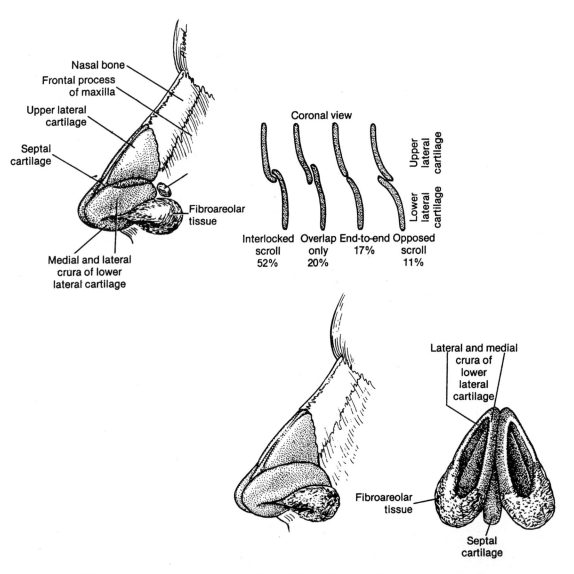

Fig. 40-1. Cartilages of the nose. Relationships of the caudal edge of the upper lateral cartilage to cranial edge of the lateral crus of the lower lateral cartilage. (Redrawn from Drumheller GW: *Anat Rec* 176:321, 1973.)

lying the skin of the vestibule thus contribute to the dome of the vestibule by providing the skeletal support for it. The width of the vestibular dome and any irregularity in it is usually reflective of the underlying anatomy of the lower lateral cartilage.

The medial crus enters the skin of the columella, where it articulates loosely with the medial crus of the opposite side. Posterior to the columella the vestibule's skin forms the membranous portion of the nasal septum and prevents fusion of the crura with the cartilaginous part of the nasal septum. Within the nares the skin of the vestibule abruptly changes at the limen vestibuli from a stratified nonkeratinizing type to the typical respiratory ciliated columnar epithelium.

NASAL MUSCLES

The nasal muscles include the procerus, nasalis (including both transverse and alar parts), levator labii superioris alaeque nasi, depressor septi, and the anterior and posterior dilator naris (Fig. 40-2). The procerus (along with the action of the forehead muscles) elevates the skin over the dorsum of the nose, whereas the nasalis acts as a compressor of the naris. Dilatation of the nostrils is accomplished by the dilators and the levator labii superioris alaeque part of the quadratus labii. Individuals with a well-developed depressor septi draw the nasal tip downward when smiling widely. Such individuals should have this muscle transected during rhinoplasty to help prevent migration of the nasal tip downward postoperatively, a common cause of "polly beak" deformity following rhinoplasty.

NASAL CAVITIES

The key to the nasal cavities is the underlying bony framework. Beyond the soft tissue of the nose the nasal cavities begin at the piriform aperture, as just described, and end at

the posterior choanae. Other limiting boundaries of the nasal cavities are the roof, floor, septal wall, and lateral wall.

Roof

The roof of the nasal cavity is formed anteriorly by the nasal bones, the nasal spine of the frontal bone, and the floor of the frontal sinus (Fig. 40-3). In its more horizontal midpart, the roof is formed by the cribriform plate of the ethmoid bone. Posteriorly the roof slopes down to the posterior choana along the anterial wall of the sphenoid sinus and the body of the sphenoid bone.

The cribriform plate is very thin and is penetrated by olfactory filaments carrying the meninges along with them. The subarachnoid space and endocranial cavity are intimately associated with the bone, making them particularly vulnerable during nasal and ethmoid surgery.

Floor

Approximately three fourths of the floor of the nasal cavity is formed by the palatal process of the maxillary bone. Posteriorly the remaining part is formed by the horizontal process of the palatine bone.

Nasal septum

The principal parts of the nasal septum are the vomer, perpendicular plate of the ethmoid bone, and quadrilateral cartilage. Additional bony reinforcements to the septum are the nasal crest and the anterior nasal spine formed by the midline fusion of the palatal processes of the maxillae. The membranous septum and columella divide the anterior part of the nasal cavities. The septum is seldom located completely in the midline, having deflections of varying degrees on all or portions of the bony or cartilaginous partitions. There may be expression from the septum into the nasal passage, particularly at the junction of the quadrilateral cartilage with the nasal crest. These "spurs" may be large enough to partially obstruct the nasal passage.

Lateral wall

The lateral wall of the nasal cavity is formed by the contribution of several bones: the nasal surface of the maxilla, inferior concha, superior and middle conchae of the ethmoid bone, and perpendicular plate of the palatine bone (see Fig. 40-3). The horizontally-aligned conchae each form a passage, or meatus, between the lateral nasal wall and the scroll-like edge of the medially projecting concha. Each meatus is named after the concha that forms its roof. In addition, a number of important landmarks are located in relation to the meatus as well as the openings of the paranasal sinuses and the nasolacrimal duct. Posterosuperior to the superior concha is the space known as the *sphenoethmoid recess* which is the drainage site of the sphenoid sinus (Fig. 40-4).

Inferior to the superior concha in the superior meatus, there are usually one or two openings for the posterior ethmoid air cells.

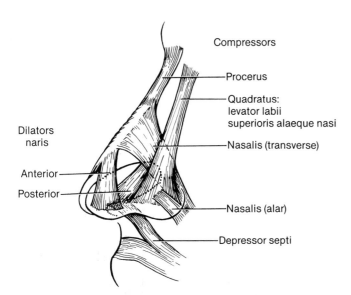

Fig. 40-2. Muscles of the nose.

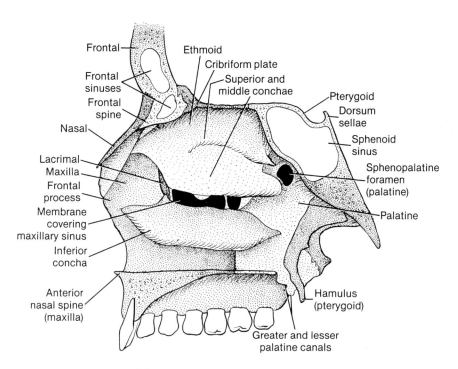

Fig. 40-3. Bones of the lateral wall of nasal cavity.

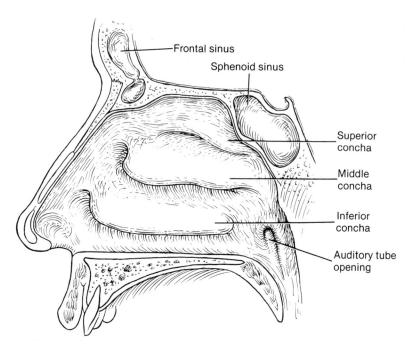

Fig. 40-4. Mucosal landmarks of the nasal cavity.

The posterior end of the middle concha points to the opening of the sphenopalatine foramen in the upper part of the vertical plate of the palatine bone. The sphenopalatine foramen actually represents a gap in the fusion between the sphenoid, palatine, and ethmoid bones rather than a specific opening in one of the bones. As described later, it transmits a neurovascular bundle to the nasal mucosa and is thus an important landmark for topical anesthetic administration or other clinical procedures.

The most complex of the three meatus lies deep to the middle concha. Elevation of the middle concha usually reveals a rounded prominence, the ethmoid bulla, which over-

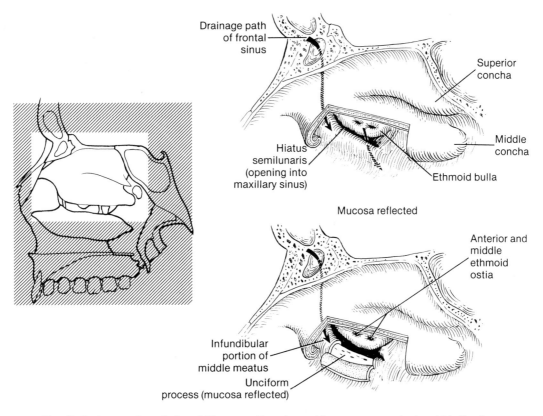

Drainage path
of frontal
sinus

Superior
concha

Middle
concha

Hiatus
semilunaris
(opening into
maxillary sinus)

Ethmoid bulla

Mucosa reflected

Anterior and
middle
ethmoid
ostia

Infundibular
portion of
middle meatus

Unciform
process (mucosa reflected)

Fig. 40-5. Osseous boundaries of hiatus semilunaris, unciform process, and ethmoid bulla. *Inset,* Area of nasal cavity magnified.

lies a slit-like opening—the hiatus semilunaris (Fig. 40-5). One to three openings on the surface of the bulla represent the drainage sites of the middle and anterior ethmoid cells. The hiatus semilunaris is in fact the opening of the maxillary sinus. Inferiorly the bony margin of the hiatus semilunaris is formed by the unciform process of the ethmoid bone; therefore, enlarging the hiatus semilunaris to place a drainage cannula is impossible without fracturing either the bulla or the unciform process. However, one should note that inferior to the unciform process to the level of the inferior concha there is no bony wall limiting the medial part of the maxillary sinus (see Fig. 40-3). This nonbony area is approximately circular (1 to 2 cm in diameter) and is closed only by a fibrous membrane, which is, in turn, covered by the nasal mucosa.

In the anterosuperior portion of the middle meatus, the middle concha narrows into the infundibulum, where an opening can be found for the frontal sinus. The proximity of the openings of the frontal sinus, as well as the anterior and middle ethmoid sinuses to the hiatus semilunaris, facilitates the spread of a sinusitis condition by allowing a purulent discharge from these sinuses to be carried into the maxillary sinus.

The key landmark in performing an intranasal ethmoidectomy is the middle concha. The anterior and middle ethmoid air cells lie inferior to this concha and drain into the middle meatus, whereas the posterior ethmoid cells lie above the middle concha and drain into the superior meatus. The anterior and middle ethmoid cells can be surgically exenterated without disturbing the concha. The posterior cells are removed through the surgical defect created by the anterior ethmoidectomy. In addition to marking the location of the ethmoid air cells, the attachment of the middle concha is a guide to other structures that the surgeon must be concerned about when performing an intranasal ethmoidectomy. The anterior attachment lies 1 cm inferior to the cribriform plate and 1 cm medial to the lamina papyracea. The posterior end of the concha marks the posterior limit of the ethmoid pneumatization and is 1 cm inferior and medial to the optic nerve.

No sinuses empty into the inferior meatus, but that meatus is the site of the nasolacrimal duct's drainage. The opening of the nasolacrimal duct is located in the anterosuperior portion of the meatus at the point that the inferior concha contacts the lateral wall of the nasal cavity. Because the inferior meatus is a common point of entry when placing a trocar during irrigation of a maxillary sinus, the nasolacrimal duct is at risk for injury. Similarly, in performing a Caldwell-Luc antrostomy, if bone is removed too far anteriorly, there is potential for damaging the duct, resulting in epiphora.

BLOOD SUPPLY OF THE NASAL CAVITIES

The blood supply of the nasal cavity is basically derived from two sources: the ophthalmic artery—a branch of the internal carotid system—and the maxillary artery, a branch of the external carotid system (Fig. 40-6). In the orbital cavity the ophthalmic artery gives off an anterior and posterior ethmoid artery. Each artery pierces the bone on the medial wall of the orbit at the point where the lamina papyracea of the ethmoid bone articulates with the orbital portion of the frontal bone (frontoethmoid suture). There the vessels enter the ethmoid sinuses to supply the mucosa and to send important branches to the attic of the nasal cavity. The posterior ethmoid artery is distributed mainly to the region of the superior concha, whereas the anterior ethmoid supplies the more anterosuperior aspect of the nasal mucosa. In some patients these vessels require ligation to control nasal hemorrhage, so the exact locations of the anterior and posterior ethmoid foramina are of surgical interest. Kirchner and others[4] noted that the anterior ethmoid foramen was 14 to 22 mm posterior to the maxillolacrimal suture in 84% of the 80 orbits they studied. The location of the posterior ethmoid foramen was more variable, but could be found 3 to 13 mm posterior to the anterior ethmoid foramen in 86% of the observed specimens. In most cases the foramina were found either on the line of the frontoethmoid suture or slightly superior to it. The anterior and posterior ethmoid arteries are the most important surgical landmarks when performing an external ethmoidectomy. These branches penetrate from the orbit into the ethmoidal sinuses at the level of the fovea ethmoidalis, thus delineating the superior extent, or roof, of the ethmoid

sinuses. Above these arteries is the floor of the anterior cranial cavity; below them, the ethmoid air cells. The posterior ethmoid artery is also a landmark for the optic nerve. This nerve lies approximately 1 cm posterior to and on the same level as the vascular structure.

The terminal branch of the maxillary artery in the pterygopalatine fossa is the sphenopalatine artery. This artery can be ligated to control nasal hemorrhage through a transantral approach to the pterygopalatine fossa. The artery enters the nasal cavity through the sphenopalatine foramen, where it supplies the mucosa on both the lateral wall and septum (see Fig. 40-6). From the sphenopalatine foramen, branches course on the lateral wall over the posterior surfaces of both the middle and inferior meatus. A septal branch of the sphenopalatine artery ascends from the sphenopalatine foramen to the roof of the nasal cavity, follows the contour of the sphenoid bone to the nasal septum, and then courses anteriorly and inferiorly on the septum along the path of the vomer. Because the septal branch is located in the mucosa covering the face of the sphenoid sinus, this mucosa should be reflected inferiorly before the sinus is entered surgically, so as not to transect the artery.

As the vomer meets the nasal crest on the nasal floor, foramina on each side of the nasal crest merge with each other to form a single canal in the anterior maxillary palate. The canal opens onto the hard palate posterior to the central incisors; it is called the *incisive foramen*. Branches of the septal sphenopalatine arteries enter the incisive foramen from both sides of the nasal cavity and emerge as a plexus of vessels on the anterior aspect of the palate in the oral cavity.

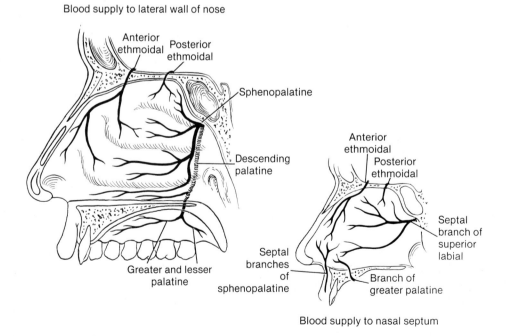

Fig. 40-6. Blood supply to the mucosa of the lateral nasal wall and nasal septum.

The anterosuperior portion of the septum is also supplied by the anterior ethmoidal artery descending from the roof of the nasal cavity. The vestibule of the nose is supplied by the terminal branches of the arteries previously discussed, as well as by nasal branches of the superior labial artery in the upper lip derived from the facial artery. The anterior portion of the nasal cavity, particularly the septum, is thus an important site of anastomosis between vessels from several sources, namely the ophthalmic, from the internal carotid system, and the maxillary and facial, from the external carotid system. Anastomosing vessels on the anterior septum, reportedly a common site of nosebleed, have been termed *Kiesselbach's*, or *Little's*, area.

Because of the various and sometimes confusing names applied to the vessels of the nose, thinking of the source of the vessels is easier than thinking of the individual names. In this simplified view there are two sources: the ethmoidal arteries in the attic of the nose and the sphenopalatine arteries arising posteriorly at the sphenopalatine foramen from the maxillary artery.

VENOUS DRAINAGE OF THE NASAL CAVITIES

The venous drainage of the nasal cavities follows the basic arterial pattern. Veins in the roof of the nasal cavity follow the ethmoidal veins into the orbital cavity, where they become tributaries of the ophthalmic veins. These usually course posteriorly into the cavernous sinuses and become part of the drainage pattern of the dural venous sinuses. The posterior portion of the nasal cavity drains via the sphenopalatine vessels into the pterygopalatine fossa and subsequently into the pterygoid venous plexus within the infratemporal fossa. The anterior portion of the nasal cavity drains into the anterior facial vein, which is a tributary of either the external or internal jugular vein. Both the pterygoid venous plexus and the ethmoidal veins have communication with the dural venous sinuses. For these reasons it is obvious that infections in the attic of the nose or nasal sinuses may spread to the adjacent orbital tissues or intracranial cavity with disastrous clinical sequelae.

INNERVATION OF THE NASAL MUCOSA

A thorough discussion of the innervation of the nasal mucosa requires specific knowledge of the osteology of the pterygopalatine fossa and the distribution of the branches of the trigeminal nerve's maxillary division. The true fibers of the maxillary nerve, which are those entering the pons in the root of the trigeminal nerve, conduct only general sensory input (touch, pain, and temperature) from the nasal, palatal, and oral mucosae and skin of the cheek. However, the terminal branches of the maxillary nerve also carry special sensory taste fibers and postganglionic, parasympathetic, secretomotor fibers. These fibers (taste and parasympathetic) join the maxillary nerve in the pterygopalatine fossa and are distributed with the various branches of the maxillary nerve from the pterygopalatine fossa to taste buds

or mucous glands in the oral or nasal mucosa. Because of the anatomic detail involved in discussing the pathways of these nerves, the subject is divided into five sections: (1) osteology of the pterygopalatine fossa, (2) maxillary division of the trigeminal nerve, (3) ophthalmic division of the trigeminal nerve, (4) parasympathetic innervation of the nasal mucosa, and (5) sympathetic innervation of the nasal mucosa.

Osteology of the pterygopalatine fossa

The following is written in a manner such that if the reader has a skull and a pipe cleaner or broom straw available, the descriptions can be followed on the specimen to clarify the complicated three-dimensional relationships of this area. The pterygopalatine fossa can be located easily on a skull specimen by removing the mandible and looking at the interval between the tuberosity of the maxilla and the pterygoid process of the sphenoid bone (Fig. 40-7). These structures form the anterior and posterior walls, respectively, of the fossa. The opening into the fossa on its lateral aspect is called the *pterygomaxillary fissure*; medially the wall of the fossa is formed by the vertical plate of the palatine bone and the sphenopalatine foramen located at the superior border of the palatine plate. If a probe is inserted into the fossa through the pterygomaxillary fissure, it exits the fossa via the sphenopalatine foramen and occupies the nasal cavity posterior to the middle concha (see Fig. 40-3). The roof of the pterygopalatine fossa is open essentially because of the inferior orbital fissure, although the greater wing of the sphenoid bone projects anteriorly into this region. Because the bony walls of the fossa are somewhat inclined, the floor of the fossa is like the apex of a cone and represents the fusion of the walls. However, the fusion is incomplete and provides an opening in the floor, leading into a canal in the palatine bone—the greater palatine canal—that terminates on the palate as the greater palatine foramen (Fig. 40-8). A lesser palatine canal, also from the floor of the fossa, traverses the pyramidal process of the palatine bone and opens slightly posterior to the greater palatine foramen; it is called the *lesser palatine foramen*.

If a skull is sectioned coronally in the exact plane of the pterygopalatine fossa, it is possible to view the anatomy of the posterior wall of the fossa. The same view can be obtained by examining the anterior surface of an isolated sphenoid bone (Fig. 40-9). When viewed in this manner, two foramina can be seen in the body of the sphenoid at the root of the pterygoid process; the foramen rotundum and the foramen of the pterygoid canal. A probe inserted into the foramen rotundum leads immediately into the middle cranial fossa, whereas a probe inserted into the pterygoid canal must transverse the entire depth of the body of the sphenoid bone before it exits the canal at the skull base near the foramen lacerum.

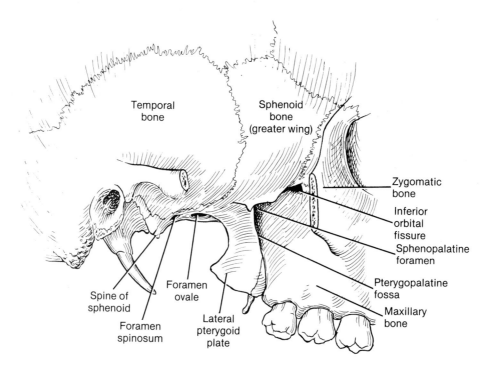

Fig. 40-7. Relationships of pterygopalatine fossa.

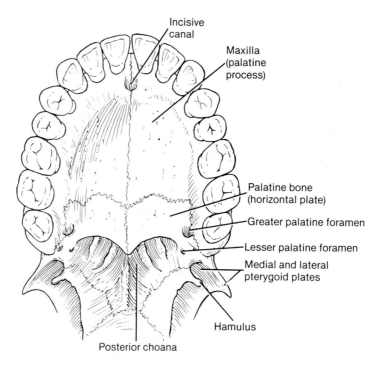

Fig. 40-8. Osseous landmarks of the hard palate.

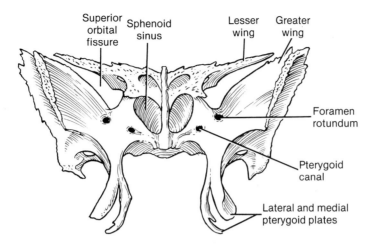

Fig. 40-9. Anterior view of isolated sphenoid bone illustrating landmarks.

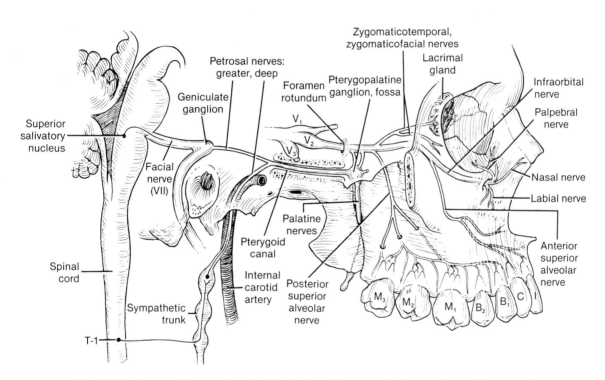

Fig. 40-10. Autonomic innervation of palatal and nasal mucosa via the seventh cranial nerve and the nerve of pterygoid canal. Distribution of secretomotor fibers via maxillary division of the trigeminal nerve.

Maxillary branch of the trigeminal nerve

The maxillary division is derived from the semilunar ganglion and exits the middle cranial fossa via the foramen rotundum. It enters the roof of the pterygopalatine fossa, traverses the inferior orbital fissure, and occupies the floor of the orbit before it comes to lie in the infraorbital groove (Fig. 40-10). Following the intraorbital groove it traverses the infraorbital canal of the maxilla and finally exits the canal via the infraorbital foramen. The nerve terminates in the skin of the face as three named branches: (1) a palpebral branch supplying the skin of the lower lid, (2) an external nasal branch supplying skin of the lateral aspect of the bridge of the nose and both the external and internal surfaces of the ala, and (3) a labial branch supplying the skin of the upper lip, the labial mucosa on the internal surface of the lip, and the labial gingiva associated with the incisors and canine teeth. The entire maxillary division may be anesthetized to perform nasal and paranasal sinus surgery by injecting a small quantity of the anesthetic agent near the vicinity of the foramen rotundum in the pterygopalatine fossa.

Needle access to the fossa is accomplished through either the greater palatine foramen or the pterygopalatine fissure, via the notch of the mandible between the coronoid process and the ramus.

Dental branches

Beginning in the pterygopalatine fossa, a number of branches arise from the maxillary division as it courses through the midface. The posterosuperior alveolar nerve arises from the maxillary nerve in the pterygopalatine fossa and exits via the pterygomaxillary fissure. The nerve penetrates the posterior wall of the maxilla as two or more filaments; it supplies the roots of the posterior teeth, including the molars and bicuspids. In addition, it supplies the buccal gingiva associated with these teeth.

After the maxillary nerve enters the infraorbital canal, a middle superior alveolar nerve is given off, which may share with the posterosuperior alveolar nerve in the innervation of the bicuspids. Slightly distal to this point is an anterosuperior alveolar nerve, which supplies the remaining teeth in the maxillary arch, namely, the incisors and canines (see Fig. 40-10).

Palatine branches

In the pterygopalatine fossa a palatine branch descends vertically from the maxillary nerve, passing through the floor of the pterygopalatine fossa, branching at the greater and lesser palatine canals, and forming the greater and lesser palatine nerves (Fig. 40-11). These nerves supply the palatal mucosa and gingiva from the region of the molar teeth anteriorly, to the area adjacent to the first bicuspid.

Nasal branches

A large medial branch of the maxillary nerve arises in the pterygopalatine fossa and enters the nasal cavity through the sphenopalatine foramen where it divides and contributes branches to the mucosa on both the lateral and septal walls of the nasal cavity. The branch on the lateral wall forms several small nerves in the mucosa, called the *posterolateral nasal nerves* (Fig. 40-12). These nerves course anteriorly in the mucosa over the middle and inferior conchae. The branch to the nasal septum leaves the sphenopalatine nerve at the foramen and follows the contour of the sphenoid bone along the roof of the nasal cavity before turning inferiorly to reach the septum. On the septum the nerve is called the *nasopalatine nerve*; it continues anteriorly as a major nerve in the mucosa, supplying branches to the septal area. Near the anterior end of the vomer the nerve enters a bony canal on the nasal floor, traverses the premaxillary palate, and exits via the incisive foramen. On the anterior aspect of the palate, the nerve supplies the mucosa and gingiva posterior to the incisor teeth (see Fig. 40-11).

Nasal branches of the ophthalmic division of the trigeminal nerve

In addition to the branches of the maxillary nerve, branches from the first division of the trigeminal nerve supply portions of the nasal mucosa. After the ophthalmic divi-

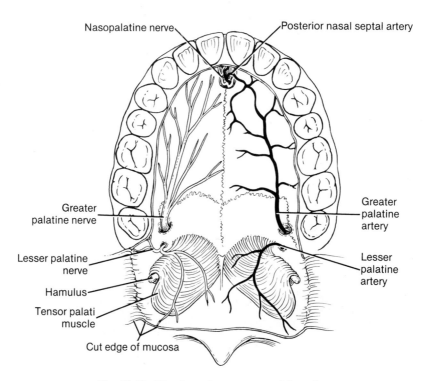

Fig. 40-11. Blood supply to mucosa of the palate.

sion of the trigeminal nerve enters the orbital cavity, it gives off several branches, among which is the nasociliary nerve. The nasociliary nerve crosses to the medial aspect of the orbit and gives off the anterior and posterior ethmoidal nerves. These nerves, accompanied by their respective vessels, enter the anterior and posterior ethmoid foramina at the frontoethmoid suture, as described before. The nerves supply the mucosa of the ethmoid sinuses, send a small twig to the dura in the anterior cranial fossa, and enter the roof of the nasal cavity. The posterior ethmoid supplies only a small area of the mucosa near the superior concha on the lateral wall and a corresponding area on the nasal septum (Fig. 40-12). After entering the attic of the nasal cavity, the anterior ethmoid nerve sends branches to the mucosa of the septum and lateral nasal wall. The nerve follows the posterior surface of the nasal bone anteriorly, as the *internal nasal nerve*, until it reaches the articulation with the upper lateral cartilage. At this point it passes between the nasal bone and the upper lateral cartilage to occupy the surface of the cartilage. Here the nerve is called the *external nasal nerve*. It provides cutaneous innervation to the skin over the dorsum and tip of the nose. Trauma to the external nasal nerve of the anterior ethmoidal undoubtedly results in hypesthesia over the dorsum after rhinoplasty.

Autonomic innervation of nasal mucosa

As already noted, an understanding of the maxillary nerve branches is important not only because of the general sensory innervation they provide, but because they also serve as conduits for the distribution of parasympathetic secretomotor fibers to the nasal, palatal, and oral mucosae.

The autonomic innervation of nasal mucosa, both parasympathetic and sympathetic, does not follow a direct path to the glands of the nasal mucosa. The parasympathetic fibers begin with the seventh cranial nerve (CN VII, the facial), but distally they use branches of the trigeminal nerve for their distribution to the individual glands. Similarly, sympathetic fibers beginning in the spinal cord have a distinct path until they reach the superior cervical ganglion. From the ganglion, postganglionic fibers may appear as diffuse plexuses on the surface of blood vessels or with branches of the trigeminal system.

Autonomic innervation, whether parasympathetic or sympathetic, requires two neurons from the central nervous system (brainstem or spinal cord) to the effector organ. In contrast, innervation of skeletal muscle requires only one neuron from the central nervous system to the motor end-plate. Thus in the autonomic pathway a ganglion, either parasympathetic or sympathetic, always intervenes between the central nervous system and the effector organ.

Parasympathetic innervation

Parasympathetic innervation of the nasal mucosa begins in the superior salivary nucleus, which is located in the brainstem at the junction between the pons and the medulla (see Fig. 40-10). Secretomotor fibers exit the brainstem at this point via the intermediary nerve. This nerve exists briefly as an independent nerve, between the brainstem and the internal auditory meatus. Within the auditory meatus its fibers join with the motor fibers of CN VII. At the anterior end of the internal acoustic canal, CN VII makes a sharp bend (genu) to follow the medial wall of the middle ear cavity. The genu

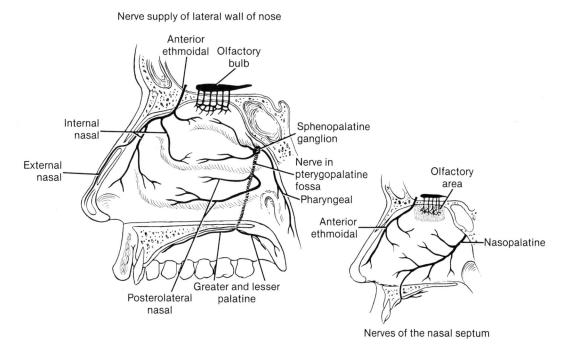

Fig. 40-12. Nerve supply to mucosa of the lateral nasal wall and nasal septum.

of CN VII is also the site of the geniculate ganglion. Although the secretomotor fibers traverse the geniculate ganglion, they do not synapse at this site because the geniculate ganglion is a sensory ganglion for other CN VII fibers. Traversing the ganglion, the fibers form an anterior branch from the ganglion, named the *greater petrosal nerve*, which penetrates the roof of the temporal bone and enters the middle cranial cavity.

On the petrous bone the greater petrosal nerve courses medially, descending on the petrous pyramid until it reaches the surface of the internal carotid artery within the foramen lacerum. The nerve continues on the lateral wall of the carotid artery until it reaches the junction between the temporal and sphenoid bones. The fibers enter the pterygoid canal of the sphenoid bone, traveling anteriorly until they exit from the canal into the pterygopalatine fossa. Crossing the fossa, the preganglionic, parasympathetic, secretomotor fibers enter the sphenopalatine ganglion to synapse with neurons, which ultimately distribute postganglionic fibers to the glands of the nasal mucosa.

Although these parasympathetic fibers begin within CN VII, after leaving the geniculate ganglion they are termed the *greater petrosal nerve* until they reach the pterygoid canal. Because these fibers are joined by sympathetic fibers (deep petrosal fibers) while they are in the pterygoid canal, the combined mixture of fibers is known as the *nerve of the pterygoid canal*, or the *vidian nerve*. The final distribution of these fibers is along the various branches of the maxillary division of the trigeminal nerve. The vidian nerve is sometimes surgically divided to reduce rhinorrhea. The vidian neurectomy is accomplished via a transantral approach to the pterygopalatine fossa, giving access to the pterygoid canal.

After synapsing in the sphenopalatine ganglion, post-ganglionic fibers course medially through the sphenopalatine foramen and follow sphenopalatine branches of the maxillary nerve, supplying both the lateral wall and septum of the nasal cavity. Thus, the posterior lateral nasal nerve and the nasopalatine nerve contain not only general sensory fibers from the nasal mucosa but both parasympathetic secretomotor fibers (to the mucous glands within the nasal mucosa) and sympathetic fibers (to the blood vessels). Similarly, the nasopalatine nerve on the nasal septum, after exiting the incisive foramen, also carries secretomotor fibers to mucous glands on the anterior portion of the palate.

The posterior parts of the hard and soft palates receive secretomotor fibers from the sphenopalatine ganglion, which follow the greater and lesser palatine nerves, respectively.

So far, three types of functional neural components have been discussed within the branches of the maxillary nerve: (1) general sensory fibers from the mucosa itself that travel back to the semilunar ganglion of the trigeminal nerve and project to the sensory nuclei of the trigeminal nerve; (2) parasympathetic secretomotor fibers; and (3) sympathetic vasomotor fibers. A fourth group of fibers carries taste from the region of the palate via the greater and lesser palatine nerves. Taste fibers do not return with the maxillary nerve; instead, they join the nerve of the pterygoid canal. In effect, they follow the pathway of the parasympathetic secretomotor fibers in a retrograde manner and eventually enter the intermediary nerve. This is accomplished by traveling posteriorly through the pterygoid canal and ascending the greater petrosal nerve to the geniculate ganglion. The taste fibers have their cell bodies within the geniculate ganglion, with central processes that project via the intermediary nerve back to the brainstem, where they make synaptic connections in the nucleus solitarius.

Although taste fibers in the palatine nerves may be few in number, they have clinical significance in Ramsay Hunt's syndrome (herpes oticus). In addition to presenting vesicles in the external acoustic meatus, patients with this syndrome may occasionally also have vesicles distributed over the region of the hard and soft palates.

Sympathetic innervation

Sympathetic fibers begin in the intermediolateral cell column of the spinal cord in the region of T-1. Traveling via the ventral roots of the spinal cord, the fibers enter the first thoracic spinal nerve. From the spinal nerve the fibers enter the first thoracic sympathetic ganglion via a white communicating ramus. The fibers do not synapse in the ganglion but ascend in the sympathetic chain to the level of the superior cervical sympathetic ganglion. This is the site of synapse and relay of postganglionic sympathetic fibers to various parts of the head, and in particular the nasal mucosa.

A large number of postganglionic fibers ascend from the superior cervical ganglion, forming the internal carotid nerve, which accompanies the internal carotid artery into the skull. After traversing the carotid canal, some of the fibers, termed *deep petrosal fibers*, leave the carotid at the posterior boundary of the sphenoid bone and enter the pterygoid canal, joining the greater petrosal nerve (see Fig. 40-10). The combination of fibers from the greater petrosal and deep petrosal nerves forms the nerve of the pterygoid canal, described previously. When the postganglionic fibers reach the pterygopalatine fossa, they do not synapse in the sphenopalatine ganglion because they are already postganglionic fibers and the sphenopalatine ganglion is a parasympathetic ganglion. The distribution of these fibers is not known precisely, but most are distributed as vasomotor fibers to the blood vessels of the nasal and oral mucosae via branches of the maxillary nerve.

PARASYMPATHETIC INNERVATION OF THE LACRIMAL GLAND

It may seem inappropriate to include the lacrimal gland in the chapter on nasal cavities, but the lacrimal gland shares its innervation pathway with the gland of the nasal and palatal mucosae. Interruption of these fibers—whether by disease, trauma, or surgical intervention, as in the case of vidian nerve neurectomy for vasomotor rhinitis—also interferes with lacrimal secretion and may require the patient to use artificial tears.

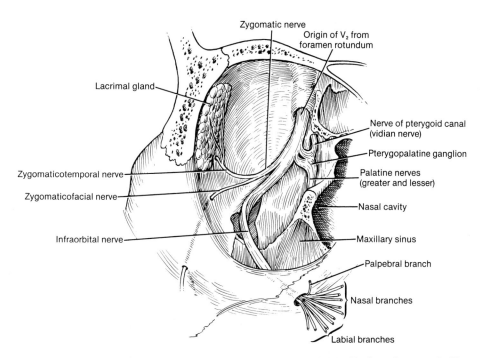

Fig. 40-13. Pterygopalatine fossa; view with orbital floor removed. Distribution of autonomic fibers via maxillary nerve. (Redrawn from Anderson JE: *Grant's atlas of anatomy*, ed 8, Baltimore, 1983, Williams & Wilkins.)

Lacrimal secretion is usually described as being of two types: basic and reflex.[5] The basic secretion contributes to a precorneal film containing a mixture of mucin and oils derived from glands in the lid and conjunctiva. Basic secretion rates are relatively constant but tend to diminish slightly with age. The oily component of the basic secretion is important in maintaining a low evaporative rate of the lacrimal secretions.

Reflex secretions are caused by direct stimulation of the lacrimal gland by parasympathetic fibers of CN VII. The afferent limb of this reflex is stimulated by several afferent mechanisms: via nasociliary branches of the ophthalmic division of the trigeminal nerve when the conjunctiva or cornea is irritated; via the optic nerve and caused by light (reflex secretion is nil in darkness or during sleep); or via cortical or hypothalamic centers in varying emotional states.

The pathway of postganglionic parasympathetic fibers to the lacrimal gland is the zygomatic branch of the maxillary nerve. Before the maxillary nerve enters the infraorbital groove, it gives off the zygomatic branch, which abruptly divides into the zygomaticotemporal and zygomaticofacial branches (Fig. 40-13). The zygomaticofacial nerve crosses the lateral portion of the orbital floor and enters the malar bone, exiting via the zygomaticofacial foramen onto the skin of the face. It provides cutaneous sensation over the malar bone. The zygomaticotemporal nerve ascends in the orbit on the lateral wall, usually penetrating the bone near the lacrimal gland, and ascends the lateral surface of the skull to become a cutaneous nerve of the scalp.

Parasympathetic fibers to the lacrimal gland are also contained in the nerve of the pterygoid canal. After synapsing in the sphenopalatine ganglion, the postganglionic fibers join the maxillary nerve and follow the zygomatic branch of it to the zygomaticotemporal nerve. Just before the point at which the zygomaticotemporal nerve leaves the orbit, the postganglionic secretomotor fibers leave the nerve and enter the substance of the lacrimal gland (see Fig. 40-13). Although a vidian nerve neurectomy is usually performed via a modified Caldwell-Luc approach, the relationship of the posterior wall of the maxillary sinus is well illustrated in Figure 40-13. The position of the opening of the pterygoid canal is always medial and inferior to the maxillary nerve and the foramen rotundum. Interestingly, it is also just medial to the sphenopalatine foramen, where it can be entered by an intranasal approach with a long, supple needle.

REFERENCES

1. Dion MC, Jafek BW, Tobin CJ: The anatomy of the nose: external support, *Arch Otolaryngol Head Neck Surg* 104:145, 1978.
2. Drumheller GW: Topology of the lateral nasal cartilages: the anatomical relationships of the lateral nasal to the greater alar cartilage, lateral crus, *Anat Rec* 176:321, 1973.
3. Hinderer KH: *Fundamentals of anatomy and surgery of the nose*, Birmingham, Ala, 1971, Aesculapius Publishing.
4. Kirchner JA, Yanagisawa E, Crelin ES: Surgical anatomy of the ethmoidal arteries, *Arch Otolaryngol Head Neck Surg* 74:382, 1961.
5. Reeh MJ, Wobig JL, Wirtschafter JD: *Ophthalmic anatomy*, San Francisco, 1981, American Academy of Ophthalmology.
6. Straatsma BR, Straatsma CR: The anatomical relationship of the upper lateral cartilage to the nasal bone and the cartilaginous septum, *Plast Reconstr Surg* 8:443, 1951.

Chapter 41

Physiology of Olfaction

Donald Leopold

The perception of odors adds a quality to life that is difficult to express. Odors are part of our everyday life, from the pleasures of perfume to the satisfactions of toast and coffee to the warnings of skunks and fire. As the molecules of substances are transported through the nose, the possibility of them being perceived occurs. The quality and intensity of that perception depends on the anatomic state of the nasal epithelium and the status of the peripheral and central nervous systems.

This chapter explores the physiology of olfaction, noting pertinent research data. The initial discussion focuses on the pathways and obstacles that odorant molecules should negotiate as they come in contact with the olfactory receptor cells. A consideration of the neural processing of odorant stimulation and the pathways projecting to the brain gives some insight into the mechanisms underlying olfactory perception. Olfactory testing explores assessment and methods of this perception. The chapter ends with a section on clinical olfactory problems in humans and includes suggestions for their diagnosis and management.

The study of olfaction poses many tantalizing questions. For example, like many animal species, do humans communicate through odorant signals (pheromones)? Why are primary olfactory receptor cells able to regenerate entirely when other special sensory primary neurons are not? Can olfactory tissue be transplanted in humans as demonstrated in rodents? The study of olfaction has attracted the attention of researchers in the fields of endocrinology, anatomy, biochemistry, and neurophysiology, and others. Through these efforts, the ability to diagnose and help individuals with chemosensory problems is improving.

ANATOMY OF OLFACTORY STIMULATION

Nasal passageways

Experiencing an odor is a result of input from the olfactory, trigeminal, glossopharyngeal, and vagus nerves. Apparently, the properties of any given odorant determine the particular "mix" of these various inputs. Olfactory nerve (cranial nerve I) stimulation, which is necessary for identification of the vast majority of odorants, depends on the odorant molecules reaching the olfactory mucosa at the top of the nasal cavity. Although molecules can reach the olfactory cleft by diffusion, essentially olfaction requires some type of nasal airflow, usually as part of respiration. While eating, there is a retronasal flow of odorant molecules that stimulate the olfactory receptors at the top of the nose, and contribute greatly to the flavor of the food.[52] This airflow can be the smallest amount of retronasal airflow generated by the mouth and pharyngeal motion.[34,263,313] Measurements in nasal models have shown this flow to be laminar at the low flow rates associated with normal breathing, and turbulent in most of the nasal cavity at high flow rates.[117,130,147,305] Additional data from a large-scale model (Fig. 41-1) indicate that at physiologic airflow rates, at least 50% of the total airflow passes through the middle and inferior meatuses, and about 15% flows through the olfactory region.[305] Using ink threads in a water flow medium through a model, Masing[235] showed that even the locus of entry through the nostril can determine the path of that flow stream through the nose (Fig. 41-2).

Mathematical models of the nose, created from digitized computed tomography (CT) anatomy slices and predicted mass transport functions, can predict odor intensity for vary-

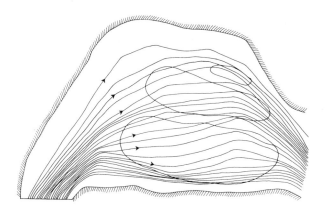

Fig. 41-1. Streamline patterns for resting inspiratory flow (250 ml/sec) through an expanded (20 × normal size) scale model of a healthy human adult male nasal cavity (sagittal view). *Lines* show the paths taken by small dust particles entering at the external nares. (From Scherer PW and others: *Otolaryngol Clin North Am* 22:265, 1989.)

ing amounts of olfactory epithelium, the character of the carrier gas, and the solubility of the odorant molecules.[129] These theoretical results show agreement with human and animal experimental data.

The effect of a rapid change in flow velocity, such as with a sniff, on the *in vivo* airflow pattern remains unknown. Scherer, Hahn, and Mozell[305] have found in their large-scale model studies that the percentage and velocity of airflow to the olfactory region is similar for various steady-state airflow rates in the physiologic range. The fact remains, however, that sniffing is an almost universally performed maneuver when a person is presented with an olfactory stimulus. It is possible that its purpose is momentarily to increase the number of olfactory molecules in the olfactory cleft by a transient change in the airflow pattern of the nose. A sniff also may allow the trigeminal nerve to alert the central olfactory neurons that an odorant is coming. Sniffing duration, flow velocity, and volume are quite different among subjects but remain remarkably constant for any one subject.[199] Furthermore, Laing[200] has shown that different sniffing paradigms do not improve a subject's olfactory perception. The naturally chosen sniff seems to be optimal for that subject's nasal anatomy.

For molecules to reach the olfactory area, they must pass through the tall but narrow nasal passageways. The epithelium lining the walls of these passageways is wet, has variable thickness, and is aerodynamically "rough." Schneider and Wolf[311] have observed that the best olfactory ability occurs when this epithelium is moderately congested, wet, and red, such as during an upper respiratory infection. Furthermore, olfactory ability appears to improve with narrowed nasal chambers,[69,366] but the changes in nasal patency that occur during the natural rhythmic engorgement and thinning of the nasal epithelium (nasal cycle)[285] do not have any effect on olfactory ability.[72,88,209]

The sorption of molecules to these mucus-lined walls extracts some of them from the air stream and increases their travel time. This process could influence the spectrum of chemicals reaching the olfactory cleft or spread their arrival over time. Moncrieff[244] described this phenomenon in the variable times required for odorants to traverse the nasal passageways of sheep. This sorption of molecules may separate or sort the odorants before they reach the olfactory mucosa. Highly-sorbable chemicals may have minimal or no odor simply because they sorb to the nasal walls before they reach the olfactory cleft, thereby accentuating the trigeminal component. Could it be that our world would smell different if we had no external nose to increase the path of the olfactory region? Does an animal with a long snout, such as the dog, smell the world differently as a result of these sorptive effects?

Olfactory mucus

After the odorant molecules reach the olfactory region, they must interact with the mucus overlying the receptor cells. The mucus apparently comes from both Bowman's glands deep in the lamina propria (only of serous type in humans)[123,155] and the adjacent respiratory mucosa (goblet cells). Researchers have observed that the supporting (sustentacular) cells of the human olfactory epithelium are not histologically equipped to secrete mucus.[155,248,249] The supporting cells of most other species, however, have secreted mucus, often in response to odorants.[110,111,123,274]

The partitioning of an odorant's molecules between the air phase and the mucus phase is most certainly another determinate of its being perceived. To reach the olfactory receptors, the odorant molecules must be soluble in the mucus but, as Laffort, Patte, and Etcheto[196] argue, not so "strongly captured" that they are unable to interact with the receptors. In addition, changes in the thickness or composition of the mucus can influence the diffusion time required for odorant molecules to reach the receptor sites.[113] Adrenergic, cholinergic, and peptidergic agents have caused these changes in the mucus overlying the olfactory receptors through their effect on the secretory activities of the mucosal glands. Moreover, these same agents have influenced the sensitivity of the olfactory receptor cells themselves.[28,112,114]

Once in the olfactory mucus-epithelial system, the rate at which the odorant is cleared also is important. Hornung and Mozell[146] have shown that 79% of a radioactively labeled odorant (butanol) remained trapped in the mucus 30 minutes after inspiratory exposure, whereas radioactively labeled octane cleared rapidly. The mucus may exert a differential role in deactivating, removing, or desorbing odorants from the olfactory area.

Olfactory epithelium

Located 7 cm inside the nasal cavity, the olfactory sensory neurons are protected in a 1-mm wide crevice of the posterosuperior nose. At the epithelial surface, these bipolar

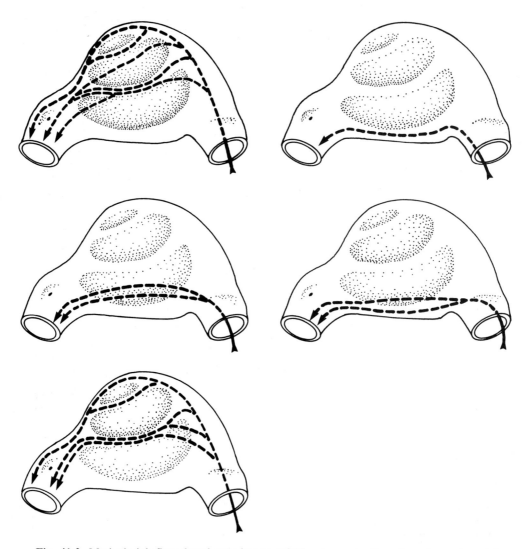

Fig. 41-2. Masing's ink flow thread experiments (1967) using water flow through nasal model (inspiration). Central and medial flow threads rise vertically into upper nasal areas, whereas dorsal, ventral, and lateral flow threads are refracted spirally and travel mainly through the lower part of the nasal cavity. (Redrawn from Masing H: *Arch Klin Exp Ohren Nasen Kehlk* 189:371, 1967.)

neurons are exposed to the outside world through their dendrites and cilia. Proximally, axons of these same neurons synapse at the base of the brain (olfactory bulb). Whereas the olfactory receptor region is a solid sheet of olfactory mucosa housed in a protected environment in human fetuses and laboratory animals, Morrison and Costanzo,[251] Naessen,[267] and Nakashima, Kimmelman, and Snow[268] have shown that there is mixing of olfactory and respiratory epithelial tissues in adult humans (Fig. 41-3). The number of these clumps of respiratory epithelium, which are found in the olfactory area, increase with age, suggesting that a loss of primary olfactory neurons at least partially explains the decreased olfactory ability associated with aging.

The human olfactory epithelium is much thicker (60 to 70 mm) than the surrounding respiratory epithelium (20 to 30 mm) and covers an area of roughly 1 square cm on each side. The epithelium is pseudostratified columnar, and it rests on a vascular lamina propria with no submucosa (Fig. 41-4). In most mammals studied, four main cell types have been identified (Figs. 41-5 and 41-6): ciliated olfactory receptors, microvillar cells, supporting (sustentacular) cells, and basal cells.[248,249,251,299] Research using immunohistochemical staining of olfactory elements continues to provide information on growth, maturation, function of specific cellular elements, and similarities with other neural tissue.* One possible use for this technique may be to clarify the etiology of the patient's olfactory dysfunction and possibly offer a prognosis regarding improvement of olfactory ability.[209,365]

The olfactory receptor neuron is bipolar and has a club-

---

* Refs. 45, 57, 314, 315, 348, 363, 364.

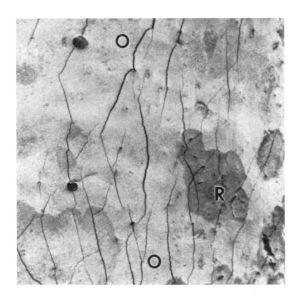

Fig. 41-3. Low magnification of the surface of the nasal cavity taken from a transition region. Patches of respiratory *(R)* epithelium *(dark areas)* can be seen within the olfactory *(O)* region. (×28.) (From Morrison EE, Costanzo RM: *J Comp Neurol* 297:1, 1990. Copyright © 1990. Reprinted by permission of Wiley-Liss, a division of John Wiley & Sons.)

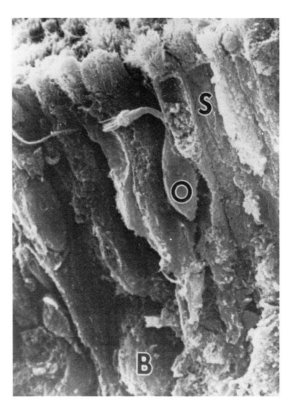

Fig. 41-5. Cross-sectional view of the olfactory epithelium showing the columnar supporting cells *(S)* that extend the full length of the epithelium. An olfactory neuron *(O)* with its dendrite and basal cell *(B)* can be seen among supporting cells. (×1241.) (From Morrison EE, Costanzo RM: *J Comp Neurol* 297:1, 1990. Copyright © 1990. Reprinted by permission of Wiley-Liss, a division of John Wiley & Sons.)

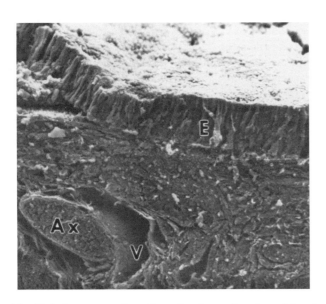

Fig. 41-4. Low-power three-dimensional scanning view of the olfactory epithelium and lamina propria. The olfactory epithelium *(E)* overlies a thick connective tissue lamina propria that contains olfactory axon fascicles *(Ax)* and blood vessels *(V)*. (×248.) (From Morrison EE, Costanzo RM: *J Comp Neurol* 297:1, 1990. Copyright © 1990. Reprinted by permission of Wiley-Liss, a division of John Wiley & Sons.)

shaped peripheral "knob" that bears the cilia (Fig. 41-7). After widening for the nucleus, it tapers to the long, thin, nonmyelinated axon that can travel several centimeters to the olfactory bulb. Bundles of these fibers form in the lamina propria and become ensheathed as a group by the plasma membranes of the Schwann cells, forming the olfactory nerve (cranial nerve I), which traverses the 15 to 20 foramina in the cribriform plate to synapse in the bulb. Allison and Warwick[12] estimate the rabbit to have about 50 million olfactory axons, whereas Jafek[155] estimates humans to have only 6 million bilaterally.

The microvillar cell occurs about one tenth as often as the ciliated olfactory neurons.[155] The cell body is flask-shaped and located near the epithelial surface, and has an apical membrane containing microvilli that project into the mucus overlying the epithelium (see Fig. 41-6).[248,249] The deep end of the cell tapers to a thin, axon-like cytoplasmic projection that proceeds into the lamina propria. Although there is no electrophysiologic evidence that these cells respond to chemical stimuli, Rowley, Moran, and Jafek[299] have hypothesized that they are a morphologically distinct class of sensory receptors. Their evidence for this is the

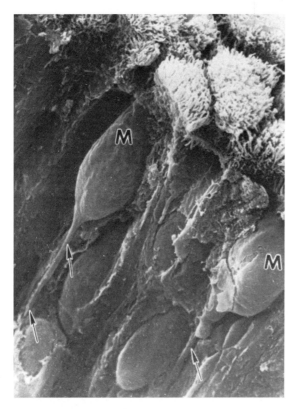

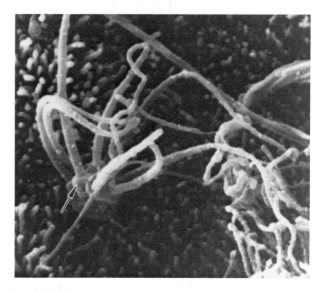

Fig. 41-7. High-power magnification of an olfactory knob with long cilia gradually tapering as they extend over the epithelial surface. At the base of individual cilia, a necklace-like structure *(arrow)* can be seen on the surface of the olfactory knob. (×14,220.) (From Morrison EE, Costanzo RM: *J Comp Neurol* 297:1, 1990. Copyright © 1990. Reprinted by permission of Wiley-Liss, a division of John Wiley & Sons.)

Fig. 41-6. Low-power magnification of fractured olfactory epithelium illustrating the axon-like processes *(arrows)* from microvillar cells *(M)*, which extend basally between supporting cells. (×3060.) (From Morrison EE, Costanzo RM: *J Comp Neurol* 297:1, 1990. Copyright © 1990. Reprinted by permission of Wiley-Liss, a division of John Wiley & Sons.)

backfilling of a cytochemical tracer macromolecule (horse-radish peroxidase) into the ciliated olfactory receptors and the microvillar cells when it is injected into the olfactory bulb.

Among these two receptor-type cells are the supporting or sustentacular cells. These tall cells have an apical membrane that joins tightly with the surface of the receptor cells and the microvillar cells. They seem positioned to separate the receptor cells from each other; however, intimate apposition between receptor cells does occur.[155,248,249] Whether this proximity allows some receptor cells to influence each other's firing patterns is unknown. Sustentacular cells do not generate action potentials, nor are they electrically coupled to each other;[108,236] thus, they do not seem to contribute directly to the olfactory transduction process and the elicitation of generator potentials by odorant stimuli.

Deep to these cells, the basal cells sit along the lamina propria. They serve as a stem cell population that can differentiate to replace the olfactory receptors lost during cell turnover or as a consequence of environmental insult.[155] This renewal of a special sensory neuron, as shown by Graziadei,[124] is not known to occur in other sensory systems. The replication cycle is between 3 and 7 weeks.[246,253] When the

new receptor cell forms, it also projects its axon to the olfactory bulb where it synapses.

The surface of human olfactory epithelium is covered with cilia, but electron microscopic studies reveal no dynein arms on these cilia.[155,249] These authors conclude from this observation that neither dynein arms nor motility is essential for human olfaction. In other animals, cilia can be differentiated on the basis of their length, motility, and response to odorant stimuli.[2,107,230,231] Different patterns of ciliary movement are a function of age and development. In the immature neuron, the cilia move rapidly and randomly, and the cell responds electrophysically to a large number of chemical stimuli. After the cell has made a central connection with the olfactory bulb, this more mature neuron exhibits longer, slower cilia motion and responds more selectively to odorants. The most mature neurons have immotile cilia.

Vomeronasal organ

Many mammals have an identifiable pit or groove in the anterior-inferior part of the nasal septum that contains chemosensitive cells. In most of these animals, a nerve can be identified connecting these cells to the central nervous system, often to an accessory olfactory bulb. In some situations, this system has been receptive to pheromones.[85] There have been recent investigations into the possibility that humans have some type of vomeronasal system. Biopsy studies of the nasal mucosa in the small pit often seen along the anterior-inferior nasal septum show olfactory-like histology, but no

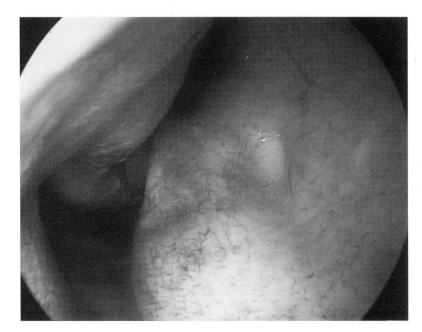

Fig. 41-8. Photograph from the right nasal cavity demonstrating the vomeronasal organ "pit" in the *right central* part of the image; it is on the anterior septum. Note the inferior turbinate and floor of the nose to the *left*.

central connection (Fig. 41-8). Electrophysiologic studies have shown negative action potentials from this vomeronasal area in response to specific chemical stimuli.[247] These same stimuli did not stimulate the olfactory system. Since no identified central brain connection seems to exist, it is possible that this system functions as a neuroendocrine system, emitting a substance in response to a specific chemical stimulus. No symptom-related importance has been determined, but prudence suggests that this anatomic area should not be disturbed during surgery unless it is necessary.[105]

Olfactory bulb

The olfactory bulb (Fig. 41-9) lies at the base of the frontal cortex in the anterior fossa. It serves as the first relay station in the olfactory pathway, where the primary olfactory neurons synapse with secondary neurons. These synapses and their postsynaptic partners form dense aggregates of neuropil called *glomeruli*. In the adult rabbit, approximately 26,000 olfactory axons enter each glomerulus, where they contact roughly 100 second-order neurons.[11] This relationship indicates a considerable convergence of information as these neurons pass from the periphery onto this first central station. (The interconnection among the various glomeruli in one bulb, the interconnections between bulbs, and the afferent and efferent connections with the brain indicate that considerable processing also occurs at the bulb level.)

The neuronal projection of the olfactory mucosa onto the bulb displays some anatomic restrictions but is not strictly point to point. In other words, a given region of the bulb receives its most dense input from a particular region of the mucosa,[279] but inputs to a particular region of the bulb converge from many areas along the anteroposterior extent of the mucosa. Conversely, a small focus in the epithelium

will project widely, but within a restrictive region of the bulb.[171] These dense and diffuse inputs possibly represent excitatory and inhibitory influences, which, as in other sensory systems, narrow the neural stimulus representation as the processing moves centrally. Alternatively, the convergence and divergence of projections from neurons in the epithelium may serve to coalesce inputs from receptor cells of sensitivity to odorants. Evidence to support this notion emerges from the coherent activation of single glomeruli or sets of glomeruli by specified odorants.[165,333] Therefore, it is clear that the microcircuitry of the bulb is specialized to narrow the spatial pattern of the glomerular activation elicited by an odorant or mixture of odorants.

Although most of the neural projections to the olfactory bulbs are ipsilateral, there are some bilateral projections, at least in the frog.[216] These projections exist in at least the mitral layer of the bulb.

Olfactory connections in the brain

Although the neural connections from the olfactory mucosa to the olfactory bulb are spatially organized to an extent, there is no spatial organization of the olfactory bulb output to the olfactory cortex.[229,319] Although complex neural branching and small fiber size have made anatomic mapping and electrical recording of specific nerve fiber tracts difficult, studies of neural function are making it clear that there may be physiologic differences among the mitral and tufted cell classes.[320]

The more central olfactory connections include the olfactory tubercule, the prepiriform cortex, part of the amygdaloid nuclei, and the nucleus of the terminal stria with further projections to a number of structures, including the hypothalamus. Although these structures receive olfactory input, they

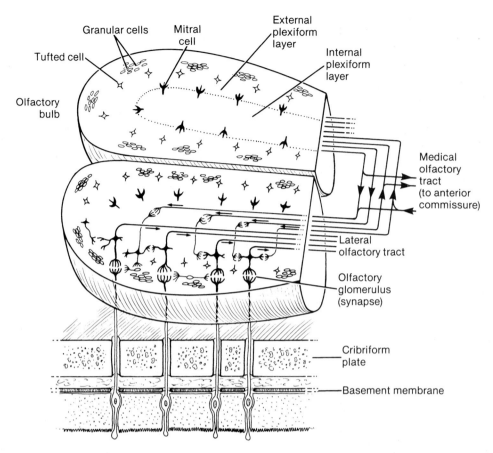

Fig. 41-9. Structure of olfactory bulbs and their neural connections to each other, the olfactory mucosa, and the brain.

also serve other functions such as food intake, temperature regulation, sleeping cycles, vision, hearing, and taste. It also is possible that these structures influence the olfactory process by efferent connections.[54,93]

Since olfactory neurons have the ability to regenerate, there has been interest in understanding this process. In addition to olfactory problems, this may be helpful for other neural areas like spinal-cord injuries. The glial cells that ensheath olfactory neurons support axonal growth of both olfactory and nonolfactory neurons.[81] Transplanting them along with nerve transplants may offer a way to ensure survival and function. Currently olfactory transplants have been done and have survived in neonatal rats.[134,135] Multiple neural pathways in the central brain from these transplants suggest potential growth in this tissue.

Common chemical sense

Free nerve endings of three cranial nerves (trigeminal—the most important, glossopharyngeal, and vagus) provide added chemoreceptivity in the mucosa of the respiratory tract.[36,39] The trigeminal nerves sense the burn of ammonia and the bite of hot pepper. In the nose, virtually all odorants stimulate olfactory and trigeminal nerves, even when no ap-

parent pungency can be perceived. The peripheral anatomic pathways for these cranial nerves have long been known; however, the central connections that allow their interaction and how they interrelate to other senses are just beginning to be determined.[36,198,264] Cometto-Muniz and Cain[53] have shown that when tested with ammonia, the common chemical sense behaves more like a total-mass detector than a concentration detector (i.e., at a given concentration the perceived magnitude increases with the time of presentation). It is even possible that the trigeminal nerve interprets pungent or chemically irritative stimuli as being painful or nociceptive in nature.

OLFACTORY TRANSDUCTION AND CODING

At each level of the olfactory system different factors control or shape how the system works. The nose has narrow passageways lined by wet mucus and swept by alternating air currents. The hydrophilic olfactory mucus presents the incoming odorant molecules with constraints of sorption, solubility, and chemical reactivity. Once the odorant molecule is dissolved in the olfactory mucus, another group of events influences whether it can interact with the olfactory receptor cells. Soluble binding proteins, like odorant-binding protein, have been described in air-breathing vertebrates, and it has been suggested that these proteins enhance the access of odorants to the olfactory receptors.[27,280,281] This is accomplished by binding and solubilizing hydrophobic odorant molecules, thus increasing their concentration in the environment of the receptor cell by as much as 1000 to 10,000 times more than their concentration in the ambient air.[322] Additionally, these same odorant-binding protein molecules may act to remove odorant molecules from the region of the receptor cell after transduction. It also is possible that air-breathing vertebrates may have in their olfactory systems a chemical-sensing system like that of unicellular and multicellular organisms. This system can produce degradative enzymes that transform stimulants into inactive products and vice versa.[46] Therefore, there are many perireceptor events occurring in the olfactory mucus before the odorant actually comes into contact with the cilia of the olfactory receptor cell.

In mammals, it is generally accepted that the actual transformation of odorant chemical information into an electrical action potential occurs as a result of specific interactions between odorant molecules and receptor proteins on the surface of olfactory cilia.[109,203] Recent evidence suggests that at least the first stages of odorant discrimination also occurs at the primary neuron level.[1,126,336] This process is probably mediated by a family of approximately 1000 seven-transmembrane domain receptor proteins that may be the actual receptors. Genes specific for these proteins have been identified, and the inability to perceive particular odorants (specific anosmia) has been associated with loss of specific genes.[20,127,290]

As this transduction process moves through the receptor cell membrane, several second messenger systems assist in depolarizing the cell and initiating the action potential. Patch clamp recordings have demonstrated that cyclic adenosine monophosphate (cAMP) and inositol phosphate (IP3) are the primary signaling pathways that can mediate olfactory transduction, depending on the species and the odorants.[1,342] With high doses of odorant, and in other parts of the olfactory pathway (like the olfactory bulb), another second messenger system involving nitric oxide (NO)/cyclic guanosine monophosphate (cGMP) has been identified.[31,62] Finally, an increase of intracellular calcium ions also have been shown to depolarize the olfactory receptor cell, and this may be an additional odorant effect.

Clinical evidence supporting the cAMP pathway comes from patients with type 1a pseudohypoparathyroidism, who not only have a deficiency in stimulatory Golf (G) proteins needed for the second messenger transduction, but also have olfactory losses.[153,350,358] This G protein appears to be exclusively localized to the olfactory epithelium.[163] The cAMP appears to be involved in the olfactory process by directly influencing an ion channel in the olfactory cilia.[65,269]

Once the peripheral olfactory receptor cells are depolarized, there begins a convergence of electrical information

towards the olfactory bulb. In the nasal cavity, a broad, genetically determined pattern of organization is emerging that becomes more specific as the information is passed through the glomeruli and mitral/tufted cells of the olfactory bulb.[250,290,336] How that electrical information is coded for the thousands of odorants that can be recognized and discriminated is just beginning to be understood. In the mid-twentieth century, Adrian[3-8] suggested several mechanisms based on his electrophysiologic recordings. Taken together, all of these mechanisms could produce different activity patterns across the mucosa, which would explain the different activity patterns he observed from anterior and posterior locations in the bulb. One mechanism is the odorant-selective sensitivity of the individual receptors, such that incoming odorants would excite different patterns of receptors along the mucosal surface. A second mechanism extends this concept, suggesting that receptors of like sensitivity will be aggregated into particular regions of the mucosa, thus giving a different spatial representation for each odorant. The final mechanism Adrian suggests proposes that each odorant, having different physiochemical properties such as solubility, would spread differentially both in time and space across the mucosal sheet. Adrian's proposals have been supported by later investigators.

The selective sensitivity of the receptor cells, Adrian's first mechanism, was clinically suspected by the existence of individuals with specific-reduced sensitivity to certain odorants.[14,15] Electrical recordings from single-receptor cells in the olfactory mucosa in animals show that each cell is tuned to different groups of chemicals; no cell responds to all odorants. However, it is difficult to classify these cells into particular types because no two cells respond to the same total group of odorants.[106,238] By studying the electrical responses of 30 receptor cells in the spiny lobster, Girardot and Derby[118] suggested that the quality part of olfactory coding is determined by the pattern of the response across the neuronal population and the intensity by the absolute magnitude. This would allow the lobster to determine whether the incoming odorant is from a friend or foe (quality) and how close he or she is (intensity). In addition, the responses of olfactory receptor neurons to chemical stimuli have added diversity since both excitatory and inhibitory responses have been measured.[66]

Several investigators have observed, as Adrian suggested, that receptor cells of like selectivity might indeed be aggregated into particular regions of the mucosa.* After surgically exposing the salamander's olfactory mucosa, the investigators puffed odorants directly onto the different regions while recording the electrical activity. Different regions gave maximal responses to different odorants.

Mozell[256-258] has analyzed the concept of spatial and temporal activity patterns. By electrically sampling olfactory nerve branches receiving input from the regions near the

---

* Refs. 172, 193, 194, 226-228, 252.

external and internal nares of the bullfrog, Mozell found each odorant produced a characteristic gradient of activity. The time interval between the responses at the external and internal nares also was measured and was found to correlate with the activity gradients. This fit in well with Adrian's theory because the molecules of different odorants spread differently across the mucosa in time and space. Later experiments, including the use of radioactive odorants, suggest that these spatiotemporal patterns result from the differential sorption of the molecules of different odorants across the mucosal sheet.[145,202,255,260,261] Furthermore, spatiotemporal patterns also have been shown in the olfactory bulb,[355] and they can be modified by early learning. It is becoming apparent that there is a great deal of learning in the early postnatal time period to establish these patterns.

The contribution made by the central nervous system towards olfactory coding and discrimination is unclear. It may be that the olfactory code is complete by the time it leaves the olfactory bulb. Alternatively, the code may need to be completed by additional central neural processing. Whatever the status of the olfactory code, it is clear that the central nervous system uses olfactory information for many purposes. One such purpose, for instance, is in the area of feeding. Glucose-sensitive cells in the lateral hypothalamus of the monkey integrate many chemosensory inputs from both endogenous and exogenous sources, whereas glucose-insensitive cells from the same area distinguish among fewer, more specific chemosensory cues to control food acquisition behavior.[168] In another area, the α-2 power on electroencephalogram (EEG) recording is increased after an unpleasant smell (valeric acid) exposure but not a pleasant exposure (phenylethyl alcohol).[30]

Where the central nervous system processes and stores the olfactory information also is unclear. Studies on laterality have suggested that humans have a better side for olfactory ability.[148,366] Zatorre and Jones-Gotman[367] have suggested that the right side is the better one, based on their observation of no deficits in olfactory identification ability in patients after left central, parietal, and posterior brain excisions. This is supported by the finding that patients with right parietal and frontotemporal lesions have difficulty with the lateralization of odorants.[23] Alternatively, Leopold and others[209] have correlated olfactory function to nasal anatomy using CT scanning. They learned that most people are only using their left side when perceiving olfactory information. Handedness may be a determinant of this trend[187] or the preferred side may be related to learning.

OLFACTORY COGNITION

Odors are understood largely on the basis of experience, and each individual develops his or her own hedonic code within cultural restraints.[90,152,221] Odor associations, once established, are notoriously difficult to erase from memory,[93,140,356] even though the incident that formed the association is forgotten or seems irrational. In one study, odor

memory was shown to last at least 1 year, whereas visual memory lasted only a few months (Fig. 41-10).[93] Interestingly, odor memory is facilitated by bilateral nasal stimulation, suggesting that people who have one-sided nasal obstruction may form poorer odor memories.[32] An odor aversion can be formed to a perfectly good food by overindulgence. Similarly, becoming ill for another reason while eating otherwise innocuous food can have the same effect.[93] This same phenomenon is used effectively in animal training, when lithium chloride, an emetic, is given with food in order to induce an aversion. For many of these reasons, the memory system that exists for odors may be distinct from other memory systems.[17,32] The exciting molecular advances made in understanding olfactory transduction and coding suggest that learning and memory also might be a ''hard-wired'' system. The adaptive ability to meet specific biologic needs, like those described above, require that no matter how the system is wired, it needs flexibility.[176]

Whether or not newborn human babies discriminate between pleasant and unpleasant odors or whether the sense of smell enters into their enjoyment of food is debatable.[93] They can, however, identify odorants having biologic meaning. Twenty-two out of 30 newborns selected the unwashed (odorous) breast when placed prone between them immediately after birth.[345] Macfarlane[224] has shown that, by the age of 6 to 10 days, infants prefer a pad from their own mother's breast as opposed to one from a strange mother. Other studies have shown that between the ages of 3 and 5 years, odor perception plays a role in a child's attachment to his mother.[303] Between the ages of 2 and 7 years, children start to show odor preferences, and these are similar to those of the adults living in the same area.[92,309,334] Nevertheless, the olfactory sensitivity of prepubescent children to specific odorants can be quite different from teenagers and adults.[184]

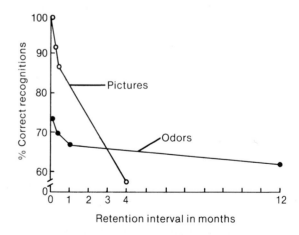

Fig. 41-10. Average percentage correct of ''old'' stimulus in pair of stimuli as function of duration of retention interval for pictures and odors. (Redrawn from Engen T: *The perception of odors.* In Birren JE, Schaie KW, editors: *Handbook of the psychology of aging,* New York, 1977, Von Nostrand Reinhold.)

All these observations of early human olfactory development have parallels in other mammals. Several researchers have suggested that this development is related to the marked growth that occurs in the neural circuitry of the olfactory epithelium and olfactory bulb from birth until adult size is reached.[241,284]

Pheromones, which are pervasive throughout the subhuman animal kingdom, are chemicals released by one member of a species and received by another member, resulting in a specific action or developmental process.[169] Thus, the male hamster knows whether the female is receptive,[63,265] and the ant knows the trail laid by a conspecific to a particular food.[49] (A more complete listing of messages that are probably conveyed among mammals by means of olfaction is in Box 41-1.)[70,266] The search for a human pheromone has been going on for many years, and various biologic odorants refined from human urine, axillary secretions, and vaginal secretions have been touted, often in the popular press, as being pheromones. Both anatomic and behavioral studies support the possibility of human communication through odorants (see the vomeronasal section above in the anatomy section); however, additional studies using double-blind techniques are needed before adequate conclusions can be made.[68,69,75,77] One example of the type of human biologic activity on which olfactory control can be exerted is menstrual cycle synchrony. Russell, Switz, and Thompson.[300] placed a mixture of alcohol and underarm secretion from one woman on the upper-lip skin of five women subjects and alcohol only on six control women subjects. Over a period of 5 months there was a statistically significant (0.01) tendency for menstrual synchrony with the woman who donated the axillary secretions among the experimental group as compared with the control group. Although this study has some methodologic problems,[77] it highlights the olfactory communication that may be going on between humans.

STIMULATION AND MEASUREMENT OF OLFACTION

For many years, the clinical evaluation of olfactory ability was simply to determine whether the patient could detect any odorant at all. However, just as this type of yes or no testing is no longer acceptable in the evaluation of vision or hearing, it also is not acceptable for olfactory evaluation. Careful clinical practice demands quantitative, repeatable tests that can be used to document olfactory ability during the course of medical management or across time. The two aspects of olfaction most commonly tested are threshold and identification ability. Of these, identification is most closely related to everyday olfactory functioning.

The measurement of the detection threshold attempts to quantify the most dilute concentration of a particular odorant that an individual can detect. Stuiver[335] estimated that the number of molecules needed to excite a single receptor is at most nine, and perhaps as few as one for mercaptans (skunk-like odorants). Stuiver further estimated that at least 40 receptors should be excited to reach the threshold level. The general format of this test is to use a series of bottles containing a range of concentrations in predetermined steps. Although pyridine and n-butyl alcohol (1-butanol) are two of the most widely used test chemicals because of their water solubility, easy identifiability, and history of successful use, phenylethyl alcohol, which has a rose like smell, may be a better choice because it has less trigeminal reactivity.[76] The odorants are presented from lowest to highest concentration until the subject correctly identifies four odorants at a given concentration. This order of presentation avoids the adaptation (i.e., the loss of sensitivity from mere stimulation) that might occur if strong concentrations were to be used first.[37] In the test situation, the subject is presented with two bottles, one containing the odorant and the other a blank. The subject is asked to choose the bottle that contains the odorant (two-alternative, forced-choice procedure).[55,219] Discretion should be used, however, in the interpretation of olfactory detection threshold scores, because the test-retest reliability of this test has been reported to be low.[141,288]

Identification tests allow the subject to smell a number of odorants and name them correctly. The test is a suprathreshold test; that is, the stimuli are presented at a concentration above threshold that the subject considers normal for that odorant. Additionally, identification tests presume normal cognitive ability. Without this ability, a low olfactory test score may be due to poor testing in someone with normal olfactory ability. Several versions of this test are available and commonly used. Cain and others[43] have developed an identification test that is administered along with a threshold test. In this test, eight common household items (e.g., baby powder, coffee, Ivory soap, and so forth) are presented to

---

Box 47-1. Types of messages conveyed by mammals by means of olfaction

Age appraisal	Individual appraisal
Alarm	Pain indication
Attention-seeking	Predator
Defense	Prey
Distress-signalling	Reproductive stage indica-
Encouraging approach	tion
Frustration	Social status appraisal
Gender appraisal	Species membership
Greeting	Gender appraisal
Gregariousness	Submission
Group membership ap-	Territory marking
praisal	Trail marking
Identification with home	Warning
range	

From Doty RL: *Experientia* 42:257-71, 1986 and Mykytowycz R: *The role of skin glands in mammalian communication.* In Johnston JW Jr, Moulton DG, Turk A, editors: *Advances in chemoreception, vol 1, Communication by chemical signals,* New York, 1970, Appleton-Century-Crofts.

the subject in screw-top jars. The subject is graded on how many of the odorants he can identify correctly.

Doty and others[74,78] have developed a method of testing identification ability using scratch-and-sniff booklets containing 40 microencapsulated odorants. This commercially available test is self-administered and can either be mailed to test subjects or used during the examination. Material accompanying the booklets allows percentile score ranking of test results by age and sex, which are known determinants of olfactory ability (see factors affecting olfactory testing). Because the subject is asked to choose the correct answer from a list of four possible answers, a chance performance would be 25% correct. Obviously, anyone scoring much less than this should be considered for malingering. The portability of the booklets, the freshness of the stimulus, and the fun of doing the test contribute to its popularity.

Another use of an identification test is to better characterize the olfactory status of the patient with an olfactory complaint. Wright[357] has applied a powerful psychophysical tool, the confusion matrix, to this task. In the Odorant Confusion Matrix, 10 single chemical odorants representing common household items (e.g., orange, vanilla, ammonia, and so forth) and one blank are presented to the subject in random order. The subject has a list of the 10 odorants, and must choose one of the words for each presentation (forced-choice). This same sequence is then repeated 9 more times, such that the group of odorants is administered 10 times. The results can then be represented on a matrix, as in Figure 41-11. Not only can the total and individual odorant percent correct scores be calculated from the diagonal, but trends showing improvement or decrement (fatigue or adapting) during the test also can be calculated. In analyzing the off-diagonal responses, the tendency for clumping or consistently responding with the same wrong answer can be determined. The 10 odorants contain four that have varying degrees of pungency. Often an individual who has minimal or no cranial nerve I olfactory ability will be able to recognize these trigeminal stimulators, and this test can measure that effect.

In other parts of the world olfactory testing also is being performed, sometimes with one of the tests noted above, and sometimes with locally designed tests. In Japan, the standard test is the T and T olfactometer, which is a rack containing eight concentrations of five different odorants. From this test, both detection and recognition thresholds can be determined and they are charted on a graph similar to an audiogram.[339] Hendriks[136] has developed a Dutch odor identification test, Geur Identificatie Test Utrecht, that has two subsets of 18 odorants each. This test has applicability for both clinical and industrial testing, and has proven useful in assessing the olfactory ability of adults in the Netherlands.

Doty and others[67] recently reviewed nine different olfactory tests, including tests of odor identification, discrimination, detection, memory, and suprathreshold intensity and pleasantness perception.[67] By using a principal components analysis, they were able to determine that most of these tests measure a common source of variance. This is borne out in clinical practice, where it is rare to find a major discrepancy between olfactory tests.

For all these olfactory tests, especially those measuring threshold, control of stimulus concentration is obviously important. In general, the two main techniques to control or vary odorant concentration are: (1) dilution of the liquid-phase odorant in varying amounts of solvent, and (2) dilution of the vapor-phase odorant with air. Racks of sniff bottles can be designed with a gradient of concentrations. Although they are conveniently portable, the liquids can become contaminated by oxidation, or the odorant concentration can be changed by oxidation or evaporation.[131] Therefore, when open-bottle tests are used, the solutions must be changed frequently. More precise control over the stimulus intensity has been achieved with a variety of olfactometers. By mixing pure air and odorized air streams, the odorant concentrations reaching the nose can be precisely controlled. Although these olfactometers are quite accurate in the control of the stimulus, their cost and size have restricted their use to research laboratories. Another variable in olfactory testing is the presentation of the odorant to the olfactory receptors. Although most techniques use the normal sniffing generated by the subject, some testing is done by puffing or blasting the odorant into the nose. These techniques should be avoided because the subject can confuse the somesthetic sensations of the blast with the odorant stimulus.[24,164] Normal sniffing is by far the easiest and most practical method, and according to Laing[200] provides optimal perception. Moreover, he has found that the first sniff provides the most significant information, and that subsequent sniffs are simply confirmatory. Optimal sniff durations of 0.39 to 0.64 seconds have been noted for cranial nerve I type odorants such as phenylethyl alcohol (rose) and propionic acid, whereas butanol, which has more trigeminal or throat sensation, requires a sniff lasting 1.63 seconds.[201] It also has been shown that although there are wide differences among individuals in sniffing technique, they consistently maintain a unique sniff pattern.[199] For these reasons most clinical olfactory testing is done using a natural sniffing technique.

In an attempt to circumvent the problems of the air stream–delivered stimulus, the Japanese have included intravenous smell testing into their olfactory evaluation.[102] In this test, the subject is asked to perceive the mercaptan (garlic) smell of injected alinamin, a thiol-type derivative of vitamin B1. The time between the injection and the recognition of the smell is designated as the latent time, and the time between the recognition and the disappearance of the smell is the duration time. They report that the latent time is influenced by olfactory acuity and that the duration time depends on adaptation to the odorant. Central olfactory disorders are suspected in patients with decreased duration times, and nonresponders to this test are said to have a poor prognosis of olfactory recovery. Although it is tantalizing

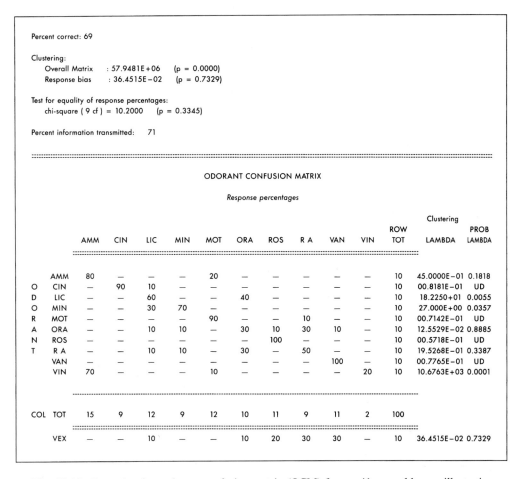

Percent correct: 69

Clustering:
Overall Matrix : 57.9481E+06 (p = 0.0000)
Response bias : 36.4515E−02 (p = 0.7329)

Test for equality of response percentages:
chi-square (9 cf) = 10.2000 (p = 0.3345)

Percent information transmitted: 71

ODORANT CONFUSION MATRIX

Response percentages

		AMM	CIN	LIC	MIN	MOT	ORA	ROS	R A	VAN	VIN	ROW TOT	Clustering LAMBDA	PROB LAMBDA
	AMM	80	—	—	—	20	—	—	—	—	—	10	45.0000E−01	0.1818
O	CIN	—	90	10	—	—	—	—	—	—	—	10	00.8181E−01	UD
D	LIC	—	—	60	—	—	40	—	—	—	—	10	18.2250+01	0.0055
O	MIN	—	—	30	70	—	—	—	—	—	—	10	27.000E+00	0.0357
R	MOT	—	—	—	—	90	—	—	10	—	—	10	00.7142E−01	UD
A	ORA	—	—	10	10	—	30	10	30	10	—	10	12.5529E−02	0.8885
N	ROS	—	—	—	—	—	—	100	—	—	—	10	00.5718E−01	UD
T	R A	—	—	10	10	—	30	—	50	—	—	10	19.5268E−01	0.3387
	VAN	—	—	—	—	—	—	—	—	100	—	10	00.7765E−01	UD
	VIN	70	—	—	—	10	—	—	—	—	20	10	10.6763E+03	0.0001
COL TOT		15	9	12	9	12	10	11	9	11	2	100		
VEX		—	—	10	—	—	10	20	30	30	—	10	36.4515E−02	0.7329

Fig. 41-11. Example of an odorant confusion matrix (OCM) from a 41-year-old man, illustrating the summary statistics and matrix display of the data. The 69% correct is an average across the diagonal. Note the 40% substitution of orange when licorice was presented, as opposed to the random responses to the orange stimulus (lambda probabilities of 0.0055 for licorice versus 0.8885 for orange). There is an impressive likelihood (lambda probability = 0.0001) for vinegar to be confused with ammonia. The Vex (*blank presentations*) indicate that no response bias exists (lambda probability = 0.7329). *Amm*—Ammonia; *cin*—Cinnamon; *lic*—Licorice; *min*—Mint; *mot*—Moth balls (napthalene); *ora*—Orange; *ros*—Rose; *r a*—Rubbing alcohol (isopropyl alcohol); *van*—Vanillin; *vin*—Vinegar; *col tot*—Column total; *vex*—Blank.

to speculate that this intravenous test directly stimulates the olfactory receptor cells through the blood stream, studies by Okabe[273] indicate that the mechanism of this test is by the discharge of alinamin's metabolic by-products from the bloodstream into the pulmonary alveoli, from where it reaches the olfactory receptors through the nasopharynx through the exhaled air stream.

A problem often encountered in testing olfactory sensitivity is that many patients confuse the loss of the sense of smell with the loss of the sense of taste. Westerman[353] has developed a simple test for such an evaluation whereby the odorant is placed on the tongue and the subject is asked to describe the flavor of the material. This test also may be used to identify malingerers because few individuals know that flavor is largely mediated through the sense of olfaction. When asked, therefore, to identify the taste of the coffee placed on the tongue, the blindfolded olfactory malingerer, who should report a bitter taste, will identify its taste as coffee, but will disclaim any ability to identify the coffee odor when it is held in front of the nose.

Objective testing of olfactory ability in humans has been developed, and is available in laboratories in the United States, Germany, and Japan. Accurate and unobtrusive delivery of the odorant molecules to the nose in warmed and humidified air is mandatory in all of these objective studies.[170,183] The most peripheral of these tests, the electro-olfactogram (EOG), is obtained by placing an electrode directly on the olfactory epithelium.[215] When an odorant stimulates the receptor cells, a slow negative shift in voltage is seen. This has been shown in multiple animals, including humans, and is thought to represent a summation of the many generator potentials from single-receptor cells.[108,274,275,325]

Although the olfactory epithelium is relatively inaccessible in the human, some researchers, including Furukawa and others,[104] have succeeded in recording these EOG potentials and have shown decreased potentials in hyposmics that are commensurate with their loss. As these researchers have said, the EOG provides the only objective method presently available for the differential diagnosis of anosmia caused by disorders of the olfactory epithelium versus the central olfactory tract.

A second objective testing method, used with success in other sensory systems such as hearing and vision, is measurement of brain-evoked potentials. In this test, the summated percutaneous brain electrical activity is averaged after multiple timed exposures to an odorant. Using this test in their research center, Kobal and Hummel[182] have succeeded in determining when the olfactory stimulation arrives at the receptors and have shown differences between pure olfactory and trigeminal stimulation. Maximal amplitudes of potentials evoked by substances that partly or exclusively excite the trigeminal nerve (high concentrations of carbon dioxide, menthol, acetaldehyde) were found at the vertex, and are defined as *chemosomatosensory-evoked potentials.* Substances that exclusively, or to a great extent, excite the olfactory nerve (hydrogen sulfide, vanillin) caused maximal responses in the parietal area and are defined as *olfactory-evoked potentials.* This would correlate best with subjective testing of odor perception. Another type of induced brain wave activity is the endogenous component, called the *contingent negative variation* (CNV).[349] They are called *endogenous* because their presence depends on subjective response strategies rather than stimulus characteristics. It would correlate best with subjective testing of odor discrimination. When the olfactory-evoked potentials and CNV are measured simultaneously, objective assessments of clinical status can be made.[19,237] When both are absent, anosmia is present. When just CNV is present, there likely is an olfactory distortion. Finally, in hyposmia, when the odorant presented is just above the discrimination threshold, the amplitude of the CNV is enhanced and the olfactory-evoked potential is undetectable. This technique is clearly a useful clinical tool, although it is not generally available.

A third objective method of testing olfactory ability uses computer technology for an on-line analysis of EEG data. This brain electrical activity monitoring (BEAM) technique can display colored topographic maps of the cortical activity while events, such as sniffing, are occurring.[83] This technique does not involve averaging of multiple trials (as does the evoked potential technique) and thus can display an individual response to a particular odorant. BEAM technology, which has already found use as a clinical tool in the diagnosis of dyslexia,[82] can illustrate different responses to various odorants and promises to be useful in clinical olfactory evaluations.[343]

FACTORS AFFECTING OLFACTORY TESTING

Age

The testing of olfactory ability in children presents special problems. Richman and others,[294,295] using an identification test designed for adults, found no consistent results in testing children under the age of 10 years, but by the age of 14 years the children's performance was equal to that of adults. By using pictures to represent the odorants instead of words, reliable results could be obtained from children as young as age 6.[293] The children who had cleft lip with cleft palate (CLP) generally did more poorly than did normal children of the same age. Boys in the CLP group were especially poor at olfactory identification. This suggests that there may be a sex bias in olfactory development or ability of children with CLP disorders. With an abbreviated odorant identification task, Richman and his colleagues have successfully tested olfactory function in children starting at age 8 years.[291]

The other popular method for testing olfactory ability in adults, the detection threshold method, has been used in 5- to 15-year-old children using a forced-choice, single-staircase method,[115] but the clinical relevance of this, especially in children, is unclear. Engen[93] found it very difficult to test a hedonic preference in children younger than 4 years of age. They answered "yes" to his query regardless of whether the question was phrased positively or negatively (i.e., both "Do you like it?" and "Do you dislike it?," yielded affirmative answers). Studies that used happy and sad faces or puppets have yielded more consistent results.[309,334]

Using a technique not often employed in testing adults, Richman and others[292] have developed a match-to-sample odorant discrimination task that has been useful in testing children as young as age 5 years. To date, this seems the most reliable way to test young children.

Testing older adults is generally only a problem if there has been a major loss of olfactory function, or if the patient has dementia. For individuals with poor olfactory ability, the testing can be boring, disheartening, and frustrating, all of which can lead to inadequate measurement of real olfactory ability. In testing olfactory ability in the demented individual, the tests used in children have been useful. Obviously, if someone is severely demented, any type of interactive testing will be futile.

Instruction

Dual thresholds exist in olfaction, one for recognition and another for identification.[339] Engen[91] showed this dual threshold by asking subjects to either detect which one of four test tubes smelled different or to identify the one test tube out of the four that contained a specific odorant. The first set of instructions consistently yielded lower absolute thresholds. The fact that two thresholds seem to be acting in olfaction could indicate the presence of different receptor types, similar to the rods and cones of the retina; on the other hand, it could also mean that a certain level of summation of peripheral events is necessary at a central locus before positive identification can be made.[259]

Satiety

Because eating is so intimately associated with aromas, one might expect the prandial state of an individual to affect the sense of smell. The testing of olfactory ability in this situation can be influenced by the pleasantness of the odor. One must be careful to focus the subject on either the detection task or the hedonic judgement because one may affect the other.[93] Cabanac[35] has shown that hunger affects judgments of pleasantness with food odorants, but not psychophysical assessments of intensity. In general, a food odor is pleasant when one is hungry and less pleasant after one has overindulged in the food. By contrast, nonfood odorants, such as laboratory chemicals, generally do not show shifts in preference judgment.[186,254]

Sex

In humans, test results averaged over many chemicals have consistently shown that females have a better olfactory ability than males, both in threshold and in identification tasks.[347] For specific odorants, however, there may be no difference.[185] In addition, the menstrual cycle influences their olfaction threshold level, being best at ovulation and poorest during menstruation.[68,77,310] The reasons for this are not simply hormonal variations because Doty and others.[77] have shown olfactory cycling even in women using oral contraceptives, whose hormone levels did not vary. In animals a clear relation exists between olfaction and sexual functioning. Pregnancy in mice can be blocked by the odor of a strange male.[33]

Adaptation and habituation

The perception of a strong odor noticeable upon entering a barn will disappear after a period of time. This adaptation response in humans, as measured by Stuiver,[335] generally occurred within 1 to 5 minutes for the chemicals studied. Data suggest that adaptation occurs both at the receptor-cell level[21,275] and more centrally.[22,191,335] Central adaptation is supported by the finding that, in humans, continued stimulation through one nostril leads to adaptation in both nostrils.[335]

Olfactory cross-adaptation is the ability of one chemical to decrease the subject's responsiveness and sensitivity to another chemical. It has been proposed that the greater the cross-adapting effect on one odorant by another, the more likely they are to share common sensory channels.[51,207,245,282,283] The manner and degree to which the odorants cause the receptors to adapt may not result from a simple mechanism because even if two different odorants are matched in subjective intensity, their cross-adapting effects may be asymmetric.[272,283] For example, pentanol seems to have a strong cross-adapting effect on propanol, whereas propanol has only a small cross-adapting effect on pentanol.[38]

Odor mixtures

Perfumers and chefs are involved in the mixing of odorants, and much of what is known in this area is in the realm of art rather than science. When two or more odorants are mixed, several sensory events may be reported.[259] First, the odorants may be discerned as being distinct. Second, an entirely new odor may develop that resembles the components but does not smell exactly like either of them. Third, one odor may mask the other. A fourth possibility, neutralization, would result if no odor were perceived, but the existence of this last phenomenon is controversial. Laing and others[197,202] have investigated the effect of odorant intensity and perceived quality when testing with mixtures. They found that the odorant with the highest intensity always predominated or was the only component perceived. Both odorants were perceived, however, when the intensities of both components were approximately equal. They also identified ''fast'' and ''slow'' odorants that are processed temporally, the fast odorants usually suppressing the slow ones.

CLINICAL OLFACTORY PROBLEMS

Decreased and distorted olfactory ability

Life for the person with anosmia has a very ''flat'' quality to it. Patients say that they select food by texture, color, and custom. Some state, for example, that they must identify sour milk by its lumpy character. Others do not use perfumes for fear of overapplication. Many express concern regarding fire and noxious or dangerous gases, and in fact most anosmic patients have been involved in at least one accident stemming from this problem. Smoke alarms are an absolute necessity for these people.

In contrast to this lack of sensory input, there are individuals who have a distorted perception of odorants or the constant perception of an odor (usually foul in character). These people are miserable and will spend a great deal of time and money trying to rid themselves of their problem, often without success. As might be expected, some of these people whose sense of smell is dysfunctional will have dietary problems such as malnutrition, obesity, and anorexia, since their food often has the same foul odor.[240,308]

Human olfactory dysfunctions

The report of the Panel on the Communicative Disorders to the National Advisory Neurological and Communicative Disorders and Stroke Council estimates that approximately 2 million American adults have disorders of taste and smell. The literature lists more than 200 conditions that have been associated with changes in chemosensory ability.[69,95,307,308,318] To better understand these clinical chemosensory problems, multiple chemosensory centers have been established over the past decade. They have had the dual role of

Table 41-1. Spectrum of olfactory loss at four chemosensory centers

Etiologic category	Goodspeed, Gent, and Catalanotto[121] (1987) (441 patients)	Davidson and others[58] (1987) (63 patients)	Leopold and others (198 patients)	Heywood and others[142] (1990) (133 patients)
Obstructive nasal and sinus disease, %	30	33	29	20
Post–upper respiratory infection, %	19	32	15	17
Head trauma, %	9	10	19	32
Aging, %	0	0	8	6
Congenital, %	0	5	8	0
Toxins, %	1	11	3	0
Miscellaneous, %	14	10	8	16
Idiopathic, %	26	0	10	10

evaluating and treating patients and integrating basic science research into the effort. Using careful histories, physical examinations, chemosensory testing, and imaging studies, these centers have categorized the majority of patients with olfactory losses into etiologic categories (Table 41-1).

Although these centers differ as to the percentage of patients placed within each etiologic category, these differences are thought to reflect the particular type of patient seen at the center and not a difference in disease pattern across the country.[142] The following sections will describe the etiologic categories in detail. Those rare patients who have a distortion of their sense of smell (parosmia or phantosmia) with no change in intensity are not included in the above classification.

Obstructive nasal and sinus disease

Total nasal obstruction, such as caused by nasal polyps (Fig. 41-12), extreme mucosal swelling (Fig. 41-13), or simply finger occlusion of the nostrils will produce anosmia. When the obstruction is released, olfactory ability should return (Fig. 41-14), although the minimal nasal opening at which this occurs is not known. The location of this opening, or the area through which air flows to get to the olfactory cleft, is thought to be medial and anterior to the lower part of the middle turbinate.[210,212] This area may function as a regulator of airflow to the olfactory cleft, and changes in its anatomy clearly affect olfactory ability. Consequently, obstruction at this area or above it by swollen mucosa, polyps, tumors, or nasal bony deformities can decrease or eliminate olfactory ability.[18,25,286] This sometimes occurs even when the lower nasal cavity appears normal. It has been known that systemic steroid management will reverse anosmia in most patients with nasal obstruction that is caused by nasal polyps and chronic rhinitis.[58,120,149,318] Although management with chronic systemic steroids has many drawbacks[317] a 1- or 2-week course may serve as a diagnostic test for nasal disease. What is still unclear is the etiology of anosmia in the rare patient with a patent nasal airway whose olfactory ability can be improved by chronic systemic steroids.[157]

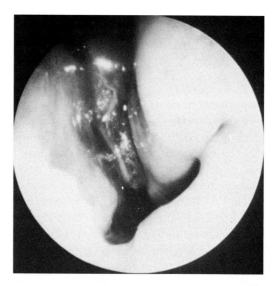

Fig. 41-12. The lower left nostril with a large polyp between the inferior turbinate and the septum.

Although several authors have proposed that traumatic nasal cavity deformity can cause olfactory loss,[29,234,328] none of these reports employed reproducible olfactory testing, nor was any meaningful change in olfactory ability brought about by surgical changes in the nasal anatomy, so the olfactory losses reported may have been caused by neural problems. In the author's experience, it is rare to identify an individual whose nasal anatomy is so deformed from external trauma that not even a small amount of air can reach the olfactory cleft. Scarring from previous surgery between the middle turbinate and the nasal septum, however, can be effective in closing off the olfactory area to airflow.

Olfactory loss following upper respiratory infection

Many people will volunteer that at one time or another they have lost their sense of smell completely during an upper respiratory infection (URI). In general, these olfactory losses are due to nasal airway obstruction and will resolve

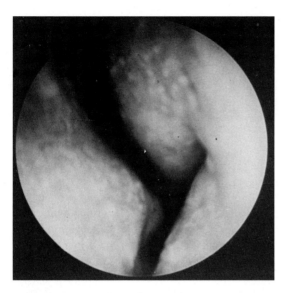

Fig. 41-13. The lower left nostril with a narrowed airway caused by mucosal edema.

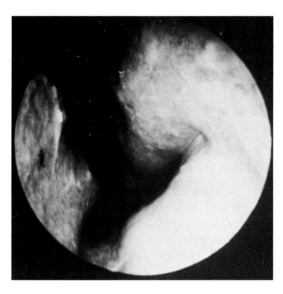

Fig. 41-14. The same patient as in Figure 41-12 after polyp removal.

when the nasal airway becomes patent again (1 to 3 days).[10] Of greater concern is the small number of patients whose olfactory ability never recovers after the other symptoms of the URI resolve. These people tend to be otherwise healthy individuals, in the fourth, fifth, or sixth decade of life, and are overwhelmingly women (70% to 80%).[58,121,136,209] The reason for this female preponderance is unclear but may relate to the fact that women tend to have more URIs.[211] Biopsies of the olfactory cleft in these patients show either decreased numbers of olfactory receptors or a complete absence of them.[160,360,361] The prognosis for recovery from this olfactory loss is generally poor. Hendriks[136] combined

several reported studies of olfactory patients and found that approximately one third of the patients recovered their olfactory ability, regardless of whether they were treated or not. Duncan and Seiden[86] have measured a light to moderate improvement in two thirds of their sample of 21 patients that takes years to occur. The problem with these studies is that an upper nasal obstruction from mucus or swollen mucosa may remain after the URI has resolved. Without concurrent imaging of the nasal cavity, it would be impossible to determine if a return of olfactory ability after a URI loss was due to clearing of the olfactory cleft or recovery of neural function.

Head trauma

A review of several large series of mostly adult head trauma patients (containing both minor and major trauma) reveals that the reported incidence of olfactory loss is between 5% and 10% (Leigh,[206] 1000 cases; Hughes,[151] 1800 cases; Sumner,[337] 1167 cases; Zusho,[371] 5000 cases). In contrast to this, the rate of olfactory loss after childhood head trauma has been reported to be 3.2% (transient) and 1.2% (permanent) (Jacobi, Rtiz, and Emrich,[154] 741 cases). The degree of olfactory loss is generally associated with the severity of the trauma; however, even minor trauma can produce total anosmia.[47,133] Most studies of patients who complain of olfactory loss after trauma find the average loss to be in the anosmic range.[58,209] Fikentscher and Mauuller,[97] who classified 77 of 122 patients as anosmic, also support this tendency for the posttraumatic loss to be complete. The degree of olfactory loss also is partly determined by the site of cranial trauma. Frontal blows most frequently cause olfactory loss; however, total anosmia is five times more likely with an occipital blow.[136,337] The onset of a traumatic olfactory loss is generally immediate, although in some instances the patient either does not appreciate the loss or does not experience the loss until months after the injury.[209,304] Recovery of olfactory function is less than 10% according to most large studies, however, Duncan and Seiden[86] showed that one third of their group of 20 patients had slight to moderate improvement in identification ability after the trauma. The quality of the returned olfactory ability is usually quite poor.

The exact injury to the olfactory system produced by trauma is unknown, although shearing of the olfactory nerves as they exit the top of the cribriform plate is a popular theory.[128] New information from biopsies of olfactory epithelium in patients who sustained a traumatically induced olfactory loss has recently become available.[158,361] After trauma the olfactory cells are generally distorted, have proliferation of axons and axon tangles in the lamina propria, and have few olfactory knobs and cilia. These findings suggest the following scenario: (1) the olfactory nerves were damaged at the time of the trauma, perhaps at the cribriform plate; (2) the normal response of the olfactory nerves is to regenerate, but the axons cannot (for some unknown reason) reach the olfactory bulb; and (3) without this connection with the bulb, the cells will not produce olfactory knobs or cilia. The key, therefore, in helping these people is to reestablish contact between the olfactory axons and the olfactory bulb. Presently, however, there is no known method to accomplish this task. Another possible area of olfactory system injury after head trauma may be in the frontal cortex. In a study of 40 patients who had traumatic total anosmia, all had major vocational problems.[346] Most of these patients showed psychosocial defects associated with frontal cortex injury. Similarly, Levin, High, and Eisenberg[218] observed impaired olfactory recognition in patients who had a traumatic hematoma or contusion in the frontotemporal region.

Aging

Although older individuals can have an olfactory loss from any of the other causes discussed here, they also can have losses caused by dementia-related diseases and from the aging process itself. In fact, in otherwise healthy individuals, deficits in balance, olfaction, and visual pursuit best discriminate between people greater than 85 years of age and less than 74 years of age.[175] Olfactory identification ability has been shown to drop sharply in the sixth and seventh decades of life such that more than one half of those aged 65 to 80 years show major olfactory declines.[332] This pattern of change with respect to age is similar to that seen for visual acuity and speech intelligibility.[79] Olfactory thresholds also have been found to decline with age, this effect being slightly less dramatic in women than in men.[40,61,332,344] From the National Geographic Smell Survey, Wysocki and Gilbert[359] have determined that the degree and rate of olfactory loss is odorant specific and varies from individual to individual. Other measured effects of aging on the sense of smell include decreased magnitude matching,[332] changes in the perception of pleasantness,[59,359] association with decreased nutritional status,[84,125] and the ability to discriminate flavor in everyday foods.[41,306]

The perceptual losses in olfactory ability that accompany aging are not surprising when the anatomic changes are noted. Bhatnagar and others[26] carefully studied olfactory bulbs from individuals aged 25 to 95 years. From a total of 50,935 mitral cells at age 25, they counted a linear decline that averaged 520 cells per year. Likewise, from a total olfactory bulb volume of 50.02 mm at age 25, they noticed a decline of 0.19 mm per year. In addition to the decline in the number of cellular elements, Liss and Gomez[222] also noted extensive degeneration in the bulb with aging.

There are at least two dementia-related diseases that are often accompanied by a smell disorder: Alzheimer's disease and Parkinson's disease. In patients with these diseases, it is likely that there has been some damage to the olfactory bulb or the central olfactory cortex and that this damage is, at least in part, responsible for the accompanying loss in olfactory detection and recognition ability.[73] Alzheimer's disease is characterized by the presence of neurofibrillary tangles and neuritic plaques in most of the central olfactory pathways.[94,179,232,195] These tangles and plaques are presumed to account for the clinical deficits of the disease.[132,278] The fact that similar pathologic changes and testing abnormalities are seen in patients with down syndrome suggests a possible genetic link.[370] Furthermore, as Pearson and others[278] have pointed out, the involvement by the olfactory system is in striking contrast to the minimal abnormality seen in other areas of the brain. This has raised the possibility that the olfactory system is the portal of entry for an environmental agent that causes the disease.[96] Recently identified abnormalities in the nasal olfactory epithelium may give additional support for this theory.[340] An alternative theory is that the olfactory system is simply attacked preferentially over other neural elements.[71] There are a number of nonmotor defects in patients with Parkinson's disease, including depression and congitive losses.[217] A reduction in the ability to detect and identify odorants is one of these defects, and the degree of this defect is related to, and may help in the diagnosis of, the clinical subtype of Parkinson's disease.[330,351] The olfactory changes have been shown to be independent of the cognitive and motor symptoms,[80] and they occur early in the disease. Neuronal losses have been identified in the olfactory bulb and tracts of individuals who died with Parkinson's disease, with a strong correlation to disease duration.[277] Because the loss of olfactory ability also occurs early in Alzheimer's disease and is not noticed by the patient, decreased olfactory ability on clinical testing ability may be an important early signal for the development of these diseases.[270]

Congenital

The usual history of the person with a total congenital loss of the sense of smell is that he or she is otherwise healthy and began to learn at about age 8 that friends, parents, and siblings could perceive something he or she could not. Most of these individuals have their other chemosensory functions intact, so that pungency, irritating odors, and tastes can be detected normally.[159] Many more people have an isolated loss of sensitivity to a particular chemical or group of chemicals (also known as a specific anosmia), for example, musks, trimethylamine (a fish-like odor), hydrogen cyanide (almond-like), butyl mercaptan (an additive to natural gas), and isovaleric acid (a locker-room odor).[13,276]

Jafek and others[159] have proposed that the pathophysiology of congenital olfactory loss is due to a degeneration or atrophy of the olfactory epithelium or the olfactory bulb late in the developmental process. They base this theory on the total lack of peripheral receptors or supporting cells and the routine finding of respiratory epithelium in olfactory cleft biopsies from people with a history consistent with a congenital loss. On olfactory testing, individuals in this congenital group scored either at or slightly better than chance performance.[58,159] Because individuals from other etiologic groups (e.g., head trauma, post-URI) have been shown to have at

ple management strategies have been proposed, often using vitamins or minerals. Vitamin A was thought to be an effective management strategy because (1) it is necessary for the repair of epithelium, (2) white rats apparently become anosmic on a diet deficient in vitamin A,[208] and (3) assays done on mammalian olfactory epithelium showed considerable amounts of vitamin A.[87] In an uncontrolled study, Duncan and Briggs[87] used Vitamin A successfully to restore at least partial olfactory ability in 50 out of 56 of their subjects. Unfortunately, other observers have been unable to reproduce their success.[136,209] B vitamins have also been tried for the management of anosmia, once again without success.[87,242]

Mackay-Sim and Dreosti[225] have shown that zinc-deficient adult mice failed to show a food odor preference. This supports the administration of oral zinc by Henkin and others[139] as a management option for losses of taste and smell associated with a zinc deficiency. It is known that severe zinc deficiency is rare and difficult to substantiate.[174] Nevertheless, occasional reports of patients who have improved on zinc therapy are available.[48,192] These reports must be evaluated, however, with the understanding that some olfactory disorders do improve spontaneously. Indeed, in a randomized, double-blind crossover study of the effects of zinc on 106 patients with taste and smell problems, Henkin and others[137] noted that zinc was no more effective than placebo. At the present time, few chemosensory centers are suggesting that zinc is useful for olfactory disorders.[318] Henkin and others[137] also have suggested, that aminophylline is useful for anosmic and hyposmic patients. This suggestion is based on the observation that cAMP plays a role in the transduction of olfactory responses. Unfortunately, corroborative data supporting its use are not available.

Once patients have been placed in one of the nonmanagable groups, they should be reassured that there are others with similar deficits. Because olfaction plays such an important role in the appreciation of foods, these patients should be counseled on possible ways to improve the variety or seasoning of their diet to enhance whatever sensory modalities remain (e.g., emphasizing the taste, color, texture, viscosity, and ''mouth feel'' of foods). Attempts should be made to ensure that the normosmic persons living with them understand the problem and can be relied on to volunteer information of social concern regarding odors. Smoke and fire detectors are mandatory. Anosmic persons living alone should elicit the confidential help of friends on matters of odor. The dangers of natural gas and liquid petroleum gas can be avoided by switching to electric appliances and nonexplosive heating or cooling fuel.[42]

The management of phantosmia is varied. In Europe, Zilstorff[368] and Fikentscher and Rasinski[98] have used topical cocaine hydrochloride directly on the olfactory mucosa; however, multiple retreatments have been required, and other clinicians have been unable to duplicate their results.[318] In addition, the author has documented the total loss of olfactory ability in one patient who used this treatment daily over several years. Neurosurgeons have done olfactory bulbectomies through a neurosurgical craniotomy approach to alleviate the phantom odor.[173,233] While the patients who have had this surgery are pleased to be rid of their phantom odor, they are left with no olfactory ability on the operated side. If both sides are operated on, they will be totally anosmic. Leopold and others[214] have successfully managed phantosmia by removing olfactory epithelium from the underside of the cribriform plate. The advantage to this procedure seems to be that the olfactory ability is not irreversibily destroyed.

SUMMARY

Although the basic mechanisms of olfaction are still being discovered, what has already been learned forms an exciting foundation for further research. The process of odorant delivery to the receptors differs from person to person and may be an adaptation to the differences in upper nasal cavity anatomy. Although the receptors regenerate throughout one's adult life, why does this process not continue after head trauma? How does the olfactory system distinguish the thousands of odorants to which humans are exposed? What is the relationship of the olfactory loss in Parkinson's disease to the progression of the disease? The answers to these questions and many others are being explored. By evaluating and diagnosing patients with olfactory problems, a better understanding of the olfactory system is being obtained, and these patients are being helped in the process.

Supported in part by NIH Grant NIDCD9 - P01 DC00220.

REFERENCES

1. Ache BW, Zhainazarov A: Dual second-messenger pathways in olfactory transduction, *Curr Opin Neurobiol* 5:461, 1995 (review).
2. Adamek GD, Mair RG, Gesteland RC: EOGs are stimulus specific during ciliary growth. Paper presented at the third annual meeting of the Association for Chemoreception Sciences, Sarasota, Fla, 1981 (abstract).
3. Adrian ED: Sensory discrimination with some recent evidence from the olfactory organ, *Br Med Bull* 6:330, 1950.
4. Adrian ED: The electrical activity of the mammalian olfactory bulb, *Electroencephal Clin Neurophysiol* 2:377, 1950.
5. Adrian ED: Psycho-physiologie, A: fonctions sensorielles, I: Olfactory discrimination, *Ann Psychol* 50:107, 1951.
6. Adrian ED: Energy into nerve impulses: the mechanism of olfactory stimulation in the mammal, *Adv Sci* 9:417, 1953.
7. Adrian ED: Sensory messages and sensation: the response of the olfactory organ to different smells, *Acta Physiol Scand* 29:5, 1953.
8. Adrian ED: The basis of sensation: some recent studies of olfaction, *BMJ* 1:287, 1954.
9. Ahlstrom R and others: Impaired odor perception in tank cleaners, *Scand J Work Environ Health* 12:574, 1986.
10. Akerlund A, Bende M, Murphy C: Olfactory threshold and nasal mucosal changes in experimentally induced common cold, *Acta Otolaryngol (Stockh)* 115:88, 1995.
11. Allison AC: The structure of the olfactory bulb and its relation to the olfactory pathways in the rabbit and the rat, *J Comp Neurol* 98:309, 1953.
12. Allison AC, Warwick PTT: Quantitative observations on the olfactory system of the rabbit, *Brain* 72:186, 1949.

13. Amoore JE: A plan to identify most of the primary odors. In Olfaction and Taste, Proceedings of the Third International Symposium, New York, 1969, Rockefeller University Press.

14. Amoore JE: *Olfactory genetics and anosmia.* In Amoore JE, editor: *Handbook of sensory physiology, vol 4, Chemical senses,* Berlin, 1971, Springer-Verlag.

15. Amoore JE: Specific anosmia and the concept of primary odors, *Chem Senses Flavor* 2:267, 1977.

16. Amsterdam JD and others: Taste and smell perception in depression, *Biol Psychiatry* 22:1481, 1987.

17. Annett JM, Cook NM, Leslie JC: Interference with olfactory memory by visual and verbal tasks, *Percept Mot Skills* 80:1307, 1995.

18. Apter AJ and others: Allergic rhinitis and olfactory loss, *Ann Allergy Asthma Immunol* 75:311, 1995.

19. Aufferman H and others: Olfactory evoked potentials and contingent negative variation simultaneously recorded for diagnosis of smell disorders, *Ann Otol Rhinol Laryngol* 102:6, 1993.

20. Axel R: The molecular logic of smell, *Sci Am* 273:154, 1995 (review).

21. Baylin F, Moulton DG: Adaptation and cross-adaptation to odor stimulation of olfactory receptors in the Tiger salamander, *J Gen Physiol* 74:37, 1979.

22. Beidler LM: *Facts and theory on the mechanism of taste and odor perception: chemistry of natural food flavors,* Chicago, 1957, Quartermaster Food and Container Institute for the Armed Forces.

23. Bellas DN, Novelly RA, Eskenazi B: Olfactory lateralization and identification in right hemisphere lesion and control patients, *Neurophysiologia* 27:1187, 1989.

24. Benignus VA, Prah JD: Flow thresholds on nonodorous air through the human naris as a function of temperature and humidity, *Percept Psychophys* 27:569, 1980.

25. Benniger MS: Rhinitis, sinusitis, and their relationships to allergies, *Am J Rhinol* 6:37, 1992.

26. Bhatnagar KP and others: Number of mitral cells and the bulb volume in the aging human olfactory bulb: a quantitative morphological study, *Anat Rec* 218:73, 1987.

27. Bignetti E and others: Purification and characterisation of an odorant-binding protein from cow nasal tissue, *Eur J Biochem* 149:227, 1985.

28. Bouvet JF, Delaleu JC, Holley A: The activity of olfactory receptor cells is affected by acetylcholine and substance P, *Neurosci Res* 5:214, 1988.

29. Bramley P: Long-term effects of facial injuries, *Proc R Soc Med* 65:916, 1972.

30. Brauchli P and others: Electrocortical and autonomic alteration by administration of a pleasant and an unpleasant odor, *Chem Senses* 20:505, 1995.

31. Breer H, Shepherd GM: Implications of the NO/cGMP system for olfaction *Trends Neurosci* 16:5, 1993 (review).

32. Bromley SM, Doty RL: Odor recognition memory is better under bilateral than unilateral test conditions, *Cortex* 31:25, 1995.

33. Bruce HM: A block to pregnancy in the mouse caused by proximity of strange males, *J Reprod Fertil* 1:96, 1960.

34. Burdach KJ, Doty RL: The effects of mouth movements, swallowing, and spitting on retronasal odor perception, *Physiol Behav* 41:353, 1987.

35. Cabanac M: Physiological role of pleasure, *Science* 173:1103, 1971.

36. Cain WS: *Olfaction and the common chemical sense: similarities, differences, and interactions.* In Moskowitz HR, Warren CB, editors: *Odor quality and chemical structure,* ACS Symposium Series No. 148, 1981, American Chemical Society.

37. Cain WS: Testing olfaction in a clinical setting. *Ear Nose Throat J* 68:316, 1989.

38. Cain WS, Engen T: Olfactory adaptation and the scaling of odor intensity. In Olfaction and Taste, Proceedings of the Third International Symposium, New York, 1969, Rockefeller University Press.

39. Cain WS, Murphy CL: Interaction between chemoreceptive modalities of odor and irritation, *Nature* 284:255, 1980.

40. Cain WS, Murphy CL: Influence of aging on recognition memory for odors and graphic stimuli, *Ann NY Acad Sci* 510:212, 1987.

41. Cain WS, Reid F, Stevens JC: Missing ingredients: aging and the discrimination of flavor, *J Nutr Elder* 9:3, 1990.

42. Cain WS, Turk A: Smell of danger: an analysis of LP-gas odorization, *Am Ind Hyg Assoc J* 46:115, 1985.

43. Cain WS and others: Clinical evaluation of olfaction, *Am J Otolaryngol* 4:252, 1983.

44. Cain WS and others: Evaluation of olfactory dysfunction in the Connecticut Chemosensory Clinical Research Center, *Laryngoscope* 98:83, 1988.

45. Carr VM and others: Developmental expression of reactivity to monoclonal antibodies generated against olfactory epithelia, *J Neurosci* 9:1179, 1989.

46. Carr WE, Gleeson RA, Trapido-Rosenthal HG: The role of perireceptor events in chemosensory processes, *Trends Neurosci* 13:212, 1990.

47. Caruso V, Hagan J, Manning H: Quantitative olfactometry in the measurement of post-traumatic anosmia, *Arch Otolaryngol Head Neck Surg* 90:500, 1969.

48. Cassirer AM: The missing zinc, *J Am Med Wom Assoc* 36:269, 1981.

49. Cavill GWK, Robertson PL: Ant venoms, attractants, and repellents, *Science* 149:1337, 1965.

50. Champion R: Anosmia associated with corrective rhinoplasty, *Br J Plast Surg* 19:182, 1966.

51. Cheesman GH, Townsend MJ: Further experiments on the olfactory thresholds of pure substances using the ''sniff-bottle method,'' *J Exp Psychol* A 8:8, 1956.

52. Chilfala WM, Polzella DJ: Smell and taste classification of the same stimuli, *J Gen Psychol* 122:287, 1995.

53. Cometto-Muniz JE, Cain WS: Temporal integration of pungency, *Chem Senses* 8:315, 1984.

54. Cooper HM and others: Neuroanatomical pathways linking vision and olfaction in mammals, *Psychoneuroendocrinology* 19:623, 1994.

55. Cornsweet TN: The staircase method in psychophysics, *Am J Psychol* 75:485, 1962.

56. Corwin J, Loury M, Gilbert AN: Workplace, age, and sex as mediators of olfactory function: data from the National Georgraphic Smell Survey, *J Gerontol B Psychol Sci Soc Sci* 50:179, 1995.

57. Crews L, Hunter D: Neurogenesis in the olfactory epithelium *Perspect Dev Neurobiol* 2:151, 1994 (review).

58. Davidson TM and others: Evaluation and treatment of smell dysfunction, *West J Med* 146:434, 1987.

59. de Graaf C, Polet P, van Staveren WA: Sensory perception and pleasantness of food flavors in elderly subjects, *J Gerontol* 49:93, 1994.

60. de Morsier G: La dysplasie of olfactogenitale, *Acta Neuropathol* 1:433, 1962.

61. Deems DA, Doty RL: Age-related changes in the phenyl ethyl alcohol odor detection threshold, *Trans Pa Acad Ophthalmol Otolaryngol* 39:646, 1987.

62. Dellacorte C and others: NADPH diaphorase staining suggests localization of nitric oxide synthase within mature vertebrate olfactory neurons, *Neuroscience* 66:215, 1995.

63. Devoir M, Chorover SL: A presumptive sex pheromone in the hamster: some behavioral effects, *J Comp Physiol* [A] 88:496, 1975.

64. Dewes W and others: MR tomography of Kallmann's syndrome, *Fortschritte auf dem Gebiete der Rontgenstrahlen und der Nuklearmedizin* 147:400, 1987.

65. Dhallan RS and others: Primary structure and functional expression of a cyclic nucleotide-activated channel from olfactory neurons, *Nature* 347:184, 1990.

66. Dionne VE, Dubin AE: Transduction diversity in olfaction *J Exp Biol* 194:1, 1994 (review).

67. Doty RL and others: Tests of human olfactory function: principal components analysis suggests that most measure a common source of variance, *Percept Psychophys* 56:701, 1994.

68. Doty RL: *Gender and endocrine-related influences on human olfac-*

tory perception. In Meiselman HL, Rivlin RS, editors: *Clinical measurement of taste and smell*, New York, 1986, MacMillan Publishing.

69. Doty RL: A review of olfactory dysfunctions in man, *Am J Otolaryngol* 1:1, 1979.

70. Doty RL: Odor guided behavior in mammals, *Experentia* 42:257, 1986.

71. Doty RL: Influence of age and age-related diseases on olfactory function, *Ann NY Acad Sci* 561:76, 1989.

72. Doty RL, Frye R: Influence of nasal obstruction on smell function, *Otolaryngol Clin North Am* 22:397, 1989.

73. Doty RL, Reyes PF, Gregor T: Presence of both odor identification and detection deficits in Alzheimer's disease, *Brain Res Bull* 18:597, 1987.

74. Doty RL, Shaman P, Dann M: Development of the University of Pennsylvania Smell Identification Test: a standardized microencapsulated test of olfactory function, *Physiol Behav* 32:489, 1984a.

75. Doty RL and others: Changes in the intensity and pleasantness of human vaginal odors during the menstrual cycle, *Science* 190:316, 1975.

76. Doty RL and others: Intranasal trigeminal stimulation from odorous volatiles: psychometric responses from anosmic and normal humans, *Physiol Behav* 23:373, 1978.

77. Doty RL and others: Endocrine, cardiovascular, and psychological correlates of olfactory sensitivity changes during the human menstrual cycle, *J Comp Physiol Psychol* 95:45, 1981.

78. Doty RL and others: University of Pennsylvania Smell Identification Test: a rapid quantitative olfactory function test for the clinic, *Laryngoscope* 94:176, 1984b.

79. Doty RL and others: Smell identification ability: changes with age, *Science* 226:1441, 1984c.

80. Doty RL and others: The olfactory and cognitive deficits of Parkinson's disease: evidence for independence, *Ann Neurol* 25:166, 1989.

81. Doucette R: Olfactory ensheathing cells: potential for glial cell transplantation into areas of CNS injury, *Histol Histopathol* 10:503, 1995 (review).

82. Duffy FH, McAulty GB: *Brain electrical activity mapping (BEAM): the search for a physiologic signature of dyslexia.* In Duffy FH, Geschwind N, editors: *Dyslexia: a neuroscientific approach to clinical evaluation*, Boston, 1985, Little, Brown.

83. Duffy FH, McAulty GB, Schachter S: *Brain electrical activity mapping.* In Geschwind N, Galibura A, editors: *Cerebral dominance: the biological foundation*, Cambridge, Mass, 1984, Harvard University Press.

84. Duffy VB, Backstrand JR, Ferris AM: Olfactory dysfunction and related nutritional risk in free-living, elderly women, *J Am Diet Assoc* 95:879, 1995.

85. Dulac C, Axel R: A novel family of genes encoding putative pheromone receptors in mammals, *Cell* 83:195, 1995.

86. Duncan HJ, Seiden Am: Long-term follow-up of olfactory loss secondary to head trauma and upper respiratory tract infection, *Arch Otolaryngol Head Neck Surg* 121:1183, 1995.

87. Duncan RB, Briggs M: Treatment of uncomplicated anosmia by vitamin A, *Arch Otolaryngol* 75:116, 1962.

88. Eccles R, Jawad MS, Morris S: Olfactory and trigeminal thresholds and nasal resistance to airflow, *Acta Otolaryngol (Stockh)* 108:268, 1989.

89. Eichel BS: Improvement of olfaction following pansinus surgery, *Ear Nose Throat J* 73:248, 1994.

90. Ellis H: *Studies in the psychology of sex, vol 4, Sexual selection in man*, Philadelphia, 1982, FA Davis.

91. Engen T: Effect of practice and instruction on olfactory thresholds, *Percept Mot Skills* 10:195, 1960.

92. Engen T: *Method and theory in the study of odor preference.* In *Human responses to environmental odors*, New York, 1974, Academic Press.

93. Engen T: *The perception of odors*, New York, 1982, Academic Press.

94. Esiri MM, Pearson RC, Powell TP: The cortex of the primary auditory area in Alzheimer's disease, *Brain Res* 366:385, 1986.

95. Feldman JI, Wright HN, Leopold DA: The initial evaluation of dysosmia, *Am J Otolaryngol* 7:431, 1986.

96. Ferreyra-Moyano H, Barragan E: The olfactory system and Alzheimer's disease, *Int J Neurosci* 49:157, 1989.

97. Fikentscher R, Mauuller H: Traumatische riechstörungen, *Z Artzl Fortbild* 79:1049, 1985.

98. Fikentscher R, Rasinski C: Parosmias: definition and clinical picture, *Laryngo Rhinotologic* 65:663, 1986.

99. Fikentscher R, Seeber H: Occupations and the sense of smell, *Z Gesamte Hyg* 35:78, 1989.

100. Frye RE, Schwartz BS, Doty RL: Dose-related effects of cigarette smoking on olfactory function, *JAMA* 263:1233, 1990.

101. Furstenberg AC, Crosby E, Farrior B: Neurologic lesions which influence the sense of smell, *Arch Otolaryngol* 48:529, 1943.

102. Furukawa M and others: Significance of intravenous olfaction test using thiamine propyldisulfide (Alinamin) in olfactometry, *Auris Nasus Larynx* 15:25, 1988a.

103. Furukawa M and others: Importance of unilateral examination in olfactometry, *Auris Nasus Larynx* 15:113, 1988b.

104. Furukawa M and others: Electro-olfactogram (EOG) in olfactometry, *Auris Nasus Larynx* 16:33, 1989.

105. Garcia-Velasco J, Garcia-Casas S: Nose surgery and the vomeronasal organ, *Aesthetic Plast Surg* 19:451, 1995.

106. Gesteland RC, Lettvin JY, Pitts WH: Chemical transmission in the nose of the frog, *J Physiol* 181:525, 1965.

107. Gesteland RC, Yancey RA, Farbman AI: Development of olfactory receptor neuron selectivity in the rat fetus, *Neuroscience* 7:3127, 1982.

108. Getchell TV: Analysis of intracellular recordings from salamander olfactory epithelium, *Brain Res* 123:275, 1977.

109. Getchell TV: Functional properties of vertebrate olfactory neurons, *Physiol Rev* 66:772, 1986.

110. Getchell TV, Getchell ML: Early events in vertebrate olfaction, *Chem Senses* 2:313, 1977.

111. Getchell TV, Getchell ML: Histochemical localization and identification of secretory products in salamander olfactory epithelium. In *Olfaction and Taste, Proceedings of the Sixth International Symposium*, London, 1977, Information Retrieval.

112. Getchell TV, Getchell ML: Regulatory factors in the vertebrate olfactory mucosa, *Chem Senses* 15:223, 1990.

113. Getchell TV, Margolis FL, Getchell ML: Perireceptor and receptor events in vertebrate olfaction, *Prog Neurobiol* 23:317, 1984.

114. Getchell ML, Zielinski B, Getchell TV: *Odorant and autonomic regulation of secretion in the olfactory mucosa.* In Margolis F, Getchell TV, editors: *Molecular neurobiology of the olfactory system*, New York, 1988, Plenum Press.

115. Ghorbanian SN, Paradise JL, Doty RL: Odor perception in children in relation to nasal obstruction, *Pediatrics* 72:510, 1983.

116. Gilchrist AG: Rehabilitation after laryngectomy, *Acta Otolaryngol* 75:511, 1973.

117. Girardin M, Bilgen E, Arbour P: Experimental study of velocity fields in a human nasal fossa by laser anemometry, *Ann Otol Rhinol Laryngol* 92:231, 1983.

118. Girardot MN, Derby DC: Independent components of the neural population response for discrimination of quality and intensity of chemical stimuli, *Brain Behav Evol* 35:129, 1990.

119. Goldwyn RM, Shore S: The effects of submucous resection and rhinoplasty on the sense of smell, *Plast Reconstr Surg* 41:427, 1968.

120. Goodspeed RB and others: *Corticosteroids in olfactors dysfunction.* In Meiselman HL, Rivlin RS, editors: *Clinical measurement of taste and smell*, New York, 1986, MacMillan Publishing.

121. Goodspeed RB, Gent JF, Catalanotto FA: Chemosensory dysfunction: clinical evaluation results from a taste and smell clinic, *Postgrad Med* 81:251, 1987.

122. Graham CS and others: Taste and smell losses in HIV infected patients, *Physiol Behav* 58:287, 1995.

123. Graziadei PPC: *The olfactory mucosa of vertebrates*. In Beidler LM, editor: *Handbook of sensory physiology*, vol 4, *Chemical senses*, part 1, Berlin, New York, 1971, Springer-Verlag.

124. Graziadei PPC: *Cell dynamics in the olfactory mucosa*. In *The ultrastructure of sensory organs*, New York, 1973, Elsevier Science Publishing.

125. Griep MI and others: Food odor thresholds in relation to age, nutritional, and health status, *J Gerontol A Biol Sci Med Sci* 50:407, 1995.

126. Griff IC, Reed RR: The genetics of olfaction, *Curr Opin Neurobiol* 5:456, 1995a (review).

127. Griff IC, Reed RR: The genetic basis for specific anosmia to isovaleric acid in the mouse, *Cell* 83:407, 1995b.

128. Hagin PJ: Post-traumatic anosmia, *Arch Otolaryngol* 85:107, 1967.

129. Hahn I, Scherer PW, Mozell MM: A mass transport model of olfaction, *J Theor Biol* 167:115, 1994.

130. Hahn I, Scherer PW, Mozell MM: Velocity profiles measured for airflow through a large-scale model of the human nasal cavity, *J Appl Physiol* 75(5):2273, 1993.

131. Haring HG: *Vapor pressure and Raoult's law deviations in relation to odor enhancement and suppression*. In *Human responses to environmental odors*, New York, 1974, Academic Press.

132. Harrison PJ, Pearson RC: Olfaction and psychiatry, *Br J Psychiatry* 155:822, 1989.

133. Hasegawa S, Yamagishi M, Nakano Y: Microscopic studies of human olfactory epithelia following traumatic anosmia, *Arch Otorhinolaryngol* 243:112, 1986.

134. Hendriks KR and others: Recovery of olfactory behavior. I. Recovery after a complete olfactory bulb lesion correlates with patterns of olfactory nerve penetration, *Brain Res* 648:121, 1994a.

135. Hendriks KR and others: Recovery of olfactory behavior. II. Neonatal olfactory bulb transplant enhance the rate of behavioral recovery, *Brain Res* 648:135, 1994b.

136. Hendriks APJ: Olfactory dysfunction, *Rhinology* 26:229, 1988.

137. Henkin RI and others: A double-blind study of the effects of zinc sulfate on taste and smell, *Am J Med Sci* 272:285, 1976.

138. Henkin RI: Drug-induced taste and smell disorders: incidence, mechanisms and management related primarily to treatment of sensory receptor dysfunction, *Drug Saf* 11:318, 1994 (review).

139. Henkin RI and others: *Treatment of abnormal chemoreception in human taste and smell*. In Norris DM, editor: *Perception of behavioral chemicals*, Amsterdam, 1981, Elsevier Biomedical Press.

140. Herz RS, Cupchik GC: The emotional distinctiveness of odor-evoked memories, *Chem Senses* 20:517, 1995.

141. Heywood PG, Costanzo RM: Identifying normosmics: a comparison of two populations, *Am J Otolaryngol* 7:194, 1986.

142. Heywood PG and others: Clinical diagnosis and treatment of olfactory dysfunction: sensorineural vs. conductive disorders. Paper presented at the Twelfth Annual Meeting of the Association for Chemoreception Sciences, Sarasota, Fla, April, 1990.

143. Hilberg O: Effect of terfenadine and budesonide on nasal symptoms, olfaction, and nasal airway patency following allergen challenge, *Allergy* 50:683, 1995.

144. Houlihan DJ and others: Further evidence for olfactory identification deficits in schizophrenia, *Schizophr Res* 12:179, 1994.

145. Hornung DE, Mozell MM: Factors influencing the differential sorption of odorant molecules across the olfactory mucosa, *J Gen Physiol* 69:343, 1977.

146. Hornung DE, Mozell MM: *Accessibility of odorant molecules to the receptors*. In Cagen RH, Kare MR, editors: *Biochemistry of taste and olfaction*, New York, 1981, Academic Press.

147. Hornung DE and others: Airflow patterns in a human nasal model, *Arch Otolaryngol Head Neck Surg* 113:169, 1987.

148. Hornung DE and others: Impact of left and right nostril olfactory abilities on binasal olfactory performance, *Chem Senses* 15:233, 1990.

149. Hotchkiss WT: Influence of prednisone on nasal polyposis with anosmia, *Arch Otolaryngol* 64:478, 1956.

150. Hudson R and others: Olfactory function in patients with hypogonadotropic hypogonadism: an all-or-none phenomenon, *Chem Senses* 19:57, 1994.

151. Hughes B: *The results of injury to special parts of the brain and skull*. In Rowbottom GF, editor: *Acute injuries to the head*, ed 4, London, 1964, Churchill Livingstone.

152. Hvastja L, Zanuttini L: Odour memory and odour hedonics in children, *Perception* 18:391, 1989.

153. Ikeda K and others: Clinical investigation of olfactory and auditory function in type I pseudohypoparathyroidism: participation of adenylate cyclase system, *J Laryngol Otol* 102:1111, 1988.

154. Jacobi G, Rtiz A, Emrich R: Cranial nerve damage after paediatric head trauma: a long-term follow-up study of 741 cases, *Acta Paediatr Hung* 27:173, 1986.

155. Jafek BW: Ultrastructure of human nasal mucosa, *Laryngoscope* 93:1576, 1983.

156. Jafek BW, Hill DP: Surgical management of chemosensory disorders, *Ear Nose Throat J* 68:398 and 400, 1989.

157. Jafek BW and others: Steroid-dependent anosmia, *Arch Otolaryngol Head Neck Surg* 113:547, 1987.

158. Jafek BW and others: Post-traumatic anosmia: ultrastructural correlates, *Arch Neurol* 46:300, 1989.

159. Jafek BW and others: Congenital anosmia, *Ear Nose Throat J* 69:331, 1990a.

160. Jafek BW and others: Postviral olfactory dysfunction, *Am J Rhinol* 4:91, 1990b.

161. Jafek BW, Murrow B, Johnson EW: Olfaction and endoscopic sinus surgery, *Ear Nose Throat J* 73:548, 1994 (review).

162. Jesberger JA, Richardson JS: Brain output dysregulation induced by olfactory bulbectomy: an approximation in the rat of major depressive disorder in humans, *Int J Neurosci* 38:241, 1988.

163. Jones DT, Reed RR: Golf: an olfactory neuron specific-G protein involved in odorant signal transduction, *Science* 244:790, 1989.

164. Jones FN: Olfactory absolute thresholds and their implications for the nature of the receptor process, *J Psychol* 40:223, 1955.

165. Jourdan R and others: Spatial distribution of deoxyglucose uptake in the olfactory bulbs of rats stimulated with two different odours, *Brain Res* 188:139, 1980.

166. Kallman FJ, Schoenfeld WA, Barrera SE: The genetic aspects of primary eunuchoidism, *Am J Ment Defic* 48:203, 1944.

167. Kanai T: Ober das Kombunerte Verkommen des partieller Reichlappendefecies met dem Eunuchoidismus, *Okajimas Folia Anat Jap* 19:200, 1940.

168. Karadi Z and others: Olfactory coding in the monkey lateral hypothalamus: behavioral and neurochemical properties of odor-responding neurons, *Physiol Behav* 45:1249, 1989.

169. Karlson P, Lauuscher M: "Pheromones": a new term for a class of biologically active substance, *Nature* 183:55, 1959.

170. Kato T and others: A device for controlling odorant stimulation and olfactory evoked responses in humans, *Auris Nasus Larynx* 22:103, 1995.

171. Kauer JS: Contributions of topography and parallel processing to odor coding in the vertebrate olfactory pathway, *Trends in Neurosciences* 14:79, 1991.

172. Kauer JS, Moulton DG: Responses of olfactory bulb neurons to odor stimulation of small nasal areas in the salamander, *J Physiol* 243:717, 1974.

173. Kaufman MD, Lasiter KR, Shenoy BV: Paroxysmal unilateral dysosmia: a cured patient, *Ann Neurol* 24:450, 1988.

174. Kay RG: Zinc and copper in human nutrition, *J Hum Nutr* 35:25, 1981.

175. Kaye JA and others: Neurologic evaluation of the optimally healthy oldest old, *Arch Neurol* 51:1205, 1994.

176. Keverne EB: Olfactory learning, *Curr Opin Neurobiol* 5:482, 1995 (review).

177. Kimmelman CP: The risk to olfaction from nasal surgery, *Laryngoscope* 104:981, 1994.

178. Kirk JM and others: Identification of olfactory dysfunction in carriers of X-linked Kallmann's syndrome, *Clin Endocrinol (Oxf)* 41:57, 1994.

179. Kishikawa M and others: A histopathological study on senile changes in the human olfactory bulb, *Acta Pathol Jpn* 40:255, 1990.

180. Kittel G, Waller G: Smell-improving effect of Cottle's septum operation, *Z Laryngol Rhinol Otol Grenz* 52:280, 1973.

181. Klingmuller D and others: Magnetic resonance imaging of the brain in patients with anosmia and hypothalamic hypogonadism (Kallmann's syndrome), *J Clin Endocrinol Metab* 65:581, 1987.

182. Kobal G, Hummel C: Cerebral chemosensory evoked potentials elicited by chemical stimulation of the human olfactory and respiratory nasal mucosa, *Electroencephalogr Clin Neurophysiol* 71:241, 1988.

183. Kobal G, Plattig K-H: Methodische Anmerkungen zur Gewinnung olfaktorischer EEG- Antworten des wachen Menschen (objektive Olfaktometrie), *EEG EMG Z Elektroenzephalogr Elektromyogr Verwandte Geb* 9:135, 1978.

184. Koelega HS: Prepubescent children may have specific deficits in olfactory sensitivity, *Percept Mot Skills* 78:191, 1994.

185. Koelega HS: Sex differences in olfactory sensitivity and the problem of the generality of smell acuity, *Percept Mot Skills* 78:203, 1994a.

186. Koelega HS: Diurnal variations in olfactory sensitivity and the relationship to food intake, *Percept Mot Skills* 78:215, 1994b.

187. Koelega HS: Olfaction and sensory asymmetry, *Chem Senses Flavor* 4:89, 1979.

188. Koizuka I and others: Functional imaging of the human olfactory cortex by magnetic resonance imaging, *ORL J Otorhinolaryngol Relat Spec* 56:273, 1995.

189. Kopala LC, Good K, Honer WG: Olfactory identification ability in pre- and postmenopausal women with schizophrenia, *Biol Psychiatry* 38:57, 1995.

190. Kopala LC, Good KP, Honer WG: Olfactory hallucinations and olfactory identification ability in patients with schizophrenia and other psychiatric disorders, *Schizophr Res* 12:205, 1994.

191. Koster EP: *Adaptation and cross-adaptation in olfaction*, Rotterdam, 1971, Bronder-Offsett.

192. Krueger KC, Krueger WB: Hypogeusia and hyposmia associated with low serum zinc levels: a case report, *J Am Med Wom Assoc* 35:109, 1980.

193. Kubie JL, Mackay-Sim A, Moulton DG: Inherent spatial patterning of response to odorants in the salamander olfactory epithelium. In Olfaction and Taste, Proceedings of the Seventh International Symposium, London, 1980, Information Retrieval.

194. Kubie JL, Moulton DG: Regional patterning of response to odors in the salamander olfactory mucosa, *Soc Neurosci Abstr* 5:129, 1979.

195. ter Laak HJ, Renkawek K, van Workum FP: The olfactory bulb in Alzheimer disease: a morphologic study of neuron loss, tangles, and senile plaques in relation to olfaction, *Alzheimer Dis Assoc Disord* 8:38, 1994.

196. Laffort P, Patte F, Etcheto M: Olfactory coding on the basis of physiochemical properties, *Ann NY Acad Sci* 237:193, 1974.

197. Laing DG and others: Evidence for the temporal processing of odor mixtures in humans, *Brain Res* 651:317, 1994.

198. Laing DG: Quantification of the variability of human responses during odor perception. In Olfaction and Taste, Proceedings of the Seventh International Symposium, London, 1980, Information Retrieval.

199. Laing DG: Characterization of human behavior during odour perception, *Perception* 11:221, 1982.

200. Laing DG: Natural sniffing gives optimum odor perception for humans, *Perception* 12:99, 1983.

201. Laing DG: Optimum perception of odor intensity by humans, *Physiol Behav* 34:569, 1985.

202. Laing DG: Coding of chemosensory stimulus mixtures, *Ann NY Acad Sci* 510:61, 1987.

203. Lancet D: Vertebrate olfactory receptor, *Annu Rev Neurosci* 9:329, 1986.

204. Lanza DC and others: The effect of human olfactory biopsy on olfaction: a preliminary report, *Laryngoscope* 104:837, 1994.

205. Lehrner JP, Kryspin-Exner I, Vetter N: Higher olfactory threshold and decreased odor indentification ability in HIV-infected persons, *Chem Senses* 20:325, 1995.

206. Leigh AD: Defect of smell after head injury, *Lancet* 1:38, 1943.

207. Le Magnen J: Analyses d'odours complexes et homologues par fatigue, *C R Acad Sci III* 226:753, 1948.

208. Le Magnen J, Rapaport A: Method of determining the role of vitamin A in the mechanism of olfaction in the white rat, *C R Seances Soc Biol Fil* 145:800, 1951.

209. Leopold DA and others: Relationship between CT scan findings and sense of smell, *Otolaryngol Head Neck Surg* 1997 (submitted for publication).

210. Leopold DA: The relationship between nasal anatomy and human olfaction, *Laryngoscope* 98:1232, 1988.

211. Leopold DA, Hornung DE, Youngentob SL: *Olfactory loss after upper respiratory infection*. In Getchell T and others, editors: *Smell and taste in health and disease*, New York, 1991a, Raven Press.

212. Leopold DA and others: The relationship between nasal anatomy and human olfaction, *Chem Senses* 12:675, 1987.

213. Leopold DA and others: Fish-odor syndrome presenting as dysosmia, *Arch Otolaryngol Head Neck Surg* 116:354, 1990.

214. Leopold DA and others: Successful treatment of phantosmia with preservation of olfaction, *Arch Otolaryngol Head Neck Surg* 117:1402, 1991b.

215. Leopold DA and others: Anterior distribution of human olfactory neuroepithelium, *Chem Senses* 20:729, 1995.

216. Leveteau J, Andriason I, MacLeod P: Interbulbar reciprocal inhibition in frog olfaction, *Behav Brain Res* 54:103, 1993.

217. Levin BE, Katzen HL: Early cognitive changes and nondementing behavioral abnormalities in Parkinson's disease, *Adv Neurol* 65:85, 1995 (review).

218. Levin HS, High WM, Eisenberg HM: Impairment of olfactory recognition after closed head injury, *Brain* 108:579, 1985.

219. Levitt H: Transformed up-down methods in psychophysics, *J Acoust Soc Am* 49:467, 1971.

220. Li C and others: Neuroimaging in patients with olfactory dysfunction, *AJR Am J Roentgenol* 162:411, 1994 (review).

221. Lindvall T, Noren O, Thyselius L: *On the abatement of animal manure odours*. In Proceedings of the Third International Clean Air Congress, Dusseldorf, 1973, VDI-Verlag.

222. Liss L, Gomez F: The nature of senile changes of the human olfactory bulb and tract, *Arch Otolaryngol* 67:167, 1958.

223. Lygonis CS: Familial absence of olfaction, *Heredity* 61:413, 1969.

224. Macfarlane A: Olfaction in the development of social preferences in the human neonate, *Ciba Found Symp* 33:103, 1975.

225. Mackay-Sim A, Dreosti IE: Olfactory function in zinc-deficient adult mice, *Exp Brain Res* 76:207, 1989.

226. Mackay-Sim A, Kubie JL: The salamander nose: a model system for the study of spatial coding of olfactory quality, *Chem Senses* 6:249, 1981.

227. Mackay-Sim A, Moulton DG: Odorant-specific maps of relative sensitivity inherent in the salamander olfactory epithelium, *Soc Neurosci Abstr* 6:243, 1980.

228. Mackay-Sim A, Shaman P, Moulton DG: Topographic coding of olfactory quality: odorant-specific patterns of epithelial responsibility in the salamander, *J Neurophysiol* 48:584, 1982.

229. Macrides F and others: Evidence for morphologically and functionally heterogeneous classes of mitral and tufted cells in the olfactory bulb, *Chem Senses* 10:175, 1985.

230. Mair RG and others: *Physiological differentiation of olfactory recep-*

tor cilia types Second Annual Meeting, American Chemical Society, vol 25, 1980 (abstract).

231. Mair RG and others: Physiological differentiation of olfactory receptor cilia during development, *Neuroscience* 7:3091, 1982.

232. Mann DM, Tucker CM, Yates PO: Alzheimer's disease: an olfactory connection, *Mech Aging Dev* 42:1, 1988.

233. Markert JM, Hartshorn DO, Farhat SM: Paroxysmal bilateral dysosmia treated by resection of the olfactory bulbs, *Surg Neurol* 40:160, 1993.

234. Martinkenas LV: Qualitative characteristics of olfactory disorders after stable nose injuries, *Vestn Otorinolaringol* 6:43, 1976.

235. Masing H: Investigations about the course of flow in the nose model, *Arch Klin Exp Ohren Nasen Kehlk* 189:371, 1967.

236. Masukawa LM, Hedlund B, Shepard GM: Electrophysiological properties of identified cells in the in vitro olfactory epithelium of the tiger salamander, *J Neuroscience* 5:128, 1985.

237. Matern G, Matthias C, Mrowinski D: Olfactory evoked potentials and contingent negative variation in expert assessment of disordered sense of smell (German), *Laryngorhinootologie* 74:118, 1995.

238. Mathews DF: Response patterns of single neurons in the tortoise olfactory epithelium and olfactory bulb, *J Gen Physiol* 60:166, 1972.

239. Mattes RD and others: Chemosensory function and diet in HIV-infected patients, *Laryngoscope* 105:862, 1995.

240. Mattes RD and others: Dietary evaluation of patients with smell and taste disorders, *Am J Clin Nutr* 51:233, 1990.

241. Meisami E: A proposed relationship between increases in the number of olfactory receptor neurons, convergence ratio and sensitivity in the developing rat, *Brain Res Dev Brain Res* 46:9, 1989.

242. Mendlesohn M: A review of olfaction, *Ear Nose Throat J* 46:583, 1967.

243. Min YG and others: Recovery of nasal physiology after functional endoscopic sinus surgery: olfaction and mucociliary transport, *J Otol Rhino Laryngol* 57:264, 1995.

244. Moncrieff RW: The sorptive properties of the olfactory membrane, *J Physiol* 130:543, 1955.

245. Moncrieff RW: Olfactory adaptation and odor likeness, *J Physiol* 133:301, 1956.

246. Monti-Graziadei GA, Graziadei PPC: Neurogenesis and neuron regeneration in the olfactory system of mammals. II. Degeneration and reconstitution of the olfactory sensory neurons after axotomy, *J Neurocytol* 8:197, 1979.

247. Monti-Bloch L and others: The human vomeronasal system, *Psychoneuroendocrinology* 19:673, 1994.

248. Moran DT, Rowley JC III, Jafek BW: Electron microscopy of human olfactory epithelium reveals a new cell type: the microvillar cell, *Brain Res* 253:39, 1982a.

249. Moran DT and others: The fine structure of the olfactory mucosa in man, *J Neurocytol* 11:721, 1982b.

250. Mori K, Shepherd GM: Emerging principles of molecular signal processing by mitral/tufted cells in the olfactory bulb, *Semin Cell Biol* 5:65, 1994 (review).

251. Morrison EE, Costanzo RM: Morphology of the human olfactory epithelium, *J Comp Neurol* 297:1, 1990.

252. Moulton DG: Spatial patterning response to odors in the peripheral olfactory system, *Physiol Rev* 56:578, 1976.

253. Moulton DG, Beidler LM: Structure and function in the peripheral olfactory system, *Physiol Rev* 47:1, 1967.

254. Mower GD, Mair RG, Engen T: *Influence of internal factors on the perceived intensity and pleasantness of gustatory and olfactory stimuli.* In *The chemical senses and nutrition*, New York, 1977, Academic Press.

255. Mozell MM: Evidence for sorption as a mechanism of the analysis of vapors, *Nature* 203:1181, 1964a.

256. Mozell MM: Olfactory discrimination: electrophysiological spatiotemporal basis, *Science* 143:1336, 1964b.

257. Mozell MM: The spatiotemporal analysis of odorants at the level of the olfactory receptor sheet, *J Gen Physiol* 50:25, 1966.

258. Mozell MM: Evidence for a chromatographic model of olfaction, *J Gen Physiol* 56:46, 1970.

259. Mozell MM: *The chemical senses, part 2, olfaction.* In *Experimental psychology*, New York, 1971, Holt, Rinehart and Winston.

260. Mozell MM, Jagodowicz M: Chromatographic separation of odorants by the nose: retention times measured across the in vivo olfactory mucosa, *Science* 181:1247, 1973.

261. Mozell MM, Jagodowicz M: Mechanism underlying the analysis of odor quality at the level of the olfactory mucosa. I. Spatiotemporal sorption patterns, *Am NY Acad Sci* 237:76, 1974.

262. Mozell MM and others: Initial mechanisms basic to olfactory perception, *Am J Otolaryngol* 4:238, 1983.

263. Mozell MM and others: Reversal of hyposmia in laryngectomized patients, *Chem Senses* 11:397, 1986.

264. Murphy C, Cain WS, Bartoshuk LM: Mutual action of taste and olfaction, *Sensory Proc* 1:204, 1977.

265. Murphy MR: Effects of female hamster vaginal discharge on the behavior of male hamsters, *Behav Neurol Biol* 9:367, 1973.

266. Mykytowycz R: *The role of skin glands in mammalian communication.* In Johnston JW Jr, Moulton DG, Turk A, editors: *Advances in chemoreception, vol 1, communication by chemical signals*, New York, 1970, Appleton-Century-Crofts.

267. Naessen R: The 'receptor surface' of the olfactory organ (epithelium) of man and guinea pig: a descriptive and experimental study, *Acta Otolaryngol* 71:335, 1971.

268. Nakashima T, Kimmelman CP, Snow JB: Structure of human fetal and adult olfactory neuroepithelium, *Arch Otolaryngol* 110:641, 1984.

269. Nakamura T, Gold GH: A cyclic nucleotide-gated conductance in olfactory receptor cilia, *Nature* 325:442, 1987.

270. Nordin S, Monsch AU, Murphy C: Unawareness of smell loss in normal aging and Alzheimer's disease: discrepancy between self-reported and diagnosed smell sensitivity, *J Gerontol B Psychol Sci Soc Sci* 50:187, 1995.

271. Ohtori N and others: Improvement of olfactory disturbance by endoscopic endonasal surgery for chronic sinusitis, *Nippon Jibiinkoka Gakkai Kaiho* 98:642, 1995.

272. O'Connell RJ, Stevens DA, Zogby LM: Individual differences in the perceived intensity and quality of specific odors following self- and cross-adaptation, *Chem Senses* 19:197, 1994.

273. Okabe E: A study of the mechanism of phleboid olfactory function, *Nippon Jibiinkoka Gakkai Kaiho* 92:111, 1989.

274. Okano M, Takagi SF: Secretion and electrogenesis of the supporting cell in the olfactory epithelium, *J Physiol* 242:353, 1974.

275. Ottoson D: Analysis of the electrical activity of the olfactory epithelium, *Acta Physiol Scand* 35(suppl 122):7, 1956.

276. Patterson PM, Lauder BA: The incidence and probable inheritance of smell blindness, *J Heredity* 39:295, 1948.

277. Pearce RK, Hawkes CH, Daniel SE: The anterior olfactory nucleus in Parkinson's disease, *Mov Disord* 10:283, 1995.

278. Pearson RCA and others: Anatomical correlates of the distribution of the pathological changes in the neocortex in Alzheimer's disease, *Proc Natl Acad Sci U S A* 82:4531, 1985.

279. Pedersen PE and others: Mapping of an olfactory receptor population that projects to a specific region in the rat olfactory bulb, *J Comp Neurol* 250:93, 1986.

280. Pelosi P: Odorant-binding proteins, *Crit Rev Biochem Mol Biol* 29:199, 1994 (review).

281. Pevsner J, Sklar PB, Snyder SH: Odorant-binding protein: localization to nasal glands and secretions, *Proc Natl Acad Sci U S A* 83:4942, 1986.

282. Pfaffmann C: *Taste and smell.* In *Handbook of experimental psychology*, New York, 1951, John Wiley & Sons.

283. Pierce JD Jr and others: Cross-adaptation of sweaty-smelling 3-

methyl-2 hexenoic acid by a structurally-similar, pleasant-smelling odorant, *Chem Senses* 20:401, 1995.

284. Pomeroy SL, LaMantia AS, Purves D: Postnatal construction of neural circuitry in the mouse olfactory bulb, *J Neurosci* 10:1952, 1990.

285. Principato JJ, Ozenberger MJ: Cyclical changes in nasal resistance, *Arch Otolaryngol* 91:71, 1970.

286. Proetz AW: *Applied physiology of the nose*, ed 2, St Louis, 1953, Annals Publishing.

287. Pryse-Phillips W: An olfactory reference syndrome, *Acta Psychiatr Scand* 47:484, 1971.

288. Punter PH: Measurements of human olfactory thresholds for several groups of structurally related compounds, *Chem Senses* 7:215, 1983.

289. Reed GF: The long-term follow-up care of laryngectomized patients, *JAMA* 175:980, 1961.

290. Reed RR: The molecular basis of sensitivity and specificity in olfaction, *Semin Cell Biol* 5:33, 1994 (review).

291. Richman RA, Wallace K, Sheehe PR: Assessment of an abbreviated odorant identification task for children: a rapid screening device for schools and clinics, *Acta Paediatr* 84:434, 1995a.

292. Richman RA and others: Olfactory performance during childhood. II. Developing a discrimination task for children, *J Pediatr* 127:421, 1995b.

293. Richman RA: Personal communication, 1991.

294. Richman RA and others: Olfactory deficits in children with cleft lip and palate, *Pediatr Res* 17:300A, 1983.

295. Richman RA and others: Olfactory deficits in boys with cleft palate, *Pediatrics* 82:840, 1988.

296. Rous J, Kober F: Influence of one-sided nasal respiratory occlusion of the olfactory threshold values, *Arch Klin Exp Ohren Nasen Kehlk* 196:374, 1970.

297. Rowe FA, Edwards DA: Olfactory bulb removal: influences on the mating behavior of male mice, *Physiol Behav* 8:37, 1972.

298. Rowe FA, Smith WE: Simultaneous and successive olfactory bulb removal: influences on the mating behavior of male mice, *Physiol Behav* 10:443, 1973.

299. Rowley JC III, Moran DT, Jafek BW: Peroxidase backfills suggest the mammalian olfactory epithelium contains a second morphologically distinct class of bipolar sensory neuron: the microvillar cell, *Brain Res* 502:387, 1989.

300. Russell MJ, Switz GM, Thompson K: Olfactory influences on the human menstrual cycle, *Pharmacol Biochem Behav* 13:737, 1980.

301. Sailer HF, Landolt AM: A new method for the correction of hypertelorism with preservation of the olfactory nerve filaments, *J Craniomaxillofac Surg* 15:122, 1987.

302. Sandmark B and others: Olfactory function in painters exposed to organic solvents, *Scand J Work Environ Health* 15:60, 1989.

303. Schall B and others: Les stimulations olfactives dans les relations entre l'enfant et la mere, *Reprod Nutr Devel* 20:843, 1980.

304. Schechter PJ, Henkin RI: Abnormalities of taste and smell after head trauma, *J Neurol Neurosurg Psychiatry* 37:802, 1974.

305. Scherer PW, Hahn II, Mozell MM: The biophysics of nasal airflow, *Otolaryngol Clin North Am* 22:265, 1989.

306. Schiffman SS: *Changes in taste and smell with age: psychophysical aspects.* In Ordy JM, Brizzeek, editors: *Sensory systems and communication in the elderly*, New York, 1979, Raven Press.

307. Schiffman SS: Taste and smell in disease. I, *N Engl J Med* 308:1275, 1983.

308. Schiffman SS: Taste and smell in disease. II, *N Engl J Med* 308:1337, 1983.

309. Schmidt HJ, Beauchamp GK: Adult-like odor preferences and aversions in three-year-old children, *Child Dev* 59:1136, 1988.

310. Schneider RA: Newer insights into the role and modifications of olfaction in man through clinical studies, *Ann NY Acad Sci* 237:217, 1974.

311. Schneider RA, Wolf S: Relation of olfactory activity to nasal membrane function, *J Appl Physiol* 15:914, 1960.

312. Schwartz BS and others: Olfactory function in chemical workers exposed to acrylate and methacrylate vapors, *Am J Public Health* 79:613, 1989.

313. Schwartz DN and others: Improvement of olfaction in laryngectomized patients with the larynx bypass, *Laryngoscope* 97:1280, 1987.

314. Schwob JE: *The biochemistry of olfactory neurons: stages of differentiation and neuronal subsets.* In Serby ML, Chodor K, editors: *Olfaction and the central nervous system*, Hillsdale, NJ, 1991, Lawrence Earlbaum Associates.

315. Schwob JE, Farber NB, Gottlieb DI: Neurons of the olfactory epithelium in adult rats contain vimentin, *J Neurosci* 6:208, 1986.

316. Schwob JE and others: Histopathology of olfactory mucosa in Kallmann's Syndrome, *Ann Otol Rhino Laryngol* 102:117, 1993.

317. Scott AE: Caution urged in treating 'steroid-dependent anosmia,' *Arch Otolaryngol Head Neck Surg* 115:109, 1989a.

318. Scott AE: Clinical characteristics of taste and smell disorders, *Ear Nose Throat J* 68:297, 1989b.

319. Scott JW: The olfactory bulb and central pathways, *Experientia* 42:223, 1986.

320. Scott JW: Organization of olfactory bulb output cells and their local circuits, *Ann NY Acad Sci* 510:44, 1987.

321. Seiden AM and others: Characteristics of patients with olfactory and taste dysfunction, *Audio Digest* 21: 1988.

322. Senf W and others: Determination of odour affinities based on the dose-response relationships of the frog's electro-olfactogram, *Experientia* 36:213, 1980.

323. Shevrygin BV: Surgical intervention on the nasal septum for the purpose of improving and preserving olfaction, *Zh Ushn Nosov Gorl Bol (Kiev)* 31:247, 1973.

324. Shevrygin BV, Maniuk MK: Anomalies in the development of the nasal cavity in children and their treatment, *Zh Ushn Nosov Gorl Bol* 6:30, 1974.

325. Shibuya T: Dissociation of olfactory neural response and mucosal potential, *Science* 143:1338, 1964.

326. Singh N, Grewal MS, Austin JH: Familial anosmia, *Arch Neurol* 22:40, 1970.

327. Skolnik EM, Massari FS, Fenta LT: Olfactory neuroepithelioma: review of world literature and presentation of two cases, *Arch Otolaryngol* 84:644, 1966.

328. Skopina EL, Tatarini TE, Batchkin IV: Significance of disorders of the respiratory and olfactory functional disturbances in forensic medical examination of nasal injuries, *Vestn Otorinolaringol* 5:40, 1979.

329. Smith DV: Assessment of patients with taste and smell disorders, *Acta Otolaryngol Suppl (Stockh)* 458:129, 1988.

330. Stern MB and others: Olfactory function in Parkinson's disease subtypes, *Neurology* 44:266, 1994.

331. Spetzler RF and others: Preservation of olfaction in anterior craniofacial approaches, *J Neurosurg* 79:48, 1993.

332. Stevens JC, Cain WS: Old-age deficits in the sense of smell as gauged by thresholds, magnitude matching, and odor identification, *Psychol Aging* 2:36, 1987.

333. Stewart WB, Kauer JS, Shepherd GM: Functional organization of rat olfactory bulb analyzed by the 2-deoxyglucose method, *J Comp Neurol* 185:715, 1979.

334. Strickland M, Jessee PO, Filsinger EE: A procedure for obtaining young children's reports of olfactory stimuli, *Percept Psychophys* 44:379, 1988.

335. Stuiver M: Biophysics of the sense of smell, doctoral dissertation Groningen, 1958, Rijks University.

336. Sullivan SL, Ressler KJ, Buck LB: Spatial patterning and information coding in the olfactory system, *Curr Opin Genet Dev* 5:516, 1995 (review).

337. Sumner D: Post-traumatic anosmia, *Brain* 87:107, 1964.

338. Suzuki M et al: MR imaging of olfactory bulbs and tracts, *Am J Neuroradiol* 10:955, 1989.

339. Tagagi SF: A standardized olfactometer in Japan, *Ann NY Acad Sci* 510:113, 1987.

340. Talamo BR and others: Pathological changes in olfactory neurons in patients with Alzheimer's disease, *Nature* 337:736, 1989.

341. Tigliev GS, Ilias MI, Dubikaitis IUV: Approach to tumors of the chiasm-sellar region with preservation of the olfactory tracts, *Zh Vopr Neirokhir Im N N Burdenko* 6:13, 1986.

342. Trotier D: Intensity coding in olfactory receptor cells, *Semin Cell Biol* 5:47, 1994 (review).

343. VanToller S: *Emotion and the brain.* In VanToller S, Dodd GH, editors: *Perfumery: the psychology and biology of fragrance*, New York, 1988, Chapman and Hall.

344. VanToller S, Dodd GH: Presbyosmia and olfactory compensation for the elderly, *Br J Clin Pract* 41:725, 1987.

345. Varendi H, Porter RH, Winberg J: Does the newborn baby find the nipple by smell, *Lancet* 344:989, 1994.

346. Varney NR: Prognostic significance of anosmia in patients with closed-head trauma, *J Clin Exp Neuropsychol* 10:250, 1988.

347. Velle W: Sex differences in sensory functions, *Perspect Biol Med* 30:490, 1987.

348. Verhaagen J and others: Neuroplasticity in the olfactory system: differential effects of central and peripheral lesions of the primary olfactory pathway on the expression of B-50 + GAP43 and the olfactory marker protein, *J Neurosci Res* 26:31, 1990.

349. Walter WG and others: Contingent negative variation: an electric sign of sensorimotor association and expectancy in the human brain, *Nature* 203:380, 1964.

350. Weinstock RS and others: Olfactory dysfunction in humans with deficient guanine nucleotide-binding protein, *Nature* 322:635, 1986.

351. Wenning GK and others: Olfactory function in atypical Parkinsonian syndromes, *Acta Neurol Scand* 91:247, 1995.

352. West SE, Doty RL: Influence of epilepsy and temporal lobe resection on olfactory function, *Epilepsia* 36:531, 1995.

353. Westerman ST: An objective approach to subjective testing for sensation of taste and smell, *Laryngoscope* 91:301, 1981.

354. Whitten WK: The effect of removal of the olfactory bulbs on the gonads of mice, *J Endocrinol* 14:160, 1956.

355. Wilson DA, Leon M: Spatial patterns of olfactory bulb single-unit responses to learned olfactory cues in young rats, *J Neurophysiol* 59:1770, 1988.

356. Wippich W, Mecklenbrauker S, Trouet J: Implicit and explicit memories of odors, *Arch Psychol (Frankf)* 141:195, 1989.

357. Wright HN: Characterization of olfactory dysfunction, *Arch Otolaryngol Head Neck Surg* 113:163, 1987.

358. Wright HN: *A clinical manifestation and its implications.* In Wysocki C, Kane M, editors: *Chemical senses*, New York, 1991, Marcel-Dekker.

359. Wysocki CJ, Gilbert AN: National geographic smell survey: effects of age are heterogenous, *Ann NY Acad Sci* 561:12, 1989.

360. Yamagishi M, Fujiwara M, Nakamura H: Olfactory mucosal findings and clinical course in patients with olfactory disorders following upper respiratory viral infection, *Rhinology* 32:113, 1994.

361. Yamagishi M, Hasegawa S, Nakano Y: Examination and classification of human olfactory mucosa in patients with clinical olfactory disturbances, *Arch Otorhinolaryngol* 245:316, 1988.

362. Yamagishi M and others: Effect of surgical treatment of olfactory disturbance caused by localized ethmoiditis, *Clin Otol* 14:405, 1989a.

363. Yamagishi M and others: Immunohistochemical analysis of the olfactory mucosa by use of antibodies to brain proteins and cytokeratin, *Ann Otol Rhinol Laryngol* 98:384, 1989b.

364. Yamagishi M and others: Olfactory receptor cells: immunocytochemistry for nervous system-specific proteins and re-evaluation of their precursor cells, *Arch Histol Cytol* 52(suppl):375, 1989c.

365. Yamagishi M and others: Immunohistochemical examination of olfactory mucosa in patients with olfactory disturbance, *Ann Otol Rhinol Laryngol* 99:205, 1990.

366. Youngentob SL and others: Olfactory sensitivity: is there laterality, *Chem Senses* 7:11, 1982.

367. Zatorre RJ, Jones-Gotman M: Right-nostril advantage for discrimination of odors, *Percept Psychophys* 47:526, 1990.

368. Zilstorff K: Parosmia, *J Laryngol Otol* 80:1102, 1966.

369. Zilstorff K, Herbild O: Parosmia, *Acta Otolaryngol Suppl* 360:40, 1979.

370. Zucco GM, Negrin NS: Olfactory deficits in Down subjects: a link with Alzheimer disease, *Percept Mot Skills* 78:627, 1994.

371. Zusho H: Post-traumatic anosmia, *Arch Otolaryngol* 108:90, 1982.

Chapter 42

Evaluation of Nasal Breathing Function with Objective Airway Testing

John F. Pallanch
Thomas V. McCaffrey
Eugene B. Kern

NASAL BREATHING FUNCTION

Disturbance in a patient's sense of well being resulting from problems with respiration can be pulmonary and nasal in origin. In optimal nasal respiration, air passes over the maximum amount of nasal mucosa with resulting humidification, cleansing, and warming but without the sensation of dyspnea. This chapter describes the assessment of *nasal* breathing function with the additional information provided by objective nasal airway testing.

The sensation of comfortable nasal breathing is a complex phenomenon. It may be influenced by several factors. There is a correlation between the amount of airflow and the symptom of nasal obstruction. Stimulation of cold receptors in the nasal vestibule and nerve endings in the nasal vestibular skin and the nasal mucosa also can play a role. In addition, the condition of the lining tissue in a dry atrophic nose can cause a sensation of disturbed nasal breathing.

Various objective tests have been used to assess the nasal airway to aid the clinician in understanding nasal breathing function. Most objective assessments of the nose measure a parameter that is directly or indirectly related to airflow. Many physiologic factors and pathologic conditions can affect the amount of airflow through the nose. The nasal pathologic conditions include mucosal hyperreactivity, septal or other structural deformities, polyps, tumors, granulations, and synechiae.

ASSESSMENT OF NASAL BREATHING FUNCTION

Patient history

The first step in assessing nasal breathing function is to obtain a thorough history. A questionnaire is sometimes used.[123] The patient is asked about the symptom of nasal obstruction. If present, the side of obstruction, severity, frequency, duration, and exacerbating factors are all recorded. Several methods have been used for recording the severity of symptoms.[1,103,126] The authors use the scale of none, mild, moderate, or severe. Sipila and others[176] used four categories for severity of symptoms, including "very patent" for the sensation that the airway was more open than normal. All of these descriptions are the patient's *subjective* evaluation of nasal breathing function.

Nasal examination

The next step in evaluating nasal breathing is to examine the nose. Methods of recording rhinoscopic findings can be detailed.[78] These methods include an assessment by the physician of the appearance of the intranasal anatomy, the cross-sectional area, and the condition of the lining tissues of the nose. It is a *subjective* assessment of anatomic factors that might affect the patient's nasal breathing.

Objective testing of the nasal airway

The final step in evaluation, *objective* measurement of the physical parameters that affect nasal breathing, is the focus of the rest of this chapter. Objective assessment can measure the intranasal anatomy, including the cross-sectional area and volume. Testing also can measure properties of the airstream through the nose, including intransnasal pressure and airflow and volume of air in each breath. Other tests have measured the blood flow in nasal mucosa and the amount of nasal sound transmitted by the airway.

Assessment of intranasal anatomy

The cross-sectional area of the nose can be assessed by computed tomography (CT), magnetic resonance imaging (MRI), fiberoptic rhinoscopy,[197] rhinostereometry, and acoustic rhinometry. Rhinostereometry uses a microscope to assess changes in nasal congestion.[104] Acoustic rhinometry gives a profile of the cross-sectional areas through the nose and the volume of the nasal cavity. Investigators[88,129] have found a correlation between cross-sectional area measured by CT scanning and by acoustic rhinometry. Hilberg and others[88] also found a correlation between volume measured by acoustic rhinometry and that measured by using a water displacement method. The application of acoustic rhinometry will be described further in subsequent sections of this chapter.

Assessment of properties of the airstream through the nose

Nasal airflow and transnasal pressure. Airflow occurs through the nose if there is a difference in pressure across the nasal airway, with the airflow occurring from the area of higher pressure to the area of lower pressure. Although the pressure outside the nose is relatively constant, the pressure in the nasopharynx changes with respiratory movement of the chest. This change creates a pressure differential (the transnasal pressure) across the nose, and air moves back and forth through the nose with the phases of respiration.

Physical factors affecting the amount of airflow. The rate of airflow through the nose depends on the length and cross-sectional area of the nasal airway, the pressure gradient across the nose, and the character of the airflow (laminar versus turbulent). The cross-sectional area of the nose is a major factor in determining airflow, with airflow increasing as the cross-sectional area increases. The cross-sectional area varies along the length of the nose. The effect of turbulence in the nasal airway has not been precisely quantified. Laminar flow occurs in a smooth-walled, straight tube at low flow rates, but turbulence occurs when irregularities are encountered in the tube, as would happen in the nose. Turbulent flow requires more energy but results in better mixing of the air, thus enhancing nasal function.

Measurement of nasal airflow, simple maneuvers. Several simple office maneuvers can be used to assess nasal airflow. At the turn of the century, methods used[64,88] included breathing on a mirror or glass plate (rhinohygrometry), assessing the sound of a forced expiration through the nose, and evaluating the pitch of the sound made by a patient humming while first one and then the other side of the nose was occluded. The mark made by warm airflow in rhinohygrometry has been quantitated.[67] Fisher and others[60] thought that acoustic rhinometry was superior to rhinohygrometry in studying the nasal cycle in children.

Another simple test is to occlude each side of the patient's nose and ask him or her to compare the nasal breathing through the two sides. To assess the effect of the nasal valve, the patient's cheek can be drawn back (like a positive Cottle sign)[86] to see whether a significant decrease in obstruction occurs. Alternatively, the patient can be asked if there is any improvement in breathing when the valve area is held open with a nasal speculum or with one of the commercially available adhesive plastic strips. These tests are easy to perform and are noninvasive, but, except for rhinohygrometry, they require subjective appraisal by the patient or clinician and thus are not easy to quantify accurately.

Measurement of peak nasal airflow. The readily available peak expiratory flow meter has been used to assess the nasal airway, and results have correlated with nasal resistance,[182] although others have stated that the method is unreliable and have recommended against its use.[45] A nasal peak inspiratory flow meter has been studied.[115] In studying children, Prescott and Prescott[155] found that peak nasal inspiratory flow measurement had the drawback of depending on the degree of cooperation of the child and on the subjective impression of the observer as to when a maximal effort had been made. Measurement of peak inspiratory flow was less sensitive than rhinomanometry for detecting changes in nasal patency after histamine challenge[26] and with increasing doses of xylometazoline.[30]

Simultaneous measurement of transnasal pressure and airflow, rhinomanometry. One of the most commonly used methods of objectively assessing the nasal airway is the simultaneous recording of the transnasal pressure and airflow. *Rhinorheomanometry, rhinomanometry, rhinometry,* and *rhinomanography* are names that have been applied to these measurements. The International Standards Committee for the Objective Assessment of the Nasal Airway has chosen the name *rhinomanometry*.[32] This technique of recording pressure and flow simultaneously over a given time interval allows for study of the relationships between pressure, airflow, and time to give an objective assessment of the passage of air through the nose. By recording pressure and flow over a given time period, mean pressure and volume of each breath can be measured. From these measurements other parameters can be calculated, which represent the relationship of these factors with each other at a single moment or during a specific time interval. An important example of the relationship of pressure and flow at a single moment is *resistance*, which is the ratio of pressure to flow, sometimes abbreviated as *NAR* or *Rn*. An example of the relationship of pressure and flow over time would be work, or mean pressure × flow. The application of rhinomanometry will be described further in subsequent sections of this chapter.

Other methods of objective assessment

Investigators have studied mucosal blood flow in the nose using laser Doppler velocimetry.[4] Manometric rhinometry[153] is a technique in which the volume of air in the nose is assessed by closing off the nose, removing a volume of air, and then recording the resultant pressure change. In forced oscillation rhinomanometry,[65,66,172] the oscillation of a loud speaker provides a complex signal of sinusoidal sound waves, which is coupled to the patient through a small mask and pneumotachometer. Nasometry measures the oral and nasal acoustic ratio across a specified frequency range. Parker and others[149] thought that this test could be performed more easily than rhinomanometry, particularly in children, because it did not require a mask or pressure cannula.

Comparison of rhinomanometry and acoustic rhinometry

Of all these methods, rhinomanometry and acoustic rhinometry are the most commonly used. With the current availability of microprocessor-assisted devices, equipment capable of rapid and sophisticated airway assessment has become readily available. Hilberg and others[88] found a correlation between cross-sectional area of the nasal airway measured by acoustic rhinometry and the area found from calculations using data from rhinomanometry. Lenders and others[118] found results from acoustic rhinometry and rhinomanometry to be abnormal in habitual snorers. Tomkinson and Eccles[185] found a correlation between the results from rhinomanometry and acoustic rhinometry in a study of healthy subjects before and after decongestion but thought the relationship was weak and that it was unlikely that they were measuring the same parameters. Investigators have found comparable results for assessing nasal challenge between acoustic rhinometry and rhinomanometry.[6,166] Cole and Roithmann[38] thought that the two techniques provided complimentary information. They noted that rhinomanometry determines nasal patency in terms more representative of how hard it is for a person to breathe, but that acoustic rhinometry might be better for studies of rapidly changing mucovascular conditions and nasal volume changes. They showed how both can give information about the site of obstruction, but believed that acoustic rhinometry might give more precise anatomic information for the nasal surgeon.

Criteria of a good airway test

A number of desirable criteria for a nasal airway test have been described.[121] These criteria include ease of performance using readily available equipment; no discomfort for the patient; no interference with the nasal anatomy or airflow; an objective means of assessment that is accurate, reproducible, and standardized; availability of normal values; use of physiologic levels of the parameters measured; and clinical usefulness. Available tests vary in their ability to fulfill these criteria.

ACOUSTIC RHINOMETRY EQUIPMENT AND METHODS

Equipment

The equipment used in acoustic rhinometry has been described by Hilberg and others.[88] By presenting a shock wave to the nasal airway and then measuring the reflected sound, a profile of the cross-sectional areas through each side of the nose may be obtained. An acoustic pulse from a spark travels through a wave tube and through a nosepiece that is in contact with the nose such that there is no noise leakage. Changes in the cross-sectional area of the nose cause changes in acoustic impedance, which affects the reflectance of the sound. A microphone detects the reflected sound, and the signal from the microphone is processed and then converted to digital data. A computer then calculates and plots an area–distance function from the data. More recently, a "continuous" noise signal has been used instead of the shock wave in some of the devices.[76]

Methods

The patient is seated, and a nosepiece on the tube is applied to the patient's nose so that there is no noise leak and no distortion of anterior nasal structures. Measurements are repeated three times to ensure reproducibility. Each measurement takes approximately 10 msec. Each side of the nose is measured separately.

Reporting results

The device calculates and displays an area–distance curve (Fig. 42-1). From this curve, a number of parameters can be calculated, including the size of the minimal cross-sectional area (MCA), location of the MCA, the cross-sectional area at various distances from the nostrils (e.g., 3.3 cm for the anterior part of the inferior turbinate and 6.4 cm for the posterior part of the nose), and the total volume (TV) of the nose. The *r.e.q.* is a parameter derived from the acoustic rhinometry data that is designed to represent a nasal resistance-like number. It is possible to have different r.e.q.'s for two nasal passages with the same MCA if the volume behind one MCA is larger than the volume behind the other. For total nasal MCA, the MCA from each side of the nose is added together.[71]

The curve usually shows two notches after the straight line corresponding to the nosepiece (see Fig. 42-1). The first dip in the curve has been called the *I-notch*.[117] The "I" stands for isthmus nasi. It occurs at the first part of the valve region. The second depression in the curve has been called

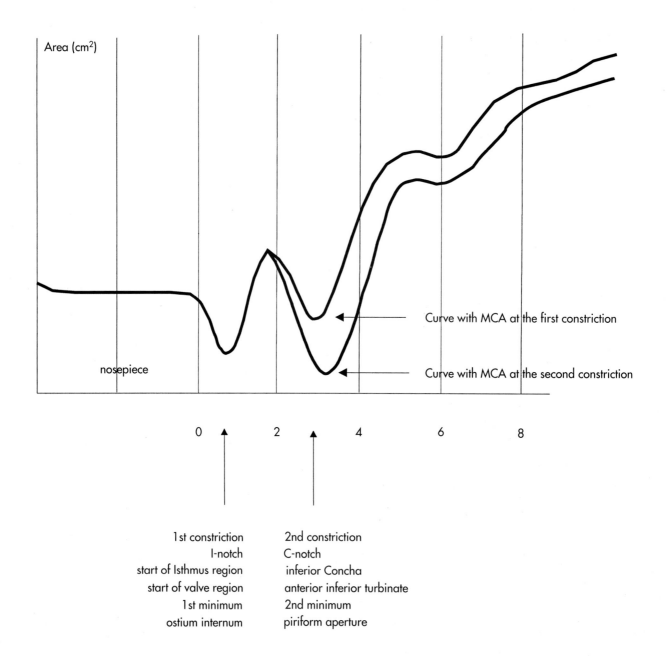

Fig. 42-1. Typical area–distance curves obtained using acoustic rhinometry. Two curves are shown with the first part overlapping. The different synonyms for the two minima on the curves are shown. The *upper curve* shows the minimal cross-sectional area (MCA) at the first constriction. The lower curve shows the MCA at the second constriction.

the *C-notch*.[117] The ''C'' stands for concha. It corresponds to the anterior tip (head) of the inferior turbinate.[117]

Lenders and Pirsig[117] stated that the part measured by the I-notch always was the narrowest segment in normal patients, with the second narrowest segment occurring at the C-notch. They called the pattern with the first notch lower than the second the *climbing W* and stated that it was present in all 134 of their normal control subjects even before decongestion. They found that the second constriction improved with congestion, but the first did not, and stated that nasal mucosa cannot be found in the first constriction. In patients with allergic rhinitis and in patients with habitual snoring,[118] the second constriction was the smallest, and they called this pattern the *descending W*.

Advantages and limitations of acoustic rhinometry

Hilberg and others[88] believed that acoustic rhinometry provided less variability of results than those obtained with rhinomanometry. Further, they noted that the method requires little cooperation by the patient, is noninvasive, and is easy to perform. Fisher and others[59] noted that acoustic rhinometry is rapid. They thought that because it required minimal cooperation from the subject, it would be particularly useful for the evaluation of children. Cole and Roithmann[38] noted that acoustic rhinometry might better assess rapid mucovascular changes like those in nasal challenge testing. Fisher and others[58] thought that acoustic rhinometry was better than rhinomanometry for showing the effect of the nasal cycle on the whole nasal cavity. The limitations of acoustic rhinometry are covered in the section on sources of variability in objective nasal airway testing.

RHINOMANOMETRY EQUIPMENT AND METHODS

Foxen and others[64] and Kosoy[112] have presented a history of the development of rhinomanometry. Rhinomanometry is the simultaneous measurement of transnasal pressure and airflow. Various types of equipment and methods have been developed to perform this measurement.

Measurement of transnasal pressure in rhinomanometry

Pressure across the nose should be measured at the front and back of the nose so that the transnasal pressure difference can be determined. Three methods of transnasal pressure detection are currently in use: anterior rhinomanometry, posterior (peroral) rhinomanometry, and postnasal (or pernasal) rhinomanometry.[34] The major difference in these three approaches is the location of the pressure detector at the back of the nose. In the anterior method, it is placed at the opening to the nostril not being tested (Fig. 42-2). In the posterior method, the pressure detector is placed in or close to the posterior oropharynx (Fig. 42-3). For the postnasal (pernasal) technique,[34] the tube is placed in the posterior nose through one of the nostrils (Fig. 42-4).

A pressure transducer, which converts pressure into an electrical signal, is connected to the tubes from the pressure detection sites for the front and back of the nose. The pressure transducer is connected to the appropriate electronic circuit, so that changes in pressure result in a corresponding change in output voltage. This voltage then is read by a recording device, usually a computer.

Measurement of nasal airflow in rhinomanometry

Airflow can be measured directly at the nasal outlet or indirectly by assessing the change in volume of the thorax with respiration. Direct measurement of airflow at the nasal

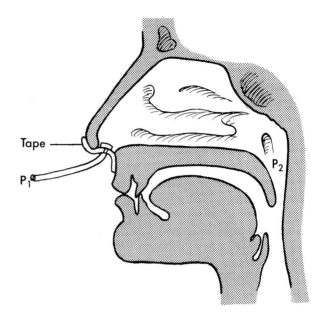

Fig. 42-2. Placement of pressure tubing for anterior rhinomanometry. Tape occludes the nostril on one side. That side acts as an extension of the tubing so that the pressure at the end of the tube (P_1) equals the pressure in the nasopharynx (P_2).

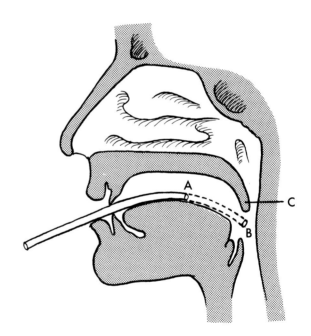

Fig. 42-3. Placement of the pressure tubing for posterior rhinomanometry. Site *A* will work as well as site *B* and avoids stimulation of the base of the tongue. The soft palate (*C*) should be relaxed.

outlet can be accomplished with nozzle or mask. Nozzles are held by the patient at the opening to either nostril. When a nozzle is used for flow detection, the large diameter tube pressing on the nose may alter the intranasal anatomic relationships and thus alter the measurements. Various masks have been used that cover all or a portion of the face (Figs

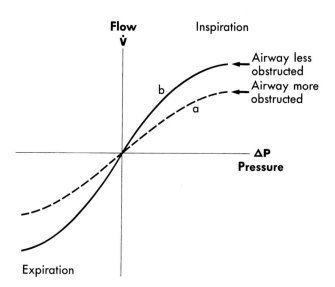

Fig. 42-9. The pressure–flow curve *(a)* for a nasal airway that is more obstructed will be closer to the pressure axis than the curve *(b)* for a less obstructed nasal airway.

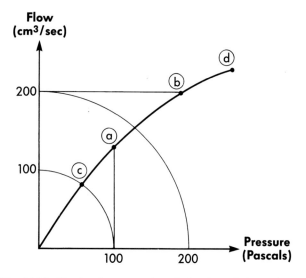

Fig. 42-10. Nasal resistance can be calculated at a designated pressure *(a)*, flow *(b)*, radius *(c)*, or maximum *(d)*.

nasal pressure–flow curve. The flow may reach a limit at which it does not increase with further pressure increase.[18] Bachmann[11] used the percent flow increase with doubling of pressure (from 150 Pa to 300 Pa) to assess the shape of the pressure–flow curve and to obtain information about the isthmus region.

Models of the pressure–flow curve. Several mathematical models of the nonlinear relationship of the pressure–flow curve have been proposed. Pallanch[142] studied the ability of a number of models to fit the data in a variety of pressure–flow curves. The best fit to the data was accom-

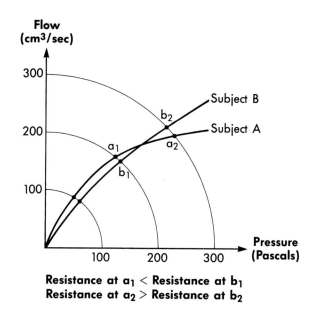

Fig. 42-11. A change in rank order of resistance values can occur when resistance is calculated at different locations on the curve, even though the same method (resistance at a designated radius) is used.

plished using the polynomial model, although the polar and geometric models also did well.

Rhinomanometric parameters—reporting values that include relationship to time

Power has been used as a parameter.[188] Power is the product of pressure and flow multiplied by a constant at a given moment. Cole and others[39] have expressed results as work. This parameter is equivalent to mean pressure multiplied by volume. Cole and others[40] found that work (in joules) per liter increased linearly with ventilation.

Rhinomanometric parameters—difference between sides of the nose

Another proposed method is to report the difference in resistance between the two sides of the nose in relation to the total airway resistance.[154] Bachmann[11] expressed the relationship between the sides of the nose by dividing the flow on the better side by the flow on the worst side. Williams and Eccles[196] found greater asymmetry in nasal resistance between the sides of the nose in patients with acute rhinitis compared with normal subjects.

Other rhinomanometric parameters recently used

Naito and others[136] described a new parameter—the acceleration change of nasal airflow in the rapid phase from inspiration to expiration. He found that this parameter and nasal resistance correlated well with patients' subjective description of nasal patency.

Comparison of the rhinomanometric parameters

With so many different parameters that can be reported, it would be useful to know if one is the best. The most useful clinical parameter would be the one that best correlates with the symptom of nasal obstruction. In a comparison of all of the previously mentioned parameters (with the exception of two) the acceleration change from inspiration to expiration[136] (and power[188]) using the same group of patients, the *resistance at maximum pressure and flow* (in normal respiration) (see Fig. 42-10) was found to be best in correlating with the symptom of obstruction.[144]

Reporting inspiratory or expiratory values

In some studies, no significant difference has been found between inspiratory and expiratory resistance values.[14,172] Others have found that inspiratory resistance is significantly lower than expiratory resistance at lower flows.[23,107,171,187] Haight and Cole,[74] on the other hand, found that during quiet respiration, the resistance was higher during inspiration. If the excursion of the pressure–flow curve is greater in the inspiratory direction and if mean or maximum resistance are being reported, this would be the case. Connell[45] thought that although expiration is important in those with pulmonary disease, it would be more logical to measure nasal patency during inspiration stating, ''Have you ever heard of a patient complaining that he cannot exhale through his nose?'' It is most common to report values obtained from inspiration.

Recommended clinical method for rhinomanometry

Recommendations of the International Committee on Standardization of Rhinomanometry

The International Committee on Standardization of Rhinomanometry[32,108,110] concluded that active anterior rhinomanometry is the preferred method of measurement. The techniques for measurement should include sealing of the pressure line to the nostril (usually with tape), a transparent face mask to ensure lack of kinking of the pressure line and no deformation of the nostrils, a linear pneumotachograph, and daily calibration. The method of decongestion of the nostrils should be specified. The patient who has rested for 30 minutes is tested in a sitting position while breathing quietly (unless a pressure of 300 cm is desired). Each measurement should be the mean of three to five recordings in each nostril. Nasal resistance is reported either at pressure of 75, 150, and 300 Pa (if reached) or at radius 2. Rhinomanometric values should be expressed in SI units, with pressure expressed in pascals and flow expressed in cm^3/sec (100 Pa = 1.0 cm H_2O; 1000 cm^3/sec = 1 l/sec). Nasal resistance is reported in Pa/cm^3/sec (0.1 Pa/cm^3/sec = 1 cm H_2O/l/sec).

Additional methods used in clinical application

Each side of the nose is measured with the mouth closed. Decongestant then is sprayed into both sides of the nose. The decongestion is reported after 5 minutes, and then after an additional 10 minutes, both sides of the nose are tested again. The results then are calculated and stored and printed by the computer.

For children, a smaller face mask can be used, but the test is performed in the same way as for adults. For patients whose chief complaint is nasal obstruction when recumbent, additional studies can be performed in the supine, right-side lying, and left-side lying positions. For patients with suspected allergic rhinitis, nasal provocation testing can be performed.

Further recommendations regarding the technique of rhinomanometry are covered in the next section.

SOURCES OF VARIABILITY IN OBJECTIVE NASAL AIRWAY TESTING

Table 42-1 shows sources of variability for objective testing of the nasal airway. There are some additional sources of variability for rhinomanometry and acoustic rhinometry.

Other sources of variability and ways to minimize them—rhinomanometry

Some variability in rhinomanometric measurements can result from movement of the nasal alae,[159] but alar dilation probably does not contribute significantly to variability of results, particularly in the normal subjects because the alar muscles tend to work toward stabilization of the vestibular wall.[74] In the patient with valve abnormality or disruption of the alar muscles (e.g., postrhinoplasty), alar collapse may cause variability. Alar movement sometimes will be revealed by looping that occurs toward the end of the pressure–flow curve.

There also are potential causes of variability from the equipment. The apparatus should first be warmed up and stable and should be properly calibrated. Rivron[158] reported the coefficient of variation of just the rhinomanometer at 3.4% by measuring a tube held in the patient's mouth. Sandham[163] reported that his early rhinomanometer had a long warm-up time, producing variation in measurements when the machine was first turned on. Potential causes of variability caused by the nozzle technique have been cited.[108] Masks have introduced some variability in results,[43,177] although Maranta and others[121a] found that different mask shapes and volumes did not change the results obtained in making rhinomanometric measurements. Visual feedback, using a real-time display of the pressure–flow curve, has been valuable to reduce variability by detecting air leaks or other artifacts.[101,163,169,177]

Other sources of variability and ways to minimize them—acoustic rhinometry

Variability in *acoustic rhinometric measurements* caused by temperature and anthropologic type are listed in Table 42-1. Other sources of variability that have been mentioned include transmission losses, response lags, and oscillation artifacts[38] and transient changes in sinus opening areas and

Table 42-1. Factors contributing to variability in objective airway testing in general and for rhinomanometry and acoustic rhinometry.

Sources of variability	Effect	References
Both rhinomanometry and acoustic rhinometry		
The nasal cycle	Causes variability in *unilateral* resistance, but *total* nasal resistance remains relatively constant	Hasegawa and Kern;[81] Heetderks[85]
Secretions	Nasal secretions can increase nasal resistance	Forsyth and others[63]
	No change caused by nose blowing	Cole and others[41]
Exercise	Exercise causes a reduction in resistance	Cole and others[41]; Forsyth and others[63]
Hyperventilation	Hyperventilation increases nasal resistance	Dallimore and Eccles;[49] McCaffrey and Kern[124]
Breathing CO_2	Breathing CO_2 decreases nasal resistance	McCaffrey and Kern;[124] Strohl and others[178]
Posture	Nasal resistance is greatest when supine and least when in the upright sitting position; pressure to specific areas of the body causes increase in resistance on the side of the pressure	Hasegawa[80] Haight and Cole[75]
Time of day	Diurnal variation in nasal resistance, highest at night and in the early morning	Schumacher[169]
Medications	Decongestant spray decreases nasal resistance	Cole and others[41]
	Increase in nasal resistance after saline spray	McLean and others;[125] Schumacher[169]
	No effect on the airway from saline spray	Cole and others[41]
	Aspirin causes a small increase in nasal resistance	Jones and others[99]
	Antihistamine treatment may increase the nasal resistance in the unchallenged nose	Havas and others[84]
Smoking	Smokers had significantly higher nasal resistance than nonsmokers	Dessi and others[50]
Height	Nasal resistance increases with height in adults	Broms;[19] Jessen and Malm;[97] Pallanch and others[145]
	No correlation between nasal resistance and height	Morris, Jawad, Eccles[131]
Age	No change in nasal resistance with increasing age in adults	Broms;[19] Jessen and Malm[97] Cole;[33] Hasegawa and others[83]
	Decrease in nasal resistance with advancing age in adults	Masing;[122] Parker and others;[148] Principato and Wolf;[156] Saito and Nishihata[162]
	Nasal resistance increases with age in children	
Acoustic rhinometry		
Temperature	1 mm shift in anatomic features for every 2.5° C difference in temperature	Tomkinson[183]
Race	MCA was significantly lower in whites and Asians than in blacks; volumes smallest in Asians, largest in blacks	Morgan and others[130]
Rhinomanometry		
Temperature	Cold air increases nasal resistance	Forsyth and others[62]
Race	Nasal resistance is greater in whites than in blacks, and intermediate in Asians	Ohki and others[139]
Humidity	No change with changes in humidity	Ivarsson and Malm[95]

pressure changes in the nose.[88] Other sources of variability will be itemized in the next section. Fisher[61] noted that such limitations dampen the original enthusiasm that acoustic rhinometry would give superior reproducibility compared with other objective tests. In addition, he noted that the repeat tests, needed to minimize these increasingly evident sources of variability, "detract from the perceived speed of acoustic rhinometry."

Operator bias

Fisher and others[61] found interobserver variation to have a "surprising effect on all parameters" and that it was in part a result of acceptance of traces of suboptimal quality. To reduce operator bias in acoustic rhinometry, Tomkinson[183] recommended maintaining a coefficient of variation of less than 20% for a reference volume at the site of interest. He also recommended[186] using the average of at least three consecutive traces because if multiple tracings are done, wider error bars can sometimes reveal areas of inaccuracy.

Angle of incidence of the wave tube

Fisher and others[61] found that an increase in the sagittal angle of the tube caused a decrease in depth of the I-notch and C-notch and shifting of both anteriorly. They found that an increase in the lateral (axial) angle caused shifting anteriorly of the I- and C-notches with a decrease in magnitude of the I-notch and changes in the wave pattern in the deeper nasal cavity. Some investigators have found it desirable to use a special stand for the patient to rest his or her head on to maintain a constant angle of incidence with the device to improve the reliability of serial measurements.[57a] Roth and others[161] demonstrated less variation and a larger cross-sectional area using a holder to stabilize the tube. In addition to increasing reliability and reproducibility of measurements, they thought the technique could save time and allow the mounting of other equipment, e.g., rhinoscopes. Fisher and others[61] thought that children would find a head holder frightening.

Avoidance of nasal tip distortion

Fisher and others[61] also found that the conical nosepiece produced a degree of deformity of the valve in many subjects. Roithman and others[160] noted that use of a nasal adapter rather than nozzles could help to avoid distortion in the compliant vestibular region, resulting in lower estimations of the MCA.

Acoustic seal with the nostril

A complete acoustic seal needs to be obtained because air leaks can cause variability. Fisher and others[61] found that where a seal was difficult to obtain (e.g., in subjects with long thin nostrils), the addition of sealant reduced the anterior cavity volume measurement. Tomkinson and others[186] found that if the air leak is small, the main effect is exaggeration of the dimension after the leak, but if the air leak is large, there will not be any useful information after the leak. Grymer and others[72] said that a leak might be indicated if a volume larger than 45 cm^3 between 9.2 and 13 cm was measured. Some testers have thought that the character of the sound of the "click" made by the device can reveal a sound leak. A layer of water-soluble jelly is recommended to provide an acoustic barrier but to allow the device to not be in firm contact with the nose to avoid distortion of the tip structures.

Size of the nosepiece

Fisher and others[61] found that with decrease in the size of the nosepiece, the I-notch deepened, and with the 8-mm (small) nosepiece, the MCA was underestimated.

No breathing or swallowing during the test

Breathing during the test causes a change in the MCA estimation[184] or a high rate of artefactual traces.[61] Swallowing also might cause variation in the results for acoustic rhinometry.[88,183] It thus is important that the patient hold his or her breath and not swallow during the measurement.

Measurement beyond a restriction

Hilberg[88] found that the area beyond a significant restriction may not be accurately estimated. They found, in general, that if the anterior area is less than 0.7 cm^2, there will be significant error for more distal (from the nosepiece) measurements. Fisher and others[59] noted that because acoustic rhinometry was less accurate in the posterior nose, it was fortunate that the rhinologist is most interested in the anterior nasal airway. Hamilton and others[76] noted that 0.7 to 0.8 cm^2 is the normal dimension for an adult nasal valve, that errors beyond this size restriction would be about 20% for nasal volume measurements, and that the error would increase with pathological restrictions or with children's noses. They also found inaccuracies in area reconstructions and distance to constrictions in measurements beyond this size constriction. They noted that the results were reproducible and so would remain useful for comparisons.

Change in geometry of the cavity measured

Tomkinson and others[186] demonstrated that the greater the magnitude of changes in cross-sectional area, the worse the estimate of the dimension of the airway. Also, the greater the rate of change of the area, the worse the estimate of airway size would be. They concluded that acoustic rhinometry was a low resolution device that may only be useful in the most anterior nasal cavity or in localizing the narrowest point or in documenting the relative changes produced by treatment.

Position or motion of the soft palate

Hilberg and others[88] noted that motion of the soft palate might cause variation in results. If the palate is elevated at the time of the test, the nasopharyngeal volume estimate will be reduced.[61]

Additional recommendations—acoustic rhinometry

Fisher and others[61] noted that for comparisons between populations (e.g., pre- and postoperative or nasal cycle studies) "great care must be taken" to ensure that all technical variables are constant. They recommended for acoustic rhinometry that all readings be taken with the tube at mid-range angles, that sealant be used if the quality of the acoustic seal is in doubt, that the patient should avoid respiration during the test, and that improved nosepieces should be used that do not enter the valve.

Other ways to minimize variability for objective testing for rhinomanometry and acoustic rhinometry

Because multiple sources of variability are potentially present, one cannot always be sure which factor is most responsible for a measured variability in results. All sources of variability should be controlled without affecting the clinical information sought. Cole[35] proposed that subjects should avoid exercise and exposure to climatic extremes for 30 minutes before testing. Patients should not be taking any interfering medications. As previously mentioned, distortion of the alae should be avoided. Measurement should be performed in a comfortable, stable, nonirritating environment. Jones and others[101] used a quiet, well-ventilated room with constant temperature and humidity, with no bright sunshine, and with the patient sitting in a comfortable chair. They recommended explaining the test procedure and the equipment first to help alleviate patient anxiety. The patient had no tobacco or coffee before the test. Knowledge of the factors that can affect variability of results allows investigators to take appropriate measures to obtain the most accurate and precise results.

WHAT IS THE ROLE OF OBJECTIVE TESTING OF THE NASAL AIRWAY?

Objective testing of the nasal airway can be used for the clinical evaluation of the symptom of nasal obstruction, for evaluation of patients with sleep apnea, for allergy challenge testing, and for pretreatment and posttreatment comparisons.

Objective testing can help in the diagnosis and treatment selection of patients with obstructive symptoms

For patients with the symptom of nasal obstruction in whom airway restriction is the suspected cause of the symptoms

If airway restriction is the suspected cause of the symptoms, objective testing results can be used with the results of history and examination to aid in the diagnosis and treatment. The method for this will be described in more detail. If there is suspicion of sinusitis or other conditions that might cause obstructive symptoms without directly restricting the airway, these are looked for before testing is done.

For patients with snoring and sleep apnea

As previously mentioned, rhinomanometry can be used to assess the change in resistance that occurs when the patient is in the supine position. This change can be more severe in the patient with sleep apnea.[3] Snoring has been decreased[152,167] by using nasal dilators to open the anterior nasal airway, implying a contributory role of nasal obstruction in causing snoring in some patients. Olsen[140] found that nasal obstruction caused by packing could cause disturbed sleep. Miljeteig and others[128] found no correlation between varying degrees of nasal resistance and amount of snoring in eight snorers who had no nasal pathology. Lenders and others[118] found that 97% of patients with habitual snoring (some with sleep apnea) had an MCA located at the C-notch (turbinate), whereas in all of their normal subjects, the MCA was located at the I-notch. Even with decongestion, the area at the C-notch of the patients who snored did not reach normal nondecongested size. They, like Blakely and Mahowald,[16] found higher than normal nasal resistance in these patients but no correlation between number of apneas and degree of nasal resistance. Petrusan[151] reported that increasing the nasal airway with a dilator can reduce the apnea index. Future studies may reveal the role of objective nasal airway testing in helping to assess the contribution of the nasal airway in patients with snoring and sleep apnea.

For challenge testing in patients with allergic rhinitis

Nasal challenge testing is performed by introducing a specific allergen into the nose to assess the pathophysiologic changes that result. This use for objective testing emerged from the desire to directly test the organ affected by allergy rather than to rely on the indirect reaction manifested by skin tests.[13,170,193] Nasal provocation testing dates from 1873.[31] A technique was sought that would be reproducible, deliver a consistent concentration of the challenging antigen, and provide objective noninvasive assessment of the response to the challenge. Provocation testing using objective testing of the nasal airway offered the promise of fulfilling these criteria. Doyle and others[51] found the intranasal allergen challenges with ragweed pollen in patients with ragweed allergy reproducibly caused an increase in nasal resistance with increasing dose of ragweed. Fireman[57] noted the advantage of rhinomanometry in providing numbers that enable calculation of percent change from a baseline value, which he noted would be difficult to assess with symptom scores alone.

Different levels indicative of a positive response have been chosen. Wang and Clement[188a] noted that an increase to 100% of baseline rhinomanometric result occurred after challenge in 94% in the early phase and 82% in the late phase, but that unilateral measurement was prefered to total measurement because it was more sensitive in the evaluation of the late phase nasal response. Pastorella and others[150] showed that an inflammatory reaction (particularly involving eosinophils) occurs after nasal challenge and is closely related to increase in nasal resistance and increase in the symptom of nasal obstruction.

More recently, acoustic rhinometry has been used for challenge testing. Lai and Corey[114] used acoustic rhinometry to show a correlation between the results of challenge testing and serum specific IgE (mRAST) results. Acoustic rhinometry and rhinomanometry have yielded comparable results in nasal challenge testing.[6,166] Lenders and Pirsig[117] thought that acoustic rhinometry could be more sensitive than rhinomanometry in detecting allergic rhinitis because it could reveal mucosal changes even when no change in resistance had occurred. Austin and Foreman[6] noted that compared with rhinomanometry, acoustic rhinometry could be more quickly performed and required minimal subject cooperation, which could be advantageous in challenge testing. Scadding and others[166] thought that acoustic rhinometry had less variability in quantifying the airway in challenge testing done in severely congested patients.

Objective testing can help in the assessment of the effect of treatment

For medical therapy

Objective testing of the nasal airway has been a useful way to assess the effect of intranasal medications because it does not rely on subjective assessment by the patient or clinician.[15,87,92,116,165] Elbrond and others[56] used acoustic rhinometry to show the change in cross-sectional area that occured in a patient with nasal polyps receiving systemic steroid treatment.

For surgical therapy

Nasal airway testing can help to objectively assess the effect of surgery on the airway. Malm[119] said that rhinomanometry has value in patients to explain why surgery has reduced or increased their nasal symptoms and that it has scientific value in "evaluating effects of certain surgical techniques." Sipila and others[174] suggested that rhinomanometry could serve as "a method of quality control" by showing how nasal obstruction was not corrected in some patients.

Change in airway dimension after surgery. Several investigators have found a significant decrease in nasal resistance in the more obstructed side of the nose after septal surgery,* and after turbinate surgery.[47,99,191] Using acoustic rhinometry, Lenders and Pirsig[117] showed an improvement in airway dimension after turbinate surgery. Grymer and others found a decrease in MCA after septoplasty,[71] after rhinoplasty, and after turbinoplasty.[70] Elbond and others[56] showed that acoustic rhinometry can document the change in the epipharynx after adenoidectomy. Kimmelman and Jablonski[111] did not find a significant decrease in total resistance in the decongested nose after septal or turbinate surgery, although there was a decrease in patients' symptoms.

Correlation with symptoms postoperatively. A number of these investigators found a postoperative improvement in symptoms associated with improvement in the nasal airway documented by objective testing.* Constantinides and others[46] did not find a correlation postoperatively between symptoms and nasal resistance after decongestion in patients who had septorhinoplasty.

Correlation with satisfaction with surgery. Patients with high preoperative resistance or low preoperative MCA were more likely to be satisfied with surgery than those with preoperatively lower resistance or higher preoperative MCA.[120,174,180] Sipila and others[174] noted that patient satisfaction was highest in patients with symptoms of obstruction whose nasal resistance was changed to "normal." Grymer and others[71] using acoustic rhinometry, found that although the MCA did not always improve with correction of septal deformities, the patient's satisfaction was correlated with the improvement in size of the MCA after surgery. They also noted a slight correlation between nasal volume and the patient's satisfaction with surgery. After turbinoplasty, Grymer and Hilberg[70] noted improvement in MCA and symptoms of patency, but they did not find a correlation between the amount of improvement in MCA and patients' satisfaction with surgery.

Criteria for surgery. Suonpaa and others[180] questioned the benefit obtained when operating on patients with preoperatively normal nasal resistance. Malm[119] suggested that it is possible to select patients for surgery on the basis of rhinomanometric data if results are from the decongested nose, if correction is done for height, and if the 95% prediction limit is used. Bachmann[11] has outlined rhinomanometric indications for and against surgery and noted that "when *constant stenosis* exists and" total flow "is below 700 cm^3/sec, then there exists a clear indication for surgery."

Recently, there has been a desire by some clinicians to have a means of obtaining an objective assessment that would demonstrate the need for surgery to managed care reviewers. This might be difficult to do meaningfully using absolute values in the highly variable environment of the nose. It might be possible to some extent in the context of a clinical algorithm that incorporates objective testing as one of the facets of the decision-making process in the selection of therapy. A clinical algorithm using objective testing will be described in a later section of this chapter.

THE ROLE OF OBJECTIVE TESTING WHEN AIRWAY RESTRICTION IS THE SUSPECTED CAUSE OF THE SYMPTOMS

Is there an abnormal airway dimension or amount of restriction that can be distinguished from normal?

For rhinomanometry

Most reports of normal resistance have been based on the values for small groups of control subjects. One goal of the International Committee on Standardization (now called

---

* Refs. 21, 68, 91, 96, 97, 112, 138, 179.

* Refs. 21, 91, 99, 120, 127, 179.

Table 42-2. Unilateral normal mean or median nasal resistance: reported adult inspiratory values

Investigator	Subject description	N	Nondecongested value*	Decongested value*	Side	Measured at
Pallanch and others[145]	Symptom-less volunteers	80	0.25	0.16	Average	Radius 1
			0.33	0.22	Average	Radius 2
			0.42	0.28	Average	Radius 3
Unno and others	No or only slight obstruction	50	0.35	—	Right	50 Pa
			0.30	—	Left	50 Pa
Kenyon[107]	Healthy	25	0.33/0.39	0.28	Average	Radius 2
Jessen and Malm[97]	Healthy	100	0.45	0.23	Average	Radius 2
			0.54	0.36	Average	150 Pa
Cole[33]	Symptom-less	1000s	Varies	0.3	Average	Mean
				0.15	(with retracted ala)	Mean
Sipila and others[174]	Healthy "Normal nasal status"	97		0.30	Average	150 Pa
				0.20	Average	Radius 2

* All values rounded off and converted to Pa/cm^3/sec. (0.1 Pa/cm^3/sec = (approximately) 1 cm H_2O/l/sec).
In some cases, the mean value is the arithmetic mean of a skewed distribution. Ranges are not shown.

the Standardization Committee on Objective Assessment of the Nasal Airway)[32,108,110] has been to establish normal values at various centers using recommended methods for consistent reporting of the results. Tables 42-2 and 42-3 present unilateral and total values for normal resistance that have been reported in the literature. Note that the values often cannot be directly compared with each other because they were obtained using different points on the pressure–flow curve.

One problem in reporting normal values is the criteria used for selection of healthy subjects. The healthy subjects in Tables 42-2 and 42-3 usually were "normal" on the basis of lack of symptoms. Szucs and others[181] concluded that lack of symptoms alone was not a sufficient criterion for the inclusion of subjects in normative studies of rhinomanometry results. Palma and others[147] recommended that subjects described as "normal" also be "rhinoscopically normal." A normal range for nasal pressure–flow curves can be shown by a shaded area on the plot of the pressure–flow curve (Fig. 42-12).[145] Although not an absolute level at which obstruction is indicated, this serves as a reference area for comparisons with a population who breathes comfortably through their nose. One problem encountered in studying a "normal" population is that resistance values are not normally, in a statistical sense, distributed.[123,145,181] For statistical analyses, transformation can be performed to normalize the distribution of the data, or nonparametric statistical methods can be used.[20,77,83,123,143]

For acoustic rhinometry

Grymer and others[72] and Lenders and Persig[117] have reported normal values for acoustic rhinometry. Lenders and Pirsig[117] found the normal MCA to be 0.73 cm^2. Grymer and others[72] reported normal MCA values for 82 subjects of 0.72 to 0.73 cm^2 before decongestion and 0.92 to 0.95 cm^2 after decongestion for the unilateral airway. For the total

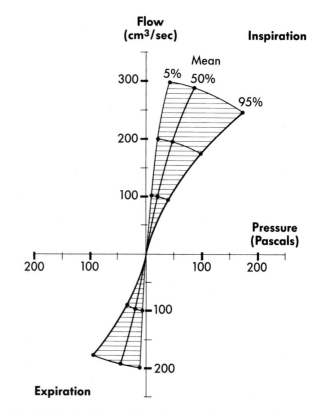

Fig. 42-12. Shaded area defined by the 5%, mean, and 95% curves representing the range in unilateral nasal pressure–flow data after decongestion in 80 healthy adults.

airway, the normal MCA was 1.46 cm^2 before decongestion and 1.88 cm^2 after decongestion. Grymer and others[72] stated that stricter criteria for normal subjects may be needed because some of the subjects in their normal group had MCAs at the anterior turbinate, whereas those in the study by Lenders and Pirsig[117] did not.

Table 42-3. Total normal nasal resistance: reported adult inspiratory values

Investigator	Subject description	N	Nondecongested value*	Decongested value*	Method	Measured at
Rundcrantz	Healthy individuals	10	0.14	—	Posterior measured	0.5 l/sec
McCaffrey and Kern[123]	Asymptomatic normal examination	23	0.22	0.15	Anterior calculated	Maximum
Connell[45]	Pedestrians on streets of New York (some children)	263 (white)	0.23	—	Anterior calculated	150 Pa
		30 (black)	0.19	—	Anterior calculated	150 Pa
Pallanch and others[145]	Symptom-less volunteers	80	0.12	0.08	Anterior calculated	Radius 2
			0.14	0.09	Anterior calculated	Radius 3
			0.16	0.10	Anterior calculated	Radius 4
			0.14	0.10	Anterior calculated	50 Pa
			0.18	0.14	Anterior calculated	100 Pa
			0.11	0.07	Anterior calculated	0.1 l/sec
			0.12	0.08	Anterior calculated	0.2 l/sec
Unno and others	No or only slight obstruction	50		0.16	Anterior calculated	50 Pa
				0.15	Posterior measured	50 Pa
Jones and others[101]	No disease normal examination	59	0.38	—	Anterior calculated	150 Pa
Jessen and Malm[97]	Healthy	100	0.19	0.11	Anterior calculated	Radius 2
			0.25	0.18	Anterior calculated	150 Pa
Cole[33,35]	Symptom-less volunteers	800	0.26	—	Posterior measured (?)	Mean
		1000s				
			0.33	—	Posterior measured (?)	150 Pa
			0.2	0.1	Posterior measured (?)	Mean
			0.25	0.12	Posterior measured (?)	150 Pa
Sipila and others[174]	Healthy	97		0.15	Anterior calculated	150 Pa
	"Normal nasal status"			0.09	Anterior calculated	Radius 2

* All values are rounded off and converted to Pa/cm³/sec. (0.1 Pa/cm³/sec = (approximately) 1 cm H_2O/l/sec).
In some cases, the value is the arithmetic mean of a skewed distribution. Ranges are not shown.

Has a correlation been found between objective test results and the symptom of obstruction?

Several methods have been used to study the correlation between the results of objective testing of the nasal airway and the symptom of nasal obstruction. One method is to determine whether there is a difference between a group of normal subjects and a group with symptoms of obstruction. Another method is to look for a correlation between symptoms and objective test results with statistical methods that consider each person studied.

Comparison of group results—normal subjects versus obstructed subjects

Both unilateral and total resistance may be related to the patient symptoms. It is not known whether unilateral or total results give the most meaningful correlation with symptoms, but McCaffrey and Kern[123] and Bachmann[11] thought the total resistance would be the most important determinant of the patient's sense of well being. Arbour and Kern[4] described the phenomenon of paradoxical nasal obstruction in which the effect of the more open side of the nose on the total resistance was the determining factor for the presence or absence of obstructive symptoms.

Unilateral airway. A significant difference has been found between median or mean resistance of the obstructed side of the nose in patients with unilateral symptoms and the unilateral resistance of a group of normal subjects.[68,123] A difference was not found with the nonobstructed side in the symptomatic patients. In patients with bilateral symptoms, the right-sided resistance for those with moderate and severe symptoms and the left-sided resistance for those with moderate symptoms was significantly greater than the median unilateral resistance for the normal patients.[123]

Total airway. Total resistance for those patients with moderate and severe bilateral symptoms and for those patients with moderate and severe unilateral symptoms was greater than the median total resistance for normal patients.[123] Lebowitz and Jacobs[116] found a correlation between symptoms and the decrease in total nasal resistance after treatment with steroid spray, but Scadding and others[165] did not.

It is apparent that there is a difference between the group

airflow restriction correlates with obstructive symptoms and those in whom it does not correlate. The first group will have the best chance of being helped by therapy that is directed at enlarging the dimension of the nasal airway, whereas the second group will not.

Testing can tell if symptoms are associated with an open (unrestricted) airway. If no airway restriction is found with testing despite the presence of symptoms, then other causes are suggested. Dry atrophic nasal mucosa also can cause the complaint of obstruction. Cole[33] thought that some patients, including those with atrophic rhinitis, may have altered nasal sensation, which they misinterpret as obstruction to airflow. Eccles[52] stated "edema or inflammation around the sensory nerve endings in the nasal mucosa may create a sensation of nasal obstruction by adversely affecting the function of the sensory receptors." Sinus disease can cause the sensation of nasal obstruction without significant restriction. Poor pulmonary function also can cause a patient to complain of nasal dyspnea. Cole[33] noted that some patients who suffer from cardiopulmonary insufficiency find any nasal resistance load intolerable. Objective testing that can verify the presence of an unrestricted airway would help the clinician avoid incorrect treatment when airway obstruction had been the suspected cause of the symptoms.

Testing can tell if symptoms are associated with a significant airway restriction. This can result in modification of the diagnosis and management and can increase confidence that intervention aimed at improving the airway will help the symptoms. Such potential changes will be demonstrated in a clinical algorithm incorporating objective testing results.

Site of sensation of obstruction

Side of sensation of obstruction. The side of greatest obstruction can be verified because a correlation has been demonstrated[58,144,175] between the side of symptoms of greatest obstruction and the most restricted airway result.

Site of sensation, vestibular skin versus caval mucosa. Some comments can be made about the cites in the nose at which symptoms occur. It has been demonstrated[22,53] that exposure to aromatic substances such as menthol, camphor, or eucalyptol caused the sensation of increased nasal patency despite no change in nasal resistance. These volatile oils increase the sensitivity of cold receptors by increasing the temperature at which they respond. By increasing cold receptor reactivity in nerve endings, the subject senses the nose is more open.

Jones and others[102] found that lidocaine injected in the nasal vestibule caused the sensation of nasal obstruction in subjects without change in nasal resistance. This finding supported their hypothesis that the amount of activity of the cold receptors affected the sensation of obstruction. They thought that cold receptors primarily reside in the vestibular skin. This was supported[27] by the finding that when an air jet was directed at the inside of the nose, the area of greatest

sensitivity to the sensation of airflow was in the nasal vestibule. Investigators have found evidence for menthol sensitive receptors in nasal mucosa also.[2,54] Most nasal mucosa is posterior to the vestibule in the cavum of the nose. Conflicting results have been obtained when the nasal mucosa was anesthetized. Jones and others[100] found that subjects reported a sensation of more patency, whereas Eccles[54] found subjects experienced a feeling of less patency. Clark and Jones[29] subsequently found that if airflow was carefully controlled, nasal mucosal anesthesia had little effect on sensation, suggesting that the most important receptors for sensation of patency are in the vestibule. Aldren and Tolley[2] concluded that both vestibular skin and caval mucosa contribute to the sensation of patency or obstruction, but the nerve endings in the vestibule have the greatest effect.

Clark and Jones[29] thought that rather than just cold receptors detecting airflow, it is more likely that flow sensation results from an interplay of "peripheral signals—tactile, thermal and perhaps chemical." Eccles[53] thought that any damage to trigeminal sensory nerve endings, whether vestibular or caval, could cause a sensation of nasal stuffiness, even though resistance is unchanged or decreased.

In the study by Wight and others,[192] radical turbinectomy resulted in a greater chance for improvement in symptoms than anterior turbinectomy, even though both resulted in decrease in resistance. There are two possible explanations for why this occurred. One is that more than airflow is involved in the experience of symptoms. It also is possible that an airflow phenomenon is occurring along the unresected portion of the turbinate, which causes persistent symptoms but is of such smaller magnitude than the larger anterior pressure drop that is not reflected in the improved resistance result. This theory would suggest that more posterior pathology, which appears to cause no significant increase in resistance, might still be important to correct to provide symptomatic relief. This speculation would be consistent with Bachmann's statement that the effect of the anatomy in the posterior sector of the nose has been undervalued.[8] Acoustic rhinometry might be able to demonstrate this[71] in future studies.

Objective testing can help to assess the accuracy of the subjective assessment of the degree of the symptoms

High threshold. If the patient's symptoms are of lower degree than the airway restriction measured by objective testing, then they have a higher threshold. An example of this is the patient who is born with a marked nasal septal deflection and is being evaluated for other problems. The clinician notes the dramatic deflection, and the patient denies being aware of it (even though the patient may be obligate mouth breathing at the time of reporting this lack of symptoms). Another example is the patient who has some symptoms, but they are much less severe than the airway restriction that is measured. This situation can be a result of the patient describing the symptoms not in terms of what the general population notices but rather in terms of what the patient is accustomed to. A patient who is accustomed to a higher level of airway restriction might say that it is causing only "mild" symptoms at a level of restriction that for another person would be "severe" obstruction. The presence of a high threshold usually does not change the approach to management of symptoms because it would still be hoped that correction of the offending pathology causing the restriction would improve the symptoms.

Low threshold. If the patient's symptoms are of higher degree than the airway restriction measured by objective testing, then they have a low threshold for the sensation of nasal obstruction. This increases concern that the condition may be harder to manage with the same degree of success that would result from treating a patient with a normal or high threshold for symptoms. The reason for this is that the symptoms in a patient with low threshold have a greater chance of being caused by factors other than airway restriction. One such possibility is that the symptoms are a result of a sensory disturbance of the nasal mucosa (e.g., some airway tissue loses some of its sensory detection with age). Thus, some patients might have decreased receptor activity, and therefore, even if the airway is unrestricted, they might not receive the receptor stimulation for the same amount of airflow and so they may sense that airflow is not adequate. If so, there is less likelihood of helping the patient's symptoms by treatment aimed at increasing the size of the airway.

It was mentioned previously that some investigators[119,127] have specified a certain level of airway restriction below which the probability of success of nasal airway surgery might decrease. Patients with a low threshold have less restricted test values and may fit into the group who are below such a level of restriction.

Has a correlation been found between objective test results and rhinoscopy?

Rhinoscopy provides a view of the condition of the nasal mucosa and the presence of excessive secretions or intranasal growths. In addition, it gives subjective appraisal of the areas of cross-sectional narrowing in the nasal airway. This appraisal can include estimation of a number of parameters, including turbinate size; turbinate-to-septum distances; width of the nostril, valve area, and floor of the nose; and diameters of the middle meatus.[78]

Correlation between rhinoscopy and objective test results

A significant correlation has been found between rhinoscopy and the results of rhinomanometry.[78,106,132] Hardcastle and others[78] thought the correlation was weak in the patients they studied, the majority of whom were normal. Huygen and others[94] thought that the correspondence between rhinoscopic findings and rhinomanometry was only reliable for large deviations in the valve region. Hardcastle and others[78] believed that the difference between results from rhinoscopy and rhinomanometry was sufficient to

suggest that they might measure different but related phenomena.

The imperfect correlation between rhinoscopy and rhinomanometry could be a result of several factors, including the variability of each technique and the limitations each might have in reflecting the actual physical parameter being assessed. Because each technique is variable, comparing them necessarily would be somewhat imprecise. An example of rhinoscopic variability can be found in the study by Keay and others,[106] who reported interobserver changes resulting from the nasal cycle.

The area of greatest constriction found by acoustic rhinometry has been found to correlate with rhinoscopy done with probes for certain anatomic features, but no study has been reported on clinician assessment of the magnitude of a rhinoscopic finding compared with the size of the restriction as measured by acoustic rhinometry.

Rhinoscopy and objective testing considered together

Rhinoscopy and objective test results can both provide information about the nasal airway. Objective testing might have some potential advantages over rhinoscopy. Hardcastle and others[79] found that the results of rhinomanometry correlated with the degree of obstruction, whereas rhinoscopy did not. Because the two modalities can provide different information, by using both, the clinician might obtain a more complete understanding of a patient's nasal airway. Bachmann[8,11] has emphasized that the two tests should be performed together because the synthesis of the simultaneous information they provide can be useful in the clinical evaluation of a patient. Objective testing results along with rhinoscopy can help to discover more about the nature of the pathology causing a patient's complaint of nasal airway obstruction.

Does the test help to identify the presence, site, type, and degree of intranasal pathology that is causing the symptoms?

Presence: What if pathology does not correlate with measured airway restriction?

In some patients, rhinoscopy may reveal suspected pathology that objective testing does not corroborate. Hypothetically, an area of pathology could be found that looked significant at a site that was not as narrow as the most critical area, so that its effect would not be reflected in the rhinomanometric results. Cole and others[42] and Chaban and others,[24] found that some of the simulated obstructions in the bony cavum of the nose that looked like impressive pathology on rhinoscopic examination produced only insignificant increases in resistance. They noted that the airstream was apparently able to find relatively nonresistive routes that were not always seen on clinical examination. Such an area might be revealed by acoustic rhinometry but not be the narrowest spot (MCA). The question of whether pathology in areas other than the smallest cross-sectional area contributes to symptoms of obstruction remains unanswered.[71] If the pathology is not causing major restriction, then management aimed at correcting that pathology to change the airway may not be appropriate.

Objective testing can lead to the discovery of pathology that is causing airway restriction by revealing abnormal findings that rhinoscopy had not found. Such a site of constriction may not have been apparent to the examiner, and so a second look is warranted.

Side as assessed by rhinomanometry or acoustic rhinometry

Rhinomanometry and acoustic rhinometry can distinguish the side with the most abnormal results. If the side of greatest restriction as measured by objective testing corresponds with the side of greatest pathology, then this is evidence that the observed pathology has the greatest effect in causing airway restriction.

Intranasal sites assessed by rhinomanometry or acoustic rhinometry

Distinction between valve and valve region. Kern[109] distinguished between the "nasal valve" and the "nasal valve area." He noted that the nasal valve was a slit-like opening between the caudal edge of the upper lateral cartilage and the nasal septum as first described by Mink and that it was only part of the nasal valve area. Mink called this slit-like opening the "ostium internum" and considered it to be the narrowest part of the nasal airway. Other synonyms are os internum, limen vestibuli, limen nasi, liminal valve, and "liminal chink." The *limen nasi* (limen vestibuli) refers to a specific anatomic ridge (boundary) on the lateral nasal wall formed by the lower end of the upper lateral cartilage, which separates the vestibule from the remainder of the nasal cavity.[90] Van Dishoeck also thought the limen nasi was the narrowest spot in the nasal airway[74] and thus would be the main determinant of the nasal resistance. Bachmann and Legler showed with plastic casts that the smallest area was at the isthmus nasi close to the pyriform aperture.[9] Shreck and others[173] found in a model based on MRI data that the greatest pressure drop occurred anterior to the inferior turbinate.

Description of valve region. Kasperbauer and Kern[105] stated that the nasal valve area (Fig. 42-14) is the functional unit that "includes the distal end of the upper lateral cartilage, the head of the inferior turbinate, the caudal septum, and the remainder of the tissues surrounding the piriform aperture" (floor of the nose, lateral fibrofatty tissue, frontal process of the maxilla). Bridger[18] described this as the "flow limiting segment," with the Mink valve as its distal orifice. Bachmann[10] described it as the "isthmus region." Other synonyms for the valve area include "valve region" and area 2.[109] In the rest of this chapter the authors will use the term *valve region* to refer to this anatomic unit to avoid

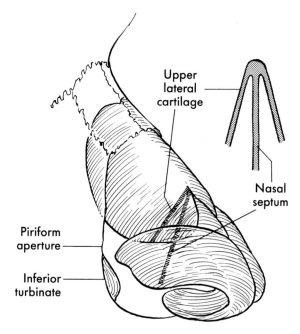

Fig. 42-14. Anatomy of the valve region.

confusion of the term *area* with the measurement of a cross-section.

The valve region is the anterior part of the nose in which the MCA occurs. Bridger and Proctor[18] using rhinomanometry and a plastic catheter passed along the floor of the nose found that instead of a solitary highest resistance point, the resistance was spread across the valve region and beyond and that only a little additional resistance was noted. Haight and Cole[74] with a similar method found that in six subjects the greatest resistance drop occurred at the anterior end of the inferior turbinate in the first few millimeters of the bony cavum. They found that the site of greatest resistance was in the same location even after decongestion. Hirschberg and others[89] extended this study to a larger group of subjects and found that before decongestion, the most restrictive portion of the nose (78% of the resistance) was in the first 4 cm, with 56% of the resistance in the first 2 cm. After decongestion, the greatest resistance (88%) was in the first 2 cm. This demonstrated that the anterior tip of the inferior turbinate was the site of most resistance in the nasal airway for some patients before but not after decongestion.

Cole and Roithmann[38] noted that the valve region is bounded by compliant and mobile as well as rigid components. This gives the valve region a dynamic character. Any change in dimension can alter cross-sectional area and thus affect airway resistance exponentially, so the effect of such changes in the valve region is greater than elsewhere in the nose. This reinforces the importance of not distorting the anterior nasal structures when performing the objective test. This region of the nose has been noted to account for half of the airflow resistance of the entire respiratory tract[38] and ensures disruption of laminar flow in the upper airways.[36] It is the most common site of pathology that causes significant obstruction.[38]

Various sites of the MCA verified by rhinomanometry and acoustic rhinometry. It would seem appropriate to designate the anatomic site of the MCA as the valve, but this would be confusing because historically the valve is the specific anatomic area described previously. Consequently, the authors use the term *MCA* to refer to the location of smallest dimension and thus greatest restriction.

Is the site of greatest constriction (MCA) located at the ostium internum as described by Mink[105,117,118,173] or in the region posterior to this[9] or at the head of the inferior turbinate at the piriform aperture?[74] It is apparent that it varies in location within the valve region.[72,89] This conclusion is supported by data from acoustic rhinometry.

There usually are two constrictions noted on the typical area–distance curve obtained with acoustic rhinometry (see Fig. 42-1). Cole and Roithman[38] noted that calibrated probes have shown that the first constriction occurs at the triangular entrance of the valve region, and the second is at the entrance of the bony cavum. They noted that the first constriction and the second can be reduced by decongestion, just as Haight and Cole[74] noted that with decongestion the resistance decreases across the nasal vestibule and the first part of the cavum. Cole[35a] noted that erectile tissue related to the valve region can be found not only in the turbinate but also in the caudal septum and lateral nasal wall. Cole and Roithman[38] thought the septal erectile body in the medial wall of the valve explained the opening of the first constriction, with decongestion noted with acoustic rhinometry.

Grymer and others[89] found that in some patients, the MCA before decongestion corresponded to the anterior tip of the inferior turbinate (second minimum). After decongestion, it shifted forward to the first minimum (ostium internum, start of valve region). The average distance to the MCA before decongestion was 2.23 cm (range, 0.6 to 3.3 cm) and after decongestion was 1.53 cm (range, 0.44 to 3.03 cm). Lenders and Pirsig[117,118] found that the MCA in 134 normal subjects always was at the first constriction and did not decrease with decongestion. Because the MCA always was at the first constriction, they called this the "I-notch" for isthmus nasi. Grymer and others[89] located the first constriction at the opening to the valve region (ostium internum) and located the MCA before decongestion at the second constriction (the anterior edge of the inferior turbinate) in the "isthmus nasi" posterior to the ostium internum. The confusion caused by association of both the first and second constrictions with the isthmus nasi can be alleviated by considering this as the "isthmus region"[10] and not a single location. Grymer had not screened his normal subject with rhinoscopy and thought that perhaps Lenders' normal patients had smaller turbinates than his because they had less prominent second

minima (C-notches). Both investigators noted that decongestion only affected the second minimum.

Lenders and Pirsig[117] described the acoustic rhinometry area–distance plot for the healthy patient as having the smallest dimension (lowest minimum) in the anterior valve region ("ascending W"), whereas a patient with mucosal disease before decongestion or a patient who has had allergen challenge might have the smallest dimension in the area of the anterior tip of the inferior turbinate ("descending W"). Grymer and others[71] found that with decongestion, the MCA moved anteriorly probably as a result of shrinkage of the inferior turbinate. When patients had severe septal deflection anterior to the inferior turbinate, no anterior shift in MCA occurred with decongestion. After correction of the septal pathology, the MCA moved anteriorly with decongestion like the normal nose.

Assessment of the valve region by rhinomanometry and acoustic rhinometry. Rhinomanometry, when performed using the pressure drop across the entire nose, primarily reflects this narrowest effective cross-sectional area of the nasal airway because the greatest part of the resistance drop occurs at the narrowest site. The authors call this assessment of the smallest dimension found by rhinomanometry the *physiologic MCA estimate*. Acoustic rhinometric measurements yield an area–distance plot that allows the measurement of the smallest cross-sectional area for the anatomic presentation of the instrument. The authors refer to this smallest dimension as determined by acoustic rhinometry as the *anatomic MCA estimate*. Acoustic rhinometry also yields the distance to the narrowest area. The results of acoustic rhinometry have been found to correlate with those from rhinomanometry.[88] The extent to which the physiologic MCA estimate and the anatomic MCA estimate are similar would reflect the extent to which acoustic rhinometry and rhinomanometry are providing a similar assessment of the nasal airway.

Stenting open the nose can help to reveal the effect of the compliant part of the valve region. Bachmann[9] noted that stenting the valve angle open may improve the airway in the case of an anterior restriction. Some authors have recommended such a maneuver to assess the function of the nasal valve. The nasal airway has been held open using tygon tubing,[14] sticks or wire,[74] a custom wire stent,[25,73] and retraction on the cheek.[158] The currently available externally applied adhesive plastic strips[167] also can be used for this purpose. If the method of retraction does not interfere with the test equipment, this can be done for either rhinomanometry or acoustic rhinometry.

Guillete and Perry[73] found a significant correlation between changes in resistance by stenting of the nares and valve pathology. If little change in resistance results with stenting, a restriction could be attributed to factors posterior to the compliant part of the valve area. Cole and Roithmann[38] stated that such alar retraction minimizes the effect of the compliant part of the valve on resistance, revealing the relative contribution of the compliant versus caval parts of the valve. They also found that a nasal dilator can open up the entire valve region back to the second constriction measured by acoustic rhinometry. They give an example of a patient with a septal deflection in the valve area in which alar retraction causes a significant reduction in resistance, whereas decongestion caused only minimal decrease. Chawdry and others[25] noted that resistance in 33 patients with structural pathology was reduced 26% by an internal nasal dilator, 41% by decongestion, and 62% by dilator and decongestion. They noted that further studies are needed to correlate these results with ''the aetiology of the nasal obstruction.'' Objective testing using a dilator might reveal valve pathology better than rhinoscopy because the introduction of the nasal speculum in the caucasian nose alters tissue relationships in this area.[38]

Such maneuvers that open the valve area mimic what a patient accomplishes with a positive Cottle sign. Heinberg and Kern[86] have noted the possibility of a false-negative Cottle sign, resulting from scar tissue immobilizing the valve.

Inspiration with maximal effort can reveal anterior pathology. Bridger[17] showed that in some patients there is a collapsible portion of the nasal airway that at high flows can restrict the amount of air flow when a critical pressure is reached. Using rhinomanometric methods, the critical pressure of collapse at maximal flow corresponded to anterior nasal pathology.[17,164] Thus some patients with valve pathology might be identified by maximal inspiration that would reveal plateauing of the pressure–flow curve.[164] This is not a routine part of rhinomanometric testing, although it is accomplished with peak flow testing.

Assessment of other intranasal sites. Cole and others[42] and Chaban and others[24] simulated septal deviations to study their effect on nasal resistance to airflow. They showed that site, size, and position of pathology can affect the magnitude of resistance to airflow. They found that only large posterior pathology would increase nasal resistance. Grymer and others[71] checked the change in cross-sectional area at 6.4 cm from the nostrils in patients with correction of posterior septal deformities and found a small (but significant) change after the operation. However, they did not find a significant difference in this dimension between patients who were satisfied compared with those who were unsatisfied with their results after surgery. They noted that most of these patients also had anterior pathology that had been corrected along with their posterior pathology. Grymer and others[72] found using acoustic rhinometry that the maximum effect of decongestion occurred in the middle part of the nose where the middle turbinate is present. Volume of the nasal airway can be measured directly with acoustic rhinometry reflecting the overall caliber of the airway along its length. The question of whether parts of the airway other than the MCA play a significant role in causing the symptom of obstruction as a result of airway restriction remains unanswered.

Objective airway testing can help to assess the accuracy of the subjective assessment of the degree of the pathology causing the symptoms

Overestimation of pathology. If the degree of airway restriction measured by objective testing is less than the degree of the pathology, then the effect of pathology was overestimated. If, before testing, the pathology had been thought to be severe, the clinician might have concluded that there was a high probability of success in modifying the airway so that the patient could breathe more freely. But if airway testing then reveals that the restriction past that pathology is minimal, then the expectations regarding the higher probability of success might be tempered.

Underestimation of pathology. If airway restriction is found to be of greater degree than the pathology, then the effect of the pathology has been underestimated. If the pathology had initially been assessed as minimal, the clinician might conclude that there was a low probability of success in modifying the airway so that the patient could breathe more freely. If airway testing reveals that the restriction past that pathology actually is dramatic, then the expectation about the probability of success in improving the airway by correcting the pathology would be raised. In other words, when the airway actually is more restricted than it appears to the clinician, then correction of the offending pathology has a greater chance of alleviating the symptoms (like a more severe conductive loss in middle ear surgery). The finding of underestimation of pathology also would cause the clinician to reexamine the nasal airway with new appreciation of the effect of the pathology noted.

PUTTING IT ALL TOGETHER, SIMULTANEOUS CONSIDERATION OF SYMPTOMS AND PATHOLOGY AND OBJECTIVE TEST RESULTS, ARRIVING AT A DIAGNOSIS AND TREATMENT PLAN

After demonstration of the information about symptoms and pathology that is revealed by objective testing, the application of objective testing in the clinical evaluation of the patient with the symptom of nasal obstruction thought to be a result of airway restriction can be examined. Although we do not have a single value from rhinomanometry or acoustic rhinometry that indicates ''significant'' restriction, the range of results from normal subjects can be used to give an idea of the extremes of possible thresholds for patients. Using these, the results of airway testing can be compared with the data from history and physical examination to arrive at a diagnosis and treatment.

Because one of the aims of clinicians is to improve the patient's sense of well being, they wish to make the most accurate diagnosis so that they can choose the best therapy to accomplish this goal. Clinicians also should counsel the patient about the relative chance of success of various therapeutic interventions. Objective airway testing, by revealing when symptoms are caused by airway restriction, can play a role in accomplishing this.

Because the patient's description of symptoms is subjective (and at varying thresholds) and because clinicians' assessment of the airway with examination is subjective, an objective assessment of the airway can provide additional information that might change the diagnosis or course of action taken in a clinical setting.[11,12] To demonstrate this, a clinical algorithm (flowchart) for the evaluation of the patient with nasal obstruction is described.

Description of the algorithm for the evaluation of the patient with the symptom of nasal obstruction thought to be caused by airway restriction

In the flowchart (Fig. 42-15), the lines and boxes that represent alternative paths determined by airway testing results are shown. All of the conditions in Figure 42-15 are after decongestion.

Definition of terms used in the algorithm

Terms used in the description of the algorithm are as follows:

1. **Symptoms:** the patient's subjective description of the sensation of obstructed nasal breathing. The flowchart includes only patients who were symptomatic at least before decongestion. If a patient has no symptoms on the day of evaluation, the patient should be reevaluated when symptoms are present.
2. **Pathology:** the physician's subjective description of the findings from intranasal examination, which are thought to be the cause of the symptoms or which are significant enough that they would be expected to cause obstruction in some patients.
3. **Airway restriction:** the amount of decrease in the dimension of the airway found by objective airway testing, e.g., rhinomanometry or acoustic rhinometry.
4. **Decongestion:** application of a decongestant spray to the patient's nasal tissues, usually done with two applications for maximal effect, using either phenylephrine or oxymetazoline (in the United States). Decongestion can be accomplished using medication or physical exercise. Jessen and Malm[97] found xylometazoline spray more effective and convenient than exercise for decongestion of the nose. Jessen and others[98] found no advantage by using a bellows device to administer decongestant. They also found that the maximal decongestant effect occurred by 10 minutes after the spray was applied. Grymer and others[72] used 0.12% ephedrine followed by xylometazoline spray. The authors have found a few patients who experienced unexpected increased nasal airway resistance after decongestion with 1% phenylephrine. Naito and others[135] found that 10% of 86 patients had a slight increase in nasal resistance after decongestion. Williams and

Eccles[196] noted that some mucosal congestion might persist after decongestion, particularly if the patient has unsuspected acute rhinitis.

Following the branches of the algorithm

The process of clinical evaluation of the patient with nasal obstruction cannot be described without some simplifications. The use of a straightforward "yes/no" binary decision tree is desirable, but in reality, clinical judgment and decisions are based on the weighting of various factors by the clinician's "neural network." In the case of the evaluation of nasal obstruction, the weighted factors that are used for this discussion are the *subjective sensation* (symptoms) noted by the patient, the *subjective observation* (pathology) of the appearance of the internal and external nose by the clinician, and *the objective airway measurements* (airway restriction). In addition, these factors are considered before and after decongestion and sometimes with stenting of the alae. These factors do not have a single "present or absent" status but rather a gradation of presence whose relative weights at the nodes of a decision tree can lead to a particular diagnosis and treatment. For the sake of a workable description of this process, the factors (symptoms, pathology, and airway results) are considered in terms of their response to decongestion (same, less, cleared) and in terms of their relevant relationships to each other in degree of presence (greater than, equal to, less than).

Other less tangible factors besides symptoms, pathology, and airway test results also might play a role in the assessment of the patient, such as the physician's observation of the general medical condition, physical conditioning, and psychological disposition of the patient, and are included in the algorithm in the context of "other causes."

Explanation of the different paths in the flowchart

Diagnoses and treatments that are shown in the algorithm are referred to in the text by text within brackets, e.g., [MEDICAL].

Initial groupings—symptoms or pathology present or absent after decongestion

The top row in Figure 42-15 shows the groupings based on the persistence of symptoms or pathology after decongestion. These are symptoms and pathology present on the same side (Path 1), symptoms present without pathology (Path 2), pathology present without symptoms (Path 3), and no symptoms or pathology present (Path 4).

Symptoms that persisted could be unchanged or decreased but still present. If the symptoms cleared completely with decongestion, it is assumed that this is, at least in part, a result of a decrease in the thickness of the mucosa that was swollen because of disease or the nasal cycle.

If pathology is still present after decongestion, it is thought the pathology does not have a mucosal component—a "structural" problem (e.g., a septal deflection, sy-

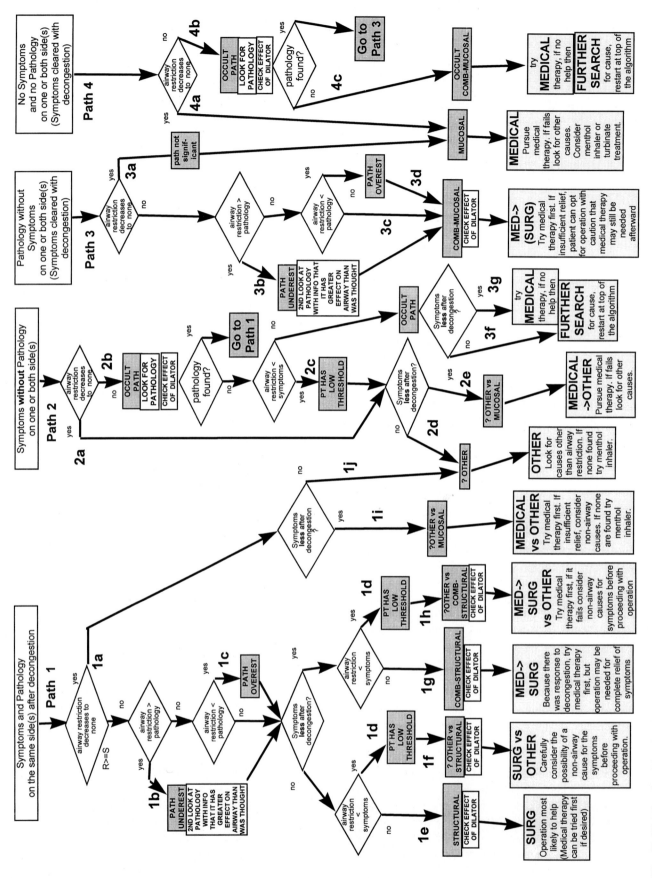

Fig. 42-15. The algorithm for the evaluation of nasal obstruction using the symptoms, pathology noted, and objective airway testing results to select diagnosis and therapy.

nechiae). For pathology to clear with decongestion, it must have been caused by mucosal swelling. Sometimes a deformity of the septum seems to disappear after decongestion. This could be either a result of septal turbinate tissue or an optical illusion. This happens when there is turbinate swelling on one side of the nose, and when the two sides of the nose are compared, it is concluded that the septum is deflected to the side of the narrowing. Then, after decongestion, the turbinate tissue has shrunk away from the septum, causing it to appear straight.

Different combinations of the conditions can be present on each side of the nose

There are a number of combinations of the presence or absence of symptoms or pathology for one or both sides of the nose. The algorithm deals only with sides of the nasal airway that have symptoms at least before decongestion. Different combinations of the conditions can be present for either side of the nose. In applying the algorithm, the clinician first considers each side of the nose. If the presence and degree of symptoms and pathology differ between the two sides of the nose, then different paths of the algorithm are followed for each side. The clinician then integrates the two results into the overall picture for that patient. The overall status of the nasal airway will lead to the predominant diagnosis and corresponding treatment.

Side of symptoms opposite side of pathology

There is one situation in which consideration of the individual sides of the nose does not adequately describe the situation. If the pathology is on the side opposite the symptoms, this raises a question about the significance of the pathology on the one side versus the symptoms on the other. With airway testing, if airway restriction is present on the side of the symptoms, this reveals that to be the side with the airway problem, and a second look is done for pathology on that side. If airway restriction is present on the side of the pathology, then symptoms the patient attributes to the opposite side could be a result of the phenomenon of paradoxical nasal obstruction.[4]

Possible diagnoses—the types of pathology that can cause the symptom of obstruction by restriction of the airway

What conditions are present that cause an airway to cross the threshold point at which the sensation of nasal obstruction occurs? The possible diagnoses used in the algorithm are shown at the end of each path in the algorithm (see Fig. 42-15) and will be described.

Structural problem [STRUCTURAL]

If symptoms and airway restriction are present and do not respond to decongestion (assuming that the patient is not someone who does not respond to decongestant spray), then the problem is considered *structural* (Paths 1e and 1f)

and unlikely to respond to medical therapy and more likely to be corrected by surgical therapy.

Combined-structural problem [COMBINED-STRUCTURAL]

If symptoms decrease with decongestion but some symptoms persist, a contribution to the problem from a structural problem and mucosal swelling is suggested. This type of combined problem is labeled *combined-structural* (Paths 1g and 1h). In the combined-structural problem, the addition of some mucosal swelling to an already present structural problem causes the symptoms to increase significantly in severity. In this case, the condition might be adequately relieved by management of the nasal mucosa with medical therapy, but the persistence of some symptoms even with decongestion suggests that if medical therapy is not an adequate solution for a given patient with this problem, then an operation might be warranted to modify the structure so that any mucosal congestion would be less likely to cause symptoms.

Combined-mucosal problem [COMBINED-MUCOSAL]

This is a combined structural and mucosal problem in which there is complete clearing of symptoms with decongestion but persistence of some airway restriction, signifying an underlying structural contribution. In the *combined-mucosal* problem (Paths 3b, 3c, 3d, and 4c), the addition of some mucosal swelling to an already present structural problem crosses the threshold for that patient, such that the symptom of nasal obstruction is present. In this case, the complete clearing of symptoms with decongestion suggests that the condition might be adequately relieved by management of the nasal mucosa with medical therapy. If medical therapy alone does not work for a given patient with this problem, then an operation might be warranted to modify the structure so that any mucosal congestion would be less likely to cause symptoms. There is a bit less certainty about the success of surgical intervention (particularly if it is for the structural part only) when the mucosal component is most significant.

Mucosal problem [MUCOSAL]

In this case, restriction is only caused by mucosal congestion (Paths 1i, 3a, and 4a), and symptoms are relieved by medicine or some other treatment of the nasal mucosa. There is no appreciable airway restriction after decongestion in a pure mucosal problem.

Other etiology [?OTHER]

When symptoms are present but no significant airway restriction is measured (Paths 1i, 1j, and 2a) or minimal airway restriction is measured (Paths 1f, 1h, and 2c), then it is suspected that the symptoms may result from a cause other than airway restriction. These may include atrophic rhinitis, inflammation, and other causes of altered nasal sensation, sinus disease, poor pulmonary function or cardiopulmonary insufficiency, or psychological effects.

Occult pathology [OCCULT PATH]

If no pathology had been noted, but significant airway restriction was measured, then the diagnosis *occult pathology* is suggested (Paths 2b and 4b). This elicits another examination of the airway to look for the cause of the restriction. This examination can include another visual examination of the intranasal appearance, and comparison of the relative opening of the airway (by patient symptom change or by airway resistance change) when the alae are held open. The alae can be held open (as described previously) with an internal or external dilator. The commonly available plastic strips that are applied to the external nose can be used for this purpose.

THE ALGORITHM SHOWS HOW OBJECTIVE TESTING CAN CHANGE THE DIAGNOSIS AND ACTION TAKEN

To arrive at a diagnosis and treatment, the relative degree of the symptoms, pathology, and airway restriction (from objective testing of the airway) are compared. In clinical assessment, nasal airway testing can verify that airway restriction resulting from observed pathology is causing symptoms, and it can help by modifying the diagnosis and management, and by modifying the expectations regarding success of management.

Objective testing can verify that symptoms are related to airway restriction

Airway testing can show the presence of airway restriction

If the results of airway testing match the patient's description of the symptoms in side and degree, it reaffirms the correctness of the diagnosis of the symptoms being caused by a restriction in the nasal airway. If the results of airway testing match the clinician's visual assessment of the airway in side and degree, it reaffirms the correctness of the diagnosis of the observed pathology causing the restriction. If airway testing results, symptoms, and pathology all match, it reinforces that the pathology is causing an airway restriction that is causing the symptoms, although such agreement does not change the course of action. It is lack of agreement that might change the action taken.

Airway testing can verify the effect of changes in the airway

Testing of the airway also can verify the effect of changes in the airway caused by either decongestion of the nasal tissues or stenting of the nasal alae. If symptoms and airway restriction are reduced by decongestion, then there is increased confidence in a diagnosis that is based on the symptoms being caused by a decrease in airflow through the nose. Further, there is increased confidence in the probability of success of therapy that will favorably modify the nasal air-

way. If the change in airway restriction is significantly more or less than the changes that occurred in the symptoms, then change in diagnosis or treatment might occur. This will be described because the algorithm is based in part on the relative endpoints of degree of symptoms and degree of airway restriction after any change resulting from decongestion.

Airway testing results can provide an objective verification of the effect of maneuvers that open the vestibule and valve area when such maneuvers decrease symptoms and a corresponding decrease in airway restriction occurs. This only changes the course of action when airway restriction persists (Paths 1e-1h and Paths 3b-3d) and the clinician wants to see how much any pathology in the compliant part of the valve region contributes to the nasal restriction, or when (Paths 2b and 4b) the measurement of an improved airway after dilation helps in the discovery of anterior pathology. The test using the dilator helps the surgeon to recognize the relative contribution of anterior pathology to the problem, which might affect the plan of action at the time of an operation by emphasizing an area to which the surgeon should pay particular attention. It also might show that the dilator could be an alternative therapeutic option.

When airway testing leads to a modification of the diagnosis and the action taken (treatment)

The selection of a diagnosis will lead to a corresponding option for treatment as shown on the flowchart (see Fig. 42-15). In the various paths of the algorithm, certain airway results can cause a change in the diagnosis and action taken (treatment).

For all paths in the algorithm—when no airway restriction is found even before decongestion

There is a potential change in diagnosis and treatment for all of the paths that can result from airway testing that is not shown on the algorithm. When airway testing reveals a widely patent, nonrestricted airway before and after decongestion, it is questionable whether any symptoms are related to nasal airway restriction and whether any pathology that was noted is causing airway impedance because no airway restriction was found. A widely patent airway measurement, even before decongestion, could change any pathway action to the action of looking for other causes [?OTHER].

The presence or absence of airway restriction after decongestion can modify the diagnosis and treatment

When symptoms are present but there is no airway restriction after decongestion (Paths 1a and 2a), the lack of any airway restriction leads one to suspect a cause for the obstruction other than airway restriction. If no pathology is noted but significant restriction is present (Paths 2b and 4b), then occult pathology is suggested. If pathology is noted but the symptoms had cleared with decongestion and no airway restriction is found (Path 3a), then the pathology may not be of significance.

In Path 1 for those patients in whom symptoms are the same after decongestion (Paths 1e and 1f versus Path 1j), the absence of airway restriction leads to a diagnosis of [OTHER] instead of [STRUCTURAL] or [?OTHER vs STRUCTURAL], changing the action taken from an operation being an option to looking for nonairway restriction causes for the symptoms with avoidance of an operation. If there is no restriction and other causes are not found, a menthol inhaler might be tried.

In Path 1 for those patients in whom symptoms are less after decongestion (Paths 1g and 1h versus Path 1i), the absence of airway restriction leads to a diagnosis of [OTHER vs MUCOSAL] instead of [COMBINED–STRUCTURAL] or [?OTHER vs COMBINED–STRUCTURAL], changing the action taken from an operation being an option if medical therapy failed to looking for nonairway restriction causes for the symptoms with avoidance of an operation if medical therapy failed. If there is no restriction and other causes are not found, a menthol inhaler might be tried.

In Path 2, no pathology is noted after decongestion. If airway restriction is absent (Path 2a), this corresponds with a lack of pathology, and the diagnosis is [?OTHER] or [?OTHER vs MUCOSAL], instead of the possibility of [OCCULT PATHOLOGY] and the consequent changes in treatment that would result if pathology was discovered. By contrast, if significant airway restriction is present and no pathology had been noted, a second look is done for pathology. If no pathology is seen, an external dilator is tried to see if it reveals pathology by causing improvement in the airway. If pathology is found, then Path 1 is followed because pathology and symptoms are now both present, and a change in diagnosis and treatment occurs because of the change to Path 1.

In Path 3, no symptoms are present after decongestion, and a corresponding lack of airway restriction (Path 3a) would correspond with this lack of restriction, leading to the conclusion that any pathology that was noted was not of significance. This would change the diagnosis from [COMBINED–MUCOSAL] to [MUCOSAL], resulting in a change in therapy from medical therapy with the cautious option of surgery (for the pathology that has possible significance because of the persistence of airway restriction) to medical therapy alone.

In Path 4, the lack of airway restriction after decongestion (Path 4a) would correspond with the absence of symptoms and pathology, and the diagnosis would be [MUCOSAL]. But if significant airway restriction is present, then one would look for [OCCULT PATHOLOGY] (Path 4b), and if it was found, the diagnosis and treatment would be changed as Path 3 was pursued. If pathology was not found, the difference in diagnosis with the presence or absence of airway restriction would be [OCCULT COMBINED–MUCOSAL] compared with [MUCOSAL], and the difference in action would change from looking for a combined–mucosal cause if medical therapy failed to medical therapy alone.

In the case of looking for a combined–mucosal cause, the persistence of significant restriction in a patient who had significant symptoms before decongestion suggests the possibility of unseen contributory pathology. An example would be prominence of bony turbinate structure, not initially noted, which could be addressed with an operation if medical therapy failed. Because no pathology had been noted (Path 4c) if medical therapy fails, the possibility of occult airway pathology causes one to restart the algorithm.

If airway restriction is present but is less in degree than the degree of the symptoms (low threshold)

In Path 1 if symptoms did not decrease with decongestion (Path 1e versus 1f), the presence of a low threshold (Path 1f) would introduce some uncertainty about whether the symptoms could be explained entirely by airway restriction, and so the diagnosis would change from [STRUCTURAL] to [?OTHER vs STRUCTURAL] and the course of action would change to a reconsideration of the possibility of other causes before proceeding with any operation.

In Path 1 if symptoms decreased with decongestion (Path 1g versus 1h), the presence of a low threshold (Path 1h) would introduce some uncertainty about whether the symptoms could be explained entirely by airway restriction, and so the diagnosis would change from [COMBINED–STRUCTURAL] to [?OTHER vs COMBINED–STRUCTURAL] and the course of action would change (if medical therapy failed) from proceeding with an operation to a reconsideration of the possibility of other causes before proceeding with any operation.

In Path 2 if no occult pathology was found and a low threshold is present (Path 2c), the diagnosis changes from the further possibility of unseen pathology [OCCULT PATH] to [?OTHER] or [?OTHER vs MUCOSAL], changing the action from further search for airway pathology to looking for nonairway (''other'') causes with a possible trial of medical treatment first if decongestion had improved the symptoms.

Airway testing can modify expectations regarding the success of treatment

The probability of success of treatment that modifies the nasal airway is related to the amount of certainty that the patient's symptoms are caused by pathology that is causing airway restriction. Because airway testing can objectively assess the amount of airway restriction, it can play a role in helping to determine the probability of success of treatment aimed at relief of airway restriction. This information is useful in treatment planning and in counseling the patient about therapeutic options. Overestimation and underestimation of pathology were described in a previous section.

Pathology underestimated

The persistence of airway restriction greater in degree than the pathology suggests that the pathology was underestimated (Paths 1b and 3b). When this occurs, there might be increased confidence that the pathology is significantly

80. Hasegawa M: Nasal cycle and postural variations in nasal resistance, *Ann Otol Rhinol Laryngol* 91:112, 1982.

81. Hasegawa M, Kern EB: Variations in nasal resistance in man: a rhinomanometric study of the nasal cycle in 50 human subjects, *Rhinology* 16:19, 1978.

82. Hasegawa M, Kern EB: Variations in nasal resistance (nasal cycle): does it influence the indications for surgery, *Facial Plastic Surg* 7:298, 1990.

83. Hasegawa M and others: Dynamic changes of nasal resistance, *Ann Otol Rhinol Laryngol* 88:66, 1979.

84. Havas TE and others: The effects of combined H_1 and H_2 histamine antagonists on alterations in nasal airflow resistance induced by topical histamine provocation, *J Allergy Clin Immunol* 78:856, 1986.

85. Heetderks DR: Observations on the reaction of normal nasal mucous membrane, *Am J Med Sci* 174:231, 1927.

86. Heinberg CE, Kern EB: The Cottle sign: an aid in the physical diagnosis of nasal airflow disturbances, *Rhinology* 11:89, 1973.

87. Hilberg O: Effect of terfenadine and budesonide on nasal symptoms, olfaction and nasal airway patency following allergen challenge, *Allergy* 50:683, 1995.

88. Hilberg O and others: Acoustic rhinometry: evaluation of nasal cavity geometry by acoustic reflection, *J Appl Physiol* 66:295, 1989.

89. Hirschberg A and others: The airflow resistance profile of healthy nasal cavities, *Rhinology* 33:10, 1995.

90. Hollinshead WH: *Anatomy for surgeons, vol 1, The head and neck*, ed 3, Philadelphia, 1982, Harper & Row.

91. Holmstrom M, Kumlien J: A clinical follow-up of septal surgery with special attention to the value of preoperative rhinomanometric examination in the decision concerning operation, *Clin Otolaryngol* 3:115, 1988.

92. Horak F and others: Effects of H1-receptor antagonists on nasal obstruction in atopic patients, *Allergy* 48:226, 1993.

93. Hoshino T and others: Statistical analysis of changes of pediatric nasal patency with growth, *Laryngoscope* 98:219, 1988.

94. Huygen PLM and others: Rhinomanometric detection rate of rhinoscopically-assessed septal deviation, *Rhinology* 30:177, 1992.

95. Ivarsson A, Malm L: Nasal airway resistance at different climate exposures: description of a climate aggregate and its use, *Am J Rhinol* 4:211, 1990.

96. Jalowayski AA and others: Surgery for nasal obstruction—evaluation by rhinomanometry, *Laryngoscope* 93:341, 1983.

97. Jessen M, Malm L: Use of pharmacologic decongestion in the generation of rhinomanometric norms for the nasal airway, *Am J Otolaryngol* 9:336, 1988.

98. Jessen M, Ivarsson A, Malm L: Nasal airway resistance after decongestion with a nasal spray or a bellows device, *Rhinology* 34:28, 1996.

99. Jones AS and others: The effect of aspirin on nasal resistance to airflow, *BMJ* 290:1171, 1985.

100. Jones AS and others: The effect of lignocaine on nasal resistance and nasal sensation of airflow, *Acta Otolaryngol* 101:328, 1986.

101. Jones AS and others: Nasal resistance to airflow (its measurement, reproducibility and normal parameters), *J Laryngol Otol* 101:800, 1987.

102. Jones AS and others: The effect of local anaesthesia of the nasal vestibule on nasal sensation of airflow and nasal resistance, *Clin Otolaryngol* 12:461, 1987.

103. Jones AS and others: Nasal airflow: resistance and sensation, *J Laryngol Otol* 103:909, 1989.

104. Juto JE, Lundberg C: An optical method for determining changes in mucosal congestion in the nose in man, *Acta Otolaryngol (Stockh)* 94:149, 1982.

105. Kasperbauer JL, Kern EB: Nasal valve physiology: implications in nasal surgery, *Otol Clin N Am* 20:699, 1987.

106. Keay D and others: The nasal cycle and clinical examination of the nose, *Clin Otolaryngol* 12:345, 1987.

107. Kenyon GS: Phase variation in nasal airways resistance assessed by active anterior rhinomanometry, *J Laryngol Otol* 101:910, 1987.

108. Kern EB: Standardization of rhinomanometry, *Rhinology* 15:115, 1977.

109. Kern EB: Surgical approaches to abnormalities of the nasal valve, *Rhinology* 16:165, 1978.

110. Kern EB: Committee report on standardization of rhinomanometry, *Rhinology* 19:231, 1981.

111. Kimmelman CP, Jablonski RD: The efficacy of turbinate surgery for the relief of nasal obstruction, *Am J Rhinol* 7:25, 1993.

112. Kosoy J: Nasal surgery and airway resistance, *Laryngoscope* 89:1655, 1979.

113. Kumlien J, Schiratzke H: Methodological aspects of rhinomanometry, *Rhinology* 17:107, 1979.

114. Lai VWS, Corey JP: The use of acoustic rhinometry to quantitatively assess changes after intranasal allergen challenge, *Am J Rhinol* 8:171, 1994.

115. Larsen K, Kristensen S: The peak flow nasal patency index, *ENT J* 71:23, 1992.

116. Lebowitz RA, Jacobs JB: Rhinomanometric and clinical evaluation of triamcinolone acetonide and beclomethasone diproprionate in rhinitis, *Am J Rhinol* 7:121, 1993.

117. Lenders H, Pirsig W: Diagnostic value of acoustic rhinometry: patients with allergic and vasomotor rhinitic compared with normal controls, *Rhinology* 28:5, 1990.

118. Lenders H, Schaefer J, Pirsig W: Turbinate hypertrophy in habitual snorers and patients with obstructive sleep apnea: findings of acoustic rhinometry, *Laryngoscope* 101:614, 1991.

119. Malm L: Rhinomanometric assessment for rhinologic surgery, *Ear Nose Throat J* 71:11, 1992.

120. Marais J and others: Minimal cross-sectional area, nasal peak flow and patients' satisfaction in septoplasty and inferior turbinectomy, *Rhinology* 32:145, 1994.

121. Maran AG and others: A method for the measurement of nasal airway resistance, *J Laryngol Otol* 85:803, 1971.

121a. Maranta CA, Scherrer JL, Simmen D: The mask: style and volume do not influence rhinomanometry, *Rhinology* 33:84, 1995.

122. Masing H: Rhinomanometry: different techniques and results, *Acta Otorhinolaryngol Belg* 33:566, 1979.

123. McCaffrey TV, Kern EB: Clinical evaluation of nasal obstruction, *Arch Otolaryngol* 105:542, 1979.

124. McCaffrey TV, Kern EB: Response of nasal airway resistance to hypercapnia and hypoxia in man, *Ann Otol Rhinol Laryngol* 88:247, 1979.

125. McLean JA and others: The effects of topical saline and isoproterenol on nasal airway resistance, *J Allergy Clin Immunol* 58:563, 1976.

126. Meltzer EO: Evaluating rhinitis: clinical, rhinomanometric, and cytologic assessments, *J Allergy Clin Immunol* 82:900, 1988.

127. Mertz JS and others: Objective evaluation of anterior septal surgical reconstruction, *Otolaryngol Head Neck Surg* 92:308, 1984.

128. Miljeteig H, and others: Snoring and nasal resistance during sleep, *Laryngoscope* 103:918, 1993.

129. Min YG, Jang YJ: Measurements of cross-sectional area of the nasal cavity by acoustic rhinometry and CT scanning, *Laryngoscope* 105:757, 1995.

130. Morgan NJ and others: Racial differences in nasal fossa dimensions determined by acoustic rhinometry, *Rhinology* 33:224, 1995.

131. Morris S, Jawad MSM, Eccles R: Relationships between vital capacity, height and nasal airway resistance in asymptomatic volunteers, *Rhinology* 30:259, 1992.

132. Naito K and others: Nasal resistance, sensation of obstruction and rhinoscopic findings compared, *Am J Rhinol* 2:65, 1988.

133. Naito K and others: Nasal patency: subjective and objective, *Am J Rhinol* 3:93, 1989.

134. Naito K and others: Computer averaged nasal resistance, *Rhinology* 27:45, 1989.

135. Naito K, Cole P, Humphrey D: Comparison of subjective and objective nasal patency before and after decongestion of the nasal mucosa, *Am J Rhinol* 5:113, 1991.

136. Naito K and others: New aerodynamic aspects of nasal patency, *Rhinology* 33:26, 1995.

137. Niinimaa V and others: Oronasal distribution of respiratory airflow, *Respir Physiol* 43:69, 1981.

138. Nofal F, Thomas M: Rhinomanometry evaluation of the effects of pre- and post-operative SMR on exercise, *J Laryngol Otol* 104:126, 1990.

139. Ohki M, Naito K, Cole PL: Dimensions and resistances of the human nose: racial differences, *Laryngoscope* 101:276, 1991.

140. Olsen KD, Kern EB, Westbrook PR: Sleep and breathing disturbance secondary to nasal obstruction, *Otolaryngol Head Neck Surg* 89:804, 1981.

141. O'Neill G, Tolley NS: Theoretical considerations of nasal airflow mechanics and surgical implications, *Clin Otolaryngol* 13:273, 1988.

142. Pallanch JF: Nasal resistance: a comparison of the methods used for obtaining normal values and a comparison of proposed models of the transnasal pressure-flow curves, thesis, University of Minnesota, Rochester, Minn, 1984, Mayo Graduate School of Medicine.

143. Pallanch JF: Statistical distribution of nasal airway data in the evaluation of nasal surgery patients, *Facial Plastic Surg* 7:283, 1990.

144. Pallanch JF: Comparison of the relative strength of correlation of various rhinomanometric parameters with the symptom of nasal obstruction, thesis, St Louis, 1995, Triologic Society.

145. Pallanch JF and others: Normal nasal resistance, *Otolaryngol Head Neck Surg* 93:778, 1985.

146. Pallanch JF, McCaffrey, Kern EB: Clinical application of computerized rhinomanometry, *Rhinology Suppl* 14:91, 1992.

147. Palma P, Papalexiou A, Sulsenti G: Nasal resistance in healthy subjects. Presentation at Plenary Session on Rhinomanometry, 13th Congress European Rhinologic Society, London, June 1990.

148. Parker LP and others: Rhinomanometry in children, *Int J Pediatr Otorhinolaryngol* 17:127, 1989.

149. Parker AJ and others: A comparison of active anterior rhinomanometry and nasometry in the objective assessment of nasal obstruction, *Rhinology* 28:47, 1990.

150. Pastorello EA and others: Comparison of rhinomanometry, symptom score, and inflammatory cell counts in assessing the nasal late-phase reaction to allergen challenge, *J Allergy Clin Immunol* 93:85, 1994.

151. Petruson B: Increased nasal breathing decreases snoring and improves oxygen saturation during sleep apnoea, *Rhinology* 32:87, 1994.

152. Petruson B, Theman K: Clinical evaluation of the nasal dilator Nozovent. The effect on snoring and dryness of the mouth, *Rhinology* 30:283, 1992.

153. Porter M and others: Manometric rhinometry: a new method of measuring nasal volume, *Rhinology* 33:86, 1995.

154. Postema CA and others: The lateralization percentages as a measure of nasal flow asymmetry in active anterior rhinomanometry, *Clin Otolaryngol* 5:165, 1980.

155. Prescott CA, Prescott KE: Peak nasal inspiratory flow measurement: and investigation in children, *Int J Pediatr Otorhinolaryngol* 32:137, 1995.

156. Principato JJ, Wolf P: Pediatric nasal resistance, *Laryngoscope* 95:1067, 1985.

157. Reeves HM and others: Quantitative measurement of nasal-airway resistance, *Arch Otolaryngol* 92:573, 1970.

158. Rivron RP: Cross-sectional area as a measure of nasal resistance, *Rhinology* 28:257, 1990.

159. Rivron RP, Sanderson RJ: The voluntary control of nasal airway resistance, *Rhinology* 29:181, 1991.

160. Roithmann R and others: Acoustic rhinometry in the evaluation of nasal obstruction, *Laryngoscope* 105:275, 1995.

161. Roth and others: A head and tube stabilizing apparatus for acoustic rhinometry measurements, *Am J Rhinol* 10:83, 1996.

162. Saito A, Nishihata S: Nasal airway resistance in children, *Rhinology* 19:149, 1981.

163. Sandham A: Rhinomanometric method error in the assessment of nasal respiratory resistance, *Rhinology* 26:191, 1988.

164. Santiago J and others: The nasal valve: a rhinomanometric evaluation of maximum nasal inspiratory flow and pressure curves, *Ann Otol Rhinol Laryngol* 95:229, 1986.

165. Scadding GK and others: Clinical and physiological effects of fluticasone propionate aqueous nasal spray in the treatment of perennial rhinitis, *Rhinology Suppl* 11:37, 1991.

166. Scadding GK, Darby YC, Austin CE: Acoustic rhinometry compared with anterior rhinomanometry in the assessment of the response to nasal allergen challenge, *Clin Otolaryngol* 19:451, 1994.

167. Scharf M, Brannen D, McDannold M: A subjective evaluation of a nasal dilator on sleep and snoring, *ENT J* 73:395, 1994.

168. Schumacher MJ: Advances in tests for the evaluation of rhinitis, *Immunol Allergy Clin North Am* 7:15, 1987.

169. Schumacher MJ: Rhinomanometry, *J Allergy Clin Immunol* 83:711, 1989.

170. Schumacher MJ, Pain MCF: Nasal-challenge testing in grass-pollen hay fever, *J Allergy Clin Immunol* 64:202, 1979.

171. Schumacher MJ and others: Computer-aided rhinometry: analysis of inspiratory and expiratory nasal pressure-flow curves in subjects with rhinitis, *Comput Biol Med* 15:187, 1985.

172. Shelton DM and others: Comparison of oscillation with three other methods for measuring nasal airways resistance, *Respir Med* 84:101, 1990.

173. Shreck S and others: Correlations between flow resistance and geometry in a model of the human nose, *J Applied Physiol* 75:1767, 1993.

174. Sipila JI and others: Rhinomanometry before septoplasty: an approach to clinical material with diverse nasal symptoms, *Am J Rhinol* 6:17, 1992.

175. Sipila J, Suonpaa J, Laippala P: Sensation of nasal obstruction compared to rhinomanometric results in patients referred for septoplasty, *Rhinology* 32:141, 1994.

176. Sipila J and others: Correlations between subjective sensation of nasal patency and rhinomanometry in both unilateral and total nasal assessment, *ORL* 57:260, 1995.

177. Solow B, Greve E: Rhinomanometric recording in children, *Rhinology* 18:31, 1980.

178. Strohl KP and others: Alae nasi activation and nasal resistance in healthy subjects, *J Appl Physiol* 52:1432, 1982.

179. Sulsenti G, Palma P: Nasal valve surgery through hemitransfixion incision: functional results assessed by rhinomanometry, *Facial Plastic Surg* 7(4):315.

180. Suonpaa JT, Sipila JI, Laippala PJ: Do rhinomanometric findings predict subjective postoperative satisfaction? Long-term follow-up after septoplasty, *Am J Rhinol* 7:71, 1993.

181. Szucs E, Kaufman L, Clement PA: Nasal resistance—a reliable assessment of nasal patency? *Clin Otolaryngol* 20:390, 1995.

182. Taylor G, MacNeil AR, Freed DLJ: Assessing degree of nasal patency by measuring peak expiratory flow rate throughout the nose, *J Allergy Clin Immunol* 52:193, 1973.

183. Tomkinson A: The reliability of acoustic rhinometry, *J Laryngol Otol* 109:1234, 1995 (letter).

184. Tomkinson A, Eccles R: Errors arising in cross-sectional area estimation by acoustic rhinometry produced by breathing during measurement, *Rhinology* 33:138, 1995.

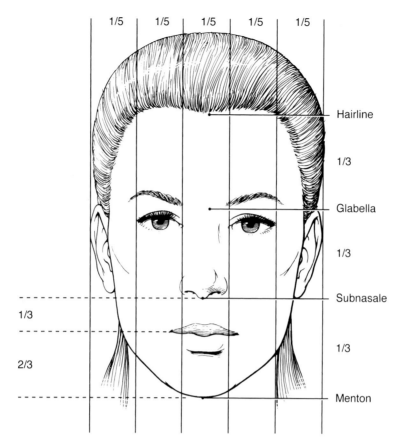

Fig. 43-1. The facial thirds and fifths.

hump. The supratip is a point just cephalic to the nasal dome. The tip-defining point is the anteriormost projection of the nose. The columellar point is the anteriormost projection of the columella. The mucocutaneous junction of the upper and lower lips are the superior and inferior vermilion borders, respectively. The labrale superius and inferius represent the anteriormost projections of the upper and lower lips, respectively. The mentolabial sulcus is the posteriormost point between the lower lip and chin. The pogonion is the anteriormost projection of the chin, and the menton is the inferiormost projection of the chin. The cervical point is the junction of the tangents to the neck and the submental area, whereas the gnathion is the intercept of the subnasale to pogonion line with the cervical point to menton line. The tragion is the point at the supratragal notch. The Frankfort horizontal plane is determined by the tragion to infraorbital rim line.

METHODS OF FACIAL ANALYSIS

Patient examination

Complete regional examination of the head and neck is the foundation of facial analysis. This encounter is usually the only time the physician can analyze the dynamics of the face with expression. Close examination will provide much information, including an estimate of skin thickness and elasticity, the amount of facial musculature used in expression, nasal tip and alar support, palpable hard-tissue abnormalities, and evidence of hypertrophic scars or keloids. The physical examination should not be shortened when a patient presents for aesthetic surgery; rather, the examination should be comprehensive and directed because a patient with vertigo is examined differently, although no less completely, than a patient with laryngeal cancer.

Photography

At a preoperative visit, the surgeon should take photographs in standard views. Each operative procedure demands a specific set of photographic views.[25] For nasal surgery, the standard views include frontal, both laterals, both obliques, basal, and lateral smiling views. Lateral views should be oriented with the Frankfort plane parallel to true horizontal. The film, lighting, magnification, and background should be consistent so that preoperative and postoperative photographs are comparable. Before the operation, the surgeon should examine and discuss the photographs with the patient and mentally plan the surgery. At this time, lines, angles, and ratios can be drawn and examined if desired.

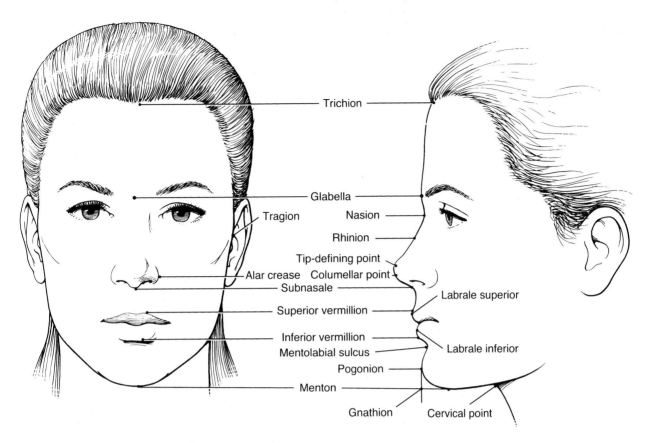

Fig. 43-2. Landmarks for facial analysis.

Computer imaging

Multiple authors have designed computer analysis systems for use with data points obtained from photographs or patients,[5,11,27] yet these systems are cumbersome and are not widely used in clinical practice. Recently developed computer-imaging systems that allow the surgeon to alter the patient's image on the screen have proven useful.[16,20] Imagers use video or digital camera images that are displayed on a monitor. The image is then altered using various software packages (Fig. 43-3). Some computer-imaging systems also can provide a slide or photographic image from the altered image. The digitized images can be stored on a video drive as a cataloging system.

The advantages of computer imaging are that it gives the patient a realistic view of anticipated postoperative results, the image facilitates better patient-physician communication on the desired outcome, and ancillary procedures that may enhance the postoperative result can be visualized, so that the patient can judge their impact before the actual operation.[20] One of the best examples of this last type of interaction is the rhinoplasty patient who also may benefit from chin augmentation. Surgeons can experiment with different surgical options and further develop the aesthetic goals and the surgical plan.[16]

Some disadvantages of computer imaging include over-zealous or idealized image alteration that shows a result that is unobtainable. There is potential legal risk in showing the patient an altered idealized image as an implied guarantee of the surgical result. The surgeon should be conservative in the imaging session so as not to give the patient unrealistic expectations. Some surgeons have the patient sign a legal disclaimer to avoid legal action or implied guarantee of a postoperative result.[4,20] During imaging, the surgeon should emphasize that the true result depends on the patient's healing characteristics and cannot be entirely predicted. Finally, the cost of the imaging system and the imaging session is another disadvantage.

Other methods of facial analysis

Hard-tissue cephalometric analysis has been used for facial plastic surgery. Its clinical application is useful to oral surgeons and orthodontists but is limited in the field of otorhinolaryngology.

FACIAL ANALYSIS

General considerations

The spectrum of variations in the face are enormous. Obvious variations secondary to gender, race, and overall facial symmetry should be considered. Harmony of the various facial features is important in planning any changes. The

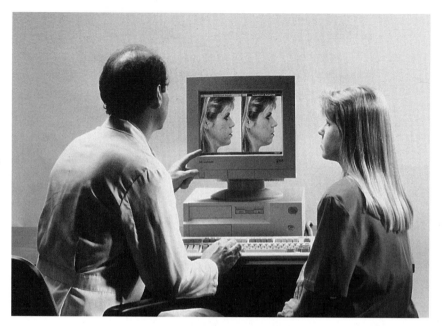

Fig. 43-3. A computer imaging session with the doctor, patient, and imaging system.

overall facial harmony and sexual identity should be preserved with any surgical intervention. Facial asymmetries should be pointed out before surgical intervention so that the patient understands that they were not caused by the surgical procedure. Some asymmetries cannot be corrected surgically.

The patient's skin type should be evaluated and analyzed. Patients with fine, light skin with a paucity of underlying subcutaneous tissue tend to show even minor subcutaneous or hard-tissue irregularities. Every minor contour abnormality demands fastidious attention during the operation. However, patients with thick, oily, sebaceous skin tend to heal with more perceptible scars, but the skin thickness hides major underlying structural changes. Somewhere between these two skin types lies the ideal skin type for aesthetic procedures.

The aging process, especially of the facial skin, is variable and should be taken into account. Skin aging depends on various intrinsic and extrinsic influences, including genetics, sun exposure, smoking history, radiation exposure, and the level of use of the facial musculature. Aging results in a progressive decrease in the thickness and elasticity of the skin. Heavy wrinkles or rhytids form at ligamentous retaining points and occur at areas of repeated facial musculature activity. Standard structural changes of the face occur as a person ages. The skull becomes thinner and smaller with resultant increased laxity in the overlying skin and soft-tissue envelope. Beginning at age 20 to 25, the eyebrows slowly and steadily descend from a position above the supraorbital rim.[3,8] Brow descent or ptosis, combined with excess skin of the upper eyelids (dermatochalasis) and weakening of the underlying orbital septum, results in the typical appearance of the aging eye. The weakened orbital septum and excess skin laxity of the lower lids allows herniation of orbital fat and results in palpebral "bags."

The cartilaginous skeleton of the nasal tip weakens and broadens, causing tip ptosis, lengthening of the nose, and occasionally increasing airway obstruction. With progressively increasing skin laxity, resorption of subcutaneous fat, and resorption of alveolar bone, a relative excess of the skin and soft-tissue envelope of the lower face and the temporal region develops. These events lead to descent of the chin pad, loss of delineation between the jawline and the neck, and a characteristic jowled "turkey gobbler" neck. As aging progresses, the hyoid bone and larynx descend, making the middle and lower neck appear more prominent.[8] The anterior edges of the platysma muscles lose tone and separate, creating the anterior banding characteristic of the aging neck. Submental fat may prolapse between these bands, resulting in further loss of the cervicomental angle.[10] Some patients develop a relative underprojection of the chin or the malar eminences secondary to redistribution of the overlying skin, subcutaneous fat, and the underlying buccal fat pad. The descent of the neck mass and progressive absorption of the buccal fat pad and subcutaneous fat result in an increase in melolabial fold definition and obvious hollowing in the infraorbital region.[8] Perioral hard tissues also resorb, especially in the edentulous patient, causing a relative excess of the skin and soft-tissue envelope.

Once all of the general considerations have been taken into account, site-specific examination can proceed. A useful technique in considering the face is to divide the head and neck into aesthetic units (Fig. 43-4).[12] The nose, lips, cheeks, and ears can be considered separately. The forehead and eyes complex and the chin and neck complex are best considered as paired units because each of these two groups of

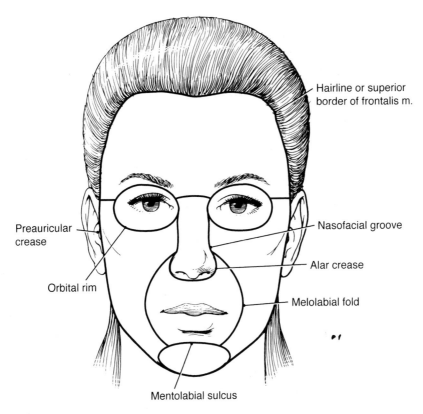

Fig. 43-4. The aesthetic units of the face.

structures are especially intimately related in the overall facial aesthetics.

Forehead and eyes

The forehead is bordered by the hairline superiorly, the nasion and the supraorbital rims inferiorly, and the superior aspect of the zygomatic arch laterally. The shape of the forehead can be sloped, flat, or curved.[18] In women, a convex shape is optimal, whereas in men, a slight amount of supraorbital bossing is desirable. The eyebrows ideally rest just above the supraorbital rim in women, with a peak in the arch between the lateral limbus and lateral canthus of the eye (Fig. 43-5). In men, the brow should be relatively straight and rest at or slightly below the supraorbital rim. The medial and lateral extent of the brow rests on the horizontal. The medial extent of the brow is to a vertical line from the medial canthus. The lateral extent of the brow is medial to a line from the inferior alar crease through the lateral canthus.[18]

The width of each eye is equal to the interchantal distance (about 30 to 35 mm). Ideally, the lateral canthus is about 2 to 4 mm higher than the medial canthus in women, whereas the two points are in a more horizontal plane in men. The supratarsal crease lies 7 to 10 mm from the inferior border of the upper lid margin, and the inferior border of the upper lid overhangs the superior border of the iris by 2 to 3 mm.[9] The peak of the upper lid lies just medial to the pupil. The lower lid ideally sits at or 1 mm above the lower border of

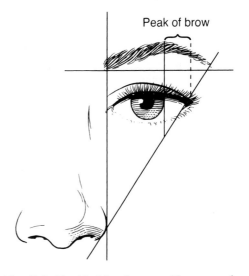

Fig. 43-5. The ideal female eye and brow complex.

the iris. Up to 10% of the healthy population have scleral show (sclera visible between the lower lid border and the lower border of the iris) unrelated to lower lid laxity.[13] This is usually secondary to relative hypoplasia of the inferior orbital rim and maxilla, resulting in poor lower lid support.

Surgical interventions to alter the forehead are usually directed at correcting the ptotic brow, glabellar frown lines, and horizontal forehead rhytids. The position of the hairline is important in planning a forehead-lift. In the female patient with a high frontal hairline, consideration should be given to a pretrichial incision. In women with a low hairline, the endoscopic or coronal brow-lift are used. Men with male pattern baldness can undergo an endoscopic brow-lift, or a midforehead brow-lift if they have deep horizontal forehead creases. Brow asymmetry secondary to facial paralysis is best managed with a midforehead brow-lift or direct brow-lift.[21] Dermatochalasis and fat herniation are managed with blepharoplasty. Senile ptosis, entropion, ectropion, and excessive lower lid laxity should be identified preoperatively and corrected at the time of blepharoplasty. If the lower lid pulls 6 mm or further from the globe on the lid distraction test or does not snap back to the globe immediately after the snap test, then lower lid shortening should be considered at the time of blepharoplasty to prevent ectropion (Fig. 43-6).

Nose

The nose is the key to facial aesthetics because of its central position in frontal view and its prominence in profile view. Minor asymmetrics and variations are more conspicuous. Multiple angles and measurements describe the nose's width, length, projection, and rotation. In general, the nasal dorsum follows a smooth curve downward from the medial aspect of the brows and straight to the supratip region (Fig. 43-7). The widest point of the nose is the alar base, which is about one intercanthal width. In profile, the dorsum should be straight, although a slight elevation at the nasal bones is acceptable (Fig. 43-8). The tip should show a double break, and 2 to 4 mm of columellar show is ideal. In the base view, the nose approximates an equilateral triangle with a columella to lobule height ratio of 2:1 (Fig. 43-9). The ideal tip width is 70% to 75% of the entire base width.[18]

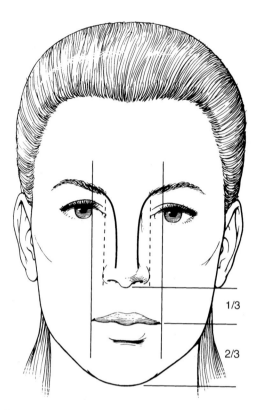

Fig. 43-7. Frontal view of the nasal dorsum with measurements of the alar base and the oral commissure.

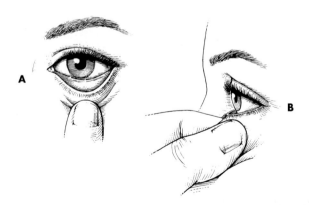

Fig. 43-6. A, In the snap test, the lower lid should immediately snap back to the globe on release. Mild laxity is shown if the lid returns slowly, and moderate or severe laxity is shown if the lower lid returns only after a blink or should be pushed back to position against the globe. **B,** The lower lid distraction test should allow the lower lid to pull less than 6 mm from the globe. Any greater distraction indicates lower lid laxity.

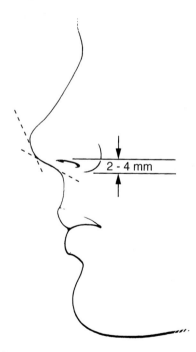

Fig. 43-8. Lateral view of the ideal nose. Note the double break (*dotted lines*) in the tip and 2 to 4 mm of columella.

Several angles are important in assessing the nose. The nasofrontal angle is measured with the lines formed from the nasion to the glabella and from the nasion to the supratip (Fig. 43-10). The ideal nasofrontal angle is 115° to 130°. The illusion of nasal shortening is produced by deepening the angle, whereas the illusion of nasal lengthening is produced by making the angle more shallow.[18] The nasofacial angle is measured by drawing a vertical line tangent to the glabella and pogonion and drawing a line along the dorsum (Fig. 43-11). The ideal nasofacial angle is 36°, and a range of 30° to 40° is acceptable. This angle measures nasal tip projection.[12] Tip projection is defined as how far the tip-defining point extends from the ala. Multiple measurements of tip projection have been described, although the description by Goode is most simple to apply.[18] Goode's method is to draw a line from the nasion to the posteriormost aspect of the ala. A perpendicular line is then drawn from this to the tip-defining point. The ratio of length (the nasion to the ala) to projection (the vertical line to the tip-defining point) that is most ideal is 0.55 to 0.60, which corresponds to a nasofacial angle of about 36°. When a hump is present, it should be transected by the dorsal line.[1] Men can tolerate slightly greater tip projection than women can.

The nasolabial angle is the major measure of tip rotation (Fig. 43-12). This angle is measured by a line from the subnasale to the superior vermilion and by a tangent of the columella from the subnasale. The ideal range of the nasolabial angle is 90° to 100° in men and 100° to 110° in women. Shorter people can tolerate greater tip rotation than taller people. The nasolabial angle may be blunted by an enlarged nasal spine. Also important to measurement of the nasolabial angle is the position of the dentition, the maxilla and the mandible, and the lips. Significant abnormalities in these areas should be addressed before or at the time of rhinoplasty.

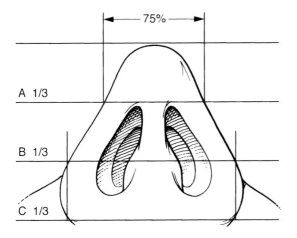

Fig. 43-9. Base view of the nose shows the ideal columella to lobule height ratio and the ideal tip to base ratio.

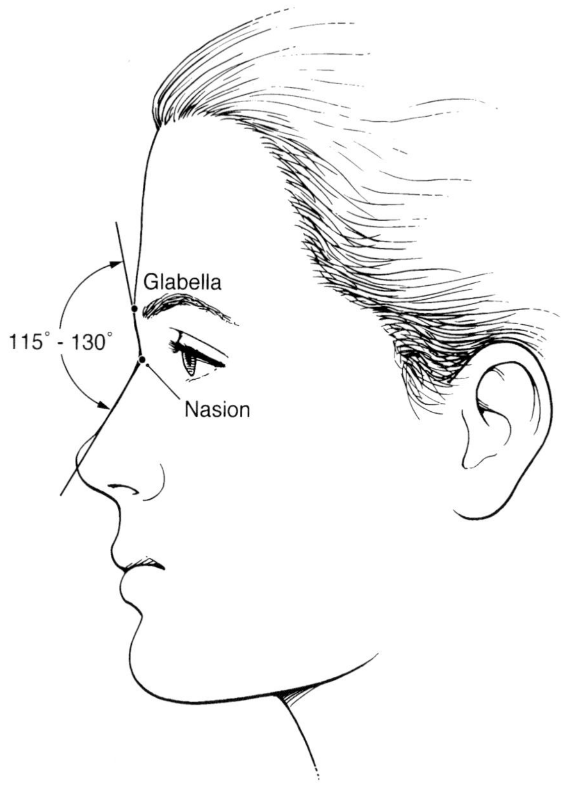

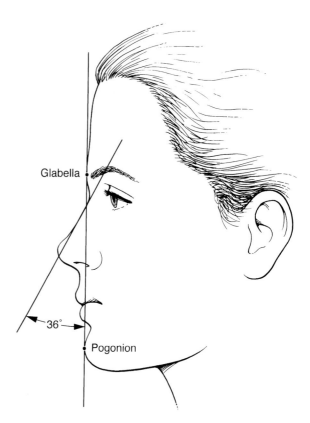

Fig. 43-10. The nasofrontal angle.

Fig. 43-11. The nasofacial angle.

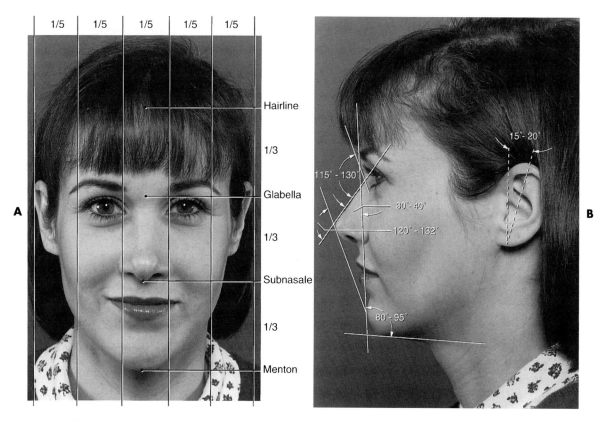

Fig. 43-16. A, The frontal view of a female shows some of the highlights of facial analysis and proportions. **B,** Facial analysis on the lateral view.

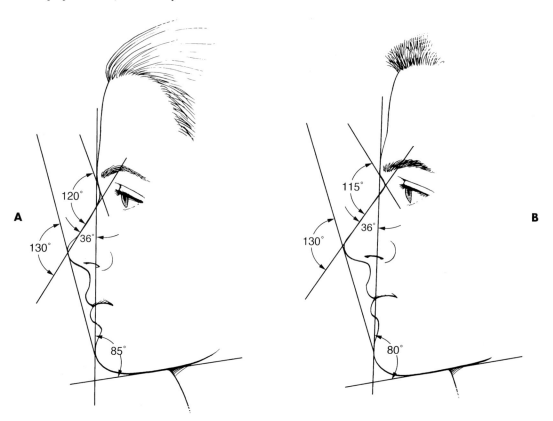

Fig. 43-17. The ideal aesthetic triangle of Powell and Humphries for **A,** a female and **B,** a male.

mental angle is 120° to 132°. Analyzing each of the angles and lines of the aesthetic triangle separately and together allows better understanding of the interplay between the forehead, nose, lips, chin, and neck in the profile view.

CONCLUSIONS

Critical review and analysis of preoperative and postoperative photographs will provide the surgeon with invaluable information and help to refine the inherent aesthetic sense necessary for success in facial plastic surgery. Computerized facial analysis systems facilitate the analysis process and improve patient-physician communication. As the cost of the computer systems and digital photography systems decrease, their use will be more widespread in facial plastic surgery. One day these computerized systems will represent the standard for facial analysis, and they will replace the need for slide or photographic documentation in a hard copy format.

ACKNOWLEDGMENT

The authors thank John Hagen for the hand-drawn illustrations, Jim Tidwell for the computer-drawn illustrations, and Randy Fravert for manuscript preparation.

REFERENCES

1. Aufricht G: Rhinoplasty and the face, *Plast Reconstr Surg* 43:219, 1969.
2. Dedo DD: A preoperative classification of the neck for cervicofacial rhytidectomy, *Laryngoscope* 90:1984, 1990.
3. Gonzales-Ulloa M, Florez ES: Senility of the face: basic study to understand its cause and affects, *Plast Reconstr Surg* 36:239, 1965.
4. Gorney M: Preoperative computerized video imaging, *Plast Reconstr Surg* 78:268, 1986.
5. Hilger PA and others: A computerized nasal analysis system, *Arch Otolaryngol Head Neck Surg* 109:653, 1983.
6. Hinderer UT: Malar implant for improvement of the facial appearance, *Plast Reconstr Surg* 56:157, 1975.
7. Larrabee WF: Facial analysis for rhinoplasty, *Otolaryngol Clin North Am* 20:653, 1987.
8. Larrabee WF, Caro I: The aging face, *Postgrad Med* 74:37, 1984.
9. Larrabee WF, Makielski KH: *Surgical anatomy of the face*, New York, 1993, Raven Press.
10. Larrabee WF, Makielski KH, Cupp C: Facelift anatomy, *Facial Plast Surg Clin North Am* 1:135, 1993.
11. Larrabee WF, Maupin G, Sutton D: Profile analysis in facial plastic surgery, *Arch Otolaryngol Head Neck Surg* 111:682, 1985.
12. Larrabee WF, Sherris DA: *Principles of facial reconstruction*, New York, 1995, Lippincott-Raven.
13. Mackinnon SE and others: The incidence and degree of scleral show in the normal population, *Plast Reconstr Surg* 80:15, 1987.
14. Martin JG: Racial ethnocentrism and judgement of beauty, *J Soc Psychol* 63:59, 1964.
15. Millard DR: Adjuncts in the augmentation mentoplasty and corrective rhinoplasty, *Plast Reconstr Surg* 36:48, 1965.
16. Papel ID, Parks RI: Computer imaging for instruction in facial plastic surgery in a residency program, *Arch Otolaryngol Head Neck Surg* 114:1454, 1988.
17. Peck H, Peck S: A concept of facial aesthetics, *Angle Orthod* 40:284, 1970.
18. Powell N, Humphries B: *Proportions of the aesthetic face*, New York, 1984, Thieme-Stratton.
19. Quatela VC, Cheney ML: *Reconstruction of the auricle*. In Baker SR, Swanson NA, editors: *Local flaps in facial reconstruction*, St Louis, 1995, Mosby.
20. Schroenrock LD: Five year facial plastic experience with computer imaging, *Facial Plast Surg* 7:18, 1990.
21. Sherris DA, Larrabee WF: Anatomic consideration in rhytidectomy, *Facial Plast Surg* 12, 1996.
22. Sherris DA, Larrabee WF: Expanded polytetrafluoroethylene augmentation of the lower face, *Laryngoscope* 106:658, 1996.
23. Simons RL: Adjunctive measures in rhinoplasty, *Otolaryngol Clinic North Am* 8:717, 1975.
24. Simons RL, Lawson W: Chin reduction in profileplasty, *Arch Otolaryngol Head Neck Surg* 101:207, 1975.
25. Tardy ME: *Principles of photography in facial plastic surgery*, New York, 1992, Thieme-Stratton.
26. Tolleth H: Concepts for the plastic surgeon from art and sculpture, *Clin Plast Surg* 14:585, 1987.
27. Toriumi DM, Maupin G, Larrabee WF: *Computerized three dimensional facial analysis*. In Strucker FJ, editor: *Plastic and reconstructive surgery of the head and neck*. Proceedings of the Fifth International Symposium, Philadelphia, 1991, Mosby.

Chapter 44

Manifestations of Systemic Diseases of the Nose

Thomas J. McDonald

The incidence of systemic diseases affecting the upper airway appears to be increasing, but in fact it is not. The diagnosis is being made earlier and more easily. The reasons for this are the heightened index of suspicion for these diseases on the part of otolaryngologist, earlier dialogue between colleagues, technologic advances such as the use of endoscopy in the outpatient setting when patients are first being seen, perinuclear antineutrophilic cytoplasmic antibody (p-ANCA) and cytoplasmic antineutrophilic cytoplasmic antibody (c-ANCA) testing, and, of course, the important use of an early biopsy.

Other advances include improved methods of staining and culturing of biopsy materials, as well as more accurate morphologic examination of the tissue. Finally, these diseases are being managed better due to early interaction with colleagues in other specialties such as pulmonary medicine, nephrology, and rheumatology.

This chapter describes three categories of diseases: (1) granulomatous diseases, including Wegener's granulomatosis and sarcoidosis; (2) infectious diseases, including tuberculosis, typical and atypical, and fungal diseases; and (3) lymphomas, specifically T-cell lymphoma.

GRANULOMATOUS DISEASES

Wegener's granulomatosis

Wegener's granulomatosis (WG) is now considered a relatively common disease of the upper airway. There was a tendency for it to be overlooked in the past, but now its detection is much earlier and management is much better. It is appropriately named for Friedrich Wegener, who in 1939 first described necrotizing granulomas and vasculitis of the upper and lower respiratory tract, occurring either together or as separate components.[22] It should be classified not only as a granulomatous disease but also viewed as a vasculitis and an autoimmune disease.

Formerly several diseases (e.g., WG, lymphomas, carcinomas, and destructive infectious disorders such as fungal infections and tuberculosis) were often called lethal midline granuloma. This is a clinical term and should be abandoned because now these diseases are known to be individual entities separable clinically, morphologically, and with diagnostic studies. Specific identification is vital because the management strategies are different for each disorder.

Clinical aspects of Wegener's granulomatosis

There are three main forms of WG: types 1, 2, and 3.[15] Type 1 is the limited form of WG. Typically, the patients present with symptoms of an upper respiratory tract infection persisting for several weeks, which is unresponsive to antibiotics and associated with serosanguineous nasal drainage and pain. The pain is especially severe over the dorsum of the nose. Of particular note is the expression of very large nasal crusts in both sides of the nose. There is no disease other than WG with such severe crusting.

Some patients with the limited form have systemic vasculitis characterized by night sweats, migratory arthralgias, generalized weakness, and moderately profound malaise. Nasal examination shows diffuse crusting of the nose and nasopharynx bilaterally. When the crusts are removed the mucosa is very friable. Septal perforations are less common as the disease is diagnosed earlier. Flexible or rigid endoscopic examination is invaluable in determining the extent of the intranasal lesions.

Type 2 indicates a sicker patient with more systemic symptoms. Nasal involvement is similar to the patient with type 1 disease, but other organs are involved. Pulmonary involvement is typified by hemoptysis and the finding of cavitating lesions on chest radiographs.

Type 3 is widely disseminated with involvement of multiple organs including airway, pulmonary, renal, and sometimes cutaneous lesions. Cutaneous involvement is typified by tick-bite–like lesions of the lower limbs. Some patients have moderate-sized cutaneous ulcerations over the back or chest. Renal involvement in the early stage is typified by hematuria and abnormal urinary sediment leading to progressive renal failure.

Wegener's granulomatosis involvement of other head and neck sites

Orbital involvement occurs either alone or in conjunction with nasal involvement. Nasolacrimal duct obstruction due to ethmoid and nasal disease, nonspecific episcleritis bilaterally, and bilateral or unilateral proptosis due to extension of disease into the orbit or pseudotumor of the orbit itself are common forms of orbital involvement.[3,11] Otologic involvement including unilateral or bilateral serous otitis media, with or without mastoiditis, occurs. This can occur alone or in conjunction with fairly profound unilateral or bilateral sensorineural hearing loss. Oropharyngeal involvement is not common, but when present, is characterized by diffuse upper and lower gingival lesions and diffuse minor salivary gland involvement accompanied by ulcerations throughout the oral cavity.

Subglottic involvement with or without nasal involvement

Subglottic involvement with or without nasal involvement is very common in WG, occurring in about one fifth of the author's Mayo Clinic experience with 500 patients. It is a capricious form of involvement because patients may present to the otolaryngologist with symptoms of asthma but normal flow volume studies. The finding of a very short segment of upper tracheal stenosis on endoscopy may suggest the diagnosis of WG.[5,10]

Diagnosis of Wegener's granulomatosis

The typical history and characteristic findings on clinical evaluation and endoscopy, as well as the presence of mild to moderate anemia associated with an elevated erythrocyte sedimentation rate are all suggestive of the clinical diagnosis of WG. An abnormal urinary sediment with elevated serum creatinine levels reflect early or advanced renal involvement. Cavitating lesions on pulmonary roentgenograms indicate pulmonary involvement. The importance of a careful biopsy cannot be overstressed. Preferably performed under topical anesthesia with intravenous sedation, the nasal crusts are removed and up to seven or eight pieces of tissue removed

from all turbinates. This tissue is sent for stains and culture, including those for acid-fast and fungal organisms.

Antineutrophilic cytoplasmic antibody

The discovery of ANCA has prompted research activity that has enhanced our understanding of the pathogenetic mechanisms of WG, microscopic polyangiitis, and related small vessel vasculitides.[18] The detection of ANCA is based on indirect immunofluorescent findings. With this method, the crucial distinction is made between coarse granular, c-ANCA and p-ANCA staining on ethanol-fixed neutrophil cytocentrifuge preparations. The characteristic c-ANCA pattern (formerly termed *ACPA*) is caused by antibodies against proteinase 3 and neutral serine protease present in the azurophilic granules of neutrophils.

The p-ANCA fluorescence represents an artifact of ethanol fixation that allows the rearrangement of positively charged granule constituents around and on the negatively charged nuclear membrane. Circulating antibodies against myeloperoxidase (MPO), elastase, cathepsin G, lactoferrin, and lysozyme have been identified as the cause of the p-ANCA phenomenon. The high specificity of c-ANCA for WG has been confirmed in large studies. In fact, it is so specific that it may in some cases preclude the need for biopsy, although the author feels that histopathologic confirmation of clinical impressions is important. However, in certain clinical situations, (e.g., subglottic stenosis in which sufficient biopsy material is difficult to obtain or is contraindicated because of the possibility of precipitating the need for a tracheostomy) the use of the c-ANCA test is extremely helpful.

A negative c-ANCA test does not exclude the diagnosis of WG. The sensitivity of the test is limited and depends on the extent and activity at the time the study is done. Its specificity is greater than 90% during the systemic vasculitic phase of the disease, but only about 65% in patients with predominantly granulomatous disease manifestations limited to the upper or lower respiratory tract, or both. In patients with no signs of disease activity (complete remission), the sensitivity is about 30%.

Cytoplasmic antineutrophilic cytoplasmic antibody testing as a predictor of relapse

Although titer changes in c-ANCA parallel disease activity changes in more than 85% of patients, the predictive value of a c-ANCA titer increase as an indicator of imminent relapse is controversial. Nevertheless, it is appropriate to interpret a c-ANCA titer increase as an ominous sign that necessitates the close monitoring of the patient.

Perinuclear antineutrophilic cytoplasmic antibody

Because of its lack of sensitivity and disease specificity, p-ANCA is not as useful as c-ANCA testing. It has been useful, however, in certain autoimmune diseases including inflammatory bowel disease, autoimmune liver disease, and rheumatoid arthritis. Additionally, p-ANCA with MPO as the target antigen has been found to be closely associated with microscopic polyangiitis for which the main manifestation is alveolar hemorrhage.

Disorders mimicking Wegener's granulomatosis

Two clinical situations are commonly confused with WG. The first is due to previous or ongoing nasal substance abuse.[2] This problem classically presents in a patient as an isolated, large septal perforation. The edges of the perforation are characteristically inflamed and crusty, and there is usually no history of external or intranasal trauma or previous surgical procedures involving the septum. With the exception of patients who admit to a chronic factitial habit, isolated septal perforations with totally normal nasal mucosa and normal nasopharyngeal mucosa are often due to substance abuse. Careful questioning will usually elicit a history of cocaine abuse, and it should be considered the diagnosis, even if the abuse was "discontinued years ago." The differentiating signs are the presence of normal mucosa throughout the upper airway, nonspecific biopsy results, normal results of blood tests, and a negative ANCA result.[15]

Histopathology of Wegener's granulomatosis

In WG there is characteristically vasculitis necrosis with an inflammatory background.[12] The vasculitis typically involves medium and small vessels including arteries, arterioles, capillaries, venules, and veins. The large vessels are rarely affected. There may be simply a mural cellular infiltrate or fibrinoid necrosis. More frequently, an intramural eccentric necrotizing granulomatous lesion is found. The capillaritis may be neutrophilic or, rarely, granulomatous. The necrosis is granulomatous in nature. There are also small microabscesses that enlarge and coalesce until the typical necrosis has developed.

The necrotic center is surrounded by palisading histiocytes and scattered giant cells. The cellular infiltrates are mixed, consisting of lymphocytes, plasma cells, scattered giant cells, and eosinophils.

Treatment of Wegener's granulomatosis

The current standard regimen for treatment of WG is oral cyclophosphamide, (2 mg/kg/day) and prednisone (1 mg/kg/day) for 1 month.[16] The prednisone is then tapered to alternate days throughout the following 2 months and then discontinued once a complete response is determined. Cyclophosphamide is continued for 6 months to 1 year. After disappearance of symptoms it is tapered gradually over several months. If relapse occurs, the standard protocol is reinitiated.

Trimethoprim - sulfamethoxazole. Trimethoprim - sulfahoxazole has several applications. First, all patients undergoing treatment with cyclophosphamide and prednisone also should be treated with trimethoprim-sulfamethoxazole (Bactrim or Septra, 1 DS). Second, when immunosuppressive therapy is discontinued, the patient should be continued indefinitely on trimethoprim-sulfamethoxazole because the author believes that it may prevent remission. The third application of this medicine is in patients with biopsy-proven but very limited disease (e.g., confined completely to the nose) where trimethoprim-sulfamethoxazole can be used alone. The results in a small group of patients with this type of limited disease is very encouraging.[8,20]

The mechanisms by which trimethoprim-sulfamethoxazole affects the course of WG are not clear. It may affect an antimicrobial agent or an infectious process that otherwise triggers an autoimmune cascade of WG, although so far the author has not identified a precise organism consistently. It may, on the other hand, have an immunomodulatory affect on neutrophils, macrophages, and lymphocytes.

Plasma exchange and intravenous immunoglobulin. Patients with generalized disease who do not respond to immunosuppressive therapy are challenging. Intravenous immunoglobulin (IVIG) has been tried in several patients with some good results. Plasma exchange has also been used, but its benefits seem to be limited to the dialysis-dependent patient population.

Surgical reconstruction. Contrary to some published statements, the author believes that surgical intervention used to restore function is appropriate when the disease is in remission. This includes tympanoplasty or correction of saddle nose deformity, as well as upper tracheal reconstruction.

Sarcoidosis

Sarcoidosis is a chronic systemic granulomatous disease capable of involving almost any organ in the body.[15] It is of immense interest to the otolaryngologist because of its predilection to involve many head and neck organs, including the eye (episcleritis, uveitis), various neuropathies (sudden deafness, unilateral or bilateral facial palsy), salivary glands (parotid swelling), the oropharynx (tonsillar hypertrophy), and larynx (epiglottic swelling and subglottic stenosis).

Nasal involvement

Nasal involvement in sarcoidosis can be external or internal. Externally, sarcoidosis may present as a raised, papular lesion on the nose. Several of these lesions may coalesce to form bluish-red swellings. The lesions are firm and elastic when palpated and extend deeply to involve the entire thickness of the dermis.

Another form of nasal sarcoidosis is called *lupus pernio*. This describes chronic, violoceous cutaneous lesions with a predilection for cold-sensitive areas such as the nose, cheeks, ears, and fingers.[1] Intranasal involvement is characterized by diffuse nasal crusting or a vasomotor-like appearance to the nasal mucosa, causing diffuse mucosal swelling.

Diagnosis

There are three criteria necessary to make the diagnosis of sarcoidosis. (1) The patient's clinical and radiographic presentation must be compatible with sarcoidosis; (2) nasal biopsy material should demonstrate noncaseating granulomas, and (3) other causes for granulomatous changes need to be excluded. Bronchoalveolar lavage (BAL) provides important insights into the pathogenesis of sarcoidosis. Studies suggest that the disease begins in the lungs with an alveolitis that consists mainly of T cells. These T cells elaborate chemotactic factors that attract monocytic cells, which ultimately transform into epithelial cells. These cells form the granuloma that potentially leads to fibrosis.

Patients with greater than 28% T lymphocytes in their BAL fluid have high-intensity alveolitis, and those with fewer than 28% T lymphocytes have low-intensity alveolitis. A decrease or return to a normal T-cell helper/suppresser ratio, accompanied or preceded by clinical and radiologic improvement in response to corticosteroid therapy, are very reliable prognostic signs. Gallium-67 scanning, often used in conjunction with BAL, is another useful diagnostic step. After Gallium-67 is injected intravenously, the isotope is taken up into inflammatory tissues and accumulates in involved organs. It still remains, however, nonspecific.

Angiotensin-converting enzyme, a normal constituent of the endothelium, converts angiotensin 1 and angiotensin 2. When elevated, enzyme levels do seem to correlate with the clinical activity of sarcoidosis in some patients. Therefore, it is used in the work-up of patients suspected of having sarcoidosis, but it is not diagnostic.

In many granulomatous disorders, activated T cells secrete a soluble form of interleukin (IL)-2 receptor (sIL-2R). Several studies have found that the levels of sIL-2R are markedly increased in patients with active sarcoidosis, and levels are lower in patients with inactive disease.

Other helpful laboratory studies include an increase in the erythrocyte sedimentation rate. Hypercalcemia and hypercalcuria may occur (10% of cases). Hypergammaglobulinemia has been noted in 20% to 25% of patients, primarily among blacks. Ten percent of patients with sarcoidosis have increased liver enzyme levels, particularly alkaline phosphatase. Electrocardiographic abnormalities include a prolonged P-R interval, bundle-branch block, arrhythmias, and nonspecific sinus tachycardia (ST)-segment changes.

When sarcoidosis involves leptomeninges, the cerebrospinal fluid contains increased numbers of lymphocytes and increased protein levels.

Immune aspects

Although the cause of sarcoidosis remains unknown, the disease is associated with abnormalities of cell-mediated and humoral immunity, and the disease develops as a result of an overstimulated local cellular immune response, probably because of an exaggerated T-helper cell network.[17] The migration, replication, and interaction of alveolar macrophages, T cells, B cells and mediators such as IL-1, IL-2, and type I interferon act in a synergistic manner to produce the migration of monocytes and T cells from the blood to the lung

and other parts of the airway, including the nose, leading to granuloma formation.

Management

The management of sarcoidosis is controversial, with most of the controversy centering on pulmonary involvement. Ocular involvement responds to cortisone-containing ophthalmic solutions. Involvement of the intranasal mucosa, epiglottis, and subglottis responds to aerosols containing cortisone. In more resistant cases, these areas respond to brief courses of systemic corticosteroids. Neuropathies, particularly of nerves VII and VIII, should be treated with corticosteroids, to which they usually respond.

In patients with stage 1 pulmonary involvement, management is "watchful waiting" with periodic examinations. Seventy percent of patients will show spontaneous remission. Patients in stage 2 or stage 3 who do not show improvement spontaneously or show worsening 6 months after diagnosis should be treated with prednisone (40 mg) on alternate days. The patient is examined in 3 months and the dose is altered according to response.

A subset of patients with persistently active or progressive sarcoidosis may be unresponsive to corticosteroids. Recently, low doses of methotrexate were shown to lead to improvement in symptoms, pulmonary roentgenographic changes, and improvement in function in a group of patients with progressive pulmonary and extrapulmonary sarcoidosis.

Churg-Strauss Syndrome

Churg-Strauss Syndrome (CSS) is classified as a granulomatous vasculitis. It is defined as an eosinophil-rich, granulomatous inflammation and necrotizing vasculitis of the upper respiratory tract affecting small to medium vessels associated with asthma and eosinophilia. There are three phases of the disease: (1) a prodromal phase that may persist for years; it consists of allergic disease (e.g., allergic rhinitis and nasal polyposis, frequently followed by asthma); (2) peripheral blood and tissue eosinophilia, chronic eosinophilic pneumonia, or eosinophilic gastroenteritis; and (3) a life-threatening systemic vasculitis. From the nasal point of view, it is usually associated with nasal polyps and does not have the diffuse mucosal destruction that typifies WG.

Histopathologically, CSS consists of prominent eosinophilia of vessels and perivascular tissue, accompanying leukocytes, plasma cells, and histiocytes in some patients. Vasculitis of the small arteries and veins is found in all patients, necrotizing extravascular granulomas is found in some patients, and in other patients fibrinoid necrosis of vessel wells is found. The morphologic difference between WG and CSS is that the coagulative or liquefactive necrotizing epithelioid granuloma in WG is morphologically different from the more fibrinoid, necrotizing epitheloid eosinophilic granuloma seen in CSS.

CSS responds well to corticosteroids. It does not respond

to cyclophosphamide, as does WG. As would be expected, the c-ANCA and p-ANCA tests are always negative in patients having CSS.

INFECTIOUS SYSTEMIC DISEASES

Rhinoscleroma

In 1870, von Hebra coined the term *rhinoscleroma*. The cause was ascribed to a bacteria in 1882. The specific organism has been identified as *Klebsiella rhinoscleromatis*. Rhinoscleroma is a chronic granulomatous disease of the respiratory tract. Its frequency in the United States is increasing. It was initially described as a lesion involving the nose, but now it is known to also involve the larynx, trachea, and bronchi.

Nasal involvement

Rhinoscleroma has several distinct stages of development. Initially there is a catarrhal stage, characterized by foul-smelling, purulent rhinorrhea for weeks or months. This is followed by the atrophic stage with large nasal plaques or crusts that are foul smelling and simulate the lesions in atrophic rhinitis. In the third stage, aptly named the granulomatous stage, multiple granulomatous nodules are found throughout the nose, pharynx, larynx, trachea, or bronchi. These nodules can enlarge and coalesce. During this stage, *K. rhinoscleromatis* is most frequently isolated and the pathologic changes are the most characteristic. Stage 4 consists of fibrosis and stenosis—often complete stenosis of the nostrils. Occasionally the fibrosis extends to the nasopharynx and trachea.

Diagnosis

Diagnosis depends on a high index of suspicion and the finding of coalescent, enlarged granulomatous nodules at or near the nasal vestibule, usually diffuse and bilateral. Cultures of infected tissue yield *K. rhinoscleromatis* in 98% of cases; this is diagnostic. Identification of the Mikulicz's cell in biopsy specimens is not definitely pathognomonic because this cell can be found (though rarely) in other disorders.

Histopathologic features

Rhinoscleroma is a chronic, granulomatous infection with characteristic fibrosis and eosin-staining Russell bodies. The hallmark is the vacuolated Mikulicz's cell, a large, foamy histiocyte that stains well with hematoxylin and eosin. During the granulomatous stage the histopathologic changes are most characteristic and the Mikulicz's cell is easiest to identify.

Treatment

Streptomycin (1 g/day for 4 weeks) plus tetracycline (2 g/day) is the recommended treatment regimen for rhinoscleroma. A second course of this therapy is repeated after 1 month. Even during the acute or granulomatous stage, this will give a 60% to 70% cure rate. Corticosteroids and radiotherapy are not effective.

In stage 4 of rhinoscleroma, when both nostrils are thickened and stenosed, in addition to antimicrobial therapy, the scar tissue can be "cored out" and the nose is allowed to re-epithelialize. A Silastic stent may be used.

Tuberculosis

The increase in the incidence of tuberculosis is probably due to two main factors: an increased number of refugees and the occurrence of tuberculosis infections in patients who have some form of acquired immunodeficiency syndrome (AIDS). Even in previous years when tuberculosis was common in the United States, involvement of the head and neck was relatively uncommon. As a result, physicians often fail to suspect tuberculosis, and when the disease involves the head and neck the diagnosis is often delayed.

Nontuberculous mycobacteria

The types of nontuberculous mycobacteria seen today are often called atypical.[14,21] They differ from *Mycobacterium tuberculosis* in that they are less virulent, are more likely to infect individuals who have altered host defenses, and are less susceptible to standard antituberculosis drugs. In general, infection with nontuberculous bacteria most commonly represents primary infection. The most common infections caused by these nontuberculous mycobacteria are the following: (1) corneal ulcers caused by *Mycobacterium fortuitum* in which the pathogenesis is inoculation of the eye by contaminated dust or other foreign material; and (2) cervical lymph nodes infected by nontuberculous mycobacteria. The organisms most commonly responsible for this are *Mycobacterium scrofulaceum*, *Mycobacterium szulgai*, and *Mycobacterium xenopi*.

Clinical aspects

Tuberculosis is a potentially lifelong chronic infection, caused by two species of mycobacteria: *Mycobacterium tuberculosis* and, rarely, *Mycobacterium bovis*. It almost always is initiated by inhalation of infectious material, rarely by injection, and more rarely still by cutaneous inoculation. Early in the infection, organisms in the bloodstream seek out the lymphatic system and other organs, leaving foci that may cause clinical illness after long latency periods. Mycobacteria are acid-fast, nonmotile, weakly gram-positive rods classified in the order Actinomycetales.

Nasal involvement

Nasal tuberculosis, another rare form of the disease, usually affects the anterior septum or anterior part of the turbinates; the nasal floor is spared. Perforations of the cartilaginous portion of the septum occur. In the early stage of the disease, nasal discharge, pain, and partial obstruction are characteristic symptoms. Examination shows a red, nodular thickening, with or without ulceration. The disease has a rapid course, usually resulting in either perforation of the septum or scarring. In lupus vulgaris (an indolent and chronic form of tuberculosis of the nose) scarring is more severe.

Diagnosis

A history of previous tuberculosis or the finding of active pulmonary tuberculosis is extremely helpful in making the diagnosis of tuberculosis of the nose. In the earliest stages, however, the manifestations of nasal bleeding, crusting, or draining may be nonspecific. As in the other granulomatous diseases discussed, diagnosis depends on smears and cultures for acid-fast bacilli and histopathologic examination of an adequate biopsy specimen.

Management

Current recommendations include a 2-month course of therapy with three drugs: isoniazid, rifampin, and either streptomycin or ethambutol. After daily therapy for 2 weeks, the drugs may be given twice a week if the patient demonstrates response. Later, twice weekly administration of isoniazid and rifampin is continued for 6 to 7 months. Baseline audiometric and bithermal caloric assessments should be done and repeated periodically because of the ototoxicity of streptomycin.

Histoplasmosis

Although histoplasmosis, a granulomatous fungal disease, primarily involves the larynx and tongue, it can involve any part of the head and neck, including the nose.[4,7,14]

Epidemiology

Histoplasmosis occurs most often in infants and in the elderly. Although it generally occurs equally in both sexes, elderly men are frequently affected. It has been reported in approximately 30 countries. In the United States it is endemic in the Missouri, Mississippi, and Ohio River valleys where the incidence of past and current infections has reached 85%, as determined by skin testing. Humans and animals are infected by inhalation of the fungus in dust. Soil from chicken houses or from areas contaminated by bat or bird feces is especially rich in *Histoplasma capsulatum* organisms.

Mycology

In its yeast phase the histoplasmosis cell is small (3 μm × 5 μm). In the mycelial phase, branched hyphae with projections called *tuberculate conidia* are evident. This phase occurs in the soil. The conidia contain the spores, and humans are infected by inhalation of these spores.

Nasal involvement

Nasal involvement is accompanied by pulmonary involvement and characterized by cough, chest pain, and hoarseness. Chest radiographs show either a diffuse miliary or a localized type of infiltrate. The larynx and tongue are most frequently involved. Nasal involvement consists of either nodules or ulcers composed of masses of organisms in macrophages.

Diagnosis

In addition to positive microscopic identification of the organism, skin tests are useful for diagnosis. One drawback is the high incidence of positive cutaneous responders in endemic areas. The complement-fixation test is reliable because titers persist for long periods; a titer of 1:32 is diagnostic.

Histopathologic features

Microscopically, the lesion is an epithelioid or histiocytic granuloma. The implicated organism can be identified by use of periodic acid–Schiff, Gridley, or Grocott-Gomori methenamine-silver nitrate stain. The capsule is a polysaccharide and stains poorly with hematoxylin and eosin. Organisms can be identified within the granuloma; however, fewer organisms are seen in the presence of a pronounced granulomatous reaction. In these cases, other methods of diagnosis, including culture and serology, are useful.

Treatment

The treatment for histoplasmosis is amphotericin B, in a dose of 1 mg to 10 mg per day and progressing to 1 mg/kg for a total dose of 2 g administered during a 2- to 3-month period. This treatment has decreased the mortality rate in the United States to about 50 cases per year.

Rhinosporidiosis

Although rhinosporidiosis, a fungal infection, is usually seen in Asian and African countries, the disease has been found in the United States due to increased foreign travel and more influx of refugees from Asia.[13] This disease is caused by *Rhinosporidium seeberi*, which is a fungus-like organism not yet successfully grown in culture medium or transferred from a human to an animal host.[13] The disease is contracted by immersion in contaminated waters in Asia and Africa. Initially, the nasal mucosal lesion is flat and sessile, then it enlarges to become a painless polypoid growth that actually fills the nasal cavities. Management consists of complete surgical excision. No medical management has been found to be effective. Microscopically, pseudoepitheliomatous squamous cell metaplasia overlies numerous multisized, microscopic globular cysts called *sporangia*. In an accompanying granulomatous reaction of fibrous tissue, neutrophils, plasma cells, and lymphocytes are prominent.

Mucormycosis

Mucormycosis is an opportunistic disease that is extremely important to the otolaryngologist. It is caused primarily by fungi of the order Mucorales and of the genera

Mucor, Rhizopus, and Absidia.[9] Although most commonly seen in patients with poorly controlled brittle diabetes mellitus, it can occur in any patient who is immunosuppressed and who is in a state of metabolic bankruptcy. Initially, there is facial pain, fever, bloody nasal discharge, facial swelling, and edema. The disease progresses dramatically, with facial cellulitis, gangrenous mucosal changes in the nose and paranasal sinuses, obtundation, cranial nerve palsies, vision loss, and proptosis. Sometimes a rapid course leads to intracranial extension and death. Diagnosis is suggested by the combination of a rapidly progressive infection and a black, necrotic mass of tissue filling the nasal cavity, eroding the nasal septum, and extending through the hard palate in an immunocompromised patient.

The finding of broad, nonseptic hyphae (typical of Mucorales) on tissue sections stained with periodic acid–Schiff or Grocott-Gomori methenamine-silver nitrate stain confirms the diagnosis. The prognosis is poor, with a reported death rate as high as 50%.

Amphotericin B is the only effective antifungal drug treatment. Aggressive surgical debridement, when the patient's condition allows, is also helpful, along with control of the underlying medical disorder.

PERIPHERAL T-CELL NEOPLASMS

The author has already defined the characteristics of WG, the many ways in which sarcoidosis can present, and the characteristics of nasal tuberculosis and fungal infections. This leaves the remaining lesion that causes nasal destruction, namely, T-cell lymphoma. *T-cell lymphoma* replaces previously used terms such as *midline malignant* or *polymorphic reticulosis.*

Clinical diagnosis

In contrast to the diffuse nasal mucosal ulceration that typifies WG, lymphoma lesions are more likely to be unilaterally placed in the nose, with extension into the soft tissue of the nose, upper lip, oral cavity, and maxillary sinus, with or without orbital involvement. The lesions are "explosive," rapidly progressive, and attended by such breakdown of tissue that there is considerable associated superimposed infection by gram-negative organisms, as well anaerobic organisms. Comparing and contrasting with patients having WG, the following are key points: (1) distribution of the ulceration is focal and localized and explosive in T-cell lymphomas compared with the diffuse ulceration in patients with WG; (2) the systemic features and the lung infiltrates can be similar in both, but in T-cell lymphoma otologic, tracheal, and renal involvement is extremely uncommon; and (3) the main differences are found on morphologic examination. WG is typified by the vasculitis as previously discussed in this chapter, whereas T-cell lymphomas have a polymorphic lymphoid infiltrate with angiocentric and angioinvasive features.[19] The best way to examine biopsy material is with paraffin-embedded tissue techniques. For immunohisto-

chemical studies, the phenotype of the atypical lymphoid cells in each case is assessed by using antibodies to leukocyte-common antigen CD45RB (Dako, Carpinteria, Calif.); the B-cell lineage marker CD20 (L26, Dako); the T-cell lineage markers CD3 (polyclonal, Dako), CD43 (Leu-22, Becton Dickinson, San Jose, Calif.), and CD45RO (UCHL-1, Dako); and the natural-killer marker CD57 (LEU-7, Becton Dickinson).

EBV-RNA is detected by *in situ* hybridization in paraffin-embedded tissue with a biotinylated 30-base oligonucleotide that is complementary to EBER 1, a region of the EBV genoma that is actively transcribed in latently infected cells.

Treatment

Patients with localized disease can be treated with irradiation. Patients with multiorgan involvement are best treated with the help of hematologic colleagues by using a standard leukemia protocol. Regarding prognosis, in 1996 the author reported on 30 patients with T-cell lymphoma.[6] Twelve patients died of the disease with or without disseminated lymphomas, 10 were alive and free of disease at 5 years, and six died of other causes, free of disease. Two patients were lost to follow-up.

ACKNOWLEDGMENT

The author wishes to acknowledge and thank his secretary, Kathleen Gehling, for her many years of collegiality, support, and help in preparing this manuscript.

REFERENCES

1. Arnold HL Jr, Odom RB, James WD: *Andrews' diseases of the skin: clinical dermatology,* ed 8, Philadelphia, 1990, WB Saunders.
2. Becker GD, Hill S: Midline granuloma due to illicit cocaine use, *Arch Otolaryngol Head Neck Surg* 114:90, 1988.
3. Bullen CL and others: Ocular complications of Wegener's granulomatosis, *Ophthalmology* 90:279, 1983.
4. Darling ST: A protozoan general infection producing pseudotubercles in the lungs and focal necroses in the liver, spleen, and lymph nodes, *JAMA* 46:1283, 1906.
5. Daum TE and others: Tracheobronchial involvement in Wegener's granulomatosis, *Am J Respir Crit Care Med* 151:522, 1995.
6. Davison SP and others: Nasal and nasopharyngeal angiocentric T-cell lymphomas, *Laryngoscope* 106(2):139, 1996.
7. DeMonbreun WA: The cultivation and cultural characteristics of Darling's histoplasma capsulatum, *Am J Trop Med Hyg* 14:93, 1934.
8. DeRemee RA, McDonald TJ, Weiland LH: Wegener's granulomatosis: observations on treatment with antimicrobial agents, *Mayo Clin Proc* 60:27, 1985.
9. Eisenberg L, Wood T, Boles R: Mucormycosis, *Laryngoscope* 87:347, 1977.
10. Gaughan RK, DeSanto LW, McDonald TJ: Use of anticytoplasmic autoantibodies in the diagnosis of Wegener's granulomatosis with subglottic stenosis, *Laryngoscope* 100:561, 1990.
11. Kaline PH and others: Role of testing for anticytoplasmic autoantibodies in the differential diagnosis of scleritis and orbital pseudotumor, *Mayo Clin Proc* 65:1110, 1990.
12. Klinger H: Grenzformen der periarteritis nodosa, *Franfurter Zeitschrift für Pathologie* 42:455, 1931.

13. Lasser A, Smith HW: Rhinosporidiosis, *Arch Otolaryngol* 102:308, 1976.
14. McDonald TJ: *Granulomatous diseases of the nose.* In English GM, editor: *Otolaryngology*, vol 2, Philadelphia, 1990, JB Lippincott.
15. McDonald TJ: *Vasculitis and granulomatous disease.* In McCaffrey TV, editor: *Rhinologic diagnosis and treatment*, New York, 1996, Thieme.
16. Specks U: Wegener's granulomatosis and pulmonary vasculitis, *Clin Pulm Med* 2(5):267, 1995.
17. Specks U, DeRemee RA: Granulomatous vasculitis and Churg-Strauss syndrome, *Rheum Dis Clin North Am* 16:377, 1990.
18. Specks U, Homburger HA: Anti-neutrophil cytoplasmic antibodies, *Mayo Clin Proc* 69:1197, 1994.
19. Strickler JG and others: Polymorphic reticulosis: a reappraisal, *Hum Pathol* 25(7):659, 1994.
20. Valeriano-Marcet J, Spiera H: Treatment of Wegener's granulomatosis with sulfamethoxazole-trimethoprim, *Arch Intern Med* 151:1649, 1991.
21. Waldman RH: Tuberculosis and atypical mycobacteria, *Otolaryngol Clin North Am* 15:581, 1982.
22. Wegener F: Über eine eigenartige rhinogene Granulomatose mit besonderer Beteiligung des Arteriensystems und der Nieren, *Beitr Pathol Anat* 109:36, 1939.

Chapter 45

Epistaxis

Jane M. Emanuel

The incidence of epistaxis in the general population is difficult to ascertain because the majority of episodes resolve with conservative self-treatment and go unreported. Patients who seek medical treatment for epistaxis typically fall into two general categories: those who have multiple minor episodes and those who have a single severe prolonged episode that will not stop. The former patient usually is a child or young adult who has anterior septal bleeding. The latter patient tends to be an older adult with a posterior origin of bleeding and underlying medical problems.

EPIDEMIOLOGY

Epistaxis occurs more commonly in male than female patients (58% versus 42%).[16] Juselius[16] also noted a higher incidence of epistaxis in older patients, as 71% of his patients were greater than 50 years of age. Also, epistaxis is more common in the colder months of the year, suggesting a link with decreased ambient humidity and the higher incidence of upper respiratory infections. To define etiologies of epistaxis, it is useful to separate local and systemic causes.

LOCAL CAUSES

Mechanical or traumatic causes

Acute nasal trauma, with or without nasal fracture, can produce epistaxis from intranasal mucosal lacerations. In such patients, bleeding usually lasts only a short time, with minor recurrences possible during the healing period. Extensive facial or head trauma may produce severe bleeding initially, although epistaxis weeks after injury should arouse suspicion of a traumatic aneurysm. Bleeding after septorhinoplasty, endoscopic sinus operations, or turbinate resection can result from mucosal surfaces or from a major vessel. Nasal intubations often are associated with acute epistaxis.

Chronic nasal trauma is a frequent cause of epistaxis. Habitual nose rubbing and picking may produce anterior septal irritation, superficial ulceration, and bleeding. This is a particularly common cause of epistaxis in children.

Topical steroid nasal sprays, especially the drier aerosol formulations, may produce nasal irritation and epistaxis. Chronic cocaine abuse eventually may produce tissue necrosis, crusting, and bleeding.

Septal deformity

Septal deflections and spurs also may produce nasal dryness, crusting, and subsequent epistaxis. Padgam[34] analyzed the position of bleeding points in relation to septal anatomy in patients with a septal deflection and found that the bleeding site was anterior to the deflection in 83%. In all patients in whom a spur was present on the side of the bleeding, the source was anterior or inferior to the spur. These findings refute the common suspicion that a bleeding point is hidden behind a septal spur. Padgam[34] also noted that posterior bleeding occurred only in patients with normal or widely patent nasal airways.

Septal perforations are a frequent source of chronic epistaxis. The edges of the perforation are subject to drying and crusting, resulting in friable mucosal edges and recurrent bleeding episodes.

Inflammatory disease

Inflammation of the nasal mucosa may produce epistaxis. This inflammation may be a result of viral upper respiratory infections, bacterial sinusitis, or the nasal manifestations of allergic disease. Irritant or toxic inhalants also may cause inflammation and epistaxis. Bleeding of inflammatory origin generally is a blood-streaked mucus, but it may become an active epistaxis depending on the degree of inflammation and how forcefully the patient blows his or her nose. Pad-gam[34] found a 50% incidence of nasal discharge, a 63% incidence of nasal obstruction, and a 22% incidence of sneezing in his patients with epistaxis, suggesting that inflammatory disease may be a common contributing factor in epistaxis.

Tumors

Benign and malignant neoplasms of the nose, sinuses, and nasopharynx may present with epistaxis. Recurrent bouts of epistaxis or severe episodes of bleeding should prompt evaluation for tumor via fiberoptic and radiologic examination.

Epistaxis is a frequent presenting sign of an angiofibroma, which is a benign, locally invasive, highly vascular tumor. Angiofibromas account for an estimated 0.5% of head and neck neoplasms. The tumor usually presents in the nose or nasopharynx of adolescent males, hence the common usage of the term *juvenile nasopharyngeal angiofibroma*.[3] The most common presenting signs and symptoms are epistaxis (73%) and nasal obstruction (71%).[51] Manipulation and biopsy of the mass should be avoided because of the potential for hemorrhage. Contrast computed tomography (CT) and magnetic resonance imaging (MRI) should be used for diagnosis and treatment planning.[51]

Aneurysms

Intracavernous aneurysms of the internal carotid artery may be posttraumatic or nontraumatic in origin. Epistaxis in patients with nontraumatic aneurysms is rare, but large aneurysms may be mistaken for a tumor and result in fatal hemorrhage with biopsy. Posttraumatic aneurysms more commonly cause epistaxis, often delayed an average of 7 weeks after injury. The mortality rate in these patients is approximately 50%.[40]

SYSTEMIC CAUSES

Coagulation deficits

Congenital or acquired coagulopathies may cause epistaxis that is difficult to manage until the underlying clotting disorder is corrected. Congenital coagulopathy should be suspected in the presence of a positive family history, easy bruisability, and a history of prolonged bleeding from lacerations, dental extractions, or minor trauma.

von Willebrand's disease is one of the most common congenital bleeding disorders, with epistaxis a frequent feature. The most common type of von Willebrand's disease is an autosomal dominant disorder, characterized by epistaxis (60%), easy bruising (40%), menorrhagia (35%), gingival bleeding (35%), and postoperative bleeding (20%). Laboratory evaluation includes a bleeding time, platelet count, activated partial thromboplastin time, assay of factor VIII coagulant activity, von Willebrand's factor antigen, ristocetin cofactor activity, and ristocetin-induced platelet aggregation.

The test results usually are abnormal, but as factor levels fluctuate, test results can be normal at times. Management depends on the severity of the disease and the clinical setting. Replacement therapy with cryoprecipitate and possibly platelets, sufficient to normalize the Duke bleeding time and factor VIII coagulant activity, is recommended for 7 to 10 days after major surgical procedures and 4 to 6 days after minor procedures.[54]

Acquired coagulopathies may be drug- or disease-mediated. Numerous medications affect coagulation as their intended therapeutic effect or as a side effect. Drug- or disease-mediated thrombocytopenia tends to produce spontaneous bleeding when platelet counts are between 10,000 to 20,000/mm^3. Counts below 10,000/mm^3 often are associated with severe bleeding. Vitamin K is essential for the synthesis of prothrombin and factors VII, IX, and X. Vitamin K deficiency as a result of diet, disease, or medications may produce severe or fatal bleeding. Liver disease is a common cause of impaired coagulation, with reduced levels of all coagulation factors except factor VIII. In the absence of liver disease, alcohol may be a factor in those with epistaxis. McGarry[28,29] noted that even low levels (1 to 10 drinks/week) of alcohol were associated with a prolongation of bleeding time. An association between regular high alcohol use and epistaxis has been confirmed by McGarry.[28,29]

Arteriosclerotic vascular disease

Arteriosclerotic vascular disease is a possible explanation for the higher incidence of nosebleeds seen in those of increased age. Although hypertension often is noted in the older patient with epistaxis, and although an increased blood pressure reading is noted in the acutely bleeding patient, an actual increase in frequency or severity of epistaxis in the hypertensive group has not been shown.[23,34,52]

Hereditary hemorrhagic telangiectasia

Hereditary hemorrhagic telangiectasia (Osler-Weber-Rendu disease) is an autosomal dominant disease manifested by diffuse mucocutaneous telangiectasias and arteriovenous malformations. Incidence is estimated at 1 or 2 per 100,000. A negative family history is found in 20% of patients, possibly as a result of asymptomatic relatives, incomplete penetrance, or spontaneous mutations.[37]

The angiodysplasia of hereditary hemorrhagic telangiectasia affects vessels from capillaries to large arteries, producing telangiectasias, arteriovenous malformations, and aneurysms. Localized areas in capillaries are lined by a single endothelial layer and lack elastic tissue, resulting in vessel fragility and impaired vasoconstriction. Telangiectasias occur throughout the body on mucous membranes and skin. Hereditary hemorrhagic telangiectasia also demonstrates arteriovenous fistulae and aneurysms, with locations in the lung, central nervous system, liver, and bowel often being clinically significant.[37]

Recurrent epistaxis is the most common manifestation of

hereditary hemorrhagic telangiectasia. Aassar[1] noted a 93% incidence of epistaxis, with a mean age of onset of 12 years and a mean frequency of 18 bleeding episodes per month. Other studies noted incidences of epistaxis in the 60% to 90% range. A trend toward increasing frequency and duration of epistaxis with age was noted by Aassar[1] whereas a stable pattern or spontaneous regression is noted in other studies.[37] Epistaxis is an early sign of hereditary hemorrhagic telangiectasia and may be useful as a marker in early diagnosis of children in affected families. Because a number of affected patients may be diagnosed by the otolaryngologist, referral for evaluation of possible cerebral and pulmonary arteriovenous malformations should be considered. Additional measures, such as iron and folate supplementation and avoidance of anticoagulant and antiplatelet medications, should be addressed.[37] Specific therapy of epistaxis in patients with hereditary hemorrhagic telangiectasia is discussed later in this chapter.

VASCULAR ANATOMY

The nasal cavity is a rich vascular bed, with blood supply originating from the internal and external carotid arteries.

The external carotid system divides and terminates as the superficial temporal artery and the internal maxillary (also known as the *maxillary*) artery. The internal maxillary artery passes deep to the neck of the mandible, through the infratemporal fossa, deep or superficial to the lateral pterygoid muscle. The artery then enters the pterygomaxillary fossa and terminates, dividing into the posterior–superior alveolar, descending palatine, infraorbital, sphenopalatine, pharyngeal, and pterygoid canal arteries. The descending palatine artery descends through the greater palatine canal, supplying blood to the lateral nasal wall. It also contributes to septal blood supply via the incisive foramen. The sphenopalatine artery usually divides at or near the sphenopalatine foramen, entering the nose and supplying the turbinates and lateral nasal wall and anastamosing with the ethmoid arteries. A terminal branch of the sphenopalatine artery crosses the roof of the nose to supply the nasal septum, anastamosing with the greater palatine and labial vessels in Kiesselbach's area (also known as *Little's area*) on the anterior septum. This anastomotic area is the site of most anterior epistaxis (Figs. 45-1 and 45-2).[36]

The facial artery, an earlier branch of the external carotid system, also contributes to the blood supply of Kiesselbach's area and the anterior nasal floor via the septal branch of its superior labial division.

The internal carotid artery contributes to the blood supply of the internal nose via the ophthalmic artery. The ophthalmic artery enters the bony orbit through the superior orbital fissure, dividing into a number of branches with two arteries, the anterior and posterior ethmoidal arteries, supplying the superior septum and lateral nasal wall. The posterior ethmoid artery branches from the ophthalmic artery and exits the orbit via the posterior ethmoid foramen (or foramina in 30%).[13] The distance from the optic canal to the posterior ethmoid foramen is variable, with a range of 2 to 9 mm noted by Harrison[13] and 3 to 17 mm noted by McQueen.[30] The artery crosses the ethmoid sinus, enters the anterior cranial fossa, and passes through the cribiform plate into the nose, dividing into lateral and septal branches.

The anterior ethmoid artery is larger and exits the orbit via the anterior ethmoid foramen, again crossing the ethmoid labyrinth, anterior cranial fossa, and descending via the cribiform plate. It divides into lateral and septal branches, with the septal branch anastomosing at Kiesselbach's area on the

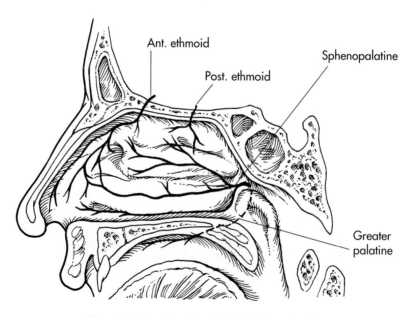

Fig. 45-1. Blood supply of the lateral nasal wall.

anterior nasal septum. The anterior ethmoid foramen is located 14 to 35 mm from the optic canal, with 96% of foramina located in the frontoethmoid suture line (see Figs. 45-1 and 45-2).[30]

MANAGEMENT OF EPISTAXIS

The vascular anatomy of the nose and clinical observation have led to the division of epistaxis into anterior and posterior locations. Anterior epistaxis has a bleeding site visible on anterior rhinoscopy and almost always originates from Kiesselbach's area on the anterior septum. The majority of bleeding sites (82% noted by Padgam) in all age groups are anterior and accessible to local treatment.

Bleeding sites not visible on anterior rhinoscopy traditionally have been assumed to originate posteriorly from the vicinity of the sphenopalatine foramen. The use of fiberoptic endoscopes continues to define this type of bleeding to more specific locations.[34]

General measures

An accurate patient history is necessary, but it may need to be done in conjunction with maneuvers to control bleeding. Specifics about location, severity, duration, and frequency of bleeding are obtained. The review of head and neck symptoms should include inquiries regarding nasal obstruction, rhinorrhea, and trauma. The history also should include questions regarding underlying medical conditions, family history, medications, tobacco use, and alcohol use to discover factors that may be causing the epistaxis or that may affect management.

A general physical examination and thorough head and neck evaluation then is performed. Anterior rhinoscopy should be done both before and after topical anesthesia and vasoconstriction. Flexible or rigid endoscopes should be used as needed for visualization of the bleeding site.

In conjunction with the physical examination, laboratory evaluation may be indicated for assessment of blood loss, fluid status, coagulopathy, or underlying systemic disease. Sinus films and CT or MRI scanning may be needed to evaluate for neoplasms and for assessment of anatomy for possible surgical access.

Treatment of anterior epistaxis

The patient with epistaxis optimally is evaluated in the seated position, with the examiner equipped with an adequate light source, suction, anesthetic solution, packing materials, and cautery available. The author has found it helpful to have an epistaxis "tackle box" stocked and ready for use at all times. The examiner and assistants should be protected with eye and face coverings, gloves, and fluid-impervious gowns. The patient's nose is examined before and after vasoconstriction. All packing and clots are removed. Although it often is tempting to leave effective packing in place, rebleeding often occurs at a time when appropriate medical care is not readily available.

Topical anesthetic and vasoconstrictor agents are applied via cotton pledgets or neurosurgical cottonoids. Topical cocaine, 4%, is excellent for this purpose, but it may not be readily available because of storage considerations. A reasonable substitute is a 1:1 mixture of oxymetazoline and xylocaine, 4%.

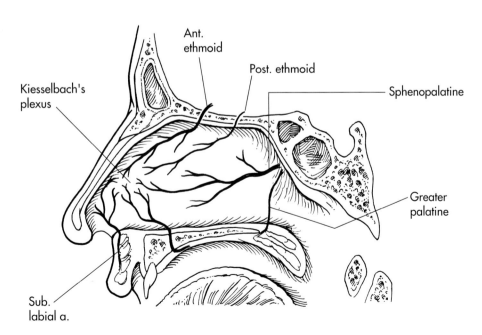

Fig. 45-2. Blood supply of the nasal septum. Kiesselbach's area (Little's area) is the site of the most anterior epistaxis episodes.

the previously placed tubing segment is placed against the anterior pack, and a C-clamp is tightened behind the tubing to maintain tension (Fig. 45-7).

The patient with posterior packing is admitted to the hospital. Most patients are treated with antibiotics to prevent sinusitis. Adequate pain control is essential. A patient-controlled analgesia pump (PCA) is an excellent method of administration.[5] Nasal packing has been shown to increase nocturnal episodes of hypoxia and may induce or exacerbate obstructive sleep apnea.[15,53] Others have noted only minimal desaturation episodes and have associated the morbidity of nasal packing to underlying diseases rather than oxygenation

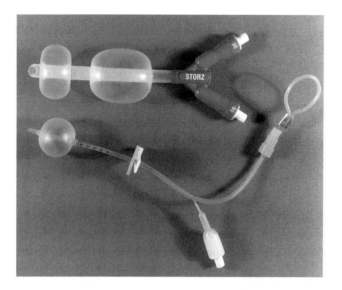

Fig. 45-5. Top, Storz Epistaxis Catheter. **Bottom,** Xomed Treace Nasal Post Pac.

drops.[23] Pulse oximetry is an effective means of monitoring oxygenation and of assessing the need for supplemental oxygen in the patient with nasal packing.[5,23]

Endoscopy cautery

Rigid and flexible endoscopes and their suction–irrigation appliances have facilitated a more precise definition of bleeding sites. A 2.7-mm or 4.0-mm 0° or 30° telescope and nasal suction is used to identify a posterior bleeding site. An irrigation device is useful for keeping the telescope lens free of blood. Topical vasoconstriction and anesthesia are induced after localization of the bleeding site. A 22-gauge spinal needle then is used to inject lidocaine and epinephrine locally. A greater palatine nerve block also may be used. An insulated suction cautery unit then is used to electrocoagulate the bleeding site. With this technique, bleeding sites have been noted and managed on the posterior nasal septum, middle meatus, inferior meatus, nasal floor, and face of the sphenoid. The success rate of posterior endoscopic cauterization is reported in the 80% to 90% range. Palatal numbness is reported as a short-term complication. Possible complications of posterior cauterization, which have not been reported, include damage to the eustachian tube orifice and the optic nerve.[26,28,33,55]

Arterial ligation

Ligation of the arterial blood supply is an effective method of epistaxis control. Ligation traditionally has been a management choice when packing has failed. Others have advocated the use of arterial ligation at an early stage in epistaxis to reduce length of hospital stay.[45] The choice of specific vessel to ligate usually is dictated by the observed site or the most likely site of bleeding based on history.

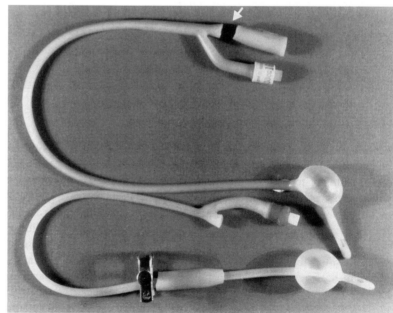

Fig. 45-6. Foley catheter preparation for use as a posterior nasal pack. Note (*arrow*) cut at drainage port (*top*) and placement of drainage port and retention with a metal C-clamp (*bottom*).

External carotid artery ligation

Ligation of the external carotid artery has been advocated by some authors because it can be performed with local anesthesia and done without specialized equipment. External carotid artery ligation (combined with anterior ethmoid ligation) was successful in 14 of 15 patients.[50] In contrast, a high rate of rebleeding with external carotid ligation (45%) was noted on long-term follow-up evaluation by Stafford and Durham.[46] Failure of this method may occur as a result of flow from anastomotic connections with the ipsilateral internal carotid or the opposite carotid system.

The external carotid artery is approached through a horizontal incision between the hyoid and upper border of the thyroid cartilage. Superior and inferior subplatysmal flaps are raised, and the sternocleidomastoid muscle is retracted posteriorly. The internal jugular vein is retracted, exposing the carotid bifurcation. Exposure of the internal carotid for several centimeters, plus dissection of the external carotid beyond its first two branches before ligation prevents ligation of the internal carotid by mistake.[24]

Internal maxillary artery ligation

Internal maxillary artery ligation has been the most popular method of arterial ligation over the past several decades. The internal maxillary artery usually is approached transantrally, although a transoral approach also has been described.[25] Preoperative radiographic assessment of antral size is necessary because a hypoplastic antrum is a contraindication to this approach.

The antrum is entered via a Caldwell-Luc approach, making a large bony opening, and a self-retaining retractor is placed. An operating microscope then is positioned. A periosteal flap then is outlined with a long guarded needle tip cautery and elevated off of the posterior antral wall. The posterior sinus wall is opened with a drill or mallet and chisel, beginning inferiorly. Pituitary ronguers then are used to remove the posterior sinus wall. The posterior periosteum is carefully opened. The vessels of the pterygopalatine fossa are dissected and elevated with blunt hooks, and two hemoclips are placed on each vessel. The internal maxillary, sphenopalatine, and descending palatine arteries should be double-clipped and not divided.[36] Gelfoam is placed over the posterior wall, and the mucosal incision is closed.[24] An antral window or middle meatal antrostomy is considered if necessary for drainage of the sinus. All nasal packing placed before the procedure then is removed to ascertain success of the procedure. Reported success rates of transantral maxillary artery ligation range from 75% to 100%.[31,42,47]

Failure of this procedure may occur as a result of the variability of arterial branching in the pterygopalatine fossa and failure to identify all branches. Complications may include infraorbital anesthesia, oroantral fistula, dental injury, sinusitis, and, rarely, blindness.[36]

Maceri and Makielski[25] advocated the transoral approach and cited its usefulness in patients with midface trauma, poorly developed maxillary antra, and maxillary tumors. Potential complications of the transoral approach include trismus, facial swelling, tongue paresthesias, and failure to control bleeding.

The sphenopalatine artery also can be approached intranasally during endoscopic visualization. An endoscopic uncinectomy may be done to facilitate exposure. Mucosa then is elevated from the lateral wall of the nose between the middle and inferior turbinates. The sphenopalatine artery is identified posteriorly as it exits its foramen. The artery then is clipped or coagulated for control of bleeding.

Ethmoid artery ligation

Ethmoid artery ligation may be indicated if the bleeding site is superior to the middle turbinate. A temporary tarsorraphy is done. An external ethmoidectomy incision is made

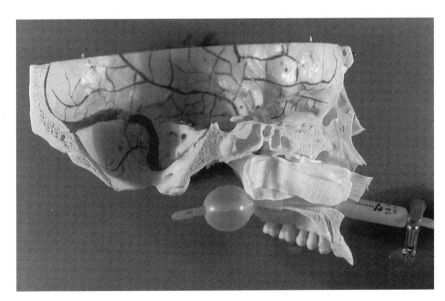

Fig. 45-7. Posterior Foley catheter balloon pack.

through skin, subcutaneous tissue, and periosteum. The periosteum is elevated to expose the frontoethmoid suture line, retracting the orbital periosteum laterally. The anterior ethmoid artery then is located an average of 22 mm from the anterior lacrimal crest (range, 16 to 29 mm).[30] The artery is double-clipped and then divided if the posterior ethmoid artery is to be ligated. The usually smaller posterior ethmoid artery then is located an average of 33 mm from the anterior lacrimal crest (range, 26 to 39 mm).[30] This artery is clipped but not divided because of the proximity of the optic nerve (3 to 17 mm). Alternately, Langer and Terry[21] described the use of a sinus endoscope and bipolar cautery to facilitate visualization in the deep dissection necessary for posterior ethmoid artery ligation.

The anterior ethmoid artery also can be approached intranasally as it crosses the ethmoid roof. An endoscopic anterior ethmoidectomy is done, and the anterior ethmoid artery is identified and coagulated with bipolar cautery.

Arterial embolization

The increasing availability of interventional radiologists has made arterial embolization an option for primary treatment of epistaxis and for surgical failures. A transfemoral route of catheterization usually is selected. Local anesthesia is administered, with sedation used in some patients. Angiography of the external and internal carotid systems is done to evaluate the vascular anatomy for any potentially dangerous anastamotic communications between the two systems. Selective angiography of the internal maxillary artery then is performed, although a bleeding site usually is not seen. Embolization of the distal internal maxillary artery then is

carried out with polyvinyl alcohol particles, gelfoam, coils, or a combination of materials. Unilateral embolization is done unless the bleeding side cannot be clearly identified, and then bilateral embolization is considered. The distal facial artery may be embolized, particularly if angiography shows major contribution to the nasal blood supply. Postoperative angiography is used to evaluate arterial occlusion. Previously placed nasal packing is removed immediately or in a delayed fashion (Fig. 45-8 A, B).

Reported success rates of embolization in control of epistaxis is 70% to 96%. The most common cause of failure is continued bleeding from the ethmoid arteries. Success, therefore, depends on accurate preembolization localization of the bleeding side and site. Recurrence is common in patients with hereditary hemorrhagic telangiectasia, but this is expected because of the nature of the disease. Short-term minor complications of embolization include facial and jaw pain, groin hematoma, and cold hypersensitivity. Potential major complications include stroke, facial paralysis, and skin necrosis. Contraindications to arterial embolization include dye allergies, severe atherosclerotic disease, and the presence of dangerous anastomotic connections between the internal and external carotid systems.[10,11,44,47,48]

TREATMENT OF HEREDITARY HEMORRHAGIC TELANGIECTASIA

Treatment of bleeding in patients with hereditary hemorrhagic telangiectasia is palliative and aimed at reasonable control of the epistaxis because the underlying defect is not curable. Multiple treatment modalities have been tried for years, including packing, cauterization, cryotherapy, estro-

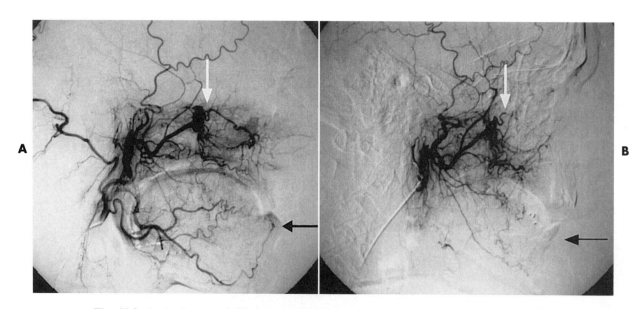

Fig. 45-8. A, Angiogram of right internal maxillary artery (*arrow*) preembolization. Note lower lip for orientation (*arrow*). **B,** Postembolization arteriogram. Note occlusion of the internal maxillary artery (*arrow*), teeth for orientation (*arrow*). (Courtesy of Patricia Thorpe, MD, Creighton University School of Medicine, Omaha, Neb.)

gen therapy, embolization, arterial ligation, and septodermoplasty. General treatment measures include humidification, topical moisturizers, iron, and folate supplementation. Current treatment of the more severe forms of the disease involves covering the nasal surface via septodermoplasty or laser coagulation of the telangiectasias. Efficacy of therapy is difficult to measure because of the variable nature and progression of the disease and the difficulty in quantitating a reduction in epistaxis.

Septodermoplasty

Septodermoplasty consists of the removal of affected septal mucosa and resurfacing the area with a graft. A lateral rhinotomy or alotomy may be used for exposure of the septum. The mucous membrane is removed using an ear currette to gently scrape it away while leaving the periosteum and perichondrium intact. The area then is grafted with a split-thickness or medium-thickness dermis or skin graft harvested from the thigh. The grafts are secured with sutures and antibiotic-impregnated packing.[24] The use of buccal mucosa as a graft material also has been reported.[43] Local pedicled flap use also has been described.[39]

Recurrent bleeding after septodermoplasty may occur as a result of regrowth of telangiectasias in the graft, graft contracture, and residual telangiectasias. Septodermoplasty may produce obstruction of the nares as a result of scarring and contracture. Crusting and dryness occur with a split-thickness skin graft, but are less of a problem when dermis is used. Septal perforation is a potential complication of septodermoplasty.[39,43]

Laser photocoagulation

Since the 1970s, laser photocoagulation has been advocated for treatment of epistaxis in patients with hereditary hemorrhagic telangiectasia. The carbon dioxide laser was initially used, but problems with intraoperative bleeding limited its usefulness. Successful management of nasal telangiectasias has been reported with use of the argon, potassium-titanyl-phosphate, and neodymium:yttrium-aluminum-garnet (Nd:YAG) lasers. Energy from these lasers is absorbed by hemoglobin, making them useful for coagulation and hemostasis. These lasers have the benefit of a flexible fiberoptic delivery system. Rigid fiberoptic endoscopes may be used to facilitate intranasal use of the laser fiber.

Telangiectasias usually are treated during topical or local anesthesia, although general anesthesia may be used if severe bleeding is anticipated. The telangiectasia is treated centripetally, working from the periphery to the center of the lesion until it blanches and flattens.[4] This approach tends to avoid active bleeding from the lesion. If bleeding occurs, the fiber may be used in a contact mode, or electrocoagulation may be needed. Levine and Mehta,[22] Rebeiz,[39] and Blitzer[4] report specifics of power and duration of laser applications for treatment of telangiectasias. Laser treatment is palliative, so repetitive treatments are needed. The majority of patients treated with laser photocoagulation had improvement in control of their bleeding, with most authors evaluating laser photocoagulation as a reasonable treatment option for this disease.[4,22,39,43]

SEPTAL HEMATOMA

Septal hematomas may result from accidental or surgical nasal trauma. Early recognition and treatment is necessary to prevent long-term functional and cosmetic deformity. Septal hematoma separates the perichondrium from the septal cartilage, compromising the vascular supply of the cartilage. The resulting cartilage necrosis may lead to septal perforation or a saddle nose deformity. Alternatively, a broadened, fibrotic septum develops, producing nasal obstruction.[20] If a hematoma progresses to an abscess, systemic complications of sepsis and meningitis may develop.

Prevention

Postoperative septal hematoma is caused by bleeding into the space created by the surgical dissection. Prevention of postoperative hematoma depends on good hemostasis before closure and on obliteration of the dead space created by elevation of the mucoperichondrium during the septoplasty. Postoperative nasal packs are used to maintain approximation of the septal flaps, but they usually are removed within 24 to 48 hours postoperatively. Bleeding then may occur with removal of the packs. Septal splints are another common method used to compress the nasal septum and may be left in place for a longer time. Splints tend to only compress the anterior portion of the septum. ''Quilting'' mattress sutures may be placed through the septal flaps and cartilage using an absorbable suture on a $\frac{1}{2}''$ straight needle (SC-1 nasal septal cutting, 4-0 plain gut).

With any of these methods, care should be taken to avoid mucosal necrosis with excessively tight sutures or packing. A method of suction drainage to remove fluid and coapt the mucosal flaps to prevent septal hematoma has been advocated by Carraway.[6]

Diagnosis and management

Early diagnosis and management of septal hematoma is essential. Unfortunately, recognition often is delayed. Kryger and Dommerby[20] found patients delayed treatment of septal hematoma from 0 to 9.6 days from trauma to the first doctor visit. They also found delay from the first medical examination to the specialist's examination to range from 0 to 12.1 days.

The diagnosis of septal hematoma should be suspected in any patient who complains of progressive nasal obstruction after nasal trauma or surgery. Frank epistaxis is uncommon in patients with septal hematoma. Evaluation for septal hematoma requires a thorough intranasal examination with a nasal speculum and adequate lighting.

A septal hematoma presents as a large, soft, dark red, or bluish mass, obstructing one or both nares. In patients with

anterior nares, posterior displacement and removal via the oropharynx may be used. Rarely, a lateral rhinotomy may be needed for removal of a very large rhinolith.[7]

Animate foreign bodies

Maggots, leeches, intestinal worms, and insects have been reported in the nasal cavity. These infestations are more commonly found in tropical or warm, dry climates. Animate foreign bodies tend to be seen in patients with poor hygiene and are associated with poor sanitation. Patients with unhealthy noses, such as with ozena, are more susceptible to these problems than healthy patients.

Myiasis (infestation with fly larvae) results from the deposition of fly ova in the human nose. The ova hatches, producing a larval infestation of the nose. The larvae initiate an inflammatory reaction that may range from a mild localized region to massive areas of destruction. Meningitis or sepsis may result. Recommended management consists of instillation of a weak solution of chloroform followed by removal of the larvae.[2,41]

Ascaris lumbricoides is one of the most common intestinal parasites found in humans. Infestation occurs via ingestion of mature eggs in fecally contaminated food. The larvae hatch in the small intestine, where they penetrate the mucosa and travel via blood vessels and lymphatics to the liver or heart. The larvae then move to the lung, perforate the alveolar walls, migrate up the trachea into the pharynx, and then travel back down the alimentary tract. At times during the transit, the worms may be coughed or vomited into the nose. Severe congestion and purulent rhinorrhea occurs. Diagnosis is confirmed by visualization of the 6- to 10-inch worm. The parasitic infestation is treated systemically with mebendazole. The worms should be removed from the nasal cavity.[2,41]

REFERENCES

1. Aassar OS, Friedman CM, White RI: The natural history of epistaxis in hereditary hemorrhagic telangiectasia, *Laryngoscope* 101:977, 1991.
2. Baluyot ST: *Foreign bodies in the nasal cavity*. In Paparella MM, Shumrick DA, editors: *Otolaryngology head and neck*, vol 3, Philadelphia, 1973, WB Saunders.
3. Batsakis JG: *Tumors of the head and neck*, ed 2, Baltimore, 1979, Williams & Wilkins.
4. Blitzer A: Laser photocoagulation in the care of patients with Osler Weber Rendu disease, *Oper Tech Otol Head Neck Surg* 5:274, 1994.
5. Cannon CR: Effective treatment protocol for posterior epistaxis: a 10-year experience, *Otol Head Neck Surg* 109:722, 1993.
6. Carraway JH, Mellow CG: Simple suction drainage: an adjunct to septal surgery, *Ann Plast Surg* 24:191, 1990.
7. Carder HM, Hill JJ: Assymptomatic rhinolith: a brief review of the literature and case report, *Laryngoscope* 76:524, 1966.
8. Cohen HA, Goldberg E, Horev Z: Removal of nasal foreign bodies in children, *Clin Pediatr* 32:192, 1993.
9. Das SK: Aetiological evaluation of foreign bodies in the ear and nose, *J Laryngol Otol* 98:989, 1984.
10. Elahi MM and others: Therapeutic embolization in the treatment of intractable epistaxis, *Arch Otol Head Neck Surg* 121:65, 1995.
11. Elden L and others: Angiographic embolization for the treatment of epistaxis: a review of 108 cases, *Otol Head Neck Surg* 111:44, 1994.
12. Gomes CC and others: Button battery as a foreign body in the nasal cavities. Special aspects, *Rhinology* 32:98, 1994.
13. Harrison DFN: Surgical approach to the medial orbital wall, *Ann Otol Rhinol Laryngol* 90:415, 1981.
14. Hartley C, Axon PR: The foley catheter in epistaxis management—a scientific appraisal, *J Laryngol Otol* 108:399, 1994.
15. Jensen PF and others: Episodic nocturnal hypoxia and nasal packs, *Clin Otol* 16:433, 1991.
16. Juselius H: Epistaxis: a clinical study of 1724 patients, *J Laryngol Otol* 88:317, 1974.
17. Kersch R, Wolff A: Severe epistaxis: protecting the nasal ala, *Laryngoscope* 100:1348, 1990.
18. Krempl GA, Noorily AD: Use of oxymetazoline in the management of epistaxis, *Ann Otol Rhinol Laryngol* 104:704, 1995.
19. Krespi YP, Ling EH: Laser management of anterior epistaxis, *Oper Tech Otol Head Neck Surg* 5:271, 1994.
20. Kryger H, Dommerby H: Haematoma and abscess of the nasal septum, *Clin Otolaryngol* 12:125, 1987.
21. Langer M, Terry O: The posterior ethmoid artery in severe epistaxis, *Otol Head Neck Surg* 106:101, 1992.
22. Levine HL, Mehta A: Management of nasal mucosal telangiectasias, *Oper Tech Otol Head Neck Surg* 2:173, 1991.
23. Loftus BC, Blitzer A, Cozine K: Epistaxis, medical history and the nasopulmonary reflex: what is clinically relevant? *Otol Head Neck Surg* 110:363, 1994.
24. Lore JM Jr: *An atlas of head and neck surgery,* ed 3, Philadelphia, 1988, WB Saunders.
25. Maceri DR, Makielski KH: Intraoral ligation of the maxillary artery for posterior epistaxis, *Laryngoscope* 94:737, 1984.
26. Marcus MJ: Nasal endoscopic control of epistaxis: a preliminary report, *Otol Head Neck Surg* 102:273, 1990.
27. McFerran DJ, Edmonds SE: The use of balloon catheters in the treatment of epistaxis, *J Laryngol Otol* 107:197, 1993.
28. McGarry GW: Nasal endoscope in posterior epistaxis: a preliminary evaluation, *J Laryngol Otol* 105:428, 1991.
29. McGarry GW, Gatehouse S, Vernham G: Idiopathic epistaxis, haemostasis and alcohol, *Clin Otol* 20:174, 1995.
30. McQueen CT and others: Orbital osteology: a study of the surgical landmarks, *Laryngoscope* 105:783, 1995.
31. Metson R, Lane R: Internal maxillary artery ligation for epistaxis: an analysis of failures, *Laryngoscope* 98:760, 1988.
32. Nandapalen V, McIlwain JC: Removal of nasal foreign bodies with a Fogarty biliary balloon catheter, *J Laryngol Otol* 108:758, 1994.
33. O'Leary-Stickney K, Makielski K, Weymuller EA: Rigid endoscopy for the control of epistaxis, *Arch Otol Head Neck Surg* 118:966, 1992.
34. Padgam N: Epistaxis: anatomical and clinical correlates, *J Laryngol Otol* 104:308, 1990.
35. Palmer O and others: Button battery in the nose—an unusual foreign body, *J Laryngol Otol* 108:871, 1994.
36. Pearson BW, Mackenzie RG, Goodman WS: The anatomical basis of transantral ligation of the maxillary artery in severe epistaxis, *Laryngoscope* 79:969, 1969.
37. Peery WH: Clinical spectrum of hereditary hemorrhagic telangiectasia (Osler-Weber-Rendu disease), *Am J Med* 82:989, 1987.
38. Quine SM and others: Microscope and hot wire cautery management of 100 consecutive patients with acute epistaxis—a superior method to traditional packing, *J Laryngol Otol* 108:845, 1994.
39. Rebeiz EE, Parks S, Shapshay SM: Management of epistaxis in hereditary hemorrhagic telangiectasia with neodymium:yttrium-aluminum-garnet laser photocoagulation, *Oper Tech Otol* 2:177, 1991.
40. Romaniuk CS and others: Case report: an unusual cause of epistaxis: non-traumatic intracavernous aneurysm, *Br J Radiol* 66:942, 1993.
41. Shapiro RS: *Foreign bodies of the nose*. In Bluestone CD, Stool E, Arjana SK, editors: *Pediatric otolaryngology*, Philadelphia, 1983, WB Saunders.

42. Shaw CB, Wax MK, Wetmore SJ: Epistaxis: a comparison of treatment, *Otol Head Neck Surg* 109:60, 1993.

43. Siegel MB and others: Control of epistaxis in patients with hereditary hemorrhagic telangiectasia, *Otol Head Neck Surg* 105:675, 1991.

44. Siniluoto TMJ and others: Embolization for the treatment of posterior epistaxis, *Arch Otol Head Neck Surg* 119:837, 1993.

45. Small M, Maran AGD: Epistaxis and arterial ligation, *J Laryngol Otol* 98:281, 1984.

46. Stafford P, Durham JS: Epistaxis and efficacy of arterial ligation and long-term outcome, *J Otol* 21:252, 1992.

47. Strong EB and others: Intractable epistaxis: transantral ligation vs. embolization: efficacy review and cost analysis, *Otol Head Neck Surg* 113:674, 1995.

48. Strutz J, Schumacher M: Uncontrollable epistaxis, *Arch Otol Head Neck Surg* 116:697, 1990.

49. Toner JG, Walby AP: Comparison of electro and chemical cautery in the treatment of epistaxis, *J Laryngol Otol* 104:617, 1990.

50. Waldron J, Stafford N: Ligation of the external carotid artery for severe epistaxis, *J Otol* 21:249, 1992.

51. Ward PH, Abemayor E: *Current therapy in otolaryngology—head and neck surgery,* Philadelphia 1990, Mosby.

52. Weiss NS: Relation of high blood pressure to headache, epistaxis and selected other symptoms, *N Engl J Med* 287:631, 1972.

53. Wetmore SJ, Scrima L, Hiller FC: Sleep apnea in epistaxis patients treated with nasal packs, *Otol Head Neck Surg* 98:596, 1988.

54. Williams WJ and others: *Hematology,* ed 4, New York, 1990, McGraw-Hill.

55. Wurman LH and others: The management of epistaxis, *Am J Otol* 13:193, 1992.

Chapter 46

Nasal Fractures

Timothy D. Doerr
Richard L. Arden
Robert H. Mathog

EPIDEMIOLOGY

Fracture of the nasal bones is generally considered the most common site-specific bony injury of the facial skeleton. Unfavorable changes in nasal appearance and function may occur where there is a loss of structural integrity. Therefore, the managing physician should render appropriate and timely treatment based on the nature and extent of the injury.

A high incidence of nasal fractures is well reported in both the pediatric[1,12,32,37] and adult patient populations.[33,49,66,67,70] These predominantly retrospective studies of maxillofacial trauma report that nasal bone fractures comprise 14% to 50% of all facial fractures. More precise prospective analyses of trauma—including a study of 1000 maxillofacial fractures by Lundin in 1972[43] and a comprehensive analysis of craniofacial trauma in 935 patients by Hussain and others[34] in 1994—show nasal fractures making up 39% and 45% of facial fractures respectively. Nasal fractures occur more often in male patients by approximately 2:1 and tend to have a higher incidence in the 15- to 30-year age group.[16,30,36,66] In 199 female patients, Murray and Maran[51] note a bimodal distribution with a peak in the 15- to 25-year age group and a second rise in the elderly. Similar observations of increased nasal fractures in the elderly are reported by Falcone and others,[22] and are the result of increased falls.[22] When considered collectively, most adult nasal fractures can be attributed to alterations and sporting injuries, with a lesser number resulting from motor vehicle accidents, falls, and miscellaneous causes. The number of fractures from a specific etiology varies according to the makeup and locality of the study population, with alcohol often having a contributory role.[34,51]

In children, a similar male to female ratio of at least 2:1 is reported by most authors.[1,7,19] Others, however, fail to find significant gender differences.[18] In contrast to adult nasal injuries, pediatric fractures are more likely to result from play accidents and athletics rather than fights and motor vehicle injuries.

PATHOGENESIS

Because of its prominent position, central location, and the low breaking strength of its skeletal support, the nose is particularly susceptible to fracture. Swearinger[72] determined that the nasoethmoidal complex has a maximum tolerable impact force before fracture of 35 to 80 grams. These forces are relatively small compared with those required for other fractures of the facial skeleton.[54,72] The pattern and extent of the fracture varies as a function of the site, direction, and intensity of the impact, as well as nasal bone density. In general, younger patients are more prone to fracture-dislocations of larger nasoseptal segments, whereas older patients with brittle osteoporotic bone are more susceptible to comminution.[17]

The paired nasal bones project like a tent on the frontal processes of the maxilla and join in the midline. Beneath this junction lies the nasal septum, which provides little support as a midline scaffold. The thicker, superior portion of the nasal bones joins with the nasal process of the frontal bone and is an area of relative stability. Approximately 80% of nasal fractures occur at the transition zone between this thicker proximal and the thinner distal segments in the lower one third to one half of the nasal bones.[39]

Trauma to the cartilaginous structures of the nose, by

virtue of their attachments to and interconnections with the nasal bones, is incurred either directly (usually from frontal or inferior directed forces) or indirectly (from lateral blows). The resilient properties of the upper and lower lateral cartilages, with their loose associations to bony structures, permit considerable absorption and dissipation of impact energy. As a result, dislocation, displacement, or avulsion injuries are more common than true fractures. In contrast, the cartilaginous septum is posteriorly interposed between two bony structures (the perpendicular plate of the ethmoid and the vomer), with a strong osseochondral junction. Weak areas of the cartilaginous dorsum (between the septum and upper lateral cartilages and just below the Y-shaped juncture of the upper lateral cartilages), and the weak connections between the septal cartilage and maxillary crest, account for a high incidence of fracture-dislocation of the septum following nasal trauma.[72] Most commonly, fracture lines are oriented vertically in the caudal portion of the septum and horizontally further posteriorly.[40]

The incidence of maxillofacial trauma in children is significantly less than that of adults. Social, anatomic, and developmental differences help explain this observation. Among the important physical factors in children are the small size and low weight that limit impact forces, along with increased soft tissue to shield the facial skeleton. Finally, a more stable skeletal lattice resulting from developing bone, mixed dentition, and immature pneumatization better distributes and absorbs traumatic forces.[44,71]

Despite these protective elements, the behavior of children results in nasal trauma with some frequency.* The patterns and types of injury are, however, distinct from those of adults. A child's nasal bones are small and the cartilaginous part of the nose is relatively large. In the newborn the length to width ratio of the nose is approximately 1:1, whereas in adults this ratio becomes 3:1 (Fig. 46-1).[3] Nasal injuries in younger children are more apt to occur in cartilage than in bone. The flexibility and resilience of cartilage and bone in children account for the tendency of these structures to fracture without any significant displacement (greenstick fractures). In many cases the dislocated bones and cartilage will spring back to normal position.[47]

Cartilaginous structures are able to distort and buckle with impact. This flexibility helps to explain the greater degree of force needed to cause nasal fractures following frontal and inferior blows as compared with the more common lateral blows, with which no significant soft tissue intermediary exists. These clinical observations are confirmed in cadaver experiments by Murray and others,[52] where a lateral force of 16 to 66 kilopascal (kPa) is required to cause a bony displacement of the dorsum, compared with a 114 to 312 kPa frontal force. In this model system, lateral injury patterns involve an ipsilateral fracture just above the nasomaxillary suture and a contralateral fracture immediately below the

* Refs. 12, 29, 32, 37, 67, 70.

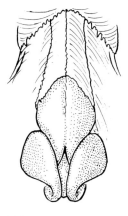
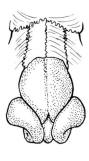

Fig. 46-1. Demonstration of relative proportions of cartilage and bones in the nose of an adult and child. In the adult, nasal bones are three times longer than their width. In the child, the length of the nasal bone nearly equals the width.

dorsum, associated with a cartilaginous septal fracture extending into the perpendicular ethmoid plate. The larger frontal forces tend to drive the caudal portions of the nasal bones posteriorly, causing an associated septal fracture in the upper part of the perpendicular plate parallel to the dorsum. These findings are consistent with an earlier report by Harrison[30] in which the pattern of septal fractures and displacement were relatively constant, irrespective of the direction of nasal trauma (frontal versus lateral). Harrison's detailed analysis of septal injuries describes the fractures as beginning just behind the nasal spine and running posteriorly approximately 2 to 3 mm above the bone-cartilage interface with the vomer, then passing backward and upward into the perpendicular ethmoid plate, and finally turning forward below the cribriform plate and the upper part of the nasal bones.[30]

Injury to the septum and the resultant effects on nasal appearance and function have been well studied. Early work by Fry[25,26] using cadaveric cartilage, and retrospective clinical data suggested that injury to the septal surface can activate interlocked stresses that will cause the cartilage to twist. Harrison[30] disputes this theory and attributes the progressing deformity to a lack of centralization of the displaced septal fracture. This latter theory is further supported by later experimental and clinical studies.[16,50,52,53]

CLASSIFICATION

As with fractures at other anatomic sites, there is no uniformly accepted classification system for nasal fractures. Most of the existing classification schema are based on the direction of the applied force and are characterized as frontal or lateral injuries of varying degrees (Fig. 46-2).* The classification systems vary greatly in complexity and range from a simple anatomically-based system suggested by Haug and

* Refs. 12, 30, 31, 63, 67, 70.

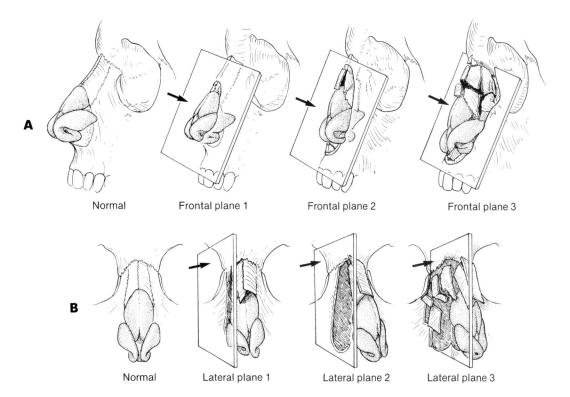

Fig. 46-2. The concept of forces of impact and levels (planes) of destruction. **A,** With frontal forces, fracture can involve (1) nasal tip; (2) nasal dorsum, septum, and anterior nasal spine; and (3) frontal processes of maxilla, lacrimal, and ethmoid bones. **B,** With laterooblique forces, fractures can involve (1) ipsilateral nasal bone; (2) contralateral nasal bone and septum; and (3) nasal bones, frontal processes of maxilla, and lacrimal bone.

Prather,[31] to more complex systems like that of Murray and others.[53] This latter system suggests seven fracture types and emphasizes the deviation of the nasal pyramid from the midline as the clinical predictor of management outcome.

One classification system that successfully addresses frontal and lateral injury patterns is that of Stranc and Robertson.[70] The less common frontal types are divided into three categories depending on the depth of the injury. Plane 1 injuries do not extend behind a line from the lower end of the nasal bones to the anterior nasal spine. In these injuries, the majority of the impact is transmitted to the lower cartilaginous vault and tip of the nasal bones. Separation and avulsion injuries of the upper lateral cartilages may occur, and occasionally posterior dislocation of the septal and alar cartilages may be encountered. Plane 2 injuries involve the external nose, the nasal septum, and the anterior nasal spine. More extensive deviation of the nasal bones, with flattening or splaying, and deviation of the septal cartilage with mucoperichondrial tears, segmental overriding, or loss of central support are seen in this classification. Plane 3 injuries extend to involve orbital and possibly intracranial structures. These injuries typically involve comminution of the nasal bones and extend to the adjacent bony structures including the frontal processes of the maxilla, ethmoid labyrinth, and lacrimal bones. Upward extensions may involve the cribriform and orbital plates of the frontal bones. Injuries to the nasal septum are severe, and they often are associated with collapse and telescoping of septal fragments.

Other classifications use subclasses to include fractures of the nasal tip and anterior nasal spine, fractures of the dorsum with or without septal deflection, and comminuted nasal fractures.[30] Courtiss[12] describes specific additional combinations of depression and twisting. Septal injuries similarly can be classified as dislocations, fractures, or fracture-dislocations.[33]

Lateral impact injuries are the more common injury pattern.[8,10] In a prospective study by Illum and others,[36] of 173 consecutive nasal fractures, 66% were of the lateral type, whereas only 13% were frontal injuries. This lateral type of injury produces a depression of the ipsilateral nasal bone and typically involves the lower half of the nasal bone, part of the nasal process of the maxilla, and a variable amount of the pyriform margin.[30] When the impact force is weak, nasal bone displacement is usually present without septal fracture. More significant forces, on the other hand, will cause medial displacement of the ipsilateral nasal bone and lateral displacement of the contralateral nasal bone. In these instances the septum is dislocated or fractured as well.

Because nasal fractures frequently occur along with other maxillofacial injuries, the complete classification should include all the known injuries. In severe trauma, the nasal fracture is often associated with a midfacial injury involving the frontal, ethmoid, and lacrimal bones.[45] Such an injury will cause distortion of the glabellar angle, displacement of the medial canthal ligaments, and possible disruption of the lacrimal collecting system. The medial wall of the orbit may be fractured and displaced, and medial rectus entrapment and enophthalmos may occur. Fractures extending to the cribriform plate can be associated with cerebrospinal fluid (CSF) leaks, disruption of olfactory function, and brain injury. Fractures extending laterally across the orbital floor may indicate a maxillary Le Fort I, II, or III fracture. An open-bite deformity and posterior maxillary displacement along with lengthening of the lower face are further indications of such fractures.

DIAGNOSTIC ASSESSMENT

History

Fractures of the nasal skeleton are associated with a history of impact to the midfacial area. The mechanism of injury is important because the location, magnitude, and direction of the blows can provide information to help anticipate and predict the extent of injury. A patient whose face strikes the dashboard in an auto accident is considered to have a potentially more significant injury than a patient assaulted with a closed fist. Consideration of the nature of the applied force with respect to force per unit of area is equally important. A narrow, solid object striking a well-defined area over the nasal dorsum will concentrate the energy of impact and result in more extensive localized injury (comminution) than an impact that delivers the same force over a greater surface area.

The appearance and function of the nose before the injury should be learned. Previous injuries to the nose may offer insight into existing deformities and nasal airway complaints. Preexisting nasal deformities are quite common; 30% of patients in a study by Mayell[46] had premorbid nasal abnormalities. Photographs of the patient taken before the injury can help provide a gross baseline of nasal contour and midline relationships. Information regarding nasal obstruction and loss of smell following nasal injury should also be obtained. A history of nasal bleeding usually indicates a mucosal laceration. The past medical history should be investigated for nasal allergy, sinusitis, illicit use of inhalant substances, previous septonasal surgery, and any systemic or localized inflammatory disorders. A regional review of systems should identify associated injury to adjacent structures. A loss of consciousness or change in mental status suggests central nervous system involvement. Changes in visual acuity, gaze restriction, diplopia, regional hypoesthesia, or epiphora warrant the examination of ocular and adnexal structures. Anosmia or hyposmia typically follows acute nasal trauma secondary to mucosal swelling, collection of blood and secretions, or internal derangements, but in-

volvement of the cribriform plate should be considered and investigated. Finally, injury to the adjacent maxilla is suggested by complaints of malocclusion and sensory deficits in the cheek and anterior dentition.

Physical examination

All nasal injuries, regardless of mechanism, warrant a thorough internal and external examination of the nose. This is especially true in children in whom greenstick fractures are common and a minimal external deformity can exist with significant internal derangements.[19] The key to a successful examination is patient comfort, adequate lighting, and proper intranasal preparation. With the patient seated in a slightly reclined position, the external nose should be examined from the frontal view and from both sides in oblique and lateral views. Changes in dorsal contour (e.g., humps and abnormal elevations or depressions) should be noted. Abnormal shortening of the nose suggests a loss of central support and telescoping of cartilaginous fragments. This often coexists with a retracted columella, an increased columellar-labial angle, and widening of the base of the nose. In frontal view, abnormal widening or flattening of the nasal root, deviations of the nasal dorsum tip deflections, or the presence of a flat, broad tip may suggest recent or past nasal injury. In the absence of other ocular findings, periorbital ecchymosis is highly suggestive of nasal fracture. In most cases posttraumatic edema masks subtle deformities, and a more accurate external examination is possible after resolution of the swelling 2 to 4 days after the injury.

If ongoing epistaxis has not necessitated earlier treatment, the internal structures of the nose are prepared for examination. All clots must be carefully removed by swab or suction and minor bleeding can usually be controlled by application of a topical vasoconstrictor. Either 0.25% phenylephrine or oxymetazoline hydrochloride administered as a spray or with soaked cotton pledgets are effective. When available, the use of 4% cocaine has the additional advantage of providing topical anesthesia. Following anesthetic effect, the bony pyramid is gently palpated to check for mobility, crepitus, and specific areas of point tenderness. Step deformities are diagnostic of old or new fracture sites.

Intranasal anatomy should be assessed using a nasal speculum and proper external lighting. Abnormal positioning, instability, or abnormal movements of the upper and lower lateral cartilages may suggest avulsion-type injuries, which often coexist with mucosal lacerations. The septum should be checked for discoloration, dislocation, and abnormal swelling. Any suggestion of a septal hematoma is investigated using direct aspiration or a mucosal incision. Because septal deviations can be found in over one half of healthy individuals, abnormal positioning alone is not indicative of septal fracture or dislocation.[35] Bimanual palpation using cotton-tipped applicators placed through each nares and against the septum, is a useful technique to confirm mobility and direct attention to the injury. Septal dislocation may or may not indicate a recent fracture in the adult, whereas a septal deformity is generally considered abnormal in children.[47,57]

Palpation of the anterior nasal spine via the sublabial route should also be performed because fractures in this area are highly correlated with significant septal trauma.[8] Finally, the ascending processes of the maxilla and adjoining orbital rim should be palpated for deformity and crepitus. Paskert and Manson[59] described a technique of bimanual examination using a finger and a Kelly hemostat to assess the stability of the frontal process of the maxilla.

Radiographic evaluation

Although long practiced as ''standard'' in many emergency rooms and trauma centers, radiographic evaluation for routine nasal fractures is now recognized as unnecessary. A number of publications demonstrate the very limited impact these radiographs have on management and outcome.* The major criticism of these radiographs is their unacceptable predictive value owing to high rates of false-negative and false-positive interpretation. In a study by deLacey and others[15] 66% (33 of 50) of healthy patients examined with a Waters' view radiograph (Fig. 46-3) had false-positive readings. These false-positive readings were the result of misinterpretation of the midline and nasomaxillary sutures, and developmental abnormalities of the nasal wall as fractures.

* Refs. 9, 15, 21, 42, 46, 55, 69.

Soft-tissue techniques on profile or lateral view are more accurate in demonstrating fractures of the anterior nasal bones, but do not provide information about lateral displacement. In addition, these views are unable to distinguish recent from old fractures.

Perhaps the greatest weakness in using plain films is their inability to evaluate the injury for appropriate management. Clayton and Lesser[9] report that 25% (7 of 28) of patients required surgical intervention on clinical grounds despite having negative radiograph reports. Conversely, in the deLacey[15] series, radiographically documented cases of nasal fracture required reduction in fewer than 10% of cases. Furthermore, a reliance on radiographs for the diagnosis of a nasal fracture may result in incomplete physical assessment, and complications like septal hematoma will go undetected. Finally, the practice of obtaining routine nasal bone radiographs for medicolegal reasons is no longer invalid.[42]

The management of nasal fractures is based solely on a clinical assessment of appearance and function, and there is no justification for routine radiographs following isolated nasal trauma. However, when associated midfacial injuries are suspected after physical assessment, a facial radiograph series should be done. Computed tomography (CT) scans can be considered when extensive fractures are present.

In a child, radiograph evaluation of nasal trauma is of even less value than in the adult. The fact that the child's nasal bones are small and unfused complicates the interpretation. Furthermore, the majority of injuries occur in the carti-

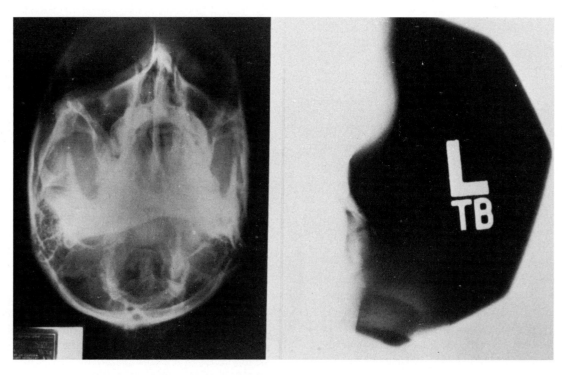

Fig. 46-3. Radiographs demonstrating nasal fracture in Waters' and lateral views. Note comminution of nasal pyramid and depression of nasal bone.

laginous skeleton, which comprises two thirds of the nasal substructure, and cannot be demonstrated by radiograph examination.

MANAGEMENT

Control of bleeding

In patients with recent nasal trauma, bleeding from the nose can be profuse and demand immediate emergency treatment. If application of a topical vasoconstrictor is not successful in controlling the area of hemorrhage, tamponade with gauze packing, balloon catheter, or nasal stent may be required. Ligation or embolization of the feeding maxillary or ethmoid vessels is rarely necessary.

Nasal packing is the most common method for controlling bleeding within the nose. The packing should be placed precisely at the bleeding sites to provide uniform pressure over the entire area. If the bleeding site is located in the anterior part of the nose, anterior packing will usually be sufficient. In such a situation, one half inch plain gauze treated with an antibiotic ointment should be layered from the floor to the roof of the nose. If the bleeding is from a more posterior site, traditional posterior packs may be necessary. Bilateral packing is important for maintaining persistent pressure over a wide area.

Packing will control nasal bleeding in most patients. After 2 to 5 days the packing can be removed, a topical and local anesthetic can be applied, and a reduction of the nasal fractures can be carried out. Occasionally, the patient will continue to bleed, which requires ligation of the internal maxillary artery or the anterior ethmoidal artery. Carotid artery ligation is seldom indicated and rarely effective in controlling persistent bleeding because of its great distance from the hemorrhage site, which permits collateral blood flow to feed the bleeding.

Timing of reduction

Significant swelling of the soft tissues of the nose and surrounding areas can preclude effective early management. Within 5 to 10 days after injury the nasal bones can become somewhat adherent and difficult to move. Fixation is usually observed within 2 to 3 weeks if the patient is young and healthy. In children, fracture fixation requires only one fourth to one half the time as in adults.[44] The surgeon must choose a time for reduction when evaluation can be accurate and the bones are still mobile. Closed reduction should be carried out within 3 to 7 days for children and within 5 to 10 days for adults.

In patients with very little swelling, early reduction can be performed. If the patient is scheduled to be in the operating room for other procedures, valuable anesthesia time can be used to complete the nasal repair. When other significant injuries exist, reduction of a nasal fracture takes low priority and surgical intervention can be delayed.

Open versus closed reduction

Closed reduction has long been practiced as standard treatment for most nasal fractures. Many authors find acceptable cosmetic and functional results using these techniques, and in those patients in whom reduction is not maintained, open reduction can be done months later by a traditional septorhinoplasty.[21,23,36,37] These authors believe that early open reduction, which requires separation of bony fragments from the periosteum, makes accurate rasping impossible. They also cite the additional cost of open reduction and the possibility that the open methods might produce undesirable sequelae as reasons against such an approach.[37]

Surgeons who favor open reduction believe that open techniques achieve better long-term results than the closed methods.[30,38,52,60,74] They suggest that open methods provide better visualization and precise repositioning of the structures. They have also observed more accurate evaluation for hematoma and improved splinting than with closed reduction.

The challenge has been to select the most conservative surgical procedure that would ultimately lead to the best long-term results. Mayell[46] reported good functional and cosmetic results in only one third of patients selected for closed reduction. Harrison's[30] retrospective review of 40 patients found only 13 perfect results.[30] Murray and others[53] offer insight into the possible cause of surgical failure following closed nasal manipulation. Prompted by a 30% to 40% failure rate in their own patients, they studied the mechanics of nasal fractures in fresh cadaver noses and found that when the nasal bones are deviated by more than one half the bridge width, there is a concomitant C-shaped fracture adjacent to the osseochondral junction of the nasal septum. They attribute late failures (deviations) to the interlocking of these fractured septal segments, which drag the mobile nasal bones toward their initially displaced position. The same authors stress the importance of reducing the septal component of an open nasal fracture when there is significant deviation of the bony dorsum to avoid subsequent deformity. A number of other surgeons recognize the advantages of open methods where there has been significant displacement of the nasal septum, bilateral fractures, or unsatisfactory reduction of the nasal and septal components following attempts with the closed approach.[10,16,33,40]

Although closed reduction of nasoseptal fractures remains the mainstay of surgical management in cases of pediatric nasal trauma, indications for open reduction do exist and are similar to those for adults. Stucker, Bryarly, and Shockley[71] point out the difficulty in determining when complete reduction has been achieved with closed techniques in children because the nasal skeleton is largely cartilaginous, making mobilization and recognition of proper positioning more challenging than in adults.[71]

Open techniques may be used when attempts at closed reduction are inadequate, but these should be guided by conservative principles that emphasize repositioning rather than excision of fractured segments. Septal cartilage in children maintains its regenerative potential, and overzealous resections around the septovomerian junction may lead to subsequent growth impairments.[62] Because cartilaginous regeneration arises from interstitial and appositional growth from the perichondrium, open approaches should emphasize preservation of intact mucoperichondrial flaps and investigation of soft tissue.[61]

Part of the difficulty in analyzing the long-term results of nasal fractures in children arises from the difficulty in differentiating the effects of the nasal injury from the surgical intervention. A comparison of cephalometric radiographs by Rock and Brain[65] of 29 adult patients who sustained nasal trauma as children demonstrated significant differences in midfacial growth (smaller forward component, greater downward component in the study group) versus matched controls. By contrast, a study by Pirsig[61] of 261 children who underwent nasal septal reconstruction (involving septoplasty and osteotomies) found no arrest in nasal growth. Similarly, the analysis by Chmielik and others[7] of nasal growth in 159 children after fracture reduction concludes that an adequate reduction (using the closed technique) causes no disturbances in nasal growth. These authors recognize, however, the potential for external nasal deformities resulting from fracture healing, which was consistent with observations by Dommerby and Tos.[18]

It appears that most nasal fractures in children should be managed by closed reduction techniques. Occasionally, conservative open reduction of the septum and nasal bones must be used when closed techniques prove inadequate to correct a severe deformity or marked nasal obstruction. The surgeon should realize that the effect of the nasal trauma if left uncorrected, or the method of open intervention (particularly if aggressive), may influence subsequent midfacial growth.

Prophylactic antibiotics and decongestants

Prophylactic antibiotics are often desirable because most nasal fractures are associated with lacerations of the mucosa or skin and with the attendant potential for bacterial contamination. The antibiotics may also afford some protection against infection if a hematoma should form. Antibiotics commonly selected include penicillin, ampicillin, or cephalosporin derivatives. Saline irrigations are also useful adjuncts to maintain humidification and to clean the mucosa. If obstruction of the nose or paranasal sinuses occurs, decongestants can be added to the medical regimen.

Anesthesia

Surgical procedures to reduce the nasal fractures can be performed in an outpatient or a hospital setting. The choice of location will often depend on the type and extent of the associated injuries, the patient's general condition, and the nature of the treating facility.

Preoperative medication should be administered according to the condition of the patient. Simple nasal fractures in adults can usually be managed with topical and local anesthetics. Using these local techniques is equivalent to using general anesthesia in regard to cosmetic and functional outcomes.[11] Although generally perceived as uncomfortable for patients, Owen, Parker, and Watson[58] administered a patient questionnaire and found that 63% of patients found the procedure no more noxious than a dental filling, and 96% would be willing to undergo the same local anesthesia if the nose was fractured a second time.[58] To further aid in the comfort of patients manipulated under local anesthesia, preoperative sedation is recommended to allay anxiety and can be supplemented intraoperatively with intravenous medications. In a child or young adult, general anesthesia usually is the procedure of choice.

When local sedation is selected, the vibrissae should be trimmed and topical anesthesia achieved through the strategic application of cotton pledgets moistened in a solution of 8 ml of 4% cocaine containing five drops of 1:10,000 epinephrine (Fig. 46-4). This solution will provide excellent vasoconstriction for the duration of the procedure. The pledgets are usually placed beneath the nasal dorsum (ethmoidal nerves), at the posterior edge of the middle turbinate (sphenopalatine nerve), along the septum, and on the floor of the nose for 10 minutes (Fig. 46-5).

After application of topical anesthesia, the surgeon should also infiltrate a local anesthetic to provide external nasal anesthesia and vasoconstriction and to supplement internal mucosal anesthesia (Fig. 46-6). A 2% solution of lidocaine containing 1:100,000 epinephrine should be injected over and beneath the bony nasal dorsum to block the infratrochlear nerve, into the infraorbital foramen bilaterally to block the infraorbital nerve, and at the base of the columella. Additional infiltration of the soft tissues of the nose may be helpful, and the addition of hyaluronidase may facilitate anesthetic dispersion and enhance the resolution of swelling.[33]

Profound local anesthesia is rarely achieved in a recently injured nose because tissue acidosis interferes with the conversion of anesthetic agents to their active state.[8] The addition of sodium bicarbonate in a 1:10 (vol:vol) dilution to the anesthetic mixture may counteract this effect, and also reduce the injection pain associated with acidic solutions.[56] Other injection techniques helpful in minimizing the pain of local injection include: (1) the use of a narrow-gauge needle (30-gauge); (2) injecting in the deep dermal-subcutaneous plane rather than within the dermis; and (3) injecting slowly to avert tissue distention, which is the primary cause of pain.[2]

An alternative technique using only topical anesthesia to manage simple fractures in the adult has been suggested by El-Kholy.[20] This technique uses a combination of topical anesthetic EMLA cream (each gram containing equal parts of lignocaine and prilocaine) applied externally plus intranasal cocainization. The cream has the advantage of good cutaneous penetration and does not require needle injections.

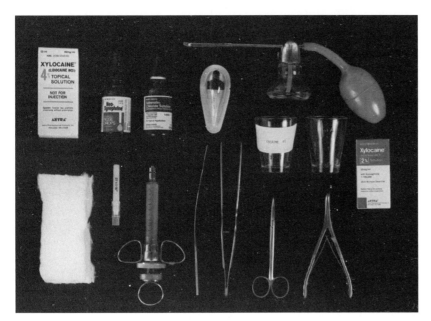

Fig. 46-4. Instruments and solutions used for anesthesia of the nose: lidocaine, 4%; phenylephrine, 0.25%; cotton; metal applicators; cocaine, 4%; epinephrine, 1:10,000; lidocaine, 2%, with epinephrine, 1:100,000; scissors; nasal forceps; nasal speculum; syringe with 27-gauge needle; medicine glasses; dropper; and atomizer.

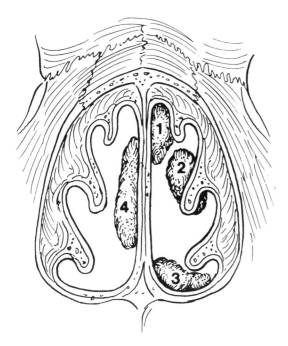

Fig. 46-5. Sites for placement of pledgets containing topical anesthetic: *1,* nasal vault; *2,* posterior portions of the middle turbinate; *3,* floor of the nose; *4,* septum.

These advantages must be weighed against the drug's availability and the need to wait 1 hour following topical application.

When general anesthesia is preferred, application of topical and locally injected anesthetics to augment visualization and control bleeding should be considered. Although most general anesthesia is safe, catecholamines can cause un-

wanted physiologic responses, and the use of these drugs should be discussed with an anesthesiologist.

REDUCTION AND FIXATION

Closed techniques

Reduction of nasal fractures requires simply reversing the direction of force that caused the fracture. Following adequate anesthesia and removal of the cotton pledgets, the nose should be evaluated for additional unsuspected anatomic alterations. Typically, fractures involving the bony nasal pyramid are reduced first, followed by reduction and then stabilization of the septum. For a simple, depressed, unilateral, nasal bone fracture, an appropriate elevator (Boies or Salinger) is inserted into the nose under the depressed fragment (Fig. 46-7) and is elevated into the proper position. The depth of insertion is determined by measuring the distance from the alar rim to the depressed segment on the external surface of the nose, and the instrument is inserted for a similar distance into the nose. The thumb is often used to mark this distance.

The force needed to reduce the depressed fracture depends on the type of fracture and the time elapsed since injury. Steady outward pressure should be applied to the nasal bone to be elevated. Because most unilateral depressed fractures involve some degree of rotation with respect to the dorsal longitudinal axis, an outward and forward movement should be applied along the posterior edge of the fractured nasal bone. The degree of elevation is controlled with external pressure by the other hand, molding the fragments into appropriate position. Tip fractures and isolated nasal bone fractures are easily managed with this technique.

Often, the side opposite the depressed nasal fracture is displaced laterally. In such a situation the depressed side

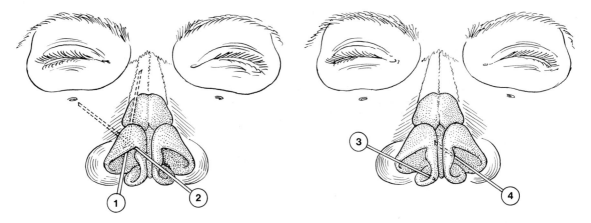

Fig. 46-6. Sites for injection of local anesthesia: *1,* above nasal bones and beneath the skin of dorsum; *2,* infraorbital nerve; *3,* greater palatine nerve at the incisive foramen; *4,* the nasal tip.

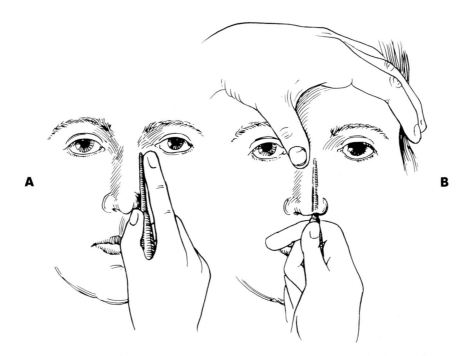

Fig. 46-7. Reduction of nasal fracture. **A,** Boies elevator is placed along the lateral wall of the nose to a point below the nasal frontal angle. Distance to ala is marked with the thumb. **B,** Elevator is placed under depressed nasal bone, lifting it into position; opposite thumb carefully exerts downward pressure on the elevated contralateral bone.

should be elevated first. Then the dorsal pyramid should be slid into the midline. Fortunately, in the newborn, twisting the nose between the fingers may be adequate to provide reduction. Many fractures will require special forceps (Fig. 46-8). For example, Walsham forceps are used to grasp and manipulate the nasal bones directly. The forceps should be inserted so one blade is beneath the bone and the other opposes the external skin surface. The depressed bone is then elevated while the opposite side is moved into position. Deformities of the bony pyramid that persist despite efforts at manual reduction often imply incomplete (greenstick) or impacted fractures, or may indicate preexisting deformities. In such cases, consideration should be given to opening the fracture line with a 3-mm osteotome.

Nasal bones that are significantly comminuted may present problems. Marked instability is best managed with internal splinting (small packing high in the nose of bacitracin-impregnated Nugauze) and an external splint such as Thermoplast or Aquaplast. The internal packing is usually left in place for 2 or 3 days and can then be replaced by small pieces of rolled Oxycel if extended internal support is needed. Care should be taken with the placement of this

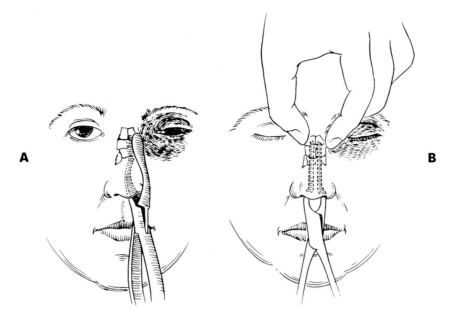

Fig. 46-8. Walsham and Asch forceps for reduction of nasal injury. **A,** Blades of Walsham forceps are used to grasp displaced bone and adjoining soft tissue, and manipulate fragments into correct position. **B,** Asch forceps are used to elevate the dorsum and disimpact the displaced septum simultaneously.

internal packing so the nasal dorsum does not widen excessively.

Nasal fractures that involve the ethmoid complex (typically caused by direct blows to the nose and its base) require additional management strategies that are beyond the scope of this chapter. These injury patterns are complex and frequently involve intracranial as well as orbital-adnexal structures. Extensive nasoethmoid fractures should not be managed by closed reduction techniques alone because these techniques frequently result in the need for secondary corrective surgery.[5,75] To correct nasal collapse and telescoping of nasofrontal-ethmoidal fracture segments, Williamson, Miller, and Sessions[75] advocate the use of an external fixation device following open reduction rather than the more conventional approach using external lead or silastic splints. Gruss[28] has classified nasoethmoid orbit fractures into five types. He advocates an open, direct approach to these fractures with meticulous reduction and fixation. There is also an important role for primary bone grafting to avoid the need for secondary corrective surgery.[24]

When external nasal compression with lead plates is chosen as a management strategy, the undersurface of the plate should be padded with a sponge-like material, such as Ivalon, and the plates positioned as far back as possible to narrow the ethmoid complex and thus support the nasal pyramid (Fig. 46-9). Excessive pressure should be avoided because skin necrosis and permanent marking of the skin may result.[48] Wadley[73] has recommended the use of intranasal silicone wedges with outside compression plates.[73] Courtiss[12] and Sear[68] prefer using spring-like clips, clamps, figure-of-

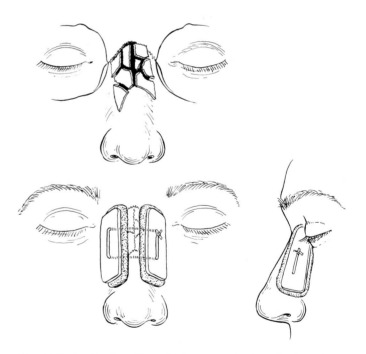

Fig. 46-9. Application of metal plates to maintain reduction of nasal dorsum. Splints can be constructed of soft metal (lead) or plastic material. Fine wire is placed mattress-suture style through splints, comminuted nasal fracture, and septum. Pressure necrosis is avoided by padding the plate and loosening transnasal wire where swelling causes excessive pressure.

seven splints, and digital compression. The efficacy of these methods is questionable.

With reduction of the external nose, the septum will often return to its preinjury position. However, the septum may not be easily reduced, or it may become further dislocated during manipulation of the external nose. If the septum is not properly reduced and stabilized, there can be a loss of dorsal support and obstruction of the nasal airways.

A dislocated septum is best managed by first elevating the nasal pyramid and then applying pressure directly to the displaced portion of the septum to move it back into its proper position. These maneuvers can be simplified with an Asch forceps, which can be used to elevate the dorsum and to reduce the septum between the arms of the instrument. The septum should be inspected carefully and any hematoma should be drained directly through a small mucosal incision. Significant lacerations and displaced mucosa should be replaced in an appropriate anatomic position.

Following the reduction of fractures of the nasal bones and septum, the internal nose should be stabilized with small amounts of packing or septal splints (Fig. 46-10 *A, B*). When the septal injury has resulted in unstable segments, polyethylene plates should be placed on both sides of the septum and sutured together loosely through the septum. A minimal amount of layered packing with bacitracin-impregnated gauze or a commercially available tampon, such as Mericel (Fig. 46-10, *C*), is applied bilaterally. Even pressure should be exerted on the septum to stabilize it in the midline without widening the external nose. Silicone rubber tubing below

the packing or prefabricated splints (Doyle) may be useful for children in whom packing is poorly tolerated.

In most patients, a tape dressing is applied to the external nose (Steri-Strips, Micropore) following application of a hypoallergenic adhesive (Mastisol). The tapes allow symmetrical swelling but resist the formation of a subcutaneous hematoma. An external splint of Thermoplast is then molded to the external nose (see Fig. 46-10, *D*).

All packing and splints are removed 5 days after the reduction. Crusts that develop on the mucous membranes should be gently removed. Normal saline douches or Ocean Mist nasal spray reduces crust formation.

The long-term outcomes from closed reduction are variable. These results reflect the heterogeneity of injury patterns, the variations in the anatomic and physiologic state of the nose prior to injury, and the mode and timing of management following the injury. The results of closed reduction as reported in many series are disappointing.[6,16,30,46,47] Murray and Maran[51] report a failure rate of 30% to 40%. In a subsequent paper the authors attribute the poor results to an unrecognized and unmanaged C-shaped septal fracture that led to the development of nasal deviation during subsequent healing.[52]

Other authors contend that closed reduction approaches afford satisfactory long-term results. Kaban, Mulliken, and Murray[37] note failure in only 2 of 55 patients, while Illum's[35] study of 106 patients reports satisfactory results with regard to appearance in 90% of patients and function in 84% of patients. A survey of patient satisfaction by Crowther and O'Donahue[13] shows similar levels of satisfaction with nasal appearance (85%) and function (79%).

When compared with most other fracture sites, the functional and aesthetic results of managing nasal fractures are less satisfying. The nose, by its location and unique anatomy, contributes to this fact. The nose is visible because it projects from the face and it possesses very little soft tissue cover capable of camouflaging bony irregularities. It also lacks the pull of strong muscles to remodel the bone once fractured, and consists of bone that heals with fibrosis and more soft tissue shrinkage.[51]

Open reduction

Open reduction requires an intimate knowledge of nasal anatomy and function in addition to rhinoplasty techniques. The patient should be informed about the procedure and its potential complications.

Two types of open reduction are performed. One type is aimed at the early correction of nasal fractures that could not be properly reduced in a closed fashion. The other type is used to correct a previously existing nasal deformity or malunion. The latter should be more properly classified as septorhinoplasty to correct an internal and external deformity.

Surgical exposure for open reduction is obtained through either intercartilaginous or intracartilaginous incisions that

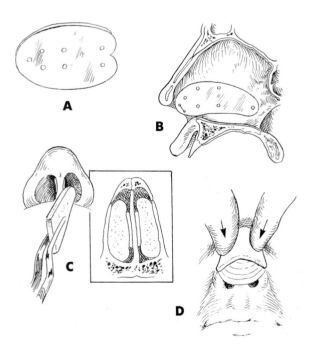

Fig. 46-10. Stabilization of septonasal structures. **A,** Polyethylene splint. **B,** Septal splint maintained in position by mattress suture. **C,** Placement of nasal tampons, correct positioning laterally adjacent to septal splint (*inset*). **D,** Application of external splint.

are extended into a hemitransfixion incision. The dorsal nasal skin is elevated from the upper lateral cartilages in the supraperichondrial plane, with further cephalad dissection proceeding in the subperiosteal plane to expose the nasal bones directly. Care should be exercised in the extent of lateral undermining, so the soft tissue is elevated only slightly beyond the fracture lines. In this way, some degree of external stabilization is afforded by the soft tissue and periosteal attachments. A small osteotome is tapped into the fracture lines and the nasal bones are gently mobilized and then moved into position as previously described (Fig. 46-11). Lateral fracture lines are easily approached through small pyriform margin incisions just anterior to the inferior turbinate attachment.

When the nasal bones are comminuted and fail to reduce properly, open reduction should be considered. In the case of open fractures, access can often be obtained through the wound itself. If additional exposure is needed, intranasal rhinoplasty incisions should be added. The goals of management include conservative débridement of any devitalized tissues, extraction of periosteum and soft tissues from the fracture sites, and proper reduction-stabilization of the fractured segments. Because the periosteal and mucosal sleeves of the bony nasal skeleton provide blood supply as well as an internal tissue splint, excessive undermining of comminuted segments should be avoided.

When confronted with closed nasal fractures that require direct access, an elective transverse incision at the nasofrontal angle can provide adequate exposure to the entire bony pyramid (Fig. 46-12 *A, B*). Alternatively, a coronal incision may be employed when extended exposure is required for repair of more severely comminuted fractures involving the nasal dorsum or frontal sinus. This latter approach can also be used to avoid a facial incision and possible scar.

Following reduction, the nasal bones can be stabilized directly with fine wires and supported with internal and external splinting (Fig. 46-12 *C, D*). Kurihara's[41] results with open reduction and interfragment wire fixation in 21 patients with comminuted nasal fractures showed no depression of the nasal pyramid after 2 years. Renner[64] suggests using slowly absorbing sutures as an alternative to wires in order to avoid the palpable mass or sharp edge occasionally encountered with wire use.

The development of versatile miniature metallic plating systems (microplates) provides the surgeon with an additional fixation option. These pliable plates can be modified to provide the desired nasal shape and give excellent fixation as well as a measure of internal support. When using these plates, precise reconstruction to more stable facial bone is critical, because any deviations in these attachments will be

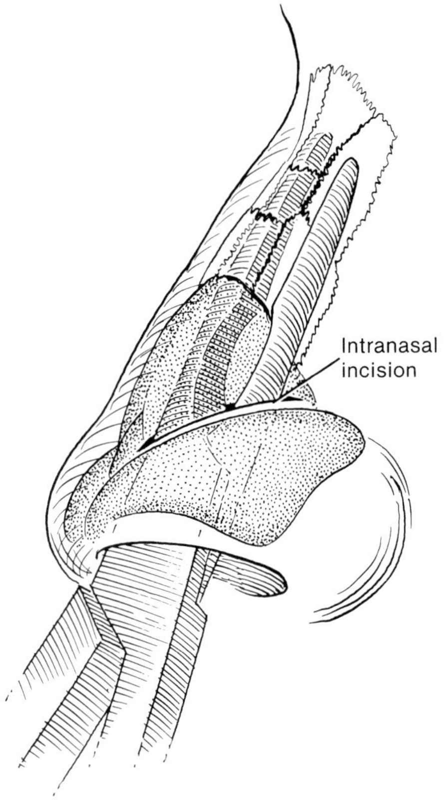

Fig. 46-11. Open reduction and manipulation of nasal bones using Lempert rongeur. After intercartilaginous incision and elevation of the dorsal skin, blades of the Lempert rongeur are inserted on each side of the depressed nasal bone and used to mobilize the bone before placing it in the correct position.

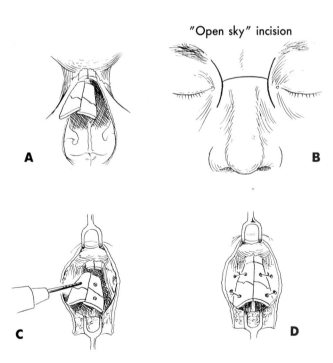

Fig. 46-12. Open management of comminuted nasal fracture. **A,** Unstable comminuted nasal fracture. **B,** Transverse nasal incision with medial orbital extensions to provide exposure to nasoethmoidal complex. **C,** Use of mini-driver to create holes for interosseous wiring. **D,** Interfragmental wiring for stabilization.

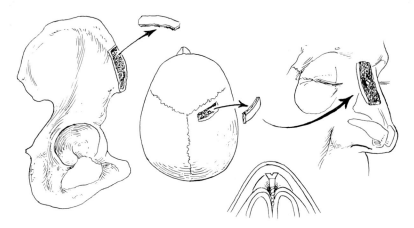

Fig. 46-13. Bone grafting of nasal dorsum. Corticocancellous grafts may be harvested from either the iliac crest or the calvarium and used to augment the bony pyramid. Stabilization can be achieved by the lag screw technique.

apparent in the reconstructed nose. Similarly, the plates and screws should be as thin and flush as possible to minimize palpation under the thin nasal skin.[64]

Although rare, there may be instances in which reduction of the remaining bone fragments fails to achieve the necessary projection and support of the nasal skeleton. In these cases, primary bone grafting should be considered (Fig. 46-13). David and Moore[14] report successful use of cantilever nasal bone grafts with miniscrew fixation using a 2-mm, countersunk, self-tapping lag screw. The authors point to the advantages of rigid stability including rapid bone healing and decreased bony resorption afforded by lag screw fixation over that of interosseous wiring.

Septal injury can also be managed using an open technique. If the septum will not stay in position after reduction, or if an obvious displacement of cartilage or bone persists, the offending pieces can be trimmed or scored and replaced in satisfactory position. The usual approach is through a Killian incision. Following elevation of a mucoperichondrium flap on one side, the fragments are visualized and repositioned. Clark[8] and Harrison[30] note good results with resection of horizontal and vertical sections of the septum compared with simple manipulative techniques (Fig. 46-14). Classic work by Fry[25,26] emphasizes the importance of scoring the concave or compressed side (Fig. 46-15). Occasionally an inferior strip of cartilage must be removed from the maxillary crest to allow the cartilage to swing back into a midline position. Even in children this method can be applied without damage to growth of the nasal skeleton.[3,4,47,57,61] When the septal reduction cannot be maintained, the suture techniques described by Wright[76] can be used (Fig. 46-16). Intranasal splints and packing can be placed to help support the repositioned septum.

A number of options are available to successfully manage nasal trauma. The methods employed need to be tailored to each patient and injury. By carefully selecting the appropri-

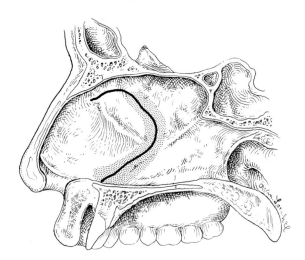

Fig. 46-14. C-shaped septal deformity (*dark line*) that may contribute to subsequent displacements of nasal contour. Resection of horizontal and vertical components along the fracture line (*stippled area*) allows proper repositioning of the septum.

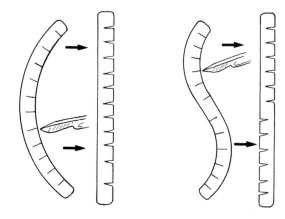

Fig. 46-15. Release of interlocked stresses of cartilaginous septum, according to Fry.[25,26] As a result of scoring with a knife, the septum should be moved to the vertical midline position.

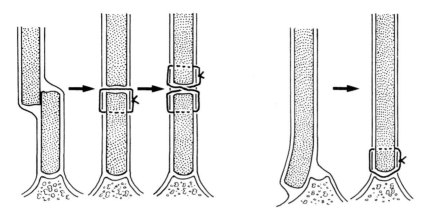

Fig. 46-16. Cartilage fixation suture described by Wright.[76] Fixation sutures should have one arm going through the fracture site. Figure-of-eight design can be used for greater stability. Sutures are also useful for maintaining septum in position on maxillary crest and anterior nasal spine.

ate intervention (Fig. 46-17), the surgeon can restore nasal function and appearance.

COMPLICATIONS

Septal hematoma

As a result of nasal trauma, bleeding can develop in the subperichondrial plane of the septum. With fractures of the septum, blood can collect on both sides of the cartilage. If the hematoma is not drained, irreversible damage can occur to the underlying cartilage. Pressure on the cartilage, coupled with a reduced blood supply from the elevated perichondrium, makes the tissues more susceptible to ischemic necrosis and infection. Irreversible damage can occur in 3 to 4 days, with loss of cartilage in important areas of the nose leading to a saddle deformity and retraction of the columella.

Although septal hematoma can occur in all age groups, it is a frequent complication of nasal injury in a child. It is suspected that the softer cartilage of children predisposes them to a more significant injury.[32]

The diagnosis of septal hematoma is made on finding persistent nasal pain and excessive swelling of the septum. Once the condition is suspected, the hematoma must be treated immediately. Following adequate topical anesthesia, one or several small incisions should be made through the mucoperichondrium to allow evacuation of the blood and prevent further accumulation.

If significant loss of cartilage exists at the time of management, Holt[33] recommends immediate autogenous auricular cartilage grafts. The perpendicular plate of the ethmoid is also a suitable implant source.[57]

To prevent further accumulation of blood, the surgeon should leave the incision on the septum open or should suture a small Penrose drain into the incision. Suction drainage from vacuum tubes can be used, but application of gentle, firm pressure from plastic splints or intranasal packing is simple and effective. Antibiotic coverage is essential to prevent infection.

Managing Nasal Trauma

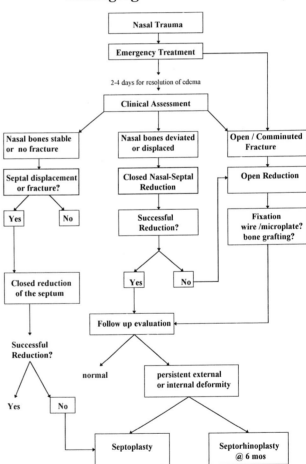

Fig. 46-17. A management algorithm for nasal trauma.

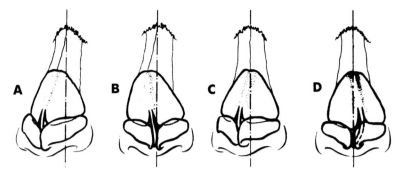

Fig. 46-18. Nasal trauma sequelae. **A,** Deviation to right bony and cartilaginous parts. **B,** Deviation of bony pyramid to right and cartilaginous part to left. **C,** Deviation of cartilaginous part to right. **D,** Deviation of cartilaginous part to left. (From Farrior R: *Management of late sequelae of nasal fractures.* In Mathog RH, editor: *Maxillofacial trauma,* Baltimore, 1984, Williams & Wilkins.)

Nasal dorsum hematoma

Hematoma can develop along the dorsum of the nose; this is usually associated with a tearing of the upper lateral cartilages from the nasal bones.[32] Because pressure necrosis of the cartilage can occur, the condition must be recognized and treated immediately. The hematoma should be evacuated through external or internal incisions, and antibiotics should be administered to prevent infection.

Infection

Although infections of the nose rarely occur following trauma, every precaution should be taken to prevent their development. Septal hematomas are particularly susceptible to this complication. Patients incapacitated by chronic disease or malnutrition are also predisposed to infection.

Early diagnosis of infection in the nose is critical. Persistent pain, swelling, and redness are important signs and symptoms. As a general rule, patients with facial trauma should be treated with prophylactic antibiotics. If infection occurs, cultures should be obtained immediately and antibiotics selected to match the sensitivity of the microorganisms. Adequate drainage is important and packing should be used sparingly.

External and internal deformities

If residual deformity or nasal obstruction persists after closed reduction of nasal fractures, open reduction should be performed as soon as possible. The fragments are carefully mobilized and then properly reduced and stabilized in position.

Patients who desire a reduction rhinoplasty when a posttraumatic deformity is being corrected will require a controlled septorhinoplasty. The ideal period for such corrective surgery is usually 3 to 6 months after injury, once all swelling has disappeared and the bones have become completely stable.[21,23,67]

In children, the timing of revision surgery is somewhat controversial. When the deformity is minimal, the surgery can be delayed until the child is 15 or 16 years of age, when facial growth is nearly complete. This is a conservative approach with little chance for additional damage to growth centers. However, if significant deformity or dysfunction exists, early precise intervention is indicated.[68] Kane and Kane[38] report that repositioning techniques in children do no harm. Bernstein[4] and Pirsig[61] found minimal problems in the development of the nose as long as the surgery is conservative and removal of tissue is minimal.

Farrior[23] characterized the deformity following nasal trauma (Fig. 46-18).[23] The common sequelae include a relative hump, a wide nasal dorsum, depression of the nasal dorsum, depression of the cartilaginous tip, deviation of the nose, splaying of the tip, saddle deformity, and columella retraction. Whether one can develop a true hump from a fracture or from altered growth centers is a matter of conjecture. Septal deflections, spurs, and complex angulations can also occur. With previous mucosal lacerations, one can expect some synechiae and intranasal scarring. Most late deformities and dysfunction must be handled with standard septorhinoplasty and soft tissue techniques.

REFERENCES

1. Anderson PJ: Fractures of the nasal skeleton in children, *Injury* 26:47, 1995.
2. Arndt KA, Burton C, Noe JM: Minimizing the pain of local anesthesia, *Plast Reconstr Surg* 72:676, 1983.
3. Bailey BJ, Caruso VH: Maxillofacial injury, *Adv Otorhinolaryngol* 23: 155, 1978.
4. Bernstein L: Early submucous resection of nasal septal cartilage, *Arch Otolaryngol* 97:273, 1973.
5. Beyer CK, Fabian RL, Smith B: Naso-orbital fractures, complications and treatment, *Ophthalmology* 89:456, 1982.
6. Bowers DG, Lynch JB: Management of facial fractures, *South Med J* 70:910, 1970.
7. Chmielik M and others: Reduction of nasal fractures in children, *Int J Pediatr Otorhinolaryngol* 11:1, 1986.
8. Clark WD: Nasal and nasal septal fractures, *Ear Nose Throat J* 62:25, 1983.

9. Clayton MI, Lesser THJ: The role of radiography in the management of nasal fractures, *J Laryngol Otol* 100:797, 1986.

10. Colton JJ, Beekhuis GJ: Management of nasal fractures, *Otolaryngol Clin North Am* 19:73, 1986.

11. Cook JA and others: A randomized comparison of manipulation of the fractured nose under local and general anesthesia, *Clin Otolaryngol* 15:343, 1990.

12. Courtiss EH: Septorhinoplasty of the traumatically deformed nose, *Ann Plast Surg* 5:443, 1978.

13. Crowther JA, O'Donoghue GM: The broken nose: does familiarity breed neglect? *Ann R Coll Surg Engl* 62:259, 1987.

14. David DJ, Moore MH: Cantilever nasal bone grafting with miniscrew fixation, *Plast Reconstr Surg* 83:728, 1989.

15. deLacey GJ and others: The radiology of nasal injuries: problems of interpretation and clinical relevance, *Br J Radiol* 50:412, 1977.

16. Dickson MG, Sharpe DT: A prospective study of nasal fractures, *J Laryngol Otol* 100:543, 1986.

17. Dingman RO: The *management of facial injuries and fractures of the facial bones*. In Converse JM, editor: *Reconstructive plastic surgery*, Philadelphia, 1964, WB Saunders.

18. Dommerby H, Tos M: Nasal fractures in children—long-term results, *ORL J Otorhinolaryngol Relat Spec* 47:272, 1985.

19. East CA, O'Donoghue G: Acute nasal trauma in children, *J Pediatr Surg* 22:308, 1987.

20. El-Kholy A: Manipulation of the fractured nose using topical local anesthesia, *J Laryngol Otol* 103:580, 1989.

21. Facer GW: A blow to the nose, *Postgrad Med* 70:83, 1981.

22. Falcone PA and others: Maxillofacial trauma in the elderly: a comparative study, *Plast Reconstr Surg* 86:443, 1990.

23. Farrior R: *Management of late sequelae of nasal fractures*. In Mathog RH, editor: *Maxillofacial trauma*, Baltimore, 1984, Williams & Wilkins.

24. Froedel JL: Management of the nasal dorsum in central facial injuries, *Arch Otolaryngol Head Neck Surg* 121:307, 1995.

25. Fry HJH: Interlocked stresses in human septal nasal cartilage, *Br J Plast Surg* 19:276, 1966.

26. Fry HJH: Nasal skeleton trauma and the interlocked stresses on the nasal septal cartilage, *Br J Plast Surg* 20:146, 1967.

27. Goode RL, Spooner TR: Management of nasal fractures in children: a review of current practices, *Clin Pediatr* 11:526, 1972.

28. Gruss JS: Naso-ethmoid-orbital fractures: classification and role of primary bone grafting, *Plast Reconstr Surg* 75:303, 1985.

29. Grymer LF, Gutierrez C, Stoksted P: Nasal fractures in children: influence on the development of the nose, *J Laryngol Otol* 99:735, 1985.

30. Harrison DH: Nasal injuries: their pathogenesis and treatment, *Br J Plast Surg* 32:57, 1979.

31. Haug RH, Prather JL: The closed reduction of nasal fractures: an evaluation of two techniques, *J Oral Maxillofac Surg* 49:1288, 1991.

32. Hinderer KH: Nasal problems in children, *Pediatr Ann* 5:499, 1976.

33. Holt GR: Immediate open reduction of nasal septal injuries, *Ear Nose Throat J* 57:343, 1978.

34. Hussain K and others: A comprehensive analysis of craniofacial trauma, *J Trauma* 36:34, 1994.

35. Illum P: Long-term results after treatment of nasal fractures, *J Laryngol Otol* 100:273, 1986.

36. Illum P and others: Role of fixation in the treatment of nasal fractures, *Clin Otolaryngol* 8:191, 1983.

37. Kaban LB, Mulliken JB, Murray JE: Facial fractures in children, *Plast Reconstr Surg* 59:15, 1977.

38. Kane AP, Kane LA: Open reduction of nasal fractures, *J Otolaryngol* 7:183, 1978.

39. Kazanjian VH, Converse JM: *The surgical treatment of facial injuries*, Baltimore, 1959, Williams & Wilkins.

40. Krause C: *Nasal fractures: evaluation and repair*. In Mathog RH, editor: *Maxillofacial trauma*, Baltimore, 1984, Williams & Wilkins.

41. Kurihara K: Open reduction and interfragment wire fixation of comminuted nasal fractures, *Ann Plast Surg* 24:179, 1990.

42. Logan M, O'Driscoll K, Masterson J: The utility of nasal bone radiographs in nasal trauma, *Clin Radiol* 49:192, 1994.

43. Lundin K and others: One thousand maxillofacial and related fractures at the ENT-clinic in Gothenburg: a two-year prospective study, *Acta Otolaryngol* 75:359, 1972.

44. Martinez SA: Nasal fractures: what to do for a successful outcome, *Postgrad Med* 82:71, 1987.

45. Mathog RH: *Post-traumatic telecanthus*. In Mathog RH, editor: *Maxillofacial trauma*, Baltimore, 1984, Williams & Wilkins.

46. Mayell MF: Nasal fractures: their occurrence, management and some late results, *J R Coll Surg Edinb* 18:31, 1973.

47. Moran WB: Nasal trauma in children, *Otolaryngol Clin North Am* 10:95, 1977.

48. Morgan RF and others: Management of naso-ethmoid-orbital fractures, *Am Surg* 48:447, 1982.

49. Muraoka M and others: Ten-year statistics and observation of facial bone fractures, *Acta Otolaryngol Suppl (Stockh)* 486:217, 1991.

50. Murray JAM: The distribution of stress in the nasal septum in trauma: an experimental model, *Rhinology* 25:101, 1987.

51. Murray JAM, Maran AGD: The treatment of nasal injuries by manipulation, *J Laryngol Otol* 94:1405, 1980.

52. Murray JAM and others: Open v closed reduction of the fractured nose, *Arch Otolaryngol* 110:797, 1984.

53. Murray JAM and others: A pathological classification of nasal fractures, *Injury* 17:338, 1986.

54. Nahum AM: Biomechanics of facial bone fractures, *Laryngoscope* 85:140, 1975.

55. Nigam A and others: The value of radiographs in the management of the fractured nose, *Arch Emerg Med* 10:293, 1993.

56. Oikarinen VJ, Ylipaavalniemi P, Evers H: Pain and temperature sensations related to local analgesia, *Int J Oral Surg* 4:151, 1975.

57. Olsen KD, Carpenter RJ, Kern E: Nasal septal injury in children, *Arch Otolaryngol* 106:317, 1980.

58. Owen GO, Parker AJ, Watson DJ: Fractured-nose reduction under local anesthesia—is it acceptable to the patient? *Rhinology* 30:89, 1992.

59. Paskert JP, Manson PN: The bimanual examination for assessing instability in naso-orbitoethmoidal injuries, *Plast Reconstr Surg* 83:165, 1989.

60. Peerless SA: Nasal and septal reconstruction in acute nasal trauma. Paper presented at the middle section meeting, American Academy of Facial Plastic and Reconstructive Surgery, Madison, Wis, January, 1984.

61. Pirsig W: Septal plasty in children: influence on nasal growth, *Rhinology* 15:193, 1977.

62. Pirsig W, Lehmann I: The influence of trauma on the growing septal cartilage, *Rhinology* 13:39, 1975.

63. Pollock RA: Nasal trauma: pathomechanics and surgical management of acute injuries, *Clin Plast Surg* 19:133, 1992.

64. Renner GJ: Management of nasal fractures, *Otolaryngol Clin North Am* 24:195, 1991.

65. Rock WP, Brain DJ: The effects of nasal trauma during childhood upon growth of the nose and midface, *Br J Orthod* 10:38, 1983.

66. Scherer M and others: An analysis of 1423 facial fractures in 788 patients at an urban trauma center, *J Trauma* 29:388, 1989.

67. Schultz RC, DeVillers YT: Nasal fractures, *J Trauma* 15:319, 1975.

68. Sear AJ: A method of internal splinting for unstable nasal fractures, *Br J Oral Surg* 14:203, 1977.

69. Sharp JF, Denholm S: Routine x-rays in nasal trauma: the influence of audit on clinical practice, *J R Soc Med* 87:153, 1994.

70. Stranc MF, Robertson GA: A classification of injuries of the nasal skeleton, *Ann Plast Surg* 2:468, 1979.

71. Stucker FJ, Bryarly RC, Shockley WW: Management of nasal trauma in children, *Arch Otolaryngol* 110:190, 1984.

72. Swearinger JJ: *Tolerance of the human face to crash impact*, Office of Aviation Medicine, Federal Aviation Administration, Civil Aeromedic Research Institute, Oklahoma City, July 1965.

73. Wadley JK: Correction of unstable nasal fractures by intranasal support, *Laryngoscope* 89:327, 1979.

74. Wexler MR: Reconstructive surgery of the injured nose, *Otolaryngol Clin North Am* 8:663, 1975.

75. Williamson LK, Miller RH, Sessions RB: Treatment of nasofrontal ethmoidal complex fractures, *Head Neck Surg* 89:587, 1981.

76. Wright W: Principles of nasal septal reconstruction, *Trans Am Acad Ophthalmol Otolaryngol* 78:252, 1969.

Chapter 47

Neoplasms of the Nasal Cavity

D. Thane Cody, II
Lawrence W. DeSanto

This chapter reviews tumors and tumor-like lesions of the nasal cavity, excluding the skin of the external nose and the nasal vestibule. These tumors embody many dissimilar pathologic conditions, and they exist in a small, intricate, highly visible anatomic region. Because of this, the head and neck surgeon should understand how the anatomy and the pathologic features of these tumors are related to their behavior, and should appreciate the considerable emotional impact that managing these tumors has on the patient. This makes diagnosis, management, and follow-up of these patients challenging.

ANATOMY

The anatomy of the nasal cavity and surrounding structures is among the most complex in the human body. Surgical management of disease in these areas necessitates knowledge of the relationships of the nasal cavity to the paranasal sinuses, nasopharynx, orbit, pterygomaxillary space, temporal and infratemporal fossa, oral cavity, basicranium, and middle and anterior cranial fossa.

The nose is divided into two cavities by the nasal septum, which comprises the quadrangular cartilage and the perpendicular plate of the ethmoid, vomer, premaxillary, maxillary, and palatine bones. Each cavity has a floor, roof, lateral wall, and medial or septal wall. Posteriorly, the nasal cavity communicates with the nasopharynx and abuts the sphenoid bone. Anteriorly, the pyriform aperture is formed by the paired nasal bones, the maxilla, and the anterior nasal spine. The lateral nasal wall is formed by the maxillary bone, the inferior nasal concha, the ethmoid bone (middle nasal concha), the perpendicular plate of the palatine bone, the lateral aspect of the medial pterygoid plate, and the lacrimal bone.

The roof of the nasal cavity is formed by the cribriform plate of the ethmoid bone.

Blood supply to the nose is provided by branches of the internal and external carotid arteries. The external carotid artery supplies blood to the nose through the facial artery and the internal maxillary artery. The facial artery provides anastamotic branches to the anterior nasal septum through the superior labial artery. It terminates in the angular artery in the nasofacial groove anastamosing with the supratrochlear, infratrochlear, and dorsal nasal branches of the ophthalmic artery; the infraorbital branches of the internal maxillary artery; and the terminal branches of the transverse facial artery. The internal carotid artery supplies the anterior and posterior ethmoid, supraorbital, supratrochlear, and infratrochlear and dorsal nasal arteries to the nose through its ophthalmic branch. In the pterygomaxillary space, anastamoses occur between internal and external carotid arteries through the foramen rotundum and the vidian canal.

The neurovascular anatomy of the pterygomaxillary space and surrounding nasal anatomy is shown in Figure 47-1. This triangular space lies between the posterior wall of the maxillary sinus and the pterygoid process of the sphenoid bone. It is bounded medially by the nasal cavity and laterally by the infratemporal fossa. It is an important distribution center for branches of the third part of the internal maxillary artery and the maxillary division of the trigeminal and the vidian nerves. It is also a pathway of spread of tumors from the nose to the orbit, temporal and infratemporal fossa, and intracranial cavity.[41]

Sensation to the external nose, face, and oral cavity is provided by branches of the trigeminal nerve (Fig. 47-2). Olfactory nerves are found in the roof of the nose, and se-

was injected into the sinus and left in place for a long time.[43]

FREQUENCY BY ANATOMIC SITE

About 55% of nasal and sinus tumors originate from the maxillary sinus, 35% from the nasal cavity, 9% from the ethmoid sinus, and 1% from the frontal and sphenoid sinuses and septum. With large tumors, the site of origin may be difficult to identify.

SIGNS AND SYMPTOMS

The signs and symptoms of benign or malignant nasal tumors are not striking. Nasal obstruction, blood-tinged mucus, and epistaxis are the most common symptoms. Early symptoms usually do not prompt medical attention, and a delay of several months between the onset of symptoms and diagnosis is common.[28] Tearing on one side may be an early symptom of a lateral nasal, medial antral, or ethmoid tumor. Facial asymmetry, loose teeth, and sensory changes around the nose are late symptoms. At times, a nasal malignant tumor is diagnosed only when a pathologist examines what is presumed to be a benign nasal polyp.

Butlin[11] described the progression of symptoms of the malignant tumors:

Sometimes the appearance of the tumor is preceded by pain, but in many instances there is no pain until the disease is advanced. The first sign of serious disease is the appearance of a swelling of the face over the antrum or of fullness and obstruction of the corresponding side of the nose. With the fullness of the nostril there may be discharge of bloody fluid. The swelling gradually increases, not only in the directions in which it first was noticed, but also up toward the orbit, down towards the mouth, and back into the sphenomaxillary fossa. The eye may be pushed up and the hard palate pushed down, but the swelling in the fossa is not so easily perceived. The nostril of the affected side often becomes completely obstructed. As the disease advances, the bony wall may be destroyed and protrusion may take place, with affection on the soft parts around the bone. The skin of the face in this way becomes adherent to the tumor and immovable over it, and the result may be a vast ulcer, with the thrusting forth of a fungous mass.

NASAL EXAMINATION

After a thorough history, observation and palpation are key in the examination of a patient with a known or suspected nasal tumor. The physician should look for facial asymmetry, ptosis, extraocular muscle palsy, tooth position and stability, and trismus and listen for obstructed nasal breathing and altered voice quality and character. The orbital bony contour, the eye, the face, the anterior wall of the maxilla, the palate, and the alveoli should be palpated and inspected. The sensory divisions of cranial nerve (CN) V are tested intraorally and on the face (see Fig. 47-2).

The nasal cavity should be examined with a nasal speculum before and after decongestion. The posterior choana, nasopharynx, and nasal cavity are then examined with a nasal endoscope. Direct extension of the tumor to the nasopharynx may be appreciated; in adenoid cystic carcinoma, vascular striations can at times be seen over the eustachian tube orifice and into the nasopharynx. When biopsied, these striations may show submucosal and perineural tumor.

The remainder of the head and neck examination is completed with careful attention to the presence of palpable neck nodes, serous otitis media, and cranial nerve deficits.

Ophthalmologic examination may be necessary in cases in which invasion into the orbit is suspected. Retinal examination may show superior retinal vein occlusion, suggesting early cavernous sinus or superior orbital fissure involvement with tumor. Fixation of the globe may occur with direct extension of a tumor into the orbit or involvement of CN III, IV, and VI in the cavernous sinus or superior orbital fissure. Tumor in the superior orbital fissure causes sensory deficit in the distribution of CN VI and spares the lower divisions. Involvement of the cavernous sinus usually affects V1 and V2 simultaneously.

RADIOGRAPHIC EVALUATION

Thorough clinical evaluation should reveal the size and extent of the tumor. Radiographic studies, including magnetic resonance imaging (MRI), magnetic resonance angiography (MRA), and computed tomography (CT), define the extent of tumor into areas that are difficult to examine, such as the pterygomaxillary space, infratemporal fossa, parapharyngeal space, sinuses, and anterior and middle cranial fossa. These studies can also provide information about the basicranium, midfacial skeleton, and regional vasculature.

High-resolution CT and MRI or MRA can be used. The information each scan can provide is complementary, and in some patients it may be useful to perform both scans. This complementary value of CT and MRI was recently recognized with the development of computer programs that render a composite scan that incorporates the data from CT and MRI in one image.

CT can aid in distinguishing tissues of markedly different densities, such as bone and soft tissue. Bone windows can further define bony anatomy. CT is less helpful in distinguishing tumor from soft tissue (other than fat, which is black), because most squamous cancers are of intermediate density. This is apparent when attempting to differentiate muscle from tumor. The addition of contrast material has helped alleviate part of this problem because tumors often enhance differently than the surrounding tissue after the administration of contrast material. Additionally, dura that is involved with tumor may be visible on contrast-enhanced CT.

MRI is poor at evaluating cortical bone and is more difficult to use because tissues of markedly different densities (e.g., bone and air) can appear the same. MRI produces images by stimulating nuclei with radiofrequencies and therefore does not subject the patient to ionizing radiation. Different pulse sequences can emphasize different tissues. Most tumors can be differentiated from fat on T1-weighted MRI: fat is white, and many solid tumors are of intermediate density. T1-weighted MRI is not as useful for differentiating muscle from tumor, but T2-weighted MRI with contrast enhancement can usually make the difference apparent. The paramagnetic contrast material gadolinium-diethylenetriaminepentaacetic acid (DTPA) is used most often. Gadolinium shortens T1 and T2 relaxation times and enhances mucosal surfaces and many tumors. In many cases, the margins of the tumor are more clearly defined from other soft tissues, including muscle. In selected cases, this allows a better idea of the extent of the margins of the tumor.[42] MRI can be used to evaluate dural involvement. Vasogenic cerebral edema secondary to brain involvement by tumor is seen with MRI. MRI can also differentiate sinus involvement with tumor from a sinus filled with secretions secondary to ostial obstruction. Secretions are dark on T1-weighted images and bright on T2-weighted images.

MRA is a noninvasive imaging technique used to selectively enhance blood flow during MRI. It helps delineate intraluminal invasion of the carotid artery and vascular anatomy in the preoperative evaluation. It can also differentiate vascular from nonvascular tumors. Although few studies have been done to determine the role of MRA in the evaluation of patients with head and neck tumors, this technique seems to provide similar information to conventional angiography without the associated risks.[19] MRA also has the advantage of providing a three-dimensional view of the vessels rather than the two-dimensional, direction-dependent view of conventional angiography. The disadvantages of MRA include the lack of interventional capabilities (e.g., embolization), an inability to visualize fine vasculature, an inability of some patients to tolerate the procedure, and effects of motion artifact on scan quality. It is contraindicated in patients with pacemakers, cochlear implants, and other metallic foreign bodies. Nasal tumors in which MRA is useful include hemangiomas, nasopharyngeal angiofibromas, and tumors thought to involve the cavernous sinus or carotid artery. Researchers at the University of Iowa[19] have developed some general indications for the use of MRA in head and neck surgery that are applicable to nasal tumors: (1) evaluation of suspected aberrant vasculature or aneurysm; (2) evaluation of tumor vascularity; (3) determination of the anatomic relationships between tumor mass and vascular structures; (4) adjunct to the preoperative estimation of great vessel involvement by adjacent malignancy; (5) back-up technique when less expensive ultrasound is indicated but not possible; and (6) occasional adjunct to the work-up of selected head and neck surgery patients with perioperative mental status changes.

Conventional radiograph angiography is another technique used to determine vascular anatomy. It has the advantage of being available in most centers, allows intervention where indicated, and provides better detail of fine vascula-

ture than MRA. Disadvantages include a 7% complication rate and a 0.7% mortality rate.[1] Complications include wound infection, hematoma, aneurysm formation, allergic reactions to contrast material, neurologic problems, and others. Conventional angiography is reported to cost about 20% more than MRI or MRA.

CT, MRI, and MRA cannot document microscopic tumor; this should be recognized when planning management of malignant disease.

CLASSIFICATION AND STAGING

The American Joint Committee on Cancer (AJCC) does not have a staging system for tumors that originate in the nasal cavity. To assist with planning management, staging systems have been developed for juvenile angiofibromas (Box 47-1). Because many tumors that present in the nasal cavity are secondary invaders from the maxillary sinus or the nasopharynx, they are included in the AJCC staging system, which is covered elsewhere in this text.

Tumors can be classified in many ways. This chapter uses the general framework of the World Health Organization (WHO). A differential diagnosis of nasal masses is presented in Box 47-2.

Box 47-1. Staging of juvenile nasopharyngeal
angiofibromas

Kadish system

A: Tumor confined to the nasal cavity

B: Tumor extension into the paranasal sinuses

C: Tumor spread beyond the nasal cavity and paranasal sinuses

Biller classification

T_1: Tumor involvement in the nasal and paranasal sinuses (except sphenoid) with or without erosion of the bone of the anterior cranial fossa

T_2: Tumor extension into the orbit or protruding into the anterior cranial fossa

T_3: Tumor involvement in the brain that is resectable with margins

T_4: Unresectable tumor

University of California Los Angeles (UCLA) modification

T_1: Tumor involvement in the nasal cavity or paranasal sinuses (except sphenoid), sparing the most superior ethmoidal cells

T_2: Tumor involvement in the nasal cavity or paranasal sinuses (including sphenoid) with extension to or erosion of the cribriform plate

T_3: Tumor extension into the orbit or extending into the anterior cranial fossa

T_4: Tumor involvement in the brain

Box 47-2. Differential diagnosis of nasal lesions

Trauma

Digital septal perforation or ulceration
Cocaine abuse

Tumor-like lesions

Mucocele
Pyogenic granuloma
Nasal polyp (allergic, antochoanal, fibrous)
Fibromatosis
Fibrous dysplasia
Giant cell granuloma
Infectious granulomas
    Rhinoscleroma
    Rhinosporidiosis
    Tuberculosis
    Leishmaniasis
    Histoplasmosis or other fungal infection
Wegener's granulomatosis
Glioma
Meningocele
Amyloid

Neoplasms

Epithelial
  Benign
    Squamous papilloma
    Inverted papilloma
    Adenoma
    Pleomorphic adenoma
  Malignant
    Squamous cell carcinoma
    Verrucous carcinoma
    Spindle cell carcinoma
    Transitional cell carcinoma
    Adenocarcinoma
      Papillary adenocarcinoma
      Sessile adenocarcinoma
      Alveolar-mucoid adenocarcinoma
        Colonic adenocarcinoma
        Mucinous adenocarcinoma
    Undifferentiated carcinomas

Soft-tissue tumors
  Benign
    Hemangioma
    Hemangiopericytoma
    Neurofibroma
    Neurilemmoma
    Myxoma
    Fibrous histiocytoma
  Malignant
    Malignant hemangiopericytoma
    Fibrosarcoma
    Rhabdomyosarcoma
    Neurogenic sarcoma
    Malignant fibrous histiocytoma
Bone and cartilage tumors
  Benign
    Chondroma
    Osteoma
    Ossifying fibroma
  Malignant
    Chondrosarcoma
    Osteosarcoma
Lymphoid and hematopoietic tumors
  Malignant lymphoma
  Plasmacytoma
Miscellaneous tumors
  Benign
    Teratoma
    Meningioma
    Odontogenic tumors
  Malignant
    Malignant melanoma
    Esthesioneuroblastoma
  Secondary invaders
    Nasopharyngeal carcinoma
    Juvenile angiofibroma
    Pituitary adenoma
    Chordoma
    Craniopharyngioma

BENIGN NEOPLASMS

Benign tumors of the nose are rare in comparison with malignant growths. The most common benign tumors (in decreasing order of frequency) are osteoma, hemangioma, papilloma, and angiofibroma. The two tumors of greatest interest are the inverted papilloma and the juvenile nasopharyngeal angiofibroma.

Inverted papilloma

Most authorities consider the inverted papilloma a true neoplasm. Other names used for this growth are *schneiderian papilloma, papillary sinusitis, polyp with inverting metaplasia, benign transitional cell growth, epithelial papil-loma, inverted schneiderian papilloma, soft papilloma, transitional cell papilloma, squamous papillary epithelioma, papillary fibroma, papillomatosis,* and *cylindrical cell carcinoma.* The microscopic features that distinguish a papilloma from an allergic or inflammatory polyp include proliferation of the squamous epithelium as extensive finger-like inversions into the underlying stroma (Fig. 47-3).

No symptoms are unique to these tumors. A history of previous operations, including polypectomy and septal or sinus surgery, is common. Suh and others[47] noted that 63% of patients who had definitive surgery for papilloma had undergone prior nasal surgery for obstruction.

Most papillomas originate from the lateral wall of the

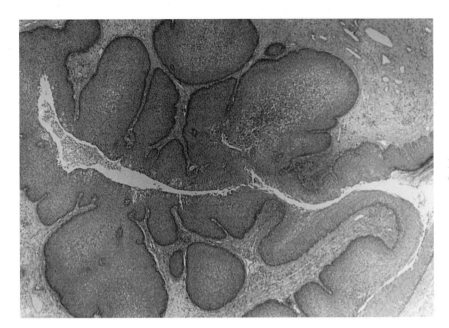

Fig. 47-3. Inverted papilloma. (Hemotoxylin-eosin stain; ×20.) (Courtesy of Dr. D. Menke.)

nose. Secondary involvement of the maxillary and ethmoid sinuses is common. Extension to the sphenoid and frontal sinuses also occurs. Radiographic studies may show bony destruction and erosion, usually in the lateral wall of the nose. Malignant change is found in about 10% of inverted papillomas (range, 0% to 56%).

Total removal is needed to avoid recurrence. The median recurrence rate with medial wall maxillectomy is 9%. Piecemeal removal by other routes yields a median recurrence rate of 43%.[40] This suggests that complete removal by transnasal excision or simple sinus surgery is not an effective form of therapy. Some authors have advocated endoscopic removal for small tumors involving the turbinate, but the recurrence rate is higher than with conventional surgery.[32]

Careful histologic study of multiple sections of the excised lateral wall of the nasal cavity is recommended to seek areas of *in situ* or invasive carcinoma.

Juvenile nasopharyngeal angiofibroma

Juvenile angiofibroma is a benign tumor typically found in young boys who have nosebleeds and nasal obstruction. Symptoms may be present for months to years. In a series of 120 male patients with angiofibroma from the Mayo Clinic, the ages at diagnosis ranged from 9 to 29 years (mean age, 15 years).[38] The site of origin of the angiofibroma has been the subject of speculation. It appears to originate in the posterior nasal cavity rather than in the nasopharynx, specifically in the posterolateral and superior nasal cavity at the point where the sphenoidal process of the palatine bone meets the horizontal ala of the vomer and the root of the pterygoid process of the sphenoid bone, near the upper margin of the sphenopalatine foramen.

At diagnosis, most of the tumors have extended beyond the nasal cavity and nasopharynx. They may push the poste-rior wall of the maxillary sinus forward and grow laterally into the pterygomaxillary fossa. Extension into the pterygomaxillary fossa can erode the pterygoid process of the sphenoid bone. Further lateral extension can fill the infratemporal fossa and produce the classic bulging cheek. Tumor can extend under the zygomatic arch and cause swelling above the arch. From the pterygomaxillary fossa, the angiofibroma can grow into the inferior and superior orbital fissures, erode the greater wing of the sphenoid bone, and leave tumor extradurally in the middle fossa. Posterior extension into the sphenoid sinus through the floor or ostium fills the sinus, pushes upward and back to displace the pituitary, and then can fill the sella turcica. Tumor in the sella or in the orbit can cause loss of vision.

The rate of growth of the angiofibroma is not known but is thought to be slow. Because the tumor is rarely seen in young adults, it is believed to spontaneously regress. Clinically, regression after incomplete removal or radiotherapy is recognized. Because regression cannot be assumed, these tumors should be managed.

Excisional biopsy confirms the diagnosis when it is in doubt. The biopsy can be taken after the patient is asleep and has been prepared for tumor removal. This avoids bleeding between biopsy and definitive management.

The radiographic findings of angiofibroma are characteristic. Holman and Miller[27] emphasized the bowing of the posterior wall of the maxillary sinus and the enlargement of the superior orbital fissure. CT is ideal for precise tumor localization. MRI also helps diagnose intracranial extension of disease. MRA may be used to determine the feeding vessels. Some have advocated conventional angiography for diagnosis and management. Angiography has the benefit of allowing embolization but carries the risk of complications. The usefulness of embolization is controversial.

The vascularity of the tumors varies. Some are very vascular, and others are fibrous. Thus, the bleeding potential of a tumor is unpredictable. The main blood supply of the angiofibroma is from the internal maxillary artery. The dural, sphenoidal, and ophthalmic branches from the internal carotid system can also contribute. Vessels sometimes carry blood supply from the thyrocervical trunk. Because of this diverse arterial input, preliminary ligation of the external carotid artery does little to decrease bleeding during excision. Ligation of the artery before definitive surgery can increase bleeding by encouraging arterial input from the less

accessible or inaccessible vessels. At times, the internal maxillary artery is pushed forward by the tumor and can be ligated during exposure of the tumor. When practical, ligation of the internal maxillary artery is worthwhile.

Other techniques have been advocated to lessen bleeding. They include electrocoagulation, interstitial irradiation, hormone therapy, cryotherapy, and irradiation. Anesthetic adjuncts, such as hypotensive techniques and hypothermia, have also been recommended. The real value of these techniques is unknown. Much of the blood loss associated with angiofibroma surgery comes from the hypervascular adja-

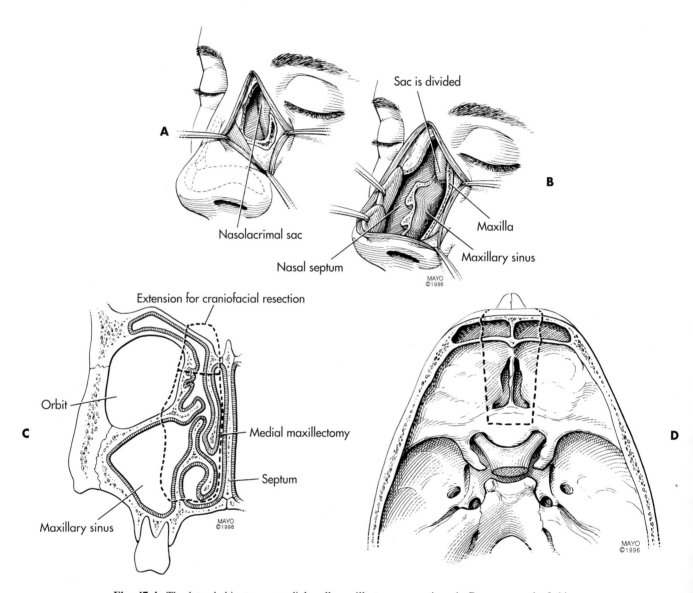

Fig. 47-4. The lateral rhinotomy, medial wall maxillectomy operation. **A,** Bony removal of rhinotomy uncovers the nasolacrimal sac and nasal bone removal. Bony removal can continue to involve more nasal bone and the face of the maxilla. **B,** The nasolacrimal duct is divided, and the maxillary sinus is opened, exposing the medial and lateral portions of the lateral wall of the nose and turbinates. **C,** Coronal section shows the extent of resection, with extension for craniofacial resection. **D,** Cuts for craniofacial resection from above.

cent bone and soft tissues during tumor exposure. Cryosurgery is impractical as an adjunct to excision for large tumors and has been abandoned, and hormones have little to support their value. Hypotensive anesthesia may be useful.

Neel and others[38] noted the survey of these tumors by Hellat[25] who found 65 techniques for tumor removal. Neel and others[38] suggested eight logical approaches: (1) through the nose, (2) through the palate, (3) through the mandible, (4) through the zygoma, (5) through the bed of the hyoid bone, (6) through the antrum, (7) combined craniotomy and rhinotomy, and (8) the lateral rhinotomy. The lateral rhinotomy is preferable because it is logical and uncomplicated. The lateral rhinotomy is an incision along the side of the nose (Fig. 47-4). An alternative is the facial degloving approach (Fig. 47-5). The rhinotomy incision provides exposure to the anterior septum. Exposure beyond that is blocked by the lateral nasal wall. Block removal of the lateral nasal wall, defined as the ''medial maxillectomy,''[46] provides access to posterior nasal septum and tumors that originate posteriorly in the nasal cavity, the pterygomaxillary space, and the nasopharynx (e.g., as angiofibromas).

Variations of the basic operation are possible. For tumors of the roof of the nose (e.g., esthesioneuroblastoma), a bilateral rhinotomy called the *superior rhinotomy* combines with anterior craniotomy *en bloc* resection of the cribriform area. In this procedure,[8] the soft tissues and the bony attachments of the nose are divided bilaterally across the nasal root, suspending the nose downward on its remaining alar and collumellar attachments. The rhinotomy exposure combined with bilateral medial maxillectomies allows *en bloc* resection of ethmoid tumors with or without intracranial extension.

The evolution of the subspecialty of skull-base surgery has increased interest in the combined intracranial-transfacial approaches to large angiofibromas. Stage 3 and 4 lesions can erode the middle cranial fossa and enter both orbital fissures, and very large tumors may approximate the cavernous sinus. Nevertheless, these tumors grow by centrifugal expansion and not by invasion. These tumors may be intracranial but are always extradural. The cavernous sinus may be compressed but is not invaded. Cranial nerve palsies are rare even with large tumors. The elaborate combined approaches are elegant but may not improve the management goal or recurrence rates.

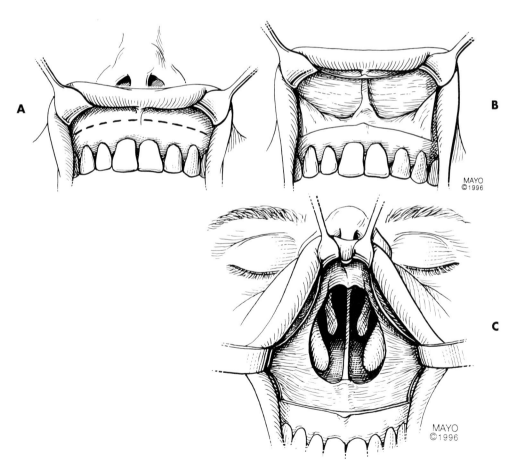

Fig. 47-5. The midfacial degloving operation. **A,** Sublabial incision. **B,** Elevation of the periosteum off the face of the maxilla. **C,** Exposure of the midfacial skeleton.

is done properly and the sequence and timing are correct, survival will be more increased for patients with tumors of comparable stages compared with survival achieved by irradiation or surgery alone.

The use of radiotherapy in combination with surgery for early curable lesions should be carefully considered in light of the long-term problems associated with combined therapy. Morita and Kawabe[37] observed that in patients who received more than 5800 rad to the eye, severe panophthalmopathy with corneal ulceration developed within 2 years. Of 21 eyes exposed to 2800 to 5400 rad, 18 experienced visual disturbances and radiation-induced cataracts.

Adenoid cystic carcinomas

Neoplasms that come from the minor salivary glands of the nose form an interesting and diverse group that comprise less than 10% of the malignant nasal tumors.

The histologic pattern of low-grade adenoid cystic carcinomas is a mixture of tubular and cribriform formations of epithelial cells with few solid cellular areas. The cribriform pattern is the classic "swiss-cheese" pattern of cells arranged in elongated tubular structures. High-grade adenoid cystic carcinoma is the pattern of the classic tumor, but solid areas of malignant cells comprise a significant volume of the tumor mass. This distinction between high and low grades is important. Vascular invasion is more common, distant metastasis more frequent, and death as a consequence of the tumor more likely in patients with a high-grade tumor.[23] Perineural invasion is common in both types, as is frequent local recurrence.

Management of adenoid cystic carcinoma is surgical resection when reasonable. The more thorough the excision, the longer a patient can expect to be free of recurrence. Although considerable pessimism exists about the curability of adenoid cystic carcinoma, ample justification for curative attempts exist. Five-year survival is not adequate to define cure. The 10-year recurrence-free rates for patients with nasal fossa tumors are about 60%, which encourages vigorous management. Some patients have a normal life span with or without recurrences, even with pulmonary metastases.

The role of radiotherapy is not clearly defined. No evidence suggests that preoperative or postoperative irradiation decreases the frequency of recurrence. With low-grade adenoid cystic carcinoma, radiotherapy is reserved for patients with recurrence and pain. The carcinoma responds to irradiation, and pain can be lessened or eliminated, although the result is seldom permanent. Some of these tumors are so extensive that no surgical procedure is feasible. In the very elderly patient with an extensive tumor but little pain, the decision not to manage may be proper.

Successful management with particle beam radiation in selected adenoid cystic tumors has been reported, but follow-up data are too short to determine how this modality will fare over the long term.

Adenocarcinomas

One method for classifying these "other" glandular carcinomas uses the same terminology as that used to describe tumors of the major salivary gland. Mucoepidermoid and acinic cell carcinoma diagnoses are used. Batsakis, Rice, and Solomon[5] described a classification based on growth forms: papillary, sessile, and alveolar-mucoid. Mucin production is variable in the first two forms, and the level of cellular differentiation may range from modest to poor.

Papillary adenocarcinomas are usually the most localized. A special type of mucus-producing papillary adenocarcinoma is described that looks like colonic carcinoma microscopically. These tumors are composed of tall columnar cells that form a single layer containing numerous goblet-shaped, mucus-producing cells (Fig. 47-6). Knowledge of this variant is important to avoid extensive evaluation of the digestive system.

A sessile adenocarcinoma has a broad surface, and the tumor cells retain little resemblance to the cells of their origin. These tumors have greater invasive properties and carry a worse prognosis than papillary adenocarcinomas.

The alveolar-mucoid variant is the most aggressive and has a poorer prognosis than papillary tumors. These carcinomas are characterized by abundant mucin in which nests of individual cells reside.

All nasal adenocarcinomas other than adenoid cystic carcinoma are considered to be relentless, aggressive tumors with a poor prognosis. An Armed Forces Institute of Pathology (AFIP) study of 50 cases suggested that the low-grade lesions can be distinguished from the other types and have a good prognosis. For the high-grade tumors, combined therapy is used, but the results of management are disappointing.[24]

Sarcomas

Sarcomas of the nasal cavity are rare. They represent 1% of head and neck sarcomas and 15% of all paranasal sinus tumors.[45] Radiation exposure has been implicated as a risk factor for the development of some sarcomas, in particular malignant fibrous histiocytoma.[31] These tumors cause late symptoms and are often so large at diagnosis that determining their exact site of origin is impossible.

Most nonrhabdomyosarcoma sarcomas are managed with surgical resection followed by radiotherapy if surgical margins are positive. In general, patients with positive margins at the time of resection will have a recurrence if no further management is used. In patients with positive margins managed with postoperative radiotherapy, about 45% will be cured. Patients with negative margins at the time of resection have a better prognosis. Patients die from local regional disease, and management of the N_0 neck is not indicated. The N+ neck should be managed with neck dissection.

Because these lesions are rare it is difficult to know how advances in skull-base surgery will change survival; how-

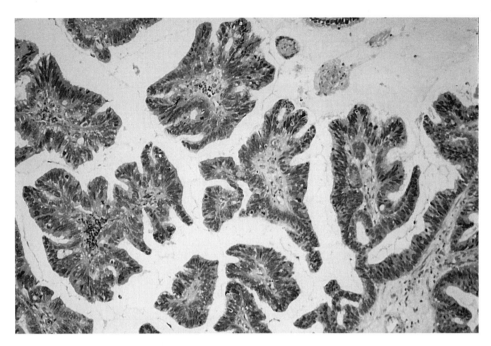

Fig. 47-6. Colonic cell carcinoma. (Hematoxylin-eosin.) (Courtesy of Dr. J. Lewis.)

ever, it is anticipated that the increased ability to obtain free margins at the skull base will improve the prognosis for patients with these tumors.

Rhabdomyosarcoma

Rhabdomyosarcoma patients are managed with multimodality therapy that includes aggressive chemotherapy, radiotherapy, and surgery. Although rhabdomyosarcoma is curable, the prognosis is not as good with sinonasal rhabdomyosarcoma when compared with other sites.[45]

Chondrosarcoma

Coates and others[16] reported on 13 nasal chondrosarcomas. The typical chondrosarcoma was low grade histologically and was a large, pale, glistening, obstructing mass. Differentiating chondromas from chondrosarcomas may be difficult for the pathologist. They are generally slow-growing lesions that metastasize late. Most originate from the posterior septum. Local excision often leads to tumor recurrence. A definitive *en bloc* excision is often curative. Patients die from uncontrolled local disease that extends intracranially. Radiotherapy does not influence tumor growth after recurrence.

Hemangiopericytoma

Nasal hemangiopericytoma is of vascular origin and can arise wherever capillaries are found. Occurrence in the nose is rare. Fewer than 20 cases involving the nasal cavity have been reported. The histopathologic features of this tumor are complex, with a single common denominator: lack of uniformity in appearance and biologic behavior. In all tu-

mors, a proliferation of capillaries is surrounded by a connective tissue sheath. Outside this sheath are tumor cells that vary in appearance. Silver stains blacken the sheath of the capillaries for easy identification and thus allow accurate demonstration of the extracapillary position of the malignant cells.[10] The biologic behavior of the tumor cannot be predicted by its histologic appearance. Nonmitotic tumors can metastasize, and metastasis can occur with a benign-looking primary tumor. Distant metastasis to lung, liver, and bone is common, but regional metastasis to lymph nodes has not been observed. The gross tumor in the nose looks benign and is described as a soft, rubbery, pale gray or tan polypoid mass. Despite the pale, avascular appearance, these tumors bleed vigorously when biopsied. Management consists of wide local excision. Irradiation decreases the size of the tumor, but cure with radiotherapy alone in other sites is rare. Recurrence after excision is frequent, but few deaths occur in the first 5 years.

Lymphomas

Malignant non-Hodgkin's lymphoma (NHL) of the sinonasal tract is rare, accounting for 0.17% of lymphomas and 0.44% of all extranodal lymphomas.[20] Most lymphomas are nasal, although at times it is difficult to identify the site of origin in large tumors. These lymphomas may be B or T cell. T-cell lymphomas of the nose are found most often in Asian males in their fifth to sixth decade. A biopsy often shows a mixed infiltrate of histiocytes, plasma cells, eosinophils, atypical lymphocytes, and other inflammatory cells, making identification of the malignant cells difficult. They are often aligned angiocentrically, with angioinvasion producing a vasculitis and necrosis. Epstein-Barr virus (EBV) has been associated with nasal T-cell lymphomas, but these patients do not have elevated levels of serum viral capsid antigen IgA antibodies as do patients with nasopharyngeal carcinoma.[15] B-cell lymphomas are less common in the nasal cavity. They do not have a propensity for angiocentricity and destroy tissue by local invasion.

Prognosis for nasal lymphomas in general is better in western than in Asian populations, better for T cell than B cell, and better with earlier stage disease, although about one half of patients will die of local or extranodal disease. Management is with multiagent chemotherapy and radiotherapy.[50]

Polymorphic reticulosis, lethal midline granuloma, idiopathic midline destructive disease, and similar terms are old nomenclature for non-healing midfacial destructive lesions that should no longer be used. These lesions often represent a T-cell lymphoma. Failure to recognize this may result in the incorrect treatment.

Malignant melanoma

Malignant melanoma is a rare nasal tumor. When it develops, it is more likely to arise from the mucous membranes of the septum and the lateral nasal wall than from the paranasal sinuses. Freedman and others[22] reviewed the Mayo Clinic experience with 56 melanomas from these sites. Lund[34] reviewed 36 patients from England.

The symptoms of melanoma are the same as those of all nasal tumors: obstruction and epistaxis. The diagnosis is usually obvious because of pigmentation, although some of the pigmented area may not be tumor. Tissue phagocytes can carry the pigment some distance from the real tumor. The distinction between tumor and submucosal benign pigmentation requires histologic study. If the diagnosis is made early enough and the tumor is completely removed, cure is possible. In the series reported by Freedman and others[22] nearly 60% of the patients were alive without disease at 5 years. The patients in the Lund[34] series did not fair as well; nearly two thirds were dead at 5 years. This difference may be related to earlier diagnosis in the former group than in the latter, or it may be the result of different management. More radiotherapy, which may have changed local resistance, was used in the series by Lund.

The incidence of local recurrence is high. Freedman and others[22] reported that 21 of 38 patients managed surgically had local recurrences. More radical excision, including removal of the eye, palate, or external portion of the nose, may not decrease the incidence of local recurrence. The tumor can be multifocal, and safe removal requires the help of a pathologist skilled in diagnosis using fresh frozen section.

The disconcerting feature of nasal melanoma is that the probability of death does not decrease with time as it does with other tumors. The recurrence curves are linear over time, whereas the risk of death with other epithelial tumors decreases greatly after a patient survives 4 or 5 years without recurrence. Death from melanoma is usually by disseminated disease. Late deaths represent silent disseminated disease held in check by a competent immunosystem. Local recurrence and even metastasis do not necessarily imply death within a short time. Patients with both have survived for several years. Vigorous secondary local excision, if possible, may be worthwhile.

Olfactory esthesioneuroblastoma

A peculiar and rare neuroepithelial malignant lesion that comes from the olfactory area of the nasal cavity is olfactory esthesioneuroblastoma. Other terms for this tumor are *esthesioneuroblastoma, olfactory esthesioneuroma, neuroblastoma*, and *olfactory neurocytoma*. The growth was described by Berger, Luc, and Richard[7]. Neuroectoderm is the presumed cell of origin because its histologic pattern is similar to that of malignant tumors of the sympathetic ganglion, adrenal medulla, and retina. McGravan[35] and Taxy and Hidvegi[48] showed neurosecretory granules of catecholamines in tumors examined by electron microscopy.

Cantrell and others[13] noted that of the 160 tumors reported since 1924, 125 have been cited in the past 15 years. This finding reflects a greater awareness of the tumor; in the past, these tumors were diagnosed as something else. Their histologic resemblance to undifferentiated small cell carcinoma can cause misdiagnosis. The histologic features that identify the esthesioneuroblastoma are undifferentiated small neuroepithelial cells arranged in compact cell aggregates consisting predominantly of densely staining cell nuclei (Fig. 47-7) surrounded by scant fibrillary cytoplasm. Occasionally cell aggregates may form pseudofibrillary cords. Mitotic figures are absent, and occasional interstitial calcification is present.

On gross examination, the tumors appear as red, polypoid masses high in the nose. The nose can bleed and become obstructed, and symptoms can be present for months or years.

The tumor can be multicentric, with separate tumors above and below the cribriform plate. Olsen and DeSanto[39] described one patient who had two separate tumors, one above and the other below the cribriform plate, with no gross or microscopic connection between the tumors.

Djalilian and others[17] found that in one of four patients, tumor in the anterior cranial cavity was present at diagnosis or developed later. They noted metastasis in 8 of 19 patients studied. Metastatic lesions in cervical lymph nodes were present in two children at diagnosis and in two adults 6 and 8 years after the nasal tumors were removed.

Surgical removal is the recommended management. Kadish, Goodman, and Wong[29] reported on a patient whose tumor responded to irradiation. Cantrell[13] and Olsen and DeSanto[39] respectively advocated combined therapy with irradiation before the surgery or after surgery. The goal of combined therapy is a decreased incidence of local recurrence. The need for combined therapy has been recently

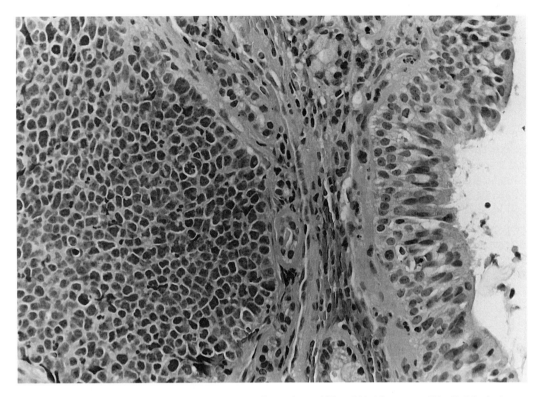

Fig. 47-7. Esthesioneuroblastoma. (Hematoxylin-eosin; ×200 ×20.) (Courtesy of Dr. D. Menke.)

questioned by Biller and others,[9] whose series of 20 patients with extracranial disease were managed by craniofacial resection without radiotherapy. One local recurrence occurred. The small recurrence rate was attributed to an adequate excision as compared with the rhinotomy alone. The combined approach permits resection of the dura over the cribriform plate, resection of the olfactory bulb, and *en bloc* resection of the ethmoid labyrinth, lamina papyracea, septum, and cribriform plate. Lateral rhinotomy may be sufficient for small tumors that originate from the lateral wall of the nose away from the cribriform area. The concept of a combined frontal craniotomy–superior rhinotomy approach, which includes the cribriform area, is sound for the superior based tumors;[14] however, with so few patients treated, the possibility that this tumor may be multicentric, and so many forms of management advocated, no reliable data exist to substantiate which management approach is best for this tumor.

Extramedullary plasmacytoma

Extramedullary plasmacytomas involving the nose and paranasal sinuses are not rare. The diagnosis is made after a thorough evaluation has failed to identify a plasma cell leukemia or multiple myeloma. Hill, Soboroff, and Applebaum[26] have summarized the clinical and diagnostic studies that should be obtained in the evaluation, including serum protein electrophoresis, total serum protein and albumin-globulin ratio, serum immunoelectrophoresis, urinary

Bence-Jones protein, bone marrow biopsy, skeletal survey, peripheral blood cell count, and differential examination and chest radiograph. Most patients with multiple myeloma will have a monoclonal gammopathy on immunoelectrophoresis and an abnormal skeletal survey. Biopsy is required to confirm the diagnosis. These tumors must be differentiated from melanoma, undifferentiated carcinoma, lymphoma, and rhabdomyosarcoma. Bleeding after biopsy may be profuse.

Radiotherapy, surgery, or both may be used to manage these tumors. They tend to be highly radiosensitive, making this form of therapy attractive for extensive lesions in which disfiguring surgery would be required. Extensive disease and bone involvement are poor prognostic signs; however, 10-year survival is still about 65%.

SECONDARY INVADERS

Pituitary adenomas

Pituitary adenomas rarely present in the nose. Involvement of the nose and paranasal sinuses occurs as a result of downward extension of a sellar tumor or from an ectopic tumor arising from remnants of Rathke's pouch. These can arise in the sphenoid bone, sphenoid sinus, nasal cavity, nasopharynx, and clivus.[30] More than half of the reported cases secrete hormones. Signs and symptoms result from the locoregional effects of the tumor or its hormonal activity. No reported cases have shown metastatic potential. Surgical removal is indicated. Incomplete removal of a large invasive tumor may be managed with postoperative radiation.

Chordomas

Chordomas are rare, slow-growing, low-grade malignancies that originate from remnants of the primitive notochord; 35% originate in the sphenoid region. They may present with symptoms related to the sinonasal tract alone in about 1% of cases or with other neurologic signs and symptoms; visual disturbance and headache are the most common. Although unusual, they should be considered in the differential diagnosis of a nasal mass. Histopathologically, they should be differentiated from chondrosarcomas. Metastasis from chordomas are rare. Patients usually die of relentless locoregional disease. Management is with surgical debulking followed with radiotherapy. Long-term survival has been achieved in some patients, although average survival is about 5 years.[12]

Other secondary invaders

Other regional tumors (e.g., nasopharyngeal carcinomas, meningiomas, odontogenic tumors, benign and malignant neoplasms of the craniofacial skeleton, tumors of the orbit, and lacrimal apparatus) can secondarily involve the nasal cavity.

MANAGEMENT

Most lesions require a biopsy to provide a histologic diagnosis. This can be done in the office with topical anesthesia using 4% lidocaine spray or topical cocaine. If necessary, a local block can be performed. Nasal masses that should not be biopsied in the office include those in the posterolateral nose that are vascular and those high in the nasal vault that have not been radiographically evaluated for intracranial extension. Fungal stains and cultures for acid-fast bacilli and fungi are obtained in appropriate cases. Management ultimately depends on the histology of the tumor, although some tumors do not behave in a predictable fashion (Box 47-3).

It is convenient when planning resection of an extensive nasal tumor to consider the direction of the approach, the soft-tissue incisions to allow access, the bony framework surgery, the resection, and reconstruction. The direction of attack may be divided into anterior midline or transfacial, paramedian or transantral, and lateral (Fig. 47-8). The choice

of the approach depends on the histology of the tumor, the origin and extent of the tumor as determined by radiographic and physical examination, the presence of regional disease, and the skills and preferences of the surgeon.

Some small benign tumors of the nasal cavity may be removed transnasally under direct vision or with endoscopic guidance. Most larger benign tumors and malignant tumors will require some type of external incision to access the nasofacial skeleton. The lateral rhinotomy incision provides good access to the medial wall of the maxilla. The incision can be extended over the brow to gain access to the ethmoid labyrinth and the fovea (see Fig. 47-8, C). This can be combined with a bicoronal or frontal craniotomy and is a good approach for tumors in the anterior ethmoid and frontal sinus and for bilateral tumors located high in the nose.[9] The standard rhinotomy incision can also be extended as a subciliary incision or subciliary plus lateral canthotomy or extended to the helical rim, sacrificing the frontal branch of the facial nerve. Appropriate craniofacial disassembly or relocation can provide access to foramen rotundum, the nasopharynx, foramen ovale, and the pterygomaxillary space if required. A lateral craniotomy can provide access to the petrous and cavernous carotid and cavernous sinus for tumors that extend into these areas. Other lateral approaches with their various modifications include the subtemporal, pterional, orbitozygomatic, infratemporal fossa, and facial translocation procedures. Paramedian approaches take advantage of the maxillary sinus to gain access to the pterygomaxillary space and sphenoid.

The limits of these resections are not yet known. Removal of a nasal tumor may be possible with bony involvement of the skull base, intracranial disease, major vessel involvement, and dural involvement. The field of skull-base surgery has extended the location of tumors that may be surgically approached and may change the probability of curable resections when tumor involves the skull base. Currently, there is not enough experience with tumors involving the basicranium and cavernous sinus and related structures to give a definitive opinion as to the indications for resection in these areas; therefore, patients with these tumors should be managed individually.

With a carefully selected operation and thorough preoper-

Box 47-3. Nasal neoplasms with unpredictable behavior

Extramedullary plasmacytoma
Fibrous histiocytoma
Giant cell tumor
Hemangiopericytoma
Teratoma

Fig. 47-8. A, Schematic representation of the possible anterior approaches to tumors involving the nasal cavity and anterior and middle fossa (*a,* transfrontal, *b,* transfacial, *c,* transseptal, *d,* transmaxillary, *e,* transoral-transpalatal, *f,* transmandibular-transhyoid). **B,** Axial representation of the extent of resection possible by using combined operations (*a,* lateral approaches, *b,* transmaxillary, *c,* anterior midline.) **C,** Some of the common incisions to gain access to the craniofacial skeleton. **D,** Some of the various osteotomies or craniotomies that may be used to approach nasal tumors and disassemble the craniofacial skeleton.

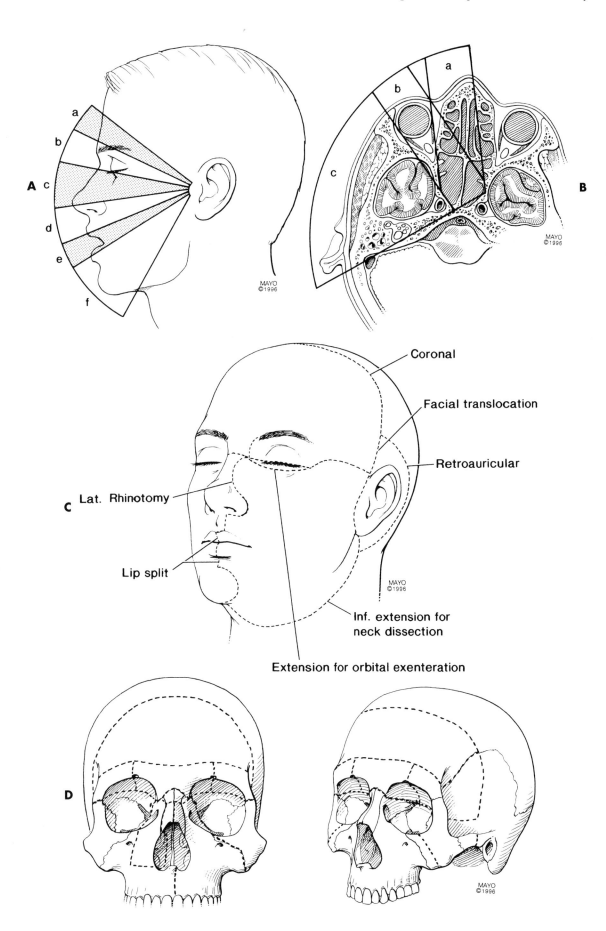

Chapter 48

Allergic Rhinitis

Richard L. Mabry

Although not so glamorous as its surgical counterparts, the management of allergic rhinitis constitutes a large proportion of the day-to-day practice of the general otolaryngologist. In addition to its primary effect, inhalant allergy of the upper respiratory tract may affect the development and clinical course of other disease states such as sinusitis, otitis media, and asthma. It has been conservatively estimated that 18% to 32% of the population of the United States[12] has clinically significant allergic rhinitis. Other statistics are equally impressive: a cost of $500 million per year in medical and drug expenses, and 28 million restricted days per year due to allergic rhinitis. Thus, the importance of allergic rhinitis should not be minimized, either by the patient or the treating physician.

THE IMMUNOLOGY OF ALLERGY

Proper diagnosis and treatment of allergic rhinitis involves an understanding of the basic mechanisms of the disease process. More detailed information on the immunology of allergy is available in textbooks devoted entirely to the subject; what is presented here is a simplified summation of this complex subject.

The primary characteristic of the immune system is the recognition of ''nonself,'' coupled with a ''memory.'' The function of the immune system involves T and B lymphocytes and soluble substances called *cytokines* that act inside and outside the immune system to affect it and a multiplicity of mediators. Gell and Coombs described four types of hypersensitivity reactions:[2] immediate, cytotoxic, immune complex, and delayed. Others have suggested the addition of two more types (stimulating antibody and antibody-dependent, cell-mediated cytotoxicity). However, allergic rhinitis involves primarily a Gell and Coombs type I immediate hypersensitivity reaction. Because various therapeutic mo-

dalities work at different points within this reaction, it is important for the clinician to have a general understanding of it.

''Allergy'' requires repeated exposures to an antigen for the formation of antibodies. In the case of respiratory allergy, this involves presentation of the relevant antigenic material from an allergen by an antigen-presenting cell (macrophage) to B lymphocytes. Each person's B cells are capable of displaying millions of uniquely configured antibody sites. These cells, under the influence of various cytokines (generated in part by T lymphocytes), produce allergen-specific immunoglobulin E (IgE). It has been estimated that a minimum of five such antigen exposures are required to produce sensitization.[4]

In type I hypersensitivity, an antigen bridges two adjacent allergen-specific IgE molecules attached to a mast cell or basophil, resulting in a dissolution of the cell and liberation of both preformed and newly formed mediators of inflammation (Table 48-1). These produce glandular stimulation, vasodilation, increased vascular permeability, and irritation, which are responsible for the typical symptoms of itching, sneezing, rhinorrhea, and congestion. The acute reaction takes place within a few minutes of the antigen-antibody reaction. About 4 to 6 hours later, under the influence of various cells and cytokines, a late-phase reaction occurs that results in a recrudescence of symptoms.

OFFENDERS AND SEASONS

The allergens that generally produce allergic rhinitis may be classed as ''seasonal'' or ''perennial'' offenders. The former group consists primarily of pollens (grasses, weeds, trees), whereas the latter include dust mites, molds, animal danders, and cockroaches. In addition to these, some patients demonstrate allergy to other unusual plants, animals, and

Table 48-1. Effects of allergic mediators produced by mast cells and basophils

Mediators	Effects
Cellular attractants	
NCF	Attracts neutrophils
ECF-A	Attracts eosinophils and monocytes
LTB4	Attracts lymphocytes
Inflammatory agents	
Histamine	Vasodilation, increased vascular permeability
PAF	Microthrombi, tissue damage
Tryptase	Proteolysis, complement activation
Kinins	Vasodilation, edema
Spasmogens, mucus secretogogues	
Histamine	Bronchial smooth muscle contraction
PGD2	Mucus secretion
LTD4	Mucosal edema

Modified from Fireman P, Slavin RG: *Atlas of allergies*, ed 2, London, 1996, Mosby-Wolfe.
ECF—Eosinophilic chemotactic factor; *LT*—Leukotriene; *NCF*—Neutrophilic chemotactic factor; *PAF*—Platelet activating factor; *PG*—Prostaglandin.

fibers. However, in the vast majority of patients, testing may be confined to a small and well-defined group of antigens.

Seasonal antigens

Seasonal antigens are pollens and the pollinating seasons for these offenders will vary significantly with the geographic area involved. As a general rule, the sequence proceeds from grasses (in the spring) to trees (in the spring, with the exception of mountain cedar in the winter), to weeds (generally pollinating in the fall). In some temperate climates, offenders elsewhere classed as seasonal may be essentially perennial offenders.

All allergens are not equipotent in their ability to produce symptoms. On a milligram for milligram basis, the most potent seasonal antigens are grasses, followed by weeds, then trees (angiosperms being more potent than gymnosperms).

Perennial antigens

As the term implies, perennial antigens are those that may be present regardless of season. These include molds, dust mites, and animal danders. This group is sometimes expanded to include dust. The composition of commercial dust antigen is highly variable (dust mites, animal danders, kapok and other fibers, insect parts, and molds), and is therefore not readily standardized between lots and manufacturers.

Despite the designation, some perennial antigens are more prevalent during certain times of year. Dust and dust mites, for instance, have a "season" which is the converse of baseball season, with symptoms beginning in the fall, peaking during the winter, and declining in early spring.

The primary dust mites in the United State are *Dermatophagoides pteronyssinus* and *Dermatophagoides farinae*. These tiny mites live on skin scales and other debris, and thrive in warm (65° to 80° F) and humid (at least 50% to 70% relative humidity) circumstances. Their allergen is found in the fecal pellets they deposit. Significant reservoirs of dust mites include bedding, mattresses and pillows, carpets, upholstered furniture, and stuffed toys.

Molds (members of the fungi imperfecta) may be an indoor or outdoor allergen. Although outdoor mold levels drop precipitously with freezing weather, indoor mold levels remain fairly constant, and may actually increase indoors when conditions of warmth and moisture are present. Significant reservoirs of mold include indoor house plants, compost piles, leaves, and refrigerator drip pans.

It is not necessary to come in direct contact with animals to be exposed to their danders. The prime example is cat dander, which is extremely light, and clings stubbornly to reservoirs such as clothing, bedding, and upholstered furniture. Studies have shown cat dander in classrooms where no cat has ever been, because of dander carried on the clothes of students. Similar problems may occur with horse dander on the clothing of trainers or riders, as well as on horse blankets.

The cockroach is an often overlooked perennial allergen. Decomposing body parts of this insect are frequently found in older homes, schools, and other buildings (even those that are clean and well maintained). Cockroach sensitivity may be a significant contributor to asthma and rhinitis.

SYMPTOMS AND SIGNS OF ALLERGIC RHINITIS

The characteristic symptoms and signs of allergic rhinitis are easily understood if one keeps in mind the effects of the mediators released by mast cells and basophils as a result of a Gell and Coombs type I reaction (see Table 48-1). These include glandular stimulation, vasodilation, increased vascular permeability, and irritation, changes that are responsible for the typical symptoms of itching, sneezing, rhinorrhea, and nasal congestion.

An allergy history includes information about the seasons or circumstances that trigger symptoms, the types of symptoms that predominate, the results of any previous allergy testing and the effect of previous treatment, as well as the presence of complicating problems such as sinusitis, asthma, otitis media, and so forth. Although an allergic history begins at the time of the first visit, it is a constantly evolving process.

The signs of allergic rhinitis include the "allergic salute," which is characterized as follows: the hand lifts the nasal tip to respond to itching while temporarily opening the airway, a transverse nasal crease appears caused by repetition of this maneuver, and facial grimacing and twitching are present due to itching membranes. The nasal turbinates are generally pale to bluish. Another characteristic sign is clear rhinorrhea. The presence of polyps does not necessarily indicate allergy.[16] Obligate mouth-breathing may result in a typical open-mouthed countenance and "adenoid facies."[8]

ADJUNCTIVE TESTS

A number of adjunctive tests have traditionally been used to confirm the clinical diagnosis of allergic rhinitis. Among these are a differential count of peripheral leukocytes, or the examination of smears of nasal secretions for the presence of eosinophils.[6] These measures have generally given way to specific diagnostic techniques that measure levels of IgE for various antigens.

The diagnosis of allergic rhinitis is made by history, and the novice rhinologist must realize that the presence of a positive test is just that—a positive test. Clinical correlation between the patient's symptoms and any postulated sensitivity to the incriminated antigens is necessary to confirm a diagnosis of clinically relevant "allergy."

Confirmatory skin testing for allergy

The gold standard of allergy testing is generally considered to be skin testing. The basis of this procedure is the reaction between antigen and sensitized mast cells in the skin, producing the classic wheal and flare skin response. This reaction begins with an acute phase that starts within 2 to 5 minutes, reaches a maximum at 10 to 20 minutes, and is characterized by vasodilation (producing erythema) and local edema (producing a wheal). It may be followed by a late phase, with further whealing and induration occuring 4 to 6 hours or more later.

A number of factors affect skin tests. In addition to the volume and potency of antigen introduced, the degree of sensitization of cutaneous mast cells, and reactivity of the skin, responses also are modified by drugs, the age and race of the patient, the area of the body injected, the distance separating individual skin tests, and the time of day of testing.[11] Skin test responses are suppressed by antihistamines and tricyclic antidepressants. The latter must be discontinued for 48 to 96 hours before skin testing. Antihistamines generally must be avoided for 48 to 72 hours, although astemizole may affect skin test results for 3 to 6 weeks after it is discontinued. To assure that skin reactivity is normal, both positive and negative controls are necessary with all skin tests.

Skin tests are generally classified as epicutaneous or intracutaneous. The former group includes scratch tests and prick-puncture testing, whereas the latter group includes both single-dilution and multiple-dilution intradermal tests.

In 1865, Blackley performed a crude scratch test on himself to show his sensitivity to rye grass, and in the early 1900s scratch tests were commonly used to diagnose immediate-type allergy. Unfortunately, these tests produced numerous false-positive reactions, and the results were highly variable and difficult to interpret, as neither the amount of antigen nor the scratch through which it was introduced were

standardized. In 1987, the American Medical Association Council on Scientific Affairs pronounced scratch testing "less reproducible than prick and puncture tests," stating that they were "no longer recommended."[1]

The most commonly applied epicutaneous test is the prick or puncture method, which was developed by Lewis and Grant in 1924 but did not gain widespread acceptance until its modification by Pepys in 1975. In this test, a drop of test extract (or control solution) is placed on the skin, then a needle or similar instrument is passed at an angle through the liquid and the skin is pricked by lifting, to elevate the dermis without producing bleeding, or is punctured by perpendicular pressure with a needle. In interpreting the test, both the wheal and surrounding erythema are evaluated and measured, and are compared with positive and negative controls, with the results graded from 0 to 4 +. Positive prick-test reactions are generally noted in patients with higher levels of allergen-specific IgE, and the test may be negative in patients with lower (but significant) degrees of atopy. Thus, prick tests are often used as a screening test, and followed by intradermal testing when indicated.

A number of variants of the prick-puncture method have been developed in an effort to standardize the test and make it more sensitive. These include standardized test instruments such as the Morrow Brown needle and the Østerballe precision needle, as well as multiple-test devices such as the Multitest and Combion tests. These latter tests are not strictly prick tests because their needles may penetrate the dermis.

The intradermal test was applied to the diagnosis of allergy by Schloss in 1912, and popularized for this purpose by Cooke in 1915. In this test, a measured amount of antigen is injected intracutaneously to form a wheal. An antigenic reaction results in significant enlargement of the wheal. Allergists who use a single-dilution intradermal testing technique measure both the wheal and erythema produced, and compare them with positive and negative controls using a grading system of 0 to 4 +, in the same way as the prick test.[13] In order to minimize the risk of systemic reaction, single-dilution intradermal testing should not be performed unless a screening-prick test for the same antigen has shown that the patient is not exquisitely sensitive to it. Although the antigen concentrations used in intradermal testing are from 1000 to 10,000 times weaker than those used for prick testing, a much greater amount of antigen is introduced with this method (Table 48-2), therefore, the risk of a systemic reaction is greater with a single-dilution intradermal test than with a prick test.

Because skin testing with prick and single-dilution intradermal techniques does not permit accurate quantitation of the patient's sensitivity, the technique of progressive-dilution intradermal testing (also known as *skin endpoint titration*) was developed. Carrying forward the work of Hansel, Herbert Rinkel perfected a system of intradermal testing in the mid-1940s using a series of fivefold dilutions of the same antigen. Testing begins with an anticipated nonreacting dose

Table 48-2. Volume and antigen dose administered per test wheal, μg

Test	Volume	Antigen concentration
Prick test	3.3×10^{-6} ml	1:10 to 1:50 (w/v)
Multitest	21×10^{-6} ml	1:10 to 1:50 (w/v)
Intradermal	0.02 ml	1:100 to 1:1000 (w/v)
Skin endpoint titration	0.01 ml	1:100 to 1:312,500 (w/v)

Modified from Gordon BR: Allergy skin tests and immunotherapy: comparison of methods in common use, *ENT J* 69:47, 1990.
w/v—Weight/volume.

and progresses to the concentration that initiates positive whealing, and then continues with the application of the next stronger concentration. This endpoint of titration indicates the relative sensitivity of the patient to the tested allergen and represents the concentration at which immunotherapy can safely be initiated, thus avoiding prolonged therapy at very low doses while providing a significant safety factor.[14]

Confirmatory *in vitro* testing for allergy

Skin testing for allergy is subject to a number of drawbacks, including the potential for production of a significant reaction, and the discomfort, however minimal, associated with the procedure. These drawbacks have led to a continued search for other diagnostic methods. Shortly after the characterization of IgE as the sensitizing factor in allergy, Wide and others[19] developed a radioimmunoassay that could detect specific IgE antibodies in serum. This assay, which they called the *radioallergosorbent test* (RAST), evolved significantly over the years that followed and has become an important tool in the diagnosis of inhalant allergy.

Although numerous variations of technology exist, the basic principle of the *in vitro* analysis of allergen-specific IgE is a ''sandwich'' technique in which allergens on a solid phase (such as a paper disk) are allowed to react with serum from the patient. Any IgE antibodies to that allergen that are present bind to the solid phase. This resultant complex is then incubated with radiolabeled rabbit antibodies to human IgE. After washing, the amount of radioactivity in the resulting sandwich of allergen/antibody/anti-IgE/radioactive marker on the disk is measured using a γ counter, and the amount of antibody present is calculated.

The modified RAST technique and scoring system of Fadal and Nalebuff (F/N mRAST) significantly improved the use of the RAST, both increasing its clinical sensitivity and bringing the classes that resulted into parallel with results from skin endpoint titration. The major changes since the development of the F/N mRAST have been in the solid phase used (cellulose, plastic, hydrophilic polymer) and in the marker used (various fluorometric techniques). If the process involves enzymatic or fluorometric processes rather than a radioactive marker, it is generally referred to as an

enzyme-linked immunosorbent assay (ELISA). Although RAST is often used as a generic term for all of these, each technology has its own characteristics, and the clinician must become familiar with the system in use in his or her practice.

Along with the popularization of the allergen-specific RAST, the measurement of total IgE has been advocated as a means of diagnosing the presence of allergy. However, it has become apparent that in some instances a high total IgE (>100 IU/ml) is not associated with true allergy, whereas in others a low total IgE may be present in patients with significant allergy. At present, it appears that the measurement of total IgE may be useful in clarifying otherwise equivocal results, but has little value when used alone.

Modern technology exists for the assay of allergen-specific IgE for numerous antigens. However, as a general rule, an assay of 8 to 15 antigens is sufficient to adequately indicate the presence or absence of significant inhalant allergy.[5] Positive responses are followed by additional testing for other relevant antigens.

A further extension of the screening concept occurs in the use of discs that have a number of antigens bound to them. These may give either a ''yes/no'' response, or a semiquantitive indication of the amount of allergen-specific IgE present. A negative response often is sufficient to rule out the presence of significant inhalant allergy. On the other hand, before treatment may be rendered, specific testing for each potentially positive antigen in the screening mix must be carried out.

Management by environmental control

The best and most desirable management of allergy is avoidance when possible. Although this must often be supplemented by pharmacotherapy, and sometimes with immunotherapy, environmental control remains the most important component of this therapeutic triad.

Printed material about specific control measures aimed at various antigens is readily available from numerous commercial sources, but must be supplemented by advice from the physician. The most ''avoidable'' antigens are the perennial offenders: dust mites, molds, and animals.[17]

House dust mites thrive in warm, moist conditions, and feed on human skin scales (such as those found in bedclothes). The antigen is found in the mite feces. Control measures include elimination of reservoirs (upholstered furniture, carpeting, stuffed animals), covering of mattresses and pillows with barrier material, control of relative humidity (below 50%), and the use of acaracides (benzyl benzoate) or preparations that denature the dust mite antigen (tannic acid). Unfortunately, no compound yet exists that both kills dust mites and renders their antigen harmless.

The major animal antigen that causes allergic problems is cat allergen, which is secreted by sebaceous glands and borne on light skin scales. Removing the cat is often a suggestion met with resistance (if not active rebellion), and other measures are often necessary. These include keeping the cat out of the bedroom, and removal of as much antigen as possible from reservoirs (furniture, carpets) by vacuuming using a high-efficiency particulate arresting (HEPA) filter vacuum. Weekly washing of the cat with copious amounts of warm water also is effective as a preventive measure.

Mold is found in many areas of the home. It requires circumstances for growth similar to the dust mite (i.e., warmth and humidity), and control of these factors also will help control indoor mold growth. In addition, such sources of indoor mold as refrigerator drip pans, stored material in basements and attics, and the soil around indoor plants should be considered in attempting to remove mold from the patient's environment.

Management by pharmacotherapy

Antigens are not always avoidable, and immunotherapy modifies the allergic response but does not always afford protection from an overwhelming antigen exposure. Therefore, symptomatic management by means of pharmacotherapy is required to some degree for every patient with allergic rhinitis. Numerous types of drugs are available for this purpose, and each has unique characteristics (Box 48-1). The physician must tailor the regimen according to the patient's symptoms and circumstances.

Box 48-1. Pharmacotherapy for allergic rhinitis

Antihistamines: rhinorrhea, sneezing, itching
  Side effects: first-generation sedation, anticholinergic effects, second-generation arrhythmias (terfenadine, astemizole), weight gain (astemizole).
Decongestants: nasal congestion
  Side effects: cardiovascular and central nervous system stimulation (potentiated by interaction with monoamine-oxidase inhibitors, tricyclic antidepressants); rebound rhinitis with topical preparations
Mast cell stabilizers: prevention/control rhinorrhea, sneezing, itching
  Side effects: local irritation
Corticosteroids: rhinorrhea, sneezing, itching, some control of congestion
  Side effects, systemic: hypothalamic-pituitary-adrenal suppression, cataracts, hypertension, hormonal irregularities, ulcer activation, osteoporosis, psychiatric aberrations, aseptic necrosis of the femoral head
  Side effects, topical: local irritation; systemic effects (with excessive use at high doses)
Anticholinergics: rhinorrhea
  Side effects, systemic: dry mouth/thick secretions, increased intraocular pressure, blurred vision, hyperthermia, tachycardia, urinary retention
  Side effects, topical: local irritation, rash

Modified from King HC, Mabry RL: *A practical guide to the management of nasal and sinus disorders,* New York, 1993, Thieme.

Antihistamines

Antihistamines act to control the "wet" symptoms of allergic rhinitis, such as rhinorrhea, sneezing, and itching membranes. Progressively more sophisticated forms have been developed since the pioneering work of Bovet and Staub in 1937. First-generation antihistamines (also called sedating preparations because of their most common side effect) act by competing with histamine for receptor sites on target organs. In addition to sedation, they may produce anticholinergic effects resulting in bladder neck obstruction and prostatism and excessive dryness of secretions. Prolonged usage of these preparations results in tachyphylaxis, or tolerance, requiring a change to a different form of antihistamine. Examples of first-generation antihistamines include chlorpheniramine, brompheniramine, triprolidine, and diphenhydramine.

Second-generation, or nonsedating, antihistamines generally have multiple actions, which often include direct effects on allergic mediators. Because they do not readily cross the blood-brain barrier, they either do not produce sedation, or do so only in large doses. Their anticholinergic effects are much less pronounced, and they are free of tachyphylaxis. However, two of these preparations (terfenadine, astemizole) have been shown to present an increased risk of cardiac arrhythmias when administered concomitantly with macrolide antibiotics and systemic antifungals. Other examples of second-generation antihistamines are loratadine, cetirizine, and acrivastine.

A third generation of antihistamines includes those that are used topically (e.g., livostin, azelastine) and "designer" antihistamines that are metabolites and congeners of existing drugs (e.g., fexofenidine) with fewer potential side effects but increased effectiveness.[15]

Decongestants

Decongestants are α-adrenergic agonists that produce vasoconstriction in the turbinates, lessening nasal congestion. When topically applied for more than 5 to 7 days they may produce a rebound rhinitis, and addiction to nose drops and sprays is a commonly encountered phenomenon in patients with chronic rhinitis. Because nasal allergy is a chronic disorder, such patients are more likely to abuse topical nasal decongestants, and must be warned of the problem.

The most common orally administered decongestants are pseudoephedrine, phenylpropanolamine, and phenylephrine. Potential side effects of these drugs are related to their vasopressor actions (which may cause elevated blood pressure, especially in patients with preexisting labile hypertension), and their central nervous system (CNS) stimulatory effects (producing insomnia and jitteriness). These stimulatory side effects are potentiated in patients taking tricyclic antidepressants or monoamine oxidase (MAO) inhibitors (in the latter case persisting for up to 2 weeks after the MAO inhibitor is discontinued).

For the management of allergic rhinitis, decongestants are often combined with either first- or second-generation antihistamines.

Mast cell stabilizers

The prototype of mast cell stabilizers, cromolyn, has been available in the United States as a topical nasal solution since 1983. In laboratory animals, cromolyn was found to stabilize mast cells, preventing the allergic reaction. Additional work has shown that in human subjects this is only one of the effects of this class of drugs, which have numerous other actions. Nevertheless, by convention, they are still referred to as *mast cell stabilizers*.

Cromolyn is most beneficial when used prior to an anticipated allergen exposure, but must be administered at least four times daily for maximum effect. Patients with severe allergic rhinitis may not respond adequately to this medication, but it is an extremely safe and often effective initial therapeutic measure.

Corticosteroids

Corticosteroid preparations are potent antiinflammatory agents, which do not prevent an antigen-antibody allergic reaction, but diminish the effects of vasoactive kinins and other mediators by decreasing capillary permeability, stabilizing lysosomal membranes, blocking the action of migratory inhibitory factor, and directly affecting phospholipase. Systemically administered corticosteroids primarily affect the late-phase allergic reaction, while topical preparations also may act on the acute phase after pretreatment for a week or longer.

Systemic administration of corticosteroids must be done with the full realization of their potential for suppression of endogenous cortisol production, as well as their possible adverse effects on many organ systems. Significant hypothalamic-pituitary-adrenal suppression may occur after approximately 5 to 7 days of the daily administration of 20 to 30 mg of prednisone or its equivalent, or occur in up to 30 days with lower doses. Adrenal recovery may occur within 1 week of discontinuing short-term, high-dose therapy, while up to 1 year or more may be required following prolonged, high-dose therapy.[18]

Potential adverse effects of systemically administered corticosteroids may be major or minor (see Box 48-1). Systemic corticosteroids in the management of allergic rhinitis may be administered orally as a tapered-dosage program (either tailored by the physician or as a commercially available item), or in the form of a repository injection. The latter should be administered with caution because although the corticosteroid effect provides relief for up to 6 weeks, virtually total hypothalamic-pituitary-adrenal suppression may occur for this same period of time.[10]

The popularization of topical nasal corticosteroid preparations during the past 15 years has greatly diminished the systemic administration of these preparations. The tendency has been for newer forms to require less frequent administration (improving patient compliance), and to have less likelihood of systemic effect (diminishing the possibility of complications associated with prolonged usage at high doses). Up to one half of all nasally administered steroids may be absorbed from the nasal mucosa. A portion of the material also is swallowed and is absorbed from the gastrointestinal tract. However, with the exception of dexamethasone, all nasal corticosteroids undergo extensive first-pass hepatic metabolism to either inactive or less active compounds. This metabolism, plus the pharmacodynamics of the individual preparation, prevents significant systemic effects from topical administration unless they are administered for prolonged periods and at higher than recommended doses (or if the patient is also using an inhaled corticosteroid preparation for lower-airway disease).

Currently, nasal corticosteroids are administered as either a pump spray (generally in an aqueous vehicle) or as a suspension dispensed in a powered fashion by a propellant (formerly a chlorofluorocarbon, now a more environmentally friendly compound). One nasal steroid in powder form (fluocortin) is under investigation. The dosage and approximate margins of safety (multiple of the maximum recommended initial dose that has been shown to result in hypothalamic-pituitary-adrenal suppression) of currently available nasal corticosteroids are listed in Table 48-3.

All topical nasal corticosteroids may cause side effects such as local nasal irritation, crusting, epistaxis, or even nasal septal perforation. The development of better pressurized delivery systems and sprays has improved this problem somewhat, as has the emphasis on advising patients of the proper way to use these sprays. This advice includes directing the tip of the nozzle toward the corner of the eye (away from the septum), and using sprays only for the duration

Table 48-3. Topical nasal corticosteroids

Preparation	Delivery	Doses/day	Margin*
Dexamethasone (Dexacort)	Prop	3	1+
Beclomethasone (Beconase, Vancenase)	Prop	2-4	5
Beclomethasone (Beconase AQ, Vancenase AQ)	Prop	2	5
Flunisolide (Nasalide, Nasarel)	Pump	2	3.5
Triamcinolone (Nasacort)	Prop	1	8
Triamcinolone (Nasacort AQ)	Pump	1	8
Budesonide (Rhinocort)	Prop	1	4
Fluticasone (Flonase)	Pump	1	8
Fluocortin (Rhinolar)	Powder	3	NA

Modified from King HC, Mabry RL: *A practical guide to the management of nasal and sinus disorders*, New York, 1993, Thieme.
Prop—Propellant-powered delivery system; NA—Not available.
* Margin of safety is the multiple or recommended initial dose required to produce HPA suppression.

recommended, with regular examinations to watch for signs of local damage.

Intraturbinal injection of repository corticosteroids has been shown to be a safe and effective means of giving relief from severe nasal allergic symptoms for a period of 4 to 6 weeks, with no significant systemic or local adverse effects. Rare instances of transient or permanent visual loss have occurred, due to retinal vasospasm or embolization.[9] However, when properly performed by the experienced clinician, the procedure is extremely useful. Nevertheless, a thorough review of proper techniques is mandatory before this methodology is employed.[7]

Anticholinergics

Because rhinorrhea is such a prominent feature of allergic rhinitis, combination preparations that contain anticholinergic drugs have been marketed for many years. Unfortunately, many of these had a profound overdrying effect, provoking nasal crusting and thickened nasal and sinus secretions. Only a few such preparations are still marketed.

Early efforts to administer topical anticholinergics included atropine in saline, compounded and administered in a spray bottle. Although often effective for up to 4 hours, a variable amount of drug was administered in each dose by this technique. In 1996, the Food and Drug Administration approved the marketing of the topical anticholinergic, ipratropium bromide, as an aqueous nasal pump spray formulation. The 0.03% strength of this drug, administered in a dose of two sprays in each nostril three times daily, produces a significant decrease in the rhinorrhea associated with symptomatic allergic rhinitis. The preparation is generally free of systemic anticholinergic effects, but offers no relief of congestion, sneezing, or itching that accompanies allergic rhinitis.

New drugs

In addition to "designer" antihistamines and more potent yet safer topical nasal corticosteroids, new antiallergy drugs are being developed to modulate the allergic reaction and inhibit the formation of vasoactive effector substances. These include leukotriene inhibitors (e.g., zileuton, a 5-lipoxygenase inhibitor), and peptides such as IgE pentapeptide and N-acetyl-aspartyl-glutamate.

Management by immunotherapy

Although not all patients with allergic rhinitis require immunotherapy, it does offer the only "cure" for this disorder. The exact mechanism through which immunotherapy is effective is still a matter of conjecture. The administration of escalating doses of an antigen to which IgE-mediated atopy exists is known to result in an eventual lowering of allergen-specific IgE, concomitant with an elevation of immunoglobulin G (IgG) and subsequent activation of allergen-specific T cells. The IgG stimulation is thought to possibly represent the formation of "blocking antibodies" that impede the allergic reaction.

Indications for immunotherapy include IgE-mediated allergy that is not readily controlled by simple pharmacotherapeutic measures, and involve symptoms that span more than one season, are severe (even for only a few weeks), and are produced by allergens that are not readily avoidable. In addition, immunotherapy should in general only be considered in patients who are likely to cooperate in a program that will span 3 to 5 years.

The technique of immunotherapy involves using doses of antigen that are as high as safely possible to administer for each reacting allergen in order to reach therapeutic levels as quickly as possible. This is best accomplished by quantitation through *in vitro* means (RAST or ELISA) or dilutional-intradermal testing (skin-endpoint titration). Progressively larger doses and more concentrated antigen solutions are employed, while always watching carefully for unacceptable local reactions (a skin wheal of 3 cm or more) or worsening of systemic symptoms following an injection. Eventually, doses of about 40 to 1000 μg of antigen (corresponding to a 1:500 weight/volume concentration of extract) should be achieved to produce long-term beneficial results.[3]

Injections are normally administered once or twice weekly until effects are noted, then once a week for a total of 1 year. Maintenance therapy is given every 2 to 3 weeks, and the total duration of therapy generally does not exceed 3 to 5 years. Although systemic reactions rarely complicate immunotherapy, which is based on the quantitative testing methods described, they remain a possibility. Thus, immunotherapy should only be administered by qualified personnel. The reader is referred to one of the numerous excellent resources on the subject for further information in this regard.[4]

CONCLUSION

Allergic rhinitis may present as a distinct clinical entity, or may coexist with other disease states such as sinusitis, polyposis, asthma, and laryngitis. The otorhinolaryngologist should be able to suspect the presence of nasal allergy based on typical history and physical examination, administer appropriate pharmacotherapy, and advise patients in proper environmental control. Testing to confirm specific inciting antigens and the administration of definitive immunotherapy may require referral, but should not be outside the abilities of the properly trained rhinologist.

REFERENCES

1. AMA Council on Scientific Affairs: In vivo diagnostic testing and immunotherapy for allergy, report 1, part 1, of the allergy panel, *JAMA* 258:1363, 1987.
2. Gell PGH, Coombs RRA, Lachman PT: *Clinical aspects of immunology*, Oxford, 1975, Blackwell Scientific Publications.
3. Gordon BR: Allergy skin tests and immunotherapy: comparison of methods in common use, *Ear Nose Throat* 69:47, 1990.
4. King HC: *An otolaryngologist's guide to allergy*, New York, 1990, Thieme.

5. King WP: Efficacy of a screening radioallergosorbent test, *Arch Otolaryngol* 108:781, 1982.

6. Krause HF: *Nasal cytology in clinical allergy.* In Krause HF, editor: *Otolaryngic allergy and immunology*, Philadelphia, 1989, WB Saunders.

7. Mabry RL: Intranasal steroids in rhinology: the changing role of intraturbinal injection, *Ear Nose Throat* 73:242, 1994.

8. Marks MB: *Stigmata of respiratory tract allergies,* Kalamazoo, Mich 1967, Upjohn.

9. McCleve D, Goldstein J, Silver S: Corticosteroid injections of the nasal turbinates: past experience and precautions, *Otolaryngol Head Neck Surg* 86:851, 1978.

10. Mikhair GR and others: Effect of long-acting parenteral corticosteroids on adrenal function, *Arch Dermatol* 100:263, 1969.

11. Nelson HS: Diagnostic procedures in allergy. I. Allergy skin testing, *Ann Allergy* 51:411, 1983.

12. NIAID Task Force Report: *Asthma and the other allergic diseases,* Washington, DC, 1979, National Institutes of Health Publication 79-387.

13. Norman PS: *In vivo methods of study of allergy: skin tests, techniques, and interpretation.* In Middleton E Jr, Ellis EF, Reed CE editors: *Allergy, principles and practice,* ed 2, St Louis, 1983, Mosby.

14. Rinkel HJ: The management of clinical allergy, part II, etiologic factors and skin titration, *Arch Otolaryngol* 77:42, 1963.

15. Simons FER, Simons KJ: The pharmacology and use of H1-receptor antagonist drugs, *N Engl J Med* 330:1663, 1994.

16. Slavin RG: Allergy is not a significant cause of nasal polyps, *Arch Otolaryngol* 118:771, 1992.

17. Squillace SP: Environmental control, *Otolaryngol Head Neck Surg* 107(suppl):831, 1992.

18. USP Drug Information for the Health Care Professional, ed 16, Rockville, Md, 1996, US Pharmacopeial Convention.

19. Wide L, Bennick H, Johansson SGO: Diagnosis of allergy by an in vitro test for allergen antibodies, *Lancet* 2:1105, 1967.

Chapter 49

Nonallergic Rhinitis and Infection

David N.F. Fairbanks
Michael Kaliner

To systematize thinking about the "stuffy nose" (nasal congestion or nasal dyspnea), it is helpful to list the various etiologic factors under four major categories as in the list below, provided one recognizes that some overlap exists between categories and that several coexisting factors may be operative in any patient.

1. Structural disorders
   a. Deformities: external, internal, congenital malformations, injuries
   b. Neoplasms and masses
   c. Foreign bodies
2. Inflammatory disorders
   a. Rhinitis/sinusitis: bacterial, viral, fungal
   b. Nasal and sinus polyposis
   c. Ozena, atrophic rhinitis
   d. Immunologic diseases: sarcoidosis, Wegener's granulomatosis, polyarteritis nodosa, midline granuloma
3. Allergic rhinitis
4. Vasomotor rhinitis (Box 49-1)

Allergists tend to classify nasal conditions as either allergic or nonallergic, the distinction being made on whether or not the patient's skin tests are positive for whatever antigens are applied.[18] "Nonallergic rhinitis" by such classification encompasses a rather broad conglomerate of disorders, some of which (e.g., structural disorders) are not at all inflammatory, which makes the suffix "—itis" not appropriate. It would be rather silly to list nasal septal deformity as a type of nonallergic rhinitis.

Infections, however, are inflammatory conditions, and

they will be discussed at the end of this chapter, but only briefly, since sinusitis is the subject of more detailed expositions elsewhere in this book.

In this chapter, the term *vasomotor rhinitis* will be applied to a group of nasal conditions that are not structural, not infectious or suppurative, not autoimmune, and not allergic in the traditional sense (i.e., not immunoglobulin E [IgE] mediated or positive for skin tests) (see Box 49-1). Technically, bacterial or viral infections and even allergies cause a vasomotor reaction in the nasal membranes, but traditionally the term *vasomotor rhinitis* excludes such entities. Some authors prefer to use *vasomotor rhinitis* to indicate only conditions of unknown etiology.[2] All classifications are arbitrary by nature. We prefer to use the term in its physiologic sense.

VASOMOTOR RHINITIS PHYSIOLOGY

Vaso refers to blood vessels; *motor* to forces; and *rhinitis* to inflammatory conditions of the nose. A brief review of nasal vascular anatomy helps one to understand this important and complex condition.

The internal part of the nose receives arterial supply from the anterior and posterior ethmoid arteries, the sphenopalatine arteries, and the greater palatine arteries. The venous drainage is less specific. In general, the venous plexuses about the head—chiefly the orbital, cavernous, and pterygoid—receive the blood from the nasal fossa and shunt it to the jugular veins in the neck. Since there are no valves in this venous system, the pressure and flow dynamics vary with the posture of the individual.

Box 49-1. Vasomotor rhinitis

1. Drug induced
   a. Antihypertensives
   b. Nose drop/spray abuse
   c. Cocaine
   d. Birth control pills
2. Pregnancy and ''premenstrual colds''
3. Hypothyroidism
4. Emotional causes
5. Temperature mediated
6. Irritative and environmental rhinitis
7. Gustatory rhinitis
8. End-stage vascular atony of chronic allergic or inflammatory rhinitis
9. Recumbency rhinitis
10. Paradoxic nasal obstruction and nasal cycle
11. Rhinitis of no airflow (laryngectomy, choanal atresia, adenoid hyperplasia)
12. Compensatory hypertrophic rhinitis
13. Eosinophilic and basophilic nonallergic rhinitis
14. Other systemic disorders: superior vena cava syndrome, Horner's syndrome, cirrhosis, uremia
15. Idiopathic rhinitis

The minute arterioles course in parallel rows in a posteroanterior direction. In contrast to the usual sequential arrangement of arteriole-capillary-venule, venous sinusoids or lakes are located between the capillaries and venules. Thus, capillary blood enters these sinusoids before it passes into the venules. The sinusoids are surrounded by fine fibrils of smooth muscle, giving them the power of vasoconstriction and vasodilation. When they fill and distend, the tissue engorges to such a degree that it is looked on as erectile tissue (Fig. 49-1). This is most striking in the inferior turbinates (Fig. 49-2) and is less so in the nasal septum and other turbinate membranes.

The smooth muscle fibers of the arterioles and venous sinusoids are innervated by the autonomic nervous system.[14] Parasympathetic stimulation results in vasodilation, which engorges the sinusoids with blood and increases congestion and mucus production. Sympathetic stimulation results in vasoconstriction, which squeezes blood out of the nasal membranes, thereby increasing nasal patency and decreasing mucus production.

CAUSES OF VASOMOTOR RHINITIS

Drug-induced rhinitis

Certain drugs, especially those that affect autonomic vascular control, may affect the vascular channels of the nose.

Antihypertensives

Sympathetic blocking agents, such as reserpine, guanethidine, hydralazine, methyldopa, propranolol, and other β-blockers, may produce a stuffy nose as a side effect. This comes from depletion of norepinephrine stores, resulting in unopposed parasympathetic vasodilation.[18] Reserpine is the most troublesome in this regard, affecting 8% of users. If this is a problem, the patient's physician can usually substitute another antihypertensive agent that causes less nasal congestion.

Nose drop/spray abuse

Decongestants are sympathomimetics that are used for their vasoconstrictive action. However, when used topically, their vasoconstriction is so intense that a semiischemic state occurs, during which time products of metabolism accumulate that are strong vasodilators. A rebound vasodilation occurs, creating congestion again. The more frequent and prolonged the use of the topical vasoconstrictors, the more profound the rebound until a loss of vascular tone ensues. The nasal congestion is often profound (Fig. 49-3). For this reason, decongestant nose drops and nose sprays should not be used for more than 3 consecutive days.

An old term for this condition is *rhinitis medicamentosa*, which is rather awkward and even comical sounding; a simpler, more descriptive term would be *rebound rhinitis*.

The treatment of rebound rhinitis requires cessation of the nose drop-spray compulsion. A short course of oral or topical corticosteroid might be very helpful. Simultaneously, the physician must address the initiating condition that led the patient to start the habit. Allergies, infections and structural abnormalities may need attention.

Infants are particularly susceptible to rebound rhinitis and may develop it after just a few days of nose drop usage. Since infants are obligate nasal breathers, a hazardous condition ensues. Fortunately, their response to withdrawal of the drops is prompt and total. Adults, on the other hand, take several days to improve even under the best of circumstances. If the habit has been well established for months or years, the nasal vasculature may have suffered such permanent changes as to require surgical therapy to the turbinates.

Cocaine

Because cocaine is also a vasoconstrictor, it is theoretically possible that a rebound rhinitis could occur from intranasal ''recreational use.''[16] As a practical matter, however, most abusers do not use it constantly. Further, ''street cocaine'' generally contains adulterants whose deleterious effects overshadow the rebound rhinitis that might result from cocaine. Common adulterants include lactose, mannitol, lidocaine, caffeine, salicylamide, heroin, camphor, talc, borax, and a variety of contaminating bacteria.[1]

These irritants cause crusting, nasal picking, and atrophic rhinitis; when the vasoconstrictive effect of cocaine is superimposed, the septal cartilage suffers from a lack of adequate blood supply, which in turn may lead to nasal septal perforation.

Birth control pills

Some women complain of nasal congestion when they are taking anovulatory drugs.[18] This condition is caused by the vasoactive effect of progesterone as described next.

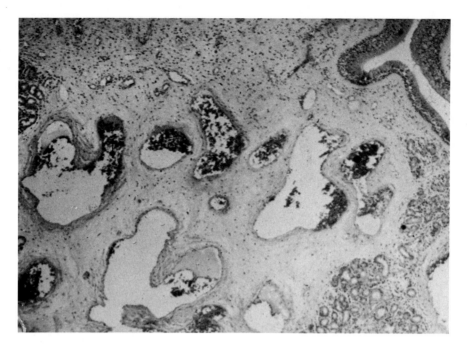

Fig. 49-1. The inferior turbinate mucosa in vasomotor rhinitis shows the cavernous venous plexus of erectile tissue.

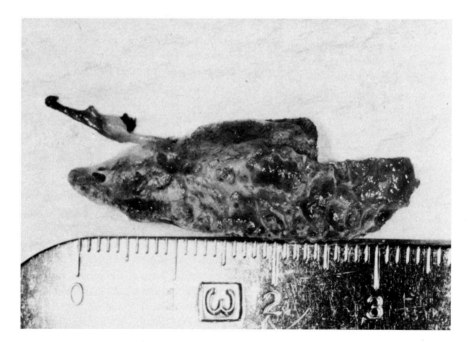

Fig. 49-2. The inferior turbinate bone in vasomotor rhinitis shows a pock-marked surface from the impression of the cavernous venous plexus.

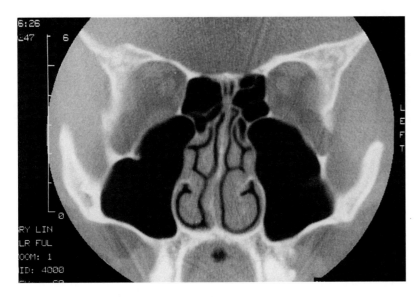

Fig. 49-3. Profound turbinate hypertrophy and nasal congestion result from rebound rhinitis of decongestant nose spray abuse.

Pregnancy and "premenstrual colds"

Most women note some degree of nasal congestion during pregnancy, and for a few it becomes quite disabling.[9,15,18] This progressively worsens throughout pregnancy in a direct relationship with the endogenous progesterone levels, which rise dramatically during the latter months. Progesterone causes vascular engorgement not only in the uterus, but also in the nose. For the same reason, some women note nasal congestion in the immediate premenstrual period, which they may mistakenly call a "cold."

Many obstetricians prefer that their pregnant patients suffer the nasal congestion rather than take drugs for it. Nevertheless, countless such patients take it on themselves to use over-the-counter antihistamines and decongestants. Many of these drugs have been widely used for many decades without proven harmful effects on the fetus, but actual experimentation in human subjects is lacking. Therefore, one cannot state that safety for use in pregnancy has been officially established. Thus the physician can offer such bits of advice, and the patient is left to make her own choice in the matter.

In general, the older antihistamine preparations such as tripelennamine (Pyribenzamine) and chlorpheniramine (ChlorTrimeton) are preferred over newer ones for patients whose condition is aggravated by a coincidental allergic rhinitis.[15,18] Topical application of corticosteroids (e.g., beclomethasone) is preferred to oral administration.[3] Orally taken decongestants such as pseudoephedrine (Sudafed, Novafed) enjoy a long safety record and may be useful for nonallergic patients, except for those who are at risk for hypertension. Elevation of the head of the bed may also be somewhat helpful. Pregnant patients who develop the nose spray habit risk a major problem with rebound rhinitis.

Extremely disabled patients may require cryosurgical treatment of the turbinates, which can be done in the office with the patient under topical and local anesthesia. The temporary effect of cryosurgery is acceptable in this instance because pregnancy is a self-limited condition.

Hypothyroidism

In up to 3% of patients with vasomotor rhinitis the diagnosis is hypothyroidism.[17] The generally hypoactive sympathetic status leads to predominance of parasympathetic activity in the nose, with vasodilation. After the endocrine abnormality is stabilized, the degree of residual change in nasal vasculature can be assessed and managed as below.

Emotional causes

Life situations that produce anxiety, hostility, guilt, or feelings of frustration and resentment can disturb the autonomic vascular balance.[18] They may cause nasal congestion and discharge by themselves, but more often they exacerbate existing nasal disease. This etiology should be considered a diagnosis of exclusion. The nasal congestion that accompanies a migraine headache is a specific example of how dysfunction in the carotid arterial system affects the nose, and it explains why so many patients with vascular headaches are certain in their own minds that they have sinus headaches.

Even if stress and anxiety cannot be eliminated, treatment directed against the nasal congestion is usually appreciated.

Temperature-mediated rhinitis

Environmental temperature exerts a vasomotor-mediated effect on nasal airway patency. In general, heat elicits vasodilation, and cool air causes vasoconstriction in much the same way that skin wastes or conserves heat. Curiously, however, a person whose feet are exposed to cold is likely to suffer nasal congestion.[11] This commonly observed phenomenon once led a public official to complain about the British House of Commons, which was so poorly heated in the winter, that it gave the members "cold feet and stuffy heads"—the worst possible combination of effects for a legislator.

These observations recall some of the old remedies for a cold: bundle up warmly with feet in a tub of hot water, a hot water bottle on the head, and a cold breeze blowing into the room through an open window. That might be good advice but only in moderation, because prolonged exposure to cold (e.g., sitting in a room at near-freezing temperatures for 60 minutes) evokes an increase in nasal airway resistance, particularly in persons with allergic rhinitis.[18]

Irritative and environmental rhinitis

Acute or chronic exposure to irritating dust (especially woodworking dust), gases (formaldehyde outgassing from particle board construction materials), chemicals (i.e., chlorophenol wood preservative, chromic acid fumes, paint and cleaning solution fumes, and vanadium), perfumes and cosmetic preparations delivered by aerosol, and other air pollutants (especially sulfur dioxide) elicits a vasomotor reaction that is not truly allergic, but one that creates nasal congestion nevertheless. The most pervasive of these is tobacco smoke, which is inhaled in much higher concentrations than any other environmental pollutant. Treatment of inhaled irritants is avoidance or air filtration. Filter masks are useful for dust at home or at work. (See the discussion of cocaine on page 911.)

Gustatory rhinitis

Some patients develop rhinorrhea when eating or drinking, especially with hot or spicy foods or beverages. This is a reflex cholinergic discharge triggered by sensory receptors on the palate, which causes nasal secretion, and sometimes flushing, tearing, and sweating. Treatment is ipratropium bromide nasal spray 0.03% (Atrovent) administered 10 minutes before meals.

End-stage vascular atony of chronic allergic or inflammatory rhinitis

Every physician who has cared for nasal disorders can recall frustrating cases in which appropriate and vigorous therapy for proven allergic rhinitis has failed to relieve nasal congestion, even though other allergy symptoms were relieved. This is because prolonged and profound parasympathetic stimulation of the nasal vascular system may lead to permanent loss of vascular tone. This phenomenon is seen not only with chronic allergies but also with chronic sinusitis. Richardson[13] reminded his audiences of this erectile nature of nasal vasculature by calling this condition *nasal turbinate priapism*. It can best be explained to patients as analogous to varicose veins.

Recumbency rhinitis

Recumbency rhinitis is a nonspecific complaint of persons who experience any form of vasomotor nasal congestion, whether acute or chronic. The hypotonic vascular bed of the nose responds to the dependent position by filling with blood in much the same way that varicose veins become engorged when the extremities are placed in a dependent position. Some investigators regard this phenomenon as a nasal reflex neurally mediated by pressure receptors in the skin.

When a person with rhinitis sleeps on his side, the dependent side becomes congested and the upper side more patent. This also explains why the person whose deviated septum obstructs the right side, for example, usually sleeps with his left side uppermost; otherwise, if he should position his more open side down, it would become congested, and then neither side would be functional.

Paradoxic nasal obstruction and nasal cycle

Eighty percent of adults experience a cyclic congestion and decongestion of the turbinates that alternates from one side to the other.[7] The mean duration of the cycle is 2.5 hours, but wide variability occurs. This is an autonomic nervous system–mediated vasomotor phenomenon. Since it is normal and physiologic, most persons are unaware of it. However, when it is superimposed on some other cause for nasal obstruction, it can be troublesome. This is especially notable in patients with one-sided nasal obstruction from long-standing deformity of the nasal septum.

With a fixed nasal obstruction, the abnormal side maintains a constant degree of resistance, and the patient may have lost awareness of it. However, the opposite or normal side has a variable resistance because of the continued fluctuations of the nasal cycle, which creates more awareness. Consequently, when the normal side is in the decongested phase of the cycle, the total nasal resistance may be within normal limits, whereas when the normal side is in the congested (turbinate engorgement) phase, the total nasal resistance may exceed the tolerable level, and the patient complains of nasal obstruction on the more normal side; hence the term *paradoxic nasal obstruction*.

Nonairflow rhinitis

Laryngectomy/tracheostomy rhinitis

When the nose has, by some structural abnormality, become excluded from the reciprocating flow of air with its cyclic variations in temperature and humidity and its effects on movement of mucus, a vasomotor reaction occurs. The vascular bed loses its tone, and the turbinates become boggy, swollen, and violaceous. This is a familiar picture to anyone who has examined the nose in a postoperative laryngectomy patient.

Choanal atresia rhinitis

The choanal atresia patient demonstrates an appearance of the nasal membranes similar to that in the laryngectomy patient, but additionally clear nasal mucus accumulates, which cannot be expelled posteriorly by the natural forces of airflow and ciliary action.

Adenoid rhinitis

To a variable extent vasomotor changes may also occur in a child whose nasopharynx is largely occluded by adenoidal hypertrophy.[14] Whether or not infection is active, the phenomenon of no airflow creates a vasomotor rhinitis with boggy, swollen turbinates and accumulations of clear, watery secretions.

Unfortunately, adenoid rhinitis may masquerade as an "allergic nose," which can lead an unwary physician and his patient on a costly, elaborate, and frustrating detour into allergy shots, dietary restrictions, and environmental prohibitions. The embarrassment of the physician is minor compared with the hostility of the parents when they insist on an adenoidectomy and find that it cures the "allergy."

Compensatory hypertrophic rhinitis

Anatomists have long been aware that when a nasal septum is deformed toward one side, the excess space created in the opposite nasal cavity becomes occupied by overgrowth of one or more of the nasal turbinates (Fig. 49-4). It is possible this occurs to protect the more patent side from excess nasal airflow with its drying and cooling effects.

When the middle turbinate participates in this event, it may become curled and redundant in the middle meatus, or an ectopic sinus cell may develop (20% of adults have such a cell [Fig. 49-5]). The inferior turbinate is most commonly involved. The turbinate becomes thicker and more spongy (see Fig. 49-2) and arches further medially into the airway. Also, the mucosa hypertrophies, and a deep vascular bed develops with an exaggerated expansile capacity.

These changes are not spontaneously reversible, and they should be corrected in conjunction with any nasal septal surgery that is performed. Otherwise, the patient will complain that the septal surgery only partially relieved obstruc-

tion on one side of the nose, although significant obstruction persists bilaterally.

Eosinophilic and basophilic nonallergic rhinitis

Eosinophilic nonallergic rhinitis and *basophilic nonallergic rhinitis* are terms applied to clinical conditions of unknown etiology with symptoms suggestive of allergic rhinitis but in which immunoglobulin E (IgE) tests are normal and skin tests to allergens appropriate for the geographic area are negative.[2] Cytology of nasal mucosal smears determines how the condition is named. The eosinophilic group has been termed nonallergic rhinitis with eosinophilia syndrome (NARES).

NARES patients suffer repetitive sneezing attacks, profuse rhinorrhea, and itching in the nose or eyes. They are exquisitely sensitive to environmental stimuli such as smoke, chemical odors, perfume, and changes in posture or weather (temperature and barometric pressure). Attacks can occur anytime of day but are usually worse on arising in the morning. There is no seasonal pattern, and congestion is not generally a complaint.

Neither antihistamines nor decongestants provide significant relief of symptoms, but nasal steroids usually produce a dramatic improvement, and eosinophilia diminishes. Response to steroids suggests to some investigators that these conditions could be caused by unrecognized allergens.

Other systemic disorders

Superior vena cava syndrome (periorbital erythema/edema, nasal stuffiness, headache, and progressive facial swelling) may so mimic allergy symptoms that patients are referred for allergy workups.[17] All of the head and neck venous vasculature is distended, including that of the nasal mucosa. Usually, a chest x-ray film will reveal a mass (97%

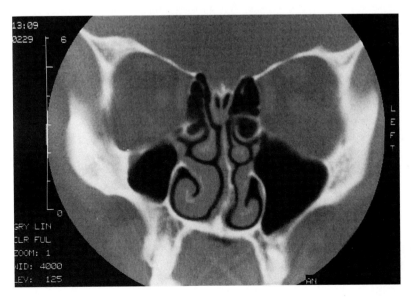

Fig. 49-4. Compensatory inferior turbinate overgrowth of bone and mucosa fills space created by a septal deformity.

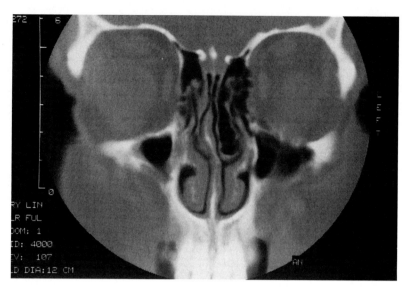

Fig. 49-5. Compensatory middle turbinate overgrowth with ectopic ethmoid sinus cell.

chance of malignancy) encroaching on the vena cava in the superior mediastinum.

Horner's syndrome (unilateral hyperemia, swelling, hypersecretion, miosis, and nasal obstruction) derives from interference with sympathetic innervation. It suggests neoplasm in the neck or a stellate ganglion block.

Cirrhosis and uremia also produce some degree of nasal congestion.

Idiopathic rhinitis

Unfortunately, some patients with either nasal congestion or rhinorrhea defy diagnosis despite thorough investigation. Empiric therapeutic trials are then offered with topical ipratropium, atropine, or cromolyn and with nonspecific measures discussed below.

DIAGNOSIS

History taking requires an awareness not only about nasal disorders per se, but also about systemic disorders with nasal manifestations, as noted in the previous list and box (see Box 49-1 and Chapter 44).

Vasomotor rhinitis is often a diagnosis of exclusion, and necessarily so because other causes of nasal obstruction are far more prevalent. Allergic rhinitis is the most common cause of chronic nasal congestion; the common cold predominates as the most frequent cause of acute complaints.

Sinusitis (acute and chronic) is associated with nasal congestion. The patient's history is vital. A thorough examination of the nasal passages (including the nasopharynx) before and after application of a topical nasal decongestant may reveal the diagnosis.

When nasal examination shows only boggy, swollen membranes of the inferior turbinates (see Fig. 49-3), it is a nonspecific finding. Typically, allergic rhinitis exhibits a pale or bluish diffusely swollen mucosa; irritation or nose spray abuse creates beefy red membranes; sinusitis exhibits either pale or reddish membranes. These color variations are often rather subtle.

The nature of the secretions is more helpful: yellow pus suggests bacterial infection; bloody or crusty secretions and ulcerations suggest bacterial infections, neoplasm, or granulomatous disease; clear secretions suggest either allergy or viral infection; and nasal smears with large numbers of eosinophils suggest allergy or NARES—as opposed to neutrophils, which suggest infection.

The response of the nasal membranes to topical (nose spray) vasoconstriction helps to differentiate a vasomotor rhinitis (which should show a considerable decongestive response) from structural deformities, neoplasms, polyps, sarcoidosis, or the bony turbinate overgrowth of compensatory hypertrophy—all of which should show a limited response. Additionally, many patients with long-established nose spray abuse will demonstrate little vasoconstrictive response to the nose spray used during the examination.

Sarcoidosis (Fig. 49-6), granulomatous disorders, polyps, and tumors are identified by tissue biopsy. Sinus x-ray films are useful not only to detect sinus infections, but also to document structural abnormalities of the septum and turbinates (see Figs. 49-4 and 49-5). Hypothyroidism is detected with thyroid function tests.

Sometimes a presumptive diagnosis is best verified or rejected by the response to empiric therapy (e.g., administration of corticosteroids). The more dramatic the response, the more likely that allergy or infection is the primary etiologic factor. Sarcoidosis may respond somewhat, but the various types of vasomotor rhinitis will respond only to the extent that allergy or inflammation is a coexisting element.

Patients who show little response to corticosteroids, either by mouth or by topical spray, will likely find allergy shots a disappointing mode of therapy, even if skin tests are quite positive for inhalant allergies. Golding-Wood[4] has reminded us that some have extended the use of the term ''allergy''

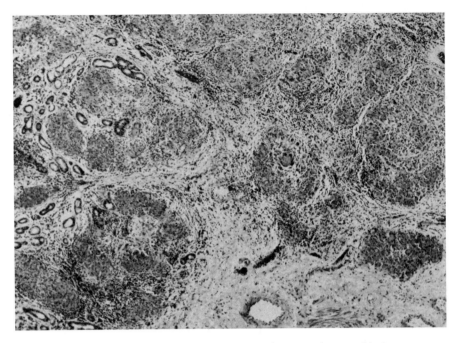

Fig. 49-6. The inferior turbinate mucosa demonstrating sarcoidosis.

to embrace a variety of hyper reactions irrespective of antigen and antibody. It may reasonably be objected that such devices imperil verbal precision and do not serve to clarify concepts.

NONSURGICAL MANAGEMENT

Wherever specific therapeutic suggestions could be made for specific disorders, they were mentioned in the preceding paragraphs. The following self-help measures are nonspecific and apply to most cases of chronic long-standing nasal congestion.

1. Sleep with head of the bed tilted upward 30°. This is accomplished not with pillows, but rather with a few bricks, blocks, or books placed under each bedpost at the head of the bed.
2. Establish a regular and vigorous exercise program that might help to reestablish vasomotor tone and control. Vigorous exercise is the body's most efficient homeostatic control to reduce nasal congestion.[11]
3. Avoid known irritating inhalants, especially tobacco smoke.
4. Try oral decongestants, such as pseudoephedrine, phenylephrine, and phenylpropanolamine. Since these drugs are sympathomimetic, caution is exercised for their use in patients with hypertension, cardiac arrhythmias, or glaucoma.
5. Oral antihistamines, like corticosteroids, are helpful to the extent that allergy plays a role in the condition.
6. Anticholinergics are helpful for rhinorrhea of various etiologies. Ipratropium bromide nasal spray 0.03% (Atrovent) has proven safe and effective for short- or

long-term treatment of nonallergic rhinitis.[5] Rhinorrhea, and to some extent congestion, is improved. Even for the common cold (virus rhinitis) it is useful. Oral anticholinergics, like antihistamines, can cause troublesome drying effects.

7. Combination remedies are extensively marketed for the stuffy/runny nose. They are likely to contain decongestants, antihistamines, anticholinergics, and/or anti-inflammatory agents in any combination. This "shotgun" approach to therapy may be helpful in combined-etiology conditions, but it can also generate needless side effects.
8. Sleep and work in a cool-air (but not cold) environment, keeping the body (especially the feet and head) warm.[11]

Well-established cases of vasomotor rhinitis are often refractory to medical management and may respond best to surgery of the nasal turbinates.

SURGICAL MANAGEMENT

Middle turbinates do not often compromise the airway unless there is a coexistent nasal septal deformity or an ectopic ethmoid cell has grown into the turbinate. In either instance, surgery may be required.

Inferior turbinates are more often at fault. They have been subjected to a wide variety of treatments by surgeons throughout the history of rhinology. Following is a partial list of various turbinate treatment methods with brief comments on the limitations of each.

1. *Inferior turbinate injection with corticosteroids* is used primarily for seasonal allergy treatment and for

weaning the rebound rhinitis patient off nose sprays. This method of treatment provides temporary relief of symptoms. The technique requires a nonforceful injection of small particle-size preparations such as triamcinolone acetonide or diacetate (Kenalog, Aristocort) or prednisolone tebutate (Hydeltra-TBA) into multiple sites along the turbinate with a small-bore needle. The medication is injected only after a topical vasoconstrictor has been applied so as to limit the chance of a direct intravascular injection, which can embolize into orbital vessels and (rarely) create visual loss.[8]

2. *Inferior turbinate injection with caustic agents* has been largely abandoned because of intensely painful reactions. This method provides only very brief relief, if any.

3. *Turbinate displacement ("out-fracture")* is easy and simple but fails to remove thickened membrane and bone. "Green-stick" effect occurs unless the fracture is created from underneath the turbinate at the apex of the meatus where turbinate bone inserts into the lateral nasal wall.

4. *Electrical or chemical surface cautery* creates damage to surface rather than to the vascular bed where it is needed. It gives only very temporary relief, if any.

5. *Electrical submucosal cautery* creates an intensive reaction that can lead to bone sequestration. More commonly, it fails to remove thickened bone (see Fig. 49-2) that occupies much of the airway. This gives only partial or temporary relief.

6. *Cryosurgery of the turbinates*[10] causes submucosal destruction at the cost of surface destruction. Also,

this method fails to remove thickened bone and gives only partial, temporary relief. Septal perforations may occur.

7. *Laser turbinectomy* is the equivalent of cryoturbinectomy.

8. *Total turbinectomy* results in a loss of functioning nasal membranes needed to warm and moisturize air. Atrophic rhinitis may result.

9. In *partial turbinectomy* (i.e., of the anterior end or the inferior margin), results and complications depend on the amount that is resected.

10. *Submucous resection* of the turbinate bone (Figs. 49-2, 49-7, and 49-8) affords the removal of disordered tissue (e.g., thickened, spongy, space-occupying bone and hypervascular submucosa) while sparing the surrounding normal physiologically functioning tissue and produces consistent, long-lasting, and predictably favorable results.[6]

Because of bleeding that occurs with turbinate surgery, most of these operations are performed in an operating room, and nasal packing may be required postoperatively.

INFECTIOUS RHINOSINUSITIS

The most common cause of nonallergic rhinitis is infection in the upper respiratory tract. The nose is continually exposed to a myriad of infectious organisms: viruses, bacteria, and fungi. Several endogenous factors protect the nasal mucosa from infection. The submucosal glands produce a thick layer of tenacious mucus that entraps microorganisms. Cilia of the mucosal epithelium then propel the mucus and the entrapped organisms into the nasopharynx where they are swallowed. This prevents penetration of these microorganisms into the nasal epithelium.

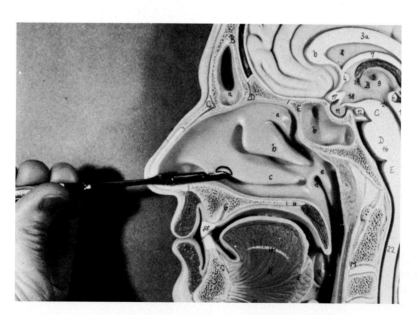

Fig. 49-7. Submucous resection of the inferior turbinate begins with excision of a crescent of hypertrophic mucosa at the anterior end.

Additionally, the nasal glands produce a series of enzymes, antibodies, and other naturally protective proteins that inactivate or kill many viruses, bacteria, and fungi. The antimicrobial properties of glandular secretions may represent the single most important function of nasal secretions.[12]

Viral infections account for about six "colds" per year in young children. The frequency diminishes throughout life, so that older adults suffer only two or three "colds" per year. In the United States, the common cold is most prevalent between the months of September and March. During a typical cold season, at least three fourths of all families will experience a "cold" in at least one family member.

The common cold can be produced by any of more than 200 different species of viruses within the following groups: picornavirus (including rhinovirus, enteric cytopathic human orphan (ECHO) virus, Coxsackie virus), adenovirus, reovirus, orthomyxovirus, paramyxovirus, and coronavirus. Of these, the rhinovirus group produces the greatest proportion of colds. Such viruses are spread through person-to-person contact with secretions from the nose, mouth, or eyes. A person may inhale virus-laden droplets from another person's sneeze, or more commonly, a person may become infected by touching a hand or object (e.g., a door handle, telephone, or handkerchief) that has been contaminated by someone with a cold. The person then touches his own eye, nose, or mouth, and the virus has been spread.

The nasal examination of a cold sufferer reveals diffusely swollen, erythematous mucosa with a watery mucous discharge, a picture not easily distinguished from an acute allergic attack, except by cytology. A common cold lasts about 1 week, but in 5% to 10% of sufferers it can persist up to 3 weeks. Viruses impair ciliary activity of the nasal mucosa, which makes the sufferer more susceptible to secondary bacterial infections of the respiratory tract. Bacterial sinusitis follows a "cold" in about 0.5% to 10% of cases.

There is no specific therapy for the common cold. Symptoms are somewhat alleviated with the self-help remedies suggested for vasomotor rhinitis. Rest, increased fluid intake, and air humidification seem to be helpful, as are a variety of over-the-counter medications selected to treat specific individual symptoms. Ipratropium bromide nasal spray is also helpful.

The influenza viruses produce a more debilitating illness than do the rhinoviruses. Fever may be more pronounced (and may last up to a week); there may be necrosis of the ciliated epithelial layer of the mucosa; systemic symptoms such as lethargy, fatigue, and myalgias are usually troublesome; and secondary bacterial infections are more common.

Viruses A, B, or C of the orthomyxovirus group cause influenza. Unlike for the common cold, immunization is available for influenza, although the selection of viruses used in the annual influenza vaccine (in advance of the influenza outbreak) still remains an art rather than a pure science. Since there is significant mortality associated with influenza (over 10,000 deaths per year), the vaccine is recommended for patients who are elderly, immunosuppressed, or debilitated with pulmonary, cardiac, or other systemic diseases.

SUMMARY

The nasal vasomotor reaction creates nasal congestion because of dilation of the highly vascular bed of the nasal mucous membranes, especially those of the inferior turbinates. This may aggravate the nasal obstruction of a patient with a structural deformity. Vasomotor reaction is also the physiologic mechanism by which allergies and infections of the nose cause nasal congestion, or it may be caused by a variety of unrelated nasal or systemic disorders that give rise to vasomotor rhinitis (see Box 49-1).

When examination reveals a specific diagnosis, the treatment should be specific. However, a variety of nonspecific remedies (as detailed above) can also be helpful where a specific etiology is not apparent.

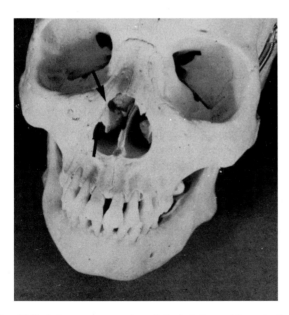

Fig. 49-8. Submucous resection of the inferior turbinate includes removal of bone in the anterior portion, especially all traces of its insertion into the lateral nasal wall (*arrows*). This maximizes expansion of the airway in its narrowest area.

REFERENCES

1. Fairbanks DNF, Fairbanks GR: Cocaine uses and abuses, *Ann Plast Surg* 10:452, 1983.
2. Georgitis JW: Helping the patient with nonallergic rhinitis, *J Respir Dis* 10:72, 1989.
3. Gluckman JL: The clinical approach to nasal obstruction, *J Respir Dis* 4:13, 1983.
4. Golding-Wood PH: Vidian neurectomy and petrosal neurectomy, *J Otol Laryngol* 75:232, 1961.
5. Grossman J, Banov C, Boggs P: Use of ipratropium bromide nasal spray in chronic treatment of nonallergic perennial rhinitis alone and in combination with other perennial rhinitis medications, *J Allergy Clin Immunol* 95:1123, 1995.

septal cartilage is preferred to indiscriminate excision. The classic submucous resection, which involved radical excision of septal bone and cartilage, has largely been supplanted by more well-crafted procedures favoring structural reconstruction and tissue preservation. Submucous resection is used more sparingly, usually a compliment to other techniques. The choice to perform a submucous resection or septoplasty is no longer controversial. Contemporary septal surgery incorporates both techniques, a blending of conservation septal surgery and the judicious resection of nonsupporting septal components. An important axiom is that the nasal septum is composed of bone and cartilage components that require different methods for correction of the deformity. If the septal deformity is located in a region of the septum that does not support the nose, the deformed segment can usually be resected. If the deformity involves a supporting septal component, other techniques (e.g., realignment, structural reconstruction, cartilage replacement) are preferred.

ANATOMY

The nasal septum is an integral part of the nose with functional and aesthetic significance. The septum divides the nasal chamber into two cavities, lends shape and support to the middle nasal vault, aids in the regulation of air flow through the nose, and helps to support the columella and nasal tip. Because the nasal septum is the cornerstone of nasal support, a thorough understanding of its anatomy, physiology, and relationship to the surrounding interconnected nasal anatomy is critical.[63]

The nasal septum is composed of cartilage and bone that is primarily covered by respiratory mucous membrane. The septum is commonly divided into anterior (dorsal), posterior, caudal, and cephalic parts (Fig. 50-1). The components of the nasal septum include the nasal spine of the frontal bone, the keel-shaped undercarriage of the joined nasal bones, the perpendicular plate of the ethmoid, the vomer and crest of the sphenoid, the nasal crest of the palatine bone, the nasal crest of the maxilla and premaxilla, the quadrangular cartilage, the upper lateral cartilage, the membranous septum, and the columella (Fig. 50-2). Unlike the external nose, where most anatomic structures are paired, the septal components are largely singular except for the vomer, which may be bilaminar owing to its embryologic origin.[17] The vomer and the perpendicular plate of the ethmoid and maxillary crest are the components of the bony septum of principal interest to the surgeon. Most of the remainder of the septum, the anterior and caudal portion, is cartilaginous and is formed by the quadrangular cartilage.

The bony septum

Along the nasal floor, small perpendicular projections known as nasal crests rise from the palatine and maxillary bones. They form the maxillary crest, the most inferior part of the bony septum. The maxillary crest extends nearly the

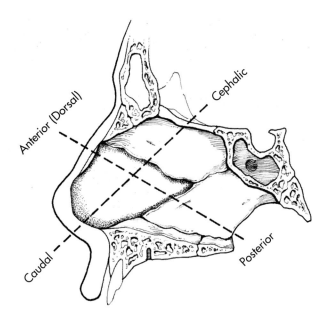

Fig. 50-1. Commonly accepted directional terminology useful in describing nasal anatomy.

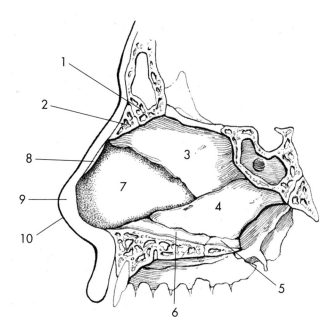

Fig. 50-2. Anatomy of the typical nasal septum.

full length of the palate and ends in a nasal spine. Posteriorly, the maxillary crest articulates with the vomer. Forward of its articulation with the vomer, the upper free borders of the maxillary crest are partially separated, thus presenting a pedestal to support the quadrangular cartilage. The vomer is the seat of the bony septum, articulating above with the perpendicular plate of the ethmoid, below with the maxillary crest, behind with the crest of the sphenoid, and in front with the quadrangular cartilage. Its free (posterior) border is concave and forms the posterior boundary of the choanae. The wings of the vomer are not uncommonly deviated or projected into the nasal cavity as spurs, either alone or in concert with enlarged and deviated crests of the maxilla.[63]

Lying between the cribiform plate above and the vomer below, the perpendicular plate of the ethmoid fuses with the crest of the sphenoid posteriorly. The anterior (dorsal) margin of the ethmoid plate is grooved to receive the nasal process of the frontal bone and the keel-shaped undercarriage of the joined nasal bones. The ethmoid plate usually makes up a large part of the nasal septum, although its contribution to nasal support is nominal. The thickness of the perpendicular plate of the ethmoid varies considerably and is sometimes rudimentary in an otherwise normal nose.[57] A thin or dehiscent ethmoid plate often coexists with a septal cartilage of substantial thickness. Some patients have a disproportionately wide perpendicular plate, measuring up to 5 or 6 mm, particularly when pneumatized. Significant deviations of the ethmoid plate contribute to posterior airway obstruction and require segmental excision or realignment after fracture. Careful manipulation of the ethmoid plate is required to avoid a rare but potentially catastrophic fracture of the cribiform plate, with the potential for cerebrospinal fluid leak and olfactory nerve injury.

The quadrangular cartilage

The quadrangular (septal) cartilage is the most important surgical component of the nasal septum. The caudal portion of the cartilage rests on the support of the anterior nasal spine and maxillary crest. The cartilage and its bony pedestal are held in close approximation by dense investing fibrous attachments, some of which cross over to join adjacent fibers to form a joint-like capsule (Fig. 50-3). The most caudal portion of the quadrangular cartilage extends beyond the nasal spine. At the caudal margin of the septum, three angles can be identified: the anterior, midseptal, and posterior angles (Fig. 50-4). The relative length of the quadrangular cartilage, the specific configuration of these angles, and the size of the nasal spine cause anatomic variation in the columella and upper lip.[63]

The posterior border of the quadrangular cartilage slants upward as it extends cephalad in the trough of the vomer. The posterior margin of the quadrangular cartilage extends into the vomer and perpendicular plate of the ethmoid for a variable distance posteriorly, in a tongue-and-groove relationship. As with all cartilage and bone, articulation is indirect, held by fibrous communications that invest the bone and cartilage. The cephalic extent of the quadrangular cartilage varies according to the general development of the nose; it often extends further posterior in patients with a dominant cartilage structure. The septal cartilage is often thickest at its cephalic border where it abuts the ethmoid plate, although the thickness of the septal cartilage and that of the bony septum do not seem to correlate.

Below the osseocartilaginous junction, the upper lateral

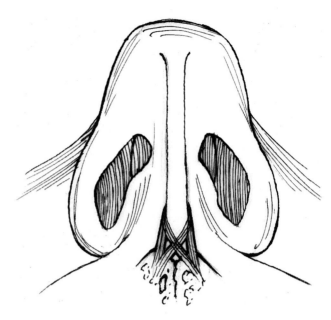

Fig. 50-3. Fibrous attachments between the caudal septum and the premaxillary bones. The cartilage is held in close approximation by a dense fascial sheath, which extends around and under the cartilage from one mucosa to the other to form a joint-like capsule.

cartilages join the anterior margin of the nasal septum to form a smooth cartilaginous vault. The upper lateral cartilages are typically described as paired triangular structures that attach centrally to the nasal septum and laterally to the frontal process of the maxilla by dense connective tissue. In reality, the nasal septum and upper lateral cartilages are not separate entities but are fused to form a unified structural arch (Fig. 50-5). Embryologic evidence supports the concept that the entire nasal structure derives from the cartilaginous nasal capsule of the chondrocranium.[17] Gradual cartilage resorption results in distinct nasal cartilages separated by fibrous tissue. Specifically, fibrous ingrowth results in separation of the upper lateral cartilages from the frontal process of the maxilla laterally, and from the caudal nasal septum and lower lateral cartilages inferiorly. In most cases, the upper lateral cartilages extend laterally to the nasal bone suture line and no further. Embryologically, the nasal bones are laid down over the nasal septum and upper lateral cartilages in an overlapping configuration. A groove on the anterior (dorsal) margin of the septal cartilage accepts the keel-shaped undersurface of the joined nasal bones. The combined attachment of the nasal septum and upper lateral cartilages to the undersurface of the nasal bones forms an articulation of substantial strength, often termed the *keystone area* of nasal support[29] (Fig. 50-6).

The nasal valve

At the midpoint of their articulation with the nasal septum, the upper lateral cartilages extend from the dorsal margin of the septum and gently curve toward the pyriform aper-

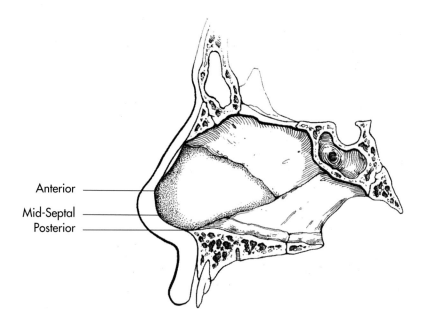

Anterior
Mid-Septal
Posterior

Fig. 50-4. At the caudal end of the normal septum, three separate angles can be identified: the anterior septal angle; the midseptal angle; and the posterior septal angle.

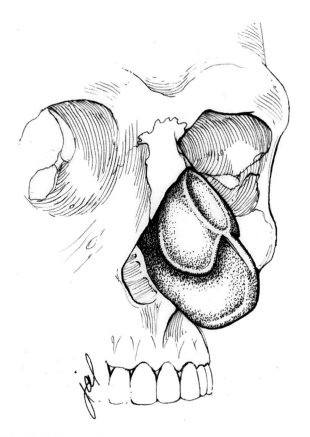

Fig. 50-5. The cartilaginous nasal vault. The nasal septum and upper lateral cartilages are fused to form a unified structural arch. In the distal few millimeters, the upper lateral cartilages depart from the septum and end in free edges.

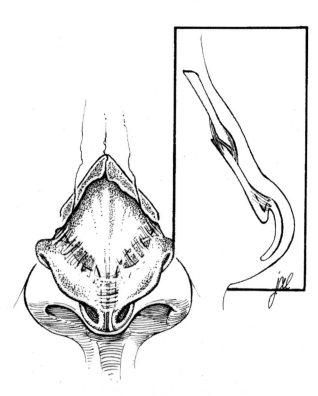

Fig. 50-6. A frontal view shows the attachment of the upper lateral cartilages and nasal septum to the undersurface of the nasal bones. This articulation is often referred to as the keystone area of nasal support. **Inset,** A cross-section shows attachment of the upper lateral cartilage to the undersurface of the nasal bone and the overlap of the upper and lower lateral cartilages.

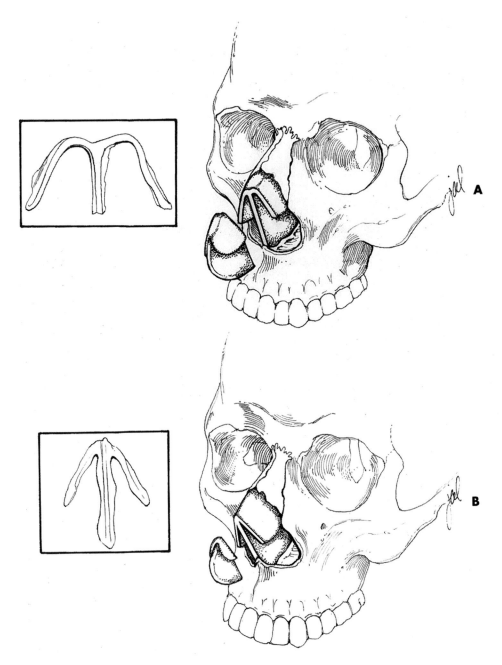

Fig. 50-7. A, A cross-section through the midpoint of the cartilaginous nasal vault. **Inset,** Note the trapezoidal configuration of the middle vault of the nose. The upper lateral cartilages extend from the dorsal margin of the septum and gently curve toward the pyriform aperture. **B,** A cross-section through the cartilaginous nasal vault at the internal valve angle. **Inset,** Note the rather acute relationship between the nasal septum and the distal upper lateral cartilages.

ture.[64] This alignment frequently establishes a trapezoidal configuration to the middle nasal vault (Fig. 50-7, *A*). Advancing from the osseocartilaginous junction toward the caudal margin of the upper lateral cartilages, the dorsal margin of the middle nasal vault narrows (Fig. 50-7, *B*). The junction between the nasal septum and the caudal upper lateral cartilage forms the nasal valve angle, which widens and narrows under the influence of the nasal musculature during respiration. The nasal valve angle is the narrowest portion of the nasal cavity; it is normally 10° to 15° in white patients[37] (Fig. 50-8). When negative inspiratory pressures are generated during nasal breathing, the nasal valve narrows, increasing nasal resistance and slowing the velocity of the airstream.[7,11] If the nasal valve is narrowed by deformities of the adjoining nasal septum, it is predisposed to collapse prematurely, resulting in symptoms of nasal blockage. Even

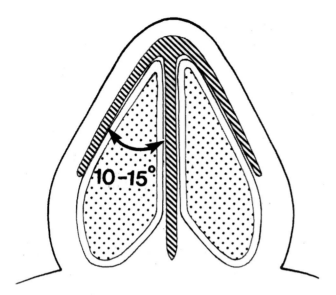

Fig. 50-8. The nasal valve angle is formed at the junction of the nasal septum and the distal upper lateral cartilage. It typically measures 10° to 15° in the leptorrhine nose.

minor changes in the shape or cross-sectional area of the nasal valve may produce clinical symptoms of nasal obstruction.

The membranous septum and columella

The membranous septum exists between the caudal end of the quadrangular cartilage and the columella. It is formed by bilateral layers of vestibular skin and an intervening layer of subcutaneous areolar tissue. The membranous septum is extremely mobile, which is confirmed by displacement of the columella in a longitudinal or transverse direction. The columella is composed of the paired medial crura, to which transverse ligamentous attachments densely adhere, and is bound in a tight skin envelope virtually devoid of subcutaneous fat along the medial nostril walls. The medial crura footplates flare to accommodate the septum and overlap it for several millimeters, but attachment of the medial crura to the caudal septum is not direct.[17]

Blood supply and innervation

The mucoperichondrial and mucoperiosteal lining of the septum contains its blood and nerve supply. Blood is supplied predominately by four paired arterial vessels. The upper nasal septum is supplied by anastomotic branches of the anterior and posterior ethmoid arteries. The posterior and inferior septum is perfused by a major division of the sphenopalatine artery, whereas the caudal septum and columella are supplied by the septal branch of the superior labial artery. The venous system generally parallels the arterial system, except for an important posterior communication with the cavernous sinus. As with cartilage elsewhere, blood vessels do not penetrate the cartilage, rather the cartilage is

immersed in the nutrient milieu of the investing perichondrium. This unique anatomic arrangement is important surgically because it results in an avascular plane for dissection between the septal cartilage and the mucoperichondrium. Lymphatic drainage of the nose occurs anteriorly or posteriorly. Lymph from the anterior nasal cavity follows the venous drainage, coursing to the submental and submandibular lymph nodes. In contrast, the posterior nasal lymphatics are drained by retropharyngeal lymph nodes, which in turn empty into the upper division of the internal jugular chain. The anterior ethmoid nerve, the nasopalatine nerve, and a terminal branch of the anterior superior alveolar nerve innervate the nasal septum, which is covered by moist respiratory mucosa that is responsive to pain and noxious agents but is virtually insensitive to the perception of airflow.[11] In contrast, the nasal vestibule is lined with dry, hair-bearing skin. This skin has a dense distribution of tactile receptors and seems to be responsible for most of the nasal sensation of airflow.[10,34,35] Teleologically, placing the sensing element at the start of the airflow system seems rational. This maximizes the opportunity for necessary adjustments in the depth and rate of respiration based on the airflow information coming from the nose.[10]

The line of nasal support

Only the portion of the nasal septum anterior to the pyriform aperture supports the nose. Supporting and nonsupporting parts of the nasal septum are divided by an imaginary vertical line dropped from the dorsal osseocartilaginous junction to the anterior nasal spine. Septal components posterior to this line contribute little to nasal support and can be sacrificed with less concern than anterior structures (Fig. 50-9). The surgical implication of this relationship is clear. Anterior septal components are critical to nasal support and should be structurally restored, and not sacrificed, when deformed. During septal surgery, it is best to preserve a stable and continuous strut of cartilage that extends uninterrupted from the osseocartilaginous junction to the anterior nasal spine.[38]

NASAL PHYSIOLOGY AND THE AIRWAY
Normal nasal function

The caudal nasal septum is the initial contact point in creating air turbulence and divides the inspired air column precisely. As part of the nasal valve area, the nasal septum also helps to configure the inspiratory air currents, changing them from a column to a sheet of air, thereby giving them shape, velocity, and direction (Fig. 50-10). Substantial deviation of the nasal septum alters the nose's normal air flow patterns, and turbulence is created. In addition to causing symptoms of nasal blockage, septal deviation can result in drying, crusting, and bleeding on the side with increased flow. The degree of airflow obstruction from septal deviation depends on the site of the lesion. Anterior deviations have

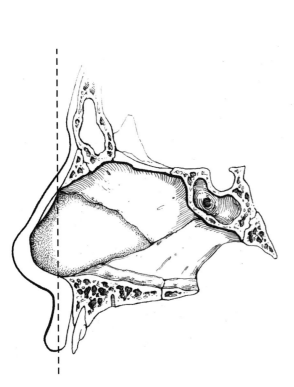

Fig. 50-9. The line of nasal support. The septal skeleton forward of this imaginary line, dropped from the osseocartilaginous junction to the nasal spine, provides the principal support of the external nose. In contrast, posterior septal components contribute little to overall nasal support.

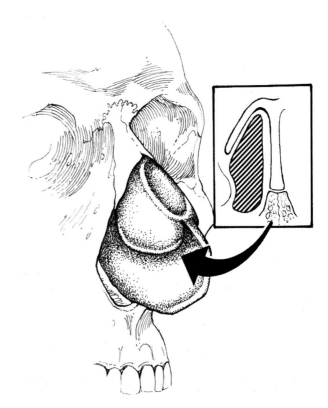

Fig. 50-11. The nasal valve area. The functional unit includes the nasal septum, upper lateral cartilage, pyriform aperture, and anterior head of the inferior turbinate.

a major effect on airflow, whereas small or posterior deviations have minimal effects.[30] This is because anterior deviations of the nasal septum often impinge on the nasal valve area, which is a bottleneck for airflow and is complex anatomically and physiologically. Sometimes, the severely deviated septum may encroach on the infundibular region of the lateral nasal wall, creating a mechanical obstruction that inhibits mucociliary function and predisposes to the development of recurrent sinusitis.

The shape and position of the nasal septum only partially aid in maintenance of an efficient nasal airway. The region of the nasal valve is of vital concern. The nasal valve refers to the cross-sectional area of the nasal cavity bordered by the junction of the caudal margin of the upper lateral cartilage and the nasal septum. Typically, a 10° to 15° angle is circumscribed by this relationship. The nasal valve is only a portion of the larger functional unit, the nasal valve area, which includes the nasal septum, upper lateral cartilage, pyriform aperture, and anterior head of the inferior turbinate[37] (Fig. 50-11). The nasal valve area is the narrowest and most flexible portion of the nasal airway. It is the primary inflow regulator and accounts for most of the inspiratory resistance to airflow. During respiration, negative inspiratory pressure is transmitted from the nasopharynx to the nasal valve area, which then actively narrows. As nasal airflow increases, the

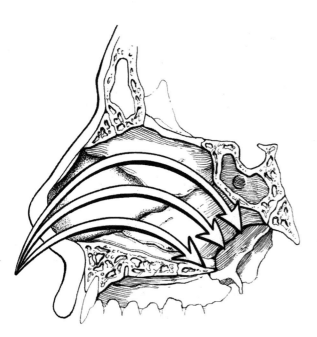

Fig. 50-10. The direction of airflow during normal nasal respiration.

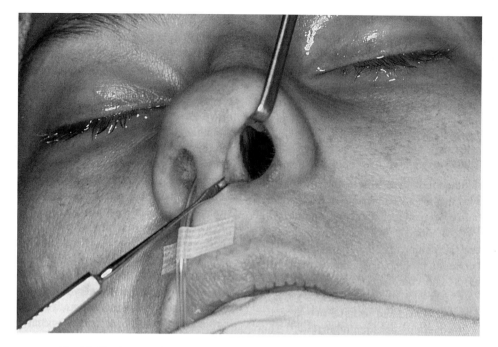

Fig. 50-13. Intranasal examination shows the resting position of the nasal valve.

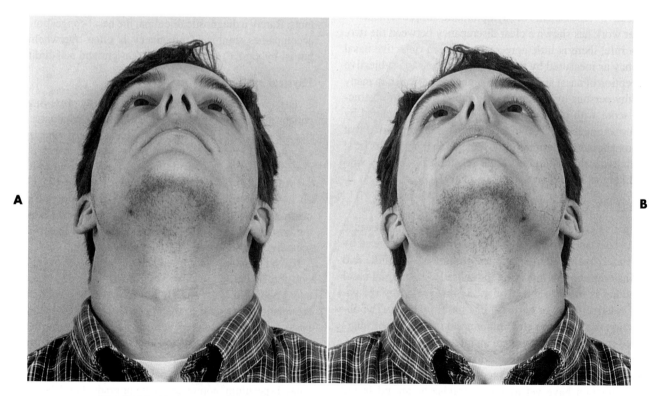

Fig. 50-14. Alar margin collapse. **A,** Basal view of the nose during quiet breathing. **B,** Collapse of the nose on deep inspiration resulting from insufficient support of the alar margin and lateral nasal sidewall.

It is important to determine whether the bony septum deviates, influencing an otherwise straight septal cartilage, or whether the cartilage itself is bent, bowed, or twisted. Sometimes, both conditions coexist.[63] The color and appearance of the respiratory mucous membrane also are considered. Pale, boggy mucosa and a thin watery discharge are typical findings in allergic rhinitis. Congested, hyperemic mucosa is suggestive of illicit drug use, vasomotor rhinitis, or the habitual use of decongestant nose drops.[3]

The entire examination is then repeated after topical vasoconstriction. Mucosal shrinkage provides visual access to previously concealed areas, particularly the posterior nasal septum and lateral nasal walls. An improved understanding of the nature and severity of septal obstruction is often now possible. Particular attention is again directed to the nasal valve area as it relates to complaints of nasal obstruction. The amount of mucosal shrinkage in response to vasoconstriction is estimated and serves as a measure of potential response to medical therapy. Finally, intranasal palpation with the thumb and forefinger yields useful information about the caudal septal segment and the size and position of the nasal spine. Downward pressure on the nasal tip highlights the anterior margin of the septal cartilage, showing any crooked nose deformity and detailing the configuration of the middle nasal vault. Transillumination of the septum is valuable in determining the quantity and location of residual septal cartilage in patients at risk for cartilage loss. Alternatively, the nasal septum can be palpated using a cotton-tipped applicator after insufflation of a topical anesthetic. When indicated, more exhaustive procedures are performed, including fiberoptic nasopharyngoscopy. Plain radiographs and direct coronal computed tomography (CT) scans may complement the examination but are infrequently required. Their value is primarily in the evaluation of congenital nasal obstruction, complex nasal trauma, and coexisting medical conditions.

NASAL SEPTAL DEFORMITY

The intrinsic properties of septal cartilage

To understand the pathogenesis of a septal deformity and to conceptualize its rational management, the biomechanical properties of septal cartilage should be understood. The mechanical properties of a material are described by the relationship between a force applied to a specimen and its resultant deformation as a function of time. Although many engineering materials have a linear force-deformation relationship, the mechanical properties of biologic materials are often more complex and subject to change within the living organism.

Septal cartilage has elastic flexibility and can be bent repeatedly without suffering permanent injury or damage. However, if externally applied forces are of sufficient magnitude to exceed the strength of the cartilage, fracture occurs and permanent deformity ensues. Minor, seemingly inconse-

quential injuries, can result in permanent bending and warping of septal cartilage. Even microtrauma sustained in childhood, often overlooked, can result in substantial deviation of the nasal septum as growth accentuates the deformity.

Insight into the biologic behavior of septal cartilage and its response to injury is provided by Gibson and Davis[22] and Fry.[21] Fry suggested that septal cartilage has an intrinsic tension, the result of a built-in system of interlocking stresses that contribute to cartilage ''memory.'' Mostly, septal cartilage lies straight, the effect of balanced tension created by the even distribution of internal stresses. If one side of cartilage is interrupted by partial-thickness injury or incisions, an imbalance occurs, and the opposite side assumes dominance. Microfractures sustained early in life simulate partial-thickness cuts. These often result in unfurling of septal cartilage on the side of injury and may lead to substantial deviation of the septum as growth accentuates the deformity (Fig. 50-15). The origin of intrinsic cartilage stress, although not fully understood, has been attributed to the histologic lamination of chondrocytes at the periphery of the septal cartilage. More recent evidence, however, suggests that cartilage tension is the product of cellular and molecular events that govern the composition and arrangement of the extracellular matrix.[48]

Although valuable, intrinsic tension cannot be used as the sole basis for the correction of a septal deformity. The straightening effect of partial-thickness incisions on the concave side of deviated cartilage is unpredictable and influenced by confounding factors. The magnitude, arrangement, and distribution of intrinsic cartilage stresses vary among different areas of the septum and among septa in different patients.[48] Furthermore, the effect of fibrous ingrowth into fracture lines, contracture of the investing perichondrium, and the calcification or thickening of injured cartilage should be factored into the surgical equation for straightening septal cartilage.[63] Generally, full-thickness incisions created on the concave side, carried to but not through the opposite mucoperichondrium, are most effective in dispelling cartilage tension and are more reliable than partial-thickness cuts for straightening bent cartilage[48] (Fig. 50-16).

Developmental deformity of the septum

Many deformities of the nasal septum occur without antecedent injury and are classified, often inaccurately, as a developmental flaw. Most suspected developmental abnormalities of the nasal septum are explained by injuries that occured in infancy or childhood, which seem inconsequential and are easily overlooked. Minor trauma frequently results in microfracture or partial-thickness injury to one side of septal cartilage. This leads to unfurling of the fractured cartilage surface, which spreads out under the influence of the now dominant opposite side. Bending of the cartilage away from the side of injury often results. As fibrous healing fills the microfracture, permanence is established. When early life trauma results in gradual bending and deviation of septal cartilage, asymmetric growth of the entire nasal structure can occur. This fact becomes important if correction of the problem is attempted.[57]

Partial-thickness injuries (microfractures) of the septum are believed to be common in the neonatal period.[13,33,40] Many of these injuries can be linked to undue labor or birth trauma, not surprising considering the cartilaginous nasal tip is the most projected facial structure and is subject to extraordinary compression and rotational forces during birth.[57] The direction of septal deviation in neonates often correlates with the presentation of the fetal head in the pelvis. For example, if the head presents in the left occipitoanterior position, rotation of the head toward the midline will displace the septal cartilage to the left of the vomer.[33] Although parturition trauma is the predominate cause of neonatal septal deformity, some injuries may result from forces applied to the nose during the late months of intrauterine life.[40] In support of this notion, by Cottle[13] observed nasal septal deformity in neonates born by cesarean section.

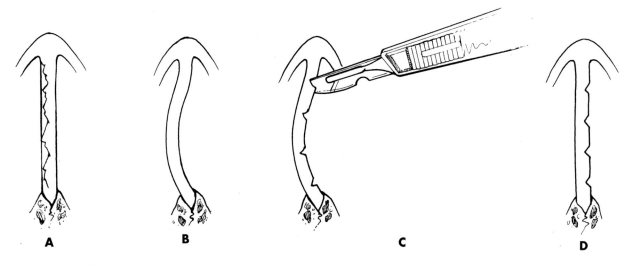

Fig. 50-15. The effect of minor trauma, or microfracture, on the shape of septal cartilage. **A,** Partial-thickness injury or fracture to one side of the septal cartilage. **B,** The cartilage bends away from the side of injury under the influence of the now dominant, opposite side. **C,** To straighten deviated cartilage, partial-thickness incisions are made on the concave cartilage surface, opposite the side of original fracture or injury. **D,** Successful realignment of the cartilage.

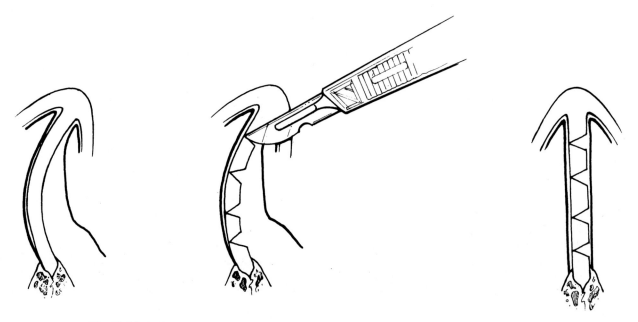

Fig. 50-16. Full-thickness incisions through cartilage, stopping short of the opposite mucoperichondrium, are clinically more reliable for long-term straightening of substantially deviated cartilage.

Pure developmental deformities of the nasal septum unrelated to trauma also occur. Most are thought to arise from the disproportionate growth of septal cartilage relative to the available space in which it grows. Confined to a restricted space, such a cartilage bends, and by doing so, generates intrinsic cartilage tension that results in a permanent deformity. A second common flaw in the developmental process leads to a deviation (bending) of the perpendicular plate of the ethmoid. This condition is easily recognized as soon as the cartilaginous septum is separated from the ethmoid plate and vomer during surgery. At this time, the cartilage can be seen to move to a more midline position, revealing the ethmoid plate as the source of the deformity.

Traumatic (acquired) deformity of the septum

Many adults acquire a deviation of the nasal septum as a consequence of nasal trauma.[55] When a force impacts the caudal septum, the compact septal cartilage is compressed from anterior to posterior, along its major axis. If the cartilage is firmly entrenched in the vomeral sulcus, the bony septum limits posterior displacement, and the incompressible cartilage is prone to fracture under stress. If the vomeral sulcus is shallow, a subluxation is likely, and the septal cartilage is displaced into the nasal floor (Fig. 50-17). Caudal impact results in vertically oriented fractures, extending from the floor of the nose toward the nasal dorsum. When extraordinary force is applied, multiple fractures may extend through the anterior (dorsal) margin of the septal cartilage,

culminating in a zigzag (sigmoid) deformity of the middle vault and lower nose (Fig. 50-18). Such anterior (dorsal) deformities of the septum are difficult to repair using standard septoplasty techniques and often require an external rhinoplasty approach. Severe caudal trauma creates an overlap of the septal fragments with subsequent shortening and thickening of the nasal septum. Frontal nasal trauma may cause fracture of the delicate caudal portion of the nasal bones, separating them from the thicker bone of the frontonasal region. Splaying of the displaced nasal fragments results in a widening of the upper nasal third but has little effect on the cartilaginous septum, providing that it remains firmly attached to the undersurface of the joined nasal bones. If injury to the keystone area is great, however, it dramatically increases the risk of a postinjury saddle deformity. A lateral blow to the nose often results in a unilateral, depressed nasal fracture, although a greater force may displace the entire bony pyramid, including the bony septum. Fracture and displacement of the ethmoid plate are frequently accompanied by displacement of the posterior septal cartilage, which remains firmly attached by way of strong fibrous connections. Most patients experience maximal deviation in the region of the bone-cartilage junction. Sometimes, the caudal septum

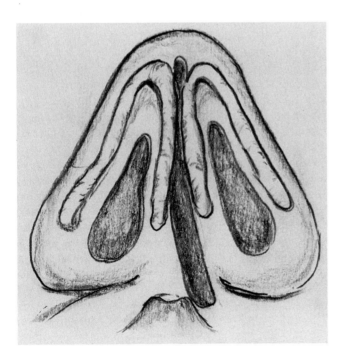

Fig. 50-17. Subluxation of the quadrangular cartilage into the nasal floor after trauma. (From Ridenour BD: *Nasal fracture.* In Gates G, editor: *Current therapy in otolaryngology—head and neck surgery,* St Louis, 1994, Mosby. Used with permission.)

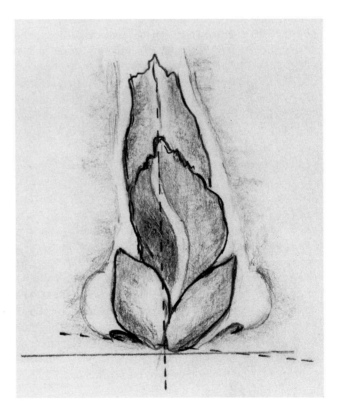

Fig. 50-18. A caudal blow to the nose may result in an S-shaped deformity of the anterior (dorsal) cartilaginous septum and middle nasal vault. (From Ridenour BD: *Nasal fracture.* In Gates G, editor: *Current therapy in otolaryngology—head and neck surgery,* St Louis, 1994, Mosby. Used with permission.)

is forced in the opposite direction, creating a caudal obstruction on one side of the nose and a posterior obstruction on the other.

NASAL SEPTAL RECONSTRUCTION

Surgical indications

Patients are considered for surgery when a septal deviation results in nasal blockage or has an undesired effect on the appearance of the nose. The goals of surgery are to enhance nasal breathing and restore aesthetic form using methods that preserve and rectify the structure of the nose. Septal reconstruction may be performed as a singular procedure or as part of a more comprehensive septorhinoplasty operation. Occasionally, septal reconstruction may be an important aspect of the management of recurring sinusitis and is helpful in controlling epistaxis and nonobstructive snoring. Septal surgery is not indicated in healthy patients who are asymptomatic.

Septal reconstruction

Deformities of the nasal septum are usually managed by resection, structural realignment, or camouflage. Septal components are gradually dissected, individually analyzed, and corrected according to the nature, severity, and location of the deformities. If a septal deformity is located in a region of the septum that does not provide major nasal support, it can usually be safely resected. Septal components more critical to nasal support should be structurally restored rather than sacrificed when deformed.

Most deformities can be corrected by elevating an ipsilateral mucoperichondrial flap, disarticulating the bone-cartilage junction, and isolating the bony septum by elevation of bilateral mucoperiosteal flaps. Bony obstruction is generally managed by resection, whereas cartilage obstruction is managed with techniques favoring structural reconstruction and tissue preservation. Deviated cartilage is incised, shaved, sliced, or morselized until sufficiently weakened to allow it to passively rest in a midline position. If a segment of cartilage is severely bent, bowed, cupped, or twisted, the deformed portion can usually be resected, provided it is not in a region of the septum that provides major nasal support. A continuous L-shaped strut of straight cartilage should be preserved, extending along the dorsal edge from the osseocartilaginous junction to the septal angle and downward along the caudal edge to the anterior nasal spine (Fig. 50-19). The mobilized septum is secured to the periosteum of the nasal spine, while the dissected cartilage is stabilized in the midline by suturing the two mucoperichondrial flaps together using a transseptal mattress suture.

This procedure will correct most deformities of the nasal septum. A major deformity of the L-shaped strut is a more complex problem. The dorsal segment of the L-shaped strut supports the upper lateral cartilages and provides the anterior projection of the nose. The caudal segment supports the nasal

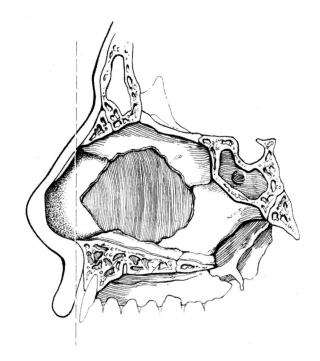

Fig. 50-19. The cartilaginous septal L-shaped strut. When possible, a continuous L-shaped strut of straight cartilage is preserved, which extends uninterrupted from the osseocartilaginous junction to the nasal spine.

tip via the interdomal ligament[32] and provides shape for the columella and upper lip. Resection of a deformed portion of the L-shaped septal strut may create a structural deficiency that may result in dorsal saddling, a crooked nose, a loss of tip projection, a retraction of the columella, or nasal valve collapse. Similarly, the physical properties of septal cartilage prohibit excessive mobilization (e.g., crosshatching), which may lead to cartilage weakening, instability, and new displacement in areas of major nasal support. Deviated segments of the L-shaped septal strut can usually be corrected with supporting grafts of bone or cartilage without compromise of nasal function rather than with techniques designed to weaken septal cartilage. Bilateral mucoperichondrial flaps are raised to abolish soft-tissue tension and permit a correct analysis of the cartilage deformity. The open rhinoplasty (external) approach allows unmatched visualization of the anterior (dorsal) septal segment and nasal valve regions for direct suturing of grafts and manipulation of the nasal septum from above (open approach) and below (hemitransfixtion).

Occasionally, patients have septal deviations of extreme magnitude that are not correctable by standard techniques such as cartilage incision, resection, structural realignment, or camouflage. In these cases, the severity of the deformity warrants radical resection of the deformed segment of septal cartilage followed by its modification and re-insertion (extracorporeal septoplasty).[26,39,54,68] Alternatively, major supporting segments of the nasal septum can be replaced with autologous cartilage harvested from the posterior inferior portion of septal cartilage or from rib cartilage (subtotal reconstruction).[6,65] Extracorporeal and subtotal reconstruction of the nasal septum requires significant dissection of the septal cartilage and its supporting structures. These techniques are accompanied by a certain degree of risk and should be reserved for severe problems in which the septum is not successfully corrected by standard septoplasty techniques.

The basic technique

Certain surgical principles are basic to all septoplasty procedures. They have proven safe, reliable, and effective in the correction of most uncomplicated septal deformities. The major steps involve the following standard surgical maneuvers, usually but not always in this sequence[63]:

1. Access to the septum through a gently curved mucosal incision, placed just behind to the caudal margin of the septal cartilage
2. Elevation of an ipsilateral continuous mucoperichondrial and mucoperiosteal flap to initiate exposure of the septal cartilage and bony septum
3. Disarticulation of the bone-cartilage junction, preserving a strong anterior attachment in the keystone area
4. Mobilization of the septal cartilage from the maxillary crest (if deviated), which is increased by removal of a narrow inferior strip of cartilage along the crest
5. Isolation of the bony septum between bilateral mucoperiosteal flaps posteriorly with resection of the deviated portions of bone that cause obstruction
6. More extensive exposure of the maxillary crest and vomer when large cartilage or bone spurs are present, carefully elevating the mucoperiostium over as much of the maxillary crest and vomer as is required and using a small osteotome to tangentially excise bony spurs
7. Gradual dissection and realignment of the septal cartilage while maintaining septal support, preserving at least an L-shaped strut of cartilage from the osseocartilaginous junction to the anterior nasal spine
8. Suture fixation of the caudal septum to the nasal spine periosteum
9. Stabilization and alignment of dissected septal components and apposition with a running transseptal mattress suture

Anesthesia and analgesia

With few exceptions, surgery is performed on an outpatient basis using a combination of monitored intravenous sedation, topical anesthesia, and local infiltration. When properly administered, monitored anesthesia provides complete patient comfort, little bleeding, and shortened recovery time. Anxious adolescents and some adults will find the process difficult and are better served by a general anesthetic.

Topical anesthesia and vasoconstriction are achieved by placing one or more cottonoid pledgets soaked in a 4% to 5% cocaine solution in each nasal cavity. The mucoperichondrium is infiltrated with a standard solution of 1% lidocaine with epinephrine, using a 27-gauge needle. Accurate infiltration beneath the perichondrium permits hydraulic dissection and simplifies subsequent flap elevation. A spinal needle is generally required to reach the far posterior mucoperiosteum covering the bony septum. Additional infiltration is sometimes needed at the nasal spine, along the nasal floor, and beneath the mucosa of the inferior turbinate. Sufficient time, usually about 10 minutes, is allowed to achieve maximal vasoconstriction. Final inspection and palpation of the septum are performed during this time, and the surgical plan is confirmed.

Incision and flap elevation

Elevation of the mucoperichondrium is begun through a gently curved vertical incision just cephalic to the caudal end of the septal cartilage. If the caudal septum is significantly weak or deformed, a hemitransfixion incision is preferred to provide adequate access. The side used for flap elevation is based on the surgeon's preference. Elevation of the concave side is technically easier to perform and favors incisional methods of cartilage straightening.[43] Elevation of the convex side is often advantageous when resecting fracture angulations, cartilage subluxations, and septal spurs with a large cartilaginous component. Most deformities of the septum can be adequately corrected through either side of the nose. The submucoperichondrial plane is located by sharp knife incision, with the proper plane for dissection distinguished by the bluish hue of the cartilage surface. The flap is developed with a blunt or semisharp elevator under direct observation as the dissection glides over the septal cartilage. Dissection posteriorly is beneath the submucoperiosteal plane to form a continuous ipsilateral mucoperichondrial and mucoperiosteal space. In traumatically deformed noses, fibrous adhesions often connect the two mucoperichondrial flaps through gaps in the cartilage. If fracture adhesions, cartilage overlaps, or scarring interferes, the dissection is slowed to avoid tearing the flap. It is sometimes helpful to look into the nose and control the progress of the elevator by watching its movements beneath the mucous membrane. An endoscope may facilitate flap elevation in some patients and can be used throughout the procedure for precise evaluation of the deformity.[23]

Disarticulation of the osseocartilaginous junction

After elevation of the mucoperichondrium, the septum is visually inspected, and the posterior edge of the septal cartilage is disarticulated from the ethmoid plate and vomer using the tip of an elevator. A strong bone-cartilage attachment is maintained superiorly in the keystone area to prevent postoperative saddling of the nasal dorsum (Fig. 50-20). Simple disarticulation of the septal cartilage from the bony septum often allows the cartilage to return to a straight midline position. If not, it may be displaced laterally along the maxillary crest, which is corrected by resecting a narrow horizontal strip of cartilage at the level of the crest. Fibrous attachments are divided along the maxillary crest to allow the cartilage to passively rest in the midline. If cartilage deformity persists after these initial maneuvers, further corrective measures are required.

Bony obstruction

Most bony septal deformities are managed by resection of the obstructing component. Fracture and realignment without bone removal is a less reliable method. Bone is removed in stepwise increments using a biting forcep until the deviated bone is removed and the airway is free of obstruction. If bone is required as a graft material, larger pieces are obtained using heavy scissors or a small osteotome. Bending, rocking, or twisting of the perpendicular plate of the ethmoid is cautiously avoided. Enlarged or deviated bony spurs are excised along the maxillary crest and vomer using a micro-osteotome or rongeur. Elevation of the mucoperiosteum along the maxillary crest and vomer is facilitated by developing one or more inferior tunnels[14] or by making a sharp knife incision as the mucoperichondrial flap inserts along the maxillary crest.

Cartilage deformity

These surgical steps are routine in most patients and they are often all that is required to establish a functional nasal airway. At this juncture in the operation, the alignment of the septum is visually inspected and palpated before further surgery is considered. If septal alignment is adequate and the nasal airway is satisfactory, the mobilized caudal septum is secured to the periostium of the nasal spine and the mucosal flaps are coapted with a running quilting transseptal suture of absorbable gut. If the airway remains compromised, further steps to straighten the septal cartilage are necessary.

If warped, cupped, or twisted cartilage is confined to a region of the septum that does not provide major nasal support, the deformed segment can usually be resected. The segment of cartilage to be removed is outlined with a knife down to but not through the opposing mucoperichondrium. Fibrous attachments are sharply divided at the maxillary crest, and a small blunt elevator is passed across the cut edge of cartilage to dissect the opposite mucoperichondrium. Only small segments of cartilage are removed, and as much septal cartilage as possible is retained. An L-shaped strut of cartilage, at least 1.5 cm in width, is retained to support the nose (Fig. 50-21).

Sharply buckled or angled septal cartilage may result from traumatic fracture lines. Such fracture angulations require re-creation of the fracture to mobilize and release cartilage segments for repositioning. Vertical, horizontal, and oblique angulations can be corrected by direct wedge excision of the fracture line (Fig. 50-22). Cartilage resection is tapered toward the dorsal and caudal margins of the quadrangular cartilage to preserve the nasal support. The remaining

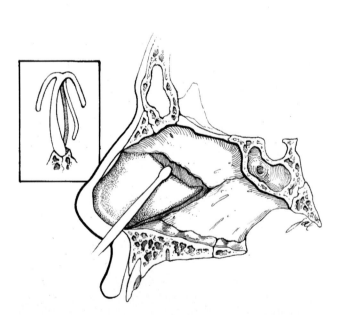

Fig. 50-20. Disarticulation of the cartilaginous septum from the bony septum. Note a strong anterior bone-cartilage attachment is preserved to support the nose. **Inset,** The ethmoid plate and vomer are isolated with the speculum after elevation of bilateral mucoperiosteal flaps.

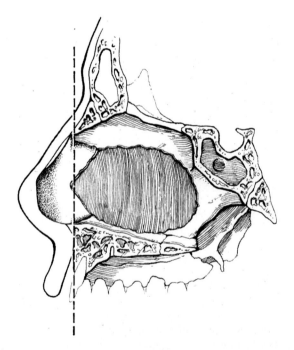

Fig. 50-21. Maximal resection of septal cartilage permissible during septoplasty. A sturdy L-shaped strut of straight cartilage is retained to support the nose, measuring at least 1.5 cm in width.

cartilage segments are securely attached to the contralateral mucoperichondrium and are sutured to prevent slippage or overlap using a quilting suture.[69] In some cases, it may be possible to correct fracture angulations of the septum without resection of cartilage.[24] A parasagittal incision is made through the line of angulation in the cartilage to re-create the fracture and release the cartilage segments. The deviated portion of cartilage is then grasped and actively repositioned into the midline. Once the cartilage is repositioned, it is maintained in the midline by suturing the two mucoperichondrial flaps together in the midline with an absorbable suture.

If a large segment of cartilage is noticeably bowed or curved, the cartilage tension should be released over a broader area. Mild bending or bowing of septal cartilage is improved by making a series of crosshatched partial-thickness incisions on the concave surface (Fig. 50-23). This usually results in an immediate release of built-in cartilage tension and improved straightness of the septum. However, if the cartilage is severely deformed, then full-thickness checkerboard (crosshatching) incisions are made in the areas of greatest cartilage deformity. The incisions are made in a crossing pattern to break the cartilage tension while preserving the opposite, undissected mucoperichondrium. Full-thickness incisions are most effective in dispelling cartilage tension, providing long-term straightening of even severe deformities. Similar to all incisional techniques, cross-hatching and checkerboarding weaken the physical structure of septal cartilage, risking unpredictable healing, deformity, and a loss of nasal support. Techniques designed to break the spring of the cartilage should be used with caution in areas of the septum that provide nasal support. If supporting segments of septal cartilage are weakened, they can be supported with straight pieces of septal cartilage or ethmoid bone inserted as a sandwich or batten graft.

Alignment and stabilization of dissected components

If the caudal segment of the septum is repositioned, it is secured to the periosteum of the nasal spine with a lasting suture. Further fixation sutures are sometimes required to preserve the realignment of dissected septal components and to prevent slippage or overlap.[69] All intranasal incisions, including any tears in the mucosa, are closed with a 4-0 or 5-0 absorbable suture. A running quilting suture is used to coapt the septal flaps, close the dead space, provide hemostasis, and stabilize the septal components. An angled (bayonet-style) needle holder improves visualization for placement of all septal sutures (Fig. 50-24).

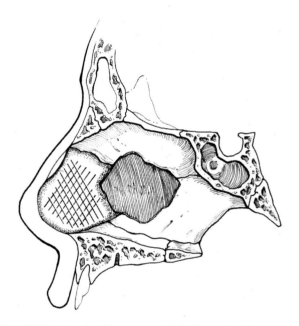

Fig. 50-23. Crosshatching or partial-thickness incisions on the concave surface of deviated cartilage improves straightness.

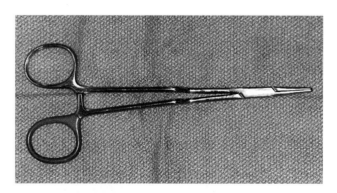

Fig. 50-24. An angled (bayonet-style) needle holder provides better direct visual placement of all septal sutures.

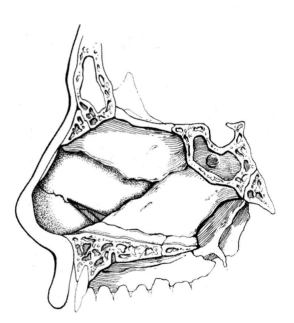

Fig. 50-22. Correction of a vertical angulation of the septal cartilage. Fracture angulations can be corrected by direct wedge resection, oriented along the direction of fracture.

Small Telfa rolls may be placed in each nostril to lightly splint the nose for 24 to 72 hours. Nasal packs are not relied on to control bleeding or to stabilize the reconstructed septum. Septal splints are rarely necessary except when synechiae have been opened or excised.

Reconstruction of the L-shaped septal strut

Substantial weakness or deformity of the supporting dorsal and caudal (L-shaped) struts requires careful management. Simple resection of the deformed portion is not recommended because of the inevitable loss of nasal support, and techniques that weaken the septal cartilage often result in long-term deformity or nasal collapse. To avoid these potential problems, deformed segments of the L-shaped strut should be reconstructed, reinforced, or braced with structural grafts of autologous bone and cartilage. This can usually be accomplished without a loss of nasal support and with preservation or improvement of nasal form.

The caudal segment

Traumatic or developmental dislocations of the caudal septum are usually corrected by freeing cartilage at the maxillary crest (Fig. 50-25). An inferior triangle of cartilage may require resection to mobilize the caudal edge. The septal cartilage is then secured to the anterior nasal spine periosteum in the midline. When dislocation of the caudal segment results from a fracture angulation, the fracture line is excised to create a caudal "swinging door" segment. Still attached to the opposite mucoperichondrium, the mobilized segment is positioned in the midline and secured with suture.[46] The repositioned cartilage can be further straightened by conservative crosshatching or morselization.

Although effective in straightening cartilage, these maneuvers may weaken the strength of the caudal septal strut. Instability of this strut risks a loss of nasal tip projection. Ethmoid bone sandwich grafts are sometimes needed to achieve long-term support of the nasal tip.[47] To place these grafts, the caudal septum is exposed via an endonasal or open approach raising bilateral mucoperichondrial flaps. Grafts of thin ethmoid bone are positioned on one or both sides of the caudal strut and secured with one or more transseptal mattress sutures. Because ethmoid bone is strong and thin, a straight and stable caudal strut is constructed without sacrifice of the nasal airway. If ethmoid bone is absent or insufficient, thin segments of straight septal cartilage can be substituted.

The dorsal segment

Deformities of the dorsal septal margin are significant when they contribute to a crooked nose appearance or result in nasal blockage caused by narrowing of the nasal valve area. Deviations of the dorsal strut should be altered in a way that will not compromise nasal support or the nasal airway. Absolute correction of the deformity is often difficult because of the structural complexity of the region and the highly visible, well-defined contours of the nasal dorsum.

Exposure of the dorsal segment requires division of the upper lateral cartilages from the nasal septum without violating the intranasal mucosa. The open approach provides di-

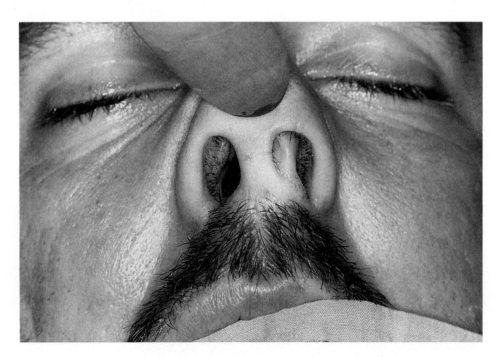

Fig. 50-25. Traumatic dislocation of the caudal nasal septum into the left nares.

rect visualization of this dissection and allows the surgeon to work from above and below. Once the septum is released from the upper lateral cartilages, the degree of angulation of the dorsal margin of the septal cartilage becomes apparent. If the septum is drawn from the midline by an asymmetry of the bony pyramid of the nose, osteotomies are required for straightening. A significant residual deviation of the dorsal border of the nasal septum will be noted in many cases after osteotomies are complete. The residual deviation may be corrected using such techniques as cartilage shaving, vertical incisions, planoconvex spreader grafts, or camouflage onlay grafting. If the patient suffers from nasal airway obstruction, more aggressive maneuvers may be required to provide adequate nasal function.

Ethmoid bone-stenting grafts may be used to structurally align the dorsal segment.[66] Thin rectangular grafts measuring 5 to 12 mm in length and 3 to 5 mm in width may be sutured on opposite sides of the dorsal septum to assure straightening (Fig. 50-26). In the absence of suitable ethmoid bone, thin straight grafts of septal cartilage are used. Before suturing the grafts in place, the deviated cartilage may be vertically incised on the concave surface to release the memory of the cartilage. Any residual concavity can be corrected with a small unilateral spreader graft placed between the

upper lateral cartilage and the stented septum (Fig. 50-27). Alternatively, the residual defect may be camouflaged using an onlay cartilage graft. After all the grafts are in good position, the upper lateral cartilages are re-attached with mattress sutures to the nasal septum. The stable construct of the sandwich grafts promotes reliable healing and a straight appearance of the cartilaginous dorsum (Figs. 50-28 and 50-29).

Subtotal reconstruction of the nasal septum

The primary indication for subtotal septal reconstruction is severe deformities of the dorsal and caudal (L-shaped) struts not correctable using standard techniques (Fig. 50-30). The deformities may involve any portion of the dorsal and caudal struts. These deformities may cause a shortened nose, narrowed nasal airway, crooked nose, saddle nose, or loss of tip projection. In this technique, a major supportive portion of the nasal septum is replaced with an autologous cartilage graft harvested from another region of the nasal septum[6,65] or from rib cartilage.[9]

The septum is dissected from below (hemitransfixtion) and above (open approach), elevating bilateral mucoperichondrial flaps. The upper lateral cartilages are separated from the nasal septum without violating the underlying mucosa. This wide exposure of the septal cartilage allows care-

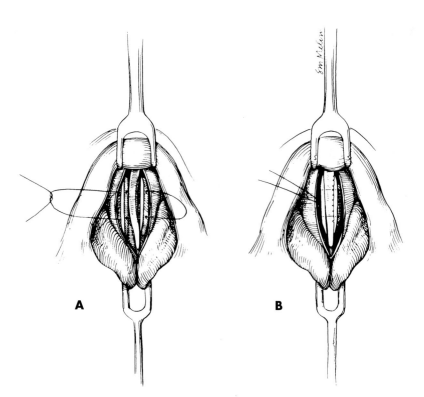

Fig. 50-26. Ethmoid bone-stenting grafts. **A,** Thin ethmoid bone grafts are applied on opposite sides of a C-shaped segment of anterior (dorsal) septal cartilage. **B,** Suturing of the grafts forces the cartilage into a straight orientation. (From Toriumi DM, Ries WR: Innovative surgical management of the crooked nose, *Facial Plast Surg Clin North Am* 1:6378, 1993. Used with permission.)

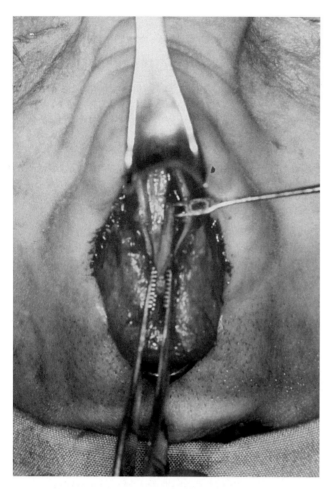

Fig. 50-27. A Planoconvex spreader graft. After application of bilateral ethmoid bone-stenting grafts, any residual concavity of the middle nasal vault can be corrected with a unilateral spreader graft, placed between the upper lateral cartilage and the stented septum.

ful assessment of the deformity (Fig. 50-31). The portion of the nasal septum that requires reconstruction is identified and removed. With an extreme deformity, most of the septal cartilage may be resected[65] (Fig. 50-32). The supporting portions of the septum are then restored with a cartilage replacement graft harvested from the posteroinferior nasal septum when there is sufficient septal cartilage to create a stable L-shaped septal strut with a width of at least 1.5 cm. If the shape, strength, or quantity of septal cartilage is insufficient, a center cut section of rib cartilage is carved to reproduce the septal plate[9] (Fig. 50-33). In the future, engineered cartilage replacement grafts may present a useful alternative to rib cartilage.[52,53]

The cartilage graft is positioned between the mucoperichondrial flaps and fixed to the cartilage remnant at the osseocartilaginous junction with lasting mattress sutures. The graft is positioned in the midline to create a dorsal and caudal (L-shaped) strut (Fig. 50-34). The profile should be smooth and straight and should not project above the level of the

nasal tip. The caudal strut of the graft is sutured between the medial crura to act as a strut.[65] The graft is fixed to any cartilage remnant at the anterior nasal spine or to the spine itself (Fig. 50-35). Adequate graft length prevents an overly short or rotated nose, but the graft should not extend caudally beyond the medial crura. The final position of the graft is determined by assessing the nasal length and projection. Adjustments are made when necessary to alter columella retraction, the height of the nasal dorsum, tip projection, or the length of the nose. Once the graft is properly positioned, the upper lateral cartilages are sutured to the dorsal margin of the graft and the tip support mechanisms are restored. The mucoperichondrial flaps are apposed with a running transseptal quilting suture. Excellent long-term results can be achieved (Figs. 50-36 and 50-37).

COMPLICATIONS OF SEPTAL SURGERY

Most complications that result from septal reconstruction relate to the inherent risks posed by nasal surgery. Others can be attributed to incorrect evaluation or a failure on surgical correction. The former includes such problems as bleeding, infection, intranasal adhesions, transient hypesthesia of the lip or palate, and allergic reactions. These are common problems of moderate consequence.[56]

Patient dissatisfaction after septal surgery is common and is often the result of an incorrect evaluation. Not all patients with obstructed breathing and some degree of septal deviation are candidates for septal surgery. Often, the contributions of mucosal disease, nasal valve narrowing, alar margin collapse, and coexisting medical illness are inadequately respected. Septoplasty, although conceptually simple, remains technically difficult.[24] The surgeon walks a fine line between inadequate mobilization, which risks failure caused by temerity, and excessive mobilization, which can lead to instability, new displacement, or nasal collapse. Many septoplasty techniques weaken the support of the nose; the septal cartilage is dissected, incised, morselized, mobilized, and resected to permit it to assume passively a nonangulated conformation.[24] As a consequence, the septal cartilage may be weakened beyond its physical tolerance, predisposing to new deformity, a crooked nose appearance, or nasal collapse. To avert these complications, the surgeon should avoid excessive weakening or resection of supporting anterior septal components. Autologous grafts of thin bone or cartilage are sometimes needed to shore up or straighten cartilage in areas of major septal support. The goal is to create a straight and sturdy L-shaped septal strut that extends uninterrupted from the osseocartilaginous junction to the nasal spine.

The long-term incidence of postoperative perforation of the nasal septum is between 0 and 5% after conservation septoplasty but is conspicuously higher after submucous resection.[4,18,50,61,67] Nasal septal perforation stems from surgically induced trauma that results in devitalized tissue within a scarred surgical bed. Risk factors include submucous resection, prior nasal surgery or trauma, advanced age, poor nutri-

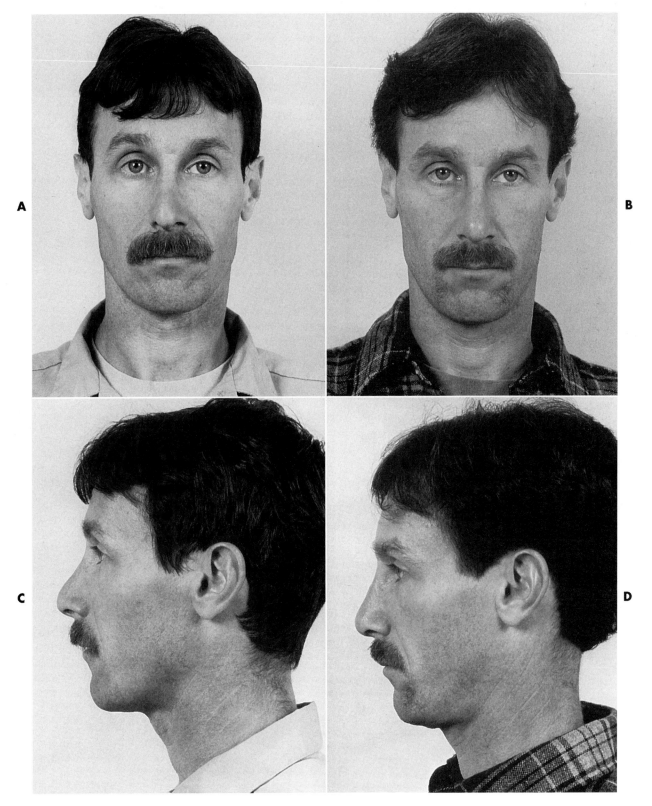

Fig. 50-28. Patient with a C-shaped deformity of the anterior (dorsal) nasal septum. After sequential medial and lateral osteotomies, bilateral ethmoid bone-stenting grafts were used to correct the deformity. **A** and **C,** Preoperative views. **B** and **D,** One-year postoperative views.

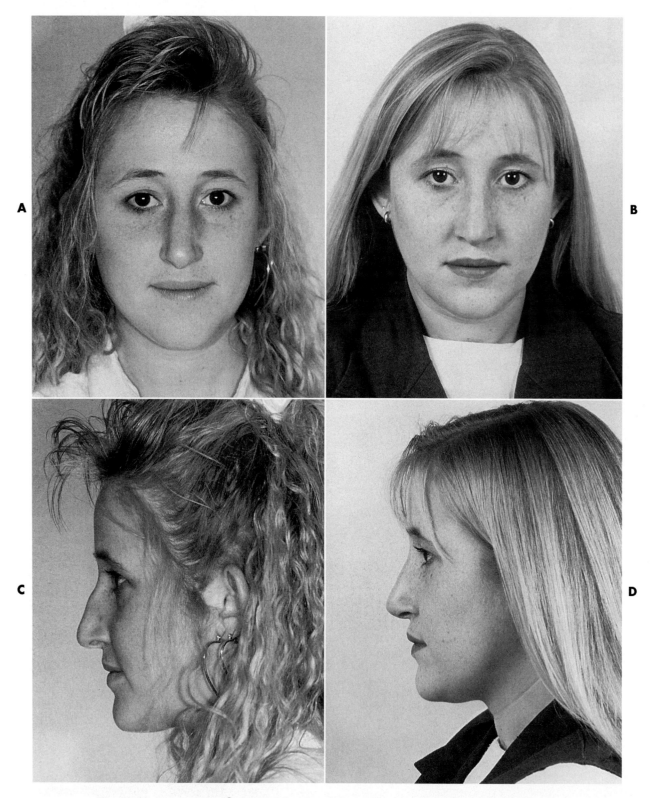

Fig. 50-29. Patient with a C-shaped deformity of the anterior (dorsal) nasal septum. A unilateral planoconvex spreader graft and lateral onlay graft were used to camouflage the deformity. **A** and **C,** Preoperative views. **B** and **D,** Three-year postoperative views.

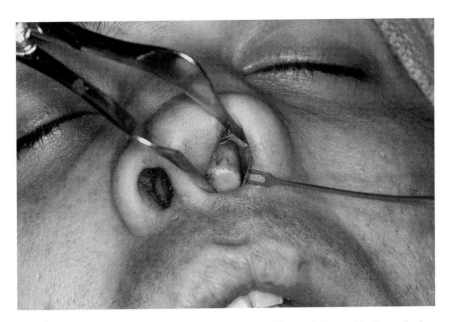

Fig. 50-30. Deviation of the nasal septum in all planes with nasal airway blockage. Such severe deformity is difficult to fully correct using standard septoplasty techniques.

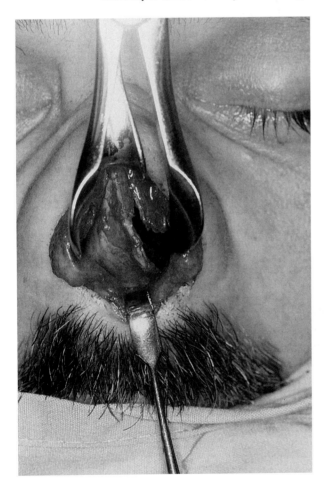

Fig. 50-31. Complete dissection of the septal cartilage and its supporting structures through the external (open) rhinoplasty approach. Marked deviation of the cartilage is seen in all planes.

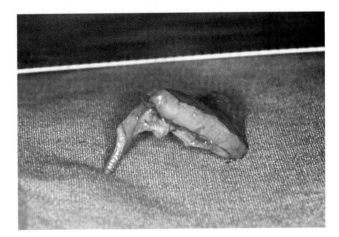

Fig. 50-32. Subtotal resection of the quadrangular (septal) cartilage. The cartilage is calcified, thickened, and deviated in all planes. (Same cartilage as shown in Figure 50-31.)

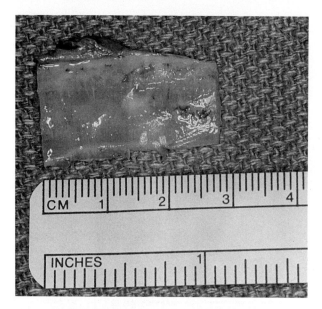

Fig. 50-33. A center-cut section of rib cartilage used to reproduce the septal plate.

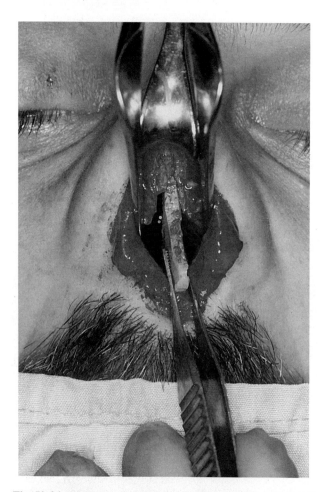

Fig. 50-34. Major septal replacement with a graft of center-cut rib cartilage. The graft is positioned precisely in the midline and sutured to a remnant of cartilage at the osseocartilaginous junction.

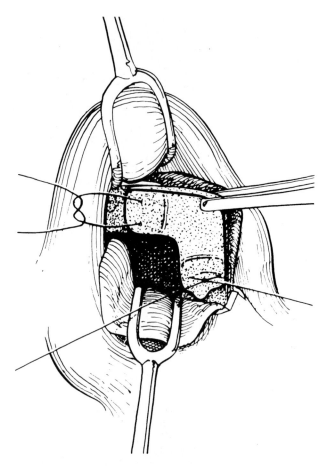

Fig. 50-35. Partial replacement of the septal L-shaped strut (anterior septal angle and caudal segment) with an autologous cartilage graft. The graft may be taken from the posteroinferior region of the nasal septum or from another source (rib). Note how the graft is sutured to cartilage remnants at the osseocartilaginous junction and nasal spine. (From Toriumi DM, Ries WR: Innovative surgical management of the crooked nose, *Facial Plast Surg Clin North Am* 1:6378, 1993. Used with permission.)

tion, and medical conditions such as diabetes and hypertension, which adversely effect the microcirculation. General preventive measures include cautious resection of septal components, fastidious subperichondrial flap elevation, precise alignment of mucosal tears, obliteration of dead space, atraumatic handling of tissues, and avoidance of cautery on mucosal flaps. Tight suturing of septal splints and heavy nasal packing also increase the risk of perforation and should be avoided.

Although a rare complication of septal surgery, injury to the cribiform area can result in cerebrospinal fluid leak, olfactory nerve injury, pneumocephalus, intracranial hemorrhage, and injury to the frontal lobe.[42] Most of these injuries are caused by injudicious twisting or levering of the ethmoid plate while it is still attached to the cribiform region. To prevent injury, it is best to separate the bony septum from the cribiform area using a pair of heavy scissors or to resect the bony septum in stepwise fashion using small biting for-

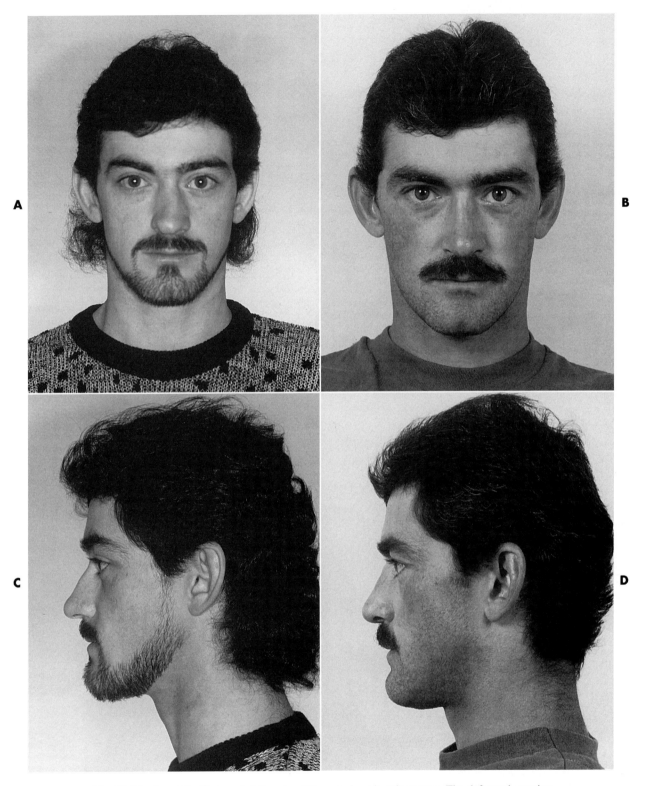

Fig. 50-36. A notable C-shaped deformity of the anterior (dorsal) septum. The deformed anterior portion of the septal L-shaped strut was replaced with a graft of autologous rib cartilage. A lateral onlay camouflage graft was used to correct a residual deformity of the upper lateral cartilage. **A** and **C,** Preoperative views. **B** and **D,** One-year postoperative views.

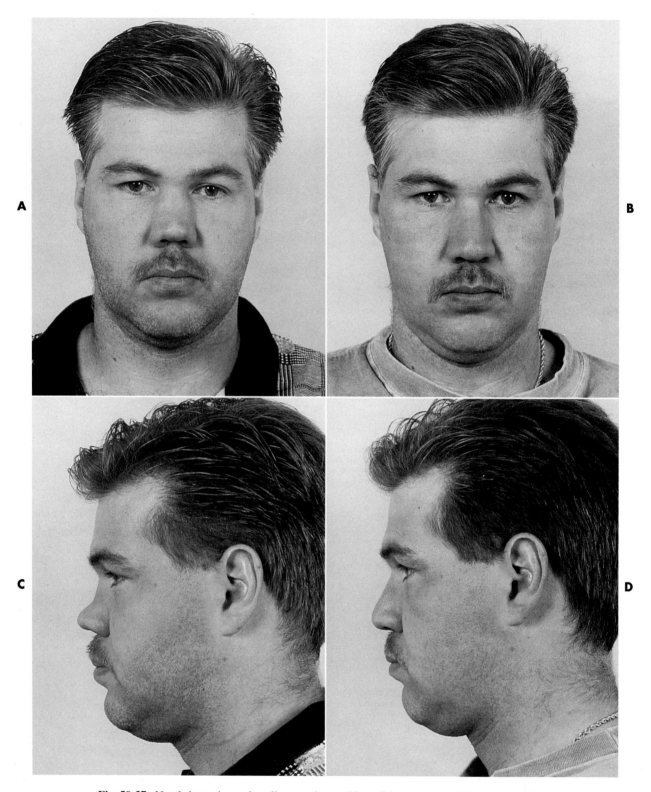

Fig. 50-37. Nasal shortening, columella retraction, and loss of dorsal support. Major septal replacement was carried out using an autologous rib cartilage graft shaped to reproduce the quadrangular cartilage. Note that adequate graft length prevents an overly short or rotated nose. **A** and **C,** Preoperative views. **B** and **D,** One-year postoperative views.

ceps. Intracranial infection may complicate cribiform fracture or may occur after local infection by direct invasion of venous communications between the mucoperiosteum and the cavernous sinus. Although rare in the era of antibiotics, intracranial infection after nasal surgery can be fatal.[44]

REFERENCES

1. Adams W: The treatment of the broken nose by forcible straightening and mechanical apparatus, *BMJ* 2:421, 1875.
2. Asch M: Treatment of nasal stenosis due to deflective septum with and without thickening of the convex side, *Laryngoscope* 6:340, 1899.
3. Becker GD, Radford ER: *Allergic rhinitis*. In Gates G, editor: *Current therapy in otolaryngology—head and neck surgery,* St Louis, 1994, Mosby.
4. Bewarder F, Pirsig W: Long-term results of submucous septal resection, *Laryngol Rhinol* 57:922, 1978.
5. Boenninghaus G: Bemerkungen zum aufsatze loewes: zur chirurgie der nasenscheidewand, *Monatsschr Ohrenh* 34:287, 1900.
6. Briant TDR, Middleton WG: The management of severe nasal septal deformities, *J Otolaryngol* 14:120, 1985.
7. Bridger GP: Physiology of the nasal valve, *Arch Otolaryngol Head Neck Surg* 92:543, 1970.
8. Broms P, Jonson B, Malm L: A pre- and postoperative evaluation in functional septoplasty, *Acta Otolaryngol (Stockh)* 94:303, 1982.
9. Candiani P and others: Anatomical reconstruction versus camouflage of the inferior two thirds of the nasal septum, *Ann Plast Surg* 34:624, 1995.
10. Clark RW, Jones AS: Nasal airflow receptors: the relative importance of temperature and tactile stimulation, *Clin Otolaryngol* 17:388, 1992.
11. Clarke RW and others: The role of mucosal receptors in the nasal sensation of airflow, *Clin Otolaryngol* 17:383, 1992.
12. Cole P: Some aspects of temperature, moisture and heat relationships in the upper respiratory tract, *J Laryngol Otol* 67:449, 1953.
13. Cottle M: Nasal surgery in children: effect of early nasal injury, *Eye Ear Nose Throat Monthly* 30:32, 1951.
14. Cottle MH and others: The ''maxilla-premaxilla'' approach to extensive nasal septum surgery, *Arch Otolaryngol Head Neck Surg* 60:301, 1958.
15. Cottle MH, Loring RM: Newer concepts of septum surgery: present status, *Eye Ear Nose Throat Monthly* 27:403, 1948.
16. Courtiss EH, Goldwyn RM: The effects of nasal surgery on airflow, *Plast Reconstr Surg* 72:9, 1983.
17. Daniel RK, Letourneau A: Rhinoplasty: nasal anatomy, *Ann Plast Surg* 20:5, 1988.
18. Fjermedal O, Saunte C, Pedersen S: Septoplasty and/or submucous resection? 5 years of nasal septum operations, *J Laryngol Otol* 102: 796, 1988.
19. Fomon S and others: Plastic repair of the deflected nasal septum, *Arch Otolaryngol Head Neck Surg* 55:141, 1946.
20. Freer OT: The correction of deflections of the nasal septum with a minimum of traumatism, *JAMA* 38:636, 1902.
21. Fry H: Interlocked stress in human nasal septal cartilage, *Br J Plast Surg* 19:276, 1966.
22. Gibson T, Davis WB: The distortion of autologous cartilage grafts: its cause and prevention, *Br J Plast Surg* 10:257, 1958.
23. Giles WC and others: Endoscopic septoplasty, *Laryngoscope* 104:1507, 1997.
24. Godfrey NV: Sagittal section septoplasty: an intrinsically stabilized septoplasty, *Plast Reconstr Surg* 93:188, 1994.
25. Goldman IB: New technique in surgery of the deviated nasal septum, *Arch Otolaryngol Head Neck Surg* 64:183, 1956.
26. Gubisch W: The extracorporeal septum plasty: a technique to correct difficult nasal deformities, *Plast Reconstr Surg* 95:672, 1995.
27. Hamilton L: Nasal airway resistance: its measurement and regulation, *Physiologist* 22:43, 1979.
28. Hardcastle PF, White A, Prescott RJ: Clinic and rhinometric assessment of the nasal airway: do they measure the same entity? *Clin Otolaryngol* 13:185, 1988.
29. Hinderer KH: *Fundamentals of anatomy and surgery of the nose,* Birmingham, Ala, 1971, Aesculapius Publishing.
30. Huygen PLM and others: Rhinomanometric detection rate of rhinoscopically-assessed septal deviations, *Rhinology* 30:177, 1992.
31. Ingals EF: Deflections of the septum narium, *Arch Laryngol* 3:291, 1882.
32. Jancke JB, Wright WK: Studies on the support of the nasal tip, *Arch Otolaryngol Head Neck Surg* 93:458, 1971.
33. Jazbi B: Diagnosis and treatment of nasal birth deformities, *Otolaryngol Clin North Am* 19:125, 1977.
34. Jones AS and others: The effect of local anesthesia of the nasal vestibule on nasal sensation of airflow and nasal resistance, *Clin Otolaryngol* 12:461, 1989.
35. Jones AS and others: The effect of lignocaine on nasal resistance and nasal sensation of airflow, *Acta Otolaryngol (Stockh)* 101:328, 1986.
36. Jones AS, Willatt DJ, Durham LM: Nasal airflow: resistance and sensation, *J Laryngol Otol* 103:909, 1989.
37. Kasperbauer JL, Kern EB: Nasal valve physiology: implications in nasal surgery, *Otolaryngol Clin North Am* 20:699, 1987.
38. Killian G: Die sumucöse Fensterresektion der Nasenscheidewand, *Arch Laryngologie Rhinologie* 16:362, 1904.
39. King ED, Ashley FL: The correction of the internally and externally deviated nose, *Plast Reconstr Surg* 10:116, 1952.
40. Kirchner J: Traumatic nasal deformity in the newborn, *Arch Otolaryngol Head Neck Surg* 62:139, 1955.
41. Krieg R: Resection der cartilago quadrangularis septi nasem sur heilung der scoliosis septi, *Medicinishes Cocrespondenz blatt Wurtenburgishen Artzlicken Verein Stuttgart* 56:201, 1886.
42. Lawson W, Kessler S, Biller JF: Unusual and fatal complications of rhinoplasty, *Arch Otolaryngol Head Neck Surg* 109:164, 1983.
43. Lawson W, Reino AJ: Correcting functional problems, *Facial Plast Clin North Am* 2:501, 1994.
44. Maniglia AJ: Fatal and major complications secondary to nasal and sinus surgery, *Laryngoscope* 99:276, 1989.
45. Mertz JM, McCaffrey TV, Kern EB: Objective evaluation of anterior septal surgical reconstruction, *Otolaryngol Head Neck Surg* 92:308, 1984.
46. Metzenbaum M: Replacement of the lower end of the dislocated septal cartilage versus submucous resection of the dislocated end of the septal cartilage, *Arch Otolaryngol Head Neck Surg* 9:282, 1929.
47. Metzinger SE and others: Ethmoid bone sandwich grafting for caudal septal defects, *Arch Otolaryngol Head Neck Surg* 120:1121, 1994.
48. Murakami W, Wong L, Davidson J: Application of the biomedical behavior of cartilage to nasal septoplastic surgery, *Laryngoscope* 92: 300, 1982.
49. Negus V: Observation on the exchange of fluid in the nose and respiratory tract, *Ann Otol Rhinol Laryngol* 66:344, 1957.
50. Peacock MR: Sub-mucous resection of the nasal septum, *J Laryngol Otol* 95:341, 1981.
51. Peer LA: An operation to repair lateral displacement of the lower border of the septal cartilage, *Arch Otolaryngol Head Neck Surg* 25:475, 1937.
52. Pirsig W and others: Cartilage transformation in a composite graft of demineralized bovine bone matrix and ear perichondrium used in a child for reconstruction of the nasal septum, *Int J Pediatr Otorhinolaryngol* 32:171, 1995.
53. Puelacher WC and others: Design of nasoseptal cartilage replacements synthesized from biodegradable polymers and chondrocytes, *Biomaterials* 15:774, 1994.
54. Rees T: Surgical correction of the severely deviated nose by extramucosal excision of the osseocartilaginous septum and replacement as a free graft, *Plast Reconstr Surg* 78:320, 1986.
55. Ridenour BD: *Nasal fracture*. In Gates G, editor: *Current therapy in otolaryngology—head and neck surgery,* St Louis, 1994, Mosby.

56. Schwab J-A, Pirsig W: Complications of septal surgery, *Facial Plast Surg* 13:3, 1997.

57. Sessions RB, Troost T: *The nasal septum.* In Cummings CW, editor: *Otolaryngology—head and neck surgery,* vol 1, St Louis, 1993, Mosby.

58. Sheen JH: Spreader graft: a method of reconstructing the roof of the middle nasal vault following rhinoplasty, *Plast Reconstr Surg* 73:230, 1984.

59. Sipila J, Suonpaa J, Laippala P: Evaluation of nasal resistance data in active anterior rhinomanometry with special reference to clinical usefullness and test-retest analysis, *Clin Otolaryngol* 17:170, 1992.

60. Smith M: Abusive rhinology, *Br J Clin Pract* 13:458, 1957.

61. Stoksted P, Vase P: Perforations of the nasal septum following operative procedures, *Rhinology* 16:123, 1978.

62. Swift AC, Cambell IT, Mckown TM: Oronasal obstruction, lung volumes, and arterial oxygenation, *Lancet* 1:73, 1988.

63. Tardy ME: *Rhinoplasty: the art and the science,* Philadelphia, 1997, WB Saunders.

64. Toriumi DM: Management of the middle nasal vault in rhinoplasty, *Operative Techniques in Plastic and Reconstructive Surgery* 2:16, 1995.

65. Toriumi DM: Subtotal reconstruction of the nasal septum: a preliminary report, *Laryngoscope* 104:906, 1994.

66. Toriumi DM, Ries WR: Innovative surgical management of the crooked nose, *Facial Plast Surg Clin North Am* 1:6378, 1993.

67. Tzadik A, Gilbert SE, Sade J: Complications of submucous resections of the nasal septum, *Arch Oto Rhino Laryngol* 245:74, 1988.

68. Vilar-Sancho B: Rhinoseptoplasty, *Aesthetic Plast Surg* 8:61, 1984.

69. Wright WK: Principles of nasal septum reconstruction, *Trans Am Acad Ophthalmol Otolaryngol* 73:252, 1969.

SUGGESTED READINGS

Cottle MH and others: The "maxilla-premaxilla" approach to extensive nasal septum surgery, *Arch Otolaryngol* 60:301, 1958.

Fry H: Interlocked stress in human nasal septal cartilage, *Brit J Plast Surg* 19:276, 1966.

Gubisch W: The extracorporeal septum plasty: a technique to correct difficult nasal deformities, *Plast Reconstr Surg* 95:672, 1995.

Kasperbauer JL, Kern EB: Nasal valve physiology-implications in nasal surgery, *Otolaryngol Clin North Am* 20:699, 1987.

Killian G: Die sumucöse Fensterresektion der Nasenscheidewand, *Arch Laryngologie Rhinologie* 16:362, 1904.

Metzenbaum M: Replacement of the lower end of the dislocated septal cartilage versus submucous resection of the dislocated end of the septal cartilage, *Arch Otolaryngol* 9:282, 1929.

Sessions RB, Troost T: *The nasal septum.* In Cummings CW, editor: *Otolaryngology—head and neck surgery,* vol 1, St Louis, 1993, Mosby.

Tardy, ME: *Rhinoplasty: the art and the science,* Philadelphia, 1997, WB Saunders.

Toriumi DM: Subtotal reconstruction of the nasal septum: a preliminary report, *Laryngoscope* 104:906, 1994.

Toriumi DM, Ries WR: Innovative surgical management of the crooked nose, *Facial Plast Surg Clin* 1:6378, 1993.

Chapter 51

Rhinoplasty

M. Eugene Tardy, Jr.
James Alex
David A. Hendrick

SURGICAL PHILOSOPHY

Aesthetic and reconstructive rhinoplasty, universally acknowledged as the most elegant but most difficult of all plastic surgical procedures, soon approaches the one hundredth anniversary of its modern development. Although certain refinements in technique gained progressive acceptance during the first three-quarters of the twentieth century, the fundamental operation remained a primarily *tissue reduction* procedure, characterized by various degrees of excision (often rather profound) of the fundamental nasal anatomic components.

In the past 15 years a striking revolution has occurred in the fine points of analysis and technique, guided by surgeons devoted to tissue reorientation and augmentation rather than resection, individualization of technique rather than a lockstep approach, and atraumatic tissue dissection in proper nasal cleavage planes. A more thorough understanding of and respect for the long-term surgical outcome now dominates and guides the selection of the surgical technique because surgeons no longer are content with satisfactory short-term results at the expense of risking future visual and functional misadventures. Thus all modifications to nasal structures should factor in the dynamic effects each maneuver exerts upon the immediate overall nasal appearance, in the nasal airway, and the anticipated control of the vagaries of healing nasal tissues. Clearly the surgically altered nose continues to be modified by the healing process and certain inexorable aging phenomena during the lifetime of the patient. Thus it is seldom possible to designate a "final result" following nasal surgery.

The philosophy, approaches, and graduated techniques presented in this chapter seek to document and validate the long-term virtues of accurate detailed analysis and planning, atraumatic and conservative surgical techniques devoted to tissue repositioning and reorientation, and methods of exercising the highest control over the healing process.

PREOPERATIVE PATIENT ASSESSMENT

Anatomic evaluation

The final result of any rhinoplasty procedure is the consequence of the individual patient's anatomy (Fig. 51-1 and Plates 5 and 6) as much as the surgeon's skill. No two noses are ever quite alike; it follows then that no single, standard procedure suffices to reconstruct every nose pleasingly. The ability to diagnose the possibilities and limitations inherent in each patient is an absolute prerequisite to achieving outstanding results. Sometimes patients with minimal deformities (a small hump, a minimally bulbous tip, a slightly overwide nose) are the best candidates for near-perfect surgical results (Fig. 51-2). Because the initial problem is minimal, this group of patients often expects and even demands perfection. More dramatic surgical results are possible in patients who demonstrate significant departures from an aesthetic ideal (a large hump; an elongated, drooping nose; a twisted nose); these patients might tolerate possible minor imperfections that result because the overall improvement is dramatic (Fig. 51-3). It is the fundamental responsibility of the surgeon to balance the wishes and desires of the patient with what is realistically possible given the anatomic limitations (or possibilities) inherent in each individual nose.

The quality of the skin is an essential indicator of the surgical outcome and plays a significant role in preoperative

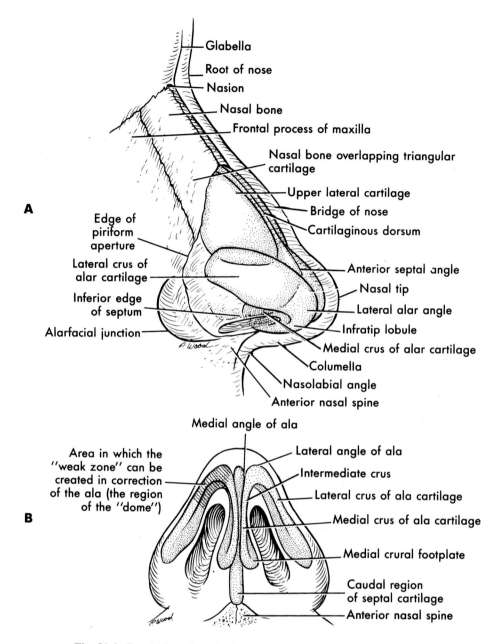

Fig. 51-1. Practical nasal surgical anatomy. **A,** Lateral view; **B,** base view.

planning. Extremely thick skin, rich in sebaceous glands and subcutaneous tissue, is the least ideal skin type for achieving desirable refinement and definition. Care should be taken not to overreduce the bony-cartilaginous skeleton in thick-skinned patients in a futile attempt to produce a much smaller nose. Failure of thick skin to contract favorably in this situation may lead to excess soft-tissue scar, an amorphous nasal appearance, and even the dreaded soft-tissue "polly beak" (Fig. 51-4).

Extremely thin skin, often pale, freckled, and nearly translucent, also should be recognized and respected for its inherent limitations. Although ideal for achieving critical defini-

tion, thin skin with sparse subcutaneous tissue provides almost no cushion to cover even the most minute of skeletal irregularities or contour imperfections, and therefore demands near-perfect surgery to achieve the desired natural result. Occasionally patients with this anatomic condition demonstrate an undesirable progressive skin retraction and unattractive shrinkage over several years, rendering the nose unnatural and angular.

The ideal skin type falls somewhere between these two extremes, being neither too thick and oily nor too thin and delicate. It possesses enough subcutaneous tissue to provide a satisfactory cushion over the nasal skeleton but still allows

Text continued on p. 955

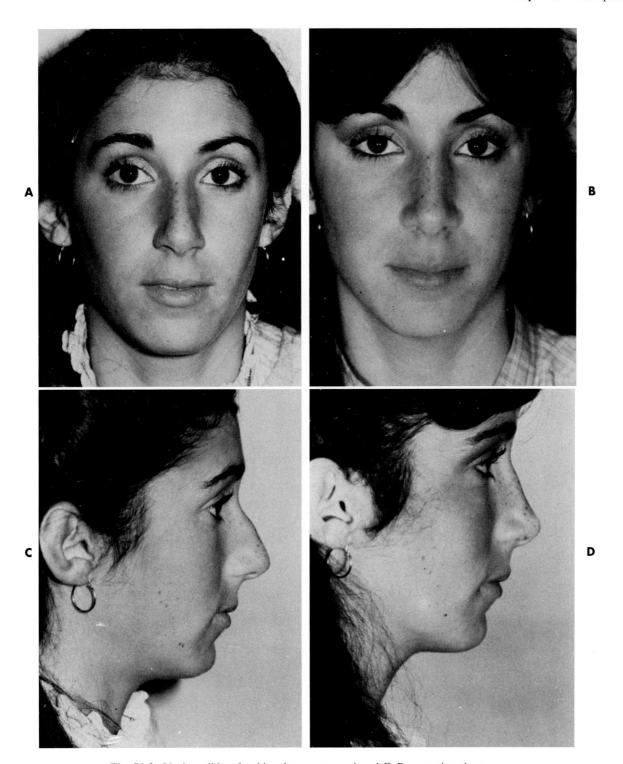

Fig. 51-2. Ideal candidate for rhinoplasty surgery. **A** and **C,** Preoperative views.
B and **D,** Postoperative views.

Continued

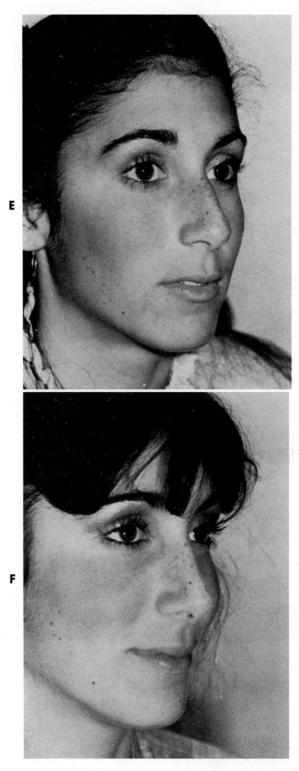

Fig. 51-2, cont'd. **E** and **F,** Pre- and postoperative views.

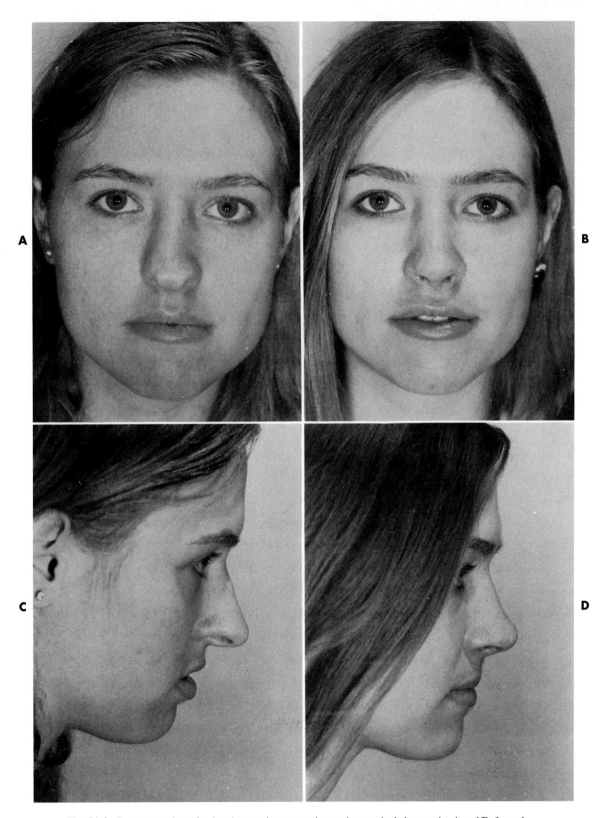

Fig. 51-3. Reconstruction of twisted nose, demonstrating major surgical changes in, **A** and **B,** frontal, and, **C** and **D,** lateral views.

Continued

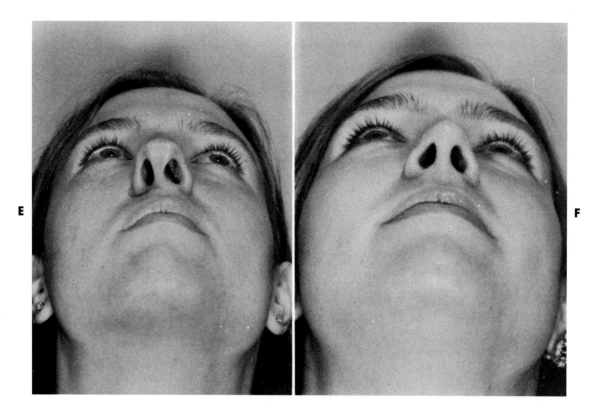

Fig. 51-3, cont'd. E and **F,** Base views.

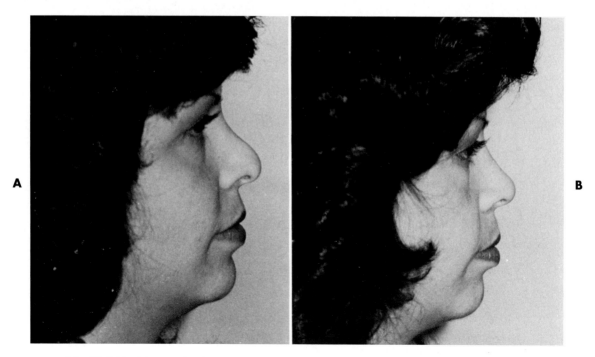

Fig. 51-4. Revision repair of patient referred with typical soft-tissue ''polly beak'' deformity. Supratip scar carefully excised with restoration of appropriate tip–supratip relationship. Cartilage only graft covers dorsum to smooth and improve contour of nasal skeleton. **A,** Preoperative view; **B,** postoperative view.

critical definition to become apparent in a relatively short time after surgery. Evaluation of skin type is made by inspection and palpation—rolling the skin over the nasal skeleton and gently pinching it between the examining fingers.

A critical factor in assessing the candidate for rhinoplasty is the inherent strength and support of the nasal tip, referred to as the *tip recoil*. Finger depression of the tip toward the upper lid provides a quick and reliable test of the ability of the mobile tip's structures to spring back into position (Fig. 51-5). The tip that possesses weak, somewhat flail alar cartilages does not tolerate an extensive sacrifice of tissue well and may require the addition of supportive struts to improve its long-term stable support. These weak tips often are accompanied by thin alar sidewalls and thin skin (Fig. 51-6). If the recoil is instantaneous and vigorous, and the tip cartilages resist the deforming influence of the finger, more definitive tip surgery usually may be performed without fear of substantial loss. The size, shape, attitude, and resilience of the alar cartilages may be estimated by palpation or ''ballottement'' of lateral crus between two fingers surrounding its cephalic and caudal margins. During this assessment the surgeon makes the all-important decision about whether to enhance, reduce, or carefully preserve the tip projection that exists preoperatively. Any asymmetry of the alar cartilages must be carefully noted for later correction.

A surprising amount of diagnostic information may be gained by palpating the internal vestibules of the nose with the thumb and forefinger surrounding the columella. Otherwise undetected twists and angulations of the nasal septum, which may significantly influence the final functional and aesthetic appearance, may be discovered. The width and length of the columella and the medial crura it contains are determined. Short medial crura will probably require supportive cartilaginous struts to lengthen the columella and aid in

rotation, if desirable; extremely flaring or overlong medial crura invite reduction in width and length as well as repositioning. Information about the potential of the tip to undergo desirable cephalic rotation is gained by the exploring fingers, which determine whether the tip-lip complex is tethered by muscle and its inadequate length. It is also important to determine whether the central skeletal component of the nose (the quadrangular cartilage) is overlong and might interfere with satisfactory tip rotation (Fig. 51-7). The size and position of the nasal spine and its related caudal septal angle also must be evaluated.

The experienced surgeon accomplishes these visual and palpatory diagnostic exercises with precision and facility, often while eliciting further history from the patient. Detecting the minute but critical structural distinguishing characteristics of each individual's nasal anatomy is the first and most important step toward a splendid surgical result.

Careful examination of the nasal fossae before and after shrinkage of the mucosa and turbinates is an essential component of the initial examination. An overt, symptomatic deviation of the nasal septum is easily diagnosed; the deflected ethmoid plate, which may appear innocent but be responsible for airway blockade after infraction of the bony

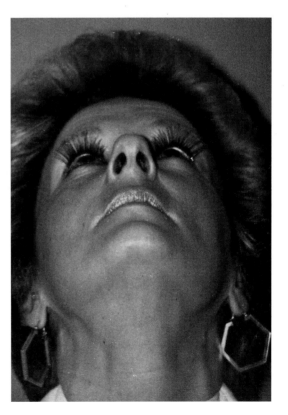

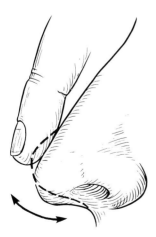

Fig. 51-5. Forceful depression of nasal tip structures, with assessment of tip recoil, guides surgeon to a better understanding of strength and integrity of tip-support mechanisms. This information is vital in selecting proper tip sculpture technique.

Fig. 51-6. A patient with thin, delicate alar sidewalls. Overaggressive excision or weakening of alar cartilages in such patients may result in progressive postoperative alar collapse and consequent nasal obstruction and asymmetry.

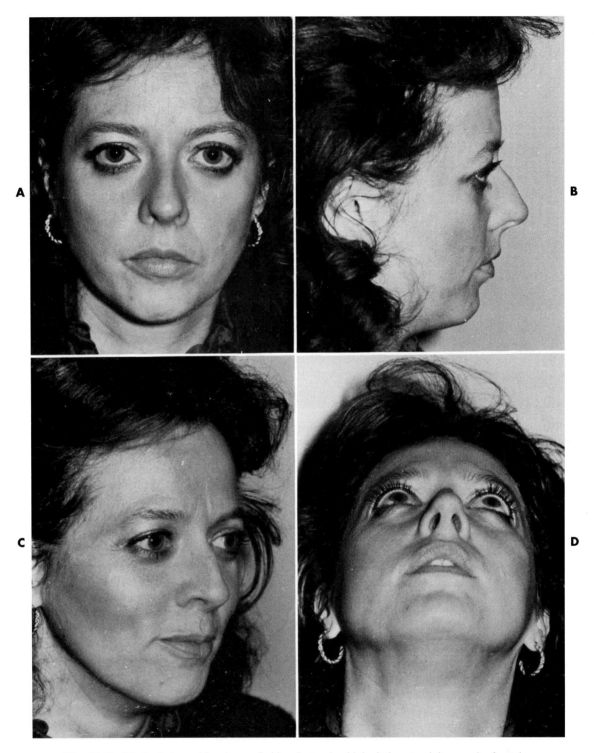

Fig. 51-11. Ideal photographic views of rhinoplasty should include, at minimum, **A,** frontal, **B,** lateral, **C,** oblique, and **D,** basal. Smiling view is often helpful. (Left oblique and lateral not shown.) In special cases close-up views may provide additional documentation.

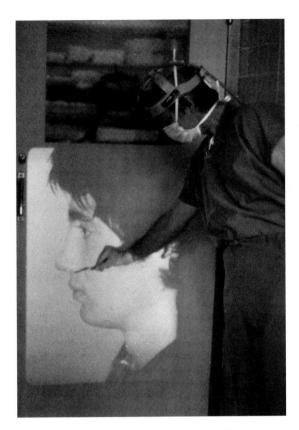

Fig. 51-12. Enlarged slide projection of patient in operating room to assist in intraoperative surgical decisions.

which at best hinders surgery. Correct anesthetic administration commonly results in a comfortable, relaxed patient and a relatively bloodless operative field, permitting precise anatomic dissection.

Just as there are a multitude of rhinoplasty techniques, so there are various approaches to nasal anesthesia. Experience suggests that a combination of monitored intravenous analgesia with local topical and infiltration anesthesia is ideal for rhinoplasty. General endotracheal anesthesia is less often employed for routine nasal surgery and is chosen only when concerns regarding patient cooperation arise.

Surgical planes

To achieve the goals of anesthesia fully, it is important to appreciate, identify, and correctly use the surgical planes of the nose. The importance of anatomic tissue planes is stressed throughout surgical training because dissection within these planes facilitates surgery with minimal bleeding and postoperative scarring.

Within the nose three distinct dissection planes can be identified. An extraperiosteal plane exists lateral and medial to the ascending process of the maxilla along the intended course of the lateral osteotomies. Infiltration of the local anesthetic on both sides of the ascending process aids remarkably in eliminating or reducing bleeding after a lateral

osteotomy (Fig. 51-14). A second plane exists in the submucoperichondrial and submucoperiosteal spaces flanking the nasal septum. Infiltration of the local anesthetic into this plane results in a hydraulic elevation of the septal flap, facilitating elevation and preservation of flap integrity (Fig. 51-15). Of greatest importance is the surgical plane occupying the immediate supraperichondrial and supraperiosteal regions over the lower and upper cartilages and nasal bones that exist just below the subcutaneous tissue layer (see Fig. 51-47). It is entered in all rhinoplasty operations. Infiltrating and operating in this plane produces a virtually bloodless field for delicate precision surgery.

A paucity of vascular and neural structures exists in these planes; anesthetic infiltration into these planes misses the vessels and nerves that lie more superficial in the subcutaneous tissue and dermis. When the anesthetic is injected into the proper planes, it diffuses more readily and requires only small amounts (usually 3.5 to 5 ml) to obtain the desired anesthetic and vasoconstrictive effects. If the infiltration is placed in the subcutaneous tissue or epithelium overlying these planes, larger quantities are needed to obtain these effects, and there is a tendency to distort and ''balloon'' the nose, creating a distortion that leads to inaccurate judgment. By identifying and using the proper dissection planes, only small amounts of anesthetic are needed to achieve maximal anesthesia and vasoconstriction with consequent minimal nasal distortion.

Preoperative medication and intravenous analgesia

Local infiltration anesthesia is administered after the patient has been sedated with preoperative medication and intravenous analgesia. It is important that the patient not receive many different families of drugs before and during surgery. Combinations of drugs, particularly when they are intermingled with intravenous medications given during surgery, are often unpredictable in their individual and combined effectiveness. Any drug reaction that may arise from the use of multiple families of pharmacologic agents is confusing to treat and may be impossible to counteract intelligently.

Close cooperation between the surgeon and anesthesiologist is important at this time as well as throughout the operation. Each is responsible for the patient's safety and well-being, and each catalyzes the operative process by a healthy respect for the other's responsibilities.

For increased comfort the patient is maintained in the reverse Trendelenburg position with the head elevated. This enhances vasoconstriction and facilitates venous and lymphatic drainage.

Topical anesthesia

Before infiltration of the local anesthetic, the nasal mucous membranes are anesthetized with a 4% cocaine solution that is color-coded to prevent the possibility of solution confusion and the inadvertent injection of cocaine. The cocaine

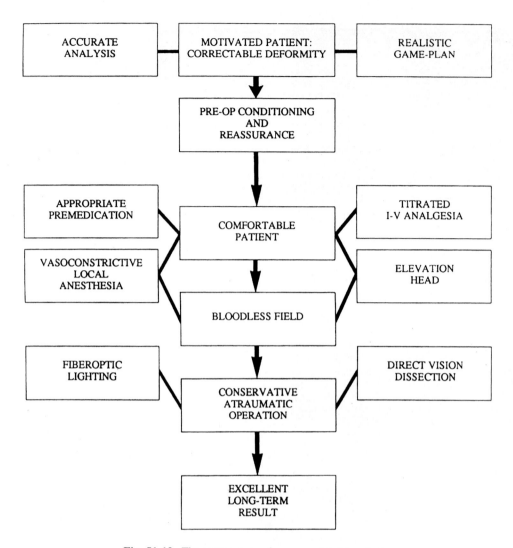

Fig. 51-13. The components of a successful rhinoplasty.

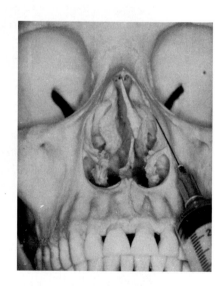

Fig. 51-14. Anesthetic infiltration of internal (medial) aspects of ascending process of maxilla as well as lateral surface creates vasoconstricted pathway for progression of lateral osteotomy, thereby reducing or eliminating bleeding and edema.

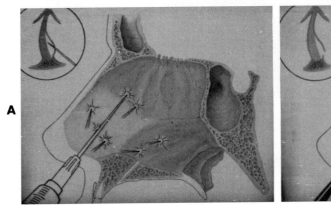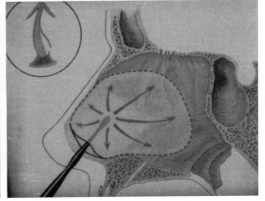

Fig. 51-15. A, Anesthetic infiltration of submucoperichondrial plane results in ''hydraulic dissection'' of mucoperichondrial flap. **B,** Facile elevation of mucoperichondrial septal flap is more easily accomplished when proper anesthetic infiltration is carried out.

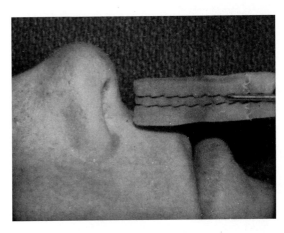

Fig. 51-16. Neurosurgical cottonoids, moistened with color-coded 4% cocaine solution, are positioned in each nasal cavity before infiltration of local anesthetic.

is deposited in each nasal fossa on a single neurosurgical cottonoid, which is wrung out to prevent any excess absorption of the drug (Fig. 51-16). It is unnecessary to anesthetize specifically precise nerves in the nose with multiple cumbersome pledgets or cotton-tipped wires, a more traditional than useful exercise.

The cottonoids further act as excellent tampons that prevent the flow of blood and nasal secretions into the pharynx. The strings attached to the cottonoids are a safety factor. They allow for ease of retrieval, prevent any accidental aspiration during the procedure, and act as an infallible reminder to remove the packing before placing the final dressing.

Infiltration anesthesia

For infiltration anesthesia 1% lidocaine with a 1:100,000 or 1:50,000 dilution of epinephrine is preferred. The weaker solution is used in older patients or in those with any question of cardiovascular or peripheral vascular disease. Both con-

centrations of epinephrine produce profound vasoconstriction if incisions are delayed for 10 to 15 minutes after the final injection. The concentration of 1% lidocaine is sufficient to produce excellent anesthesia and has an effective duration of 1.5 to 2 hours.

Except in unusual cases, a total of 3.5 to 5 ml of the solution, sparingly injected into the proper surgical planes, is sufficient to produce profound vasoconstriction and complete nasal anesthesia with no significant tissue distortion. No effort is made to block specific nerves. If septal reconstruction is required, an additional 2 to 3 ml of the anesthetic is injected into the septal mucoperichondrial and mucoperiosteal planes to aid in the hydraulic dissection of the septal flap.

The infiltration of the local anesthetic is initiated by retracting the ala cephalically with the thumb and forefinger, exposing the caudal edge of the upper lateral cartilage (specula or retractors are unnecessary and redundant at this point). A long 27-range needle is placed parallel to the long axis of the exposed upper lateral cartilage, and with a quick stabbing motion the needle penetrates the epithelium, usually with minimal sensation to the patient (Fig. 51-17, A). Any sensation of the needle stick may be masqueraded by simultaneous blunt pinching of the skin elsewhere on the nose or face, a concept referred to as *lateral inhibition.*

The needle is advanced along the lateral wall of the dorsum, hugging the perichondrium of the upper lateral cartilages and the periosteum of the nasal bones, thus remaining in the proper plane. Identification of this plane is enhanced by lifting the soft tissues overlying the nasal dorsum with thumb and forefinger.

A minimal quantity, usually less than 0.5 ml, is deposited into this plane as the needle is withdrawn to but not beyond the point of initial penetration (Fig. 51-17, B). If the nose becomes distorted during this maneuver, the needle is not in the proper plane, and the infiltration stops until the plane

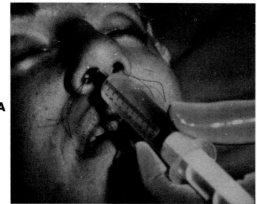

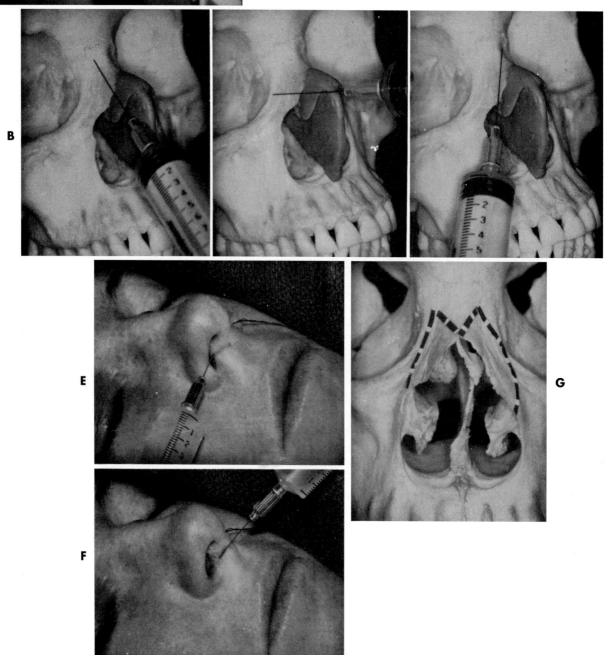

Fig. 51-17. A, Initial advancement of needle in proper plane over bony and cartilaginous vaults, with infiltration in plane between nasal skeleton and subcutaneous tissues. **B,** Infiltration of lateral wall of nose, intimate to nasal skeleton. **C,** and **D,** Rotation of needle within soft tissues to affect further anesthesia of lateral and dorsal nasal tissues. **E** and **F,** Infiltration of nasal base and floor with one-needle penetration. **G,** Intended pathway of low lateral osteotomies. Infiltration of local anesthetic should surround this pathway medial and lateral to ascending process.

is located. With alternate slight rotation of the needle laterally and medially over the dorsum (Fig. 51-17 *C, D*), the procedure is repeated until the anesthetic is deposited in the proper plane over the area to be dissected. The procedure is repeated on the opposite side. With this method only two injection penetrations are sufficient to anesthetize the nasal dorsum.

Anesthesia of the base of the nose and columella is accomplished next. The needle penetrates the skin at the junction of the floor of the right nostril and columella and is advanced to a point just beyond the left alar facial junction (Fig. 51-17, *E*). Infiltration occurs as the needle is withdrawn to the columella. Without removal the needle is rotated and advanced into the columella. Again, a small amount of anesthetic is deposited as the needle is withdrawn. Sparing the patient an additional needle prick, the needle is rotated into the right nasal base, which is anesthetized in a similar fashion (Fig. 51-17, *F*).

The technique of nasal tip anesthetic infiltration depends on the type of planned nasal tip incision. If a transcartilaginous incision is intended, the vestibular skin on the undersurface of the lower lateral cartilage is exposed and everted by pressure above the nostril. The solution is deposited along the course of the proposed incision in the natural plane beneath the perichondrium. Surgical elevation and preservation of an intact vestibular skin flap is thereby facilitated. If delivery of the alar cartilage is contemplated, the anesthetic is infiltrated in the soft tissue along the extent of the planned incision at the caudal margin of the cartilage.

The anesthetic then may be deposited along the course of the lateral osteotomies (see Fig. 51-17 *A, B*), or if desired this may be deferred until later in the operation. This delay adds a safety measure to the procedure by allowing the patient to metabolize the initial lidocaine and epinephrine before adding any further solution. The margin of the piriform aperture just above the leading anterior edge of the inferior turbinate is brought into sharp relief by surrounding it with the blades of a small nasal speculum. The needle is inserted at this site and a small amount of medication is injected. The needle is advanced lateral to and then medial to the ascending process of the maxilla along the intended path of the lateral osteotomies (Fig. 51-17, *G*), and as the needle is withdrawn, solution is deposited. Thus the path of the lateral osteotomies is surrounded by local vasoconstrictive anesthesia, a valuable adjunct to bloodless osteotomies and patient comfort. Postoperative ecchymosis is reduced to a minimum or eliminated by the latter maneuver combined with a gentle operative procedure.

When septal reconstruction is planned, anesthesia of the already anesthetized (with cocaine) septum is accomplished. Unlike the preceding steps, infiltration of a generous amount of solution into the proper septal plane is preferred. This quantity results in hydraulic dissection of the mucoperichondrium and mucoperiosteum from the cartilaginous and bony septum (see Fig. 51-15). It allows for an avascular flap eleva-

tion and may help to dissect synechiae from areas of old fractures.

With nasal shrinkage intense at this point, the cottonoids are removed temporarily. The needle is inserted with the bevel down into the mucous membrane on the side of intended mucoperichondrial flap elevation. The needle is advanced to the plane between the quadrangular cartilage and periochondrium, and with anesthetic infiltration hydraulic elevation is created. This is repeated at several other sites along the mucous membrane. The needle is then inserted beneath the mucoperiosteum overlying the bony septum on both sides, and the anesthetic is infiltrated there. Small amounts of solution also are deposited on both sides of the base of the septum at the maxillary crest–quadrangular cartilage junction. After completion of the septal anesthesia, the cottonoids are reinserted. If surgery is deliberately delayed 10 to 15 minutes, vasoconstriction will reach its maximal effectiveness and bleeding will be minimized.

This combination of monitored intravenous anesthesia and local topical-infiltration anesthesia has been repeated successfully several thousand times over the past 25 years with no serious sequelae. It ensures patient comfort, provides for constant patient monitoring, limits the number of needle penetrations, minimizes the amount of anesthetic, and prevents tissue distortion. In the vast majority of operations little if any bleeding occurs during the procedure, and postoperative ecchymosis is minimal or nonexistent. All of these factors help to permit the precise and bloodless dissection of the nasal structures, which is essential for a carefully controlled rhinoplasty operation.

Surgical landmarks

Although not strictly necessary, it can be helpful to the neophyte as well as the experienced surgeon to indicate on the external skin surface the anatomic surgical landmarks with a marking pen. These external manifestations of the nose skeleton and framework may ordinarily be judged within tolerances of 1 to 2 mm, allowing the development of critical, measured judgments about planned excisions, augmentations, and reorientation of nasal structures (Fig. 51-18). It may be helpful (particularly in a teaching environment) to mark the margins of the alar cartilages and their precise tip-defining points, as well as the preplanned amount of cephalic reduction required for refinement and definition. The caudal margins of the nasal bones and maxillary ascending processes are indicated, and the estimated extent of the bony-cartilaginous hump removal and the planned osteotomy pathways may be indicated by dotted lines. A plus (+) mark on contour depressions serves to remind the surgeon of the need for intended augmentation because small depressions may later be obscured by anesthetic infiltration and surgical edema. Skin markings are general guidelines to the intended surgical maneuvers, but may be useful in guiding the thought processes by which precise surgery is executed.

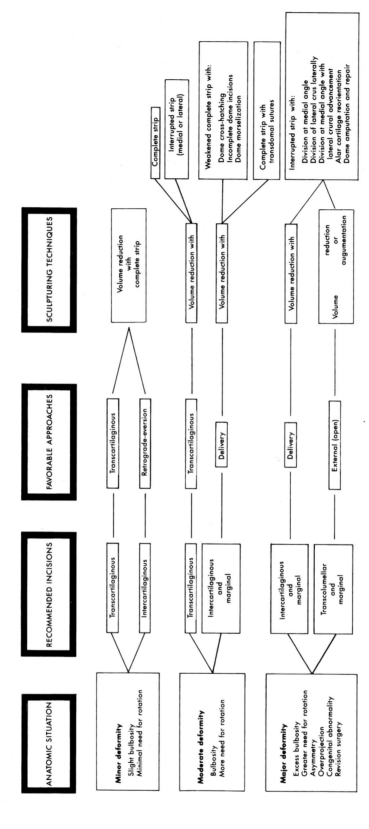

Fig. 51-21. Operative algorithm useful in selecting the incisions, approaches, and techniques employed in nasal tip surgery. In every case, the patient's anatomy dictates the selection. As the anatomic deformity worsens or becomes more abnormal, a graduated approach is taken in a stepwise fashion to correct the deformity.

ployed in nasal tip surgery are listed in Figure 51-21 and Table 51-1. Because of the amazing complexity of anatomic configurations encountered in nasal tip surgery, further modifications are frequently employed to ensure further stable refinements.

Table 51-1. Classification of surgical terms

Incisions	Transcartilaginous
	Intercartilaginous
	Marginal
Approaches	Delivery
	Nondelivery
	Cartilage-splitting
	Retrograde
	External (open)
Techniques	Volume reduction with:
	Complete strip
	Weakened complete strip
	Interrupted strip

In assessing the need for tip remodeling, the surgeon must determine whether or not the tip requires (1) a reduction in the volume of the alar cartilages, (2) a change in the attitude and orientation of the alar cartilages, (3) a change in the projection of the tip, and (4) a cephalic rotation with a consequent increase in the columellar inclination (nasolabial angle). Once these factors are accurately assessed, the most favorable incisions, the approach, and the tip-sculpture technique may be chosen (Fig. 51-22).

Ideally, conservative reduction of the volume of the cephalic margin of the lateral crus, preserving the majority of the crus while maintaining a complete (uninterrupted) strip of alar cartilage, is preferred (Fig. 51-23). This procedure is satisfactory and appropriately safe when minimal conservational tip refinement and rotation are required. As the tip deformity increases in size and complexity, more aggressive techniques are required. A philosophy of a graduated incremental anatomic approach to tip surgery is recommended. This implies that no routine tip procedure is ever used; instead *the appropriate incision(s), approach, and tip-*

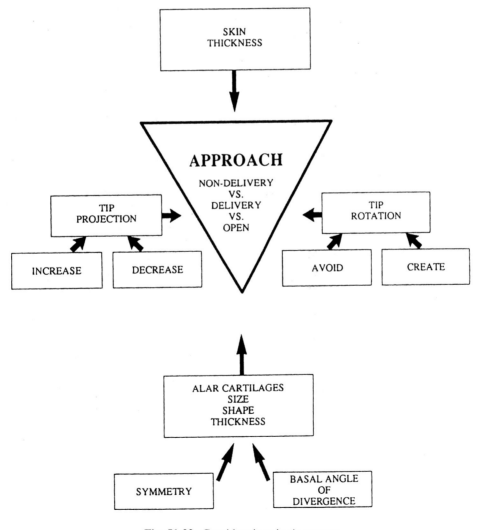

Fig. 51-22. Considerations in tip surgery.

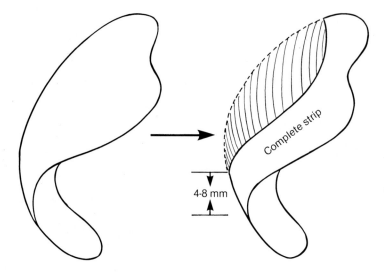

4-8 mm

Complete strip

Fig. 51-23. Maintenance of complete strip of alar cartilage after volume reduction is desirable. At least 4 to 8 mm of uninterrupted lateral crus in vertical dimension should be preserved to ensure long-term support and natural contouring.

sculpting technique is selected based entirely on an analysis of the varying anatomy encountered. Whenever possible a complete strip operation is employed, reserving more risky interrupted strip techniques for anatomic situations in which more profound refinement changes and significant rotation are desirable.

Nondelivery approaches

When the anatomic situation requires conservative or minimal tip refinement and rotation, a *nondelivery* (cartilage-splitting or retrograde-eversion) approach is preferred (Fig. 51-24). The majority of the lateral crus is left intact as a complete strip, with resection of only a few millimeters of the medial-cephalic portion of the lateral crus to effect refinement. This operation is useful in many patients because it tends to "mimic nature," disturbs very little of the normal anatomy of the tip, and therefore consistently heals predictably, with symmetry and minimal scarring (Figs. 51-25 and 51-26).

Delivery approaches

As the tip anatomy becomes more abnormal or asymmetric, more complex surgical techniques are gradually employed. In these patients, a delivery approach is recommended, allowing visual presentation of the alar cartilages as bipedicle chondrocutaneous flaps for further analysis and reconstruction (Fig. 51-27). Under direct vision, surgical modifications of varying designs can then be executed symmetrically. Greater volume reduction of the medial portion of the lateral crus is usually necessary, still maintaining a complete strip at least 5 mm wide (Figs. 51-28 and 51-29). If judged necessary, further refinement in the tip may be created by weakening the complete strip convexity with con-

servative crosshatching, gentle morselization, or incomplete noncoalescent dome incisions (Fig. 51-30). In patients with extremely thin skin, delicate alar sidewalls, and bulbous cartilage, predictable narrowing refinement may be achieved by transdomal suturing of the complete strips with a horizontal mattress suture of 4-0 clear nylon (Figs. 51-31 and 51-32). Narrowing refinement is accomplished, vital tip supports are preserved, and symmetric healing is facilitated (Fig. 51-33). Delivery approaches are indicated almost exclusively when significant defatting or scar resection is required.

In more severe tip deformities, and particularly when more significant cephalic tip rotation is indicated to improve the tip relationship to the face and nose, the surgeon must consider interrupted strip techniques for maximal results (Figs. 51-34 and 51-35). Here the residual complete strip, after volume reduction of varying degrees, is divided somewhere along its course (usually at or near the angle), excessive portions of the lateral and occasionally the medial crus are removed, and the cartilages are reconstructed so that their cut ends abut or overlap. Inherent dangers (asymmetric healing and scarring) exist whenever the complete strip is interrupted, and some tip support is almost always sacrificed, which may be compensated for by placement of a shoring cartilage strut in the columellar compartment. Interrupted strip techniques tend to foster cephalic tip rotation but are a decided liability if rotation of the tip is contraindicated. Tip rotation may be further accentuated by shortening of the caudal septum and placement of cartilage plumping grafts to efface the nasolabial angle further.

Open approach

In patients with cleft lip and nose deformities, severely asymmetric tips, and some markedly overprojecting tips with eccentric anatomy, an open (external) approach to the tip

Text continued on p. 979

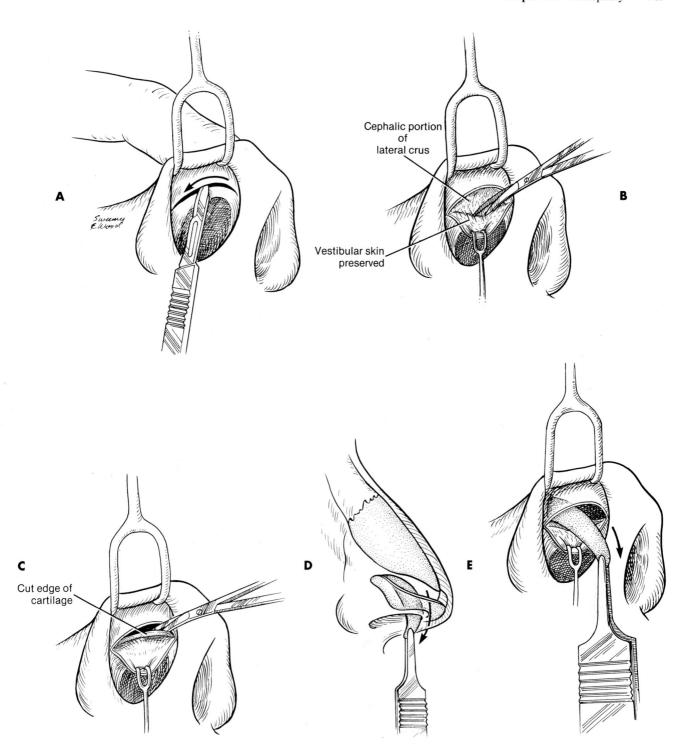

Fig. 51-24. Cartilage-splitting (transcartilaginous) nondelivery approach with preservation of generous, complete strip used on patients demonstrating satisfactory preoperative projection and minimal interdomal distance who require only minimal tip-cartilage modeling. **A,** Single incision through vestibular skin only, made several millimeters cephalic to caudal margin of lower lateral cartilage. **B,** With scissors, vestibular skin is dissected free from portion of lower lateral cartilage to be removed. **C,** Mobilization of cartilage to be excised for volume reduction of lateral crus; portion of dome and medial crus are included when indicated. **D,** Medial detachment of lateral cartilage from dome area. **E,** Volume reduction of lower lateral cartilage completed with lateral detachment; complete strip of intact residual alar cartilage remains.

Continued

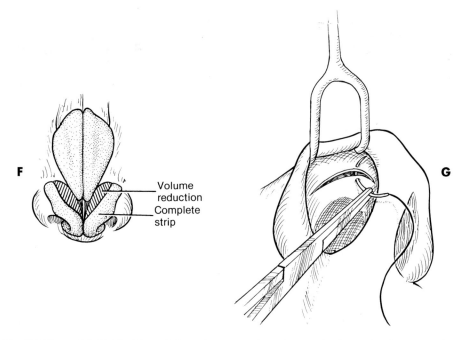

Fig. 51-24, cont'd. F, Final intended result: symmetric volume reduction and refinement of alar cartilages. Generous intact complete strip remains. **G,** Transcartilaginous incision repair with 5-0 chromic catgut.

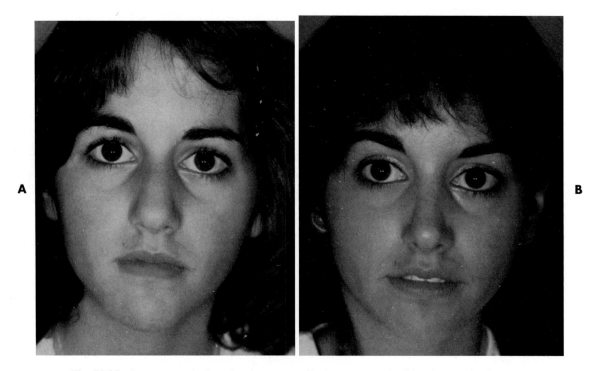

Fig. 51-25. One-year surgical result using transcartilaginous approach with volume reduction, complete strip technique. **A** and **B,** Pre- and postoperative views.

Continued

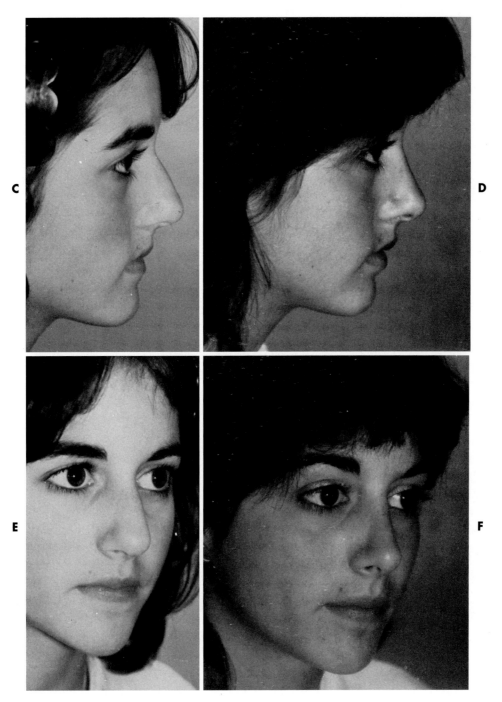

Fig. 51-25, cont'd. C to **F,** Pre- and Postoperative views.

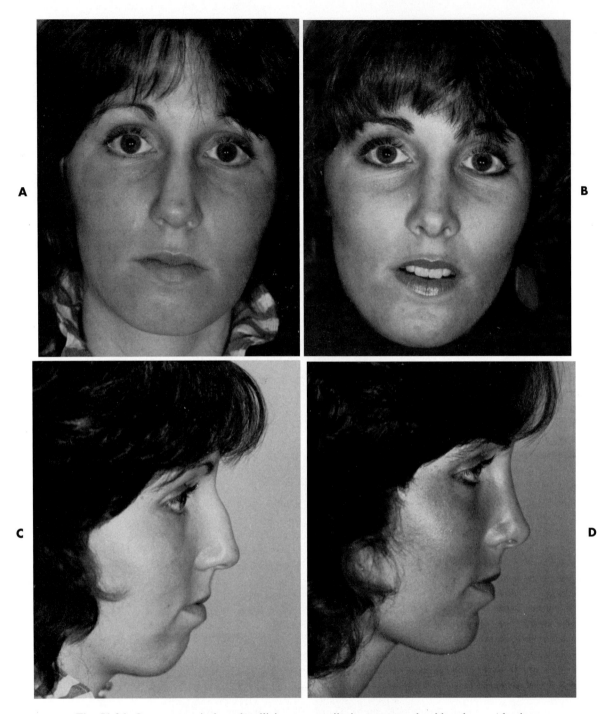

Fig. 51-26. One-year surgical result utilizing transcartilaginous approach with volume reduction, complete strip technique. Addition of chin augmentation enhances rhinoplasty result. **A** to **D,** Pre- and postoperative views.

Continued

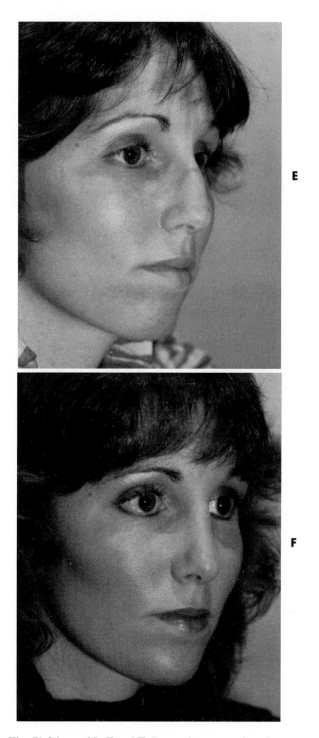

E

F

Fig. 51-26, cont'd. E and **F,** Pre- and postoperative views.

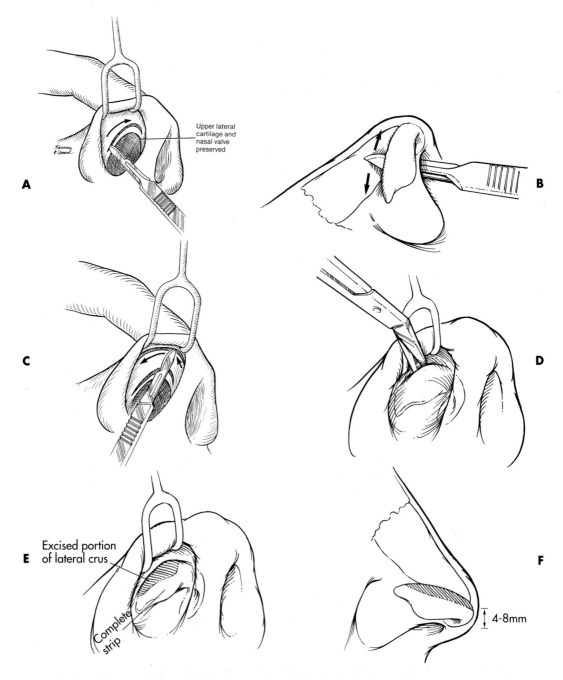

Fig. 51-27. Delivery approach to surgery of alar cartilages utilizing intercartilaginous and marginal incisions. Alar cartilages are delivered as individual bipedicle chondrocutaneous flaps for inspection and sculpturing. **A,** Intercartilaginous incision created along and above projecting rim of upper lateral cartilage. **B,** Knife elevates skin and soft tissue from cartilaginous pyramid and septal angle, dissecting in the immediate supraperichondrial plane. **C,** Curved incision created in vestibular skin precisely at caudal margin of lower lateral cartilage. **D,** Lateral crus and dome dissected free in preparation of delivery through nostril for sculpturing refinement. **E,** Cartilage remodeling, conservative excision of portion of cephalic margin lateral crus. **F,** Maximal extent of cartilage excision necessary to preserve strong, intact, complete strip (4 to 8 mm).

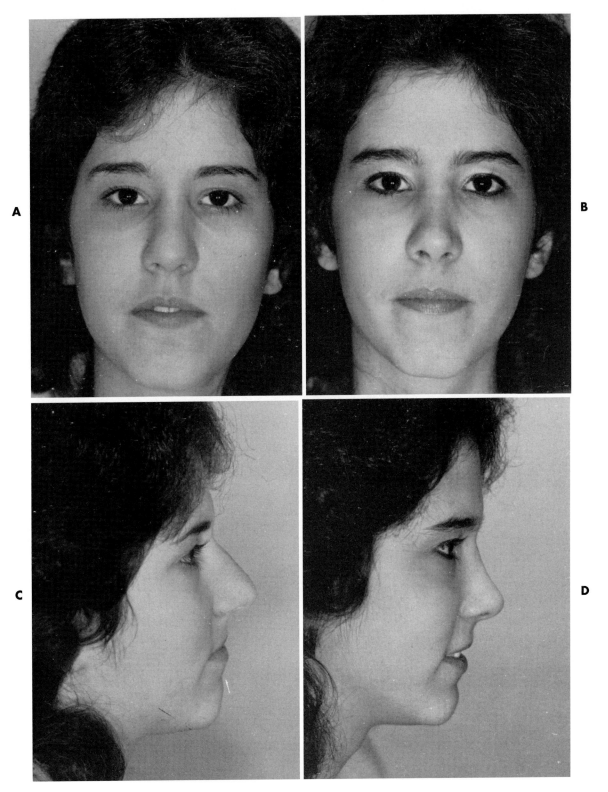

Fig. 51-28. Surgical result obtained in patient judged ideal for delivery approach with volume reduction, complete strip technique. **A** to **D,** Pre- and postoperative views.

Continued

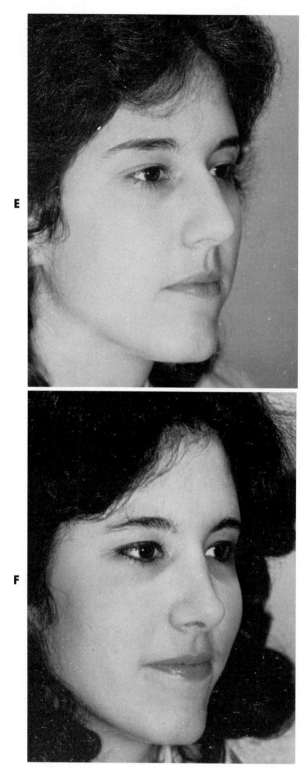

Fig. 51-28, cont'd.   E and F, Pre- and postoperative views.

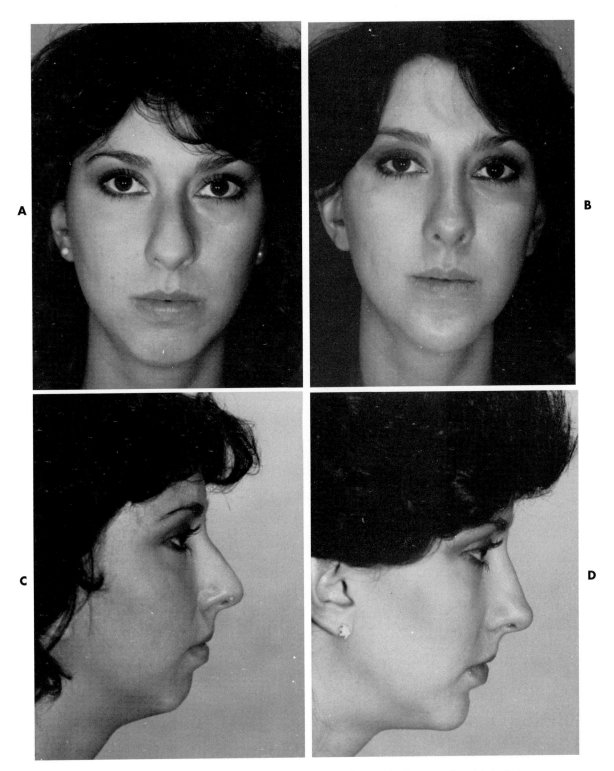

Fig. 51-29. Surgical result using delivery approach with volume reduction, complete strip technique. Generous defatting of tip carried out. Note value of chin augmentation to overall facial balance. **A** to **D,** Pre- and postoperative views.

Continued

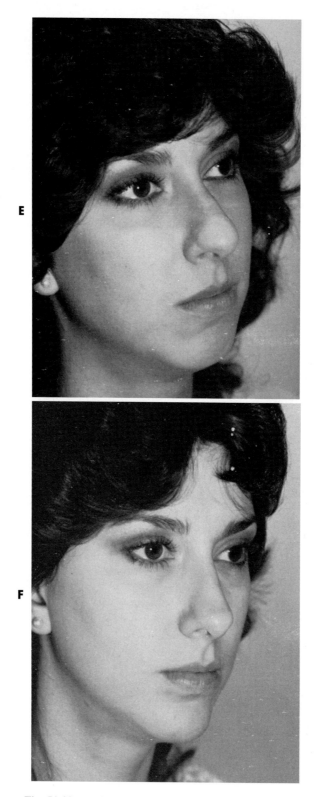

Fig. 51-29, cont'd. E and **F,** Pre- and postoperative views.

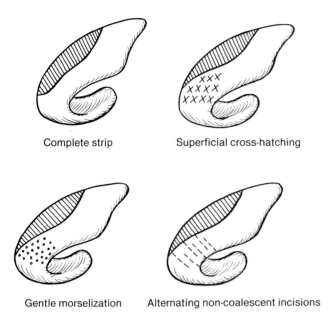

Complete strip   Superficial cross-hatching

Gentle morselization   Alternating non-coalescent incisions

Fig. 51-30. To enhance tip refinement further while maintaining tip support, the complete strip may be weakened at the dome in a variety of ways.

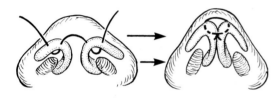

Fig. 51-31. Narrowing refinement of nasal tip in patients with delicate cartilages and thin skin may be effectively accomplished with one or more 4-0 clear nylon transdomal sutures. Suture passes through both medial and lateral crus on either side and is "test-tightened" before final securing to ensure proper suture placement and symmetric narrowing. A modest increase in projection and significant refinement of the trapezoidal tip may be realized, if desired, with transdermal suture narrowing.

Interdomal soft tissue
to be excised

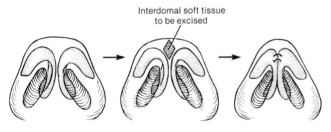

Fig. 51-32. Interdomal suturing of medial crura for modest narrowing.

may be helpful (Fig. 51-36) (Box 51-1), particularly when the variant anatomy is not clear preoperatively. Although more operative edema and scarring result from this approach, the advantages of precise direct-vision diagnosis, bimanual surgery, and extraordinary exposure render this approach useful in selected patients (Fig. 51-37).

In the open approach, the soft tissues of the nose are elevated off the underlying cartilaginous and bony skeleton to reveal the exact anatomy responsible for the nasal shape. Reduction and augmentation procedures, particularly when adding cartilage grafts to the tip and dorsum, may be effected precisely with suture control. Because both sides of the nose are viewed simultaneously, surgical symmetry may be easily achieved.

Tip projection

A final critical decision in undertaking nasal tip surgery involves the need for preservation, enhancement, or reduction of existing tip projection. Because the majority of patients undergoing a rhinoplasty demonstrate satisfactory projection, it becomes the surgeon's responsibility to ensure that the major and minor tip supports are left largely intact (or reconstructed) to prevent an eventual loss of projection. Complete strip techniques are therefore recommended whenever feasible, avoiding the complete transfixion incision, which destroys the vital support provided by the medial crural overlap of the caudal septum (Fig. 51-38). If additional projection is required, it may be achieved in a variety of ways. Autogenous cartilage struts positioned below or between the medial crura (Figs. 51-39 and 51-40) are effective in establishing permanent support and projection. Plumping grafts of cartilage fragments, introduced into the base of the columella through a low lateral columellar incision (Fig. 51-41), provide an additional platform for the tip projection resulting from the strut. Cartilage struts should be shaped with a gentle curve to match the anatomy of the curved columella, at times aiding in the creation of a distinct "double break," but should never extend to the apex of the tip skin lest a visible tent-pole appearance develop. If the medial crural footplates diverge in a widely splayed fashion, further tip projection may be gained by resecting excessive intercrural soft tissue and suturing the medial crura together. Height and contour may be added to the tip by the use of autogenous cartilage grafts from the nasal septum or auricular cartilage (Fig. 51-42). Because these grafts lie immediately subcutaneously, intimately subjacent to the skin, great care must be

Text continued on p. 986

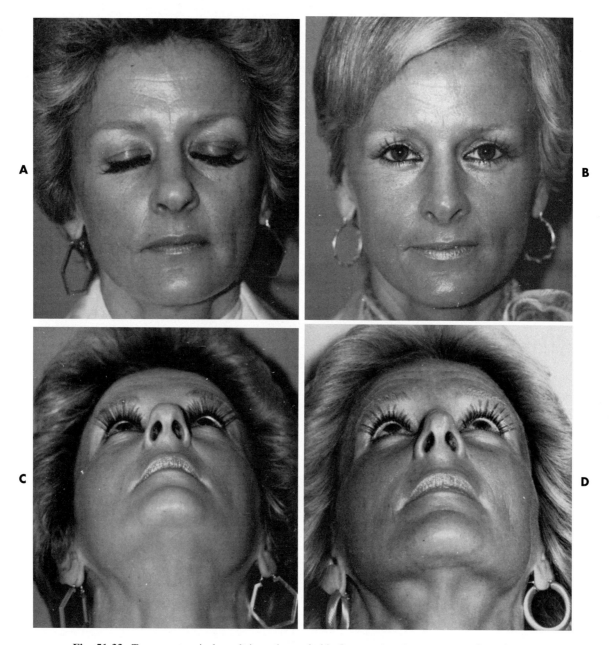

Fig. 51-33. Two-year surgical result in patient suitable for transdomal suture narrowing of nasal tip. Minimal volume reduction carried out, maintaining generous complete strip. Note permanent change from trapezoidal tip to more desirable triangular configuration. **A** and **C,** Preoperative views. **B** and **D,** Postoperative views.

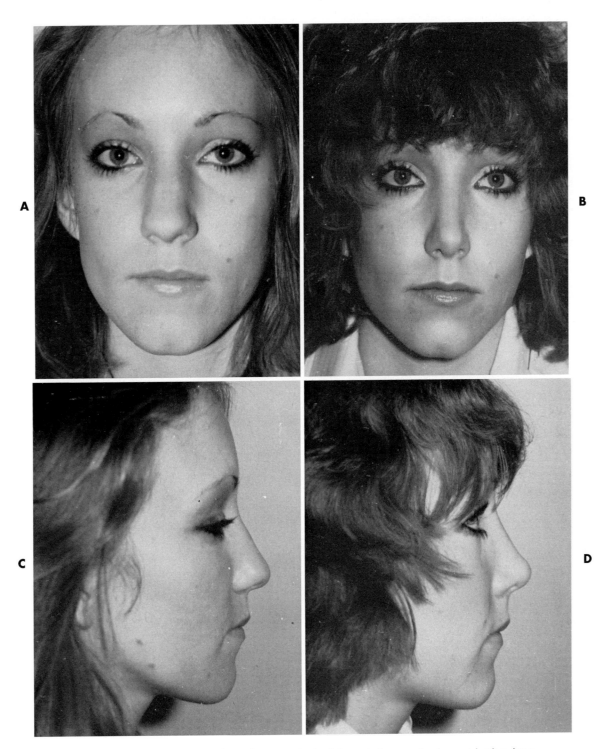

Fig. 51-34. Significant narrowing refinement obtained through the use of volume reduction, interrupted-strip technique with suture reconstitution of interrupted strip. Thick skin and subcutaneous tissue allows vertical interruption of complete strip at angle between medial and lateral crus. **A** and **C,** Preoperative views. **B** and **D,** Postoperative views.

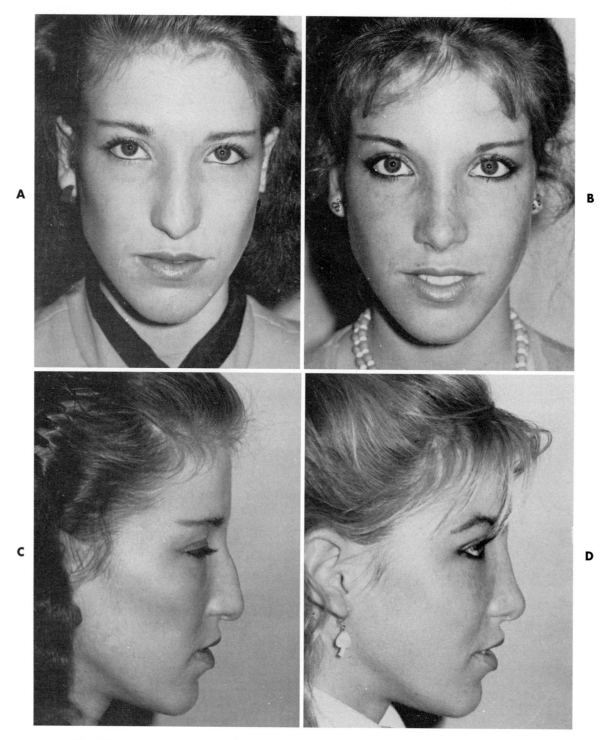

Fig. 51-35. Interrupted-strip technique chosen for patient with bulky cartilages, thick skin, and need for modest tip rotation. **A** and **C,** Preoperative views. **B** and **D,** Postoperative views.

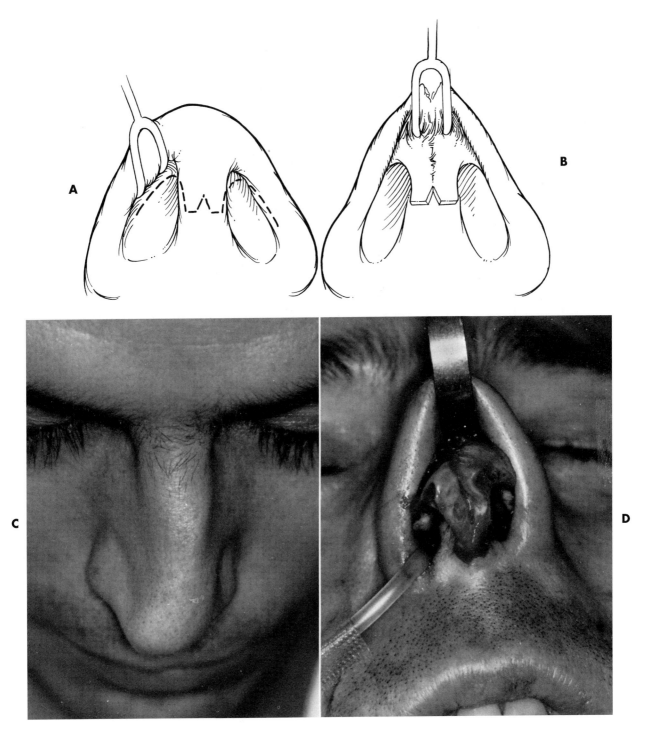

Fig. 51-36. A, Incision utilized for open (external) approach to nasal tip. **B,** Exposure of nasal tip anatomy through open approach. **C,** Dorsal view of nose characterized by asymmetric nasal tip, demonstrating *convex* left lateral crus and *concave* right lateral crus. **D,** View, through open approach, of asymmetric, twisted, and unequal lateral cartilages.

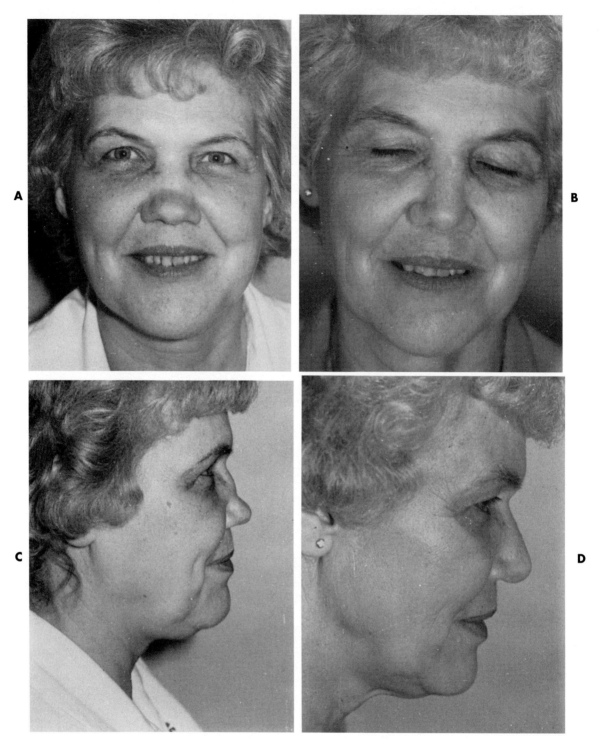

Fig. 51-37. Refinement of nasal tip combined with cartilage graft augmentation of collapsed nose through open approach; result after 3 years. **A** to **D,** Pre- and postoperative views.

Continued

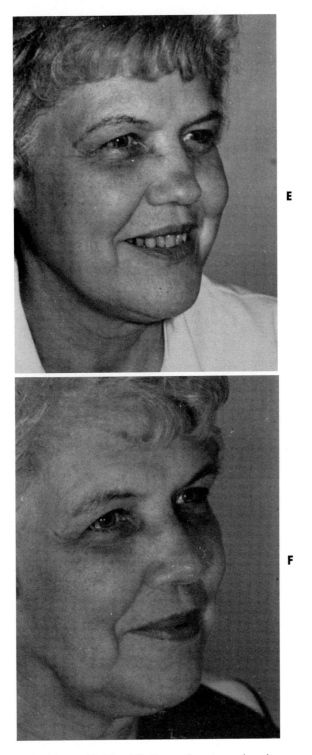

Fig. 51-37, cont'd. E and **F,** Pre- and postoperative views.

taken in their positioning. An exacting ''pocket preparation'' becomes a basic prerequisite for their use; that is, a pocket is fashioned into which the graft fits as precisely as a hand in a glove. Carved in a triangular, trapezoidal, or shield-like shape, tip grafts may accentuate favorable tip-defining points and highlights and can succeed in giving a more normal appearance to tips with congenital or postsurgical inadequacies (Fig. 51-43). For modest tip projection and symmetry improvement, cartilage tip grafts may be effectively placed, through limited marginal incisions, and precisely fashioned

in the infratip lobule. When more major tip projection and contouring is in order, tip grafts are best suture-fixated to the intermediate crura.

Cephalic rotation of the tip may increase projection by advancing the lateral crura medially and suturing them to lie above the cut ends of the medial crura. Transdomal sutures properly positioned between two complete alar cartilage strips may result in additional projection of the tip.

It should be appreciated then that nasal tip surgery is a compromise in which the surgeon gives away something to

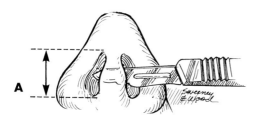

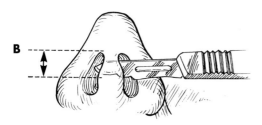

Fig. 51-38. Partial transfixion incisions are always preferable to complete-transfixion incisions, although not always feasible. Preserving medial crural footplate attachment to caudal septum maintains one vital tip-support mechanism. **A,** Complete-transfixion incision, which sacrifices medial crural footplate attachment to septum. **B,** Partial-transfixion incision, which preserves medial crural footplate attachment to septum.

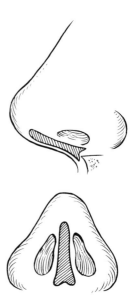

Fig. 51-39. Position of cartilaginous strut between medial crura, creating supportive influence on nasal tip support and projection.

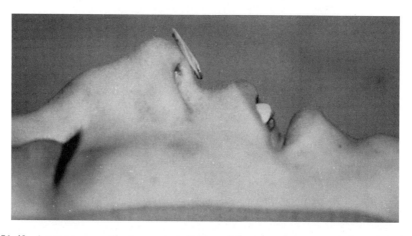

Fig. 51-40. Autogenous cartilaginous strut, fashioned from nasal septum, about to be placed in precise columellar pocket.

achieve a narrower, more defined, and stable tip component of the nose. Years of experience are required to understand and master tip surgery techniques thoroughly. Along with this invaluable insight, emphasis should always be placed on conserving tip anatomic structures and avoiding both radical excision and sacrifice of tip tissue. Compulsive long-term follow-up and evaluation of patients both by frequent examination and by review of standardized, uniform photographs facilitates the development of expertise in nasal tip surgical refinement.

SURGERY OF THE CARTILAGINOUS VAULT

The dorsal surface of the quadrangular cartilage and its related upper lateral cartilages comprise the cartilaginous vault. Ordinarily a new relationship should be established

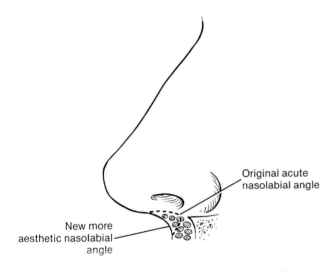

Fig. 51-41. Plumping grafts of autogenous cartilage, effective in lending support to otherwise weak tip and in effacing acute or retracted nasolabial angle.

between the tip and profile line. Reduction of the supratip area to a level that allows the leading edge of the tip to exist 1 to 2 mm above the cartilaginous profile is the usual aesthetic goal. Making this new relationship permanent requires that tip projection, whether preexistent or the consequence of tip surgery, be stable and lasting. Tip surgery then is usually performed at the outset of the operation, unless a significant overgrowth of the dorsal septum has created an anatomic variant in which this normally minor tip-support mechanism is giving greater support thrust to the tip projection "tension nose." In this latter circumstance, reduction alignment of the supratip area to eliminate this spurious support procedes tip surgery thereby allowing more accurate evaluation of the true magnitude of normal tip-support mechanisms.

Aesthetics are best served when reduction in both the cartilaginous and bony vaults results in a relatively strong, high, and straight-line profile in the male (Fig. 51-44), with the leading edge of the tip just slightly higher in the female (Fig. 51-45). In the latter circumstance a gentle slope of about 2 to 3 mm should exist between the tip-defining point and the lower extent of the cartilaginous profile. (In the final analysis, however, the "ideal" profile consists of what makes each patient content and happy.) In planning a profile alignment, the two stable reference points are the nasofrontal angle (located ideally at the level of the upper eyelid) and the tip-defining point. Reversal of the usual tip–supratip relationship (in which the supratip cartilaginous dorsum lies variably higher than the tip) is required to achieve this aesthetic ideal.

It can be appreciated then that the degree and angulation of "hump removal" depend on a variety of factors, some of which are under the control of the surgeon and some of which are not. These factors include skin thickness, the amount of bony hump relative to cartilaginous hump, the

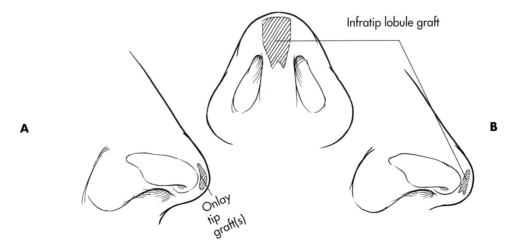

Fig. 51-42. A, Onlay tip cartilage grafts, frequently employed to enhance tip projection and contour nasal tip. **B,** Cartilage grafts, precisely positioned in infratip lobule area, enhance tip projection and aid in contouring tip anatomy. Size, shape, and length of tip may be altered to achieve a variety of favorable aesthetic contours. Grafts may be sutured in place for greater stability when employing either the open or delivery approach.

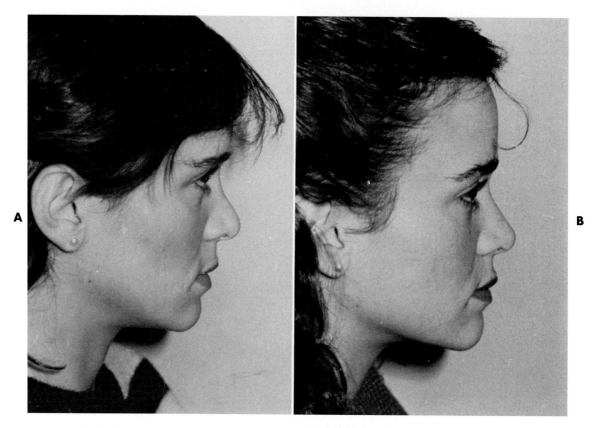

Fig. 51-43. Revision rhinoplasty patient whose appearance is enhanced and normalized with addition of nasal tip grafts as well as onlay cartilage grafts augmenting overreduced nasal dorsum. **A,** Preoperative view. **B,** Postoperative view.

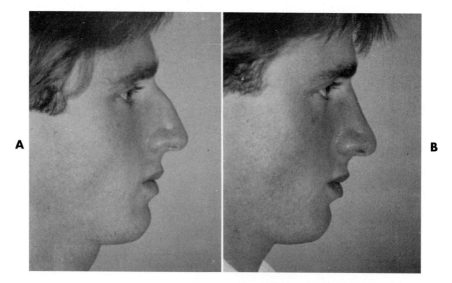

Fig. 51-44. A, Unsatisfactory male nasal profile aligned to normalize nasal proportions and improve overall facial balance and aesthetics. **B,** Straight nasal profile with strong, high dorsum provides highly desirable appearance.

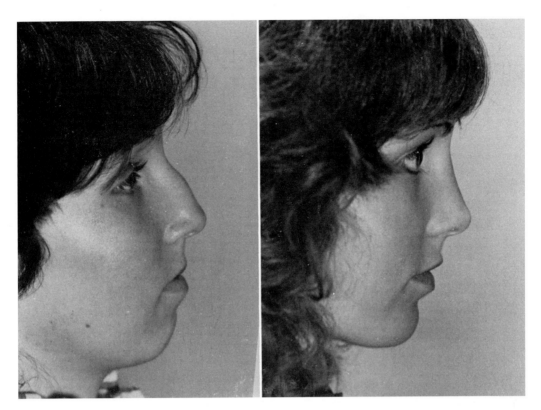

Fig. 51-45. Desirable female profile remains strong with a high dorsum, but generally is enhanced when nasal tip projection leads supratip profile by 2 to 3 mm. In addition, slightly more open nasolabial profile is desirable, accompanied by subtle columellar ''double-break'' configuration.

relative width of the nose, the inclination of the nasal tip, and, equally important, the patient's wishes regarding the desired nasal profile. In the final analysis, it is the surgeon's ability to visualize the final appearance of the nose after approximately 12 to 18 months of healing that allows exact and precise profile alignment.

Because the thickness of the overlying skin differs from that of soft tissues (thinner overlying the rhinion and thicker in the supratip area), it follows that a straight-line removal of both cartilaginous and bony hump may result in over-reduction and an unsatisfactory final profile. To accommodate this tissue thickness differential, an initial controlled incremental reduction of the cartilaginous dorsum under direct vision is preferred.

Access to the nasal skeleton is gained by elevation of the soft tissues over the cartilaginous vault by knife dissection in the precise tissue plane that is intimate to the perichondrium enveloping the upper lateral cartilages and the cartilaginous dorsum (Fig. 51-46). Respecting and using this tissue plane prevents unnecessary trauma to the more superficially located blood vessels and sensory nerves, resulting in significantly less bleeding and a reduction in healing scar. Access to the bony vault is continued by elevation of the periosteum over the nasal bones with the Joseph elevator (see Fig. 51-46, *B*), thereby exposing the entire bony-cartilaginous skeleton of the nose for inspection and direct-vision surgery. Ex-

cellent exposure may be gained during these technical maneuvers simply by carrying the medial extent of the transcartilaginous or intercartilaginous incision 4 to 6 mm around the anterior septal angle—the partial transfixion incision. The vital support relationship of the medial crural attachment to the caudal margin of the septum is thereby preserved by avoiding the more traditional complete transfixion incision.

With the Converse retractor in place, excellent exposure of the nasal dorsum is achieved, visualized best with intense fiberoptic headlighting. The stage is thus set for incremental cartilaginous profile alignment. A knife is positioned at the osseocartilaginous junction and drawn lightly down to the anterior septal angle to allow any remaining soft-tissue fibers to fall laterally, exposing the blue–white underlying cartilage clearly. Under direct vision, with the knife blade at precise right angles to the cartilaginous dorsum (quadrangular cartilage and upper lateral cartilages combined) are shaved away smoothly (Fig. 51-47)). How thick a strip (1 to 3 mm) depends on the amount of supratip reduction required to establish the new satisfactory tip–supratip relationship. After each increment is removed, the profile is inspected and palpated to ensure smoothness and a properly developing relationship to the tip. It may be helpful to depress the tip toward the lip from time to time to determine the precise degree of cartilaginous reduction. Failure to re-

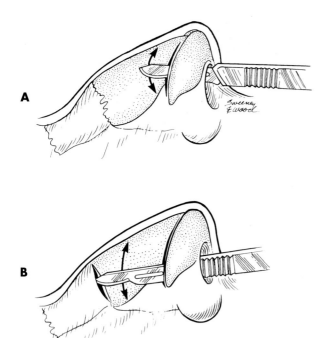

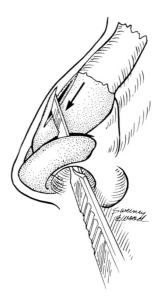

Fig. 51-46. A, Sharp knife elevation of soft tissues over cartilaginous dorsum-should be accomplished in the favorable tissue plane intimate to cartilaginous pyramid to reduce scarring and bleeding. **B,** Elevation of periosteum with knife initially followed by Joseph periosteal elevator finalizes décollement of nasal soft tissues. Inclusion of periosteum in skin flap creates additional thickness of covering skin mantle, cushioning and camouflaging any possible irregularities in bony healing.

Fig. 51-47. Increments of cartilaginous dorsum are shaved away with sharp knife under direct vision until satisfactory tip-supratip relationship is established. Except in unusual circumstances, underlying mucoperichondrium bridging upper lateral cartilages to quadrangular cartilage is always preserved.

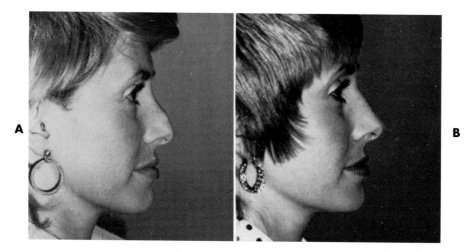

Fig. 51-48. Postoperative stigma of cartilaginous "polly beak" deformity results from inaccurate alignment or inadequate reduction of cartilaginous pyramid. **A,** Preoperative view. **B,** Postoperative view.

duce this supratip in relation to the ultimate tip projection is a common error, leading to a displeasing tip-supratip relationship, or worse, a cartilaginous "polly beak" deformity requiring revision surgery (Fig. 51-48).

In the typical rhinoplasty procedure the upper lateral cartilages are involved in surgical reduction only as a consequence of their intimate attachment as the wings of the quadrangular cartilage. As this reduction progresses, the underlying bridge of mucoperichondrium stabilizing the upper laterals to the septum may be exposed. This vital portion of the nasal lining contributes significantly to the internal nasal valve and is best left undisturbed and undivided. By gently teasing the mucoperichondrium away from the cartilages, further cartilaginous reduction may be accom-

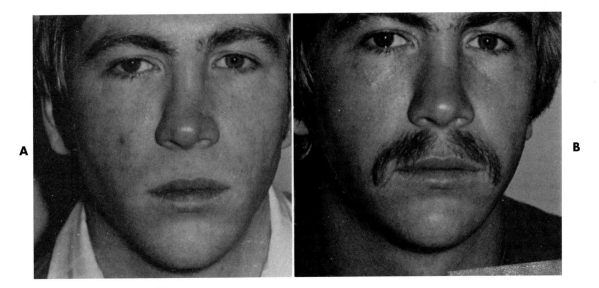

Fig. 51-49. A, Traumatic or iatrogenic avulsion of upper lateral cartilage from undersurface of nasal bones constitutes serious aesthetic and often functional deficiencies. Once airway integrity is ensured, appearance improvement is best accomplished with, **B,** thin cartilage autografts.

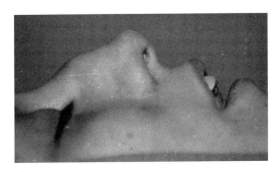

Fig. 51-50. Precision reduction of bony profile is most accurately accomplished if cartilaginous dorsum is aligned at outset of profile-alignment procedures.

plished, if necessary, without jeopardizing the mucoperichondrium to be preserved. Occasionally the caudal margin of the upper lateral cartilage, in its anatomic relationship to the cephalic margin of the alar cartilage, demonstrates a scroll-like appearance. If this redundance of cartilage contributes to excessive thickness in the middle third of the nose on frontal and oblique views, it may be resected. Except in the abnormally long, drooping nose, the length of the upper lateral cartilages plays a small role in overall nasal length and ordinarily requires no significant shortening. Of vital importance, however, is the underlapping attachment of the upper lateral cartilages to the undersurface of the nasal bones. If this critical supportive relationship is avulsed by surgical or nonsurgical trauma, repair is extremely difficult, a typical depressed-contour deformity results, and the ipsilateral airway may be compromised. Repair is often best effected by an onlay cartilage autograft (Fig. 51-49).

Alignment of the cartilaginous profile initially generates several significant advantages. The tip–supratip relationship

is established with precision (Fig. 51-50), undesirable over- or underreduction is easily prevented, and the exact amount of bony hump to be removed or reduced is clearly apparent.

SURGERY OF THE BONY VAULT

Bony profile reduction

With the tip–supratip relationship satisfactorily established, the exact degree of bony hump excess is readily apparent (see Fig. 51-50). If minimal bone requires removal to establish the predetermined desired profile, the sharp tungsten-carbide down-cutting rasp facilitates a rapid and minimally traumatic reduction. Even less trauma is created from initial hump removal by the small Rubin osteotome, sharpened to razor edge; a sharpening stone is kept on the operating table setup, allowing the critical edge on each osteotome to be honed just before its use.

As previously described, only enough periosteum to allow removal of the bony hump is elevated over the bony dorsum. Preserving the periosteum and soft-tissue attachment overlying the nasal bones and maxillary ascending processes laterally reduces trauma and bleeding and, more important, stabilizes the mobile bony sidewalls after all infractions are complete—an internal splint.

The Rubin osteotome is seated at the caudal end of the bony hump and aligned and positioned to effect removal of only that amount of bone desired to leave a high, strong profile line (Fig. 51-51). Conservatism is most important here because any further bony refinement may be further accomplished with the rasp. Progressive taps with the sound-deadened mallet force the sharp osteotome precisely through the thick nasal bones as guided by the surgeon. The vertical fin located on the handle of the Rubin osteotome serves admirably to allow exact surgical control in aligning the instrument.

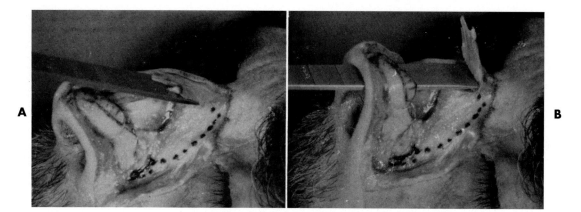

Fig. 51-51. A, Rubin osteotome seated at osseocartilaginous junction (caudal end of bony hump) in preparation for bony profile alignment. **B,** Bony hump removed symmetrically. Precision in alignment is significantly aided by vertical fin on handle of Rubin osteotome, which prevents misalignment or unwanted rotation during cephalic progression of instrument.

The detached bony fragment is then removed and inspected for asymmetries, which can provide the surgeon with clues about the need for further selective bony reduction. If irregularities of bone persist, several methods may be useful for achieving absolute smoothness. If one cut edge of nasal bone requires further reduction, it may be lowered by shaving with the sharp, thin osteotome, trimmed under direct vision with the strong double-action Becker scissors, or smoothed with the down-cutting rasp.

Before final finishing and smoothing of the bony dorsum is carried out with the rasp, it is useful to inspect the relative height of the upper lateral cartilages, trimming them under direct vision to lie at the same level or just below the level of the cartilaginous dorsum. This step is considered to be important at this stage of the procedure because upper laterals that remain too high above the cartilaginous dorsum may be caught in the teeth of the rasp, risking avulsion or displacement, a difficult complication to repair.

The nasal profile must then be critically assessed by the surgeon. The final profile must not only be aesthetically pleasing but absolutely smooth and free of irregularities. Otherwise, displeasing contour irregularities may develop months and even several years later, particularly in the relatively thin-skinned patient. Several techniques are helpful in assessing profile smoothness before completing the bony profile alignment with a finishing rasp. Palpation of the dorsum through the skin with a wet finger reveals irregularities not otherwise detectable with routine palpation. Tensing the skin over the dorsum during palpation facilitates evaluation. During internal visualization of the bony-cartilaginous dorsum, palpating the dorsum with the noncutting edge of the No. 15 Bard-Parker knife blade often allows discovery of minute irregularities that are frequently inapparent to the most critical eye. If redundant soft tissue exists beneath the skin either medially or laterally, it may be conservatively excised at this point.

Final finishing of the bony dorsum is effected with the delicate tungsten-carbide rasp, an instrument that retains its extreme sharpness for long periods without significant detectable dulling. The down-cutting rasp is preferred, preventing trauma to the soft tissues in the nasofrontal area. The rasp should be pulled firmly and obliquely down the bony dorsum, cutting bone with each stroke and eliminating excessive, overly traumatic to-and-from motions. All the products of rasping (bone fragments and ''sawdust'') must be removed by suction to prevent later irregularities.

Should overaggressive hump removal occur as the result of a maldirected osteotome, several remedies are available. The excised bony hump may be replaced after reduction in size and removal of all attached mucosa (after Skoog). Splinted in place, this bone graft can be used to reconstruct an over-reduced dorsum satisfactorily. More delicate realignment of the dorsum's irregularities (bony or cartilaginous) can be satisfactorily reconstructed with autogenous cartilage grafts from the septum, alar cartilage remnants, or auricular cartilage autografts. Reconstruction with alloplastic implants is not always recommended because autogenous tissues are always preferable in the nose.

Narrowing the nose: osteotomies

Profile alignment in the typical reduction rhinoplasty inevitably results in an excessive plateau-like width of the nasal dorsum, which requires narrowing of the bony vault for a normal, natural appearance when the patient is viewed from the front. To accomplish this narrowing, the lateral bony sidewalls (consisting of the nasal bones and the maxillary ascending processes) should be mobilized and moved medially. The upper lateral cartilages also are moved medially because of their stable attachment to the undersurface of the nasal bones.

The stage is set for precision narrowing by medial-oblique osteotomies. A 2- to 3-mm delicate, sharp microos-

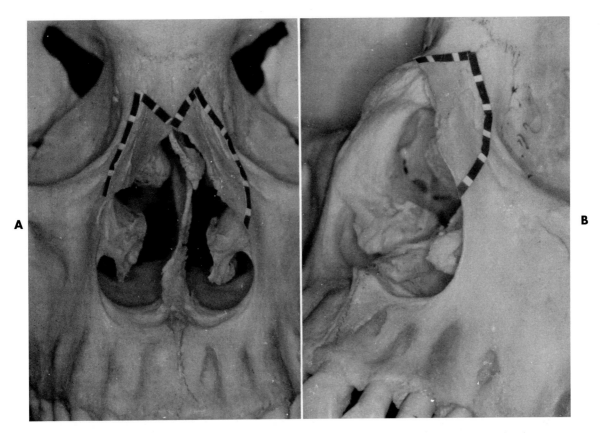

Fig. 51-52. A, Medial-oblique osteotomy is helpful, particularly in patients with heavy or previously fractured nasal bones, in creating significant and atraumatic narrowing and straightening of bony pyramid. Osteotomy pathway is directed 15° to 20° away from midline; at its most cephalic extent it establishes bony weakness, which dictates exact point of bony infraction from lateral osteotomies in majority of operations. **B,** Site and direction of medial-oblique and low lateral osteotomy.

teotome is seated at the superior extent of the bony hump removal on either side of the bony septum and advanced cephalically and obliquely at an angle of 15° to 20° outward (Fig. 51-52). Little trauma results from these medial-oblique osteotomies, which create a predetermined weakness or dehiscence at which the ultimate back-fracture occurs from the lateral osteotomies. This represents a safety factor in the osteotomy procedure, preventing the ever-present possibility of eccentric or asymmetric surgical fractures developing when only lateral osteotomies are performed. In addition, bony narrowing occurs without necessitating strong pressure to be exerted on the nasal bones to accomplish infraction, a traditional but unnecessarily traumatic maneuver.

Lateral osteotomies are reserved for last in a rhinoplasty because they may be more traumatic than the steps previously accomplished. Additional tip refinement, septal reconstruction, or alar base reduction surgery—if indicated—is completed before the lateral osteotomies are initiated.

Trauma may be significantly reduced in lateral osteotomies if 2- or 3-mm microosteotomes are employed to accomplish a controlled fracture of the bony sidewalls. No need

exists for elevation of the periosteum along the pathway of the lateral fractures because the small osteotomes require little space for their cephalic progression. Appropriately, the intact periosteum stabilizes and internally splints the complete fractures, facilitating stable and precise healing. The low-curved lateral osteotomy is initiated by pressing the sharp osteotome through the vestibule skin to encounter the margin of the piriform aperture at or just above the inferior turbinate (Fig. 51-53). This preserves the bony sidewall along the floor of the nose (where narrowing would achieve no favorable aesthetic improvement) but might compromise the lower nasal airway without purpose. The pathway of the osteotomy then progresses toward the face of the maxilla, curving next up along the nasomaxillary junction to encounter the previously created small medial-oblique osteotomy. A complete, controlled, and atraumatic fracture of the bony sidewall is thus created, allowing infraction without excessively traumatic pressure (Fig. 51-54). Immediate finger pressure is applied bilaterally over the lateral osteotomy sites to forestall further any extravasation of blood into the soft tissues. In reality, little or no bleeding occurs during micro-osteotomies because the soft tissues embracing the bony sidewalls remain essentially undamaged.

After infraction the dorsum is again palpated and inspected for any irregularities; if they exist, they are corrected under direct vision. The upper lateral cartilages are viewed to ensure that their relationship to the height of the septum is appropriate.

The fracture line of the lateral osteotomy should be as low as possible to allow a large lateral wall for infraction and to prevent the palpable step deformity that results when osteotomies are positioned too high on the nasal sidewall (nearer the dorsum). The bones should ideally be freely mo-

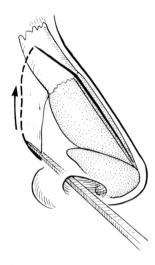

Fig. 51-53. Low lateral osteotomy is initiated at piriform aperture at or just above attachment of inferior concha to ascending process of maxilla. No incision is required for 2 or 3 mm osteotome.

bile but splinted by the undisturbed periosteum and soft tissues that remain attached to the bony fragments.

When the nasal bony sidewalls are twisted, asymmetric, or markedly irregular, further osteotomies may be required higher on the ascending process to achieve correction (Figs. 51-55 and 51-56).

GRAPHIC RECORD-KEEPING AND SELF-EDUCATION

Invaluable feedback and learning about the effectiveness of various techniques is based on studying the surgical records. When the ultimate postoperative appearance is compared side by side with a detailed graphic record of the operation, a great deal of information surfaces. There is no better method for reducing the often ardous ''learning curve'' between inexperience and experience, which is a vital ingredient for successful rhinoplasty surgery.

After each operation, a detailed visual record of the operative event is prepared, and routine as well as unique procedures are recorded in color (Fig. 51-57). This information, if desired, may be ultimately transferred to the more stylized Gunter graphic for teaching purposes (Fig. 51-58).

POSTSURGICAL CONSIDERATIONS

The care of the postrhinoplasty patient is directed toward patient comfort, reduction of swelling and edema, patency of the nasal airway, and compression–stabilization of the nose.

Whether discharged the afternoon of or the morning after surgery, *all* intranasal dressings are removed from the nose before the patient leaves. A detailed list of instructions is supplied for the patient or accompanying family member

Fig. 51-54. Following intersection of low lateral osteotomy with cephalic extent of medial-oblique osteotomy, infraction and narrowing of bony pyramid is ordinarily accomplished easily with gentle medial finger pressure. In young patients, complete fractures with total mobilization of bony pyramid is desirable. Less mobilization and even so-called greenstick fractures may be acceptable in older adult patients. Gentle pressure held over lateral osteotomy site until final splint application is effective in reducing edema and potential ecchymosis.

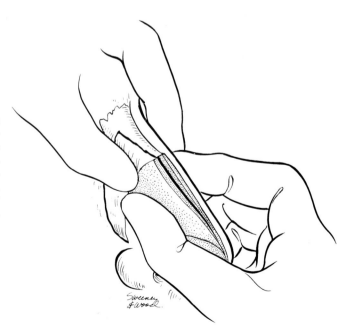

(Box 51-2); the important aspects of these "do's" and "don'ts" are emphasized. Prevention of trauma to the nose is clearly the most important consideration. Oral decongestant therapy is helpful, but the value of corticosteroids and antibiotics in a routine rhinoplasty is conjectural.

The external splint is removed by the surgeon or surgical nurse 5 to 7 days after surgery. An important consideration should be the gentle removal of the tape and splint by bluntly dissecting the nasal skin from the overlying splint with a dull instrument, without disturbing or tenting up the healing skin. Failure to follow this policy may lead to disturbance of the newly forming subcutaneous fibroblastic layer over the nasal dorsum with additional unwanted scarring and even abrupt hematoma. After cleansing of the skin with an adhesive solvent, immediate frontal and lateral photographs are taken to document the early postoperative surgical result (these early photographs may assume vital medicolegal importance if the patient's surgical result is compromised by trauma in the immediate future). Thereafter it is to the surgeon's educational advantage and the patient's best interest

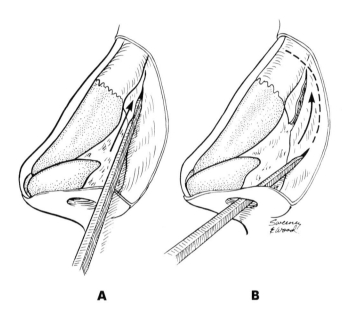

A   **B**

Fig. 51-55. A, Intermediate higher lateral osteotomies may be required in patients with extreme asymmetry of bony sidewalls; only by their use can complete and adequate mobilization be satisfactorily accomplished. **B,** The intermediate osteotomies must always be carried out before lower lateral osteotomies are completed.

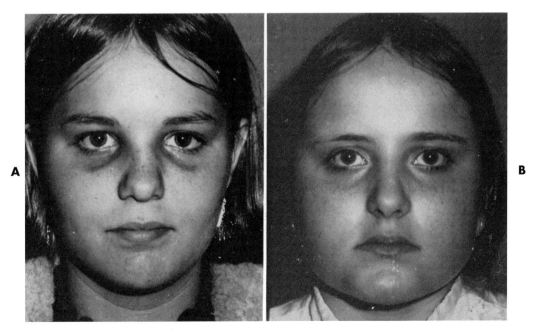

A   **B**

Fig. 51-56. Typical twisted pyramid in which double osteotomies may be helpful. **A,** Preoperative view. **B,** Postoperative view.

RHINOPLASTY DATA SHEET

NAME _____ AGE _____ DATE _____ ANEST $\Leftarrow$ Local / I-V analgesia / General

Procedure: _____

INCISIONS

TC
IC
Marginal
Transfix.
 -partial
 -complete
High septal
_____

TIP

Delivery
Non-delivery
Cart.-split
Retrograde
Complete strip
Rim strip
Lateral crural flap
Dome division
Dome suture
Soft tissue
Weir
Nostril sill
Strut
Plump _____

PROFILE

Periosteal elev.
No hump
Cart.-incremental
Bony   osteotome
         rasp
ULC's
 -lowered
 -shortened
 -divided
Procerus
Soft tissue

OSTEOTOMIES

Medial
Lateral
 -curved
 -straight
 -high
 -low
 -double R-L
 -asymmetric

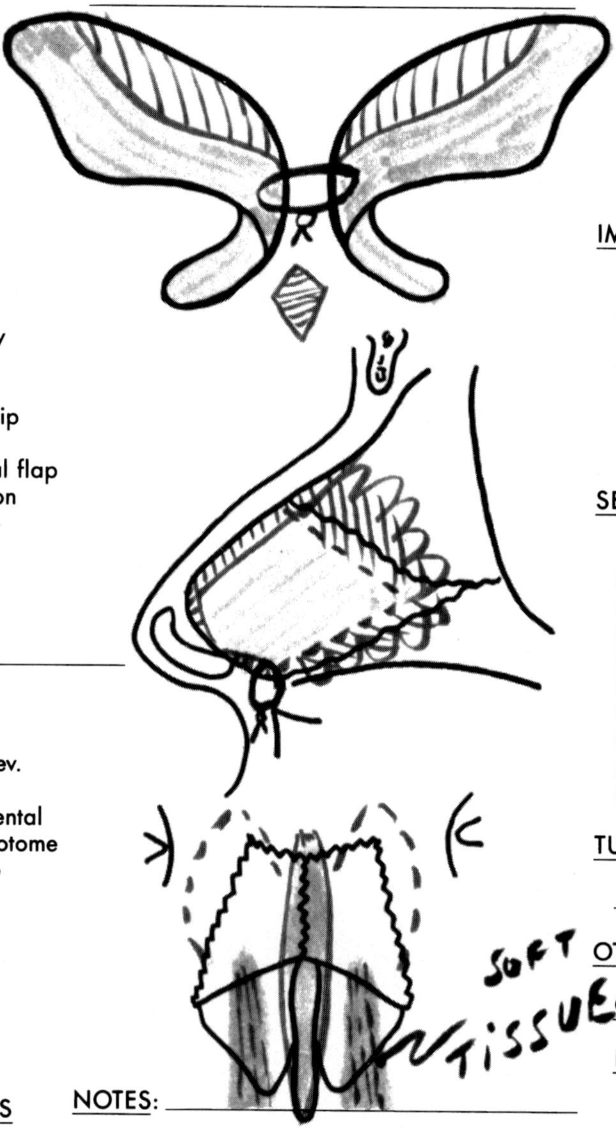

COLUMELLA

Strut
Batten
Narrowed
Implant
Trim MC
 -caudal
 -feet

IMPLANTS

None
Cartilage
Bone
Other:
_____
_____

SEPTUM

None
Dev. — R-L
Spur — R-L
Flap elev. R-L
Disartic.
Swinging door
Building blocks
Caudal resect.
Morselized
Spine

TURBINATES

_____

OTHER

CHIN: _____

LIDS:
 Upper _____
 Lower S   SM

LIFT:

SCARS:

LESIONS:

NOTES: _____
_____
_____

SOFT TISSUE

Fig. 51-57. The rhinoplasty graphic record sheet used to portray exact operative events.

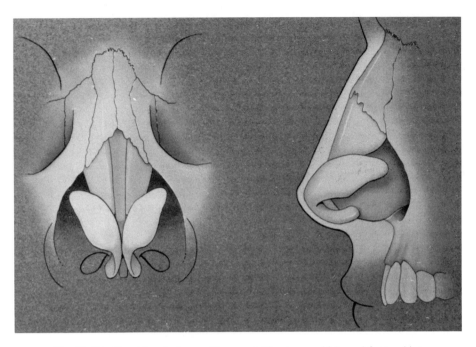

Fig. 51-58. The rhinoplasty graphic record (Gunter graphic) used for teaching.

Box 51-2. Patient instructions after nasal plastic surgery

A. Introduction

Please read and familiarize yourself with these instructions both before and after surgery. By following them carefully you will assist in obtaining the best possible result from your surgery. If questions arise, do not hesitate to communicate with me and discuss your questions at any time. Take this list to the hospital with you, and begin observing these directions on the day of surgery.

B. Instructions

1. Do not blow nose until instructed. Wipe or dab nose gently with tissues, if necessary.
2. Change dressing (if it is present) under nose as needed.
3. The nasal plaster cast will remain in place for approximately 1 week and will be removed in the office. Do not disturb it; keep it dry.
4. Avoid foods that require prolonged chewing. Otherwise, your diet has no restrictions.
5. Avoid extreme physical activity. Obtain more rest than you usually get and avoid exertion, including athletic activities and sexual intercourse.
6. Brush teeth gently with a soft toothbrush only. Avoid manipulation of upper lip to keep nose at rest.
7. Avoid prolonged telephone conversations and excessive social activities for at least 10 to 14 days.
8. You may wash your face, but carefully avoid the dressing. Take tub baths until the dressings are removed.
9. Avoid smiling, grinning, and excessive facial movements for 1 week.
10. Do not wash hair for 1 week unless you have someone to do it for you. Do not get nasal dressing wet.
11. Wear clothing that fastens in front or back for 1 week. Avoid slipover sweaters, T-shirts, and turtlenecks.
12. Absolutely avoid sun or sun lamps for 6 weeks after surgery. Heat may cause the nose to swell.
13. Don't swim for 1 month.
14. Don't be concerned if, after removal of dressing, the nose, eyes, and upper lip show some swelling and discoloration; this usually clears in 2 or 3 weeks. In certain patients it may require 6 months for all swelling to subside completely.
15. Take only medications prescribed by your physician(s).
16. Do not wear regular glasses or sunglasses that rest on the bridge of the nose for at least 4 weeks. We will instruct you in the method of taping the glasses to your forehead to prevent pressure on the nose.
17. Contact lenses may be worn within 2 or 3 days after surgery.
18. After the physician removes your nasal plaster cast, the skin of the nose may be cleansed gently with a mild soap or Vaseline Intensive Care lotion. Be gentle. Makeup may be used as soon as bandages are removed. To cover discoloration, you may use Erase by Max Factor, Cover Away by Adrien Arpel, or On Your Mark by Kenneth.
19. Don't take chances! If you are concerned about anything you consider significant, call me at [insert physician's phone number].

to arrange for visits at 1, 3, 6, 9, 12, 18, and 24 months after the operation. After that, yearly visits are helpful to review the subtle changes in nasal appearance that inevitably occur. Observing these changes, favorable as well as unfavorable, allows the surgeon to refine his or her technique both to anticipate and to control these long-term healing characteristics.

SUGGESTED READINGS

Brennan HG, Parkes ML: Septal surgery: the high septal transfixion, *Int Surg* 58:732, 1973.

Fry HJH: Nasal skeletal trauma and the interlocked stresses of the nasal septal cartilage, *Br J Plas Surg* 20:146, 1967.

Gilbert JG, Felt LJ: The nasal aponeurosis and its role in rhinoplasty, *Arch Otolaryngol* 61:433, 1955.

Goin MK, Goin JM: *Changing the body*, Baltimore, 1981, Williams & Wilkins.

Goodman WS, Charles DA: Technique of external rhinoplasty, *Can J Otolaryngol* 7:13, 1978.

Gunter JP: Anatomical observations of the lower lateral cartilages, *Arch Otolaryngol* 89:61, 1969.

Janeke JB, Wright WK: Studies on the support of the nasal tip, *Arch Otolaryngol* 93:458, 1971.

Natvig P and others: Anatomical details of the osseous-cartilaginous framework of the nose, *Plast Reconstr Surg* 48:528, 1971.

Ortiz-Monasterio F, Olmedo A, Oscoy LO: The use of cartilage grafts in primary aesthetic rhinoplasty, *Plast Reconstr Surg* 67:597, 1981.

Padovan IF: External approach in rhinoplasty, *Surg ORL Lug* 3:354, 1966.

Parkes ML, Brennan HG: High septal transfixion to shorten the nose, *Plast Reconstr Surg* 45:487, 1970.

Smith TW: As clay in the potter's hand: a review of 221 rhinoplasties, *Ohio Med J* 63:1055, 1967.

Sheen JH: Achieving more nasal tip projection by use of small autogenous vomer or septal cartilage grafts, *Plast Reconstr Surg* 56:35, 1975.

Sheen JH: Secondary rhinoplasty, *Plast Reconstr Surg* 56:137, 1975.

Sheen JH: *Aesthetic rhinoplasty*, St Louis, 1985, Mosby.

Skoog T: *Plastic surgery*, Philadelphia, 1975, WB Saunders.

Straatsma BR, Straatsma CR: The anatomical relationship of the lateral nasal cartilage to the nasal bone and the cartilaginous nasal septum, *Plast Reconstr Surg* 8:443, 1951.

Tardy ME: Rhinoplasty tip ptosis: etiology and prevention, *Laryngoscope* 83:923, 1973.

Tardy ME: Septal perforations, *Otolaryngol Clin North Am* 6:711, 1973.

Tardy ME: *Nasal reconstruction and rhinoplasty*. In Ballenger JJ, editor: *Textbook of otolaryngology*, ed 12, Philadelphia, 1977, Lea & Febiger.

Tardy ME: *Rhinoplasty in midlife*. In Symposium on the Aging Face, *Otolaryngol Clin North Am* 13:289, 1980.

Tardy ME: *Surgical correction of facial deformities*, In Ballenger JJ, editor: *Textbook of otolaryngology*, ed 12, Philadelphia, 1977, Lea & Febiger.

Tardy ME: Color monograph with Richards' manufacturing, *Rhinoplasty* 1980.

Tardy ME, Hewell TS: Nasal tip refinement—reliable approaches and sculpture techniques, *Facial Plast Surg* 1:87, 1984.

Tardy ME, Tom L: Anesthesia in rhinoplasty, *Facial Plast Surg* 1:146, 1984.

Tardy ME, Denneny JC: Micro-osteotomies in rhinoplasty—a technical refinement, *Facial Plast Surg* 1:137, 1984.

Tardy ME: *Rhinoplasty*, Baltimore, 1984, Williams & Wilkins.

Tardy ME, Denneny JC, Fritsch MH: The versatile cartilage autograft in reconstruction of the nose and face, *Laryngoscope* 95:523, 1985.

Tardy ME: *Rhinoplasty*. In Cummings CW and others, editors: *Otolaryngology—head and neck surgery*, vol 1, St Louis, 1986, Mosby.

Tardy ME, Younger R, Key M and others: The overprojecting tip—anatomic variation and targeted solutions, *Facial Plast Surg* 4:4, 1987.

Tardy ME: Transdomal suture refinement of the nasal tip, *Facial Plast Surg* 4:4, 1987.

Tardy ME, Toriumi D: Alar retraction: composite graft correction, *Facial Plast Surg* 6:2, 1989.

Tardy ME, Broadway D: Graphic record-keeping in rhinoplasty: a valuable self-learning device, *Facial Plast Surg* 6:2, 1989.

Tardy ME and others: The cartilaginous pollybeak: etiology, prevention and treatment, *Facial Plast Surg* 6:2, 1989.

Tardy ME, Schwartz MS, Parras G: Saddle nose deformity: autogenous graft repair, *Facial Plast Surg* 6:2, 1989.

Tardy ME: *Rhinoplasty: The art and the science*, Philadelphia, 1996, WB Saunders.

Webster RC: Advances in surgery of the tip: intact rim cartilage techniques and the tip-columella-lip esthetic complex, *Otolaryngol Clin North Am* 8:615, 1975.

Webster RC, Smith RC: *Rhinoplasty*. In RM Goldwyn, editor: *Long-term results in plastic and reconstructive surgery*, Boston, 1980, Little, Brown.

Wright WK: Study on hump removal in rhinoplasty, *Laryngoscope* 77:508, 1967.

Wright WK: Surgery of the bony and cartilaginous dorsum, *Otolaryngol Clin North Am* 8:575, 1975.

Wright MR, Wright WK: A psychological study of patients undergoing cosmetic surgery, *Arch Otolaryngol* 101:145, 1975.

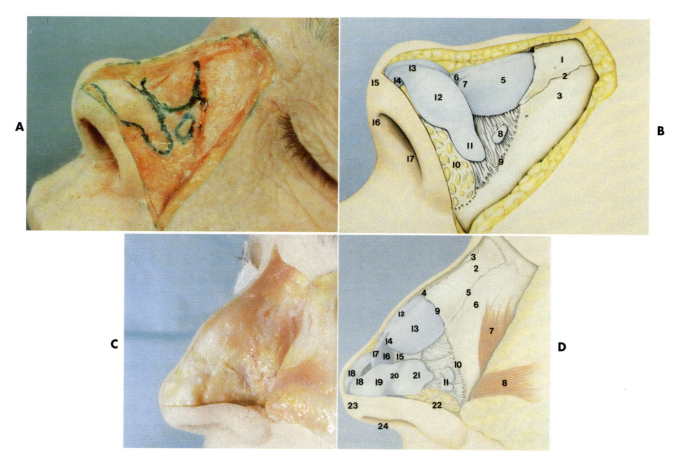

Plate 5. **B,** *1,* Nasal bone; *2,* nasomaxillary suture line; *3,* ascending process of maxilla; *4,* osseocartilaginous junction (rhinion); *5,* upper lateral cartilage; *6,* anterior septal angle; *7,* caudal free edge of upper lateral cartilage; *8,* sesamoid cartilage; *9,* piriform margin; *10,* alar lobule; *11,* lateral crus of alar cartilage—lateral portion; *12,* lateral crus of alar cartilage—central portion; *13,* tip-defining point; *14,* transitional segment of alar cartilage (intermediate crus); *15,* infratip lobule; *16,* columella; *17,* medial crural footplate. **D,** *1,* Nasofrontal suture line; *2,* nasal bone; *3,* internasal suture line; *4,* osseocartilaginous junction (rhinion); *5,* nasomaxillary suture line; *6,* ascending process of maxilla; *7,* levator labii superioris muscle; *8,* transverse nasalis muscle; *9,* cephalic portion of upper lateral cartilage (articulates to undersurface of nasal bone); *10,* piriform margin; *11,* sesamoid cartilages; *12,* cartilaginous dorsum; *13,* upper lateral cartilage; *14,* caudal free margin of upper lateral cartilage; *15,* intercartilaginous ligament; *16,* quadrangular cartilage; *17,* anterior septal angle; *18,* tip-defining point alar cartilage; *19,* lateral crus of alar cartilage; *20,* concavity ("hinge") of lateral crus; *21,* lateral aspect of lateral crus; *22,* alar lobule; *23,* infratip lobule; *24,* columella.

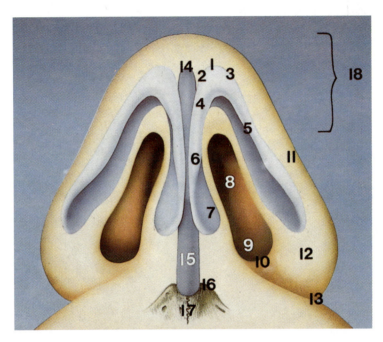

Plate 6. *1*, Apex of alar cartilage; *2*, medial angle of dome; *3*, lateral angle of dome; *4*, alar cartilage transitional segment—intermediate crus; *5*, lateral crus alar cartilage; *6*, medial crus alar cartilage; *7*, medial crural footplate; *8*, nostril aperture; *9*, nostril floor; *10*, nostril sill; *11*, lateral alar sidewall; *12*, alar lobule; *13*, alar—facial junction; *14*, anterior septal angle; *15*, caudal septum; *16*, maxillary crest; *17*, nasal spine; *18*, infratip lobule.

Chapter 52

Special Rhinoplasty Techniques

Richard T. Farrior
Edward H. Farrior

The nasal abnormalities to be addressed in this chapter are those that usually have some type of combined internal and external deformity and are often difficult to correct. The chapter will not address the standard or cosmetic rhinoplasty but rather will attempt to show some of the variations required in these problem cases.[3,13,16,17] Management is complex if the injury has been severe, such as when there has been loss of support because of hematoma or infection or if the nose has been operated on previously. In a nose requiring revision, particularly when an excessive amount of scarring has been created or an excessive amount of tissue has been removed, management may include a multitude of variables. Of the congenital anomalies, only the cleft-lip nose will be discussed.

These patients require the inclusion of all aspects of combined septorhinoplasty, with frequent extension and modification of the technique.[3,17] The use of implants is frequently required. Autogenous implants are advised; the authors use them almost exclusively because synthetic implants when utilized for the nose have been disappointing in long-term follow-up.[4,6,11,12,31] One is hopeful that Gore-Tex implants will prove the exception.

These cases are particularly challenging in regard to improving the airway and gaining maximum improvement in appearance. A form of combined septorhinoplasty to correct both the external and the nasal septal deformities in one stage is virtually essential.[1,3,16,17] These noses are often twisted, and the septum cannot be adequately straightened without correcting the external deformity. Figure 52-1 illustrates several nasal deviations and the anatomic components involved. Each of these deviations may be associated with a long side and a short side of the osseous and cartilaginous lateral nasal vaults, particularly when the deviation extends to the root of the nose and the deformity is of congenital origin. A plumb line should be dropped from the center of the glabella, and the nasal base analyzed in relation to any deviations of the lower third of the face. If present, these facial asymmetries should be pointed out to the patient preoperatively.

Often there is excessive scarring, which requires the freeing of contracting forces and tension vectors on the nasal septum. The osseous dorsum and the cartilaginous dorsum are reduced before the septal surgery is performed because these cases require extensive exposure, mobilization, and release of the tissues to allow repositioning and structural reorganization.[16] An experienced surgeon can ''take the nose apart'' and yet preserve most tissue, by ''repositioning'' rather than ''removal.''

In the traumatized nose, whether the trauma is caused by injury or previous surgery, one must determine whether tissue is simply displaced or whether it is absent.[17] Ideally, all tissue, particularly the septal cartilage, remains available for modification or for possible use as an implant. The surgeon must determine what structures can be left undisturbed and what can be retained but repositioned to ensure adequate support. In addition to the structural framework, the soft tissue may contribute to the deformity through asymmetric adhesion of the overlying skin, resulting in dimpling, or through webbing of the mucosa, causing nasal obstruction.

Revisional surgery is indicated if the nose can be functionally improved, whether or not an ideal aesthetic result can be obtained.[13,16,27,32,35]

ANALYSIS

A thorough examination using not only observation but also detailed palpation of the nose is essential in determining preoperatively what anatomic components are actually in-

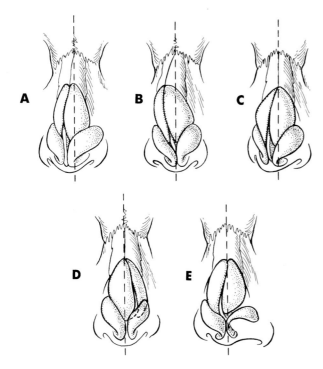

Fig. 52-1. A variety of nasal deformities, including the anatomic components involved. Each anatomic component of the deviated or twisted nose influences the remaining components, particularly those immediately adjacent, just as each step of the surgery influences the other steps. **A,** Deviation of the entire nose, including the nasal bones up to the radix. **B,** Twisted nose with the tip and caudal septum returning to the midline. The nasal bones are deviated from the midline up to the radix. The greatest convexity or concavity of the bony and cartilaginous vaults are frequently at their junction. **C,** Deviation of the cartilaginous components of the nose, including the septum, with caudal dislocation off the anterior spine. **D,** Deviation of the dorsal septum and septal angle, with the remainder of the nose in the midline. This creates distortion of the lower lateral cartilage, with actual or simulated asymmetry. **E,** Deviation of the dorsal septum and septal angle with the distortion of the entire tip of the nose and medial crura.

volved in the deformity. Experience is a great factor in being able to do this at the time of the office examination. Careful examination should be coordinated with appropriate photographs, radiograph films, and facial analysis. The preoperative findings strongly influence the selection of the most appropriate surgical approach and exposure techniques.

If previous surgery has been performed by someone else and revision is required, it is most helpful in the analysis if the previous operative report can be obtained. Even with this, it is difficult to decipher precisely how much tissue remains or how much scarring may exist. Although examination by blunt-instrument palpation is helpful, actual exploration at surgery is often required to determine the amount of tissue that remains.

Coordination of the preoperative analysis with the findings at the operative table can be accomplished through either the standard intranasal rhinoplasty approaches or the external rhinoplasty approach. The external rhinoplasty approach is particularly useful in the twisted nose and the nose requiring implant materials, but the authors use predominantly the standard rhinoplasty approaches with only occasional use of the external technique. However, for the severely deviated nose and the cleft-lip nose, the external rhinoplasty is used with increasing frequency.[17,22,32,38]

The pathologic anatomy is variable, and multiple techniques are required to achieve adequate correction. All components of the internal and external anatomy may be involved, and the influence of one component on the next must be taken into consideration in the repair.[16]

Some of the more common deformities encountered in the previously injured nose are:

1. "Relative" hump
2. Wide lateral bony vault
3. Depression of caudal nasal bone
4. Depression of cartilaginous dorsum
5. External twist and deviation
6. Splayed cartilaginous dorsum and tip
7. Loss of septal and upper lateral cartilage support
8. Saddle deformity (cartilage and/or bone)
9. Caudal dislocation of septum
10. Columella retraction with absence of cartilage
11. Flattened or asymmetric nostrils
12. Distorted or fractured lower lateral cartilages
13. Septal deflections, spurs, lamination (fibrous and cartilaginous duplication), complex angulations, and fibrous union
14. Intranasal scarring (1) at the limen vestibuli ("anterior web") and (2) on the floor of the nose
15. Synechiae
16. Septal perforations

Incisions and soft-tissue elevation

In the intranasal rhinoplasty approach to the deviated nose, a rather generous intercartilaginous incision is made bilaterally, and the soft tissue over the upper lateral cartilage is elevated. The incision is carried into a complete transfixion incision (Fig. 52-2). Alar cartilage margin incisions are made to allow delivery of the lower lateral cartilages so that they can be analyzed, especially in the face of any asymmetries, fractures, or lacerations of the cartilages. A complete transfixion incision is most often used for these deviated noses in anticipation of work on the caudal septum and anterior spine area and also to allow the insertion of a columella strut into a retrograde columella pocket. The septum is approached through this incision when correction of the caudal septum and anterior spine is required. If the caudal septum is intact and there is no dislocation, the classic Freer incision is used, leaving all anterior or caudal mucoperichondrium and cartilage undisturbed.

Although the authors generally use intranasal incisions for a deviated nose, the open or external rhinoplasty is being

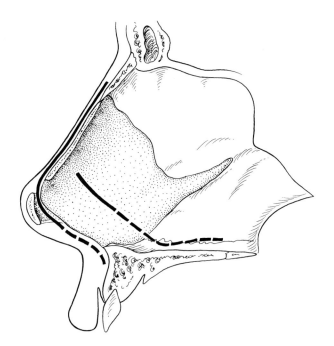

Fig. 52-2. Modified incisions for septal surgery. The dorsal elevation is carried into the transfixion incision, which may then be carried all the way to the anterior spine or only partway as a hemitransfixion incision. The intranasal or freer incision may be limited, carried to the floor, or extended along the floor as a "hockey stick" incision beneath a severe spur.

used with increasing frequency when there are severe asymmetries, deviations, and tissue deficiencies (Fig. 52-3).[17,22,32,38] The incisions measure approximately 7 mm in length and have had a variety of configurations. To have a single point at the end of this random pattern flap, the authors now use the gull-wing incision as opposed to the previous inverted gull-wing incision (Fig. 52-4 *A, B*).

Some of the indications for use of the external rhinoplasty are as follows: (1) a nasal deformity that is difficult to precisely analyze; (2) one in which there is severe asymmetry of the lateral bony walls as well as the lower lateral cartilages; (3) when tissue deficiencies exist so that it is necessary to precisely place and suture implants in position[17]; (4) congenital anomalies such as the cleft-lip nose or other deformities in which profound asymmetries exist; and (5) an extremely wide bony and cartilaginous dorsum, whether or not a hump is removed.

The external approach involves a transverse midcolumella incision in a gull-wing curve rather than at a sharp angle. The incision is then extended upward along the caudal edge of the medial crus and laterally along the caudal margin of the lateral crus (see Fig. 52-4). The elevation is initiated with sharp knife dissection, with the columella skin being elevated before the elevation is extended laterally over the lateral crura of the lower lateral cartilages. The technique allows incorporation of the various modifications the authors have developed through the years to deal with specific ana-

tomic components.[13,16] The external incision crossing the columella leaves a barely perceptible scar and offers excellent visualization via the "degloving" of the nose.

Although the caudal septum can be exposed through the external approach by spreading the medial crura, such an approach requires extensive separation of the medial crura, columella, and membranous septum, and even then the exposure for septal surgery may be limited.

Because there is only limited elevation of the skin with the intranasal approaches, the skin redrapes easily to allow precise intraoperative analysis of the resculptured nasal framework. In the external rhinoplasty, however, the soft tissue is undermined more extensively, and some distortion may result as the elevated skin is laid back down. This more extensive tissue mobilization also leads to greater tissue reaction and edema postoperatively, so that it takes slightly longer to resolve the swelling postoperatively than is the case with intranasal approaches.

Reduction of the bony and cartilaginous dorsum

It is interesting that debate remains as to whether to do the hump removal or the septal reconstruction first. Some surgeons even prefer to do the septum in an initial procedure, followed by the rhinoplasty several months later. The authors have long advocated a single-stage procedure for the twisted and combined internal–external deformity, and strongly prefer to reduce the nasal dorsum *before* performing the septal reconstruction. This allows the surgeon to know exactly how much cartilage he or she is working with beneath the dorsum.

The surgeon must first determine exactly how much, if any, hump reduction should be carried out. Often in the traumatized nose, a "relative" hump is created by loss of support and flattening in the cartilaginous portion of the dorsum. In these patients initial attention should be devoted to increasing the cartilaginous projection with combined septal surgery and nasal tip surgery.[16]

In the externally deviated nose there is usually an equality of the lateral vaults, both bony and cartilaginous. This may be corrected with an asymmetric hump removal, with more bone and cartilage being removed on the longer side (Fig. 52-5). In some patients, it is desirable to section the mucosa as well as the bone or cartilage during hump removal. This is particularly true when a large hump has been removed; the redundant mucosa beneath the dorsum can herniate upward beneath the skin and result in an undesirable dorsal fullness.

In some patients the nose should be straightened before the final trimming of the long side because it may be best to add an implant to the short side rather than additionally reducing the long side.

Revisions of the dorsal profile line often involve the simple correction of specific irregularities caused by bone spicules or prominent cartilages. The supratip area is a subject unto itself; correction of deformities there requires correc-

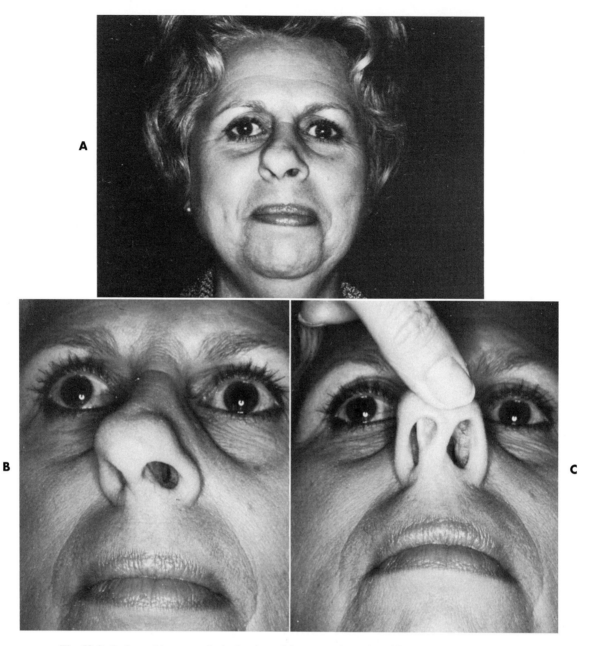

Fig. 52-3. Patient with a severely deviated nasal dorsum and tip (**A** and **B**), with dislocation of the septal cartilage into the right nasal vestibule (**C**).

tion of dorsal framework deformities and reduction of soft tissue thickening and fibrosis.

Supratip swelling that results in a fullness and rounding of the tip with healing—that is, a "polly beak" deformity—can result from several factors. The most common are excessive postoperative fibrosis between the skin and the septal angle and simply insufficient lowering of the dorsal margins of the septum or upper lateral cartilages. In correcting the polly beak deformity, the surgeon should slightly overcorrect the cartilaginous framework to allow for recurring fibrosis in the supratip area (Fig. 52-6). Any excessive

scar tissue should be removed, although it often recurs. The authors do not advocate the use of steroid injections into the supratip area.

Supratip swelling may also result from an excess of mucosa herniating upward beneath the dorsal skin (Fig. 52-7). This is likely to occur when an extensive reduction has been done and an extramucosal approach has been used, preserving all of the mucosa in the valve area.

Perhaps the most common secondary deformity of the nasal dorsum is created when too much bone has been removed, so that implants of one type or another must be

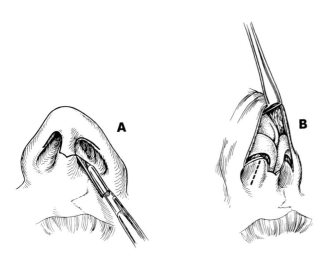

Fig. 52-4. The external (open) approach. **A,** A gull-wing incision is made, crossing the columella just above the flare of the feet of the medial crura and then extending upward along the caudal edge of the medial crura and into marginal incisions laterally using the surgical knife. The skin is further elevated using the Stevens tenotomy scissors. **B,** Excellent exposure can be obtained to the root of the nose, which assists in evaluating asymmetry of the dorsum. The caudal septum and anterior nasal spine can be approached through the external approach, or a separate hemitransfixion incision may be made as shown by the *dashed line*.

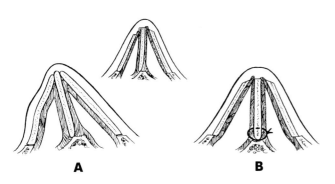

Fig. 52-5. A, Asymmetric lateral vaults, both osseous and cartilaginous, in the deviated nose. An asymmetric hump removal is used to even the lateral vaults. **B,** The corrected relationship with combined septal reconstruction. Occasionally grafts may be placed over the short side rather than reducing the long side. Insert shows deformity, which may occur with the long lateral vault remaining longer than the short after hump removal if this asymmetry is not considered.

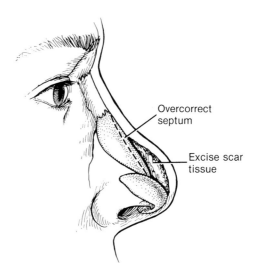

Fig. 52-6. The supratip area. The supratip may be considered the uncontrolled part of the rhinoplasty in that there is considerable variation between individuals in the amount of fibrous buildup over the septum and immediately superior to the newly projected tip. Rounding can occur even with appropriate sculpturing of the cartilaginous framework. (See also Fig. 52-42.)

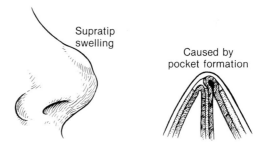

Fig. 52-7. Redundant mucosa in the supratip area. Redundant mucosa or a sealed-off pocket of mucosa anywhere along the dorsum may create simple prominence or fullness and may also lead to an inclusion cyst.

inserted. Fascia inserted beneath the skin is effective in masking slight irregularities of the dorsum.[23] This may be the only implant needed, particularly for small soft-tissue defects. The fascia temporalis is readily available for this purpose, but fascia lata can also be used.

The open rhinoplasty offers an opportunity to suture either cartilage implants or fascia implants precisely into position. When wide elevation is not required to perform

the rhinoplasty, a limited pocket is made for the implant to allow precise positioning. Draw sutures carried out through the skin aid in positioning the implant and may be left in place until the end of the procedure to stabilize the implant until the dressing is completed. For longer-term stability, the draw sutures may be secured over a thin plastic polyethylene bolus on the dorsal skin and left in place for several days.

Modification of the lower lateral cartilages

It is not the authors' purpose to discuss all aspects of surgery of the nasal tip, especially as it relates to cosmetic surgery, but rather to consider correction of severe asymmetries and deficiencies that occur in the traumatized or congenitally deformed nose. For these noses wide exposure of the lower lateral cartilages is absolutely essential and may

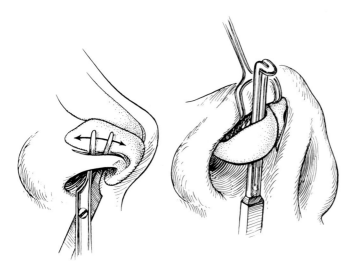

Fig. 52-8. Delivery of the lower lateral cartilages. When the lower lateral cartilages are very asymmetric or have been severely traumatized, delivery should be done to allow adequate exposure for proper modification. This modification can also be accomplished through the external rhinoplasty approach.

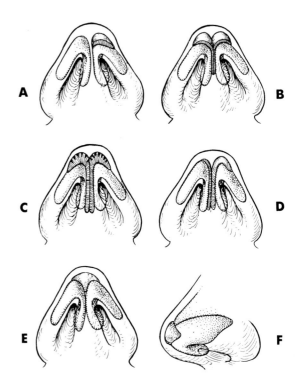

Fig. 52-9. Revisional surgery with implants for nasal tip. **A,** A simple onlay implant, which may be sutured in position to the cartilage or held in position by a draw suture through the external skin. **B,** Implant to the tip and columella, most commonly using auricular cartilage. **C,** Contouring of the implant by scoring. **D,** Asymmetric implant. **E** and **F,** Tip button with stabilization between the medial crura.

be achieved either through delivery of the cartilages (Fig. 52-8) or via the external approach.

When there are severe asymmetries of the lower lateral cartilages, management usually requires modification of the more normal cartilage as well as the more abnormal side if one is to achieve a symmetric tip. The cephalic portion of the lower lateral cartilage is an excellent implant to be used for the nasal tip to overlie angulations or fill small depressions or for splinting a cartilage by direct suturing. When more sturdy cartilage is necessary, sculptured or laminated septal or auricular cartilage is useful (Fig. 52-9). In the tip these implants may be combined and sutured directly to a columella strut or to the domes of the lower lateral cartilages. If there is marked distortion with associated soft-tissue contracture, it may be necessary to free the lateral crus of the lower lateral cartilage on the involved side of both dorsal and vestibular skin, and then advance the lateral crus into the nasal tip between the two skin layers as in the technique used in the cleft-lip nose repair (Fig. 52-10).

The septum is an ideal source of grafts to be placed in the nasal tip. Such an implant has the effect of stabilizing the medial crura and domes in proper relationship and giving some increased tip projection. This technique is useful in both severely traumatized tip and the previously operated nose, in which all too often too much tissue has been removed from the lower lateral cartilages (Fig. 52-11). The authors have used for a number of years reinforcing plates, now commonly referred to as shields. The plates should be sutured directly to the lower lateral cartilages. This may be accomplished readily through intranasal incisions (alar cartilage margin incisions) or can be placed with greater ease and less chance of dislodgment through an external rhino-

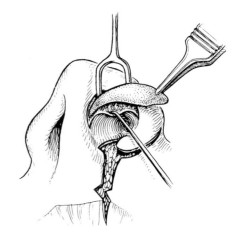

Fig. 52-10. Freeing of the alar cartilage for the cleft-lip nose or certain asymmetries of the lower lateral cartilage. The lower lateral cartilage is freed of both surface and vestibular skin, allowing the cartilage to be rotated medially to project the tip of the nose. The cartilage is then sandwiched between the two skin surfaces in the new position and held with transalar sutures tied over a flat plastic film on the external surface. This technique is used for unilateral and bilateral nasal deformities, and can be accomplished using either the intranasal or the external approach. Boluses on both surfaces are to be avoided.

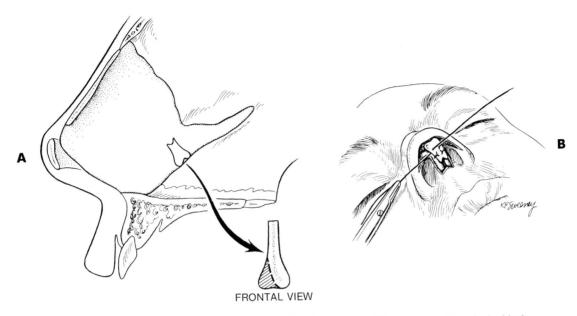

Fig. 52-11. A, Nasal tip graft (shield or plate). The lower edge of the septal cartilage is the ideal location for obtaining a tip shield. It should be modified by cutting off a portion of the thickened inferior aspect of the septal cartilage. **B,** The tip is positioned over the caudal border of the tip cartilages at their domes, preventing too much sharpness in the tip of the nose. (See Fig. 52-21.)

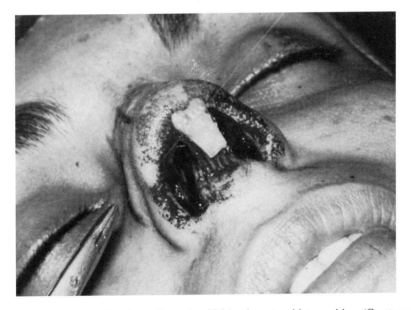

Fig. 52-12. The external rhinoplasty allows the shield to be sutured into position. (Courtesy of Dr. Calvin Johnson, New Orleans.)

plasty (Fig. 52-12). Migration of the shields has been the major problem with their use, and direct suturing will prevent this displacement. By removal of a wedge from the inferior border of the shield, two points are created along the inferior border, which assists in stabilization to prevent rotation or movement.

Septal reconstruction

The full range of septal reconstructive techniques must be used in the twisted nose. The specific techniques required are determined by the amount of cartilage that remains, and how angulated or dislocated it is (Fig. 52-13).[13,16,17]

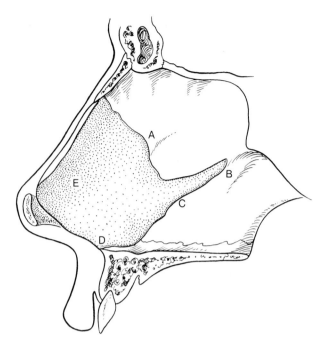

Fig. 52-13. Common sites of septal angulations and dislocations in order of frequency starting with *A. A,* Junction of the septal cartilage with the perpendicular plate of the ethmoid. Abnormalities here usually involve both cartilage and bone. *B,* Continuation of a cartilaginous spur toward the sphenoid rostrum; associated with posterior bony spurs from the vomer. *C,* Bony and cartilaginous components of an inferior spur. *D,* Caudal dislocations off of the anterior spine and maxillary crest. *E,* Area of the lumen vestibuli and anterior valve. Here buckling, when not associated with fracture lines, is frequently corrected by relieving all surrounding tension vectors. Even slight deviations here may cause significant nasal destruction. Most angulations and deviations occur at the junction of the cartilage with the bone, except where there has been a fracture of the septal cartilage.

The subject of septal surgery is discussed in detail in Chapter 50. It is impossible, however, to discuss correction of the difficult nasal deformity without addressing surgery of the involved septum. Once the incisions are made, elevation of the mucoperichondrial flaps is frequently difficult because of fibrosis through fracture sites and overlapping or lamination of the cartilage itself.

In the previously operated nose, a practical approach involves beginning the elevation of the mucoperichondrium beneath the dorsum because this area is often virginal. The elevation then proceeds downward toward the previous operative site, where cartilage and bone may have been removed.

For the severely deviated or previously operated nose, it is usually necessary to elevate the mucoperichondrium on both sides of the septal cartilage, although it is preferable whenever possible to leave it attached on one side as the bone and cartilaginous angulations are corrected. Freeing fibrous contractions and septal angulations is essential in allowing the septal framework to straighten. The extent to which cartilage and bone must be removed or repositioned is dictated by the particular deformity encountered and the direction of the angulations. Generally, incision or removal of thin strips of cartilage along the existing angulations is required to achieve straightening (Fig. 52-14). Release of all tension vectors allows a buckled septum to straighten. Determination of the final position of the septum may not be possible until osteotomies have been performed, particularly if the nasal bones and upper lateral cartilages are severely deviated from the midline. A final determination of what, if anything, more needs to be done to the septum therefore must sometimes await the completion of medial and lateral osteotomies, when the entire nose is positioned in the midline. (See Fig. 52-31 regarding deviations of the central bony complex.)

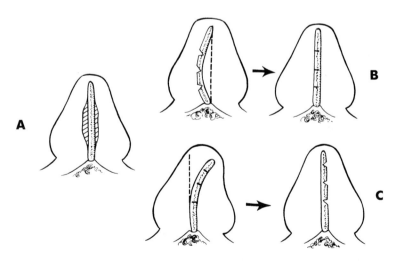

Fig. 52-14. Correcting septal curvature. **A,** Vertical shave to reduce septal thickening. The shave may also be used to reduce bowing. **B,** Removal of cartilage wedges to straighten the septum in the midline. **C,** Scoring to allow the cartilage to open and return to the midline.

Transseptal coaptation sutures, which bring the two mucoperichondrial flaps together and pass between angulations or cartilage pedicles to prevent overlap, are great aids in this surgery (Figs. 52-15 and 52-16). Polyethylene plates have been used for a number of years to stabilize the septum in the early postoperative period and also prevent the development of synechiae, particularly when turbinate surgery has been performed (Fig. 52-17). Two through-and-through sutures are always placed through the polyethylene plates. These are placed so that one arm of the suture goes between

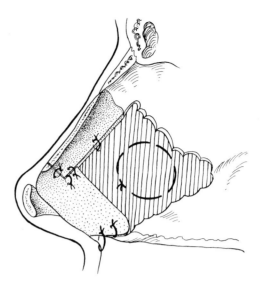

Fig. 52-16. Coaptation sutures. Further modifications of the septal reconstruction in which it has been necessary to remove a significant amount of cartilage and bone. Coaptation sutures may be either single sutures through and through the mucoperichondrium or a continuous suture passed back and forth through and through and tied to the original free end.

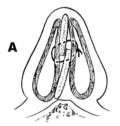 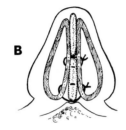

Fig. 52-15. Transseptal coaptative sutures. **A,** Whether passed through the mucoperichondrium or submucosally, simple sutures may assist in approximating the cartilage but will not prevent dislocation. **B,** Coaptation sutures through the mucoperichondrium should be passed between the cartilage pedicles or fractures to prevent the cartilage segment from overriding. Below, the suture is passed between the cartilage and bone and back through the cartilage, including the mucoperichondrium.

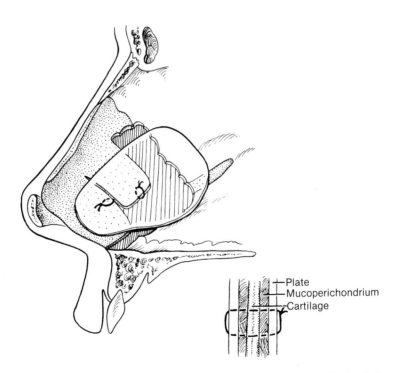

Fig. 52-17. Intranasal dressing to include polyethylene plates. The contoured polyethylene plate is inserted and removed as one piece, slightly curved or folded to pass with the edges touching the blades of the nasal speculum. The plate is used to prevent synechiae and to support the septum. At least two sutures are used to prevent flaring or opening of the plates from each other.

cartilage pedicles or beneath the septal cartilage for support. One may splint the septum further at a major angulation with a straight portion of thin perpendicular plate of the ethmoid.

When it is necessary to reposition the caudal portion of the septum, it is usually necessary to free the mucoperichondrium on both sides to release all extrinsic tension on the cartilage. The septal cartilage is then detached from the underlying anterior nasal spine, and intrinsic tension is relieved by scoring, cross-hatching, wedging, and so on. This then allows the septal cartilage to swing into the midline. Once this caudal pedicle is freed of the tension vectors, it may be maintained in the midline by sutures that go around the anterior spine or through a burr hole in the spine (Fig. 52-18). To further prevent dislocation, an additional suture may be passed through the two mucoperichondrial flaps and between the bone of the spine and the cartilage. The cartilage pedicle then is not only attached directly to the spine, but the two mucoperichondrial flaps when sutured together add further stability. When necessary, the caudal edge of the septum may be held in proper relationship to the columella with interrupted sutures or direct through-and-through septo-columellar sutures (Fig. 52-19).

The working *columella strut* is intended to give strength to the medial crura, and has also often been used as a splint

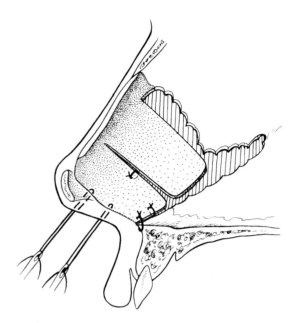

Fig. 52-19. Stabilization of the caudal septum with draw sutures through the center of the columella, reestablishing the septocolumellar relationship. At the end of the procedure the draw sutures may be removed or may be tied loosely against the columellar skin.

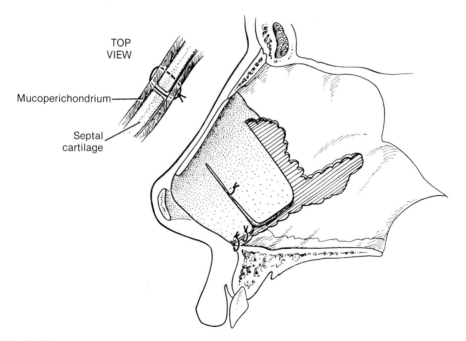

Fig. 52-18. Repositioning and suturing of the caudal septum. The dislocated septum is repositioned on the anterior spine and maxillary crest. Reconstruction is augmented by scoring or cross-hatching and proper placement of sutures such that one suture is passed submucosally around the anterior spine. The next fixation suture is passed through one mucoperichondrial flap, between the bone of the anterior spine and the septal cartilage and out through the mucoperichondrium on the other side, and then back through flap, septum, and flap to complete the loop. The other sutures are passed between the mucoperichondrial flaps and between the cartilage pedicles to prevent dislocation.

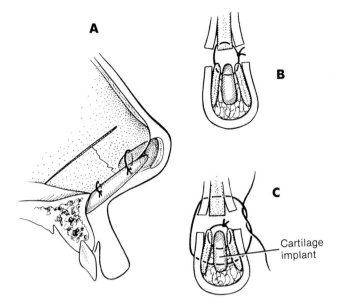

Fig. 52-20. A, Demonstrates the splinting of a horizontal fracture or angulation of the caudal septum or pedicle. Reinforcement of medial crural support. **B** and **C,** A subcutaneous suture is passed so as to suture the columella–medial crura complex subcutaneously directly to the caudal septum (**C**). This may be done with permanent sutures of clear nylon to ensure proper positioning of the medial crura and tip support.

for the caudal edge of the septum when there are horizontal angulations or fractures of the caudal margin of the septum (Fig. 52-20). The columella strut is sutured directly to the caudal septum so that the whole complex prevents caudal angulation of the septum and strengthens tip support.

The main source for the columella strut is the cartilaginous spur from the nasal septum where it is angled or dislocated from the maxillary crest. This prism-shaped inferior portion of the septum is useful because of its considerable strength (Fig. 52-21). The strut may be inserted either under direct vision in an external rhinoplasty or into a retrograde columella pocket in the intranasal rhinoplasty (Fig. 52-22). The cartilaginous strut is then sutured directly to the medial crura, and the septocolumellar draw sutures are passed to hold the strut forward in the columella (Fig. 52-23). As the sutures progress toward the tip of the nose, they pass through the columella strut and medial crura.

The septum must be considered also as an ideal donor site for cartilage and bone implants. When adequate material is available, it is an excellent implant for the nasal dorsum, for the ''working'' columella strut, for the shield implant to the tip, or as a filler for depressions in the area of the upper lateral cartilages. In the latter instance, the implant should be precisely sutured into position. This septal cartilage is a good source for spreader grafts between the septum and the

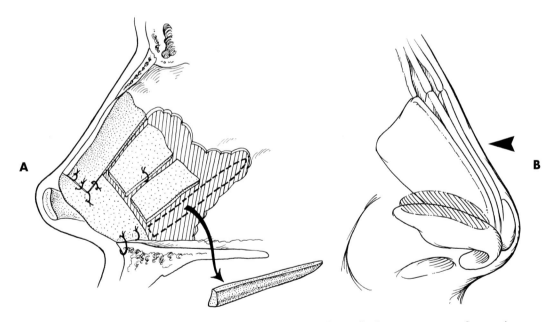

Fig. 52-21. A, Septal cartilage used for columella strut. The cartilaginous component of a spur is an excellent source of autogenous implant material. This may be long enough to extend the full length of the dorsum of the nose and is an excellent source for the working columella strut, tip implants, or shields and for fashioning of spreader grafts and battens. **B,** Collapse of upper lateral cartilages at junction with septum along dorsum *(arrow)*. Position of batten (flying buttress) for valve area.

Continued

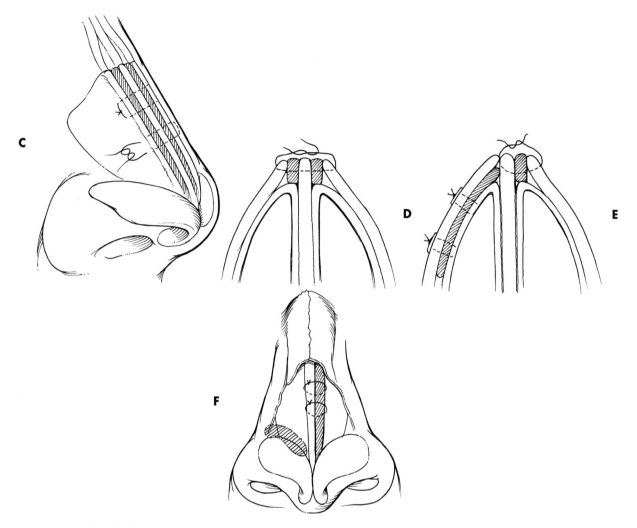

Fig. 52-21, cont'd. C, Bilateral spreader grafts being sutured in position. **D,** Spreader grafts in position, extramucosal. **E,** Spreader graft being sutured in position, *left side.* Batten graft held in position with bolus sutures over flat plastic sheeting, *right side.* **F,** Spreader and batten grafts may be used in combination, unilateral or bilateral.

upper lateral cartilages and when sculptured for battens laterally in the valve area, for a "flying buttress" effect.

Shortening the caudal septum

For the traumatized nose with a drooping tip and columella retraction, the entire septocolumellar complex must be critically evaluated. In correcting the drooping tip, the lower lateral cartilages must be rotated cephalically, and strong tip support is needed. Both the caudal septum and the soft tissue may need modification to achieve this (Fig. 52-24). Frequently there is an associated columella retraction, resulting in an acute nasolabial angle. Correction of the retraction requires straightening the caudal septum and placement of plumping grafts (Fig. 52-25). Some limited resection of the caudal edge of the septum may be necessary to remove a portion of deformed septum that is dislocated off the ante-

rior spine and projecting into one nostril. When the caudal edge of the septal cartilage is severely dislocated, it often creates distortion and retraction of the columella even though adequate cartilage is present. Straightening and repositioning of the caudal septum within the columella sometimes will correct the retraction (Fig. 52-26). Rarely is it necessary to shorten the upper lateral cartilages, although reduction of the scroll along their caudal border may be necessary to reduce excessive width in that area.

The septocolumella complex

The columella and caudal septum must often be addressed in rhinoplasty. There may be columellar retraction caused by retraction of the caudal septum as previously discussed, or there may be other abnormalities of the septum and columella that distract from the appearance of the nose. Ptotic

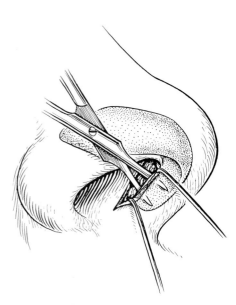

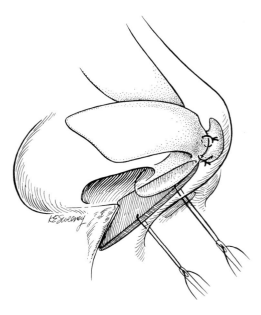

Fig. 52-22. Between two hooks the iris scissors are used to create a retrograde pocket between the medial crura and into the columella. This is done through the transfixion incision in the standard rhinoplasty. The columella strut can be placed directly between the medial crura from above in the external rhinoplasty.

Fig. 52-23. The working columella strut draw sutures. The columella strut is drawn into the retrograde pocket so as to pass in front of the anterior spine resting on the face of the maxilla. It is passed after the sutures are placed in the dome of the nose to assist in greater projection and to prevent protrusion between the medial crura. The draw sutures are removed after the strut is stabilized with sutures.

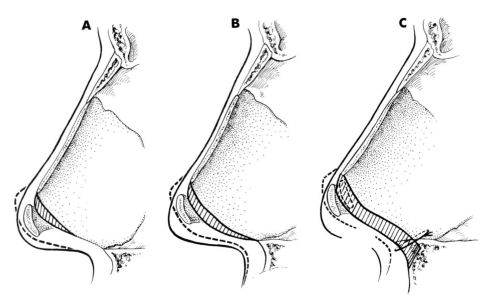

Fig. 52-24. Modifications for shortening the nose. **A,** Ideal limited shortening and elevation of the tip involving only the outer one third to one half of the caudal septum and limited transfixion incision. **B,** Shortening of the entire caudal septum with slight angulation extending to the spine. **C,** Shortening of the entire caudal inferior nose with a deepening of the nasolabial angle. The obtuse nasolabial angle is corrected. A right-angle wedge of bone is removed from the anterior spine, and a suture is passed from the cartilage to the base of the membranous columella, reinforcing the angulation and eliminating the dead space.

lower lateral cartilages with a convex caudal margin can cause increased columellar show. This may also be exacerbated by prominent caudal margin of the septum and/or excessive membranous septum. These deformities can be addressed by trimming or sculpturing as demonstrated in Figure 52-27. Other structures that may contribute to the perceived or actual abnormalities of the caudal septum and columella include either ptosis of the lateral crus or the lower lateral cartilage, causing what appears to be a retracted columella, or retraction of the ala resulting in excessive colu-

mella show. These abnormalities must be corrected when addressing the lower lateral cartilages, either through reduction or augmentation. Repositioning of the anterior maxillary spine, division of the depressor nasi muscle, sectioning of the frenulum, and defatting or augmentation of the nasolabial angle may also be necessary in addressing the caudal septum and columella.[9]

The nasal valve area

The nasal airway immediately beneath the upper lateral cartilages is of particular importance functionally. This valve area requires special consideration when there is inward collapse of the upper or lower lateral cartilages at the level of the limen vestibuli. Here it may be necessary to place cartilage implants from the auricle or the septum, shaped into an outward convexity to create a flying buttress effect. The cephalic portion of the lower lateral cartilages with its vestibular skin may be rotated into a supratip defect. Often both skin and cartilage are required, and the natural curvature of the concha of the auricle with its thin anterior skin is an ideal composite graft to use in the valve area (Fig. 52-28). Narrowing of the junction of the upper lateral cartilage and the septum adds to obstruction and requires a "spreader" graft between the upper lateral cartilages and the dorsal septum, often for the entire length. These grafts are preferably placed in a submucosal or extramucosal pocket and are sutured directly into position, which is made especially easy with the open exposure. The battens (flying buttress) cartilage implants are held precisely in position with tie-over sutures through a thin plastic bolus externally. Spreader grafts and battens may be used simultaneously. See Figures 52-21 and 52-28.

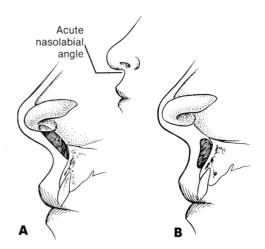

Fig. 52-25. Correction of acute septolabial angle. **A,** The columella strut adds columella fullness. **B,** When the columella strut is not required, a simple plumping graft serves as a filler and gives support to the feet of the medial crura. An implant may be necessary over the face of the maxilla and beneath the anterior spine to create fullness of the lip portion.

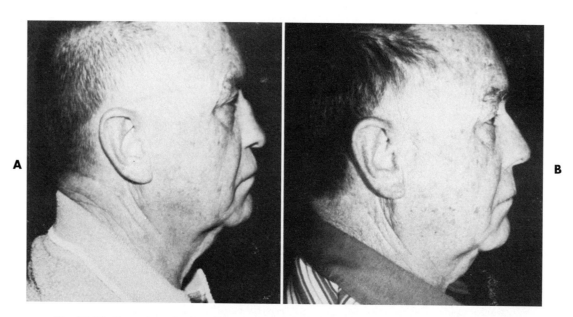

Fig. 52-26. Correction of columella retraction. **A,** Marked columella retraction and drooping tip (preoperative). **B,** After septal reconstruction with tip rotation and columella filling.

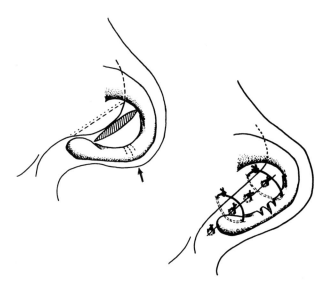

Fig. 52-27. The septocolumella complex. Apart from abnormalities of the lateral ala and its relation to the columella, this complex involves at least the caudal septum, the membranous septum, and the curvature and strength of the medial crura. The exaggerated convex caudal edge of the medial crura, as occurs in the hanging columella, may be partially sectioned to allow the crura to straighten with suturing. The caudal cartilaginous septum and membranous septum may require partial resection. The septocolumella complex is reestablished with sutures, including through-and-through septocolumella sutures. The medial crura may be approached retrograde through the transfixion incision and with subcutaneous elevation of the skin or directly by the external approach. (See also Figs. 52-20 to 52-26 and 52-41.)

Nasal osteotomies

The medial osteotomies are performed first.[15,16,17] If there is to be an intermediate osteotomy halfway between the medial and lateral osteotomies, it is done second. The lateral osteotomy is performed last (Fig. 52-29). If there is a thick plate of bone just at the upper edge of the now-open roof, it may act as a fulcrum over which the nasal bones rock outward at the nasion as the lower border is moved medially. This wedge of bone is removed with an osteotome, with an incision being made in the plane of the septum and then in the plane of the nasal bones.[15,16] Following this the medial osteotomies are extended to the radix, either in a plane paralleling the nasal septum or curving laterally toward the position where the upper end of the lateral osteotomy will be (Fig. 52-30). Extending the bone incision to the radix is considered the complete osteotomy and is often essential in a twisted nose, particularly if the deviation extends up to the radix. When this is required, the osteotome is reinserted into the medial osteotomy after completion of the medial and lateral osteotomies and carried into the firm bone of the radix, where a strong fulcrum for the osteotome is developed. The osteotome is used to fracture the nasal bone and perpendicular plate of the ethmoid toward the midline (Fig. 52-31). This is not an outfracturing maneuver but rather a fracturing of the central portion of the superior nasal complex to include the midline root of the nasal bones and perpendicular plate of the ethmoid.

In the wide flat nose in which it is not necessary to change the profile line, the flat roof of the bony vault and of the upper lateral cartilages must be narrowed. The intermediate

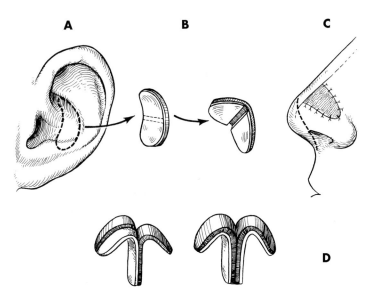

Fig. 52-28. A, Auricular cartilage may be used as a composite graft, with its attached thin anterior skin being used to open the valve areas when there is marked loss of support and intranasal contracture. The skin is excised from the central portion of the graft, which rides over the septum like a saddle, and the skin is inserted into the mucosal opening. To avoid excessive thickness in the dorsum, it may be necessary to excise a strip of cartilage along the dorsum of the septum. The skin edges are precisely sutured to the nasal mucosa. **B,** Position of spreader graft. **C,** Spreader graft being sutured in position. **D,** Batten sutured into position.

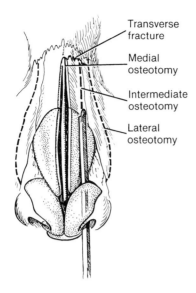

Transverse
fracture

Medial
osteotomy

Intermediate
osteotomy

Lateral
osteotomy

Fig. 52-29. Nasal osteotomies. For the deviated nose, complete medial osteotomies and low lateral osteotomies are most often used. These require the creation of a transverse fracture at the cephalic end of the osteotomies. For the wide-flaring nasal bones that might result from a previous crushing injury or large hump removal, an intermediate osteotomy is often used. This is done halfway between the medial and lateral osteotomies but is done before the lateral osteotomy is performed; the Neivert osteotome with the flat guard is used.

osteotomy is useful in narrowing such a nose (Fig. 52-32). The intermediate osteotomy is carried out through the inter-cartilaginous incision above the upper lateral cartilages. The Neivert osteotome with its flat guard, which serves as a periosteal elevator, is used to carry the osteotomy superiorly to the radix.

In the deviated nose the lateral osteotomy follows the curvature of the nasofacial groove—that is, against the face of the maxilla—and with rotation of the osteotome it curves upward to join the medial osteotomy. Provided the medial osteotomy has been done first as recommended, back fracture and bony spicules are rare.[16,42] High osteotomies—that is, away from the maxillary face—are satisfactory for some cosmetic rhinoplasties, but with deviated external noses, low complete osteotomies are advised. These require the creation of a transverse fracture that joins the medial and lateral osteotomies at their cephalic ends.

Debate still exists as to the benefits of elevating the periosteum overlying the osteotomy to preserve it or simply performing the osteotomy through the periosteum. The authors are firm believers in the subperiosteal approach. This is an avascular plane, and with minimal elevation laterally a periosteal blanket is preserved to drape over the osteotomy site. Without the periosteal elevation, the edge of the osteotome will lacerate the periosteum and perhaps traumatize the subcutaneous tissue as well. The lateral osteotomy may be performed through a horizontal intranasal incision at the piriform rim, an intraoral incision, or an alar attachment if this has been done as for the Weir procedure or for the cleft-lip nose. For the cases under discussion, in which there is often

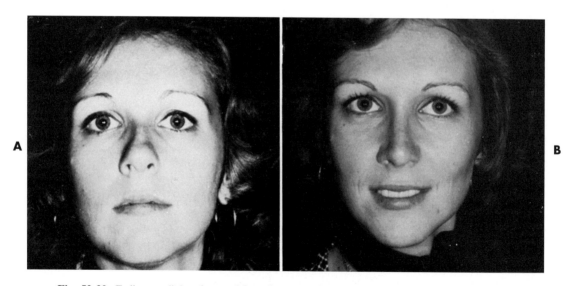

A   B

Fig. 52-30. Fading medial and curved lateral osteotomies in a twisted nose with a narrow nasal root. **A,** The narrow nasal root with deviation only in the inferior portion of the nasal bones. Dislocation of the caudal edge of the septum is also apparent in this anterior view. Fading or curved medial osteotomies combined with the slightly higher curved lateral osteotomy are advocated in such a case. **B,** Postoperative result where there was no need to fracture the narrow medial portion of the nasal bones.

Continued

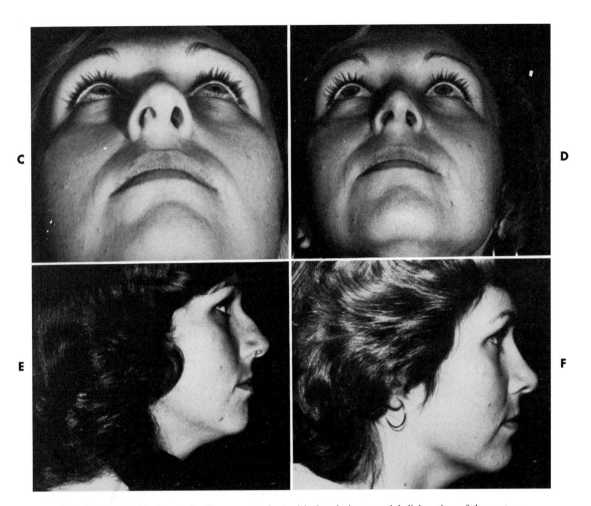

Fig. 52-30, cont'd. C and **D,** The same patient with the obvious caudal dislocation of the septum and some long-term distortion of the flare of the medial crus on the right side. The nose was adequately straightened, the tip projection maintained, and the caudal septum held in position. There is persistent flaring of the distorted foot of the medial crus. **E,** The profile also demonstrates the caudal dislocation of the septum into the right nostril, the need for conservative hump removal, tip projection, and a small chin implant. **F,** Postoperative result. (See also Figs. 52-16, 52-18, and 52-21 for management of the caudal septum.)

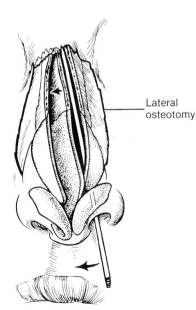

Lateral osteotomy

Fig. 52-31. Correction of central component deviation. For deviations of the entire root of the nose or the remaining central component of the nose, it is necessary to establish a firm fulcrum with the osteotome to fracture this central portion toward the midline. This difficult maneuver requires a complete medial osteotomy paralleling the septum as close as possible, as opposed to the fading medial osteotomy.

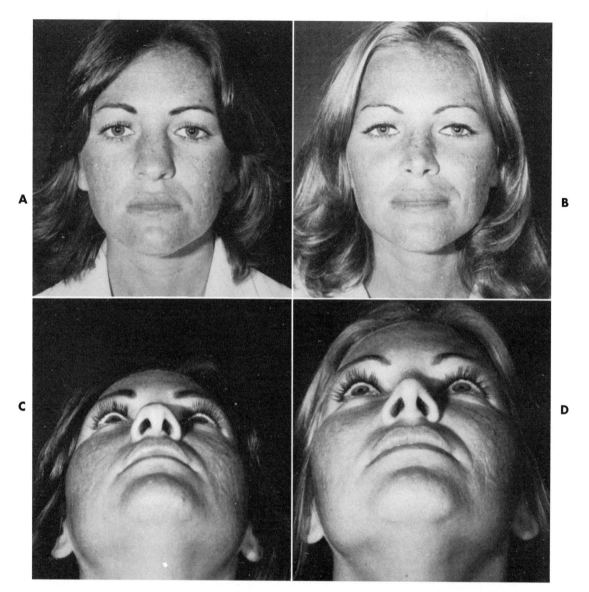

Fig. 52-32. Complete and intermediate osteotomies. **A,** This case demonstrates the flattened, wide nose with outward splaying of the nasal bones, and only minimal change in the profile is required. This patient would require narrowing of the nose, which is accomplished in many cases by the use of an intermediate osteotomy placed halfway between the complete medial and low lateral osteotomies. **B,** Results of this surgery combined with an autogenous cartilage columella implant. The cartilaginous dorsum has been narrowed without changing the profile. **C** and **D,** Basal views of the same patient before and after narrowing with tip sculpturing and increases in tip projection and columella support. (See also Fig. 52-29.)

already a great deal of intranasal scarring resulting from mucosal trauma or extensive earlier surgery, the authors prefer to approach through the buccal sulcus, avoiding additional intranasal incisions and possible circumferential scarring.

In revisional surgery when there is prominence of the previous osteotomy site, multiple osteotomies or fragmentation over this site seems to produce a more acceptable result than simply rasping the area or repeating the single osteotomy.

Making the final septal assessment

It is not until all septal reconstructive surgery and the osteotomies are completed that the final analysis of the position of the septum can be made. This position is particularly critical to the junction of the bony and cartilaginous portions of the nose, both internally and externally. At this point, the surgeon can determine whether adequate dorsal support has been maintained. Should there be any tendency for the cartilaginous dorsum to sink inward, a draw suture can be passed

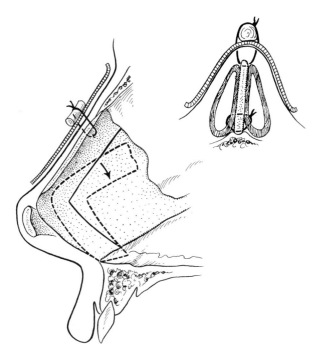

Fig. 52-33. Dorsal draw suture. If there is loss of support either from injury or surgery at the junction of the septal cartilage with the nasal bones and perpendicular plate of the ethmoid, the remaining caudal septum tilts downward *(arrows)*. A draw suture may be passed through the skin of the dorsum of the nose and then used to pick up either the septum alone or the septum with the upper lateral cartilages. The draw suture is then passed through a soft thin metal nasal splint and tied over a bolus. Dorsal draw sutures may be utilized simply to maintain the position and support while all intranasal surgery is completed and the nose is packed. The sutures are then removed. When necessary, the sutures may remain in position for 1 week, and are removed with the splint.

through the skin to pick up either the septum alone or the upper lateral cartilages and the septum along the dorsum (Fig. 52-33). The suture is passed upward through the skin and held in position while all coapting and supporting sutures are placed and packing is completed. The draw suture can then be removed. In extreme cases, the draw suture can be passed through a thin external metal splint and tied over a bolus to remain in place for a week until the splint is removed.

Intranasal dressing

The senior author is a strong proponent of precise combined internal and external splinting of the nose. Attention should be paid to carefully suturing the septal flaps and then placing a limited amount of packing in the nose. This intranasal dressing assists in preventing bleeding and postoperative edema. The use of coaptation sutures has eliminated the absolute need for packing, especially for cosmetic rhinoplasty or cases in which limited septal surgery is done. In cases in which there has been major septal reconstruction and bilateral mucoperichondrial elevation, packing and in

special instances the use of polyethylene plates may be required. With materials available at this time, packing consists of folded Telfa sheeting into which strips of nasal tampon are inserted. The strips are used because discomfort and bleeding are minimal when they are carefully removed one at a time along their long axis. Unfolding long strips of gauze or a wider wad of tampon is not advised.

IMPLANTS

Over a 30-year period the use of any synthetic material for nasal implantation has been disappointing in regard to long-term results. The authors prefer using only autogenous materials in the nose, and preferably nasal tissue.* If there is not enough material available from the nose, auricular cartilage is the second choice; it can be used for lesser defects, in which support is not a major factor. If a strong columella strut remains after septal reconstruction to assist in tip support, sculptured auricular cartilage frequently will prove to be adequate. For the severe saddle nose deformity, autogenous cancellous bone from the hip is used for the dorsum, and cartilage is used for the columella strut (Figs. 52-34 and 52-35). Homograft costal cartilage that has been irradiated to 3 million rads is readily carved and is well tolerated in the nose. The authors suggest that the reader give irradiated cartilage consideration, along with calcium triphosphate (Ossoplast).[2,41] For lamination of smaller cartilage implants and positioning of implants, tissue glue (butyl-cyanoacrylate) may prove to have a useful clinical application.[33,36,39]

Gore-Tex implants

As filler implants, increased experience is being gained with the use of laminated Gore-Tex sheeting or the thicker subcutaneous augmentation material (SAM) facial implants of Gore-Tex.

Gore-Tex ePTFE has been useful in dorsal augmentation. The tolerance of Gore-Tex as implant material has been well documented.† In addition, minimal amounts of fibrous ingrowth lead to stability of the implant but do not restrict its removal when necessary. The reinforced sheets of 4.0 to 7.0 mm are much easier to sculpt for augmentation. With these implants and the sheeting, it is important to taper the edge to ensure smooth transition to the surrounding soft tissue. This can be done through sharp beveling using a scalpel or by crushing the margins with a hemostat or needle holder.

For the saddle nose deformity in which extensive septal surgery and osteotomies are required, it is sometimes best to stage the procedure, with the implants being placed at a second operation. Extensive septal reconstruction may be essential in completely straightening the nose and in increasing the vertical height, thereby making the required size of

*Refs. 2, 4, 6, 7, 11, 12, 21, 23, 34, 41.
†Refs. 18, 24, 25, 29, 37, 40.

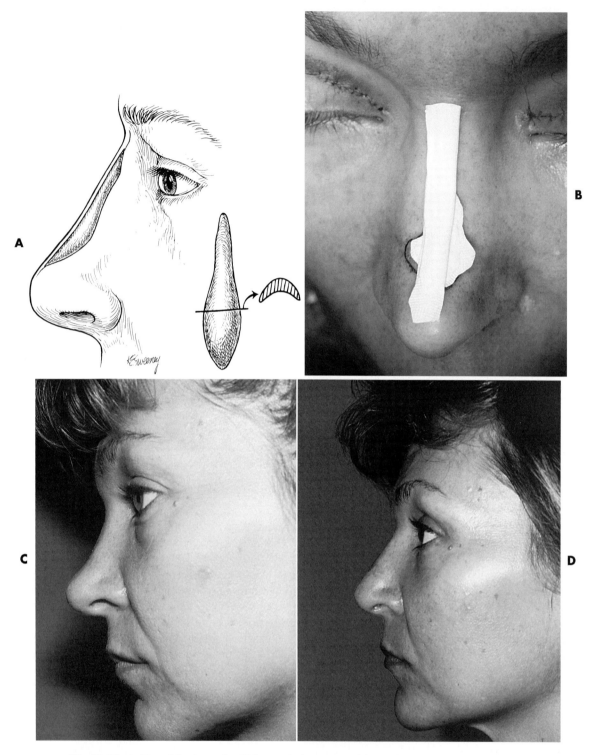

Fig. 52-34. A, Dorsal implants should be precisely contoured in three dimensions and preferably should extend the entire length of the nasal dorsum. Autogenous material is used, and when nasal tissue or auricular cartilage is not sufficient, cancellous bone from the hip is used. Iliac bone grafts have now largely been replaced by calvarial bone grafts. If iliac bone is used, more cortex is allowed to remain on the cancellous bone. **B,** Laminated Gore-Tex sheet for dorsal augmentation with tapering of the Gore-Tex margin by crushing the edge of the Gore-Tex with the hemostat and separate soft-tissue patch. **C,** Preoperative view of mild saddle-nose deformity and soft-tissue irregularity of the cartilaginous dorsum. **D,** Postoperative view with dorsal augmentation and soft-tissue filler of the left cartilaginous nasal dorsum.

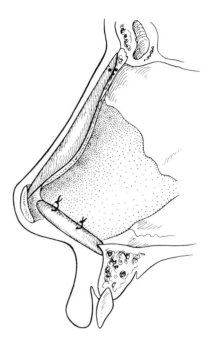

Fig. 52-35. Dorsal and columella implants. Two implants, in separate pockets, are preferred. The dorsal implant is wired to the nasal bones and passed beneath the lower lateral cartilages in the tip. For the columella strut, cartilage is preferred and can usually be obtained from the septum.

the implant smaller (Fig. 52-36). In the saddle nose the anterior valve is frequently circular rather than oval or piriform, and the septal reconstruction should be combined with intranasal Z-plasties to release the scar contractures and open the anterior valve areas.

One of the difficulties of rhinoplasty, and especially of revision rhinoplasty, is ensuring a smooth contour over the nasal dorsum. This can be especially difficult in thin-skinned patients when implants are used. Where there are skin irregularities and scarring or cicatricial adhesions to the underlying framework, it is necessary to prevent recurrence once elevated. Sculpted laminated autogenous cartilage implants of any sort may leave irregular edges or an irregular surface. One way of softening these edges and other irregularities involves draping a piece of temporalis fascia over the entire nasal framework, both bony and cartilaginous. The temporalis fascia graft can be placed through either an intercartilaginous incision or an open rhinoplasty approach. The graft is secured in position with 5-0 nylon draw sutures, which are then tied over a soft plastic bolus at the level of the nasal frontal angle at each corner and with direct suturing inferiorly, laterally, and at the dorsum. Precise, direct suturing can be accomplished through the open rhinoplasty approach. Temporalis fascia has been shown not to resorb significantly *in vivo,*[28] and donor site morbidity is minimal. This fascial graft technique is an important part of the surgical armamentarium, particularly for revision rhinoplasty, dorsal irregularities, scars, and overlying implants (Fig. 52-37). The senior

author has had experience over the past 6 years with thin 0.4-mm cardiovascular sheeting in place of the fascia and has had no reaction or extrusions (Fig. 52-37 *D, E*).

NASAL BASE MODIFICATIONS

There are numerous modifications of the Weir procedure, which involve the excision of triangles, wedges, or crescents from the alar base on either side. These are usually done to narrow the nasal base and are usually combined with procedures to increase tip projection through added columella support and lengthening. The technique used most often for the extremely wide nose combines narrowing the nasal base and reducing the length of the ala. For all of these procedures, a subcutaneous suture is placed to reduce tension on the repositioned ala and maintain it in its new position. Modification of the alar base is, of course, a major consideration in both the unilateral and the bilateral cleft-lip nasal deformity, as will be discussed later (Figs. 52-38 through 52-40).

ALAR SOFT-TISSUE SCULPTURING

The procedures described earlier may be combined with surgery for the thick inferior border of the ala, which requires excision and thinning (see Fig. 52-40). Further sculpturing may be required to arch the ala in correcting alar hooding. In sculpturing or thinning the ala or nostril margin, one should make the excision slightly toward the nostril side. This not only makes the scar less visible but also creates a more natural roll to the border. The procedure is usually combined with a columella strut or other procedure to create greater columella "show" relative to the alar margin. Other techniques may be used to create greater columella prominence, such as the use of a composite auricular graft or skin and cartilage transposition flaps from the cephalic border of the lower lateral cartilages.

THE EXTRAMUCOSAL APPROACH

Preservation of an intact mucosal lining wherever possible is an important principle, especially beneath the nasal dorsum. This is readily accomplished when the external rhinoplasty approach is used and may be achieved in the standard rhinoplasty when submucosal tunnels are created under the upper lateral cartilages. With this intranasal degloving, mucosa can be preserved to provide additional mucosa for the closure of perforations or for lengthening the nose. However, when a major reduction rhinoplasty has been performed the extra mucosa may create problems by herniating into the dorsum. Also, when there is a severely twisted nose or when there is extensive intranasal scarring and contracture, it may be necessary to completely separate the upper lateral cartilages and their mucosa from the septum. No complications have been observed when this is done, and there can be advantages in trimming the upper lateral cartilage and mucosa on the long lateral vault of the deviated nose.[8,22]

The retracted or elevated alar margin may be difficult to

Text continued on p. 1023

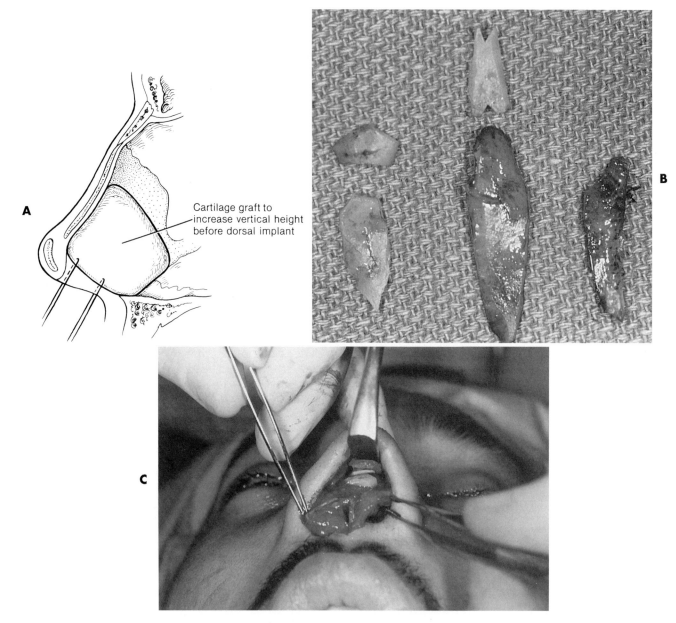

Fig. 52-36. A, The septum and the saddle nose deformity. Straightened septal cartilage can be reinserted as a large columella strut in order to increase the vertical height of the nose and provide support for the dorsal implant. **B,** Cartilage implants taken from the nasal septum. **C,** Laminated cartilage implants to be sutured in position via the open approach. Irregularities may be smoothed out by a blanket of temporalis fascia or Gore-Tex sheeting. (See also Fig. 52-37.)

Cartilage graft to increase vertical height before dorsal implant

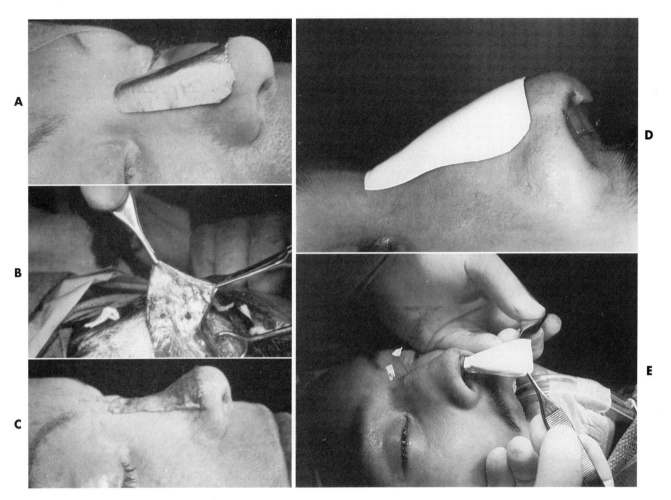

Fig. 52-37. In addressing the nose with thin skin and bony cartilaginous irregularities, such as laminated implants, a temporalis fascia graft may be useful. **A,** The template fashioned to the size of the graft to be taken. **B,** Harvesting the temporalis fascia graft through a vertical incision through a shaved portion of the temporal scalp. **C,** Facial graft draped over the nasal dorsum before insertion into the subcutaneous pocket over the nasal dorsum. **D,** Cardiovascular Gore-Tex sheeting placed as a blanket over the dorsum to smooth out any irregularities. **E,** As with temporalis fascia, Gore-Tex sheeting is carried into position with draw sutures. Inferiorly, the thin sheeting may be precisely sutured into position, especially with the open approach.

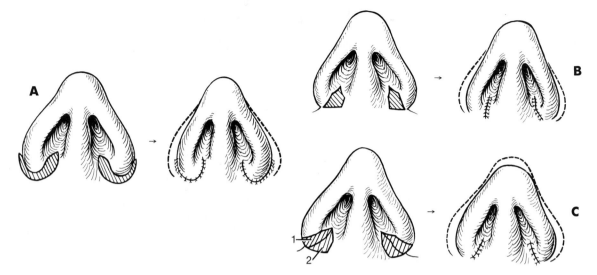

Fig. 52-38. Management of the nasal base. **A,** The authors' technique done predominantly to narrow the nasal base. The superior incision, which is the inside of a curve, is lengthened by curving to meet the outer incision in the floor of the nose and laterally. This equalizes the two sides of the excision for closure. The authors use subcuticular sutures as well as fine skin sutures. **B,** Narrowing the nasal base by excising a wedge from the floor of the nose. **C,** A commonly performed procedure that narrows the base and reduces the height of the alae.

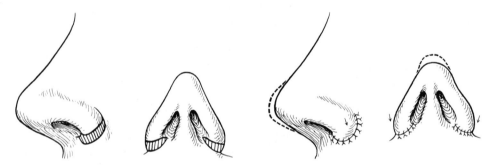

Fig. 52-39. Alar wedge excision to reduce the height of the ala and reduce tip projection. Excision of the ala laterally must be combined with other procedures for the tip and septal angle.

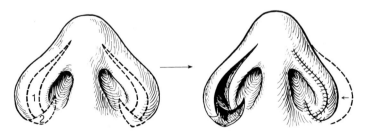

Fig. 52-40. Combined reduction and thinning of the alae. For noses with excessive thickening of the ala, a wedge of skin is removed extending toward the tip. This incision should be slightly internal or toward the nasal side of the vestibule to create a more desirable roll and hide the incision.

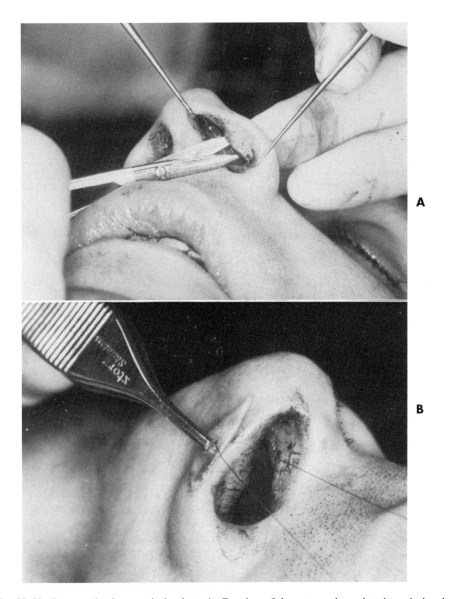

Fig. 52-41. Retrograde alar margin implant. **A,** Creation of the retrograde pocket through the alar cartilage margin incision down to the rim. **B,** The sculptured cartilage implant is brought into the pocket with draw sutures and held in position with transalar sutures tied over a tin polyethylene film. (See also Fig. 52-42.)

correct. Strips of cartilage from the cephalic segment of the lower lateral cartilages or the septum may be inserted into an incision within the vestibule of the nose to serve as a filler and support (Figs. 52-41 and 52-42). These implants are held in position with transalar monofilament nylon sutures carried over a thin plastic film on the external surface. A strip of composite graft including the thin skin of the anterior surface of the auricle may be necessary if there is a deficiency of lining skin.

THE CLEFT-LIP NOSE

The cleft-lip nasal deformity requires special attention to the asymmetric and retrodisplaced lower lateral cartilage in the unilateral cleft and to the depressed tip with a relatively short columella in the bilateral cleft. Associated with the deformity is hypoplasia of the maxilla on the cleft side or bilaterally, with midfacial hypoplasia resulting from the lack of mesodermal penetration (Fig. 52-43).

The unilateral cleft-lip nasal deformity is asymmetric and complex, and one drawing cannot bring out all three-dimensional aspects of the deformity. Major characteristics include the retrodisplacement of the lower lateral cartilage on the involved side, with an S-shaped deformity of the cartilage and soft tissue. There is thickening of the ala laterally, and the alar base is laterally and inferiorly displaced with a loss of the alar-facial angle. Classically the caudal end of the septum is dislocated toward the normal side, along with the anterior nasal spine and columella base. Internally, there is

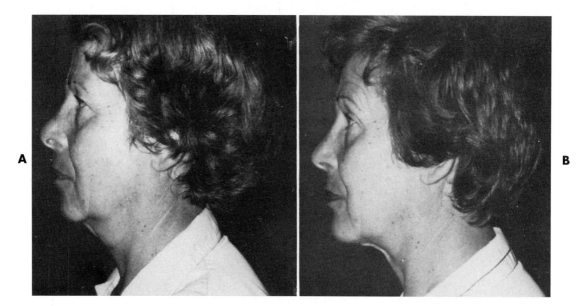

Fig. 52-42. Cephalad retraction of the alar margin. **A,** Postoperative complications: the all too frequent supratip swelling or polly-beak deformity and cephalic retraction of the lateral alar margin. **B,** Correction is accomplished by reducing the cartilaginous nasal septum and removing supratip fibrous tissue, further sculpturing the lower lateral cartilages, freeing the lateral crus, and inserting a cartilage implant retrograde along the alar margin. (See also Fig. 52-41.)

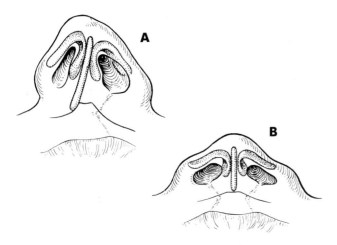

Fig. 52-43. Cleft-tip nasal deformities. **A,** Unilateral cleft-lip deformity. **B,** Bilateral cleft-lip deformity. (See also Fig. 52-10.)

often a large posterior spur extending into the cleft side. The maxilla is underdeveloped on the involved side because of the lack of mesodermal development and penetration. The dome of the lower lateral cartilage on the cleft side is depressed, resulting in a lack of tip projection on that side. There is usually an excessively wide nasal floor on the cleft side, although stenosis may occur following childhood surgical repair of the lip and nasal floor.

The bilateral cleft-lip nasal deformity is much more complex than the unilateral deformity. There is frequently underdevelopment of the entire premaxilla and prolabium, with a short caudal septum as well as a short columella. Further, in the secondary deformity, there is flattening of the ala with little tip angulation or projection and bilateral widening of the nasal floor and flattening of the alar–facial angle.

Although soft-tissue repair can be readily accomplished at the time of initial lip repair or as revisional surgery, reconstruction will always be inadequate if the asymmetry of cartilage and bone is not addressed.

The authors frequently use the external approach for both the unilateral and the bilateral cleft-lip nasal deformities.[10,141] In the unilateral cleft-lip nasal deformity, the lateral crus of the lower lateral cartilage on the cleft side is dissected free of both surface and vestibular skin, and the cartilage is advanced medially to match the normal side (Figs. 52-10 and 52-44). The position is maintained with sutures to the opposite dome to project the tip on the cleft side, along with sutures through the vestibular skin, cartilage, and surface skin (see Fig. 52-44). These transalar sutures of 5-0 monofilament nylon are tied over a thin flat plastic bolus on the surface skin side only. With the open rhinoplasty it is possible, under direct vision, to stabilize the involved lateral crus further by suturing it directly to the upper lateral cartilage or septum (Fig. 52-45). This is particularly important when the cleft side is caudally displaced, resulting in a hooding deformity.

In the unilateral cleft-lip deformity, particular attention must be paid to the dislocation of the caudal septum toward the normal side and the posterior nasal septal spur on the cleft side. All septorhinoplasty techniques may be useful in correcting the cleft-lip nasal deformity, and onlay grafts are

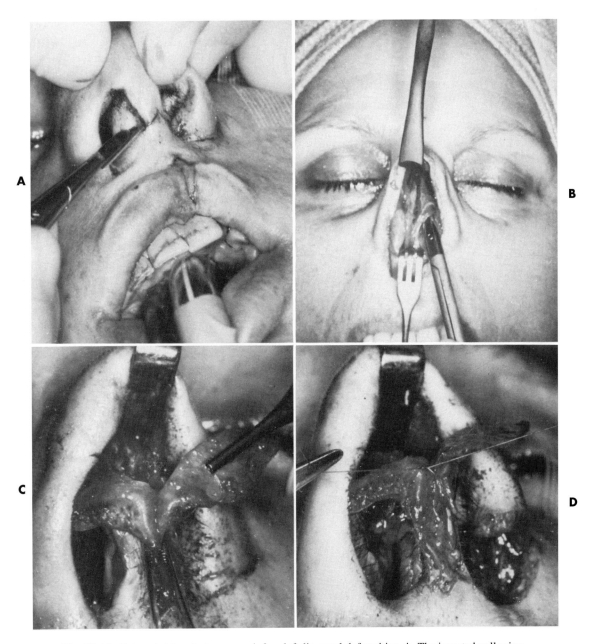

Fig. 52-44. External rhinoplasty approach for cleft-lip nasal deformities. **A,** The inverted gull-wing incision is made below the base of the medial crura. **B,** The lower lateral cartilages are dissected free of the overlying dorsal skin and underlying vestibular skin. The two lateral crura are trimmed and shaped until they are symmetric. In this case the upper lateral cartilages have been sutured under direct vision to the septum along the dorsum. **C,** Complete exposure of the lower lateral cartilage on the cleft side, freeing it of both surface and vestibular skin, allows precise repositioning and sandwiching between the two skin surfaces. **D,** The two medial crura are sutured together, recruiting the lateral crus on the cleft side to project the tip on the unilateral cleft side, or on both sides in the bilateral cleft deformity.

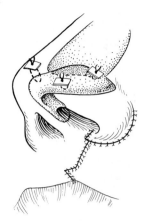

Fig. 52-45. Suturing the medial crura together in the dome, sometimes with slight overcorrection for the retrodisplaced cartilage on the cleft side. Lower lateral cartilage overlaps inferior edge of upper lateral cartilage.

frequently necessary beneath the alar base on the cleft side (Figs. 52-46 and 52-47). In the bilateral cleft-lip deformity, the cartilages can be precisely sculptured bilaterally and dissected free of both skin surfaces to allow medial recruitment and suturing to project the tip (Fig. 52-48).

Grafts are combined with high Le Fort's I osteotomies to advance the maxilla in severe deformities associated with both unilateral and bilateral cleft lip.[30] Both maxillary and mandibular osteotomies may be required. There is some choice between suspension and intermaxillary wiring and mini-plate fixation.[19,20] Occlusion must be precise and is combined with interdental splinting and fixation. Bone grafts are placed between the advanced maxilla and the pterygoid plates, over the face of the maxilla, and about the piriform rim (Figs. 52-49 and 52-50).

For the bilateral cleft-lip deformity, a variety of columella-lengthening procedures have been developed. Selection depends on the severity of the deformity and what previous surgery has been performed. The most commonly used procedures for lengthening the skin of the columella are the

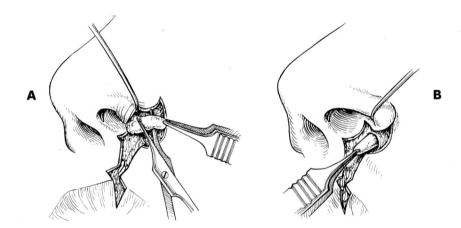

Fig. 52-46. Lateral ala thinning and placement of maxillary implants. **A,** Any excessive fibrous tissue at the alar attachment is removed subcutaneously between the vestibular skin and external skin surfaces. **B,** Through the alar incision, implant material of cartilage or bone, usually obtained from the nose, is placed over the face of the maxilla beneath the lip scar and the alar base. (See also Fig. 52-10.)

Fig. 52-47. Repositioning and suturing of the lower lateral cartilage. **A,** The alar cartilage is repositioned in a slight overcorrection. A subcutaneous suture should be used to reinforce the repositioning of the alar base in a symmetric position. **B,** A composite of the complete operation shows the septal reconstruction, correction of the distorted alar cartilage, and correction of the laterally displaced alar base. Bone and cartilage grafts are placed subperiosteally over the face of the maxilla. Fixation sutures are tied over flat, plastic boluses externally.

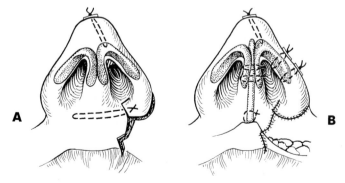

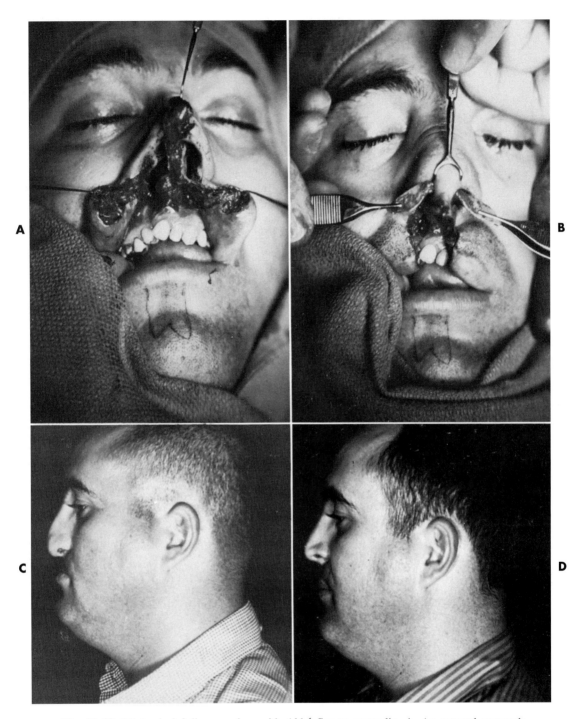

Fig. 52-48. Bilateral cleft-lip procedure with Abbé flap to upper lip. **A,** An external approach utilizing a transfixion incision. This differs from the external approach more recently popularized, in which the exposure is external to the medial crura rather than internal to the medial crura in the membranous septum. The synchronous lip repair is done with an asymmetric Abbé flap because of the stenosis on the right side. **B,** The lower lateral cartilages are presented bilaterally through the standard alar cartilage margin incisions and dissected free of both surface and vestibular skin so that they may be advanced into the tip, sutured together, and fixed between the surface and vestibular skin. **C,** Preoperative profile, demonstrating the disparity between the lips, and between maxilla and mandible, and illustrating the fact that the prolabium had been removed. **D,** Postoperative appearance. Autogenous cartilage implants have been placed in the columella, and bone and cartilage from the nose have been placed over the face of the maxilla.

Continued

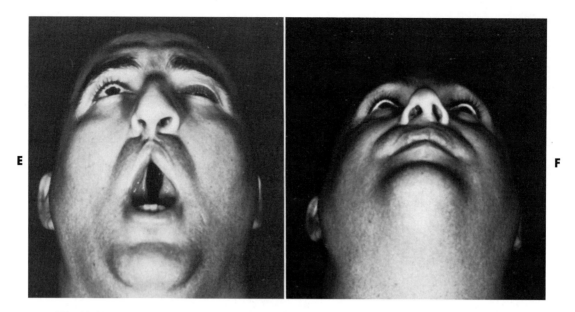

Fig. 52-48, cont'd. E, Basal view showing the absence of a prolabium, and the stenosis of the right nasal vestibule. The palate has never been repaired. **F,** Postoperative view showing the tip projection, columella lengthening, and asymmetric Abbé flap. The flap was later defatted in the floor of the right nostril.

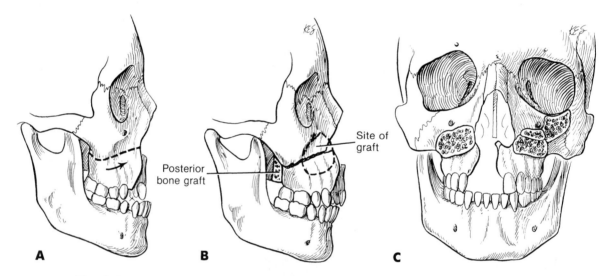

Fig. 52-49. Le Fort's I maxillary osteotomies to correct underdevelopment of the maxilla. **A,** When the deformity includes severe malocclusion, onlay grafts alone are not adequate, and a Le Fort I osteotomy should be performed. **B,** Bone grafts are placed posteriorly between the maxilla and the pterygoid bones. **C,** Onlay grafts over the face of the maxilla may be required as well. Maxillary repositioning must be coordinated with an orthodontist; there must be preoperative planning and placement of an intradental splint.

forked flap of Millard (Fig. 52-51)[26] and the advancement flap from the floor of the nose of Brauer and Cronin (Fig. 52-52).[5] Both of these procedures provide augmentation of the columella and, when combined with techniques to project the domes of the lower lateral cartilages, result in a marked improvement in the patient's appearance.

When stenosis of the nasal airway is present, the above techniques can be used for managing the lower lateral cartilage and septal and alar deformities, but the alar attachment must be displaced laterally to open the airway. The floor is widened with a V to Y advancement laterally (Fig. 52-53).

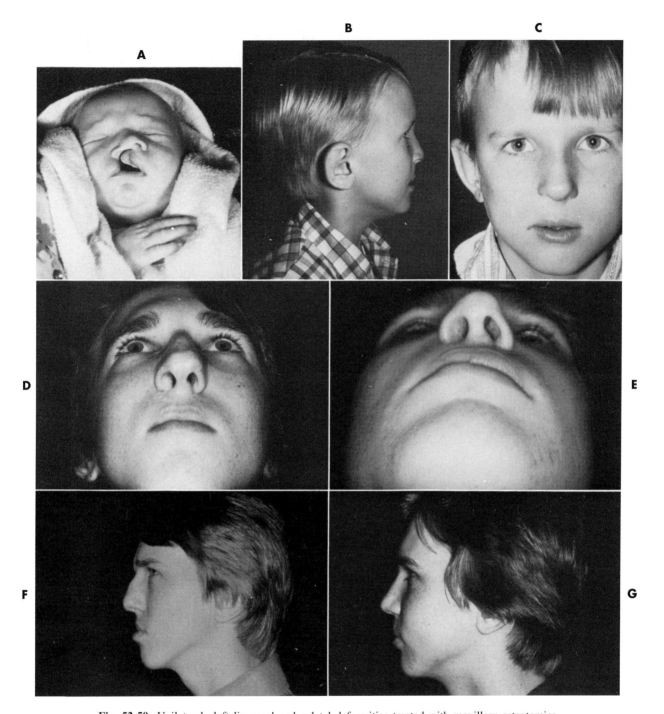

Fig. 52-50. Unilateral cleft lip nasal and palatal deformities treated with maxillary osteotomies. The senior author performed the original repair of the unilateral cleft lip and palate. The preoperative photography (**A**) demonstrates the severity of the deformity and emphasizes the lack of mesodermal penetration in the right maxilla. **B** and **C,** Early postoperative results after lip and palate repair that reveal interval profile with satisfactory nasal appearance and maxillary and mandibular relationships. **D** and **E,** A later result showing the changes that have occurred in the nasal base with correction of the caudal septal dislocation. **F** and **G,** Preoperative and postoperative appearances following a Le Fort's I osteotomy and autogenous bone implants along with a revision rhinoplasty at 18 years of age.

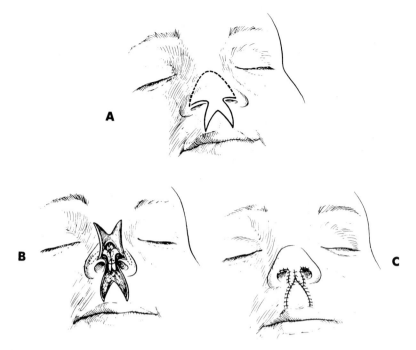

Fig. 52-51. Millard's forked flap technique for lengthening the columella. **A,** Each flap should be carefully designed for proper length and width. Modifications may be necessary, depending on the degree and location of the lip scarring. **B,** Millard's technique should be combined with an external rhinoplasty approach to increase nasal tip projection. **C,** The lip flaps are advanced upward to augment the columella.

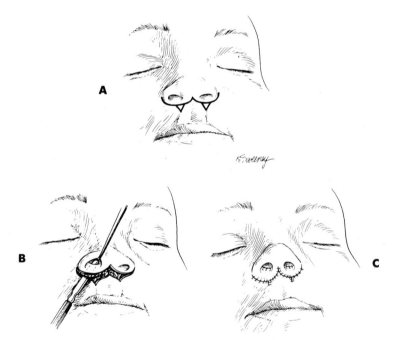

Fig. 52-52. The Cronin technique for lengthening the columella. **A,** Incisions are made beneath the nasal sills bilaterally. **B,** The nasal sills are dissected free bilaterally and advanced medially to elongate the columella. The Burow triangles may be excised in the bilateral cleft-lip scars. A columella strut should be sutured into position to maintain the tip projection. **C,** The incisions are closed, advancing the nasal sill tissue upward to augment the columella.

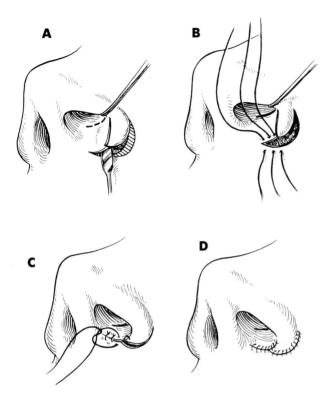

Fig. 52-53. Correction of nostril stenosis by increasing the width of the nasal floor. **A,** A laterally based V incision is made across the nasal sill, and a crescent of skin is excised laterally. **B,** The alar base is advanced laterally. **C,** The nasal sill is closed, advancing the alar base as a V to Y. **D,** The alar–facial incision is closed.

SUMMARY

This chapter is intended to emphasize the great variety of nasal and nasal septal deformities that can occur and the many surgical techniques that may be required to correct them. The combined internal and external deviations, dislocations, and twists require combined internal and external surgical correction. To achieve adequate correction, the surgeon's armamentarium must include the full spectrum of advanced and sophisticated techniques for septal reconstruction and corrective rhinoplasty.

The stigma of the cleft lip is often accentuated by a residual nasal deformity. As soft-tissue techniques improve, it is often the nasal deformity that draws attention to the lip. Because of the distortions created by a lack of mesodermal penetration, there will frequently be persistent nasal deformities no matter how well the lip and nasal abnormalities are repaired at the time of primary repair. The cleft-lip nasal deformity presents unique surgical problems, which may be very difficult to solve. Use of both intranasal and external rhinoplasty techniques has been discussed.

The patient with a severe nasal deformity should not leave the surgeon's care breathing less well than he or she did before the operation. These patients with complicated nasal deformities deserve the surgeon's critical attention to func-

tion as well as appearance during the planning of surgical correction. In the majority of cases the aesthetic appearance is markedly improved even when a major reorganization of the nasal framework is required.

REFERENCES

1. Becker OJ: Problems of septum in rhinoplastic surgery, *Arch Otolaryngol* 53:622, 1951.
2. Bull TR, MacKay IS: Augmentation rhinoplasty, *Facial Plast Surg* 1(2):125, 1984.
3. Converse JM: Corrective surgery of nasal deviations, *Arch Otolaryngol* 52:671, 1950.
4. Converse JM, Becker OJ, Peer LA: Implants in nasal plastic surgery: a panel discussion, *Trans Am Acad Ophthalmol Otolaryngol* 59:522, 1955.
5. Cronin TD: Lengthening columella by use of skin from nasal floor and alae, *Plast Reconstr Surg* 21:417, 1958.
6. Dingman RO: The use of iliac bone in the repair of facial and cranial defects, *Plast Reconstr Surg* 43:117, 1969.
7. Dingman RO, Walter C: Use of composite ear grafts in correction of the short nose, *Plast Reconstr Surg* 43:117, 1969.
8. Fairbanks D, Fairbanks G: Nasal septal perforation: prevention and management, *Ann Plast Surg* 5(6):452, 1980.
9. Farrior EH, Farrior RT: *The septocolumella complex.* In Stucker FJ, editor: *Reconstructive surgery of the head and neck: proceedings of the international symposium,* ch 1, Philadelphia, 1991, Mosby.
10. Farrior RT: The problem of the unilateral cleft-lip nose, *Laryngoscope* 72(3):289, 1962.
11. Farrior RT: Implant materials in restoration of facial contour, *Laryngoscope* 76(5):934, 1966.
12. Farrior RT: Synthetics in head and neck surgery, *Arch Otolaryngol* 84: 82, 1966.
13. Farrior RT: Modifications in rhinoplasty: where and when, *Trans Am Acad Ophthalmol Otolaryngol* 78:341, 1974.
14. Farrior RT: *The cleft-lip nose (septorhinoplasty and combined lip repair).* In Sisson GA, Tardy EM, editors: *Plastic and reconstructive surgery of the face and neck: proceedings of the second international symposium,* vol 1, New York, 1977, Grune & Stratton.
15. Farrior RT: The osteotomy in rhinoplasty, *Laryngoscope* 88(9):1449, 1978.
16. Farrior RT: *Corrective and reconstructive surgery of the external nose.* In Naumann HH, editor: *Head and neck surgery,* Stuttgart, 1980, Thieme.
17. Farrior RT: *Management of the late sequelae of nasal fractures.* In Mathog RH, editor: *Maxillofacial trauma,* Baltimore, 1984, Williams & Wilkins.
18. Farrior EH, Hall PJ, Farrior RT: The use of Gore-Tex ePTFE in rhinoplasty. Presented to Southern Section of American Academy of Facial Plastic and Reconstructive Surgery. January, 1992, Birmingham, Ala.
19. Farrior RT: The cleft lip nose: an update, *Facial Plast Surg* 9(4):241, 1993.
20. Farrior RT, Pennington JH: In Stucker FJ, editor: *Plastic and reconstructive surgery of the head and neck: proceedings of the fifth international symposium,* ch 129, Philadelphia, 1991; Mosby.
21. Gibson T, Curran C, Davis WB: The long-term survival of cartilage homografts in man, *Br J Plast Surg* 11:177, 1958.
22. Goodman WS: Recent advances in external rhinoplasty, *J Otolaryngol* 10:433, 1981.
23. Guerrerosantos J: Temporoparietal free fascia grafts in rhinoplasty, *Plast Reconstr Surg* 11(3):491, 1984.
24. Maas CS, Gnepp DR, Bumpous J: Expanded polytetrafluoroethylene (Gore-Tex) in facial augmentation. Presented before American Academy of Facial Plastic and Reconstructive Surgery. January, 1992, Beverly Hills, Calif.

25. Matsumoto H and others: A new vascular prosthesis for small caliber artery, *Surgery* 74:519, 1973.

26. Millard DR: Columella lengthening by a forked flap, *Plast Reconstr Surg* 22:454, 1958.

27. Millard DR: Secondary corrective rhinoplasty, *Plast Reconstr Surg* 44:545, 1969.

28. Miller TA: Temporalis fascia grafts for facial and nasal augmentation, *Plast Reconstr Surg* 81:524, 1988.

29. Neel HB: Implants of Gore-Tex, *Arch Otolaryngol* 109:428, 1983.

30. Obwegeser HL: Surgical correction of small or retroplaced maxillae, "the dish face deformity," *Plast Reconstr Surg* 43:351, 1969.

31. Peer LA: Fate of autogenous septal cartilage after transplantation in human tissue, *Arch Otolaryngol* 34:697, 1941.

32. Rees TD, Krupp S, Wood-Smith D: Secondary rhinoplasty, *Plast Reconstr Surg* 46:332, 1970.

33. Sachs ME: Enbrucrilate as cartilage adhesive in augmentation rhinoplasty, *Arch Otolaryngol* 3:389, 1985.

34. Sheen JH: Achieving more nasal tip projection by the use of a small autogenous bone or cartilage graft, *Plast Reconstr Surg* 56:35, 1975.

35. Sheen JH: Secondary rhinoplasty, *Plast Reconstr Surg* 56:137, 1975.

36. Staindl O: Indications of the fibrin sealant in facial plastic surgery, *Facial Plast Surg* 2(4):323, 1985.

37. Stoll W: The use of polytetrafluoroethylene for particular augmentation of the nasal dorsum, *Esthet Plast Surg* 15:233, 1991.

38. Strezlow VV: External septorhinoplasty approach to septal surgery, *Facial Plast Surg* 2(1):65, 1984.

39. Vinazzer H: Fibrin sealing: physiologic and biochemical background, *Facial Plast Surg* 2(4):291, 1985.

40. Waldman RS: Gore-Tex for augmentation of the nasal dorsum: preliminary report, *Ann Plast Surg* 26:520, 1991.

41. Walter C, Brunt PB: Tricalciumphosphate as an implant material: preliminary report, *Br J Plast Surg* 35:510, 1982.

42. Wright WK: General principles of lateral osteotomy and hump removal, *Trans Am Acad Ophthalmol Otolaryngol* 65:854, 1961.

SUGGESTED READINGS

Broadbent TR, Woolf RM: Anatomy of a rhinoplasty—saw technique, *Ann Plast Surg* 13(1):67, 1984.

Broadbent TR, Woolf RM: Basic anatomy: clinical application in rhinoplasty, *Ann Plast Surg* 13(1):76, 1984.

Converse JM: *Reconstructive plastic surgery*, vols II and III, Philadelphia, 1964, WB Saunders.

Converse JM and others: *Deformities of the nose. In Reconstructive plastic surgery*, vol 2, Philadelphia, 1964, WB Saunders.

Denecke HJ, Meyer R: *Plastic surgery of the head and neck, corrective and reconstructive rhinoplasty*, New York, 1967, Springer-Verlag.

Diamond H: Rhinoplasty techniques, *Surg Clin North Am* 51:317, 1971.

Herber SC, Lehman JA: Orthognathic surgery in the cleft lip and palate patient, *Clin Plast Surg* 20(4):755, 1993.

Johnson CM, Toriumi DM: *Open structure rhinoplasty*, Philadelphia, 1990, WB Saunders.

Joseph J: Nasenplastik und sonstige Gesichtplastik: nebst einem Anhang über Mammaplastik und einige weitere Operationen aus dem Gebiete der ausseren Korperplastik, Leipzig, 1931, Kabitzsch.

Meyer R: Correction of rhinoplasty complications. Transactions of the Vth International Congress on Plastic and Reconstructive Surgery, Melbourne, 1971, Butterworth.

Meyer R: *Secondary and functional rhinoplasty, the difficult nose*, Orlando, Fla, 1988, Grune & Stratton.

Rees TD, Guy CL, Converse JM: Repair of the cleft lip nose: addendum to the synchronous technique with full thickness skin grafting of the nasal vestibule, *Plast Reconstr Surg* 37:47, 1966.

Rees TD, Wood-Smith D: *Rhinoplasty. In Cosmetic facial surgery*, Philadelphia, 1973, WB Saunders.

Tardy ME, Brown RT: *Surgical anatomy of the nose*, New York, 1990, Raven Press.

Chapter 53

Revision Rhinoplasty

J. Regan Thomas
Gregory H. Branham

This chapter covers a variety of postsurgical problems that present frequently after rhinoplasty. No discussion within the context of a single chapter can deal with every possible event related to nasal surgery. However, there are general categories of surgical problems that represent more common entities that occur after rhinoplasty. With the realization that these categories are represented clinically by different degrees of severity or by variations of the basic category, it is possible to suggest steps to correct complications.

Revision rhinoplasty is contrasted as much as possible with those problems related to inadequate preoperative evaluation. For example, a secondary revision of the nasal profile that was not adequately reduced in the initial surgery is not correction of a complication. It is an incomplete correction of the profile or a misjudgment of the amount of correction required at the time of the initial surgery. Proper initial evaluation and preoperative assessment are tremendously important steps in rhinoplasty. It is important, however, to differentiate incomplete corrections from complications which have occurred despite adequate preoperative assessment of nasal anatomic structures or aesthetic goals.

Revision surgery is occasionally required under the care of experienced surgeons. Rhinoplasty is often characterized as the most demanding and difficult facial plastic procedure. It is an operation in which millimeters make a difference, therefore revisions will be required from time to time. Prevention is the key to avoiding revision. The knowledge of anatomic variations that are more likely to be at risk for postoperative sequelae is a hallmark of the proficient surgeon. Corrections in revision rhinoplasty may require dealing with various degrees of scarring, asymmetries, or other irregularities of the healing process. These technical difficulties are compounded typically by the patient's inability to comprehend the complexities encountered in revision surgery. Patients' expectations are usually greater than the results that can realistically be attained. The surgeon should counsel the patient to expect improvement rather than perfection.

This chapter is divided into sections: the lower third of the nose (nasal tip area); and the upper two thirds of the nose. Some revision surgery may require work in both areas. However, the preoperative evaluation and operative steps are divided into tip structure strategies and nasal dorsum, bony or cartilaginous corrective surgical consideration (Fig. 53-1).

LOWER ONE THIRD OF THE NOSE AND NASAL TIP

Knowledge of the anatomic factors contributing to tip shape and support is essential to correction of tip abnormalities. Frequently, the goals of reconstructive surgery in the nasal tip are focused on reconstructing tip structures back to normal anatomy. Two categories of considerations in revision rhinoplasty exist. The first includes situations that were unrecognized or not accurately addressed in the primary rhinoplasty. The second category is composed of iatrogenically-created asymmetric relationships of tip anatomic structures. These deformities include unequal division or resection of cartilage, formation of bossae or angulations, and asymmetric placement of sutures and tip grafts. Scar contracture or unfavorable fibrosis and healing also may contribute to these nasal tip abnormalities.

Soft tissue consideration

Various skin reactions may occur postoperatively. Fortunately, most are reversible and do not present long-term problems.

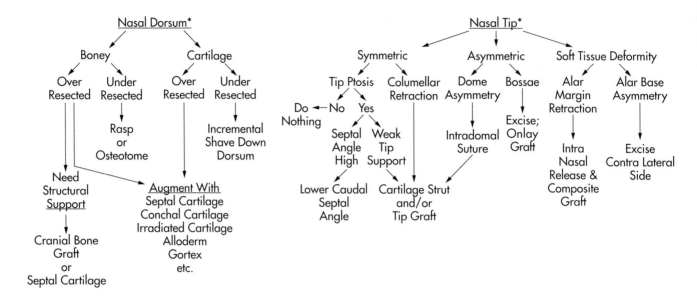

*Each Component Should be Considered Separately

Fig. 53-1. Algorithm: revision rhinoplasty.

Some patients are allergic to adhesives or tape. The patient will develop an eczematoid skin reaction with a rash or, at times, drainage and crusting beneath the tape. Treatment is tape removal, topical corticosteroids, and gentle cleansing (Fig. 53-2).

Postsurgical hyperpigmentation usually appears 2 to 3 weeks postoperatively in susceptible patients. Ultraviolet (UV) light exposure exacerbates this tendency, so patients should be advised to avoid UV exposure and to use sunscreen skin protection factor of 15 or higher. Hydroquinones are effective in treating hyperpigmentation and should be used as soon as the condition is recognized.

A similar condition is postoperative telangiectasia formation in the overlying skin of the nose. Certain patients may have a greater propensity for this skin reaction and UV exposure should be avoided. Persistent telangiectasis can be treated using a variety of methods, including microcautery or lasers.

The nasal alae

Precision in nostril sill or alar base resection is required to maintain symmetry.[15] Secondary surgery may require unilateral or asymmetric revision to reapproximate a symmetric appearance. Skeletal facial asymmetry may contribute to the difference in the alar appearance. Some asymmetry of position and placement cannot be corrected and this information should be conveyed to the patient preoperatively.

Alar margin retraction

Aggressive resection of the lateral crura of the lower lateral cartilages may cause weakening or collapse of the lateral margins of the nose. This may result in airway obstruction

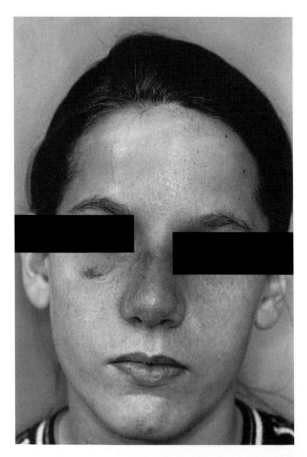

Fig. 53-2. Allergic skin reaction from paper tape used with a nasal splint.

in addition to an asymmetric appearance of the lateral nasal tip complex.

Avoiding this sequelae depends on recognition of the potential for alar margin weakness. Thin, weak lower lateral cartilages should not be used for tip procedures, which divide the lateral crura or aggressively resect significant cephalic portions. The margin is then free to contract superiorly and may collapse on inspiration.

Correction may be achieved by reconstituting cartilaginous strength to the lateral crura, usually with a cartilage graft. Auricular or septal autogenous cartilage are the donor sites of choice. Auricular cartilage may be preferable because it more closely resembles alar cartilage in thickness and flexibility. In addition to recontouring the alar margin, the graft will support the airway by preventing collapse on inspiration.[6]

In more severely retracted alar margins, soft tissue also may be needed in the form of a composite graft.[14] A vestibular skin incision is made over the internal alar surface several millimeters cephalic to the retracted alar margin. Scissor dissection is used to create a fusiform tissue void slightly larger than the amount needed to correct the retraction. A composite graft of skin and cartilage is harvested from the auricle and sutured into the tissue void created by the dissection. This graft unfurls the retracted margin and corrects the alar retraction (Fig. 53-3).

Loss of tip support

Tip support deficiencies after rhinoplasty contribute to a variety of nasal tip malpositions. Related structures and adjacent nasal anatomy may be affected. The supratip fullness is commonly referred to as *polly beak*. This condition may be caused by a loss of tip support or by a residual overprojection of the dorsal septal height (Fig. 53-4).

Postoperative tip ptosis must be differentiated from undercorrected long lateral crura and structurally-compromised alar cartilage components. Patients with undercorrected lower lateral crura must be treated using techniques to shorten the crura in accordance with the nasal tip tripod theory. Elongated lateral crura (uncorrected) will tend to push the tip complex downward, creating tip ptosis.

Patients with structurally-weakened or -compromised tip support mechanisms represent the result of violating key supportive architecture of the nasal tip. Tip support mechanisms vary from patient to patient in terms of relative contribution to overall tip support. There are major and minor support mechanisms. Major support mechanisms include the inherent size and strength of the medial and lateral crura: the projection of the septal angle, the attachment of the medial crura, and the caudal septum as well as the fibrous connections between the upper and lower lateral cartilages. Minor support mechanisms vary with the nose. Postrhinoplasty loss of tip support is predictably a function of the loss of one or more of these structural support mechanisms.

When the surgeon wants to maintain tip position during the initial rhinoplasty, these structures should be preserved. If they are violated and the loss of tip support results, then revision techniques to reestablish tip position and support are required.

The common steps used in many rhinoplasty techniques frequently disrupt anatomy contributing to tip support. For example, transcartilaginous and cartilage delivery techniques disrupt the attachments between the upper and lower cartilage. Lowering the cartilaginous dorsum or altering the caudal angle or caudal end of the septum may contribute to loss of support. Certain transfixion incisions interrupt the attachments of the upper lateral cartilages at the septal angle. If the incision is carried inferiorly enough, the attachments of the feet of the lower lateral cartilages are divided away from the septum. When an unacceptable amount of tip support is lost, revision surgery requires structural augmentation, which generally is accomplished through cartilage columellar struts, cartilage tip grafts, or both.

Columellar struts

Columellar struts provide additional tip support and tip projection. A well-placed strut that is sutured into place will also strengthen weak medial crura, straighten buckled crura, and aid in gaining tip symmetry. Septal cartilage is the ideal material to use for a strut because of its strength, resiliency, and relative straightness. If septal cartilage is not available, then auricular cartilage is an excellent alternative.

The strut is sutured into position between the medial crura. The length of the strut is important. Precision is required to ensure the effectiveness of the technique. The base of the strut should extend inferiorly to the maxillary spine. However, it should not be placed directly against the spine to avoid clicking back and forth across the spine or healing asymmetrically to one side of the spine. Superiorly the strut should extend to the level of the cartilage domes. Care must be taken to not extend the strut beyond the level of the domes or it may be visible postoperatively.

Tip grafts

Tip grafts may be used in a variety of sizes and thicknesses. Onlay and camouflaging grafts may be used to conceal irregularities. However, in nasal tips that require more support or projection, shield grafts are generally used. A strut graft is usually also used in combination with the shield tip graft. Although tip grafts can be placed through endonasal approaches, the authors typically use an open rhinoplasty approach for tip graft placement. The graft is fashioned from either septal (preferred) or auricular cartilage. The graft is carved to the appropriate shape and length and sutured to the caudal markings of the medial crura with 6-0 clear polypropylene sutures.

In addition to providing projection, tip grafts can establish definition in an amorphous tip or in thick-skinned patients.

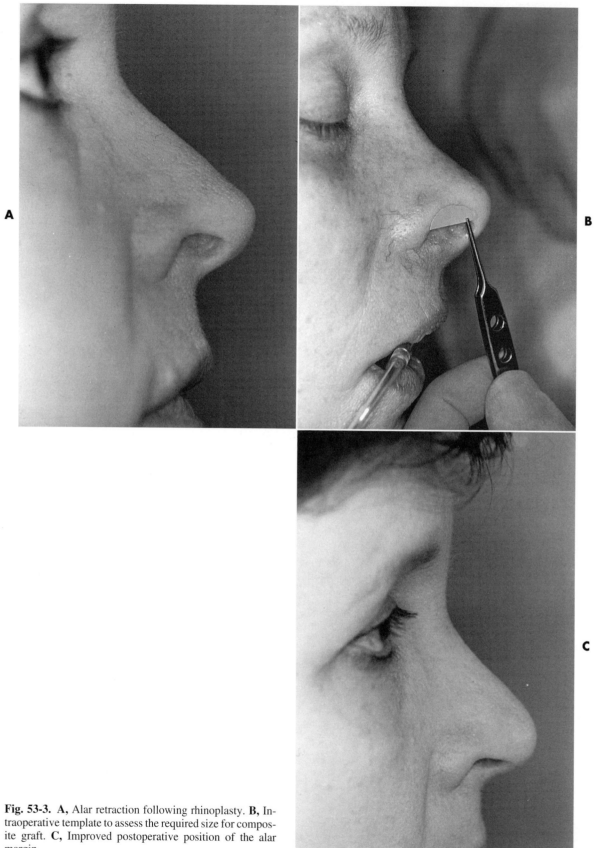

Fig. 53-3. A, Alar retraction following rhinoplasty. **B,** Intraoperative template to assess the required size for composite graft. **C,** Improved postoperative position of the alar margin.

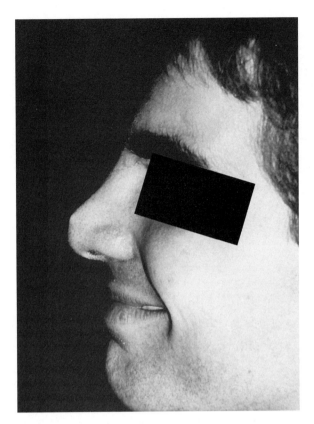

Fig. 53-4. A septal angle projection following the loss of tip support.

Dorsal length also may be enhanced, depending on placement of the graft.

Columellar retraction

Shortening or retraction of the columella also may be seen as a component of tip support loss. Mild-to-moderate columellar retraction can be improved with the columellar strut and shield tip graft. Placement of the strut anterior or caudal to the medial crura will give the columella a stronger, less retracted appearance. Likewise, an extended shield graft running inferiorly along the leading edges of the medial crura will strengthen and straighten the retracted columellar region.

Tip asymmetry and bossae

Tip asymmetry is a challenge to the rhinoplastic surgeon whether encountered in primary or secondary procedures. Asymmetries may be congenital, developmental, or related to trauma or surgery of the nasal tip. Bossae or corner-like deformities of the lower lateral cartilages are infrequently found after previous surgical procedures.

Unequal healing or fibrosis, unequal taping or nasal dressing, and asymmetric cartilage excision or suturing are factors frequently considered as contributing to postoperative tip asymmetries. Bossae are sharp angulations or corner-like projections, usually near or at the cartilaginous dome region. Bossae may develop following any type of lower lateral cartilage technique and are seen following intact strip techniques as well as divided dome procedures.

Treatment of tip asymmetries by the authors is most frequently accomplished through an external or open rhinoplasty approach. The lower lateral cartilages are dissected and asymmetries and irregularities inspected directly. Depending on the problem, the lower lateral cartilages are trimmed, augmented, or grafted to gain a symmetric appearance. The domes or intradomal region is typically sutured to maintain position.

If a bossa is present, the apex of the bossa is excised and the free margins are repositioned and sutured into a normal anatomic relationship. A thin onlay graft of cartilage is added over the repair to further mask and camouflage the area (Fig. 53-5).

UPPER TWO THIRDS OF THE NOSE: BONY NASAL VAULT

Surgical correction of the nasal tip is generally performed with the supratip and dorsal profiles adjusted to match the new tip projection. There are circumstances under which one might wish to reverse the order of surgery. For example, a large bony or cartilaginous hump will significantly alter tip support and tip projection. In such cases in which the dorsal projection is grossly disproportionate to the tip, correction of the hump deformity will release tension from the tip and allow better assessment of the tip projection. Regardless of the order in which these are performed, the ultimate goal is a harmonious transition from a straight dorsum to a slight (1 to 2 mm) supratip depression to a refined and symmetric nasal tip.

Dorsal profile irregularities after primary rhinoplasty exist as an excess of tissue remaining (undercorrected) or an excess of tissue excised (overcorrected). Undercorrection of the upper bony component of the nasal dorsum results in a persistent nasal hump, whereas undercorrection of the cartilaginous nasal dorsum (cartilaginous septum and upper lateral cartilages) results in a classic polly beak deformity.

Overresection of the bony and cartilaginous components of the nasal dorsum results in a concave *retrussé* look that was trendy in the 1950s and 1960s. The rhinoplastic surgeon should avoid techniques that yield anything other than a straight, strong profile giving a classic, natural look. Marked overresection of the nasal dorsum will result in a saddle nose deformity that significantly impairs nasal airway function and aesthetics.

Meticulous attention to detail and precise determination of the amount of bony and cartilaginous dorsum to be resected can prevent the need for revision rhinoplasty, but it is better to leave too much than to initially overresect.

When resecting the nasal dorsum it is essential to vary the amount of tissue resected to compensate for the varying

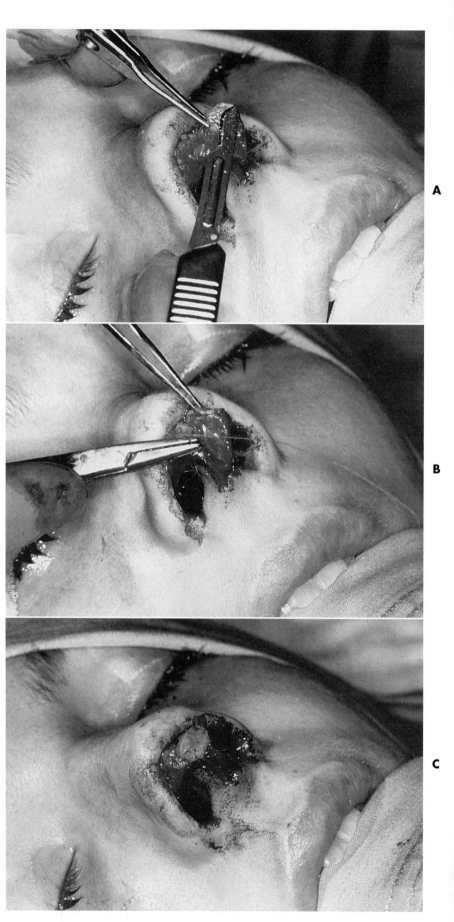

Fig. 53-5. **A,** A bossa of the lower left lateral cartilage. **B,** Cartilage edges are realigned and sutured. **C,** A thin cartilage onlay graft is sutured into position to camouflage the repaired cartilage.

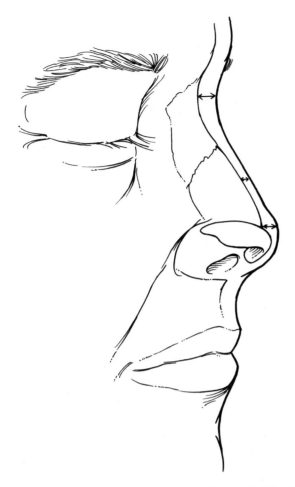

Fig. 53-6. The thickness of the nasal skin varies greatly. The skin is thinnest at the rhinion and becomes thicker over the supratip area and above the nasion. These variances in thickness must be considered in planning how much dorsum to resect in rhinoplasty.

thickness of the soft-tissue envelope overlying the dorsum. The skin is typically thinnest at the rhinion and gradually becomes thicker and more sebaceous as it descends to the nasal tip (Fig. 53-6). This is true in primary and revision rhinoplasty and failure to follow this principle frequently leads to revision rhinoplasty. Excess of bony or cartilaginous dorsum should be excised after careful analysis.

Occasionally persistent supratip fullness is present that can be attributed to soft-tissue excess or persistent supratip edema. Judicious injection of the supratip area with Triamcinolone Acetonide can be helpful in ameliorating this problem. Some surgeons advocate injection 2 weeks postoperatively whereas others prefer a measured, less aggressive approach. Time will improve the problem and the patient should be encouraged to wait.

The overreduced dorsum

The overreduced dorsum presents a challenge; correction requires augmentation of the nasal dorsum with grafts or implants. The ideal reconstruction of the nasal dorsum al-

lows for bony reconstruction of the upper bony dorsum and cartilaginous reconstruction of the lower cartilaginous dorsum. However, this approach is not possible using a single implant or graft, and the perfect material for nasal dorsal augmentation does not exist.

Although many alloplastic materials have been advocated for correction of these deformities, autogenous tissue is preferable. The choice of materials and techniques used by the authors depends on whether the augmentation is needed for structural support or to fill a nonstructural soft- or hard-tissue void. For nasal defects that are not structurally significant, the authors prefer autogenous septal cartilage when available. Conchal cartilage provides an acceptable alternative.

Conchal cartilage also is an excellent graft material for batten grafts to the nasal valve area, reconstruction at the lower lateral cartilages, and composite grafts for correction of alar retraction. However, conchal cartilage is not ideal as septal cartilage for dorsal nasal augmentation or as a columellar strut as it lacks the necessary stiffness to provide adequate structural support.

Most alloplastic materials are not suitable for use in the dorsum because the risk for extrusion is high. Expanded polytetrafluoroethylene (PTFE-GoreTex) has shown some initial promise, however data concerning long-term results are not available with this material.[7,10,11] Although it is not stiff enough to provide structural support, it can be used like conchal cartilage to fill small nasal dorsal defects. Irradiated homologous cartilage also has been advocated in the past for use in nasal dorsal augmentation. However, some laboratory studies indicate this material is resorbed over time.[8,16]

Significant bony defects are best reconstructed with autogenous bone. The authors have found autogenous calvarial bone grafts to be an excellent material that, when properly immobilized using a lag screw technique, provides structural reconstitution of the bony nasal dorsum (Fig. 53-7).[2,9,12]

The calvarial bone grafts are harvested from the outer table parietal bone taking care to avoid the sagittal sinus. The bone grafts are outlined using a saw down to the level of the diploë. The outer edge of the incision is then beveled using a large cutting burr. This allows the grafts to be undermined in the diploë using a right angled saw blade. Once the graft is fully undermined it can be harvested easily.

This method is an effective way to harvest split calvarial grafts with less attendant morbidity than the more conventional method of harvesting the full thickness of calvarium and then replacing the outertable and using the inner table as graft material.

Once harvested, the grafts are fashioned to the appropriate size using a cutting burr. The graft should be beveled on the edges to provide a smoother contour. The graft should not be too wide and it should not extend beyond the lower lateral cartilages, but its tip should be buried under the lower lateral cartilages using an interdomal suture.

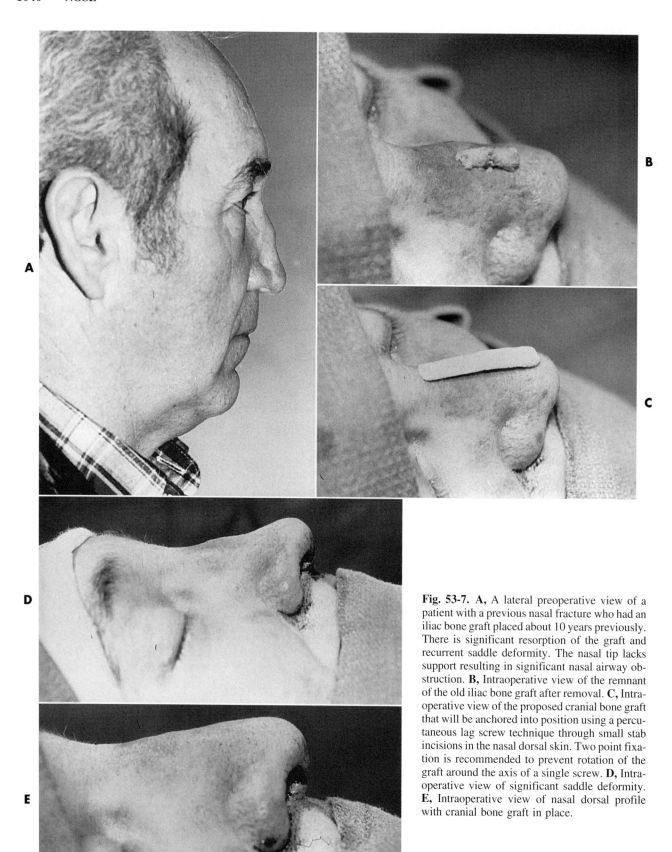

Fig. 53-7. A, A lateral preoperative view of a patient with a previous nasal fracture who had an iliac bone graft placed about 10 years previously. There is significant resorption of the graft and recurrent saddle deformity. The nasal tip lacks support resulting in significant nasal airway obstruction. **B,** Intraoperative view of the remnant of the old iliac bone graft after removal. **C,** Intraoperative view of the proposed cranial bone graft that will be anchored into position using a percutaneous lag screw technique through small stab incisions in the nasal dorsal skin. Two point fixation is recommended to prevent rotation of the graft around the axis of a single screw. **D,** Intraoperative view of significant saddle deformity. **E,** Intraoperative view of nasal dorsal profile with cranial bone graft in place.

Cartilaginous nasal vault

The cartilaginous nasal vault consists of the septum and the paired upper lateral cartilages and their attachments to the bony vault. Disruption of the relationships of the structures that comprise the cartilaginous vault can create major dysfunction of the nasal valve and result in nasal airway obstruction.[5] It is therefore critical to maintain their integrity in primary rhinoplasty and to reconstitute that relationship in revision rhinoplasty.

Deformities of the upper lateral cartilages associated with previous rhinoplasty most commonly involve overresection or avulsion of their attachments to the bony vault. Avulsion of the upper lateral cartilages typically occurs during rasping of bony nasal dorsum resulting in an inverted V deformity that gives a pinched appearance to the middle third of the nose.[3]

If the dorsal edge of the upper lateral cartilages is resected lower than the dorsal septal cartilage, then the upper lateral cartilages will collapse inward creating a narrowed nasal vault and airway obstruction at the nasal valve. As a result, the septal cartilage becomes solely responsible for dorsal projection and a sharp, unsightly, artificial looking ridge is apparent along the dorsum (Fig. 53-8).

This deformity is corrected with placement of spreader grafts (Fig. 53-9). These are struts of septal cartilage that are interposed between the septum and the dorsal edge of the upper lateral cartilages. They also can be interposed between the nasal bones and bony septum to widen the entire dorsum. Excessive resection of the cephalic border of the lower lateral cartilages may disrupt the proper relationship of these cartilages to the lower lateral cartilages. This disruption results in a pinched nasal valve area externally. This nasal valve problem is typically manifested by a positive Cottle's sign and nasal valve collapse on deep inspiration.[4,17]

This deformity can be corrected with the placement of batten grafts in the external valve area. The batten graft is formed as a wafer of conchal cartilage and is placed with the convex surface facing outward.[13]

Revision surgery of the bony pyramid often requires osteotomies to straighten the pyramid. Medial osteotomies are performed in the same manner as in primary rhinoplasty and fade to meet the lateral osteotomy superiorly. The lateral osteotomy is a low curved osteotomy performed in a similar fashion as in a primary rhinoplasty. Pitfalls include entering an old fracture line that may not be ideally placed. Also,

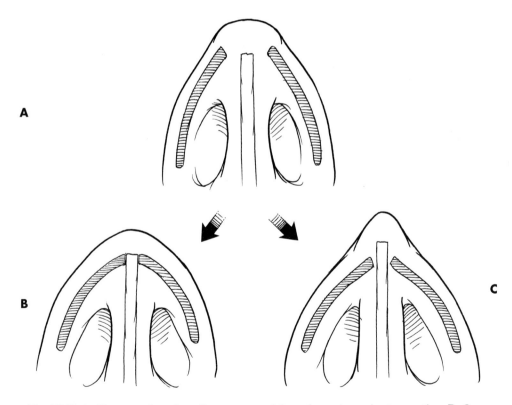

Fig. 53-8. A, The upper lateral cartilages separated from the septum prior to resection. **B,** Overresection of the upper lateral cartilages resulting in an inward collapse of the cartilages onto the septum. This creates a narrowed and incompetent nasal valve and a dorsal nasal profile that is determined by the projection of the septal cartilage. The nose appears narrowed with a sharp ridge along the dorsum. **C,** The upper lateral cartilages and the septum at the same level form a stable structural arch that allows the nasal valve to remain functional.

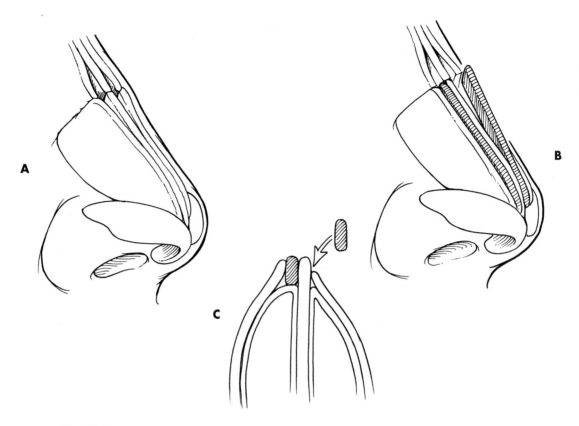

Fig. 53-9. A, An overly-narrowed nose with inward collapse of the upper lateral cartilages (see Fig. 53-8, *B*), can be corrected by interposing spreader grafts between the upper lateral cartilages and the septum, thus widening the valve area and improving nasal function and appearance (**B, C**).

because the bone may have healed asymmetrically, intermediate osteotomies may be necessary to correct these asymmetries. Osteotomies should proceed from medial to intermediate to lateral, because it is extremely difficult to perform an intermediate osteotomy on an unstable bone. Thus, the decision to perform intermediate osteotomies should be made prior to lateral osteotomy. The authors prefer to perform the lateral osteotomies after the incisions are closed so that pressure can be applied and the nasal dressing placed immediately to minimize swelling and ecchymosis.

REFERENCES

1. Arden RL, Crumley RL: Cartilage grafts in open rhinoplasty, *Facial Plastic Surgery* 9:285, 1993.
2. Cheney ML, Gliklich RE: The use of calvarial bone in nasal reconstruction, *Arch Otolaryngol Head Neck Surg* 121:643, 1995.
3. Constantian MB: The incompetent external nasal valve: pathophysiology and treatment in primary and secondary rhinoplasty, *Plast Reconstr Surg* 93:919, 1994.
4. Constantian MB: The middorsal notch: an intraoperative guide to overresection in secondary rhinoplasty, *Plast Reconstr Surg*, 91:477, 1993.
5. Constantinides MS, Adamson PA, Cole P: The long-term effects of open cosmetic septorhinoplasty on nasal air flow, *Arch Otolaryngol Head Neck Surg* 122:41, 1996.
6. Glasgold MJ, Glasgold AI: Tip grafts and their effects on tip position and contour, *Facial Plastic Surgery Clinics*, 3:367, 1995.
7. Godin MS, Waldman SR, Johnson CM Jr. The use of expanded polytetrafluoroethylene (Gore-Tex) in rhinoplasty: a 6 year experience, *Arch Otolaryngol Head Neck Surg* 121:1131, 1995.
8. Kridel RW, Konior RJ: Irradiated cartilage grafts in the nose: a preliminary report, *Arch Otolaryngol Head Neck Surg* 119:24, 1993.
9. Maniglia AJ, Swim S: Parietal bone graft and titanium plate fixation in nasal reconstruction, *Laryngoscope* 103:1066, 1993.
10. Miloro M: Gore-Tex for nasal augmentation, *Plast Reconstr Surg* 95:1334, 1995.
11. Owsley TG, Taylor CO: The use of gore-tex for nasal augmentation: a retrospective analysis of 106 patients, *Plast Reconstr Surg* 94:241, 1994.
12. Romo T, Jablonski RD: Nasal reconstruction using split calvarial grafts, *Otolaryngol Head Neck Surg*, 107:622, 1992.
13. Stucker FJ, Hoasjoe DK: Nasal reconstruction with conchal cartilage: correcting valve and lateral nasal collapse, *Arch Otolaryngol Head Neck Surg* 120:653, 1994.
14. Tardy ME, Genack SH, Murrell GL: Aesthetic correction of alar columellar disproportion, *Facial Plastic Surgery Clinics* 3:395, 1995.
15. Tardy ME, Patt BS, Walter MA: Alar reduction and sculpture: anatomic concepts, *Facial Plastic Surgery* 9:295, 1993.
16. Welling DB and others: Irradiated homologous cartilage grafts: long-term results, *Arch Otolaryngol Head Neck Surg* 114:291, 1988.
17. Zijlker TD, Quaedvlieg PC: Lateral augmentation of the middle third of the nose with autologous cartilage in nasal valve insufficiency, *Rhinology* 32:34, 1994.

Chapter 54

Reconstructive Rhinoplasty

C. Rose Rabinov
Roger L. Crumley

Reconstruction of nasal defects is a common procedure for facial plastic surgeons. Such defects may result from trauma, tumor resection, prior aesthetic rhinoplasty, or congenital deformities. Planning for reconstruction of distorted or missing tissues of the nose should consider both form and function. Systematic evaluation of nasal defects involves perception of the nose as a three-layered structure: (1) a cover of skin and subcutaneous fibrofatty tissue, (2) an underlying bony and cartilaginous framework, and (3) a soft-tissue lining of vestibular skin and nasal mucosa. Defects may involve any combination of these layers. The choice of tissue for reconstruction is generally determined by which elements are missing. The primary reconstructive goal is that each component be restored as closely as possible to its original anatomic state for optimal functional and aesthetic outcome.

The outermost to innermost layer is evaluated in terms of options for restoration. Although each layer is discussed separately, defects usually involve multiple levels, and a combination of reconstructive procedures may be required. Regional nasal characteristics and involvement of adjacent structures require further specific consideration.

COVER (EXTERNAL) LAYER

The nose has been described as being composed of concave and convex surfaces separated by ridges and valleys.[9] These surfaces, known as aesthetic or topographic subunits, include the tip, the dorsum, the paired side walls, alar lobules, soft triangles, and the columella. When a defect involves greater than 50% of a subunit, replacement of the entire subunit is often better than replacement of only a part. Placement of scars along contour lines recreates normal highlights and landmarks. Although this may require some

healthy tissue to be discarded, the outcome is often improved.

Just as the contour of the nasal surface varies, nasal skin texture and thickness also demonstrates regional variation. Skin over the upper half of the nose is thin and nonsebaceous, whereas that over the tip and alar lobules is thicker, and contains sebaceous glands. Caudally, over the alar margins and columella it again becomes quite thin and shiny. Nasal skin mobility also varies. Skin over the upper half of the nose is freely movable, whereas that over the caudal half is firmly adherent to underlying cartilage and fibrofatty tissues. These tissue differences should be considered when reconstruction is planned.

Options for repairing defects involving skin alone include healing by secondary intention, primary closure, skin grafting, and local and regional flap coverage. The choice of method is best guided by evaluation of location and depth of the wound. Healing of superficial wounds by secondary intention on concave surfaces may result in a satisfactory aesthetic outcome. For example, this method is a good choice for wounds of the medial canthal region where advancement of local tissue may distort the eyelids. However, when wounds on convex surfaces heal by secondary intention, the result is often a flattened or depressed scar. Similarly, primary closure may be used for a small defect of the mobile skin over the nasal dorsum, whereas closure of a similar defect over the tip region may result in alar retraction or asymmetry.

Full-thickness skin grafts (FTSGs) are useful in the reconstruction of superficial defects involving convex surfaces of the nose. This is especially true in the areas of the tip and alar lobules where tissue mobility is limited for the creation of local flaps. Donor sites for FTSGs include the preauricu-

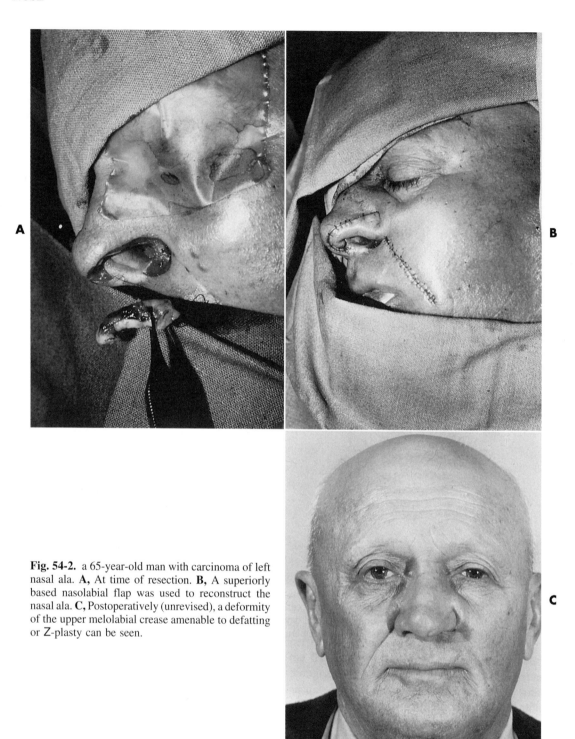

Fig. 54-2. a 65-year-old man with carcinoma of left nasal ala. **A,** At time of resection. **B,** A superiorly based nasolabial flap was used to reconstruct the nasal ala. **C,** Postoperatively (unrevised), a deformity of the upper melolabial crease amenable to defatting or Z-plasty can be seen.

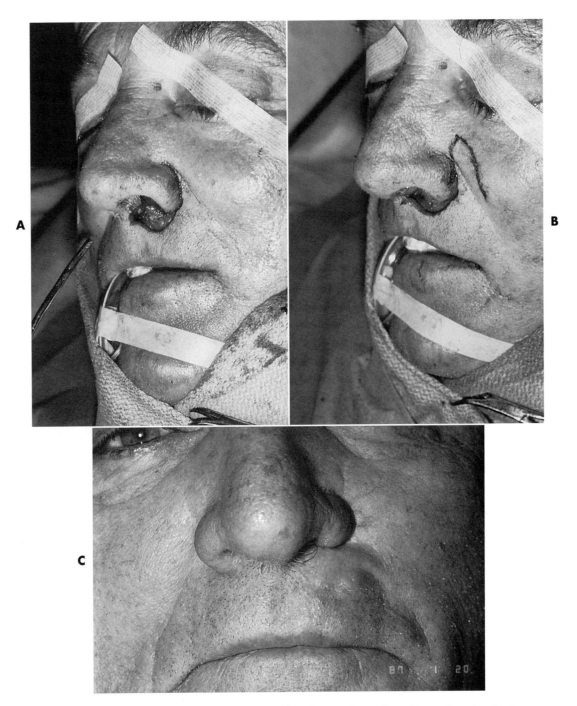

Fig. 54-3. A 74-year-old man with squamous cell carcinoma of upper lip and floor of nasal vestibule. **A,** After cancer excision. **B,** The inferiorly based nasolabial fold is marked. **C,** The postoperative result at 5 months. The patient subsequently underwent Z-plasty to restore the melolabial crease.

The forehead flap is versatile when used for nasal reconstruction, and it can be combined with cheek advancement, cervical rotation, or Karapandzic type flaps for larger defects that extend laterally or involve the upper lip. In cases of total or near-total nasal loss the forehead flap is combined with cartilage or bone grafting for restoration of a stable structure (Fig. 54-4).

FRAMEWORK

When nasal defects extend more deeply to include skeletal supporting structures, functional issues become more important. Strength and stability of the bony cartilaginous framework are of primary consideration. Without adequate support, contracture of the overlying soft-tissue envelope

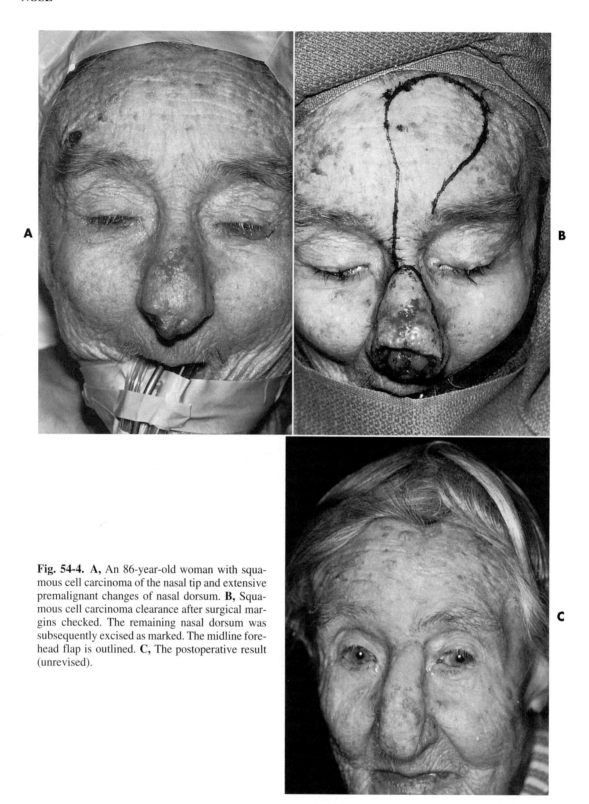

Fig. 54-4. A, An 86-year-old woman with squamous cell carcinoma of the nasal tip and extensive premalignant changes of nasal dorsum. **B,** Squamous cell carcinoma clearance after surgical margins checked. The remaining nasal dorsum was subsequently excised as marked. The midline forehead flap is outlined. **C,** The postoperative result (unrevised).

may occur, resulting in an abnormal contour and possible airway stenosis. A solid skeletal structure is essential to achieve satisfactory aesthetic and functional results.

Grafting material for skeletal reconstruction should ideally be compatible with the host tissues, easily shaped, and resistant to infection, resorption, and extrusion. Replacement of missing tissue with similar tissue is usually the best option for accurate reproduction of the rigid nasal dorsum and strong but flexible tip-alar complex. Autogenous cartilage and bone are the natural choices for this purpose. When these tissues are not available, alternative materials should be substituted. Some surgeons advocate using alloplastic implants when autogenous bone or cartilage are unavailable, although such scenarios are infrequent.

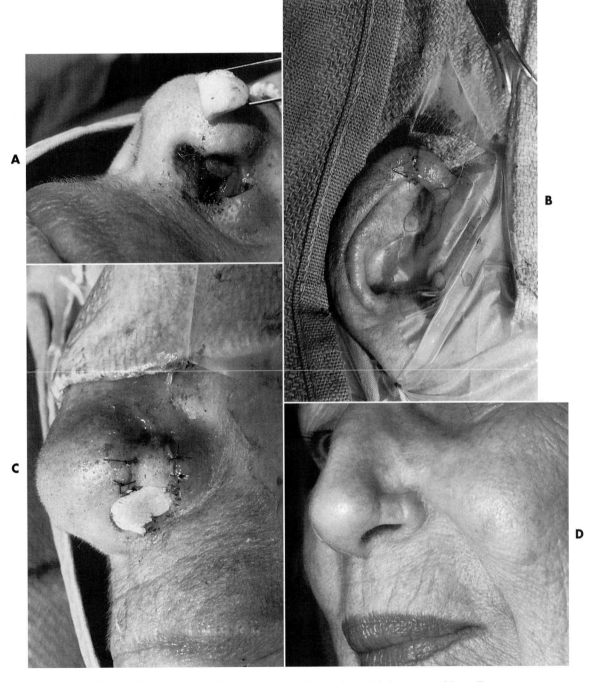

Fig. 54-5. **A,** The composite graft reconstructive technique in an elderly woman with small squamous cancer of left nasal ala. **B,** The donor defect is closed at the superior portion of the auricle. **C,** The immediate postoperative result and **D,** the healed defect at 1 year.

Solid medical grade silicone rubber, polytetrafluorethylene carbon, and polyamide mesh are among the alloplastic (synthetic) materials that have been used for restoration of tip, alar, and septal defects and for saddle deformities.[6,16,25] Advantages of these materials include their ready availability and lack of donor site morbidity. Current alloplasts, however, lack the composition and stability necessary for permanent structural support and are better used as onlay grafts for contour deficiencies. Further disadvantages include a high extrusion rate, foreign body reaction, and susceptibility to infection.[1] These disadvantages relegate alloplastics to a secondary role at this time.

Homograft tissues may also be used for nasal skeletal reconstruction. Biologic implants (e.g., irradiated cartilage, demineralized bone) have been used for support in total nasal reconstruction and in cases of severe saddle deformity. As with alloplasts, these materials are easily obtained and readily sculptured. They are, however, associated with a low rate of infection and extrusion. The main disadvantages of homografts are a high rate of resorption, occasional warping, and a tendency to become mobile over time.[15]

Autogenous cartilage and bone are the most appropriate and useful materials for reconstruction of the nasal framework. Cartilage may be used alone or in a composite graft of skin and cartilage depending on the need.[21,26] Composite grafts have been used to open stenosis of the nasal airway, to repair alar retraction after rhinoplasty, and to perform columellar and alar reconstruction after tissue loss (Fig. 54-5).

Composite grafting is a relatively simple, one-stage procedure. Grafts may be harvested from the conchal bowl, helical rim, or root of the helix with minimal donor site deformity. Survival of free composite grafts is unpredictable and depends on nutrients from the recipient bed until ingrowth of new blood vessels occurs. Viability of the graft depends on the successful transfer of fluids and nutrients from serum imbibition in the recipient site immediately after placement. Inosculation occurs over the next 24 hours, and vascular ingrowth occurs in 3 to 5 days. The successful survival of the graft depends on a recipient site with good blood supply, meticulous hemostasis, and careful immobilization of the graft. In addition, graft size is critical in survival; grafts larger than 2 cm in diameter are prone to fail.

Autogenous cartilage may also be used as a free graft without attached soft tissue. The most common donor sites include the nasal septum, auricular concha, or costal cartilage. Cartilage grafts have been used for multiple purposes, including increased tip support, rebuilding of missing or weakened alar cartilages, and dorsal augmentation (Fig. 54-6).[2] In addition, autogenous cartilage is especially useful in managing nasal valve collapse when used as battens or spreader grafts.[31]

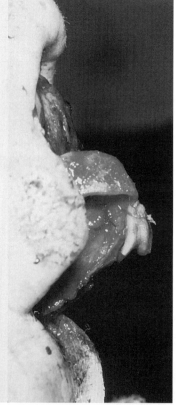

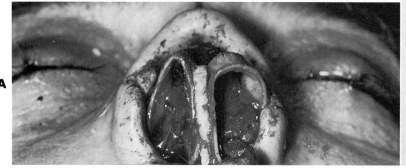

Fig. 54-6. A, A patient after subtotal lower nasal resection. Tip reconstruction with a columellar strut, conchal cartilage graft, and lower lateral cartilage reconstruction from additional pieces of auricle cartilage was tailored to restore contour of alar cartilage. **B,** The additional onlay graft for improved tip contour was sutured before forehead flap placement.

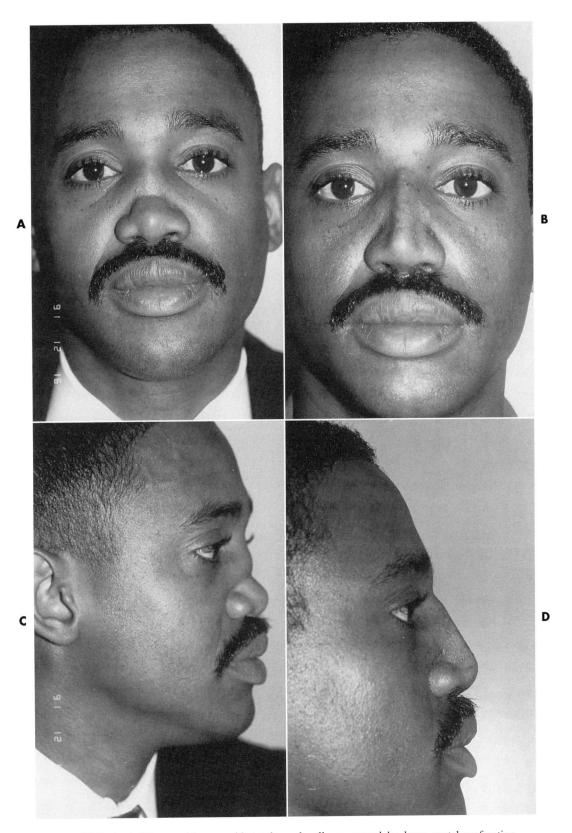

Fig. 54-7. **A,** A 27-year-old man with total nasal collapse caused by large septal perforation. **B,** The patient is seen after an L-shaped double calvarial bone graft. Lag screw fixation through the dorsal skin was used for approximately 6 weeks postoperatively. **C,** Preoperative right lateral view and **D,** postoperative right lateral view.

Continued

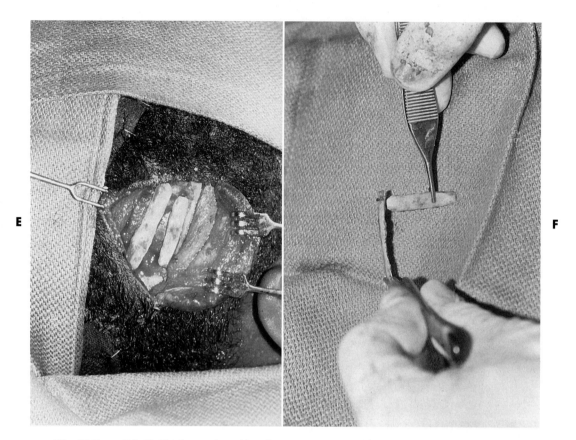

Fig. 54-7, cont'd. E, The harvesting of two bone grafts forms an L-shaped bone graft. **F,** The L-shaped bone graft is secured and ready for implantation. Fixation was with one microplate, lag screw dorsally, and wire to anterior nasal spine.

Reconstruction of the bony nasal framework is commonly required in major facial trauma. When severe comminution or loss of bone is present, grafting is necessary to recreate the projection and shape of the nasal dorsum and base. Although the iliac crest and rib have been used, calvarial bone is currently the donor site of choice[14] because of the easy access and low morbidity of the donor site and the decreased graft resorption noted with this membranous bone.[12] Harvest is most often done from the parietal region using outer cortical bone contoured to reconstruct the nasal dorsum or used as an L-shaped strut when dorsal and columellar support are needed (Fig. 54-7). Such a reconstruction is often combined with cartilaginous grafts for alar reconstruction and a forehead flap for external coverage.

Proper fixation of bone grafts is imperative for reestablishment of a stable skeletal structure. In addition, rigid fixation results in less resorption of the graft.[28] Dorsal grafts are cantilevered to the nasal process of the frontal bone, whereas lateral grafts are fixed to the maxilla (see Fig. 54-7). Miniplates or lag screws are usually used for this purpose.[17,24] Repair of nasal skeletal defects in this manner yields satisfactory functional and cosmetic results. The main disadvantage of using autologous bone grafts is their rigidity, which distorts the natural flexibility of the distal segment of the nose.

INNER LINING

The vestibular lining should be reconstructed when nasal defects involve full-thickness loss. Without replacement of the lining, contraction and fibrosis may result in stenosis and inadequate nasal airway. The restoration of this thin, vascular lining is best accomplished using similar tissue.

When a defect is limited to the alar margin, adjacent nasal lining may be advanced caudally as a bipedicle flap. Any remaining alar cartilage is also advanced toward the rim margin to maintain structural support. A hinge flap of septal cartilage with its contralateral mucosa attached is then used to repair the defect at the donor site.[8] When more extensive tissue loss occurs or when the existing vestibular lining is severely scarred, this method of repair is usually not possible. Other options include skin grafting of the undersurface of the covering flap, a turn-over flap to provide lining, and placement of a second local flap or composite graft (Fig. 54-8). Although these methods usually provide adequate in-

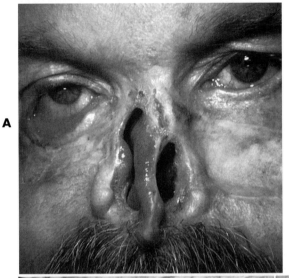

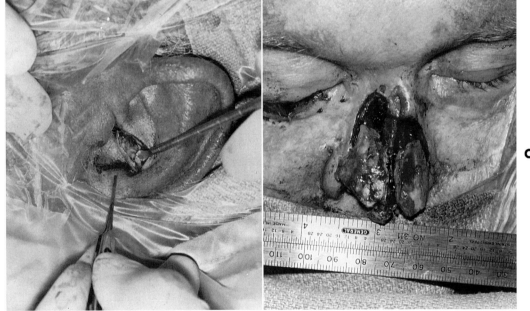

Fig. 54-8. A, A 45-year-old man after subtotal rhinectomy. **B** and **C,** Bilateral concave conchal cartilage grafts were harvested for internal and intermediate layer reconstruction of the lower nose.

Continued

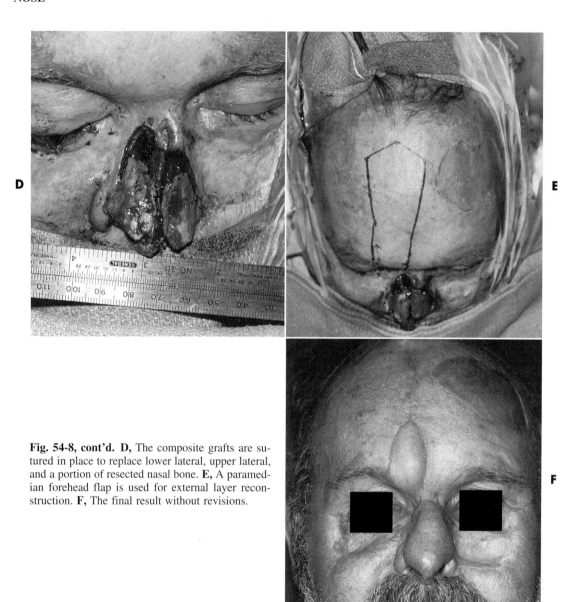

Fig. 54-8, cont'd. D, The composite grafts are sutured in place to replace lower lateral, upper lateral, and a portion of resected nasal bone. **E,** A paramedian forehead flap is used for external layer reconstruction. **F,** The final result without revisions.

ternal coverage, postoperative shrinkage of a skin graft or unnatural bulkiness of a flap may cause nasal obstruction.

CONCLUSIONS

The evaluation of nasal defects is best carried out systematically. The three-layered approach to this assessment allows surgery to be planned based on precise information regarding the amount and type of tissue requirements. Reconstructive procedures may then be selected and tailored to the specific defect and patient.

REFERENCES

1. Adams JS: Grafts and implants in nasal and chin augmentation: a rational approach to material selection, *Otolaryngol Clin North Am* 20: 913, 1987.
2. Allcroft RA, Friedman CD, Quatella VC: Cartilage grafts for head and neck augmentation and reconstruction, *Otolaryngol Clin North Am* 27: 69, 1994.
3. Antonyshyn O and others: Tissue expansion in head and neck reconstruction, *Plast Reconstr Surg* 82:58, 1988.
4. Apesos J, Perofsky HJ: The expanded forehead flap for nasal reconstruction, *Ann Plast Surg* 30:411, 1993.
5. Becker FF, Adham RE: *Melolabial flaps.* In Baker SR, Swanson NA, editors: *Local flaps in facial reconstruction*, St Louis, 1995, Mosby.
6. Beekhuis GJ: Polyamide mesh used in facial plastic surgery, *Arch Otolaryngol Head Neck Surg* 106:642, 1980.
7. Bouton FE: Aesthetic aspects of nasal reconstruction, *Clin Plast Surg* 15:155, 1988.
8. Burget GC: Aesthetic restoration of the nose, *Clin Plast Surg* 12:463, 1985.
9. Burget GC, Menick FJ: The subunit principle in nasal reconstruction, *Plast Reconstr Surg* 76:239, 1985.
10. Burget GC: Aesthetic reconstruction of the tip of the nose, *Operative Techniques in Plastic and Reconstructive Surgery* 2:55, 1995.

11. Burget GC: Personal communication (Dr. Rabinor), *Rhinoplasty* Atlanta, Ga, March, 1996.

12. Citardi MJ, Friedman CD: Nonvascularized autogenous bone grafts for craniofacial skeletal augmentation and replacement, *Otolaryngol Clin North Am* 27:891, 1994.

13. Cupp CL, Murakami CS: Flap necrosis and pincushioning, *Operative Techniques in Otolaryngology—Head and Neck Surgery* 4:82, 1993.

14. Day TA and others: Calvarial bone grafting in craniofacial reconstruction, *Facial Plast Surg Clin North Am* 3:241, 1995.

15. Donald PJ: Homographic cartilage in facial implantation, *Facial Plast Surg* 8:157, 1992.

16. Flowers RS: Nasal augmentation, *Facial Plast Clin North Am* 2:339, 1994.

17. Frodel JL: Primary and secondary nasal bone grafting after major facial trauma, *Facial Plast Surg* 8:194, 1992.

18. Giebfried JW and others: Reconstruction of nasal defects with a nasolabial island flap, *Arch Otolaryngol Head Neck Surg* 113:295, 1987.

19. Johnson TM and others: The rieger flap for nasal reconstruction, *Arch Otolaryngol Head Neck Surg* 121:634, 1995.

20. Kazanjian VH: Repair of nasal defects with median forehead flap, *Surg Oncol Obstet* 83:37, 1946.

21. Konior RJ: Free composite grafts, *Otolaryngol Clin North Am* 27:81, 1994.

22. Kroll SS: Forehead flap nasal reconstruction with tissue expansion and delayed pedicle separation, *Laryngoscope* 99:448, 1989.

23. Larrabee WF Jr, Sherris DA: *Nose. In Principles of facial reconstruction,* Philadelphia, 1995, Lippincott-Raven.

24. Maniglia AJ, Swin S: Parietal bone graft and titanium plate fixation in nasal reconstruction, *Laryngoscope* 103:1066, 1993.

25. Mass CS and others: Comparison of biomaterials for facial bone augmentation, *Arch Otolaryngol Head Neck Surg* 116:551, 1990.

26. Maves MD, Yessenow RS: Use of composite auricular grafts in nasal reconstruction, *Dermatol Surg Oncol* 14:994, 1988.

27. Millard RD: Aesthetic reconstructive rhinoplasty, *Clin Plast Surg* 8:169, 1981.

28. Phillips JH, Rahn BA: Fixation effects on membranous and endochondral bone graft resorption, *Plast Reconstr Surg* 82:872, 1988.

29. Shumrick KA, Smith TL: The anatomic basis of forehead flaps in nasal reconstruction, *Arch Otolaryngol Head Neck Surg* 118:373, 1992.

30. Tardy ME Jr and others: Full-thickness skin graft reconstruction of nasal tip defects, *Facial Plast Surg* 9:269, 1993.

31. Teichgraeber JF, Wainwright DJ: Treatment of nasal valve obstruction, *Plast Reconstr Surg* 93:1174, 1994.

PART FOUR

PARANASAL SINUSES

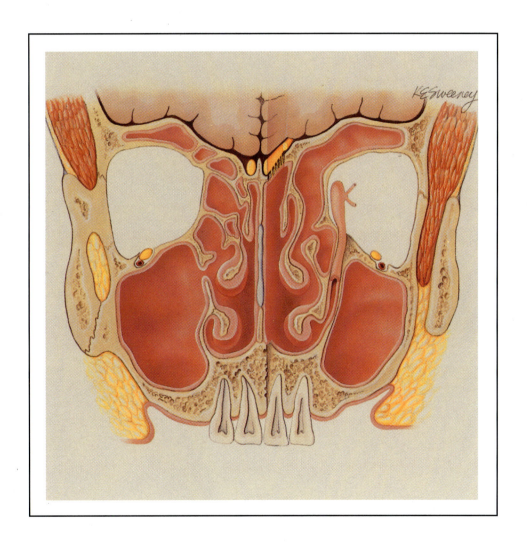

Chapter 55

Anatomy

Daniel O. Graney
Dale H. Rice

The clinical significance of the paranasal sinuses is well known to anyone who has sufferred from acute or chronic sinusitis. The functional significance of the sinuses has, however, eluded physiologists and physicians alike since the sinuses were first described some 1800 years ago. Blanton and Biggs[1] reviewed several theories related to the function of the sinuses and concluded that most are conjecture. These theories claim that sinuses (1) impart resonance to the voice, (2) humidify and warm the inspired air, (3) increase the area of the olfactory membrane, (4) absorb shock applied to the head, (5) secrete mucus for keeping the nasal chambers moist, (6) provide thermal insulation for the brain, (7) contribute to facial growth, (8) represent vestigial structures, and (9) lighten the bones of the skull. No substantive laboratory studies document any of these hypothetic sinus functions. However, the sinuses do seem to form a collapsible framework to help protect the brain from frontal blunt trauma.

Each of the four pairs of sinuses is named after the skull bones in which it is located: maxillary, ethmoid, frontal, and sphenoid. During the development of a sinus, however, pneumatization may involve adjacent bones—for example, the maxillary sinuses invading the zygomatic bones, or the ethmoid complex invading the frontal, sphenoid, and maxillary bones. The size of the sinuses depends particularly on the age of the individual, especially until late puberty; the sinuses may be asymmetric in the same individual.

The sinuses are similar in the sense that they all contain air and are lined by the typical respiratory mucosa composed of ciliated, pseudostratified columnar, epithelial cells. Interspersed among the columnar cells are goblet-type mucous cells. Because the mucosa is attached directly to bone, it is frequently referred to as a *mucoperiosteum*. Although it is somewhat thinner, the mucoperiosteum of the sinuses is continuous with that of the nasal cavities through the various ostia of the sinuses.

To facilitate discussion, each sinus is described separately, including descriptions of its development, anatomic relationships, blood supply, and innervation.

MAXILLARY SINUSES

Development

The maxillary sinus begins as a bud in the lateral wall of the ethmoid portion of the nasal capsule in approximately the third month of fetal life. At the base of the middle concha, the developing uncinate process of the ethmoid projects medially, forming a groove between it and the lateral nasal wall—the infundibulum,[10] or uncibullous groove.[4] This is the site of the original maxillary sinus cell or bud. Enlargement of this cell occurs slowly throughout fetal life, and the size of the sinus at birth is estimated at 6 to 8 cm³.[7] By 4 to 5 months after birth, the maxillary sinus can be readily seen radiographically, in a standard anteroposterior view, as a triangular area medial to the infraorbital foramen. After birth, growth of the maxillary sinus continues rapidly until about 3 years of age, and then slowly progresses until the seventh year (Fig. 55-1). At this time, another acceleration in growth occurs until about the age of 12 years. By then pneumatization has extended laterally as far as the lateral wall of the orbit and inferiorly to the point where the floor of the sinus is level with the floor of the nasal cavity. Thereafter, modest enlargement occurs until the adult size is attained in the late teens.[2,5,7,9] However, it is important to note that much of the growth occurring after the twelfth year is

1059

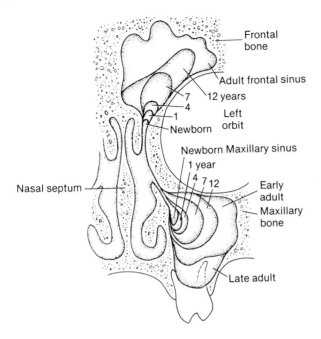

Fig. 55-1. Developmental stages of maxillary frontal sinuses.

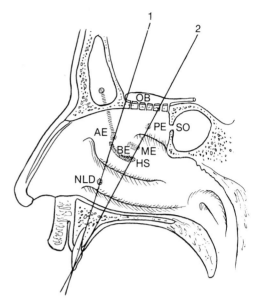

Fig. 55-2. Sagittal section of head, illustrating position of ostia of paranasal sinuses and sectioning planes of Figure 55-3. *Section 1: OB*—olfactory bulb; *SO*—sphenoid ostium; *PE*—posterior ethmoidal ostium; *ME*—middle ethmoidal ostium; *BE*—ethmoidal bulla; *HS*—hiatus semilunaris. *Section 2: OB*—olfactory bulb; *AE*—anterior ethmoidal ostium; *NLD*—nasolacrimal duct.

related to an invasion of the alveolar process after the eruption of the secondary dentition. Thus in the adult, the floor of the maxillary sinus is usually 4 to 5 mm inferior to the floor of the nasal cavity.[10]

The maxillary sinus occupies the body of the maxilla and is approximately 15 ml in volume. The average dimensions are 34 mm anteroposteriorly, 25 mm transversely, and 33 mm in height.[7,10] When viewed from above in a transverse section, the sinus appears triangular, with its base formed by the lateral wall of the nasal cavity and its apex projecting into the zygomatic process. The anterior wall corresponds to the facial surface of the maxilla and the posterior wall to the infratemporal surface of the maxilla. Its roof is the orbital surface of the maxilla, which is about twice as wide as the floor, formed by the alveolar process of the maxilla. The limits of the maxillary floor are usually marked anteriorly by the first bicuspid and posteriorly by a small recess posterior to the roots of the third molar. Recesses within the sinus occur variably and when present are described as *zygomatic, palatine, anterior* (to the nasolacrimal duct), and *alveolar.*

The maxillary ostium is located within the infundibulum of the middle meatus, with accessory ostia occurring in 25% to 30% of individuals.[7,10] Its shape and size vary from a small, narrow slit to a large, oval opening, depending on the anatomy of the ethmoid bulla and uncinate process of the ethmoid bone (Figs. 55-2 and 55-3). Its average diameter is 2 to 4 mm. Embryology thus mandates that the ostium be within the infundibulum usually where it passes under the bulla ethmoidalis (Fig. 55-4).

Because of these bony limitations, it is impossible to enlarge the opening without fracturing bone. Inferior to the uncinate process the medial wall of the maxillary sinus is usually membranous, consisting only of a reduplication of the mucosae of the sinus and lateral nasal wall, the so-called *fontanella.* This also may be the site of an accessory maxillary ostium.

Blood supply

The major blood supply of the maxillary sinus is via branches of the maxillary artery, although the facial artery may make a small contribution. Distribution of the maxillary arterial branches is essentially topographic and includes the infraorbital, greater palatine, posterosuperior, and anterosuperior alveolar arteries and the lateral nasal branches of the sphenopalatine artery.

Venous drainage may occur anteriorly via the anterior facial vein into the jugular vein or posteriorly via tributaries of the maxillary vein, which parallel the branches of the maxillary artery. After the maxillary vein joins the superficial temporal vein in the substance of the parotid, they form the retromandibular vein, emptying into the jugular system. However, in the region of the infratemporal fossa, the maxillary vein communicates with the pterygoid venous plexus, an abundant plexus of veins intertwining the pterygoid muscles, which in turn has anastomoses with the dural sinuses through the skull base. These vessels are responsible for the spread of infection from the maxillary sinus to the interior of the cranium and the resulting meningitis or phlebitis.

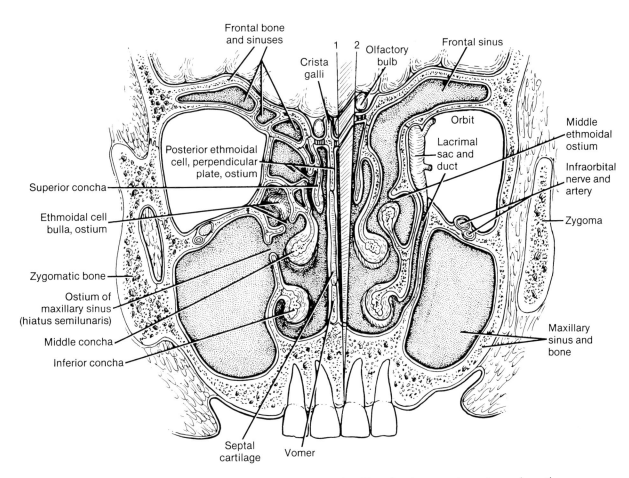

Fig. 55-3. Coronal section of head to illustrate relationships of ostia to nasal conchae and meati (see Figure 55-2 for planes of sections 1 and 2).

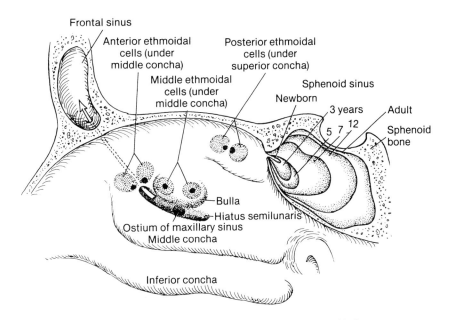

Fig. 55-4. Developmental stages of ethmoid and sphenoid sinuses.

The venous drainage of the sinus follows the pattern of the nasopharynx and nasal cavity. It drains into the maxillary vein and pterygoid venous plexus.

Innervation

The first and second divisions of the trigeminal nerve supply the mucosa of the sphenoid sinus. The posterior ethmoid nerve from the nasociliary branch of the ophthalmic division supplies the superior portion, and the sphenopalatine branches of the maxillary division supply the floor of the sinus.

REFERENCES

1. Blanton PL, Biggs NL: Eighteen hundred years of controversy: the paranasal sinuses, *Am J Anat* 124:135, 1969.
2. Caffey J: *Pediatric x-ray diagnosis*, Chicago, 1967, Mosby.
3. Kasper KA: Nasofrontal connections: a study based on one hundred consecutive dissections, *Arch Otolaryngol* 23:322, 1936.
4. Libersa C, Laude M, Libersa J-C: The pneumatization of the accessory cavities of the nasal fossae during growth, *Anat Clin* 2:265, 1981.
5. Maresh MM: Paranasal sinuses from birth to late adolescence, *Am J Dis Child* 60:58, 1940.
6. Myerson MC: The natural orifice of the maxillary sinus. I. Anatomic studies, *Arch Otolaryngol* 15:80, 1932.
7. Schaeffer JP: *The nose, paranasal sinuses, nasolacrimal passageways, and olfactory organ in man*, New York, 1920, McGraw-Hill.
8. Shapiro R, Janzen AH: *The normal skull: a roentgen study*, New York, 1960, Paul B. Hoeber, Inc.
9. Torrigiani CA: Lo sviluppo cells cavita accessorie delle fosse nasali nell uomo, *Arch Ital Anat Embriol* 12:153, 1914.
10. Van Alyea OE: *Nasal sinuses: an anatomic and clinical consideration*, ed 2, Baltimore, 1951, Williams & Wilkins.

SUGGESTED READING

Blitzer A, Lawson W, Friedman WH: *Surgery of the paranasal sinuses*, Philadelphia, 1985, WB Saunders.

Chapter 56

Radiology of the Nasal Cavity and Paranasal Sinuses

Patrick J. Oliverio
S. James Zinreich

Radiologic examination of the sinuses is designed to give information that is complementary to clinical findings. Traditionally, conventional radiography was the modality of choice to examine the paranasal sinuses. The standard radiographic sinus series consists of four views: lateral view, Caldwell view, Waters view, and submentovertex or base view.[42] The lateral view shows the bony perimeter of the frontal, maxillary, and sphenoid sinus. The Caldwell view (Fig. 56-1) shows the bony perimeter of the frontal sinus. The Waters view (Fig. 56-2) shows the outlines of the maxillary sinuses, some of anterior ethmoid air cells, and the orbital outline. The submentovertex view evaluates the sphenoid sinus and the anterior and posterior walls of the frontal sinuses.

Standard radiography may be accurate in showing air and fluid levels in the frontal, maxillary, and sphenoid sinuses, but they significantly underestimate the degree of chronic inflammatory disease present. Furthermore, the superimposition of fine bony structures precludes the accurate evaluation of the anatomy of the osteomeatal channels.[56-60,63]

COMPUTED TOMOGRAPHY

Computed tomography (CT) is currently the modality of choice in the evaluation of the paranasal sinuses and adjacent structures.[56-60,63] Its ability to optimally display bone, soft tissue, and air facilitates accurate depiction of anatomy and extent of disease in and around the paranasal sinuses.[56-59,63] In contrast to standard radiography, CT can clearly show the fine bony anatomy of the osteomeatal channels.

Many authors stress the importance of initially perform-

ing CT after a course of adequate medical therapy to eliminate changes of mucosal inflammation and to better evaluate the underlying anatomic structures. To minimize mucosal edema and allow an improved display of the fine bony architecture, some authors also suggest routine management with a sympathomimetic nasal spray before scanning to reduce nasal congestion.[1]

Technique

Imaging in the coronal plane is recommended (Fig. 56-3). The coronal plane optimally shows the osteomeatal unit, the relationship of the brain and ethmoid roof, and the relationship of the orbits to the paranasal sinuses.[56-60,63] Coronal images correlate with the surgical approach and, therefore, should be obtained in all patients with inflammatory sinus disease who are surgical candidates.[42]

In patients who are intubated or have tracheostomy sites, it is not technically feasible to position them for coronal scans. Also, young children, patients with severe cervical arthropathy, and patients who are otherwise debilitated usually will not tolerate the examination. In such patients, thin section, contiguous axial images with coronal reconstructions are performed.

Direct axial images are recommended to complement the coronal scans when severe disease in the sphenoid and posterior ethmoid sinuses is present and surgical management is contemplated. Spiral CT technique can aid the evaluation of the pediatric and debilitated patients and afford additional data to improve the quality of multiplanar reconstructed images.

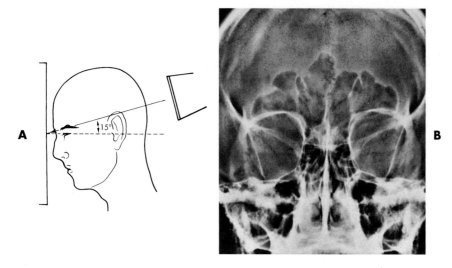

Fig. 56-1. The modified Caldwell view. **A,** Positioning diagram. **B,** Sample radiograph.

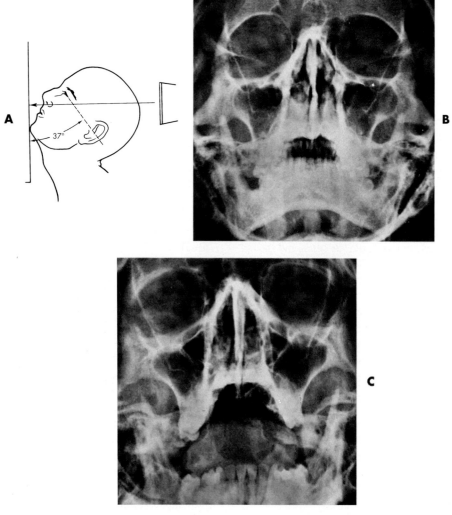

Fig. 56-2. The modified Waters view. **A,** Positioning diagram. **B,** Sample closed-mouth radiograph. **C,** Sample open-mouth radiograph.

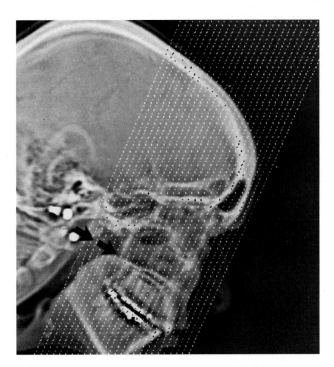

Fig. 56-3. Lateral computed tomography shows the patient's position during the examination. *Dotted lines* represent the scanner gantry angulation, which should be as perpendicular as possible to the hard palate *(arrows).*

Scanning is performed from the anterior wall of the frontal sinus through the posterior wall of the sphenoid sinus. Contiguous 3-mm thick images are obtained. Scanning with contiguous images is important to avoid loss of information through "skipped" areas.[30] The field of view is adjusted to include only the areas of interest. This helps reduce artifact from the teeth and associated metallic restorations and helps magnify the small structures of the nasal cavity and adjacent paranasal sinuses.[56]

Windows are chosen to highlight the air passages, the bony detail, and the soft tissues. A window width of 2000 Hounsfield units with a level of −200 Hounsfield units is the most advantageous.[56-59,63]

Sagittal reconstructions can be obtained for a morphologic orientation. Various distances and angles can be measured to aid in the passage of instruments during surgery. Axial reconstructions can be helpful in displaying the position of the internal carotid arteries and optic nerves with respect to the bony margins of the posterior ethmoid and sphenoid sinuses.

Originally, the exposure settings for sinus CT were 125 kVp and 450 mAs (scan time, 5 seconds). Babbel and others[1] showed that images are not compromised with 200 mAs (scan time, 2 seconds), whereas Melhem and others[30] showed no significant loss of diagnostic quality with 160 or 80 mAs. Recommended exposure settings are 125 kVp and 80 to 160 mAs.

Radiation exposure

The radiation exposure (dose) a patient receives is known as the *radiation-absorbed dose.* The radiation-absorbed dose measures the total energy absorbed from the radiation by a substance and is expressed in Grays (Gy). Gy is the radiation needed to deposit energy of 1 J in 1 kg of tissue (Gy = 1 J/kg). Formerly, radiation-absorbed dose was expressed in ionizing radiation units (rad), which measure the amount of radiation needed to deposit energy of 100 ergs in 1 g of tissue. The conversion of rad to Gy is 100 rads = 1 Gy.[3,8]

A more useful term is *radiation dose equivalent*, which considers the quality factor (Q) of the radiation (radiation dose equivalent = radiation dose absorbed × Q). Q accounts for differing biologic effectiveness of different forms of ionizing radiation. For radiographs, Q = 1; thus, the radiation-absorbed dose is equal to the radiation dose equivalent, which is measured in sieverts (Sv), formerly measured in the roentgen equivalent unit rem. Therefore, for diagnostic radiographs, 1 Gy = 1 Sv, and 1 Sv = 100 rem.[3,8]

Radiation dose equivalent depends on the kVp and mAs. For a given kVp, radiation dose equivalent will vary linearly with the mAs. At 125 kVp, the radiation dose equivalent for a CT slice is approximately 1.1 to 1.2 cSv/100 mAs (1.1 to 1.2 rem/100 mAs). The actual dose will vary slightly among machines. The radiation dose equivalent for a CT slice can be considerably reduced using a low mAs technique.

In contiguous CT, the dose delivered to a particular region scanned (i.e., the paranasal sinuses) is approximately equal to the dose per slice. The dose will be less than the dose per slice if there is a gap between slices, and the dose will be higher if there is overlap between slices.

The *effective dose equivalent* refers to the fraction of the total stochastic risk of fatal cancers and chromosomal abnormalities in a particular organ or tissue when the body is uniformly irradiated.[3,8] A system of weighing factors considers the individual sensitivity of the major tissues and organs of the body.[3,8] For a given examination, the effective dose to the patient will be less than the dose (radiation dose equivalent) received by the area scanned.

MAGNETIC RESONANCE

Although magnetic resonance imaging (MRI) better visualizes soft-tissue than does CT,[56,57] it does not visualize cortical bone. Because cortical bone and air have no mobile protons, they yield no MRI signal, resulting in an inability to discern the intricate anatomic relationships of the sinuses and their drainage portals. Thus, MRI is not a reliable operative road map to guide the surgeon during functional endoscopic sinus surgery (FESS).

The side-to-side cyclic variation in the thickness of the nasal mucosa is known as the *nasal cycle* (Fig. 56-4). The signal intensity of the mucosal lining of the nasal cavity and ethmoid sinuses varies with the nasal cycle.[22,61] During the edematous phase of the nasal cycle, the mucosal signal inten-

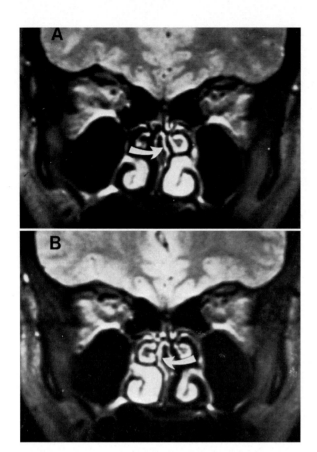

Fig. 56-4. A, Coronal magnetic resonance images of a healthy volunteer. **B,** Motion of the nasal cycle is seen.

sity on T2-weighted images in these two areas appears similar to mucosal inflammation,[1,59] which limits the usefulness of MRI (see Fig. 56-2). Interestingly, cyclic variation of the mucosal signal does not occur in the frontal, maxillary, or sphenoid sinuses. Increased mucosal thickness and increased signal on T2-weighted images are always abnormal.[22,61]

With respect to sinus imaging, MRI has proven most helpful in the evaluation of regional and intracranial complications of inflammatory sinus disease and their surgical management, in the detection of neoplastic processes, and in improved display of anatomic relationships between the intra- and extraorbital compartments. For example, MRI is helpful in diagnosing fungal concretions, which often show low or no signal on T2-weighted images.[41,43,44,62] MRI also is useful in the evaluation of mucoceles and cephaloceles.[51]

The standard protocol to evaluate the paranasal sinuses with MRI includes sagittal and axial T1-weighted images and axial T2-weighted images. After intravenous administration of gadolinium-diethylenetriaminepentaacetic acid (DTPA), axial and coronal T1-weighted images can be obtained.

OSTEOMEATAL UNIT AND SINUS PHYSIOLOGY

For a clear understanding of the regional anatomy and the importance of the anterior ethmoid sinus structures, it is critical to understand (1) the flow pattern of the mucous blanket coating the major sinuses (mucociliary clearance) and (2) the concept that inflammatory sinus disease is largely the result of compromise of the drainage portals (osteomeatal channels) of the individual sinus cavities.

The mucosal lining of the paranasal sinuses is made up of a ciliated cuboidal epithelium. In turn, a mucous blanket is found on the surface. The cilia are in constant motion and act in concert to propel the mucous in a specific direction. The pattern of flow is specific for each sinus and will persist even if alternative openings are surgically created in the sinus.[20,31,45,53] Therefore, FESS has gained widespread acceptance because it restores drainage of the sinuses through their anatomic drainage pathways.

In the maxillary sinus, the mucous flow originates in the antral floor with the flow being directed centripetally toward the primary ostium. This pattern of mucous movement persists even after a nasal antrostomy is created.*

In the frontal sinus, mucous flows up along the medial wall, laterally across the roof, and medially along the floor. As the flow approaches the medial aspect of the floor, some is directed into the primary ostium while the remainder is recirculated. The cleared mucous travels down the frontal recess and into the middle meatus, where it joins the flow from the ipsilateral maxillary sinus.*

The posterior ethmoid and sphenoid sinus clear their mucous into the sphenoethmoidal recess. The flow enters the superior meatus and subsequently the nasopharynx.

Thus, there are two main osteomeatal channels: (1) The anterior osteomeatal unit includes the frontal sinus ostium, frontal recess, maxillary sinus ostium, infundibulum, and middle meatus. (2) The posterior osteomeatal unit consists of the sphenoid sinus ostium, sphenoethmoidal recess, and the superior meatus. These channels provide communication between the ipsilateral frontal, anterior ethmoid, and maxillary sinuses. Radiology of the anatomy should show these osteomeatal channels.

Normal anatomy

Understanding of the anatomy of the lateral nasal wall and its relationship to adjacent structures is essential[13,14,60] (Fig. 56-5). The lateral nasal wall contains three bulbous projections: the superior, middle, and inferior turbinates (conchae). The turbinates divide the nasal cavity into three distinct air passages: the superior, middle, and inferior meati. The superior meatus drains the posterior ethmoid air cells and, more posteriorly, the sphenoid sinus (through the sphenoethmoidal recess). The middle meatus receives drainage from the frontal sinus (through the nasofrontal recess), maxillary sinus (through the maxillary ostium and subsequently

* Refs. 23, 31, 32, 40, 45, 53, 63.

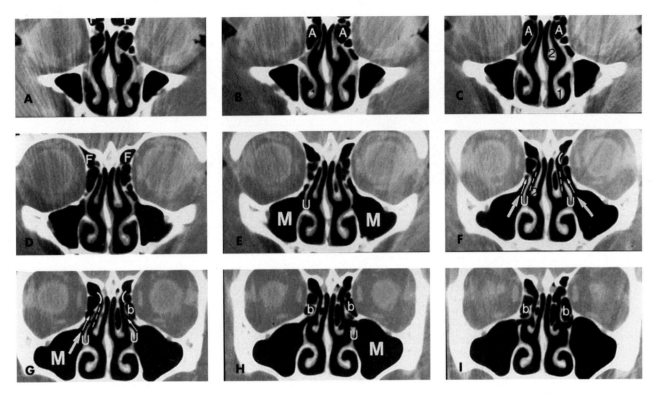

Fig. 56-5. A to **I,** Coronal computed tomography (CT) of paranasal sinus anatomy and thin-section coronal CT images of a cadaver. The frontal sinus *(F)*, the agger nasi cell *(A)*, ethmoid bulla *(b)*, the maxillary sinus *(M)*, the basal lamella *(black arrow)*, the sphenoid sinus *(S)*, the inferior turbinate *(1)*, the middle turbinate *(2)*, and the superior turbinate *(3)* are seen. The anterior osteomeatal unit is shown in images **F** to **H**. The frontal recess *(small curved lines)*, the middle meatus *(dashed lines)*, the infundibulum *(small arrows)*, and the primary ostium of the maxillary sinus *(large white arrows)* are seen.

the ethmoidal infundibulum), and the anterior ethmoid air cells (through the ethmoid cell ostia). The inferior meatus receives drainage from the nasolacrimal duct, a structure usually identifiable on coronal sections.

On CT, the first coronal images display the outline of the frontal sinuses (Fig. 56-6). The frontal sinuses are funnel-shaped. Their aeration varies among patients. They can be small and only occupy the diploic space of the medial frontal bone, or they can be large and extend through the floor of the entire anterior cranial fossa posteriorly to the planum sphenoidale. In general, a central septum separates the left and right sides; however, several septa are often present. The floor of the frontal sinus slopes inferiorly toward the midline.

Close to the midline, the primary ostium is located in a depression in the floor. The frontal recess is an hourglass-like narrowing between the frontal sinus and the anterior middle meatus through which the frontal sinus drains[58] (Fig. 56-7).

Anterior, lateral, and inferior to the frontal recess is the agger nasi cell. The agger nasi cell is an ethmoturbinal remnant, which is present in nearly all patients. It is aerated

and represents the most anterior ethmoid air cell. It usually borders the primary ostium or floor of the frontal sinus; thus, its size may directly influence the patency of the frontal recess and the anterior middle meatus. The frontal recesses are the narrowest anterior air channels and are common sites of inflammation. Their obstruction subsequently results in loss of ventilation and mucociliary clearance of the frontal sinus.

The uncinate process is a superior extension of the lateral nasal wall (medial wall of the maxillary sinus).[57,58] Anteriorly, the uncinate process fuses with the posteromedial wall of the agger nasi cell and the posteromedial wall of the nasolacrimal duct. The uncinate process has a free (unattached) superoposterior edge. Laterally, this free edge delimits the infundibulum (Fig. 56-8), which is the air passage that connects the maxillary sinus ostium to the middle meatus. Posterior to the uncinate is the ethmoid bulla, usually the largest of the anterior ethmoid cells. The uncinate process usually courses medial and inferior to the ethmoid bulla. The ethmoid bulla is enclosed laterally by the lamina papyracea.

The gap between the ethmoid bulla and the free edge of the uncinate process defines the hiatus semilunaris. Medi-

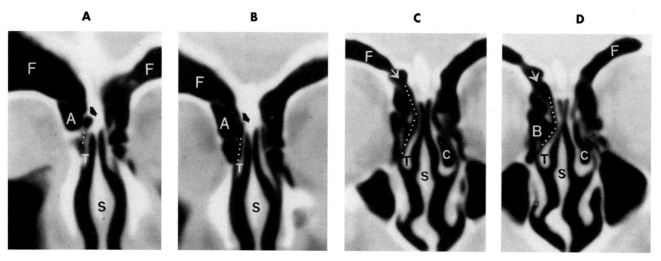

Fig. 56-6. Anatomy of the frontal sinus. Coronal computed tomography of the frontal sinuses from **A,** anterior to posterior **D,** show the relationship between the frontal sinus *(F)* and the middle meatus *(dotted line).* Note that there is a bony strut *(heavy black arrow)* separating the frontal sinus and the anterior middle meatus. This separation is lost on the more posterior images, revealing the position of the frontal recess *(white arrow).* Note the position of the agger nasi cell *(A)* and its relationship to the frontal recess. The nasal septum *(S),* the ethmoid bulla *(B),* the middle turbinate *(T),* and the concha bullosa *(C)* are also seen.

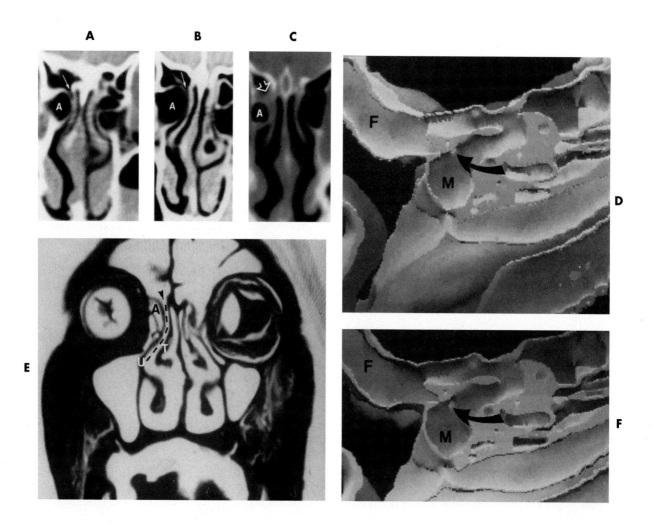

ally, the hiatus semilunaris communicates with the middle meatus, the air space lateral to the middle turbinate.[57,58] Laterally and inferiorly, the hiatus semilunaris communicates with the infundibulum, the air channel between the uncinate process and the inferomedial border of the orbit. The infundibulum serves as the primary drainage pathway from the maxillary sinus.[57,59]

The structure medial to the ethmoid bulla and the uncinate process is the middle turbinate. Anteriorly, it attaches to the medial wall of the agger nasi cell and the superior edge of the uncinate process. Superiorly, the middle turbinate adheres to

the cribriform plate. As it extends posteriorly, the middle turbinate emits a laterally coursing bony structure, the basal or ground lamella, that fuses with the lamina papyracea posterior to the ethmoid bulla. The basal lamella demarcates the anterior ethmoid sinus from the posterior ethmoid sinus.

In most patients, the posterior wall of the ethmoid bulla is intact, and an air space is usually found between the basal lamella and the ethmoid bulla. This air space, the sinus lateralis, may extend superior to the ethmoid bulla and communicate with the frontal recess (Fig. 56-9). Dehiscence or total absence of the posterior wall of the ethmoid bulla is common

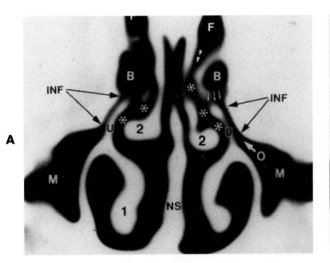 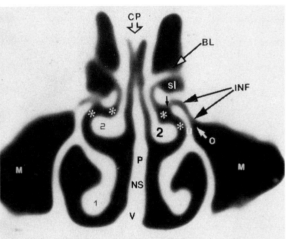

Fig. 56-8. Anterior osteomeatal channels. Coronal computed tomography through the anterior ethmoid sinuses shows the air passages intercommunicating the frontal sinus *(F)*, anterior ethmoid sinus, and maxillary sinus *(M)*. The primary ostium *(O)* of the maxillary sinus communicates with the infundibulum *(INF)*, which is bordered medially by the uncinate process *(U)* and laterally by the orbit. In turn, the infundibulum communicates with the middle meatus *(asterisks)* through the hiatus semilunaris *(most medial white arrow* in **A,** *black arrow* in **B).** The frontal recess *(white arrowheads)* is patent. The ethmoid bulla *(B)* is usually the largest air cell in the anterior ethmoid sinus. Note the vertical attachment of the middle turbinate *(2)* to the cribriform plate *(CP)* and its lateral attachment to the lamina papyracea, the basal lamella *(BL).* The air space between the basal lamella and the ethmoid bulla is the sinus lateralis *(sl).* The inferior turbinate *(1),* the nasal septum *(NS),* the vomer *(V),* and the perpendicular plate of the ethmoid bone *(P)* are also seen.

Fig. 56-7. Anatomy of the frontal recess. **A** and **B,** Coronal computed tomography (CT) reveals a patent frontal recess *(white arrow)* despite the presence of a large agger nasi cell *(A).* **C,** Coronal CT in a different patient with an obstructed right frontal recess and mucoperiosteal thickening in the right frontal sinus *(open arrow).* An agger nasi cell *(A)* is seen. **D,** Density-reversed coronal CT in a cadaver optimally shows the position of the frontal recess *(arrowhead).* Also note the relationship between the middle turbinate *(T),* the uncinate process *(U),* the agger nasi cell *(A),* and the middle meatus *(dashed line).* **E** and **F,** Three-dimensional CT with a sagittal cut–plane view of the paranasal sinuses shows the position of the frontal recess *(curved arrow)* and shows that its shape is that of an hourglass narrowing between the frontal sinus *(F)* and middle meatus *(M).*

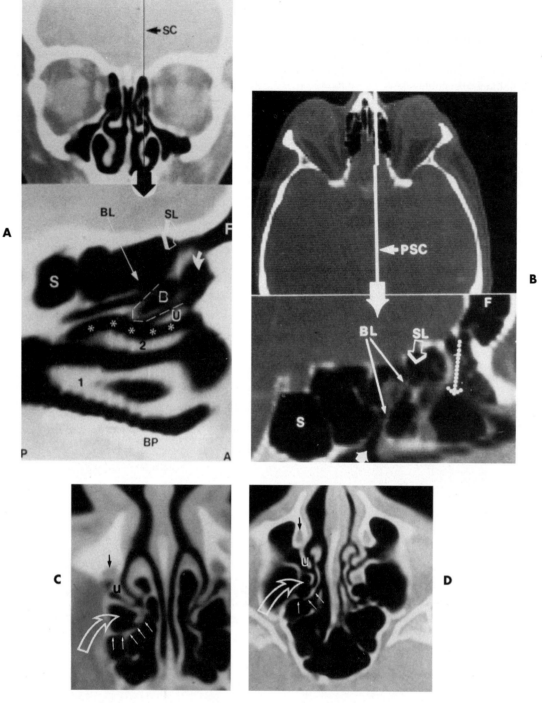

Fig. 56-9. Anatomy of the basal lamella and sinus lateralis. **A,** Sagittal reconstructed plane *(SC)* from direct coronal computed tomography (CT) data and **B,** sagittal reconstructed plane *(PSC)* from direct axial computed tomography data show the outline of the basal lamella *(BL)* and the position of the sinus lateralis *(SL)* in between the basal lamella and the ethmoid bulla *(B)*. The position of the hiatus semilunaris *(dashed U-shaped line* in **A**), the frontal recess, and the anterior middle meatus *(curved arrow* in **A** and *dotted line* in **B**) are noted. The frontal sinus *(F)*, sphenoid sinus *(S)*, uncinate process *(U)*, middle meatus *(asterisks)*, inferior turbinate *(1)*, middle turbinate *(2)*, bony palate *(BP)*, and middle meatus-nasopharynx junction *(heavy white arrow* in **B**) are shown anterior *(A)* and posterior *(P)*. **C** and **D,** Axial computed tomography images show the orientation of the uncinate process *(u)* and its association with nasolacrimal duct *(small black arrow)*. Note the attachment of the basal lamella *(small white arrows)* to the lamina papyracea. The ethmoid bulla *(curved arrow)* is the air cell anterior to the basal lamella; in both of these patients, the posterior wall of the air cell is incomplete, providing direct communication between the ethmoid bulla and the sinus lateralis.

and may provide communication between these two usually separated air spaces.

The posterior ethmoid sinus consists of air cells between the basal lamella and the sphenoid sinus. The number, shape, and size of these air cells vary significantly among persons.[54,56,58,59]

The sphenoid sinus is the most posterior sinus. It is usually embedded into the clivus and bordered superoposteriorly by the sella turcica. Its ostium is located medially in the anterosuperior portion of the anterior sinus wall, which in turn communicates with the sphenoethmoidal recess into the posterior aspect of the superior meatus. The sphenoethmoidal recess lies just lateral to the nasal septum and can sometimes be seen on coronal images but is best seen in the sagittal and axial planes[56-58] (Fig. 56-10).

The relationship between the aerated portion of the sphenoid sinus and the posterior ethmoid sinus needs to be accurately represented so the surgeon can avoid operative complications. Usually in the paramedian sagittal plane, the sphenoid sinus is the most superior and posterior air space. More laterally, the sphenoid sinus is located more inferiorly, and the posterior ethmoid air cells become the most superior and posterior air space. This relationship is well seen on axial and sagittal images. The number and position of the septa of the sphenoid sinus vary. Some septa can adhere to the bony wall covering the internal carotid artery, which frequently penetrates the sphenoid sinus.

Anatomically, the paranasal sinuses are in close proximity to the anterior cranial fossa, cribriform plate, internal carotid arteries, cavernous sinuses, the orbits and their con-

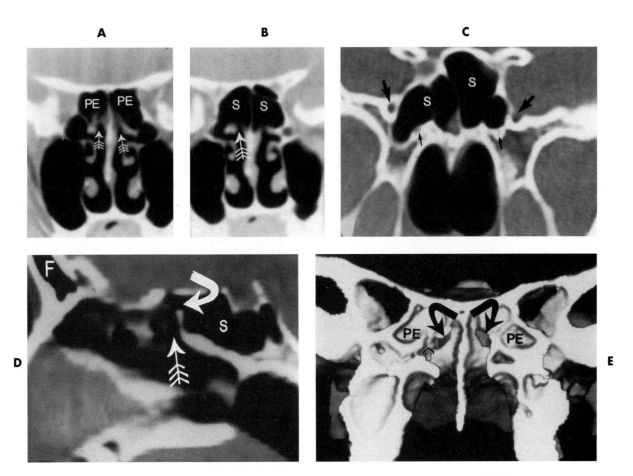

Fig. 56-10. The sphenoid sinus anatomy. **A** and **B,** Coronal computed tomography (CT) shows the boundary between the posterior ethmoid sinus *(PE)* and the sphenoid sinus *(S)*. This boundary is best recognized by the position of the sphenoethmoidal recess *(feathered arrows)*. **B,** The coronal image is likely through the anterior sphenoid sinus when only the inferior edge of the sphenoethmoidal recess is identified. **C,** Coronal CT through the sphenoid sinus *(S)* shows the number and orientation of septa within the sinus and the relationship to the foramen rotundum *(heavy black arrow)* and vidian canal *(fine black arrow)*. **D,** Paramedial sagittal CT shows the position of the sphenoid sinus ostium *(curved arrow)* and the sphenoethmoidal recess *(feathered arrows)*. The frontal sinus *(F)* and sphenoid sinus *(S)* are seen. **E,** Three-dimensional CT with a coronal cut–plane view through the posterior aspect of the posterior ethmoid sinus *(PE)* reveals the orientation of the sphenoethmoidal recess *(open arrow)* and position of the sphenoid sinus ostia *(curved arrows)*.

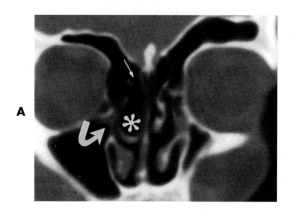
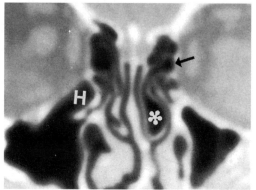

Fig. 56-11. The concha bullosa in two patients. **A,** The coronal computed tomography (CT) shows a prominent right concha bullosa *(asterisk)* with communication to the frontal recess *(small arrow)*. Note the obstruction of the right middle meatus *(curved arrow)*. **B,** The coronal CT shows a left-sided concha bullosa *(asterisk)* with communication to the sinus lateralis *(small arrow)*. Note the contralateral Haller cell *(H)*.

tents, and the optic nerves as they exit the orbits.[6,15,16,28,29] The surgeon should be cautious when maneuvering instruments in the posterior direction to avoid inadvertent penetration and drainage of these structures.[16,28,57,63]

Anatomic variations and congenital abnormalities

Although the nasal anatomy varies significantly among patients, certain anatomic variations are common in the general population and are often seen more frequently in patients with chronic inflammatory disease.[4,25,40,56-58,63] The significance of an anatomic variant is determined by its relationship with the osteomeatal channels and nasal air passages. The ability of the variation to obstruct the air passages implies a role in the recurrence of sinusitis. The most common variations are discussed in the following paragraphs.*

Concha bullosa

Concha bullosa is defined as an aeration in a middle turbinate (Fig. 56-11). Concha bullosa may be unilateral or bilateral. Less frequently, aeration of the superior turbinate may occur, whereas aeration of the inferior turbinate is infrequent. A concha bullosa in the middle turbinate may enlarge to obstruct the middle meatus or the infundibulum. The air cavity in a concha bullosa is lined with the same epithelium as the rest of the nasal cavity; thus, these cells can undergo the same inflammatory disorders experienced in the paranasal sinuses. Obstruction of the drainage of a concha can lead to mucocele formation.

Nasal septal deviation

Nasal septal deviation is an asymmetric bowing of the nasal septum that may compress the middle turbinate laterally, narrowing the middle meatus (Fig. 56-12). Bony spurs are often associated with septal deviation, which may

* Refs. 4, 5, 27, 40, 55-58, 63.

Fig. 56-12. The nasal septal deviation with spurring. The coronal computed tomography shows deviation of the nasal septum toward the right side with a right-sided cartilaginous nasal spur *(asterisk)*. Note the ipsilateral concha bullosa *(arrow)*. Both of these anatomic variants contribute to marked narrowing of the right nasal cavity and ethmoid passages.

further compromise the ostiomeatal unit. Nasal septal deviation is usually congenital but may be a posttraumatic finding in some patients.

Paradoxic middle turbinate

The middle turbinate usually curves medially toward the nasal septum. However, its major curvature can project laterally and, thus, narrow the middle meatus and infundibulum. This variant is called a *paradoxic middle turbinate* (Fig. 56-13). The inferior edge of the middle meatus may assume various shapes with excessive curvature, which in turn may obstruct the nasal cavity, infundibulum, and middle meatus.

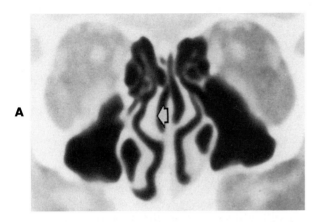

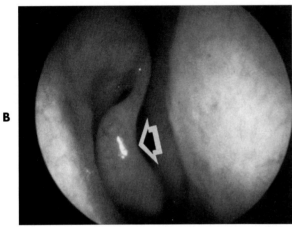

Fig. 56-13. The paradoxic middle turbinate. **A,** The coronal computed tomography (CT) shows bilateral paradoxic middle turbinates. The right side is highlighted *(solid arrow).* **B,** The endoscopic view correlates with the CT findings *(arrow).*

Variations in the uncinate process

The course of the free edge of the uncinate process varies. In most cases, it extends slightly obliquely toward the nasal septum with the free edge surrounding the inferior or anterior surface of the ethmoid bulla, or it extends more medially to the medial surface of the ethmoid bulla.

Sometimes, the free edge of the uncinate adheres to the orbital floor or inferior aspect of the lamina papyracea, which is termed an *atelectatic uncinate process* (Fig. 56-14). This variant is usually associated with a hypoplastic, and often opacified, ipsilateral maxillary sinus resulting from closure of the infundibulum. It is important to note this variant when planning surgery because the ipsilateral orbital floor will be low-lying as a result of potentially compromising the infundibulum, although this occurs infrequently.

Haller cells

Haller cells are ethmoid air cells that extend along the medial roof of the maxillary sinus (Fig. 56-15). Their appearance and size vary. They may cause narrowing of the infun-

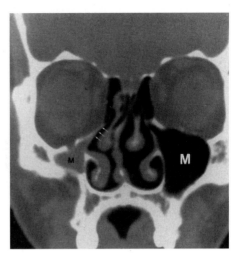

Fig. 56-14. The atelectatic uncinate process. The coronal computed tomography shows that the right uncinate process is apposed to the inferomedial aspect of the orbit *(arrows).* The resultant obstruction of the infundibulum is usually the cause of the prominent inflammatory process in the ipsilateral maxillary sinus *(small black M).* Note that this is associated with hypoplasia of the ipsilateral maxillary sinus compared with its counterpart *(large white M).*

dibulum when they are large. Haller cells may exist as discrete cells or they may open into the maxillary sinus or infundibulum.

Onodi cells

Onodi cells are rare. They are lateral and posterior extensions of the posterior ethmoid air cells. They extend the paranasal sinus cavity very near the optic nerves as they exit the orbits. These cells may surround the optic nerve tract and put the nerve at risk during surgery.

Giant ethmoid bulla

The largest of the ethmoid air cells, the ethmoid bulla may enlarge to narrow or obstruct the middle meatus and infundibulum.

Extensive pneumatization of the sphenoid sinus

Pneumatization of the sphenoid sinus can extend into the anterior clinoid processes and clivus, surrounding the optic nerves. When this occurs, the risk of damage to the optic nerves is increased during surgical exploration (Fig. 56-16).

Medial deviation or dehiscence of the lamina papyracea

Medial deviation or dehiscence of the lamina papyracea may be a congenital finding or the result of prior facial trauma. Regardless, the intraorbital contents are at risk during surgery because of the common dehiscences in the area and the ease of confusing this medial bulge with the ethmoid bulla. Excessive medial deviation and bony dehiscence tend to occur most often at the site of the insertion of the basal

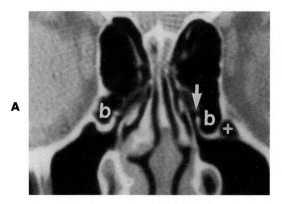
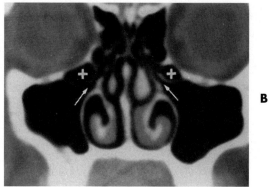

Fig. 56-15. A Haller cell. **A,** Note the left Haller cell (*plus sign*) with the ethmoid bulla ostia (*b*) located medially opening into the infundibula. **B,** Bilateral Haller cells (*plus sign*). Note their close proximity to the uncinate process and their influence on the infundibula (*small arrows*).

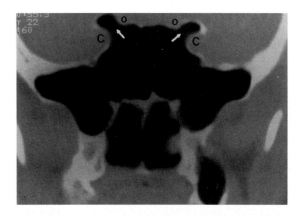

Fig. 56-16. Extensive pneumatization of the sphenoid sinus. Coronal computed tomography shows pneumatization of both anterior clinoid processes (*arrows*) and their relationship to the optic nerves (*o*) and internal carotid arteries (*C*). The presence of anterior clinoid process pneumatization is an important indicator of optic nerve vulnerability during functional endoscopic sinus surgery.

lamella into the lamina papyracea, thus rendering this portion of the lamina papyracea to be most delicate.

Aerated crista galli

Aeration of the crista galli, a normally bony structure, can occur. When aerated, these cells may communicate with the frontal recess. Obstruction of this ostium can lead to chronic sinusitis and mucocele formation. It is important to recognize this entity preoperatively and to differentiate it from an ethmoid air cell to avoid extension of surgery into the cranial vault.

Cephalocele

Preoperative CT is useful to assess for congenital abnormalities, such as cephaloceles[24] (Figs. 56-17 and 56-18), which may be spontaneously present or may result from previous ethmoid or sphenoid sinus surgery. Their presence

needs to be considered when dealing with an isolated soft-tissue mass adjacent to the ethmoid or sphenoid roof, especially if complemented by adjacent bone erosion. The differential diagnosis includes mucocele, neoplasm, cephalocele, and less likely, a polyp associated with an adjacent bony dehiscence. Coronal CT will best display the extent of bony erosion and sagittal and coronal MRI will be helpful in narrowing the differential diagnosis.

Asymmetry in ethmoid roof height

It is important to note any asymmetry in the height of the ethmoid roof. The incidence of intracranial penetration during FESS is higher when this anatomic variation occurs. Intracranial penetration is more likely to occur on the side where the position of the roof is lower.[10]

INTERPRETATION OF IMAGES

Using a systematic approach is helpful when interpreting sinus CT studies. While reading from anterior to posterior, a mental checklist of important structures to be evaluated and commented on should be made. The reporting system includes three steps.

1. Identify and describe the important structures of the paranasal sinuses including the frontal sinus, the frontal recess, the agger nasi cell and anterior ethmoid sinus, the ethmoid roof, the ethmoid bulla, the uncinate process, the infundibulum, the maxillary sinus, the middle meatus, the nasal septum and nasal turbinates, the basal lamella, the sinus lateralis, the posterior ethmoid sinus, and the sphenoid sinus.
2. Evaluate the critical relationships when planning surgery. The symmetry of the ethmoid roof should be noted. If not recognized, discrepant heights of the ethmoid roof may lead to inadvertent penetration of the cranial vault during FESS.

   Careful attention should be paid to the status of the lamina papyracea, and any dehiscence or excessive

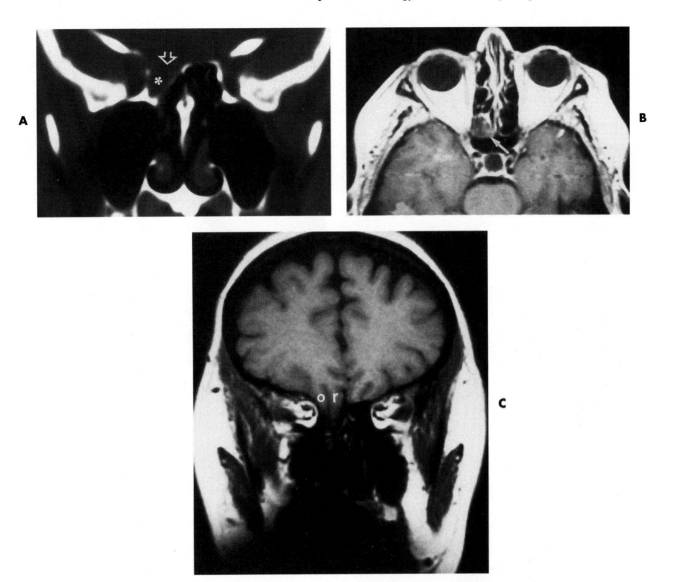

Fig. 56-17. A to **C,** Computed tomography and magnetic resonance imaging display of an encephalocele. **A,** Coronal computed tomography through the posterior ethmoid sinus shows erosion of the roof of the posterior ethmoid sinus *(open arrow* and *asterisk).* **B,** Axial T1-weighted magnetic resonance imaging shows an isolated soft-tissue mass within the posterior ethmoid sinus *(arrow),* which on **C,** coronal T1-weighted magnetic resonance image is confirmed to be an encephalocele. The gyrus rectus *(r)* and gyrus orbitales *(o)* are noted.

medial deviation of this bone should be reported. The relationship of the sphenoid sinus and posterior ethmoid air cells with the internal carotid artery and optic nerves should be noted. Findings that put either of these structures at increased risk during endoscopic surgery should be conveyed to the referring surgeon. In particular, extensive expansion of the sinuses around the internal carotid artery or the optic nerve and bony dehisences adjacent to either structure should be noted. The incidence of bony dehiscence around the presellar and juxtasellar portions of the internal carotid artery is 12% to 22%.[9,17] The carotid canal frequently penetrates the aerated portion of the sphenoid sinus; in many cases, the sphenoid sinus septa will adhere to the bony covering of the carotid canal. The surgeon needs to be aware of this variation to prevent fracture of the sphenoid sinus septum–carotid canal junction and avoid puncturing the carotid canal.

The relationship between the posterior paranasal sinuses and the optic nerves is important to note to avoid operative complications (Fig. 56-19). Delano, Fun, and Zinreich[9] classified the relationship into four categories. Type 1 includes optic nerves coursing adjacent to the sphenoid sinus without indentation of the

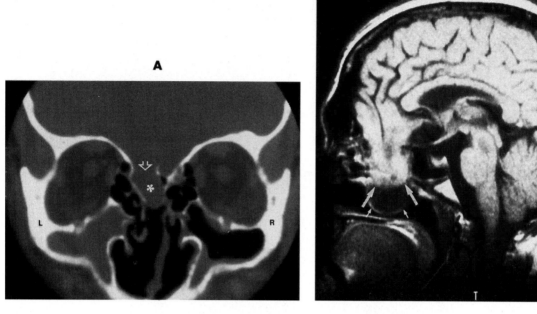

Fig. 56-18. Computed tomography (CT) and magnetic resonance imaging appearance of an encephalocele. **A,** The coronal CT through the posterior ethmoid sinus shows wide erosion of the ethmoid sinus roof *(open arrow)* with a soft-tissue mass penetrating into the ethmoid sinus *(asterisk)*. **B,** T1-weighted sagittal magnetic resonance image shows the outline of the brain tissue *(large arrows)* and meninges and cerebrospinal fluid *(small arrows)*.

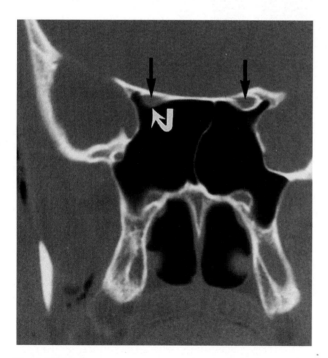

Fig. 56-19. Relationship of optic nerves to sphenoid sinus. Type three optic nerves *(black arrows)* course through the sphenoid sinus with greater than 50% of the nerves surrounded by air. Note that there is dehiscence of the bone covering the right optic nerve *(curved white arrow)*. This increases the risk of optic nerve damage during functional endoscopic sinus surgery.

wall or contact with the posterior ethmoid air cell. This type is most common and occurs in 76% of patients. Type 2 nerves course adjacent to the sphenoid sinus causing indentation of the sinus wall, without contact with the posterior ethmoid air cell. Type 3 nerves course through the sphenoid sinus with at least 50% surrounded by air. Type 4 course adjacent to the sphenoid sinus and posterior ethmoid sinus. In this study, the optic nerve was dehiscent in all cases in which it traveled through the sphenoid sinus (type 3) and in 82% of cases in which the nerve impressed on the sphenoid sinus wall (type 2). Delano, Fun, and Zinreich[9] also found that 85% of optic nerves associated with a pneumatized anterior clinoid process were of type 2 or 3 and 77% were dehiscent. Therefore, the presence of anterior clinoid process pneumatization is an important indicator of optic nerve vulnerability during FESS because of frequent associations with bony dehiscence and type 2 and 3 configurations[9].

3. Evaluate the bony outline of the nasal cavity and paranasal sinuses. Prominent thickening of the bone outlining the paranasal sinuses occurs, especially in patients who have undergone several surgical procedures and in those with repeated exacerbations of chronic inflammation (Fig. 56-20). Similar changes occur in patients with Wegener's granulomatosis. These patients suffer with a prolonged chronic inflammation and no

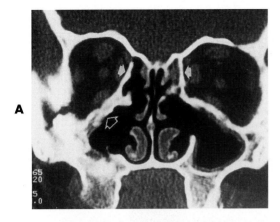

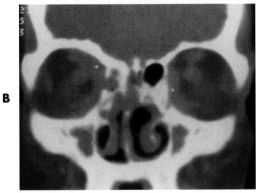

Fig. 56-20. Osteitis of the paranasal sinus walls. **A,** Coronal computed tomography (CT) through the ethmoid sinus shows bilateral antrostomies, uncinectomies, and partial anterior ethmoidectomies. Note the pronounced thickening of the orbital floors bilaterally but more severely on the right side *(open arrow)*. There is marked thickening of the lamina papyracea bilaterally *(solid arrows)*. These changes are occasionally seen in patients who have undergone multiple surgical procedures in this area. **B,** Coronal CT through the anterior ethmoid sinus in a patient with Wegener's granulomatosis shows diffuse, pronounced bony thickening of the perimeter of the maxillary sinuses and lamina papyracea and the presence of soft-tissue masses *(asterisks)* within the orbits.

previous surgery. Unfortunately, no pathophysiologic explanation of this finding exists; however, this change is directly related to the underlying inflammatory process and periosteal stimulation.

Bone erosion or absence of bone may have three causes. Bone may have been removed during a previous surgical procedure, and therefore, a dehiscence is noted. Evidence of prior surgery should be looked for on CT and established through a proper medical history. These changes may also be caused by the erosion secondary to a mucocele or neoplasm. The associated mass will be a clue as to the cause, and MRI may distinguish between these processes. Bony dehiscences may also be developmental; in the absence of prior surgery or additional pathology, this possibility should be considered.

RADIOGRAPHIC APPEARANCES OF INFLAMMATORY SINUS DISEASE

Acute sinusitis

Acute sinusitis is usually caused by bacterial superinfection of an obstructed paranasal sinus. The obstruction is often the result of apposition of edematous mucosal surfaces from an antecedent viral upper respiratory tract infection. The edema disrupts the normal mucociliary drainage pattern of the sinus, and obstruction of the sinus ostium results. The accumulation of fluid within the sinus predisposes to a bacterial superinfection. The bacterial pathogens most often responsible include S*treptococcus pneumoniae, Haemophilus influenza,* β-hemolytic streptococci, and *Moraxella catarrhalis.*[5,11,51] Acute sinusitis only rarely results from a pure viral infection. Acute sinusitis usually only involves a single sinus; the ethmoid sinus is the most common location.[11,25] The risk of regional and intracranial complications is increased with involvement of the frontal, ethmoid, and sphenoid sinuses.[25]

Radiographically, the hallmark of acute sinusitis is an air-fluid level (Fig. 56-21). However, the radiologic findings in acute sinusitis may be nonspecific, with smooth or nodular mucosal thickening or complete opacification of the sinus. On MRI, the findings include watery secretions with hypointense signal on T1-weighted images and hyperintense signal on T2-weighted images.

An air-fluid level is not a pathognomonic sign of acute sinusitis. This finding is mimicked by acute blood within the sinus in patients with a history of recent trauma.

Chronic sinusitis

Chronic sinusitis is diagnosed when the patient has repeated bouts of acute infection or persistent inflammation.[11,25] The responsible pathogens include *Staphylococcus, Streptococcus, Corynebacterium, Bacteroides, Fusobacterium,* and other anaerobes.[5] Anaerobes are more commonly involved in chronic sinusitis than in acute sinusitis.[11,25] The radiographic findings vary. Signs suggestive of chronic sinusitis include mucosal thickening or opacification, bone remodeling and thickening caused by osteitis from adjacent chronic mucosal inflammation, and polyposis.[11,12,51] The anterior ethmoid air cells are the most common location involved with chronic sinusitis.

Opacification of the OMU predisposes to the development of sinusitis. Zinreich and others[56,58,63] found middle meatus opacification in 72% of patients with chronic sinusitis; 65% of these patients had mucoperiosteal thickening of the maxillary sinus.[56,58,63] All of the patients with frontal sinus inflammatory disease had opacification of the frontoethmoidal recess.[56,58,63] Frontal sinus opacification involving the OMU without frontal, maxillary, or anterior ethmoid sinus inflammatory disease was rare.[56,58,63] Yousem, Kennedy, and Rosenberg[55] found that when the middle meatus

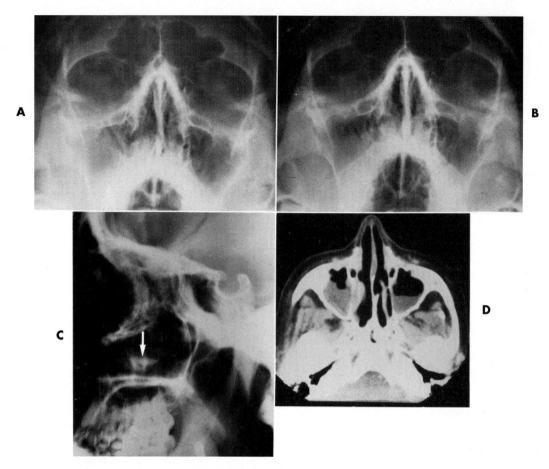

Fig. 56-21. Maxillary sinus air-fluid level. **A,** Waters view (patient prone) with right maxillary sinus opacity. **B,** The same patient in upright position shows the air-fluid level. **C,** The lateral view with maxillary sinus air-fluid level *(arrow).* **D,** Computed tomography shows bilateral maxillary sinus air-fluid levels.

was opacified, associated inflammatory changes occurred in the ethmoid sinuses in 82% of patients and in the maxillary sinuses in 84%.[55] Bolger, Butzin, and Parsons[5] found that when the ethmoid infundibulum was free of disease, the maxillary and frontal sinuses were clear in 77% of patients.

Babble and others[2] reviewed 500 patients with screening sinus CT and defined five recurring patterns of inflammatory sinonasal disease,[2] including infundibular, OMU, spheno-ethmoidal recess, sinonasal polyposis, and sporadic or un-classifiable disease. The infundibular pattern (26% of patients) referred to focal obstruction within the maxillary sinus ostium and ethmoid infundibulum that was associated with maxillary sinus disease. The OMU pattern (25% of patients) referred to ipsilateral maxillary, frontal, and anterior ethmoid sinus disease (Fig. 56-22). This pattern was caused by obstruction of the middle meatus. The frontal sinus was sometimes spared because of the variable location of the nasofrontal duct insertion in the middle meatus. The sphenoethmoidal recess pattern (6% of patients) resulted in sphenoid or posterior ethmoid sinus inflammation caused by

sphenoethmoidal recess obstruction. The sinonasal polypo-sis pattern (10% of patients) was caused by diffuse nasal and paranasal sinus polyps. Associated radiographic findings included infundibular enlargement, convex (bulging) eth-moid sinus walls, and attenuation of the bony nasal septum and ethmoid trabeculae.[2,13,39]

When sinus secretions are acute and of low viscosity, they are of intermediate attenuation on CT (10 to 25 Houns-field units). In the more chronic state, sinus secretions be-come thickened and concentrated, and the CT attenuation increases with density measurements of 30 to 60 Hounsfield units[43] (Fig. 56-23).

On MRI, the appearance of chronic sinusitis varies be-cause of the changing concentrations of protein and free water protons.[41,43] Initially, watery secretions on MRI ap-pear as hypointense on T1-weighted images and hyperin-tense on T2-weighted images.[41,43] According to Som and Curtin,[43] when sinonasal secretions become obstructed, two important physiologic events occur: the number of glycopro-tein-secreting goblet cells in the mucosa increases, and the

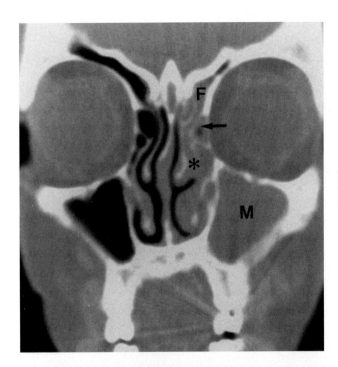

Fig. 56-22. OMU pattern of sinusitis. Inflammatory changes obstruct the left middle meatus *(asterisk)* with resulting opacification of the left maxillary *(M)*, frontal *(F)*, and anterior ethmoid *(arrow)* sinuses.

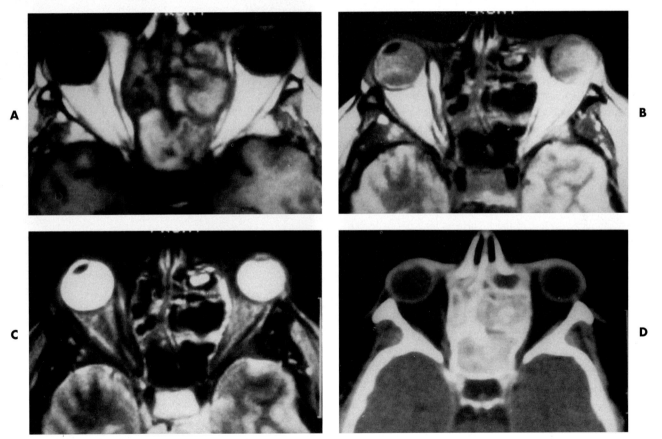

Fig. 56-23. Chronic sinusitis. **A,** Axial T1-weighted proton density. **B,** Axial T2-weighted (T2W) proton density. **C,** Magnetic resonance (MR) scan. **D,** Computed tomography (CT) scan. The expanded ethmoid and sphenoid sinuses are opacified (**A**). However, if a proton density and T2W series were the only MR scans taken, the dried secretions easily seen on CT (**D**) could be mistaken for aerated sinuses in **B** and **C**.

mucosa resorbs free water. This results in a transition from a thin serous fluid, to a thicker mucous, and ultimately to a desiccated stone-like plug. As the protein concentration increases, the signal intensity on T2-weighted images decreases. These charges are presumably caused by cross-linking that occurs between glycoprotein molecules. Som and Curtin[42,43] describe four patterns of MRI signal intensity that can be seen with chronic sinusitis: (1) hypointense on T1-weighted images and hyperintense on T2-weighted images with a protein concentration less than 9%; (2) hyperintense on T1-weighted images and hyperintense on T2-weighted images with total protein concentration increased to 20% to 25%; (3) hyperintense on T1-weighted images and hypointense on T2-weighted images with total protein concentration of 25% to 30%; and (4) hypointense on T1-weighted images and T2-weighted images with a protein concentration greater than 30% and inspissated secretions in an almost solid form. MRI of inspissated secretions (i.e., those with protein concentrations greater than 30%) may have a pitfall in that the signal voids on T1- and T2-weighted images may look identical to normally aerated sinuses.[41,43]

Certain anatomic variants, as described, have been implicated as causative factors in the presence of chronic inflammatory disease. Stammberger and Wolfe[46] and Lidov and Som[26] found that a large concha bullosa can produce signs and symptoms by narrowing the infundibulum. However, Yousem, Kennedy, and Rosenberg[55] found that the presence of a concha bullosa did not increase the risk of sinusitis. This was corroborated by Bolger, Butzin, and Parsons,[5] who found that a concha bullosa, paradoxic turbinates, Haller cells, and uncinate pneumatization were not significantly more common in patients with chronic sinusitis than in asymptomatic patients. Yousem, Kennedy, and Rosenberg[55] found that nasal septal deviation and a horizontally oriented uncinate process were more common in patients with inflammatory sinusitis. Although these variants may not necessarily predispose to sinusitis, the size of a given anatomic variant and its relationship to adjacent structures are important in the development of sinusitis.[54]

Fungal sinusitis

Fungal sinusitis may be suspected clinically when the patient fails to respond to standard antibiotic therapy. Although fungal infection in the paranasal sinuses is uncommon, the fungal pathogens most commonly encountered are *Aspergillus* species, mucormycosis, and *Candida* species.[54,55] Although mucormycosis and *Aspergillus* are part of the normal respiratory flora,[25] their involvement in the paranasal sinuses can often be differentiated clinically. *Aspergillus* sinusitis usually occurs in a noninvasive, saprophytic form in an otherwise healthy patient. Allergic fungal sinusitis usually occurs in patients with a history of atopy or asthma. This entity and marked nasal and sinus polyposis are associated. This process may expand the sinuses border-

ing the orbits, thus causing exophthalmos or optic nerve compression.[34] The invasive form of *Aspergillus* infection can occur in immunocompromised hosts.[25] The involvement is much more extensive than that in the allergic or saprophytic forms, and deep extension into the mucosa and bone often occurs.

Mucormycosis is caused by various genera (*Rhizopus, Mucor, Absidia*) of the family Mucoraceae. Spores of these

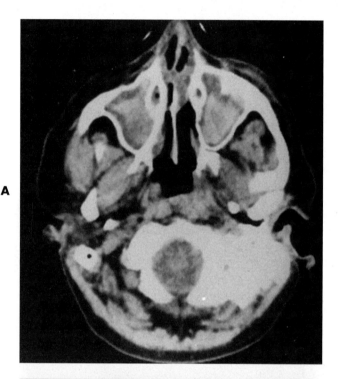

A

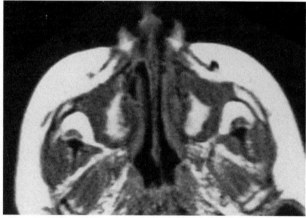

B

Fig. 56-24. A, Axial computed tomography. Central areas of increased attenuation in both maxillary sinuses are separated from the sinus walls by a thin zone of low attenuation (mucoid) material. This is consistent with desiccated sinus secretions, mycetoma, and hemorrhage. **B,** T1-weighted (T1W) magnetic resonance imaging. The central areas of the antra have high T1W signal intensity with surrounding low signal intensity material, which is diagnostic of hemorrhage with inflammation.

organisms are ubiquitous in the environment, and organisms are part of the normal respiratory flora. Infection only occurs in immunocompromised hosts; patients with poorly controlled diabetes account for 50% to 75% of cases.[7,43,62]

On imaging, the presence of an air-fluid level is uncommon. The maxillary and ethmoid sinuses are the most common sites of involvement.[43] Imaging findings vary depending on the aggressiveness of the fungus. Nonspecific mucosal thickening or sinus opacification may occur. The allergic form of *Aspergillus* is associated with recurrent sinonasal polyps. With more invasive fungi, sinus opacification with a central mycetoma and associated bony thickening or erosion may occur.[43] With mucormycosis and invasive *Aspergillus*, vascular invasion may occur, leading to intra- and extracranial thrombosis and infarction.

Several imaging characteristics suggest fungal sinusitis[43,44,62] (Fig. 56-24). On CT, a focal hyperdense lesion may be seen with surrounding hypodense mucoid material. On MRI, low signal intensity on T1-weighted images and a signal void on T2-weighted images have been found in many patients with fungal sinusitis, possibly because of the presence of paramagnetic metals (iron, manganese). Although the MRI appearance is similar in chronic bacterial infection caused by desiccated secretions, the decreased signal is not as pronounced as it is in fungal disease.

According to Som and Curtin,[41,43] two other circumstances suggest the presence of fungal infections: soft-tissue changes in the sinus with thickened, reactive bone and localized areas of osteomyelitis. Also suggestive of fungal infection is the association of inflammatory sinus disease with involvement of the adjacent nasal fossa and the soft tissues of the cheek. These signs of aggressive infection are atypical for bacterial pathogens.

Allergic sinusitis

Allergic sinusitis occurs in 10% of the population.[13] It typically produces a pansinusitis with symmetric involvement.[2] CT often shows a nodular mucosal thickening with thickened turbinates.[13] Air-fluid levels are rare unless bacterial superinfection occurs.[12]

Granulomatous sinusitis

Although many granulomatous diseases involve the sinonasal cavity, Wegener's granulomatosis and idiopathic midline granulomas are the most commonly encountered.

Complications of inflammatory sinus disease

Mucous retention cyst

Mucous retention cyst is a small cyst that most commonly occurs in the maxillary sinus floor in patients with a history of inflammatory disease. In occurs in 10% of the population. It is the result of inflammatory obstruction of a seromucinous gland within the sinus mucosal lining.[13,42] On CT (Fig. 56-25), this will appear as a homogenous, well-circumscribed hypo- to isodense mass. On MRI, it is usually hypointense on T1-weighted images on T1-weighted images and hyperintense on T2-weighted images (Fig. 56-26).

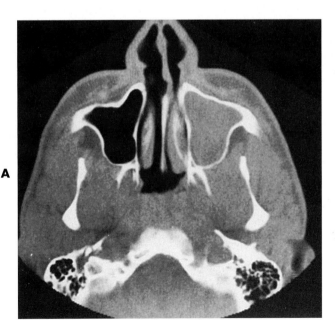 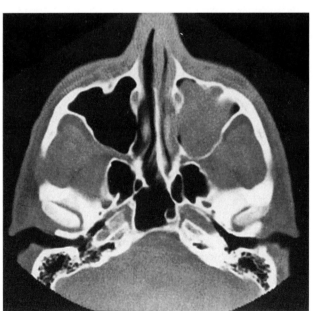

Fig. 56-25. Axial computed tomography scans **A,** in the midsinus and **B,** in the upper portion of the left maxillary sinus. In **A,** the sinus appears to be opacified. However, in **B,** air can be seen outlining the upper surface of a large retention cyst or polyp.

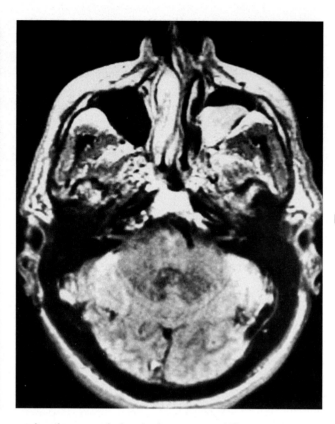

Fig. 56-26. Axial proton density magnetic resonance imaging scans **A,** low in the antrum and **B,** higher in the antrum show a retention cyst in the left antrum. If the contour of the upper surface is not clearly noted on all scans, this cyst could be mistaken for an air-fluid level.

Mucocele

Mucocele is a dilated mucous-filled sinus that is lined by mucous membrane. It is the result of a chronically obstructed sinus ostium with enlargement of bony walls caused by mucous secretions filling the sinus cavity.[39,43] It is most commonly caused by inflammatory obstruction of the ostium but also can be secondary to trauma, tumors, or surgical manipulation[12]; 66% of mucoceles occur in the frontal sinuses, and 25% and 10% occur in the ethmoid and maxillary sinuses, respectively.[25] On CT (Fig. 56-27) mucocele appears as a hypodense, nonenhancing mass that fills and expands the sinus cavity. On MRI, the appearance varies because of alterations in protein concentration of the obstructed mucoid secretions.

An infected mucocele, a mucopyocele, may show rim enhancement.[2]

Inflammatory polyps

Polyps in the paranasal sinuses result from local upheaval of the sinus mucosa with mucous membrane hyperplasia secondary to chronic inflammation.[2,25] Allergic sinusitis often plays a role in the formation of polyps. If large or numerous, polyps can cause local problems as a result of obstruction of the important osteomeatal channels, including the sinus ostia. On CT and MRI, polyps are often indistinguishable from mucous retention cysts (Fig. 56-28).

Orbital complications

About 3% of patients with sinusitis (most commonly children) have some form of orbital involvement; manifestations may be the first sign of sinus infection. Complicated sinusitis is the most common cause of orbital infection in 60% to 84% of cases.[6,36,50,52] The ethmoid sinuses are the most common origin, followed by the frontal, sphenoid, and maxillary sinuses in decreasing order. The ethmoid and maxillary sinuses are present at birth and therefore are the source in younger children. The frontal sinuses are usually detectable radiographically after 6 years but are not usually significant sources of infection until after 10 years. The sphenoid sinuses also develop late and are rarely implicated in pediatric patients.

Most authors recommend CT when clinical evidence of postseptal infection is present (i.e., when exophthalmos and limited eye movement are present) or when there is failure to improve with antibiotics.[2,13] Because the disease can be more aggressive in pediatric patients, CT should be considered when clinical evidence of preseptal inflammation is present.

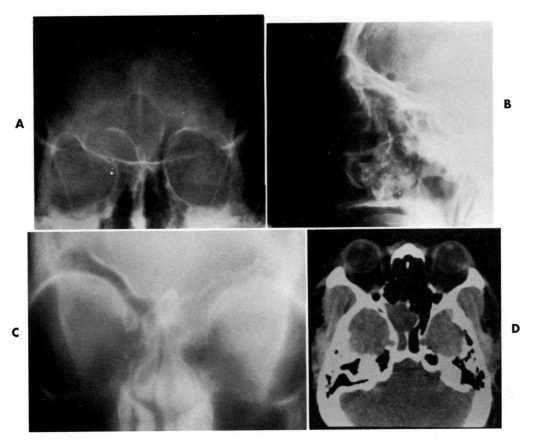

Fig. 56-27. Sinus mucoceles. **A,** Frontal view of right frontal-ethmoid sinus mucocele. Right orbital border is expanded. **B,** Lateral view of same patient with expansible change in frontal sinus and ethmoidal expansion. **C,** Frontal tomogram of another patient with left ethmoid sinus mucocele. Note expansible thinning of ethmoidal cells and orbital roof thinning. **D,** Right sphenoid sinus mucocele with expanded thinning of septum.

Preseptal orbital edema is a common finding in sinusitis, especially in children. CT reveals diffuse soft-tissue density and thickening of the preseptal soft tissues. At this stage, swelling and redness of the eyelids occur but not exophthalmos or limited eye movement. As infection spreads from the ethmoid sinus to the orbit, the orbital periosteum becomes inflamed, thickened, and elevated, with accumulation of an inflammatory phlegmon. On CT, this appears as an ill-defined, slightly enhancing mass on the sinus and orbital sides of the lamina papyracea. It is limited laterally by the periosteum; however, in more advanced cases, it merges with a thickened and enhancing medial rectus muscle, which is displaced laterally. Subsequently, liquefaction may occur in the subperiosteal compartment to form an abscess, which will be evident on CT as regions of low density, sometimes with an enhancing rim. CT findings of low-attenuation material surrounded by an enhancing rim suggest an abscess rather than a phlegmon, although the distinction between them can be difficult, given the continuum existing between these two states.

Rare orbital complications of paranasal sinus infection include superior ophthalmic vein thrombosis, cavernous sinus thrombosis, and blindness.[38] Superior ophthalmic vein thrombosis is suspected on CT when enlargement of this vessel (best seen on coronal scans) is asymmetric with a relative lack of normal enhancement, although thrombus within the lumen can be hyperdense. MRI may show these changes more accurately. Magnetic resonance angiography, especially phase-contrast techniques, can establish the presence of superior ophthalmic vein thrombosis.

Cavernous sinus thrombosis will be evident as fullness of the affected side with convexity of the lateral margin of the cavernous sinus (instead of the normal, slightly concave margin). Gadolinium-enhanced, axial and coronal MRI would be expected to be more sensitive to the presence of cavernous sinus thrombosis than would CT.

Permanent loss of vision is a rare complication of sinusitis, although recent studies report about a 10% incidence in patients with postseptal infection.[34,36,50,52] Mechanisms for loss of vision may be optic neuritis as a reaction to adjacent infection. Ischemia secondary to thrombophlebitis, arteritis,

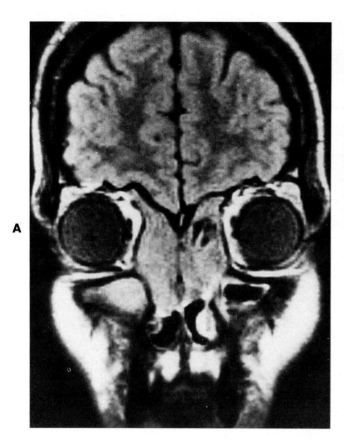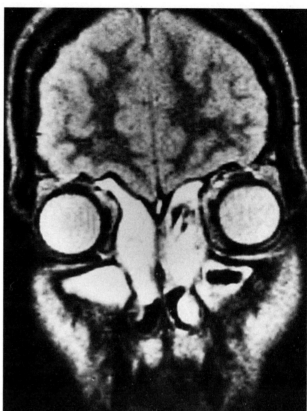

Fig. 56-28. Polyposis and sinusitis. **A,** Coronal proton density image and **B,** T2-weighted magnetic resonance imaging scans show bilateral nasoethmoid expansile masses causing hypertelorism. These masses have the same signal intensities as the mucosal thickening in the left antrum and the material in the right antrum, namely an intermediate signal intensity in **A** and a high signal intensity in **B.**

or pressure on the central retinal artery also may result in blindness.

RADIOGRAPHIC EVALUATION OF PATIENTS AFTER FUNCTIONAL ENDOSCOPIC SINUS SURGERY

Expected findings

Postoperative evaluation of patients is similar to preoperative evaluation. Ideally, patients should be followed with coronal CT. Because a surgical procedure was performed, the type and extent of surgery should be established. Subsequently, the emphasis is on the anatomy. The presence or absence of important structures should be identified and mentioned. The nasal cavity and paranasal sinus boundaries and important anatomic relationships should be inspected (Fig. 56-29). Areas of bony thickening of dehiscence should be noted.

The following merit close scrutiny on follow-up CT:

Frontal recess

The frontal recesses should be identified to determine their patency. Postoperatively, recurrence of disease is caused by persistent obstruction in this area, which is the narrowest channel within the anterior ethmoid complex and is difficult to access surgically. Therefore, the frontal recess is most likely to be affected with inflammatory disease in a patient who underwent previous surgery in the paranasal sinuses. The agger nasi cell (if it remains) should be noted because its persistence may continue to narrow the frontal recess.

Ostiomealal unit

The extent of the excision of the uncinate and removal of the ethmoid bulla should be noted. The course of the infundibulum should be examined for persistent anatomic narrowing. The outline of the middle turbinate should be examined to determine whether a middle turbinectomy has been performed. If so, careful attention should be paid to the vertical attachment of the middle turbinate to the cribriform plate and to the attachment of the basal lamella to the lamina papyracea. Traction on the vertical attachment and basal lamella of the middle turbinate during the course of middle turbinectomy can fracture the lamina papyracea or the cribriform plate. Breaks in the continuity of the laminal papyracea and ethmoid roof are easily seen on coronal images.

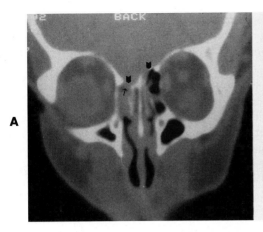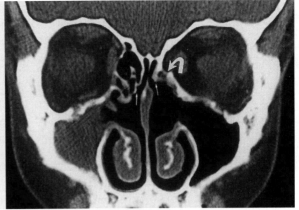

Fig. 56-29. Anatomic landmarks to be evaluated in patients after functional endoscopic sinus surgery. **A,** Coronal computed tomography (CT) image through the anterior ethmoid sinuses shows a prominent asymmetry in the position of the roof of the ethmoid sinuses *(solid arrowheads)*. The intracranial penetration *(fine black arrow)* is usually on the side where the roof is lower in position. **B,** Coronal computed tomography image through the anterior ethmoid sinus in a patient after bilateral uncinate resections and partial middle turbinectomies *(fine white arrows)*. If there is an intraorbital complication during such a surgical procedure, it usually involves the lamina papyracea at the attachment of the basal lamella *(curved arrow)*.

Lamina papyracea

The course of the lamina papyracea should be inspected to evaluate the integrity of this structure. Postoperative dehiscences are commonly found posterior to the nasolacrimal duct and may be caused by the uncinate resection.

Ethmoid roof

Asymmetry in position of the roof of the ethmoid sinus should be noted. Intracranial penetrations are usually on the side where the position of the roof is lower.

Sphenoid sinus area

The margins of the sphenoid sinus should be evaluated for bony dehiscence or cephalocele.

Operative complications

The incidence of FESS-related complications is related to the use of instruments, the patient's underlying anatomy, the overall health of the patient, the extent of disease, and the experience of the surgeon.*

The field of view available to the surgeon during FESS is quite small, and variant anatomy can make surgical landmarks difficult to identify. The surgeon's view is limited to the surface mucosa and does not extend beyond the mucosa directly in view. The presence of various anatomic variants can contribute to surgical complications if not noted prospectively.[16] As stated, because an accurate surgical road map is needed, all patients scheduled to undergo FESS should undergo preoperative coronal CT.

*Refs. 15, 16, 28, 29, 35, 47, 48.

Brisk bleeding in the operative field and extensive nasal polyposis can hinder visibility and predispose the patient to operative complications.[16] Standard surgical techniques and microscope-assisted surgery can be used when problems arise. However, they have many of the same complications.

In general, complications can be divided into minor and major.[15,16,28,47,48] Minor complications include periorbital emphysema, epistaxis, postoperative nasal synechiae, and tooth pain. Although these can commonly occur, they are usually self-limited and do not require postoperative radiologic evaluation.

Major complications are rarer but can be severely devastating or fatal.[29] A preexisting loss of integrity of the lamina papyracea can permit intraorbital fat to herniate into the ethmoid sinuses. Preexisting dehiscence of the lamina papyracea may be caused by prior trauma or erosion from chronic sinus disease. Disruption of the lamina papyracea can occur during resection of the middle turbinate if the ground lamella is resected back to its attachment to the lamina papyracea (Fig. 56-30).

The medial rectus muscle, superior oblique muscle, or other orbital contents can be directly damaged if preexisting or intraoperative disruption of the lamina papyracea occurs.[35] Injuries to the orbital contents may result in postoperative diplopia, which can be caused by muscle entrapment among bone fragments or direct muscle laceration, or it may occur secondary to nerve injury. Clinically, subconjunctival hemorrhage is often associated with extraocular muscle damage.[35] If intraorbital and intraocular pressure builds up as a result of an expanding hematoma or air being forced into the orbit from the nasal cavity (through a dehiscent

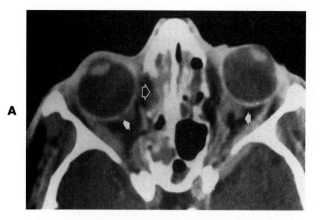

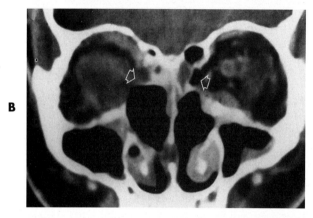

Fig. 56-30. Orbital complications from functional endoscopic sinus surgery. **A,** Axial and **B,** coronal computed tomography images in a patient who was found to be blind after undergoing bilateral anterior ethmoidectomies, partial bilateral middle turbinectomies, and bilateral uncinate resections. Note the defects in the lamina papyracea bilaterally *(open arrows)* and the severed bilateral optic nerves *(solid arrows).*

lamina papyracea), then visual impairment or blindness secondary to ischemia can result.[35]

Temporary or permanent blindness caused by injury of the optic nerve can occur during posterior ethmoidectomy if the bony limit of the sinus is violated[15,29,35,48] (see Fig. 56-29). Trauma to the vascular supply to the optic nerve also can result in visual loss.

Perforation of the cribriform plate can lead to intracranial hematoma or infection.

Massive hemorrhage from direct injury to major vessels can occur. Laceration of the internal carotid artery has been reported and is often fatal.[15,16,29] Emergent angiography with balloon occlusion of the lacerated artery has been performed. Patients who report severe postoperative headache or photophobia or who have signs that suggest subarachnoid hemorrhage should undergo noncontrast head CT. If subarachnoid blood is found, cerebral angiography is recommended to detect vascular injury.[15,16,47]

Injury to the nasolacrimal duct can result during anterior

enlargement of the maxillary ostium in the middle meatus. Injury to the membranous portion of the duct may be self-limited and remit by spontaneous fistulization into the middle meatus. Stenosis or total occlusion of the nasolacrimal duct can result from more severe injury.[35]

Postoperative cerebrospinal fluid (CSF) leak is another major complication of FESS.[28,29,35,48] These leaks occur after inadvertent penetration of the dura. Extension of the injury to involve the cribriform plate, fovea ethmoidalis, anterior cranial fossa, and the skull base has been reported. Secondary nasal encephalocele or deep penetration of the cerebrum can be seen after violation of the cranial vault.[51] A CSF leak may not become clinically apparent for up to 2 years after surgery.[15,16] CSF leaks will often close spontaneously with conservative measures (e.g., lumbar drain).[15,16] However, if they persist, radiologic workup is indicated.

In many institutions, a radionuclide CSF study is the initial radiologic screening examination in such patients.[4,33] Before beginning the study, the otolaryngologist places three to four absorbent pledgets on each side of the nasal cavity and notes their location within the nasal cavity. Next, 400 to 500 Ci of indium-111 (^{111}In)–labeled DTPA is placed in the subarachnoid space by the neuroradiologist through a cervical or lumbar puncture.

The patient undergoes imaging with a γ camera at multiple intervals up to 24 hours. Any position or activity known to provoke the leak is encouraged. Although images of the head and neck are obtained, evidence of the leak is unusual on these images. Rather, indirect signs of leaking are sought. Images over the abdomen are done to search for activity in the bowel, which indicates that the patient is swallowing CSF as it leaks into the nasal cavity (Fig. 56-31).

At 24 hours, the nasal pledgets are removed and assayed. The results are compared with ^{111}In activity in a serum sample drawn at the same time. A ratio of pledget activity to serum activity is determined and expressed in terms of counts/g. Pledgets showing activity 1.5 times greater than serum activity are positive. It is then possible to predict the general area of the leak based on which pledgets show increased activity. If none of the pledgets have increased activity but activity over the abdomen is increased, the radionuclide test is considered positive.

When the radionuclide test is positive (directly or indirectly), a contrast CT cisternogram in the coronal and axial planes is done to define the anatomy and to pinpoint the site of leakage. This CT scan can help the surgeon plan further therapy to correct the leak.

COMPUTER-ASSISTED SURGERY

Kennedy and others[19] showed that the number of major surgical complications (e.g., death, orbital and intracranial damage) is increasing with the increasing numbers of FESS.[19] Although CT provides a road map for the surgeon, the information that is provided is remote. The surgeon

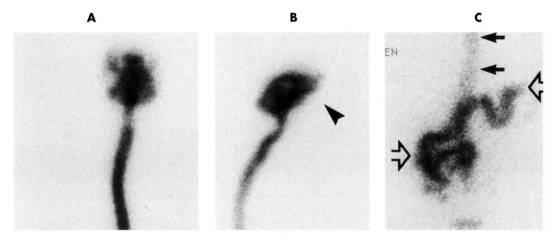

Fig. 56-31. A cerebrospinal fluid (CSF) leak seen after functional endoscopic sinus surgery. Indium-111 pentetic acid cerebrospinal fluid study in the **A,** Anteroposterior (AP) and **B,** lateral projections shows normal activity in the subarachnoid spaces. No activity is seen within the paranasal sinuses or nasal cavity *(black arrowhead).* **C,** Delayed AP image of the abdomen shows abnormal bowel activity because of swallowed secretions from occult CSF leakage *(open arrows).* Residual activity within the subarachnoid space is noted *(black arrows).*

should mentally transfer information from the image to the operative site.

Given the extreme variations in anatomy, extensive inflammatory disease, and at times the copious amount of intraoperative bleeding that makes landmarks difficult to identify, it is not surprising that inadvertent injuries to the orbital and intracranial compartments occur.

Thus, there is a need for an objective and interactive correlation of the image data with the anatomic findings at the time of surgery. Over the past 5 years, this goal has been achieved with an ISG Allegro multimodality computer (ISG Technologies, Mississauga, Ontario, Canada) using a mechanical sensor manufactured by Farro Medical Technologies and more recently using the Pixys infrared sensor technology.[64] Prior to CT, 5 to 10 external markers are placed on the patient's face. These markers are used to register the data in the computer so that they can be applied to the patient *in vivo* on the surgical table. With the registration complete and the patient immobilized, the mechanical arm holding a probe can be placed into the nasal cavity. The tip of the probe is the location of the sensor. Axial, coronal, and sagittal reformatted images at the tip of the sensor are generated by the computer, and the location of the sensor in the patient is shown by cross hairs on these images. The Pixys sensors may be directly placed on the surgeon's instrument. Furthermore, additional sensors may be directly attached to the patient's head through a headband. Thus, two sets of sensors are available: one follows the position of the surgeon's instrument, and the other updates the computer with the patient's head motions. This new sensor technology allows this instrumentation to be used during surgery with general or local anesthesia. Hopefully, the probe will confirm the location of specific anatomic structures and avoid penetration of

the ethmoid roof and lamina papyracea. It can easily identify the relationship of the sphenoid sinus to the optic nerves and carotid canals. The accuracy of this device is within 2 mm.[64]

Several groups have attempted to improve sensor technology and the computer software that supports the system. In the near future, use of this technology is expected to become widespread.

CONCLUSIONS

Coronal CT is the imaging modality of choice in patients with sinus disease. CT provides an initial screening of these patients and can display anatomic causes of recurrent sinusitis when they exist. CT is essential for planning surgery, and it provides an operative road map for subsequent FESS. Interactive image-guided computer-assisted surgery is promising for objectively and directly integrating the imaging information with the endoscopic view and will thus improve the accuracy and safety of the operative management of patients undergoing sinus surgery.

Close cooperation between the radiologist and otolaryngologist before surgery may bring to light imaging findings predisposing the patient to operative complications. When complications occur, the radiologist can provide assistance in evaluation using CT, MRI, and nuclear medicine studies.

REFERENCES

1. Babbel R and others: Optimization of techniques in screening CT of the sinuses, *Am J Roentgenol* 157:1093, 1991.
2. Babbel R and others: Recurring patterns of inflammatory sinonasal disease demonstrated on screening sinus CT, *AJNR Am J Neuroradiol* 13:903, 1992.
3. Beck T: Personal communication, Radiation Physicist, Dept. of Radiology, The Johns Hopkins Hospital, Baltimore, Md.
4. Benson ML, Oliverio PJ, Zinreich SJ: *Techniques of imaging of the*

nose and paranasal sinuses. In *Advances in otolaryngology—head and neck surgery*, vol 10, St Louis, 1996, Mosby (in press).

5. Bolger W, Butzin C, Parsons D: Paranasal sinus bony anatomic variations and mucosal abnormalities: CT analysis for endoscopic sinus surgery, *Laryngoscope* 101:56, 1991.

6. Buus D, Tse D, Farris B: Ophthalmic complications of sinus surgery, *Ophthalmology* 97:612, 1990.

7. Centeno R, Bentson J, Mancuso A: CT scanning in rhinocerebral mucormycosis and aspergillosis, *Radiology* 140:383, 1981.

8. Curry TS, Dowdey JE, Murry RC: *Christensen's physics of diagnostic radiology*, ed 4, Philadelphia, 1990, Lea & Febiger.

9. Delano M, Fun FY, Zinreich SJ: Optic nerve relationship to the posterior paranasal sinuses: a CT anatomic study, *AJNR Am J Neuroradiol* 17:669, 1996.

10. Dessi P and others: Difference in height of the right and left ethmoidal roofs: a possible risk factor for ethmoidal surgery. Prospective study of 150 CT scans, *Laryngol Otol* 108:261, 1994.

11. Evans F and others: Sinusitis of the maxillary antrum, *N Engl J Med* 293:735, 1975.

12. Gullane P, Conley J: Carcinoma of the maxillary sinus: a correlation of the clinical course with orbital involvement, pterygoid erosion or pterygopalatine invasion and cervical metastases. *J Otolaryngol* 12: 141, 1983.

13. Harnsberger R: *Imaging for the sinus and nose.* In: *Head and neck imaging handbook,* St Louis, 1990, Mosby.

14. Hosemann W: *Dissection of the lateral nasal wall in eight steps.* In Wigand ME, editor: *Endoscopic surgery of the paranasal sinuses and anterior skull base,* New York, 1990, Thieme.

15. Hudgins P: Complications of endoscopic sinus surgery: the role of the radiologist in prevention, *Radiol Clin North Am* 31:21, 1993.

16. Hudgins P, Browning D, Gallups J: Endoscopic paranasal sinus surgery: radiographic evaluation of severe complications, *AJNR Am J Neuroradiol* 13:1161, 1992.

17. Johnson DW and others: The unprotected parasphenoidal carotid artery studied by high-resolution computed tomography, *Radiology* 155:137, 1985.

18. Jones DJ, Wall BF: Organ doses from medical x-ray examinations calculated using Monte Carlo techniques, NRPB-R186 (HMSO, London), National Radiological Protection Board, 1985.

19. Kennedy D and others: Complications of ethmoidectomy: a survey of fellows of Otolaryngology—Head & Neck Surgery. Otolaryngology—Head & Neck Surgery (in press).

20. Kennedy DW, Zinreich SJ: The functional endoscopic approach to inflammatory sinus disease: current perspectives and technique modifications, *Am J Rhinol* 2:89, 1988.

21. Kennedy DW, Zinreich SJ, Hassab MH: The internal carotid artery as it related to endonasal sphenoethmoidectomy, *Am J Roentgenol* 4:7, 1990.

22. Kennedy D and others: Physiologic mucosal changes within the nose and ethmoid sinus: imaging of the nasal cycle by MRI, *Laryngoscope* 98:928, 1988.

23. Kennedy DW and others: Functional endoscopic surgery: theory and diagnostic evaluation, *Arch Otolaryngol Head Neck Surg* 111:576, 1985.

24. Laine FJ, Kuta AJ: Imaging the sphenoid bone and basiocciput: pathologic considerations, *Semin Ultrasound CT MR* 14:160, 1993.

25. Laine F, Smoker W: The ostiomeatal unit and endoscopic surgery: anatomy, variations, and imaging findings in inflammatory diseases, *Am J Roentgenol* 159:849, 1992.

26. Lidov M, Som P: Inflammatory disease involving a concha bullosa (enlarged pneumatized middle nasal turbinate): MR and CT appearance, *AJNR Am J Neuroradiol* 11:999, 1990.

27. Mafee M: Preoperative imaging anatomy of the nasal-ethmoid complex for functional endoscopic sinus surgery, *Radiol Clin North Am* 31:1, 1993.

28. Maniglia A: Fatal and major complications secondary to nasal and sinus surgery, *Laryngoscope* 99:276, 1989.

29. Maniglia A: Fatal and other major complications of endoscopic sinus surgery, *Laryngoscope* 101:349, 1991.

30. Melhem ER and others: Optimal CT screening for functional endoscopic sinus surgery, *AJNR Am J Neuroradiol* 17:181, 1996.

31. Messerklinger W: *Endoscopy of the nose,* Baltimore, 1978, Urban & Schwartzenberg.

32. Messerklinger W: Zur Endoskopietchnik des mittleren Nassenganges. *Arch Otorhinolaryngol* 221:297, 1978.

33. Mettler FA, Guiberteau MJ: *Essentials of nuclear medicine imaging,* ed 3, Philadelphia. 1991, WB Saunders.

34. Moloney J, Badham N, McRae A: The acute orbit, preseptal, periorbital cellulitis, subperiosteal abscess, and orbital cellulitis due to sinusitis, *J Laryngol Otol* 12:1, 1987.

35. Neuhaus R: Orbital complications secondary to endoscopic sinus surgery, *Ophthalmology* 97:1512, 1990.

36. Osguthorpe J, Hochman M: Inflammatory sinus diseases affecting the orbit, *Otolaryngol Clin North Am* 26:657, 1993.

37. Panje WR, Anand VK: *Endoscopic sinus surgery indications, diagnosis, and technique.* In Anand VK, Panje WR, editors: *Practical endoscopic sinus surgery,* New York, 1993, McGraw-Hill.

38. Patt B, Manning S: Blindness resulting from orbital complications of sinusitis, *Otolaryngol Head Neck Surg* 104:789, 1991.

39. Scuderi A and others: The sporadic pattern of inflammatory sinonasal disease including postsurgical changes, *Semin Ultrasound CT MR* 12: 575, 1991.

40. Shankar L and others: *An atlas of imaging of the paranasal sinuses,* 1994, Imago Publishing.

41. Som P: Imaging of paranasal sinus fungal disease, *Otolaryngol Clin North Am* 26:983, 1993.

42. Som P: *Sinonasal cavity.* In Som P, Bergeron T, editors: *Head and neck imaging,* St Louis, 1991, Mosby.

43. Som P, Curtin H: Chronic inflammatory sinonasal diseases including fungal infections: the role of imaging, *Radiol Clin North Am* 31:33, 1993.

44. Som P and others: Hypointense paranasal sinus foci: differential diagnosis with MR imaging and relation to CT findings, *Radiology* 176: 777, 1990.

45. Stammberger H: *Functional sinus surgery,* Philadelphia, 1991, Mosby.

46. Stammberger H, Wolf G: Headaches and sinus disease: the endoscopic approach, *Ann Otol Rhinol Laryngol Suppl* 134:3, 1988.

47. Stankiewicz J: Complications of endoscopic intranasal ethmoidectomy, *Laryngoscope* 97:1270, 1987.

48. Stankiewicz J: Complications in endoscopic intranasal ethmoidectomy: an update, *Laryngoscope* 99:668, 1989.

49. Vinning EM, Kennedy DW: Surgical management in adults: chronic sinusitis, *Immunology and Allergy Clinics of North America* 14:97, 1994.

50. Walters E and others: Acute orbital cellulitis, *Arch Ophthalmol* 94: 785, 1976.

51. Weber A: Inflammatory diseases of the paranasal sinuses and mucoceles, *Otolaryngol Clin North Am* 21:421, 1988.

52. Weber A, Mikulis D: Inflammatory disorders of the paraorbital sinuses and their complications, *Radiol Clin North Am* 25:615, 1987.

53. Wigand ME, Steiner W, Jaumann MP: Endonasal sinus surgery with endoscopic control: from radical operation to rehabilitation of the mucosa, *Endoscopy* 10:255, 1978.

54. Yousem D: Imaging of sinonasal inflammatory disease, *Radiology* 188: 303, 1993.

55. Yousem D, Kennedy D, Rosenberg S: Ostiomeatal complex risk factors for sinusitis: CT evaluation, *J Otolaryngol* 20:419, 1991.

56. Zinreich S: Imaging of chronic sinusitis in adults: x-ray, computed

tomography, and magnetic resonance imaging, *J Allergy Clin Immunol* 90:445, 1992.

57. Zinreich S: Imaging of inflammatory sinus disease, *Otolaryngol Clin North Am* 26:535, 1993.

58. Zinreich S: Paranasal sinus imaging, *Otolaryngol Head Neck Surg* 103: 863, 1990.

59. Zinreich S, Abidin M, Kennedy D: Cross-sectional imaging of the nasal cavity and paranasal sinuses, *Operative Techniques in Otolaryngol Head Neck Surg* 1:93, 1990.

60. Zinreich SJ, Benson ML, Oliverio PS: *Sinonasal cavities: CT normal anatomy, imaging of the osteomeatal complex, and functional endo-scopic surgery*. In Som P, Curtin H, editors: *Head and neck imaging*, ed 3, St Louis, 1996, Mosby.

61. Zinreich SJ and others: MR imaging of normal nasal cycle: comparison with sinus pathology, *JCAT* 12:1014, 1988.

62. Zinreich S and others: Fungal sinusitis: diagnosis with CT and MR imaging, *Radiology* 169:439, 1988.

63. Zinreich S and others: Paranasal sinuses: CT imaging requirements for endoscopic surgery, *Radiology* 163:769, 1987.

64. Zinreich S and others: Frameless stereotaxic integration of CT imaging data: accuracy and initial applications, *Radiology* 188:735, 1993.

Chapter 57

Management of Thyroid Eye Disease (Graves' Ophthalmopathy)

Douglas A. Girod

In 1835, Robert Graves described a clinical syndrome that included such symptoms as hypermetabolism, diffuse enlargement of the thyroid gland, and exophthalmos. Although others also had recognized this entity, it was Graves who defined the thyroid as playing a central role in the disease. Graves' disease is now recognized as a multisystem disorder characterized by one or more of the following: (1) hyperthyroidism associated with diffuse hyperplasia of the thyroid gland, (2) infiltrative ophthalmopathy (leading to exophthalmos), and (3) infiltrative dermopathy (localized pretibial myxedema). Recent work has helped to establish Graves' disease as an autoimmune process targeted at the thyroid-stimulating hormone (TSH) receptor in the thyroid.[42,53,56] In addition, retroocular fibroblasts have been found to play a key role in the development and progression of the ophthalmopathy seen in some Graves' patients.[2,3]

Despite these advances in the understanding of Graves' disease pathogenesis, only limited progress has been made in the management of the disease. Therapy is still primarily directed at the manifestations of the disease in a palliative fashion rather than at preventing the underlying destructive autoimmune process. This chapter will focus on the evaluation and management of the ophthalmic manifestations of Graves' disease.

PATHOPHYSIOLOGY

Extensive research in recent years has led to important insights into the pathologic mechanisms involved in Graves' disease and Graves' ophthalmopathy. As the understanding progresses, so should the ability to deal with this challenging disorder.

Graves' disease

Current theory describing the development of Graves' disease involves autoreactive T cells, which arise through either an escape from clonal deletion, failure of suppressor T cell activity, or through molecular mimicry to become reactive to TSH receptors.[7] Subsequent thyroid damage from any etiology (chronic thyroiditis, radiotherapy, smoking, drugs, and so on) results in the release of the thyroid autoantigen (TSH receptors). As the autoimmune process amplifies, T lymphocytes are activated, and humoral immunity produces antibodies to the TSH receptor that are stimulatory, resulting in hyperthyroidism. In some patients, underlying chronic thyroiditis may dramatically reduce thyroid reserve or TSH receptor blocking antibodies may be present, resulting in the "euthyroid" patient with Graves' disease.

Graves' ophthalmopathy

The extraocular muscles are the site of the most clinically evident changes in patients with Graves' ophthalmopathy. Although the muscles are enlarged on computed tomography (CT) scan, the myocytes themselves appear fairly normal histopathologically.[35] There is an associated intense proliferation of perimysial fibroblasts and dense lymphocytic infiltration. Early reports of circulating autoantibodies against eye muscle antigen *in sera* from patients with Graves' ophthalmopathy led to the theory that the disease was a result of an autoimmune response directed against the extraocular eye muscle fibers.[41] This theory began to lose favor as study of these autoantibodies proved them to be neither tissue- or disease-specific. The lack of histologic evidence of cytotoxicity against eye muscle *in vivo* also argues against this theory.

Attention has now focused on the retrobulbar fibroblast as playing a key role in the pathogenesis of Graves' ophthalmopathy. These fibroblasts have several capabilities that place them at the center of the changes seen in the eye. They secrete a range of glycosaminoglycans (predominately hyaluronate), the deposition of which is a hallmark of Graves' ophthalmopathy and causes interstitial edema as a result of its intensely hydrophyllic nature. These cells also can produce major histocompatibility complex class II molecules, heat shock proteins, and lymphocyte adhesion molecules, which allow them to act as target and effector cells in the ongoing immune process in those with Graves' ophthalmopathy.[31] In addition, autoantibodies against fibroblast antigens have been found in a majority of patients with Graves' ophthalmopathy. These antibodies share some characteristics with TSH receptor antibodies (TRAbs).[3] More recently, probes to TSH receptor messenger ribonucleic acid (mRNA) have labeled mRNA within the retrobulbar fibroblasts of Graves' ophthalmopathy patients.[7] Thus, the "fibroblast antigen" may be similar to all or part of the TSH receptor and therefore represents a shared thyroid–eye antigen. Such an antigenic similarity would explain the immune cross-reactivity between these two seemingly unrelated tissue sites.

Lymphocytes also are active in the ongoing immune process of Graves' ophthalmopathy. Orbital lymphocyte infiltrates have been found to be primarily T cells, including CD4+ (T helper cells) and CD8+ (T suppressor and cytotoxic cells). Cytokines released by T cells have been shown to induce fibroblast proliferation and collagen and glycosaminoglycan deposition. Recently, Grubeck-Loebenstein and others[27] cultured retrobulbar suppressor and cytotoxic T cells out of tissues removed at the time of orbital decompression and found them capable of targeting the retrobulbar fibroblasts. Interactions with fibroblasts resulted in pronounced T cell cytokine production and fibroblast proliferation without evidence of fibroblast cytotoxicity. Thus, the T cell–retrobulbar fibroblast interaction may be responsible for the clinical manifestations of Graves' ophthalmopathy.

Burch and Wortofsky[7] have proposed a hypothetical sequence of events that lead to the initiation and progression of Graves' ophthalmopathy based on an extensive review of the recent literature (Fig. 57-1).

EPIDEMIOLOGY/ETIOLOGY

An accurate estimate of prevalence for Graves' ophthalmopathy is difficult to determine and depends in part on the diagnostic criteria used to define the presence of ophthalmopathy. For example, "lid lag" and "stare" are nonspecific signs and can be seen with thyrotoxicosis stemming from etiologies other than Graves' disease. In an exhaustive review of the literature, Burch and Wartofsky[7] found an incidence of ophthalmopathy in patients with Graves' disease of 10% to 25% if these nonspecific signs were excluded and 30% to 45% if lid findings were included as diagnostic criteria. When intraocular pressure on upgaze or CT findings also were included, the incidence increased to nearly 70%. Fortunately, the most severe form of Graves' ophthalmopathy with optic nerve involvement and visual impairment occurs in only 2% to 5% of patients with Graves' disease.[46,68]

EFFECTS OF GENETICS AND GENDER

The role of genetic predisposition and major histocompatibility complex (MHC) antigen patterns in those with Graves' ophthalmopathy has been extensively studied but remains poorly characterized.[7] Ethnicity appears to play some role, as Tellez and others[65] found that Europeans with Graves' disease were six times more likely to develop ophthalmopathy than Asian patients with Graves' disease. More important are the influences of gender on the development of Graves' disease and the associated ophthalmopathy. A strong 3:1 female-to-male preponderance exists for Graves' disease,[48,66] which decreases to about 2:1 for those with Graves' ophthalmopathy. Overall, male patients with Graves' disease have a higher incidence of ophthalmopathy that is more severe and tends to develop later in life.[7]

EFFECTS OF TOBACCO

Several studies have reported an increased incidence of goiter in tobacco smokers compared with nonsmokers, attributing this to thiocyanate, a known goitrogen, which is present in inhaled tobacco smoke.[10,16] Studies also have reported an association between smoking and the incidence and severity of Graves' ophthalmopathy.[4,65] This relationship was not found in patients with other forms of thyroid disease and suggests the tobacco effects are specific for Graves' disease. It is possible that the decrease in female preponderance in Graves' ophthalmopathy, especially in the more severe forms, may be a reflection of the higher incidence of smoking among male patients rather than a true gender difference.[7]

EFFECTS OF THYROID STATUS

The role of thyroid hormonal status in the development and severity of Graves' ophthalmopathy has been particularly difficult to ascertain because of the overlap of thyrotoxicosis with antithyroid therapy in this patient population. Thyrotoxicosis alone is thought to have little direct effect on the autoimmune process. It serves as a fairly poor marker for disease severity because the prevalence and course of hyperthyroidism correlate poorly with that of Graves' ophthalmopathy.[7] An improvement in eye status with maintenance of euthyroidism during antithyroid therapy may be more a reflection of improving immune function than a decreased circulating thyroid hormone.

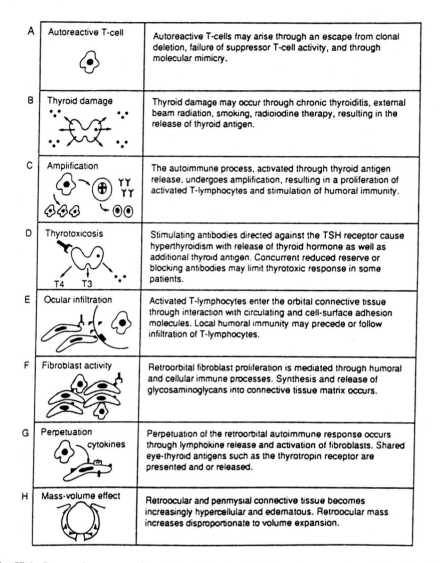

A	Autoreactive T-cell	Autoreactive T-cells may arise through an escape from clonal deletion, failure of suppressor T-cell activity, and through molecular mimicry.
B	Thyroid damage	Thyroid damage may occur through chronic thyroiditis, external beam radiation, smoking, radioiodine therapy, resulting in the release of thyroid antigen.
C	Amplification	The autoimmune process, activated through thyroid antigen release, undergoes amplification, resulting in a proliferation of activated T-lymphocytes and stimulation of humoral immunity.
D	Thyrotoxicosis	Stimulating antibodies directed against the TSH receptor cause hyperthyroidism with release of thyroid hormone as well as additional thyroid antigen. Concurrent reduced reserve or blocking antibodies may limit thyrotoxic response in some patients.
E	Ocular infiltration	Activated T-lymphocytes enter the orbital connective tissue through interaction with circulating and cell-surface adhesion molecules. Local humoral immunity may precede or follow infiltration of T-lymphocytes.
F	Fibroblast activity	Retroorbital fibroblast proliferation is mediated through humoral and cellular immune processes. Synthesis and release of glycosaminoglycans into connective tissue matrix occurs.
G	Perpetuation	Perpetuation of the retroorbital autoimmune response occurs through lymphokine release and activation of fibroblasts. Shared eye-thyroid antigens such as the thyrotropin receptor are presented and or released.
H	Mass-volume effect	Retroocular and perimysial connective tissue becomes increasingly hypercellular and edematous. Retroocular mass increases disproportionate to volume expansion.

Fig. 57-1. Proposed sequence of events leading to the initiation and progression of Graves' ophthalmopathy based on the current literature. (From Burch HB, Wartofsky L: Graves' ophthalmopathy: current concepts regarding pathogenesis and management, *Endocr Rev* 14:747, 1993.)

Elevated circulating TSH levels appear to promote eye disease in Graves' patients. Hamilton and others[30] and others have reported an increased incidence of progressive ophthalmopathy with the hypothyroidsm, which followed antithyroid therapy. Tamaki and others[64] described a marked improvement in eye status and a reduction of circulating TRAb in two patients receiving thyroid hormone replacement during antithyroid therapy. The mechanism by which elevated TSH achieves its influence is not clear, but it may serve to upregulate TSH receptors (apparent autoantigens, to be discussed) in thyrocytes[34] and possibly lymphocytes.[23]

NATURAL HISTORY

On summarizing the available literature on the natural history of Graves' ophthalmopathy, Burch and Wartofsky[7] noted the disease tended to progress through a phase of rapid progression (6 to 24 months), followed by a prolonged plateau phase with subsequent slow but incomplete regression of eye changes. Lid retraction and soft tissue changes, such as chemosis and eyelid edema, tended to be short-lived with improvement or resolution over 1 to 5 years (60% to 90%). Ophthalmoplegia resolved incompletely and less rapidly, although 30% to 40% of patients showed some improvement in ocular motility without specific therapy. Proptosis is the eye finding least likely to improve or resolve spontaneously (10%). Trobe[67] reviewed 32 patients with untreated Graves' optic neuropathy and found that vision improved spontaneously in most, but 21% had a final visual acuity of 20/100 or worse, with five patients progressing to near blindness. Facing potential loss of sight, it is not surprising that attempts at medical and surgical intervention, some of them heroic, have occurred for the past 80 years.

CLINICAL FEATURES

Thyroid disease

The patient with Graves' ophthalmopathy will most commonly present to the endocrinologist for management of thyroid disease or to the ophthalmologist for evaluation of eye complaints. A thorough history, examination, and high level of suspicion are required to make the diagnosis. Classically, the patient is hyperthyroid with the expected hypermetabolic findings at the time of presentation with eye disease. However, in a review of more than 800 cases from the literature, Burch and Wortofsky[7] found that 20% of patients presented with eye disease before any manifestation of hyperthyroidism, 39% presented concurrently with thyroid and eye disease, and 41% presented with eye disease after clinical hyperthyroidism already was evident. In 80% of the patients in whom both diseases eventually manifested, both became clinically evident within 18 months of each other, although some patients either may never demonstrate thyroid and eye disease or many years may separate the two.

Pretibial myxedema

Pretibial myxedema or thyroid dermopathy is the localized thickening of the skin, usually in the pretibial area. It occurs in 0% to 4.3% of patients with Graves' disease but at a higher rate (12% to 15%) in patients with Graves' ophthalmopathy[20,43] and usually is a late manifestation. Conversely, almost all patients with pretibial myxedema have Graves' ophthalmopathy, although the dermopathy may precede the ophthalmopathy. Symptomatic lesions consist of shiny, erythematous to brown plaques, nodules, or areas of nonpitting edema, which most commonly occur in the anterior or lateral aspects of the leg or at sites of old or recent trauma. Involvement of other body sites is rare. Almost all patients have high circulating levels of TRAbs, although the true pathogenesis of the dermopathy is not understood. Pretibial myxedema usually is of cosmetic importance only, but if the feet or hands become massively swollen, it can cause functional difficulties.

GRAVES' OPHTHALMOPATHY

As described previously, Graves' disease occurs more commonly in women and over a broad age range (16 to 81 years), with a mean age in the fifth and sixth decade.[11,25,73] Eye involvement in those with Graves' disease is bilateral in the majority of patients although 5% to 14% of patients will have unilateral disease depending on the method of detection.[7] With careful testing (i.e., CT scan) 50% to 90% of these patients will have changes in both eyes. In contrast, major asymmetry in the extent of eye involvement is common. Thus, Graves' ophthalmopathy remains the most common etiology of "unilateral" proptosis in adults.[8]

Ophthalmopathy classification

The spectrum of eye changes ranges from eyelid retraction (resulting in the appearance of a "stare"), to proptosis, corneal exposure and ulceration, diplopia, and loss of vision.

Table 57-1. Detailed classification of the eye changes of Graves' disease

Classes	Grades	Ocular symptoms and signs
0		No signs or symptoms
1		Only signs, no symptoms (signs limited to upper lid retraction and stare, with or without lid lag and proptosis
2		Soft-tissue involvement with symptoms and signs
	o	Absent
	a	Minimal
	b	Moderate
	c	Marked
3		Proptosis 3 mm or more in excess of upper normal limit, with or without symptoms
	o	Absent
	a	3 to 4 mm increase over upper normal
	b	5 to 7 mm increase
	c	8 or more mm increase
4		Extraocular muscle involvement (usually with diplopia, other symptoms or signs)
	o	Absent
	a	Limitation of motion at extremes of gaze
	b	Evident restriction of motion
	c	Fixation of a globe or globes
5		Corneal involvement (primarily a result of lagophthalmos)
	o	Absent
	a	Stippling of cornea
	b	Ulceration
	c	Clouding, necrosis, perforation
6		Sight loss (caused by optic nerve involvement)
	o	Absent
	a	Disc pallor or choking, or visual field defect: vision 20/20 to 20/60
	b	Same, but vision 20/70 to 20/200
	c	Blindness, i.e., failure to perceive light, vision less than 20/200

A clinical classification system for eye involvement by Graves' disease was proposed by Werner,[76] approved by the American Thyroid Association (ATA), and subsequently modified in 1977. The ATA's detailed classification is shown in Table 57-1. This classification is strictly clinical and has been helpful for reporting purposes. Unfortunately, the disease does not necessarily progress systematically through the classes and may skip one or more classes entirely. In addition, the classification system has been criticized for not considering disease activity (stable or rapidly progressing), which is critical for making patient treatment decisions.[71]

In response to these deficiencies and several other proposed classification schemes, an international *ad hoc* committee representing the American, European, Asia-Oceanic, and Latin America Thyroid Associations recommended in 1992 a new characterization of Graves' ophthalmopathy, which is shown in Table 57-2. This system is recommended for use in attempting objective clinical assessment and docu-

Table 57-2. Characterization of Graves' ophthalmopathy: recommendations of an international *ad hoc* committee*

Category of disease	Objective criteria monitored
Eyelid	Maximal lid fissure width
	Upper lid to limbus distance
	Lower lid to limbus distance
Cornea	Exposure keratitis assessed by rose bengal or fluorescein staining (indicate presence or absence)
Extraocular muscles	Single binocular vision in central 30° of vision (indicate presence or absence, with or without prisms)
	One or more of the following measurement techniques:
	Maddox rod test
	Alternate cover test
	Hess chart measurements
	Lancaster red-green test
	Optional
	Intraocular pressure in downward gaze
	CT or MRI
Proptosis	Exophthalmometer reading (CT or MRI measurement may also be used for measurement)
Optic nerve	Visual acuity
	Visual fields
	Color vision
Activity score	Sum of one point each for any of the following:
	Spontaneous retrobulbar pain
	Pain with eye movement
	Eyelid erythema
	Eyelid edema or swelling
	Conjunctival injection
	Chemosis
	Caruncle swelling
Patient self-assessment	Satisfaction with the following (indicate change with therapy in each using a scale such as: greatly improved, improved, unchanged, worse, much worse):
	Appearance
	Visual acuity
	Eye discomfort
	Diplopia

* Consensus of an 18-member *ad hoc* committee comprised of representatives from the American, European, Asia-Oceanic, and Latin America Thyroid Associations (From 1992 Classification of eye changes of Graves' disease, *Thyroid* 2:235).
CT—Computed tomography; MRI—Magnetic resonance imaging.

menting disease activity, as in clinical studies. The older ATA classification system is still used for educational purposes and clinical evaluation.

Eye findings

Lid lag and the appearance of a "stare" are seen in the mildest form (ATA class I disease) of eye involvement by Graves' disease. This is thought to occur initially as the result of an increased sympathetic sensitivity to catecholamines as seen with those with hyperthyroidism.[9] As the disease progresses and the lymphocytic inflammatory reaction infiltrates the extraocular muscles and orbital fat, the fibroblasts proliferate and deposit glycosaminoglycans, predominately hyaluronic acid.[57,59] The resulting muscle and fat enlargement combines with interstitial edema to cause an increase in intraocular pressure.

Intraocular pressure is increased in primary gaze (straight ahead) and even more so in upward gaze (supraduction). This increase in intraocular pressure can lead to a misdiagnosis of glaucoma, with a subsequent delay in appropriate therapy.[25] Over time, increases in intraocular pressure also produce conjunctival chemosis, excessive lacrimation, periorbital edema, and photophobia (ATA class II disease).

As enlargement of orbital muscle and fat progresses, the volume of the orbital contents increases. The orbital cavity has four fixed bony walls with an average volume of 26 ml.[26] In healthy people, the globe takes up 30% of this volume, with retrobulbar and peribulbar structures taking up the remaining 70% of the volume. With nowhere else to expand, an increase of only 4 ml in the volume of the orbital contents will result in 6 mm of proptosis (ATA class III disease).

As the extraocular muscles become increasingly enlarged by edema and infiltration, they also become dysfunctional, resulting in reduced ocular mobility and diplopia (ATA class IV disease). Over time, the inflammatory response provokes the deposition of collagen by the fibroblasts, replacing the normally elastic muscles of the eye and ultimately causing a permanent fibrotic, restrictive ophthalmoplegia.

Progressive proptosis also dramatically interferes with the protective mechanisms of the cornea, causing exposure, dessication, irritation, and ultimately, ulceration (ATA class V disease). Corneal ulceration becomes a vision-threatening problem, with a risk of permanent corneal scarring, and requires immediate attention.

In its most severe form, Graves' ophthalmopathy involves the optic nerve to impair vision (ATA class VI disease). Optic nerve involvement typically presents as a painless gradual loss of visual acuity or visual field,[46] although it can occur precipitously over days to weeks. Although originally thought to be caused by ischemia or venous congestion of the nerve as a result of increased intraocular pressure, there now is convincing evidence to support crowding and compression of the optic nerve at the orbital apex by the enlarged extraocular muscles as the etiology of nerve dysfunction.[54]

Optic nerve function is measured in several ways, one or all of which may be impaired. In one study of 31 patients with optic nerve involvement,[25] visual acuity was 20/25 or worse in 100% of eyes; color vision was decreased in 64%; and visual fields were decreased in 70%, with inferior scotomata and cecocentral scotomata defects most common. Impaired visual fields or color vision also may be found in patients with normal visual acuity.[11]

Clinical evaluation

Differential diagnosis

Graves' ophthalmopathy presents a spectrum of clinical manifestations that are reminiscent of other clinical entities. Eye changes range from minimal—requiring a detailed eye examination or CT scan to identify—to dramatic, disfiguring, and vision-threatening changes that eclipse the manifestations of the underlying thyroid disease. The high prevalance of asymmetric eye involvement also may lead the clinician to suspect a unilateral disease process rather than a systemic one. Although the differential diagnosis for proptosis is extensive (Table 57-3), most other disease entities have only superficial similarities to Graves' ophthalmopathy and can be quickly ruled out. Most importantly, the clinician should maintain a high degree of suspicion if the diagnosis of Graves' ophthalmopathy is to be made in a timely fashion.

Thyroid function

A full endocrinology workup is essential in the diagnosis and management of Graves' disease. Laboratory testing should include thyroid function tests and a TSH level. In some apparently euthyroid patients, more detailed dynamic testing of thyroid function may be required to uncover thyroid dysfunction. These studies include the suppression of radioiodine uptake with T3 to assess for non–TSH-mediated thyroid stimulation, the thyrotropin-releasing hormone (TRH) stimulation test to determine the presence of low-grade suppression of the hypothalamic–pituitary axis, and TSH stimulation tests of thyroid reserve. Serologic evaluation for evidence of thyroid autoimmunity also can be performed, including microsomal antibody, thyroglobulin antibody, and TRAb assays. Overall, with sufficient scrutiny, most if not all patients with euthyroid ophthalmopathy can be shown to have some degree of thyroid dysfunction.[7]

Eye evaluation

A thorough examination by a skilled ophthalmologist is critical for the diagnosis and management of Graves' ophthalmopathy. Serial eye examinations are required to monitor disease activity, progression, and response to therapy. The eye examination should include attention to soft tissue changes, including lid edema and retraction, chemosis, scleral injection, documentation of proptosis (Hertle exophthalmometer), and intraocular pressure in primary and upward gaze (Schiøtz tonometer), limitation of ocular motility, strabismus and visual function in the form of acuity (Snellen's wall chart), color vision (Ishihara's color plates), and visual fields (Goldmann perimetry).

Imaging studies

CT scans of the orbit can be helpful in the diagnosis of Graves' ophthalmopathy in the euthyroid patient and are essential if surgical intervention is being considered. Typical findings include a twofold to eightfold enlargement of the

Table 57-3. Differential diagnosis of proptosis

Endocrine
  Graves' ophthalmopathy
  Cushing's syndrome
Orbital neoplasms
  Primary neoplasms
  Hemangioma
  Lymphoma (may be systemic)
  Optic nerve glioma
  Choroidal melanoma
  Lacrimal gland tumors
  Meningioma
  Rhabdomyosarcoma
Extension of paranasal sinus tumors
Metastatic disease
  Malignant melanoma
  Breast carcinoma
  Lung carcinoma
  Kidney
  Prostate
Inflammatory
  Orbital pseudotumor
  Orbital myositis
Granulomatous
  Sarcoidosis
  Wegener's granulomatosis
Infectious
  Orbital cellulitis
  Syphilis
  Mucormycosis
  Parasitic (trypanosomiasis, schistosomiasis, cystocercosis, echinococcal disease)
Vascular
  Carotid-cavernous fistula
Miscellaneous
  Lithium therapy
  Cirrhosis
  Obesity
  Amyloidosis
  Dermoid and epidermoid cysts
  Foreign body

extraocular muscle bodies, sparing the tendinous portions (Fig. 57-2). The changes will be bilateral in 90% of patients, although asymmetry in the extent of involvement is the rule. The medial and inferior rectus muscles are involved most commonly, although any or all of the muscles may be enlarged.[36] The orbital and extraocular muscle volume may be estimated using CT images.[21,22,28] Although estimates of extraocular muscle volume have correlated with the presence of optic neuropathy, subsequent studies have not found a correlation between muscle volume estimates and the severity of optic neuropathy or the effectiveness of decompression,[25,29] thus limiting the usefulness of these estimates.

Ultrasound (orbital echography) has been reported to be reliable and effective in evaluating extraocular muscle size.[15] Although not as beneficial in the initial diagnosis and surgical planning as the CT scan in those with Graves' disease, it is proposed as an inexpensive, noninvasive

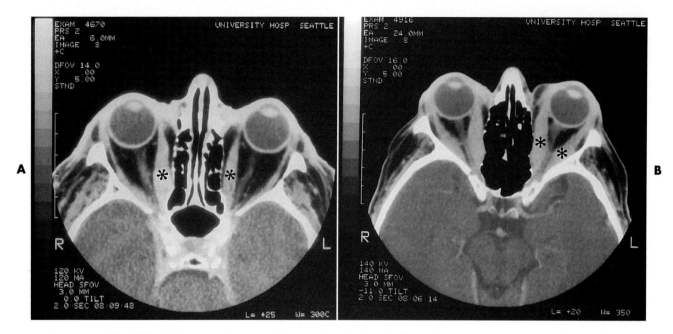

Fig. 57-2. Axial computed tomography scans through the orbits in two patients with Graves' ophthalmopathy, demonstrating **A,** medial rectus muscle enlargement *(asterisks)* with normal lateral rectus muscle size and **B,** medial and lateral rectus muscle enlargement *(asterisks)* with orbital apex crowding, causing optic neuropathy.

method for monitoring response to therapy (steroids or radiation).

Magnetic reasonance imaging (MRI) of the orbits has proven excellent for the evaluation of the soft tissues of the orbit. Recent studies have suggested that T2-weighted MRI images may provide a sensitive measure of active inflammation in the orbit, giving much needed information on disease activity.[33,37] Unfortunately, MRI provides little detail of the bony anatomy of the orbit, which is required if the possibility of surgical intervention is being entertained.

Management of Graves' ophthalmopathy

A multispecialty team approach for the treatment of patients with Graves' disease and Graves' ophthalmopathy is recommended because of the multiple organ systems involved and the variety of diagnostic and theraputic modalities needed to provide optimal care of this complex entity. Team members representing endocrinology, radiology, nuclear medicine, radiotherapy, ophthalmology, otolaryngology—head and neck surgery, and neurosurgery will be involved to varying degrees. A coordinating member of the team (usually the endocrinologist for Graves' disease and the ophthalmologist for Graves' ophthalmopathy) is critical for maintaining records, tracking disease progression, and providing continuity of care for long periods.

Medical therapy

Thyroid therapy. The management of the thyroid in those with Graves' disease remains somewhat controversial, and a complete discussion is beyond the scope of this chap-

ter. The impact of thyroid management on Graves' ophthalmopathy is only now becoming clear. As previously discussed, the correlation between the severity of hyperthyroidism and the prevalence or course of Graves' ophthalmopathy is poor at best. For patients with thyrotoxicosis, the thyroid may be managed with either antithyroid drugs (i.e., propylthiouracil and methimazole), radioiodine ablation (iodine-131), or thyroidectomy (usually subtotal). Reports on the effect of each of these modalities on the development or progression of ophthalmopathy are conflicting in the literature, although in a recent prospective study, Tallstedt and others[63] randomized 168 patients into groups receiving either antithyroid drugs, radioiodine ablation, or surgery. There was no difference in the rate of new onset or progression of existing ophthalmopathy between the antithyroid drug and surgery groups (10% to 16%), but the radioiodine ablation group showed a higher incidence (33%) of these problems.

One possible mechanism for the increase in those with ophthalmopathy receiving radioiodine ablation includes transient hypothyroidism and the release of thyroid antigens, promoting an acceleration of the autoimmune process. In support of this hypothesis, investigators have found that TRAb levels briefly decrease and then show a sustained increase after iodine-131 ablation for Graves' disease.[6] Although after thyroidectomy, TRAb levels showed a transient increase followed by a gradual decrease.[5] Potentially least concerning were TRAb levels, which gradually declined after antithyroid therapy alone. Thus, it would seem that radioiodine ablation of the thyroid may not be the best option for the management of thyrotoxicosis in patients with Graves' disease. As mentioned previously, thyroid hormone replacement and suppression during antithyroid drug therapy or after radioiodine or surgical ablation (before the onset of measurable hypothyroidism) appear to result in a decrease in the prevalence or progression of ophthalmopathy in those with Graves' disease and therefore should be considered.[64]

Local therapy. The majority of patients with Graves' ophthalmopathy will experience a self-limited disease course requiring only local measures for symptomatic relief. Corneal exposure and drying respond well to eye drops and nocturnal taping of the eyelid. Some have found the use of diuretics useful in decreasing swelling. Sunglasses help with photophobia, and prisms may help with mild strabismus. Topical guanethidine eye drops have been found to reduce lid retraction and lid lag, reportedly by sympathetic blockade of Muller's muscle in the upper lid, but they are poorly tolerated and rarely used.

Steroid therapy. High-dose corticosteriods (prednisone, 80 to 100 mg/day) are commonly used as the first-line management of more severe Graves' ophthalmopathy. High doses are maintained for 2 to 4 weeks, followed by a slow taper over several months. Patients experience rapid relief of pain, erythema, and conjunctival edema and improved vision. Trobe, Glaser, and Laflamme reported a 48% success rate after 2 months of therapy. Unfortunately, steroids may only be temporizing, with recurrence of visual loss on taper. Improvement in proptosis and ophthalmoplegia also may be seen with corticosteroid therapy but generally are less so and are more likely to recur on steroid withdrawal. The multiple side effects of steroid therapy are well known and include glucose intolerance, weight gain, psychosis, peptic ulcer disease, and osteoporosis with vertebral fracture. Thus, corticosteroid therapy should be considered temporizing, while awaiting either regression and stabilization of disease or definitive therapy.

Immunosuppression with cyclosporine also has been evaluated for those with Graves' ophthalmopathy and been found to be less effective than prednisone in single-agent therapy.[7] The beneficial effects of both drugs appear to be additive, and maintenance cyclosporine therapy may be corticosteroid-sparing. Careful drug level monitoring is necessary to avoid nephrotoxicity. Other common side effects include hypertension, liver enzyme elevation, gum hypertrophy, and paresthesias. Plasmapheresis to remove circulating antibodies and other immunomodulatory drugs also have been used, but the results suggest further evaluation before widespread use.

Radiotherapy

Radiotherapy to the orbit has been used for patients with Graves' ophthalmopathy by delivering 20 Gy in 10 fractions over 2 weeks. The fractions are delivered to a field just behind the lateral canthus to spare the cornea and lens. In a review of the literature, Sautter-Bihl and Heinze[58] found a good-to-excellent response overall in 35% to 92% of patients and improvement of impaired visual acuity in 33% to 85% of patients treated with orbital radiation. The mechanism of action of radiation to the orbit is thought to be, in large part, an effect on the lymphocytes infiltrating the orbital muscles and fat during the inciting stages of the disease. Thus, patients treated early in the course of the disease with pronounced soft tissue involvement are most likely to benefit. Proptosis, ophthalmoplegia, and optic neuropathy are less responsive, and patients with long-standing stable disease are not likely to benefit. The portion of the radiation dose delivered to the lens is less than 5% and has not been reported to be harmful.

Surgical therapy

Indications for surgical decompression of the orbit have evolved over the years and have included cosmetic management of proptosis, lid lag, and stare and the management of optic neuropathy.[9,11,18,24] New-onset strabismus after orbital decompression has been reported in as many as 30% to 64% of the patients, suggesting that patient selection should be done with caution.[24,61] As a result, many centers perform orbital decompression primarily in the setting of optic nerve involvement combined with failure to respond or inability to tolerate steroid therapy or for the relapse of symptoms with the taper of steroid therapy.[25,46] Radiotherapy generally is reserved for those who cannot tolerate, refuse, or fail surgical decompression, although some still advocate primary radiotherapy.[55,69]

The goal of surgical decompression of the orbit is simply to expand the bony orbital confines to make room for the increased volume of the orbital contents. Surgical decompression was first described by Dollinger,[12] who advocated removal of the lateral orbital wall for decompression into the temporal fossa (Krönlein's procedure). Twenty years later, Naffziger[52] reported removal of the orbital roof with decompression into the anterior cranial fossa via a transcranial approach. Decompression into the paranasal sinuses was first advocated by Sewell,[60] who described decompression into the ethmoid air cells, and Hirsch,[32] who later reported inferior decompression into the maxillary sinus by removal of the orbital floor. Walsh and Ogura[72] combined the inferior and medial approaches into a single transantral decompression of two orbital walls using the Caldwell-Luc approach (Fig. 57-3). This approach is extracranial, decompresses two walls of the orbit into the largest empty space, and allows gravity to aid in the expansion of orbital contents into the paranasal sinuses. For these reasons, it has become the most widely used technique.

Predicting the results of transantral decompression in patients with severe Graves' ophthalmopathy remains a challenge. In a retrospective analysis of 428 patients, Fatourechi and others[17] reported that young men with long-standing eye symptoms were likely to have more severe initial proptosis. Only the severity of the initial proptosis and longer postoper-

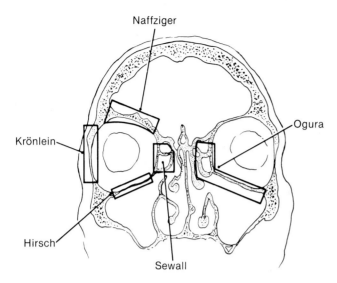

Fig. 57-3. Diagram of a coronal section through the skull and paranasal sinuses showing portions of the orbit removed for various methods of orbital decompression.

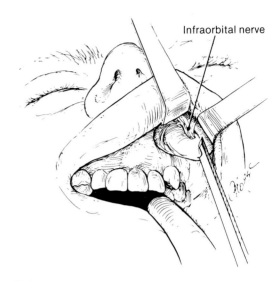

Fig. 57-4. Sublabial buccogingival incision that exposes the anterior wall of the maxillary sinus. An osteotome is used to create the antrostomy.

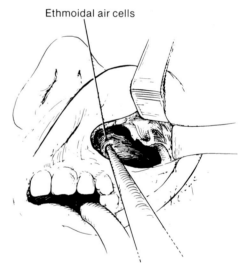

Fig. 57-5. Ethmoidal cells are entered with a curette and subsequently removed by curettage and bone-biting forceps.

ative follow-up period correlated with greater recession of proptosis after decompression. Failure of corticosteroid or orbital radiotherapy did not affect the degree of recession of proptosis or improvement in visual acuity. A greater degree of recession of proptosis postoperatively was associated with better visual acuity but also with a greater likelihood of persistent strabismus. Patient satisfaction with postoperative eye appearance was associated only with procedures performed for cosmetic indications.

Transantral orbital decompression

Surgical technique. The transantral decompression (Walsh-Ogura method) of the orbital floor and medial wall is performed during general anesthesia with an oral Ray endotracheal tube secured in place. The eyes are protected with topical ointment and are not taped to allow examination of the pupil during the procedure. Intravenous broad-spectrum antibiotics and high-dose corticosteroids (dexamethasone, 8 to 10 mg) are given before starting the surgery. A curved sublabial incision with a standard Caldwell-Luc antrostomy and ethmoidectomy is performed (Fig. 57-4). Care is taken to identify and preserve the inferior orbital nerve in its bony canal. An extensive ethmoidectomy should be performed while preserving the lamina papyracea, middle turbinate insertion, and fovea ethmoidalis (Fig. 57-5). The remaining mucosa is then carefully stripped from the maxillary sinus roof, keeping in mind that the inferior orbital nerve will be partially or completely dehiscent in 29% of patients.[39] The bone of the maxillary sinus roof (orbital floor) medial to the infraorbital nerve is then carefully removed (Fig. 57-6). This maneuver can be performed using a drill with cutting or diamond burrs or with small osteotomes, as long as the underlying periorbita is not violated. Some surgeons find the operating microscope useful at this stage of the procedure.

The lamina papyracea (medial orbital wall) then is gently fractured medially and removed up to the posterior ethmoid neurovascular bundle, preserving the periorbita. A No. 12 scalpel blade is used to make incisions in the posterior-to-anterior direction through the periorbital fascia, which allows the immediate herniation of orbital fat through the incision and into the sinuses (Fig. 57-7). This process is begun medial and superior to avoid the loss of visualization as the fat herniates from the orbit. The number of incisions required is determined intraoperatively by assessing the degree of residual proptosis after each incision. Calcaterra and Thompson[9] recommend operating on the more severe eye first with

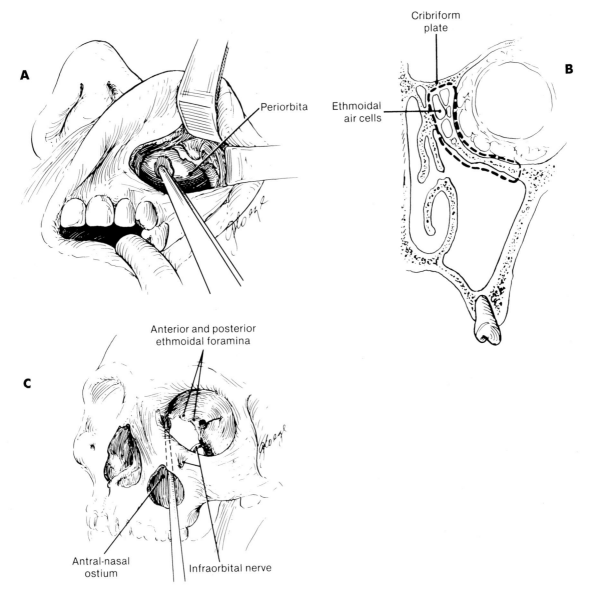

Fig. 57-6. A, Removal of the floor of orbit after egg-shell fracturing of bone. **B,** Coronal section of paranasal sinuses showing the extent of bone removal. **C,** View of the skull showing completion of ethmoidectomy and removal of the lamina papyracea.

planned incomplete recession because an additional 1 to 2 mm of recession develops during the first 3 months after surgery. The less severe eye then is decompressed to match the position of the first eye. Four to six incisions in the periorbita usually will be adequate.[75] Finally, a large nasoantral window is created, and the sinus is packed with a large penrose drain coated in antibiotic ointment and brought out through the nose for removal the next day. The sublabial incision then is closed with absorbable suture. The patient is maintained on antibiotics and corticosteroids intravenously overnight and then orally on discharge from the hospital.

Immediately after surgery all patients (unless medically contraindicated) are maintained on high-dose corticosteroids

with a slow taper. The rate of steroid taper is determined by the clinical response to the surgery. In one study, steroid use was discontinued in 80% of patients within 2 months of surgery.[25]

Surgical outcome. Results of transantral orbital decompression surgery depend on the indications for the operation. For those with optic neuropathy, Walsh-Ogura decompression was effective in improving vision in 92% of patients (Fig. 57-8). Equally important, these patients had stabilization of their disease with successful taper of steroid therapy. Major improvement in proptosis in the range of 1 to 12 mm can be achieved (Fig. 57-9, *A*), with an average improvement of 3.4 to 5.3 mm.[24,25,73,74] This decrease in

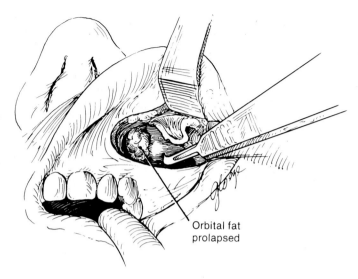

Orbital fat
prolapsed

Fig. 57-7. Radial incisions in the intact periorbita with a scalpel, permitting prolapse of orbital fat into the sinuses.

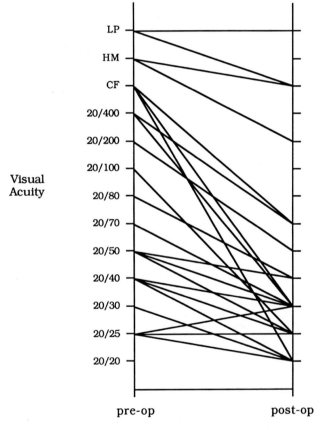

Fig. 57-8. Preoperative *(left)* and postoperative *(right)* best corrected visual acuity for 36 eyes in 20 patients undergoing transantral orbital decompression for Graves' optic neuropathy. *CF*—Counts fingers; *HM*—Hand motion; and *LP*—Light perception. (From Girod and others: Orbital decompression for preservation of vision in Graves' ophthalmopathy, *Arch Otolaryngol Head Neck Surg* 119:229, 1993.)

proptosis is of functional and cosmetic benefit and is not seen with either medical or radiotherapy. Major reduction in intraocular pressure (100% of patients, Fig. 57-9, *B*), improvement of extraocular motility (36%), and improvement of strabismus (47%) are other benefits of decompression.

Transantral decompression failed to stabilize the disease in 3% to 8% of patients who underwent surgery for severe ophthalmopathy.[24,25] In this setting, repeat CT scanning with coronal cuts can be helpful to assess the adequacy of the decompression and to decide between further surgery using the same approach or via a lateral or superior approach[19] or proceeding with radiotherapy.

The earlier the diagnosis of Graves' optic neuropathy is made and intervention initiated, the better the outcome. When preoperative visual acuity was limited to detecting hand motion or worse, decompression provided little improvement in vision (see Fig. 57-8).[25] When visual acuity allowed counting fingers or better, all patients experienced a favorable outcome.

Ocular dysmotility and strabismus remain a major problem in surgical patients despite decompression. Extraocular motility was impaired (primarily in supraduction) in 92% of patients undergoing decompression; only one third showed improvement, and 9% experienced a worsening of motility postoperatively.[25] Strabismus (diplopia) was present preoperatively in 67% to 85% of patients and in 71% to 80% of patients postoperatively.[24,25] Once the eye disease was stable, 70% of patients underwent extraocular muscle surgery to correct diplopia, and some were able to be corrected with prisms alone. One long-term follow-up evaluation (average, 8.8 years) of 355 decompression patients reported only 17% having double vision most or all of the time.[24]

Transantral decompression for cosmetic indications

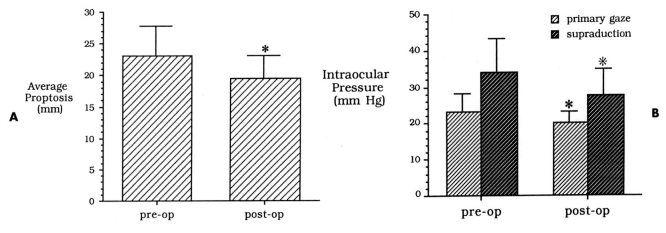

Fig. 57-9. A, Preoperative *(left)* and postoperative *(right)* average proptosis for the 36 eyes undergoing decompression in Figure 57-8. **B,** Intraocular pressure in the same eyes in primary gaze and upward gaze before and after decompression surgery. *$P < 0.05$.

should be evaluated carefully because it carries the risk of lower patient acceptance of side effects than when vision is threatened. Fatourechi and others[18] reviewed the outcomes of 34 patients who underwent transantral decompression for cosmesis and noted a dramatic improvement in proptosis (average, 5.2 mm) but no major change in asymmetry between the eyes. Postoperative diplopia developed in 73% of patients who did not suffer from diplopia preoperatively. Half of the patients underwent subsequent extraocular muscle surgery and eyelid surgery. On long-term follow-up evaluation (average, 12 years after surgery) of 29 patients, 82% reported they were satisfied with their current eye status. Thus, decompression surgery for cosmetic indications may be appropriate in a select group of patients who are willing to undergo subsequent eye muscle surgery for diplopia.

Surgical complications. Patients uniformly complain of hypoesthesia in the distribution of the inferior orbital nerve immediately after decompression as a result of intraoperative stretching of the nerve with retraction. This resolves spontaneously over several months in more than 95% of patients. In one large series, Garrity and others[24] reported other infrequent complications, including sinusitis (4%), lower eyelid entropion (9%), cerebrospinal fluid leaks (3%), and frontal lobe hematoma (0.2%). Blindness from nerve injury or orbital hemorrhage is rare but occurs.[24,51] Although theoretically possible, orbital infection has not been reported.

Modifications of transantral orbital decompression. The transantral orbital decompression has held up well to the test of time since its description in 1957. Only in the past several years have advances in surgical technique and instrumentation led to the description of major modifications to the Walsh-Ogura operation. A transorbital approach using a modified blepharoplasty (subcilliary) incision provides excellent exposure to the anterior orbital floor and decreases the risk to the infraorbital nerve.[46] This approach

also provides access for a lateral orbital wall decompression without disrupting the orbital rim or canthal tendon, thus providing a three-wall decompression.[1] This method is reported to have a lower incidence of postoperative strabismus, although the reason for this is unclear. Others have reported using the transconjuctival approach for the antral–ethmoidal decompression.[44] The major criticism of these anterior approaches is limited exposure to the medial orbit, which can restrict the degree of decompression around the orbital apex as is required in patients with optic neuropathy.

With the rapid development and dissemination of endoscopic instrumentation and techniques for transnasal paranasal sinus surgery, it is expected that some surgeons have extended this technology to include antral–ethmoidal decompression of the orbit. Despite concerns about adequate anterior orbital floor access, Kennedy and others[38] reported equivalent results with transantral decompression and endoscopic decompression. Metson and others[50] reported an average 3.2 mm reduction of proptosis with an endoscopic decompression alone and 5.6 mm when combined with a percutaneous lateral orbital wall decompression via the upper lid crease. In addition, Metson and others[49] have successfully performed endoscopic and combined endoscopic and lateral wall decompressions during local anesthesia, which has the advantage of avoiding general anesthesia, avoiding the morbidity of a Caldwell-Luc antrostomy, and permitting intraoperative monitoring of visual function, critical for surgery on an only-seeing eye. In this setting, if both eyes are to be decompressed, they are done so in stages.

For a more thorough optic nerve decompression, Khan and others[40] have described a combined transconjunctival–endoscopic decompression of the orbit. The addition of a small medial external skin incision also aided the retraction of the orbital contents to allow the dissection of the medial wall beyond the posterior ethmoidal neurovascular bundle up to the optic canal.

As many otolaryngologists are now becoming facile with endoscopic techniques, it seems likely that this approach to orbital decompression will gain in popularity, providing further information on long-term efficacy.

Other approaches for orbital decompression.   A modification of the Walsh-Ogura method called the *three-wall orbital decompression* refers to the addition of the lateral wall decompression to the standard antral–ethmoidal decompression. This addition can be achieved by any combination of approaches, including a modified blepharoplasty incision, a sublabial or transconjunctival incision plus an anterior orbitotomy, or through a bicoronal forehead flap. The advantage of the three-wall decompression is allowing the further enlargement of the orbital volume by expansion into the temporal fossa and the paranasal sinuses. As mentioned previously, Metson, Dallow, and Shore[50] were able to increase the recession of proptosis from an average of 3.2 mm to 5.6 mm with the addition of the lateral decompression to the endoscopic antral–ethmoid decompression. Other authors prefer the bicoronal approach[45,70] to the three-wall decompression, even for unilateral decompressions. Although dramatic decompression is reported (average, 7.5 mm), a high complication rate can be expected, including infraorbital hypesthesia (70%), supraorbital hypesthesia (60%), and frontalis palsy (30%).[45]

A two-wall decompression of the superior–lateral orbit may be achieved through a bicoronal incision with subsequent frontal craniotomy[47,52] or a lateral rim approach.[14] This allows decompression of the orbital contents into the anterior cranial fossa and temporal fossa. Expansion of orbital contents into the empty paranasal sinuses with the help of gravity would be predicted to provide a more adequate decompression, although in a cadaveric study, Stanley and others[62] found the superior–lateral decompression to be as effective as the antral–ethmoidal decompression in withstanding intraocular pressure increases and in allowing orbital recession. The craniotomy approach has the advantages of direct access to the optic canal for superior decompression and of potential additional medial orbital wall decompression via the ethmoid sinuses. The orbital rim approach has the advantage of less dural exposure and the ability to advance the superior orbital rim with plates, screws, and bone grafts to further increase orbital volume.[14] Because the superior–lateral decompression is a more involved procedure with the violation of the cranial cavity, irrespective of the approach, most centers reserve it for recalcitrant patients in whom antral–ethmoidal decompression has failed.

Classical descriptions of orbital decompression always have referred to the removal of one or more orbital bony walls. Trokel, Kazim, and Moore[69] have reported successful decompression of the orbit strictly by the removal of orbital fat via superior and inferior orbitotomies without any bone removal. This procedure was reserved primarily for cosmetic indications in patients with inactive disease. An average reduction in proptosis of 1.8 mm was achieved, although patients with large amounts of fat seen by CT scan and with greater preoperative proptosis had more dramatic reductions. Importantly, there were no new long-term motility problems commonly reported with bony orbital decompression for cosmesis, which may be an important decompression option for cosmetic indications in an attempt to reduce postoperative strabismus and the need for subsequent eye muscle surgery.

Ancillary procedures.

Extraocular muscle surgery.   Extraocular motility problems resulting from Graves' ophthalmopathy are not likely to resolve spontaneously with disease regression and are mostly refractory to medical management. It also is the manifestation of eye involvement most likely to develop or worsen after orbital decompression. Although disturbing, this is not surprising because irreversible extraocular muscle fibrosis is seen late in the disease. In one study, up to 70% of decompression patients ultimately underwent eye muscle surgery for strabismus once the eye disease was stable.[24]

The indications for eye muscle surgery are diplopia in the primary and reading positions, with the goal being to restore single vision in these positions. It is unlikely that eye muscle surgery will achieve single vision in all positions because of the baseline restrictive ophthalmoplegia induced by the disease. Dyer[13] reviewed 290 patients with Graves' ophthalmopathy requiring eye muscle surgery and found 59% required a single surgery, 30% required two procedures, and 12% required three or more procedures to achieve single vision in the primary and reading positions.

The timing of eye muscle surgery is critical for predictable results. Patients not requiring orbital decompression for Graves' ophthalmopathy should manifest stable disease with corticosteroid administration for 6 months to avoid subtle changes in the muscles over time. If these patients have serious proptosis, orbital decompression should be considered before eye muscle surgery, which may exacerbate the proptosis and corneal problems.[13] In addition, a decompression is likely to alter the position of the globes and thus disturb the gaze and therefore should be completed before eye muscle surgery. Because recession of the globe is progressive for several months after an orbital decompression, it is advisable to delay eye muscle surgery for 2 to 3 months.

Eyelid surgery.   Surgery on the eyelids may be required early or late in the management of Graves' ophthalmopathy. Early in the disease, a lateral tarsorrhaphy may be needed to urgently provide corneal coverage and protection as a temporizing measure while medical therapy is instituted. Late in the course of the disease, eyelid surgery may be indicated for cosmesis and corneal protection in patients with permanent lid retraction. Multiple upper eyelid procedures have been described, including excision or recession of Müller's muscle, levator aponeurosis transection or recession with or without scleral grafts, and levator myotomy.[7] Similar procedures have been described for the lower lid. In the overall rehabilitation of the eye, eyelid surgery should be delayed for 1 year after control of the hyperthyroidism and at least 6 months after the eye disease stablizes.

SUMMARY

Although recent studies on the etiology of Graves' disease suggest a common thyroid–eye antigen (TSH receptor), this difficult and debilitating disease is still not preventable. Further advances in the identification of the specific autoantigenic site in the eye and the thyroid and in antigen-specific immunotherapy are necessary before a major shift in management can occur. Until that time, therapy for Graves' disease and the associated Graves' ophthalmopthy will remain palliative. A team approach to these patients is warranted given multiple organ system involvement and the complexity of manifestations encountered. Only through close collaboration between team members can optimal therapy be provided.

REFERENCES

1. Antoszyk JH, Tucker N, Codere F: Orbital decompression for Graves' disease: exposure through a modified blepharoplasty incision, *Ophthalmic Surg* 23:516, 1992.
2. Bahn RS and others: Human retroocular fibroblasts *in vitro*: a model for the study of Graves' ophthalmopathy, *J Clin Endocrinol Metab* 65: 665, 1987.
3. Bahn RS, Heufelder AE: Retroocular fibroblasts: important effector cells in Graves' ophthalmopathy, *Thyroid* 2:89, 1992.
4. Bartalena L and others: More on smoking habits and Graves' ophthalmopathy, *J Endocrinol Invest* 12:733, 1989.
5. Bech K and others: The acute changes in thyroid stimulating immunoglobulins, thyroglobulin, and thyroglobulin antibodies following subtotal thyroidectomy, *Clin Endocrinol (Oxf)* 16:235, 1982.
6. Bech K, Madsen N: Influence of treatment with radioiodine and propylthiouracil on thyroid stimulating immunoglobulins in Graves' disease, *Clin Endocrinol (Oxf)* 13:417, 1980.
7. Burch HB, Wartofsky L: Graves' ophthalmopathy: current concepts regarding pathogenesis and management, *Encocr Rev* 14:747, 1993.
8. Calcaterra TC, Hepler RS, Hanafee WN: The diagnostic evaluation of unilateral exophthalmos, *Laryngoscope* 2:231, 1974.
9. Calcaterra TC, Thompson JW: Antral-ethmoidal decompression of the orbit in Graves' disease: 10-year experience, *Laryngoscope* 90:1941, 1980.
10. Christensen SB and others: Influence of cigarette smoking on goiter formation, thyroglobulin, and thyroid hormone levels in women, *J Clin Endocrinol Metab* 58:615, 1984.
11. DeSanto LW: The total rehabilitation of Graves' ophthalmopathy, *Laryngoscope* 90:1652, 1980.
12. Dollinger J: Die drickentlastung der augenhokle durch entfernung der ausseren obitalwand bei hochgradigen exophthalmus und koneskutwer hornhauter kronkung, *Dtsch Med Wochenschr* 37:1888, 1911.
13. Dyer, JA: *Ocular muscle surgery.* In Gorman CA, Campbell RJ, Dyer JA, editors: *The eye and orbit in thyroid disease,* New York, 1984, Raven Press.
14. Elisevich K and others: Decompression for dysthyroid ophthalmopathy via the orbital rim approach, technical note, *J Neurosurg* 80:580, 1994.
15. Erickson BA and others: Echographic monitoring of response of extraocular muscles to irradiation in Graves' ophthalmopathy, *Int J Radiat Oncol Biol Phys* 31:651, 1995.
16. Ericsson UB, Lindgarde F: Effects of cigarette smoking on thyroid function, the prevalence of goitre, thyrotoxicosis and autoimmune thyroiditis, *J Clin Endocrinol Metab* 229:67, 1991.
17. Fatourechi V and others: Predictors of response to transantral orbital decompression in severe Graves' ophthalmopathy, *Mayo Clin Proc* 69: 841, 1994.
18. Fatourechi V and others: Graves' ophthalmopathy. Results of transantral orbital decompression performed primarily for cosmetic indications, *Ophthalmology* 101:938, 1994.
19. Fatourechi V and others: Orbital decompression in Graves' ophthalmopathy associated with pretibial myxedema, *J Endocrinol Invest* 16: 433, 1993.
20. Fatourechi V, Pajouhi M, Fransway AF: Dermopathy of Graves' disease (pretibial myxedema), *Medicine (Baltimore)*, 107:257, 1994.
21. Feldon SE, Weiner JM: Clinical significance of extraocular muscle volumes in Graves' ophthalmopathy: a quantitative computed tomography study, *Arch Ophthalmol* 100:1266, 1982.
22. Forbes G and others: Ophthalmopathy of Graves' disease: computerized volume measurements of the orbital fat and muscle, *Am J Neuroradiol* 7:651, 1986.
23. Francis T and others: Lymphocytes express thyrotropin receptor specific mRNA as detected by the PCR technique, *Thyroid* 1:223, 1991.
24. Garrity JA and others: Results of transantral orbital decompression in 428 patients with severe Graves' ophthalmopathy, *Am J Ophthalmol* 116:533, 1993.
25. Girod DA, Orcutt JC, Cummings CW: Orbital decompression for the preservation of vision in Graves' ophthalmopathy, *Arch Otolaryngol Head Neck Surg* 119:229, 1993.
26. Gorman CA: The presentation and management of endocrine ophthalmopathy, *Clin Endocrinol Metab* 7:67, 1978.
27. Grubeck-Loebenstein B and others: Retrobulbar cells from patients with Graves' ophthalmopathy are CD8+ and specifically recognized autologous fibroblasts, *J Clin Invest* 93:2738, 1994.
28. Hallin ES, Feldon SE: Graves' ophthalmopathy: I. Simple CT estimates of extraocular muscle volume, *Br J Ophthalmol* 72:674, 1988.
29. Hallin ES, Feldon SE, Luttrell J: Graves' ophthalmopathy: III. Effect of transantral orbital decompression on optic neuropathy, *Br J Ophthalmol* 72:683, 1988.
30. Hamilton RD and others: Ophthalmopathy of Graves' disease: a comparison between patients treated surgically and patients treated with radioiodine, *Mayo Clin Proc* 42:812, 1967.
31. Heufelder AE, Bahn RS: Modulation of Graves' orbital fibroblast proliferation by cytokines and glucocorticoid receptor agonists, *Invest Ophthalmol Vis Sci* 35:120, 1994.
32. Hirsch O: Surgical decompression for malignant exophthalmosis, *Arch Otolaryngol Head Neck Surg* 51:325, 1950.
33. Hosten N and others: Graves' ophthalmopathy: MR imaging of the orbit, *Radiology* 172:759, 1989.
34. Huber GK and others: Positive regulation of human thyrotropin receptor mRNA by thyrotropin, *J Clin Endocrinol Metab* 72:1394, 1991.
35. Hufnagel TJ and others: Immunohistochemical, ultrastructural studies of the exenterated orbital tissues of a patient with Graves' disease, *Ophthalmology* 91:1411, 1984.
36. Jelks GW, Jelks EB, Ruff, G: Clinical and radiographic evaluation of the orbit, *Otolaryngol Clin North Am* 21:13, 1988.
37. Just M and others: Graves' ophthalmopathy: role of MR imaging in radiotherapy, *Radiology* 179:187, 1991.
38. Kennedy DW and others: Endoscopic transnasal orbital decompression, *Arch Otolaryngol Head Neck Surg* 116:275, 1990.
39. Kent KJ, Merwin GE, Rarey KE: Margins of safety with transantral orbital decompression, *Laryngoscope* 98:815, 1988.
40. Khan JA and others: Combined transconjunctival and external approach for endoscopic orbital apex decompression in Graves' disease, *Laryngoscope* 105:203, 1995.
41. Kodama K, and others: Demonstration of a circulating autoantibody against soluble eye-muscle antigen in Graves' ophthalmopathy, *Lancet* 2:1353, 1982.
42. Kosugi S and others: The extracellular domain of the TSH receptor has an immunogenic epitope reactive with Graves' sera but unrelated to receptor function as well as epitopes having different roles for high

affinity TSH binding, the activity of thyroid stimulating antibodies, *Thyroid* 1:321, 1991.

43. Kriss JP: Pathogenesis and treatment of pretibial myxedema, *Endocrinol Metab Clin North Am* 16:409, 1987.

44. Kulwin DR, Cotton RT, Kersten RC: Combined approach to orbital decompression, *Otolaryngol Clin North Am* 23:381, 1990.

45. Leatherbarrow B, Lendrum J, Mahaffey PJ: Three wall orbital decompression for Graves' ophthalmopathy, *Eye* 5:456, 1991.

46. Lindberg JV, Anderson RL: Transorbital decompression: indications and results, *Arch Ophthalmol* 99:113, 1981.

47. MacCarty CS and others: Ophthalmopathy of Graves' disease treated by removal of roof, lateral walls, and lateral sphenoid ridge: review of 46 cases, *Mayo Clin Proc* 45:488, 1970.

48. Marcocci D and others: Studies on the occurrence of ophthalmopathy in Graves' disease, *Acta Endocr (Copenh)* 120:473, 1989.

49. Metson R and others: Endoscopic orbital decompression under local anesthesia, *Otolaryngol Head Neck Surg* 113:661, 1995.

50. Metson R, Dallow RL, Shore JW: Endoscopic orbital decompression, *Laryngoscope* 104:950, 1994.

51. Mourits MP, and others: Orbital decompression for Graves' ophthalmopathy by inferomedial, by inferomedial plus lateral, and by coronal approach, *Ophthalmology* 97:636, 1990.

52. Naffzinger H: Progressive exophthalmos following thyroidectomy: its pathology and treatment, *Ann Surg* 94:582, 1931.

53. Nagy E and others: Graves' IgG recognizes linear epitopes in the human thyrotropin receptor, *Biochem Biophys Res Commun* 188:28, 1992.

54. Neigel JM and others: Dysthyroid optic neuropathy: the crowded orbital apex syndrome, *Ophthalmology* 95:1515, 1988.

55. Pigeon P and others: High voltage radiotherapy and surgical orbital decompression in the management of Graves' ophthalmopathy, *Horm Res* 26:172, 1987.

56. Rees Smith B, McLachlan SM, Furmaniak J: Autoantibodies to the thyrotropin receptor, *Endocrinology* 9:106, 1988.

57. Riley FD: Orbital pathology in Graves' disease, *Mayo Clin Proc* 47:974, 1972.

58. Sautter-Bihl ML, Heinze HG: Radiotherapy of Graves' ophthalmopathy, *Dev Ophthalmol* 20:139, 1989.

59. Sergott RC, Glasner JS: Graves' ophthalmopathy: a clinical, immunologic review, *Surv Ophthalmol* 26:1, 1981.

60. Sewell EC: Operative control of progressive exophthalmosis, *Arch Otolaryngol Head Neck Surg* 24:621, 1936.

61. Shorr N, Neuhaus RW, Baylis HA: Ocular motility problems after orbital decompression for dysthyroid ophthalmopathy, *Ophthalmology* 89:323, 1982.

62. Stanley RJ and others: Superior and transantral orbital decompression procedures. Effects on increased intraorbital pressure and orbital dynamics, *Arch Otolaryngol Head Neck Surg* 115:369, 1989.

63. Tallstedt L and others: Occurrence of ophthalmopathy after treatment for Graves' hyperthyroidism, *N Engl J Med* 326:1733, 1992.

64. Tamaki H and others: Improvement of infiltrative ophthalmopathy in parallel with a decrease of thyroid-stimulating antibody activity in two patients with hypothyroid Graves' disease, *J Endocr Invest* 12:47, 1989.

65. Tellez M, Cooper J, Edmonds C: Graves' ophthalmopathy in relation to cigarette smoking and ethnic origin, *Clin Endocr (Oxf)* 36:291, 1992.

66. Teng CS and others: Thyroid-stimulating immunoglobulins in ophthalmic Graves' disease, *Clin Endocr (Oxf)* 6:207, 1977.

67. Trobe JD: Optic nerve involvement in dysthyroidism, *Ophthalmology* 88:488, 1981.

68. Trobe JD, Glaser JS, Laflamme P: Dysthyroid optic neuropathy. Clinical profile, rationale for management, *Arch Ophthalmology* 96:1199, 1978.

69. Trokel S, Kazim M, Moore S: Orbital fat removal. Decompression for Graves' orbitopathy, *Ophthalmology* 100:674, 1993.

70. van der Wal KG and others: Surgical treatment of proptosis bulbi by three-wall orbital decompression, *J Oral Maxillofac Surg* 53:140, 1995.

71. Van Dyk HJL: Orbital Graves' disease. A modification of the ''NO SPECS'' classification, *Ophthalmology* 88:479, 1981.

72. Walsh TE, Ogura JH: Transantral orbital decompression for malignant exophthalmos, *Laryngoscope* 67:544, 1957.

73. Warren JD, Spector JG, Burde R: Long-term follow-up and recent observations on 305 cases of orbital decompression for dysthyroid orbitopathy, *Laryngoscope* 99:35, 1989.

74. Weisman RA, Osguthorpe JD: Orbital decompression in Graves' disease, *Arch Otolaryngol Head Neck Surg* 120:831, 1994.

75. Weisman RA, Savino PJ: Management of endocrine orbitopathy, *Otolaryngol Clin North Am* 21:93, 1988.

76. Werner SC: Classification of the eye changes of Graves' disease, *J Clin Endocrinol Metab* 29:982, 1969.

77. Werner SC: Modification of the classification of the eye changes of Graves' disease: recommendations of the ad hoc committee of the American Thyroid Association, *J Clin Endocrinol Metab* 44:203, 1977.

Chapter 58

Infection

Jonas T. Johnson
Berrylin J. Ferguson

Humidification, filtering, and temperature regulation are important functions of the nose and paranasal sinuses. The nose and paranasal sinuses are connected through the various sinus ostia and are lined with ciliated stratified columnar epithelium, containing goblet cells.

Inflammation causes increased secretions and edema in the sinonasal mucosa. With progression of the inflammatory components, secretions may be retained within the paranasal sinuses because of altered ciliary function or because of obstruction of the relatively small sinus ostia. The antigravitational placement of the ostia, particularly in the maxillary sinus, also contributes to poor drainage. Sinus obstruction leads to a reduction in the partial pressure of oxygen within the sinuses and to a relatively anaerobic environment. These factors create a milieu ideally suited for the growth of bacterial pathogens.

An inflammatory insult, such as an acute exacerbation of allergic rhinitis or a viral upper respiratory tract infection, frequently precedes purulent sinusitis. These inflammatory changes and retained secretions serve as an excellent medium for a bacterial superinfection.

In a landmark study, Gwaltney and others[18] studied 31 healthy adults 2 to 3 days after the onset of a self-diagnosed cold. Computed tomography (CT) abnormalities were detected in 27 subjects (87%). After resolution of all symptomology, 79% of subjects had resolution of CT findings without treatment. These data suggest that CT is too sensitive as a stand-alone criterion to use to diagnose bacterial sinusitis.

A sudden onset of purulent sinusitis in normal sinuses without a predisposing inflammatory episode is unusual except when a massive bacterial inoculation of the sinuses occurs during swimming or when there is direct spread of infection into the maxillary sinus as a consequence of a dental infection or dental manipulation. The proximity of the maxillary tooth roots to the antrum may allow the direct extension of a periapical abscess into the sinus, or the maxillary sinus may be entered during root canal therapy.

Because the lining of the nose and paranasal sinuses is in continuity, inflammation of the nasal cavity usually is associated with inflammation of the sinus lining. Consequently, viral rhinosinusitis may occur without the development of a bacterial infection. Distinguishing between generalized inflammation of the mucous membranes and bacterial sinusitis is important because the treatment of these two conditions is different.

PATHOGENESIS

Studies clearly have shown that no correlation exists between the growth on cultures obtained from the nose or nasopharynx and the bacteriology of material obtained with sinus aspiration or open antrostomy.[2,17,54] Orobello and others[40] reported that a strong association exists between culture obtained from the middle meatus and the maxillary (83%) and ethmoid (80%) sinuses when undertaken using endoscopic techniques. *Streptococcus pneumoniae* and *Haemophilus influenzae* have been implicated as the primary pathogens in acute bacterial sinusitis.[13,17,19,54] Other important pathogens include *Moraxella catarrhalis* and viruses.[17,19,54]

An increasing effort has been made to identify anaerobic bacteria in those with acute sinusitis because the reduced oxygen pressure and lowered pH present in an obstructed sinus would be expected to facilitate the growth of anaerobic bacteria, although anaerobic organisms have been identified in fewer than 10% of patients with acute purulent sinusitis.[2,6,18,23] In contrast, anaerobic bacteria appear to play an important role in those with chronic paranasal sinusitis.[15,25,49] The most commonly isolated anaerobic bacteria in patients with chronic sinusitis are *Veillonella, Peptococcus,* and *Corynebacterium acnes*. Brook[4] demonstrated anaerobic bacteria in the sinus aspirate of 100% of 40 children studied with chronic sinusitis, whereas 14 patients (38%) had mixed aerobic organisms.

BACTERIAL INFECTION

Acute sinusitis

The presence of nasal congestion and rhinorrhea for 7 to 14 days suggests acute bacterial sinusitis (Fig. 58-1). Nasal examination reveals edema, hyperemia, and frequently purulent debris.

Acute sinusitis may be thought of as an abscess or empyema. Treatment should be aimed at providing adequate drainage and eradication of local and systemic infection. In most patients, drainage of the involved sinuses can be accomplished medically. Topical vasoconstrictors and systemic decongestants frequently provide adequate drainage so that antibiotics can effectively treat the infection. The antibiotic used should be directed toward the more commonly encountered organisms such as *S. pneumoniae, H. influenzae,* and *M. catarrhalis*. The increasing frequency of lactamase-producing organisms identified in patients with

sinusitis should influence the choice of antibiotic, especially in those with refractory or recurrent cases.

When a patient fails to improve in 3 to 5 days or continues to have symptoms beyond 10 to 14 days, it usually is found that drainage has been inadequate or a resistant organism has emerged. Under these circumstances, another course of antibiotic therapy is appropriate. The use of a drug effective against the β lactamase-producing bacteria should be considered. If signs and symptoms persist, sinus secretions should be obtained for Gram's stain, culture, and sensitivity studies. When the infection continues to worsen despite appropriate antibiotic therapy or when a complication develops, surgical drainage of the affected sinuses is required.

A number of techniques may be effectively used to establish drainage in those with acute maxillary sinusitis. The mucosa of the middle turbinate and middle meatus should first be vasoconstricted, and the intended puncture site should be anesthetized. Either the canine fossa or the inferior meatus are ideal puncture sites. The contents of the maxillary sinus then can be displaced by passing a trocar into the maxillary sinus and by irrigating with normal saline. The contents of the sinuses will flow out through the natural ostium.

The traditional approach to empyema of the frontal sinus that fails to respond to conservative therapy is to trephine the sinus, which is accomplished through an incision made in the medial aspect of the upper eyelid, exposing the floor of the frontal sinus. The bone is removed with a cutting drill; specimens are obtained for culture and sensitivity; and the sinus is irrigated. In patients in whom the frontal sinus is involved bilaterally, the intersinus septum can be taken down. A catheter is placed through the wound into the frontal sinus to allow irrigation with a decongestant–antibiotic solution (e.g., neosynephrine, $\frac{1}{4}$%, with bacitracin), which is undertaken twice daily until free flow of the irrigating solution through the nasal frontal duct into the nose is achieved. Unfortunately, it often takes 7 to 10 days to restore function of the nasal frontal duct.

Management of acute frontal sinusitis with restoration of integrity of the nasal frontal duct using endoscopic sinus surgical techniques[43] is an ideal alternate to trephination because it avoids an external incision.

Empyema of the ethmoid or sphenoid sinuses that fails to respond to medical therapy may require surgical drainage, which can be accompanied endoscopically in most patients. An external surgical approach, such as external sphenoethmoidectomy, is an alternative for surgeons who are not familiar with internasal surgery.

Chronic sinusitis

Chronic paranasal sinusitis is characterized by persistent suppuration lasting beyond the acute stages of infection. An arbitrary temporal definition has little real value, although sinus symptoms lasting more than 6 to 12 weeks can be considered chronic. Critical to the treatment of the patient with chronic sinusitis is a thorough search for underlying

Acute Bacterial Sinusitis

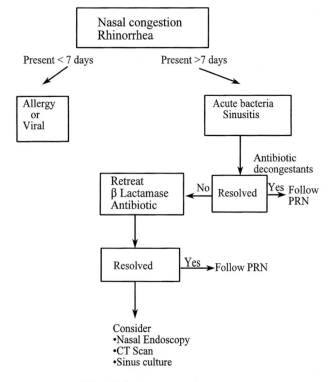

Fig. 58-1. Acute bacterial sinusitis.

etiologic factors that are manageable. If, for example, unrecognized or uncontrolled nasal allergy causes the chronic sinusitis, the benefits of surgery alone usually are limited in extent and brief in duration. Allergic patients should be identified, and every effort should be made to treat the underlying allergies with appropriate desensitization. Topical steroids applied through nasal inhalers usually provide some degree of temporary control, particularly during peak periods of exposure to allergen. Systemic steroids usually are effective in reducing nasal polyposis, but the well-known side effects preclude their use as long-term therapy. When nasal polyposis is severe and refractory to medical therapy, surgical removal of the polyps and the mucosa from which they originate (i.e., ethmoid or maxillary sinus mucosa) prevents recurrence for months or years, although if the underlying allergies remain, the polyps usually will recur.

The initial treatment of a patient with chronic sinusitis should include antibiotics, intranasal steroid sprays, and decongestants. If the patient fails to respond to medical management, surgical intervention aimed at débriding the diseased mucous membrane and at establishing improved drainage from the sinuses is required. Most authorities now agree that a sustained effort at medical management with antibiotics, steroid sprays, and decongestants should be undertaken before surgery is deemed necessary.

SINUSITIS IN CHILDREN

At birth, the paranasal sinuses are incompletely developed. The maxillary sinus is a small air cell attached to the lateral wall of the nose, and the ethmoidal labyrinth is just beginning to pneumatize. The frontal sinus does not develop until the age of 6 to 8 years; the sinuses do not complete their development until well into adolescence. The variability that occurs in the rate of pneumatization frequently creates confusion in the examination of children with purulent nasal discharge.

Wald and others[54] outlined the pathophysiology of sinusitis in children. Symptoms in young children usually include halitosis, nasal discharge, and a cough that is characteristically protracted. In older children, a history of antecedent upper respiratory tract infection usually exists. Subsequently purulent rhinorrhea, nasal obstruction, and periorbital pain may develop. Exudate draining from the middle meatus in association with an upper respiratory tract infection and pain indicates acute paranasal sinusitis.[23]

The diagnosis may be confirmed radiographically. The presence of fluid or clouding of the sinuses correlates well with purulent sinusitis. Completely opaque sinuses will contain pus on aspiration in 80% to 88% of patients.[2,34,53] Sinuses that demonstrate thickened mucous membranes with central aeration contain pus on aspiration 50% of the time.[2] The interpretation of sinus radiographs in children should be undertaken with some caution because asymmetry of sinus development may lead to misinterpretation.[5]

Children rarely develop allergic nasal polyps before age 10 years,[44] therefore the presence of nasal polyps in young children requires evaluation for cystic fibrosis.

Aspiration of an infected maxillary sinus in children usually requires a general anesthetic. Indications for sinus aspiration include a failure to respond to antibiotics and decongestants, evidence of sinusitis in an immunosuppressed patient, or the development of a complication of sinusitis.

FUNGAL SINUSITIS

Fungal sinusitis is categorized into five manifestations: invasive, chronic invasive, mycetoma, saprophytic, and allergic fungal sinusitis. Failure to categorize the manifestation and to instead use the general term of *fungal sinusitis* results in confusion because the prognosis and therapy of each manifestation of fungal sinusitis is different. These manifestations have distinctive histopathologies that also reflect the immunologic status of the host. Prognostic and therapeutic differences exist depending on which fungal species is responsible, but these differences, depending on the fungal species, are of less importance than the manifestation of the fungal sinusitis as categorized along the immunologic spectrum (Table 58-1).

Invasive fungal sinusitis

Invasive fungal sinusitis almost always is confined to the patient with altered host defenses such as a patient undergoing transplantation (bone marrow, liver, lung, and so on), a diabetic patient, a patient with primary or acquired immunodeficiency (immunoglobulin deficiency, systemic prednisone, and so on), or the patient with leukemia. As the name implies, on histopathologic inspection, the fungus can be

Table 58-1. Classification of fungal sinusitis along an immunologic spectrum

Classification	Immunologic status	Prognosis	Therapy
Invasive	Compromised	Guarded	Reversal of immunocompromise; surgery; antifungal agents
Chronic invasive	Normal	Fair	Surgery; antifungal agents
Mycetoma	Normal	Good	Surgery
Saprophytic	Normal	Excellent	Removal
Allergic	Atopic	Excellent	Surgery; steroids; immunotherapy

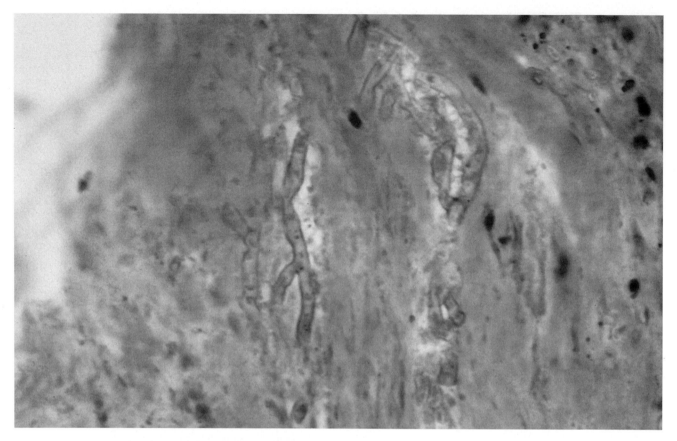

Fig. 58-2. Histopathologic section demonstrating invasive fungal sinusitis on frozen section in a patient with leukemia. Subsequent cultures grew out an *Aspergillus* species. Note that some of the hyphae appear swollen, suggesting mucormycosis; this is an artifact of the frozen section. The 45° branching typical of *Aspergillus* species and septated hyphae are present.

seen within and invading tissue (Fig. 58-2). Invasive fungal sinusitis is suspected when the immunocompromised patient develops a fever and localization of symptoms to the paranasal sinus area, such as orbital swelling, facial pain, or nasal congestion. Nasal endoscopy may show necrosis of the nasal mucosa, indicative of mucormycosis, and in rare situations actual hyphae. It is more usual to note only edema and changes indistinguishable from nonfungal causes of sinusitis. Anesthesia of the nasal mucosa or cheeks, independent of topical anesthetics, is suspicious for mucormycosis. The oral cavity always should be examined for invasion through the hard palate from the sinuses. If the diagnosis is suspected, a sinus CT should be obtained. Changes seen on sinus CT or plain radiographs usually are indistinguishable from bacterial sinusitis, although they may show bony erosion or soft-tissue invasion. Unfortunately, abnormal imaging studies are common in this compromised population. Up to 42% of patients with leukemia in one series had abnormal sinus radiographs.[28]

Biopsy of the suspected tissue for pathology and culture is critical to making the diagnosis. Histopathology with special stains for fungus establish the diagnosis of invasive fungal sinusitis. Cultures should be obtained, preferably before the initiation of systemic antifungals, which decrease the likelihood of the culture growing. It is critical that the diagnosis, once suspected, be made as quickly as possible. Therefore, a frozen section of the pathologic specimen or evaluation of the material submitted for culture by special fungal stains, such as Calcofluor white (Fig. 58-3) should be requested, and if either of these is positive for fungus, appropriate antifungal therapy and extended surgical resection can be initiated without delay. Neither frozen section of the involved tissue or special stains for fungus will definitively distinguish between fungal species, although mucormycosis can be suspected if the fungal elements seen are broad ribbon-like (10 to 15 μm), irregular, and rarely septated (Fig. 58-4). The artifacts of frozen section may cause *Aspergillus* hypha elements to appear swollen and similar to mucormycosis. Generally, on permanent histopathologic sections, the distinction between mucormycosis and *Aspergillus* species can be made. The *Aspergillus* species demonstrate more narrow hyphae with regular septations and 45° branching on histopa-

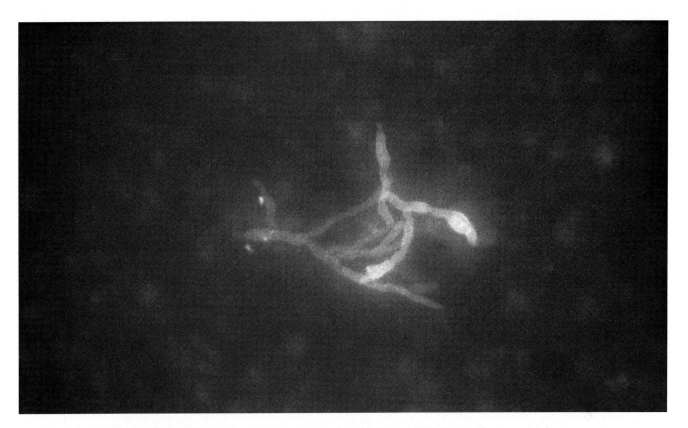

Fig. 58-3. Calcofluor white stain demonstrating hyphal elements. This immunofluorescent stain can be used for immediate identification of fungal elements.

thology (Fig. 58-5). Cultures are important for distinguishing *Aspergillus* species from less common pathogenic fungal species, which also are septated, such as *Fusarium, Alternaria, Pseudallescherii boydii*, and so on. *Aspergillus* species are the most virulent and frequent species found in those with invasive fungal sinusitis, although every year, additional previously nonpathogenic fungi are reported as causing invasive disease, and this trend will continue as the at-risk population of immunocompromised patients continues to grow. The pseudohyphae of *Candida* infections are distinct from the fungal species with true hyphae, although the ubiquity of *Candida* presence requires either a large number of organisms present on culture or deep and not superficial invasion of the tissues to distinguish saprophytic *Candida* growth from invasive *Candida* fungal infection.

Fungal infections in the at-risk population of severely neutropenic patients, such as those in the bone marrow unit, can be reduced by eliminating the source of fungal exposure using high-efficiency particulate air filter systems and by eliminating fungal sources such as potted plants.

Therapy

Therapy of invasive fungal sinusitis requires reversal of the underlying predisposing condition, appropriate systemic antifungal therapy, and surgical débridement. Of these, the most important is reversal of the underlying cause of immunocompromise.[42] Invasive fungal sinusitis in the immunocompetent patient is exceedingly rare and generally is less fulminant, although occasionally lethal. These cases are classified as chronic invasive fungal sinusitis.[33,38]

For the majority of patients with invasive fungal sinusitis, systemic amphotericin B continues to be the drug of choice at intravenous doses of 0.8 to 1.5 mg/kg/day to a total dose of up to 3 g. Nephrotoxicity is the major dose-limiting toxicity and can be reduced with sodium loading. Fever, chills, nausea, and hypotension frequently accompany the first few doses. These toxicities can be reduced or eliminated with the use of amphotericin B lipid complex, which is amphotericin B delivered through liposomes. These liposomes have an affinity for the reticuloendothelial system and so bypass toxicities otherwise imparted to other tissues by amphotericin B. Unfortunately, liposomal amphotericin B is not yet approved by the Food and Drug Administration and is only available on a compassionate use basis.[52] Certain fungi also respond to other antifungal agents, and occasionally other antifungal agents are the drug of choice. Approximately half the cases of invasive *Aspergillus* infections in one series were salvaged with itraconazole.[47] Table 58-2 lists various fungal agents and the antifungal drugs of choice.

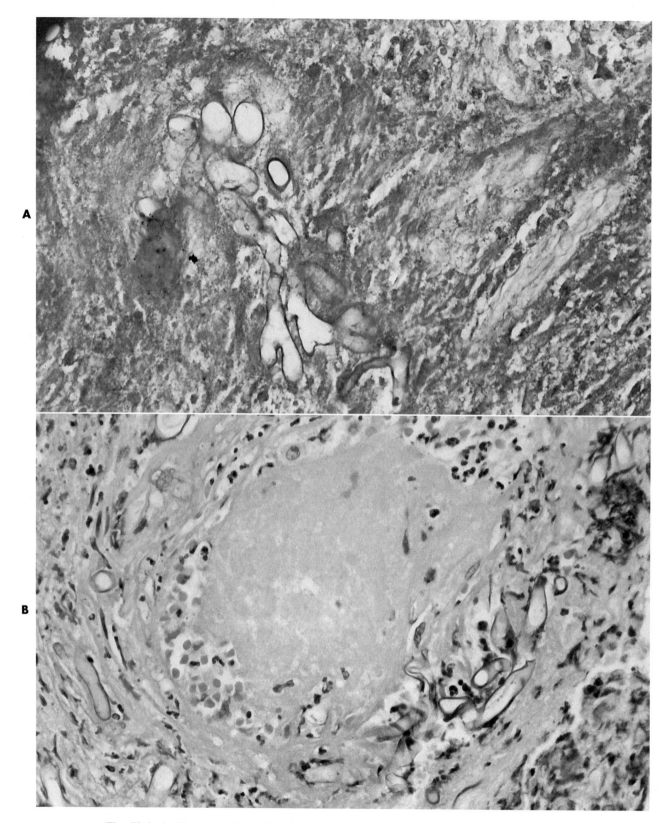

Fig. 58-4. A, Mucormycosis on histopathologic section demonstrating broad hyphae. (Periodic acid–Schiff stain.) **B,** The hyphae of mucormycosis can be seen invading the vessel wall. The vessel is thrombosed. (Hematoxylin-eosin stain.)

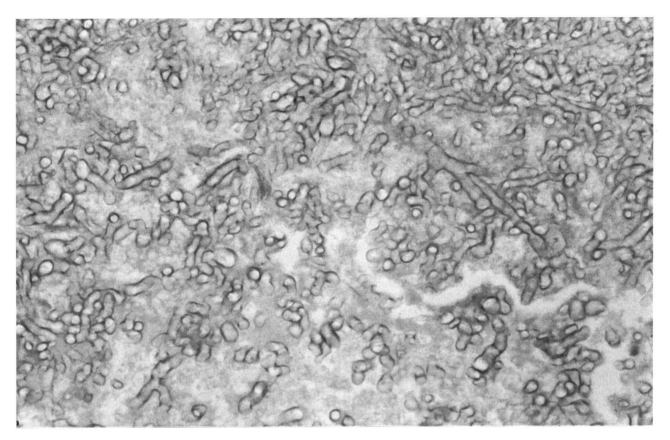

Fig. 58-5. Mycetoma showing hyphae of *Aspergillus*. The entire speciman was composed of a tangled mass of hyphae. No tissue invasion was seen.

Table 58-2. Choice of antifungal drug for invasive fungal sinusitis

Infection	Dosage	Alternatives
Aspergillus	Amphotericin B 1–1.5 mg/kg, IV	Itraconazole 200 mg twice daily, PO
Candidiasis	Amphotericin B 0.5–1.0 mg/kg, IV	Fluconazole 400–800 mg, IV, or four times daily, PO
Mucormycosis	Amphotericin B 1.0–1.5 mg/kg, IV	No dependable alternative
Pseudallescherii	Ketoconazole 400–800 mg/day, PO; or itraconazole, 200 mg twice daily, PO	Miconazole 600 mg every 8 hours
Sporotrichosis	Amphotericin B 0.5 mg/kg/day, IV	Itraconazole 200 mg twice daily, PO

The Medical Letter 38:10, 1996.
IV—Intravenous; PO—By mouth.

Aspergillus

The *Aspergillus* species most commonly responsible for invasive disease in this country is *Aspergillus fumigatus*. *Aspergillus flavus* is commonly associated with the more indolent chronic invasive fungal disease seen primarily in those in the Sudan, but it also can be responsible for fulminate invasive disease regardless of geographic location.[7] Therapies and prognosis do not differ among *Aspergillus* species. *Aspergillus* species can be angioinvasive, but it is not the obliterative invasion seen with mucormycosis. Hem-

orrhagic infarcts can be seen if there is cerebral involvement.[14]

Mucormycosis

Mucormycosis is a term that is commonly used to designate all fungal species within the order Mucorales in the class of the Zygomycetes. The most virulent and common species is *Rhizopus oryzae*. *Mucormycosis* has earned the reputation as the most acutely fatal fungal infection known to humans. It is rapidly growing, and within 24 hours, cul-

sinusitis, nasal obstruction and rhinorrhea are unusual findings.

A frontoethmoidal mucocele on radiographic examination consists of clouding of the sinus, loss of the typical scalloped outline of the frontal sinus, and sclerosis of the surrounding skull.

Sphenoethmoidal mucocele

Sphenoethmoidal mucoceles have been well described.[10,30,46] These lesions may cause subtle symptoms initially. Headache with occipital, vertex, or deep nasal pain may accompany various ophthalmologic complaints, such as diplopia, visual field disturbance, and globe displacement. Pituitary disturbances are unusual but have been described. Diagnosis of a sphenoethmoidal mucocele is made based on an adequate index of suspicion and the characteristic radiographic findings.

Frontoethmoidal and sphenoethmoidal mucoceles require surgical removal. A sphenoethmoidal mucocele should be opened widely into the nasal cavity. Frontal sinus mucoceles should be removed completely, and the frontal sinus should be obliterated.

Orbital complications

The spread of infection to involve the orbital structures is the most common complication of sinusitis. Because the orbital contents are separated from the ethmoidal labyrinth only by the thin lamina papyracea, direct extension of infection into the orbit is common. In addition, the ethmoidal veins may become thrombophlebitic, resulting in the spread of infection into the orbit. The first indication of orbital involvement usually is inflammatory edema of the eyelids. With progression of the cellulitis, erythema, progressive proptosis, and fever (to 101° F) occur. Early in the process, extraocular muscle function and results of funduscopic examination usually are normal, but as the cellulitis progresses, chemosis increases, ophthalmoplegia may develop, and funduscopic examination may show mild vascular congestion. Although the fever may increase to 102° to 104° F, the patient usually is not particularly toxic. As the disease progresses, an abscess may form along the lamina papyracea or within the periorbita.

The following classification of orbital involvement caused by ethmoid sinusitis was developed by Chandler[8] to aid in the correlation of physical findings with orbital disease:

1. Inflammatory edema—lid edema; no limitation of extraocular movement with normal acuity;
2. Orbital cellulitis—diffuse edema of orbital contents; no discrete abscess formation;
3. Subperiosteal abscess—purulent collection beneath periosteum of lamina papyracea; displacement of globe downward and laterally;
4. Orbital abscess—purulent collection within orbit; pro-

ptosis and chemosis with ophthalmoplegia and decreased vision; and

5. Cavernous sinus thrombosis—bilateral eye findings; prostration; meningismus.

This represents a clinical approach to orbital inflammation aimed at predicting pathology. Today, modern imaging allows the practitioner to improve his or her diagnostic accuracy.

Purulent frontal sinusitis also may result in orbital complications. The floor of the frontal sinus frequently is the path of least resistance for the infection because it usually is the thinnest wall. An abscess along the orbital roof causes inferolateral displacement of the globe. When the infection spreads to become osteomyelitis of the frontal bone, a subperiosteal abscess develops over the anterior surface. This overlying soft tissue swelling is called *Pott's puffy tumor.* As the osteomyelitis of the frontal bone advances, there usually is sequestration of necrotic bone through a cutaneous fistula in the upper lid.

Orbital inflammation and cellulitis may be adequately treated with sinus drainage and intravenous antibiotics. The patient should be hospitalized and carefully observed for evidence of a developing orbital abscess or cavernous sinus thrombosis. When an abscess develops within the confines of the orbit, drainage is mandatory. Failure to recognize and drain an orbital abscess may lead to permanent orbital sequelae and intracranial complications. Surgical intervention usually is required if:

1. Orbital cellulitis continues to progress despite adequate levels of an appropriate intravenous antibiotic;
2. Physical signs (e.g., fever, erythema, edema, protosis) regress slightly for 2 or 3 days and then stabilize or exacerbate;
3. Definite evidence of an abscess on ultrasound examination or CT scan exists; or
4. Loss of visual acuity occurs.

Surgical treatment should include adequate drainage of the infected sinus (frontal sinus trephination or ethmoidectomy) and drainage of the orbital abscess. The latter should be approached directly through an eyelid or Sewell incision overlying the anticipated abscess site. Most abscesses are found along the lamina papyracea or frontal sinus floor, but if the infection has extended through the periorbita, it should be widely opened to ensure adequate drainage. A drain should then be left in place until no further drainage occurs.

Schramm, Myers, and Kennerdell[45] described the clinical characteristics of 134 patients with orbital complications of acute sinusitis whose cases were reviewed retrospectively. The patients ranged in age from 5 weeks to 66 years, but 75% were less than 16 years of age. More than 80% of the patients had symptoms of an upper respiratory tract infection in the 2 weeks preceding hospitalization. Cultures were obtained from the conjunctival nose and nasopharynx, blood, tissue aspirate, and sinus if surgery was undertaken. In children, *H. influenzae* and *S. pneumoniae* were most commonly cultured from blood of sinus drainage. Conjunctival cultures were frequently misleading. Similarly, nose and nasopharyngeal cultures rarely correlated with the results of percutaneous aspiration or culture of the sinus at surgery. Organisms most commonly cultured in adults included *S. pneumoniae* and microaerophilic *Streptococcus*.

The evaluation of these patients included careful physical examination, sinus radiographs, an ultrasonic B scan, and CT scanning. The B scan proved to be 90% effective in detecting abscesses in the anterior orbit or along the medial wall. CT scanning was more accurate and more valuable in identifying the posterior extension of the abscess.

All patients were hospitalized and treated with intravenous antibiotics. Ninety-seven patients (72%) responded to antibiotic therapy alone, and another nine patients responded after irrigation of the sinus. Twenty-eight patients (21%) required surgical drainage of an orbital abscess. Incision and drainage were required more commonly in adults than in children. Thirteen of 33 patients 16 years or older required surgery, whereas only 3 of 46 patients less than 4 years of age were treated surgically.

Cavernous sinus thrombosis

Differentiating orbital cellulitis or abscess from a developing cavernous sinus thrombosis may be difficult but is of vital importance because of the life-threatening nature of the latter. Infections of the paranasal sinuses or orbits may spread readily to the cavernous sinus because the absence of valves in the orbital veins allows blood to flow either toward or away from the cavernous sinuses.

The most important clinical signs of a developing cavernous sinus thrombosis include bilateral orbital involvement, rapidly progressive severe chemosis and ophthalmoplegia, severe retinal engorgement, fever to 105° F, and prostration. Even with rapid recognition and treatment, the condition may progress to loss of vision, meningitis, and even death. The thrombosis usually can be detected on CT scanning. Treatment includes intravenous antibiotics, drainage of any abscess, and orbital decompression if visual acuity decreases. Many physicians advocate heparinization to minimize the progression of thrombosis.

Intracranial complications

The precise incidence of intracranial complications of paranasal sinusitis is not known, although sinusitis is reported to be the source of 35% to 65% of subdural abscesses.[22,24,27] Infection may gain access to the intracranial space by direct extension through a defect in the posterior wall of the frontal sinus caused by trauma or the infection itself. Retrograde thrombophlebitis of the valveless ophthalmic vessels also may offer a route of transmission for infected material into the intracranial cavity. The subdural space may be involved even when no infection of the inter-

vening tissues exists.[27] The arachnoid is a good barrier to bacterial invasion, but thrombosis of dural vessels may lead to focal cerebral abscess, seizures, and neurologic deficits. Meningitis rarely develops in adults, but bacterial meningitis frequently occurs in infants.

Septic thrombosis of major dural sinuses usually results in massive cerebral edema and infarction, which rapidly progresses to decreased mentation, coma, and death.

Evidence of nuchal rigidity in a patient with sinusitis should alert the physician to the possibility of an intracranial complication. Patients should be hospitalized and examined carefully for evidence of progression of the disease. Intravenous antibiotics should be instituted. Signs of increased intracranial pressure manifested by headache, intractable vomiting, and deteriorating levels of consciousness should be viewed with gravity in a patient with sinusitis. The management of intracranial sepsis that develops as a complication of sinusitis requires close collaboration between the neurosurgeon and otolaryngologist. High-dose antibiotic therapy, management of increased intracranial pressure, and prevention of seizures should be instituted. Surgical drainage of an intracranial abscess when present should be planned in conjunction with the establishment of proper drainage of the involved sinus. Failure to recognize and treat the underlying sinus disease may result in recurrent or persistent intracranial disease.

REFERENCES

1. Artis WM and others: A mechanism of susceptibility to mucormycosis in diabetic ketoacidosis: transferrin and iron availability, *Diabetes* 31: 1109, 1982.
2. Axelsson A, Brorson IE: The correlation between bacteriologic findings in the nose and maxillary sinus in acute maxillary sinusitis, *Laryngoscope* 83:2003, 1973.
3. Boelaert JR and others: The role of desferrioxamine in dialysis-associated mucormycosis: report of three cases and review of the literature, *Clin Nephrol* 29:261, 1988.
4. Brook L: Bacteriologic features of chronic sinusitis in children, *JAMA* 246:967, 1981.
5. Caffey J: *Pediatric x-ray diagnosis*, ed 7, Chicago, 1977, Mosby.
6. Carenfelt C and others: Bacteriology of maxillary sinusitis in relation to the quality of the retained secretion, *Acta Otolaryngol* 86:298, 1978.
7. Chakrabarti A, Sharma SC, Chander J: Epidemiology and pathogenesis of paranasal sinus mycoses, *Otolaryngol Head Neck Surg* 107:745, 1992.
8. Chandler JR, Langenbrunner DJ, Stevens ER: The pathogenesis of orbital complications in acute sinusitis, *Laryngoscope* 80:1414, 1970.
9. Chinn RYW, Diamond RD: Generation of chemotactic factors by *Rhizopus oryzae* in the presence and absence of serum: relationship to hypha damage mediated by human neutrophils and effects of hyperglycemia and ketoacidosis, *Infect Immun* 38:1123, 1982.
10. Close LG, O'Conner WE: Sphenoethmoidal mucoceles with intracranial extension, *Otolaryngol Head Neck Surg* 91:350, 1983.
11. Corey JP, Delsupehe KG, Ferguson GJ: Allergic fungal sinusitis: allergic, infectious, or both? *Otolaryngol Head Neck Surg* 113:110, 1995.
12. Evans C: Aetiology and treatment of fronto-ethmoidal mucocele, *J Laryngol Otol* 95:361, 1981.
13. Evans FO and others: Sinusitis of the maxillary antrum, *N Engl J Med* 293:735, 1975.
14. Fernando SSE, Lauer CS: Aspergillus fumigatus infection of the optic

nerve with mycotic arteritis of cerebral vessels, *Histopathology* 6:227, 1982.

15. Frederick J, Braude AL: Anaerobic infection of the paranasal sinuses, *N Engl J Med* 200:135, 1974.

16. Gale GR, Welch A: Studies of opportunistic fungi. I. Inhibition of *R. Oryzae* by human sera, *Am J Med Sci* 45:604, 1961.

17. Gwaltney JM, Sydnor A, Sande MA: Etiology and antimicrobial treatment of acute sinusitis, *Ann Otol* 90(suppl 84):68, 1981.

18. Gwaltney JM and others: Computed tomographic study of the common cold, *N Engl J Med* 330:25, 1994.

19. Hamory BH and others: Etiology and antimicrobial therapy of acute maxillary sinusitis, *J Infect Dis* 139:197, 1979.

20. Handley GH and others: Bone erosion in allergic fungal sinusitis, *Am J Rhinol* 4:149, 1990.

21. Henderson LT and others: Benign mucor colonization (fungus ball) associated with chronic sinusitis, *South Med J* 81:846, 1988.

22. Hitchcock E, Andreadis A: Subdural empyema: a review of 29 cases, *J Neurol Neurosurg Psychiatry* 27:422, 1964.

23. Jannert M and others: Acute sinusitis in children: symptoms, clinical findings and bacteriology related to initial radiologic appearance, *Int J Pediatr Otorhinolaryngol* 4:139, 1982.

24. Jenkins RB and others: Intracranial extradural and subdural empyemas, *Med Ann DC* 37:472, 1968.

25. Karma P and others: Bacteria in chronic maxillary sinusitis, *Arch Otolaryngol* 105:386, 1979.

26. Katzenstein AL, Sale SR, Greenberger PA: Allergic *Aspergillus* sinusitis: a newly recognized form of sinusitis, *J Allergy Clin Immunol* 72:89, 1983.

27. Kaufman DM, Miller MH, Steigbigel NH: Subdural empyema: analysis of 17 recent cases and review of the literature, *Medicine* 54:485, 1975.

28. Kavanagh KT and others: Fungal sinusitis in immunocompromised children with neoplasms, *Ann Otolaryngol* 100:331, 1991.

29. Lowe J, Bradley J: Cerebral and orbital *Aspergillus* infection due to invasive aspergillosis of ethmoid sinus, *J Clin Pathol* 39:774, 1986.

30. Lundgren A, Olin T: Muco-phocele of sphenoidal sinus or posterior ethmoidal cells with special reference to apex orbitae syndrome, *Acta Otolaryngol* 53:61, 1961.

31. Mabry RL, Manning SC, Mabry CS: Immunotherapy in the treatment of allergic fungal sinusitis, *Otolaryngol Head Neck Surg* 116:31, 1997.

32. Manning SC and others: Culture-positive allergic fungal sinusitis, *Arch Otolaryngol Head Neck Surg* 117:174, 1991.

33. Maskin SL and others: Bipolaris hawaiiensis- caused phaeohyphomycotic orbitopathy, *Ophthalmology* 96:175, 1989.

34. McNeill RA: Comparison of the findings on transillumination, x-ray and lavage of the maxillary sinus, *J Laryngol* 77:1009, 1963.

35. Millar JW, Johnston A, Lamb D: Allergic aspergillosis of the maxillary sinuses, *Thorax* 36:710, 1981 (abstract).

36. Milosev B and others: Primary aspergilloma of paranasal sinuses in the Sudan. A review of seventeen cases, *Br J Surg* 56:132, 1969.

37. Milroy CM and others: *Aspergillosis* of the nose and paranasal sinuses, *J Clin Pathol* 42:123, 1989.

38. Morgan MA and others: Fungal sinusitis in healthy and immunocompromised individuals, *Am J Clin Pathol* 82:597, 1984.

39. Ohnishi T and others: Fronto-ethmoidal mucocele: observation of its mode of enlargement, *Rhinology* 20:213, 1982.

40. Orobello PW and others: Microbiology of chronic sinusitis in children, *Arch Otolaryngol Head Neck Surg* 117:980, 1991.

41. Reference deleted in pages.

42. Saah D and others: Rhinocerebral aspergillosis in patients undergoing bone marrow transplantation, *Ann Otol Rhinol Laryngol* 103:306, 1994.

43. Schaeffer SD, Close LG: Endoscopic management of frontal sinus disease, *Laryngoscope* 100:155, 1990.

44. Schramm VL, Effron MZ: Nasal polyps in children, *Laryngoscope* 90:488, 1980.

45. Schramm VL, Myers EN, Kennerdell JS: Orbital complications of acute sinusitis: evaluation, management, and outcome, *Trans Am Acad Ophthalmol Otolaryngol* 86:221, 1978.

46. Sellars SL, DeVilliers JC: Clinical records: the sphenoid sinus mucocoele, *J Laryngol Otolaryngol* 95:493, 1981.

47. Sharkey PK and others: Itraconazole treatment of phaeohyphomycosis, *J Am Acad Dermatol* 23:577, 1990.

48. Shugar MA, Montgomery WW, Hyslop NE: Alternaria sinusitis, *Ann Otol* 90:251, 1981.

49. Su WY and others: Bacteriological study of chronic maxillary sinusitis, *Laryngoscope* 93:931, 1983.

50. Sugar AM: *Agents of mucormycosis and related species.* In Mandell GL, Bennnett JE, Dolin J, editors: *Principles and practice of infectious diseases*, ed 4, New York, 1995, Churchill Livingstone.

51. Sugar AM: Mucormycosis, *Clin Infect Dis* 14(suppl 1):S126, 1992.

52. Tkatch L, Kusne S, Eibling D: Successful treatment of zygomycosis of the paranasal sinuses with surgical debridement and amphotericin B colloidal dispersion, *Am J Otolaryngol* 14:249, 1993.

53. Vusrinen P, Kauppila A, Pulkkinen K: Comparison of results of roentgen examination and picture and irrigation of the maxillary sinuses, *J Laryngol* 76:359, 1962.

54. Wald E and others: Acute maxillary sinusitis in children, *N Engl J Med* 304:749, 1981.

55. Zinreich SJ and others: Fungal sinusitis: diagnosis with CT and MRI imaging, *Radiology* 169:439, 1988.

SUGGESTED READING

Majumdar B, Bull PD: The incidence and bacteriology of maxillary sinusitis in nasal polyposis, *J Laryngol Otol* 96:937, 1982.

Chapter 59

Neoplasms

Ernest A. Weymuller, Jr.

True neoplasms of the paranasal sinuses are uncommon in the general population. The most common are squamous cell carcinomas, which occur with a frequency of less than 1 : 200,000 per year.[2] Because sinus malignancy initially mimics benign disease, the diagnosis usually becomes evident only after an advanced stage has been reached, thus explaining the relatively poor prognosis. Additionally, as indicated by Ketcham,[30] "no one physician, no matter how intense his interest or ideal his patient referral patterns might be, can accumulate the experience to make him a paranasal sinus (cancer) specialist."

This chapter first discusses material common to all sinus tumors: anatomy, symptoms, physical findings, diagnostic assessment, and surgical options. Although these lesions are rare, numerous histologic subtypes must be differentiated and are discussed individually because management varies significantly among them (Fig. 59-1).

ANATOMY

Assessment and surgical management of this group of tumors demands an intense personal effort to understand the complex anatomy of the sinuses and skull base. Such knowledge is best obtained through anatomic dissection and repeated review of the anatomy of the human skull. It may be helpful to have a skull available in the operating room for inspection during complex resections, especially those that approach or traverse the skull base.

Pertinent to this discussion are the structures contiguous to each of the sinuses, because they define the extent of disease and determine the design of therapy.

Maxillary antrum

The most significant structures prognostically are above and behind the maxillary antrum. Superiorly is the orbit and the ethmoid sinus. The posterior border approaches the pter-

ygoid plates, the pterygoid space, and the infratemporal fossa. The other boundary areas are more easily resected *en bloc* and thus are less worrisome when involved. Anteriorly is the canine fossa, inferiorly the alveolus, and medially the nasal cavity.

Ethmoid sinus

As with the antrum, the least worrisome areas of spread from the ethmoid sinus are inferiorly into the antrum or medially into the nasal cavity. Of much greater concern is spread superiorly, where the fovea ethmoidalis and the cribriform plate provide little barrier to intracranial spread. Evidence of intracranial spread requires consideration of an anterior craniofacial resection. The lateral wall consists of the thin bone of the lamina papyracea, which also provides little resistance to neoplastic invasion.

Sphenoid sinus

Located in the center of the head, the sphenoid sinus relates to very complex and vital structures. For this reason, complete resection of a malignant tumor involving the sphenoid sinus is usually not possible. The optic nerve and the pituitary gland are superior, and the internal carotid artery and the cavernous sinuses sit laterally. The bone of the lateral wall is usually less than 0.5 mm thick, and not uncommonly is totally dehiscent.[17] Anterior to the sinus are posterior ethmoidal cells, and inferiorly are the vidian nerve and the nasopharynx.

Frontal sinus

The least frequently involved by malignant tumor, the frontal sinus is bounded anteriorly by the soft tissues of the scalp, inferiorly by the ethmoidal cells and the orbit, and posteriorly by the anterior cranial fossa.

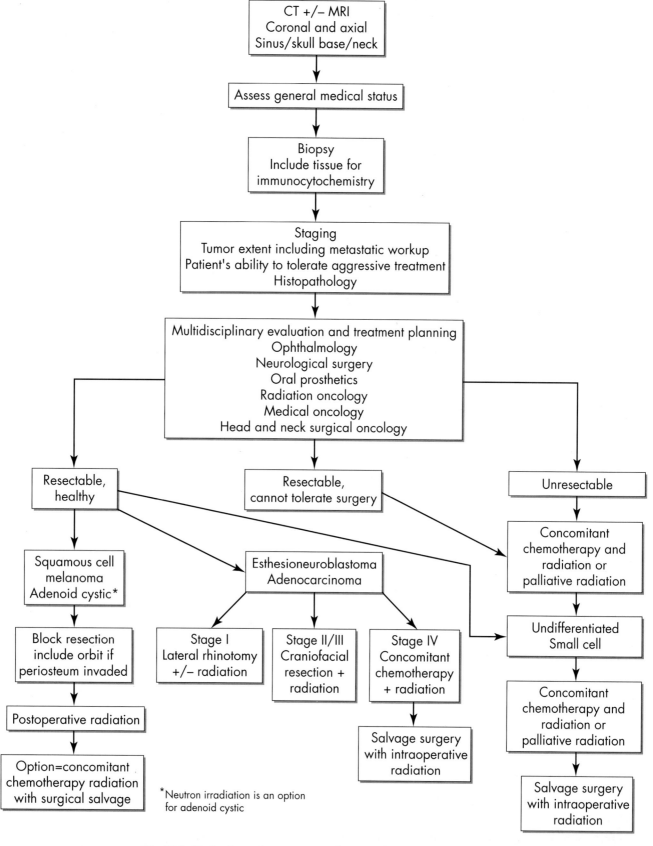

Fig. 59-1. Evaluation and management of suspected paranasal sinus cancer.

It is important to realize that all of the sinuses have venous communications with intracranial veins, which provide yet another avenue for lethal spread of neoplasm.

Lymphatics

Ohngren[45] emphasized the importance of a precise understanding of the lymphatic drainage of the nose and paranasal sinuses as a prerequisite to adequate therapy. He contested the established dictum that these tumors do not often metastasize. He held that they do metastasize but that clinical evidence of early metastasis is absent because the primary drainage is to the lateral and retropharyngeal nodes. He believed that the relative success of his therapy hinged on electrocoagulation and irradiation of the rich lymphatic channels passing from the nose and paranasal sinuses posteriorly to the retropharynx.

The following is a precise description by Ohngren[45] of the lymphatics of this region:

Ever since first demonstrated by Mascagni the regional lymph nodes of the tumors under review here have been the subject of close study by, chiefly, Simon, Sappey, Kuttner, Key, Retzius, Cuneo, Marc Andre, Most, Turner, Broekaert, Grunwald and Moore. The view I have arrived at regarding the metastasis of these tumors is the outcome of a critical study of the works by the above authors as well as of observations on my own cases.

Close anatomical investigations by the above-mentioned authors have revealed that the lymph channels from the whole of the nasal cavity inside the vestibule from the lateral as well as the medial and lower walls pass in a backward direction towards the choana running together into a plexus in the lateral part of this. From this plexus a few large lymph channels are given off backwards above as well as below the eustachian cushion towards the posterior pharyngeal wall. Here they pick up finer branches from the nasopharynx before entering the retropharyngeal space. The lateral retropharyngeal lymph nodes receive most of these lymph vessels; only small branches pass directly upwards emptying into the medial jugular glands located just below the base of the skull. From the lateral retropharyngeal lymph glands the lymph is conducted in stems of larger calibre which empty into a node belonging to the deep jugular chain and usually located at the level of the carotid bifurcation. It has generally been left to this node to determine the presence or not of metastases in the tumours we are concerned with. Obviously such methods must lead to an erroneous conception of the frequency of metastases in the case of tumors of the lateral nasal wall, since the node is nothing but a secondary localization of metastases whereas the primary metastases located in the retropharyngeal nodes have escaped the attention of the observer.

SYMPTOMS

The most common symptoms associated with malignant tumors of the paranasal sinuses are facial or dental pain, nasal obstruction, and epistaxis. These early signs represent the impact of a necrotic infected mass situated within the paranasal sinus or nose. As the disease progresses, it infiltrates adjacent structures, giving rise to additional symptoms as follows:

1. *Diplopia or vision loss* is most often a manifestation of tumor mass compressing or invading the orbit and may also result from direct involvement of the optic or oculomotor nerves at the orbital apex or the cavernous sinus.
2. *Epiphora* is caused by obstruction or infiltration of the lacrimal duct situated in the anteromedial aspect of the maxilla.
3. *Facial swelling and malocclusion* result from bone destruction and advancement of the tumor into the soft tissues of the face or mouth.
4. *Trismus* signals far-advanced tumor invading the muscles of mastication, most commonly the pterygoid muscles.
5. *Neck mass*, palpable metastatic adenopathy in the jugular chain, is another sign of advanced disease because the first-echelon nodes are located in the parapharyngeal region.
6. *Hearing loss* usually results from nasopharyngeal extension of the tumor causing serous otitis. This finding is important because nasopharyngeal extension of disease is a contraindication to surgery.
7. *Facial numbness* is a manifestation of tumor invasion of portions of the trigeminal nerve.

PHYSICAL FINDINGS

Until the tumor has infiltrated a cranial nerve or facial bones or grown sufficiently to obstruct a sinus osteum, it will silently advance in size and extent. Discovering an asymptomatic sinus tumor at an early stage is truly a rare and fortuitous event. The most common features include the following:

1. *Nasal, facial, or intraoral mass.* The intranasal mass is often necrotic, but polypoid mucosa may obscure underlying tumor tissue in the nose. Facial swelling results when an antral tumor erodes into the soft tissues of the cheek. The widening of the upper alveolar ridge or development of loose, nonvital teeth may be the earliest sign of inferior bony invasion. A palatal mass and ulceration are evidence of more advanced disease.
2. *Proptosis.* Mild protrusion of the eye may be consistent with tumor compression of the periorbita without frank invasion, but usually it reflects intraorbital tumor and implies advanced disease.
3. *Cranial nerve deficits.* The commonly involved cranial nerves are the CN II, CN III, CN IV, two branches of CN V (CN V1 and CN V2), and CN VI. Involvement of cranial nerves is a manifestation of advanced disease and indicates a poor prognosis.[29,65]

DIAGNOSTIC ASSESSMENT

The choice of diagnostic studies should be guided by the results of a thorough head and neck examination, including a careful assessment of cranial nerve function. Assuming a working diagnosis of neoplasm based on the history and physical examination, the subsequent studies are directed toward establishing the extent of the lesion and its histology.

Imaging studies

Computed tomography scan

When obvious evidence of neoplasm exists, the evaluation should move directly to computed tomography (CT) scanning. Baseline sinus radiographs are an unnecessary expense in this setting, whereas the CT scan is helpful to achieve a three-dimensional image of the lesion. Jing, Goepfert, and Close[25] have stated that CT is equal to tomography for assessment of bony involvement but superior for assessment of the soft tissue extension. Standard coronal tomography, however, has a place. CT "has been found to have limitations in the delineation of soft tissue disease in areas of high contrast in tissue density (such as dental fillings) and in the evaluation of possible intracranial tumor extension in isodense, avascular lesions."[25] CT scanning may also be misleading in evaluation of the orbital floor, where an axial CT scan may give the impression of a mass because of "partial voluming" of the thin bone.[40] CT scanning is particularly helpful for evaluation of tumor involvement of the retroorbital and orbital apex region. There should be a "central low density region of fat surrounding the optic nerve with a radial arrangement of the extraocular muscles."[40] Loss of this plane implies advanced disease because the veins in this area have direct contact with the cavernous sinus. CT scanning is also valuable in assessing infiltration of the nasopharynx, where normal anatomy consists of a very thin layer of mucosa over the medial pterygoid plate. Thickening in this region implies tumor infiltration.[40] When evaluation of intracranial extension is necessary, contrast-enhanced CT scanning may improve the definition of tumor from adjacent brain.[56]

Angiography

Angiography may be appropriate, especially if the lesion demonstrates enhancement during initial CT study or if it approximates the carotid system. It will also be necessary in the evaluation of unusual tumors involving the sphenoid sinus and skull base. In the instance of vascular tumors involving the sinuses, angiography is essential for assessment of tumor extent and delineation of feeding vessels and as an approach for embolization when it is deemed necessary and safe.[46] Digital-enhancement angiography would seem to be preferable to conventional angiography because it is more rapidly performed with less need for selective catheterization and requires smaller amounts of contrast.[56]

Ultrasound

Ultrasound B-mode scanning is helpful in assessing orbital masses but is not as precise as CT scanning in defining the borders and extent of lesions.

Magnetic resonance imaging

The impact of magnetic resonance imaging (MRI) on the preoperative assessment of tumor extent has been dramatic. The combination of CT scan to evaluate changes in the bony architecture of the cranial and facial structures with MRI to define soft tissue extent of disease has introduced a new era in planning surgery for sinus neoplasms. The particular benefit of MRI is its ability to differentiate tissue density and predict with near-perfect accuracy the difference between tumor bulk and retained secretions in the sinuses. By using T1 and T2 weighting with gadolinium dye enhancement, the experienced neuroradiologist is able to predict with considerable accuracy the true extent of the tumor. It has been our experience that surgical planning based on these two modalities has been very satisfactory.

Biopsy

Often the lesion will present a surface that lends itself to biopsy at the time of initial clinical presentation. In this instance a biopsy specimen obtained using local anesthesia and a biting punch forceps will move the diagnostic evaluation along rapidly. Infiltration of a local anesthetic containing epinephrine may decrease bleeding. Tumors contained within the sinus cavities should be biopsied transnasally because transcutaneous or transmucosal approaches may breach the margins of a later *en bloc* resection. One must be mindful of the possibility of a vascular tumor or an encephalocele when biopsying unilateral nasal masses. Usually palpation of the tumor with an instrument will demonstrate its solid nature. If the mass is soft or cystic, the patient should be asked to perform a Valsalva maneuver while the mass is being observed. Expansion of the mass implies an intracranial connection or a major venous connection. If doubt still exists, it is best to precede the biopsy with aspiration using a fine-gauge spinal needle. If the needle aspirate returns cerebrospinal fluid (CSF) or active bleeding, CT scanning and angiography should be considered before a biopsy is performed.

Aspiration cytology provides another avenue for diagnosis. Martin[41] recommended it for deep tumors of the antrum. It is particularly useful for tumors that cause proptosis and present along the medial aspect of the orbit. Because the diagnosis in this setting includes benign lesions such as an orbital pseudotumor, histologic evaluation before surgical invasion is most appropriate. When concern for damage of the orbital contents exists, the aspiration needle can be positioned using CT guidance.

If none of the preceding methods achieves satisfactory material for histologic examination, the tumor must be approached directly. A surgical procedure appropriate to the lesion must be selected (such as frontal trephination, transseptal sphenoidotomy, intranasal antrostomy, or external ethmoidectomy). The operation should be designed to avoid or minimize disruption of later *en bloc* resection. Possibly, biopsy will be the only surgical procedure carried out during the patient's treatment. In that case wide drainage of the sinus should be carried out to allow for the discharge of necrotic debris that results from subsequent radiotherapy.

SURGICAL OPTIONS

Extirpation of paranasal sinus tumors is a challenging exercise in surgical planning, which may be considered in three phases. First, one must assess the bony and soft tissue structures to be included for *en bloc* resection. Second, the approach must be designed to provide adequate exposure while preserving functional tissue and cosmetic integrity whenever possible. Third, the repair should be planned to use prosthetics or soft tissue techniques to best advantage. See Figure 59-2 for anatomic reference.

External ethmoidectomy

Indications

The most limited operation to be discussed, external ethmoidectomy (Fig. 59-3), is appropriate for removal of benign tumors of the ethmoidal region and as an approach to biopsy and drainage for tumors of the sphenoethmoidal region and the medial orbit.

Bony excision

The limits of bony resection include the medial orbital wall and the ethmoidal labyrinth.

Surgical approach

The surgical approach is through an incision on the lateral wall of the nose.

Benefits

The external ethmoidectomy approach allows excellent cosmesis and preservation of functional tissue.

Limitations

External ethmoidectomy will not provide *en bloc* excision for any but the most limited tumors (middle turbinate). Typical of any lateral nasal incision, there is a tendency to form a fistula to the nasal cavity when this area is irradiated.

Inferior medial maxillectomy

Indications

Inferior medial maxillectomy (Fig. 59-4) is designed for resection of the medial wall of the antrum and the inferior turbinate. It is most often used for management of an inverted papilloma.

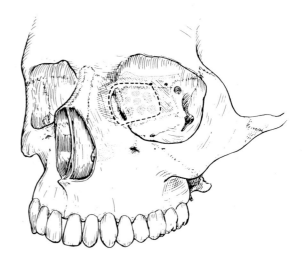

Fig. 59-3. External ethmoidectomy.

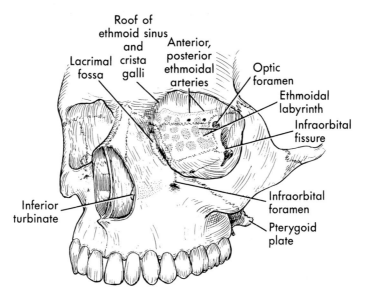

Fig. 59-2. Anatomic reference.

Bony excision

The margins extend laterally to a vertical line dropped from the infraorbital foramen, inferiorly to the floor of the nose, superiorly to the lacrimal fossa and the middle meatus, and posteriorly to the dorsal end of the inferior turbinate.

Surgical approach

A lateral rhinotomy incision is frequently used in an inferior maxillectomy. The same bony excision may be achieved through a sublabial approach, although an *en bloc* resection may be more difficult with this approach.[8]

Benefits

Inferior medial maxillectomy allows adequate exposure and resection for limited tumors while preserving functional tissue and providing a very acceptable cosmetic result.

Limitations

Inferior medial maxillectomy provides *en bloc* removal of a limited area. When an inverted papilloma is being removed, careful monitoring using a frozen section is often necessary, especially at the posterior margin.

Medial maxillectomy

Indications

Medial maxillectomy (Fig. 59-5) may be used for larger benign or intermediate tumors involving the entire lateral nasal wall but without extension to the orbit, anterior cranial fossa, lateral maxilla, or alveolus.

Bony excision

The block removed contains the lateral nasal wall, including all turbinate tissue, and the contents of the ethmoid and maxillary sinuses.

Surgical approach

An extended lateral rhinotomy incision provides excellent exposure. In some instances the same procedure may be accomplished by combining an ethmoidectomy incision with a sublabial incision.

Benefits

An *en bloc* resection may be accomplished with little cosmetic deformity resulting. Epiphora is not uncommon postoperatively as a result of division of the nasolacrimal duct.

Limitations

The posterior and superior margins of resection should be monitored using a frozen section where indicated. Removal of all turbinate tissue results in an abnormal nasal cavity, often requiring chronic management of crusting.

Radical maxillectomy

Indications

Radical maxillectomy (Fig. 59-6) is the standard operation for advanced carcinoma of the maxilla. Considerable debate exists regarding the proper application of this procedure because amount of tissue to be removed depends on a careful assessment of the extent of tumor involvement.[54,62] Another uncertainty relates to the establishment of proper indications for removal of the orbital contents in combination with radical maxillectomy.

Bony excision

Complete radical maxillectomy includes removal of the maxilla along with the nasal bone, the ethmoid sinus, and in some instances, the pterygoid plates.

Surgical approach

The Weber-Fergusson incision is used with extensions around the eyelids to preserve those soft tissues. A skin or

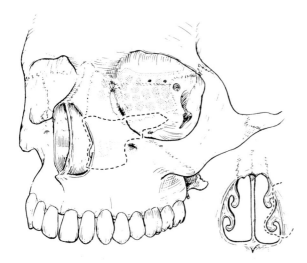

Fig. 59-4. Inferior medial maxillectomy.

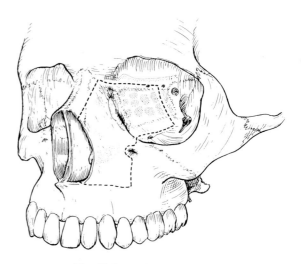

Fig. 59-5. Medial maxillectomy.

dermis graft is used to line the defect.[7] A preformed obturator can be of great assistance in the immediate postoperative period by acting as a support for packing.

Benefits

Radical maxillectomy is adequate treatment for malignant tumors confined to the maxilla and those with extension to the facial soft tissues, palate, or anterior orbit but without invasion of the ethmoidal roof, posterior orbit, or pterygoid region. When the procedure is supplemented by irradiation, one may expect a cure rate approximating 30%.[23,59,64] There is, however, continuing debate regarding the indications for resecting the orbital contents in patients with advanced paranasal sinus carcinoma. As indicated by Ketchan and Van Buren,[30] the decision to excise the orbital contents has been made on the basis of achieving an *en bloc* resection of the tumor. However, Ketcham implied that as imaging became more precise more selective resection might be possible. Perry and others[49] emphasized the impact of CT scanning on surgical planning and documented that selective preservation of the orbital contents is appropriate and achieves adequate local control in properly selected cases. This finding is consistent with the experience of Weymuller, Reardon, and Nash[66] who also could not demonstrate an improved local control rate or survival advantage when the orbital contents were included in maxillectomy procedures. This position is further supported by the experience of Larson[36] and Perry.[48]

Limitations

Even when orbital exenteration is included, a maxillectomy fails to provide an adequate resection when the tumor has escaped superiorly (ethmoidal roof) or posteriorly (orbital apex, pterygoid region). When these areas are demonstrably involved, one must decide whether to undertake craniofacial resection or use a regimen as described by Sakai and others[54] which relies on chemotherapy, curettage, and irradiation.

Craniofacial frontoethmoidectomy

Indications

Craniofacial frontoethmoidectomy (Fig. 59-7) is specifically designed to provide *en bloc* resection for tumors of the ethmoidal and frontal regions. By including exposure of the anterior cranial fossa, the procedure makes possible complete resection of the ethmoid and frontal sinuses, and dural resection may be included when necessary.

Bony excision

Resection may include the anterior cranium (including the frontal sinus), the floor of the anterior cranial fossa, the ethmoid labyrinth (and the eye when necessary), and the nasal septum. If the tumor crosses the midline, the procedure may be performed bilaterally.

Surgical approach

The craniofacial frontoethmoidectomy approach described by Johns and others[26] allows excellent exposure with preservation of the supraorbital rim to decrease the cosmetic impact of the surgery. Although removal of the eye is unpleasant to consider, Ketcham and others[29] have documented an improved survival when orbital resection is combined with craniofacial resection (57% versus 26% without exenteration).

Benefits

Craniofacial exposure provides direct visualization of the cribriform plate and the fovea ethmoidalis and the potential for *en bloc* removal. It also provides wide exposure to allow effective repair of dural tears, thus decreasing the chance of a postoperative CSF leak and intracranial infection. In

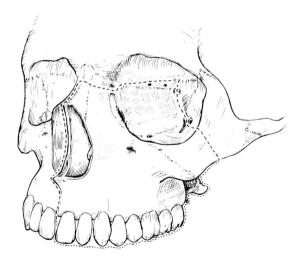

Fig. 59-6. Radial maxillectomy.

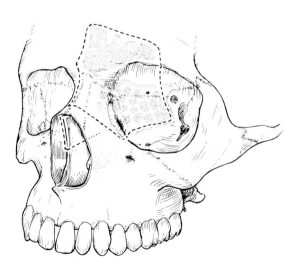

Fig. 59-7. Craniofacial frontoethmoidectomy.

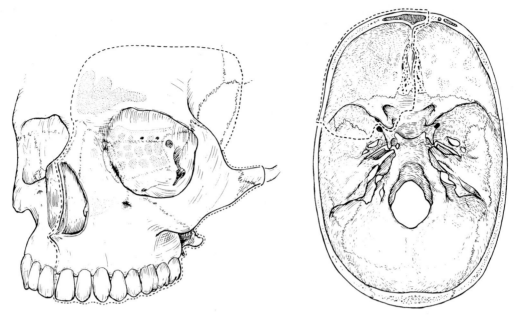

Fig. 59-8. Craniofacial resection.

addition, the exposure afforded would allow intraoperative irradiation or placement of a radioactive implant.

Limitations

If the tumor extends to the sphenoid sinus, the cavernous sinus, or transdurally, *en bloc* resection cannot be achieved.

Extended craniofacial resection

Indications

There is no one definitive extended craniofacial resection to be described (Fig. 59-8). Extensive tumors involving the anterior skull base, including certain tumors with involvement of the pterygoid plates, can be surgically approached, with the resection to include any and all of the structures outlined below. Each operation is individually tailored according to the extent and nature of the tumor to be excised.[24,60]

Bony margins

The posterior line of resection is defined by the oval foramen, the round foramen, and the internal carotid artery. The excision may extend through the sphenoid sinus and up to the contralateral optic nerve. The remaining margins are those of the craniofacial frontoethmoidectomy and the radical maxillectomy.

Surgical approach

A team including a neurosurgeon and an otolaryngologist should perform the extended craniofacial resection. A combination of bicoronal and anterior or lateral facial incisions is used for exposure. The closure is improved by including a split-galea flap to cover the dura.[55]

Benefits

Thorough exposure and complete excision of otherwise unresectable tumors are the main benefits of extended craniofacial resection.

Limitations

In discussing the limitations of the craniofacial approach Ketcham and others[29] have cited clear-cut pterygoid plate erosion and cranial nerve invasion as indicators of inoperability. Even though this operation has extended the limit of surgical resection and in so doing has resulted in numerous cures, it still must be accepted that it does not provide adequate *en bloc* resection for tumor at the orbit apex, in the nasopharynx, or deeply infiltrating the pterygoid space.

Supplemental management in extended craniofacial resection

The boundary between resectability and unresectability for advanced skull base malignancy is ill defined. For reasons of palliation or for attempted cure, it is not uncommon for extended craniofacial resection to be performed for the resection of all grossly resectable tumors, understanding that at the most central margins of the resection there is a high probability of residual microscopic disease. In this setting, consideration of supplemental therapy is appropriate and has a modest track record of success. In particular, using the surgical exposure as an opportunity to deliver localized supplemental radiation is now a well-accepted technique. Intraoperative radiotherapy of the skull base has been documented as a technique to improve local control rates.[15,51]

At the University of Washington, the institutional experience with intraoperative iodine seed implantation has been recently reviewed. Local regional control appears acceptable for tumors with a predictably long time-frame with respect to distant metastases (such as adenoid cystic carcinoma). For patients with undifferentiated carcinoma and squamous cell carcinoma, the anticipated benefit for long-term survival is less optimistic. Additionally, the institutional experience has highlighted the risk of intracranial infection when seed implantation is used after previous radiation. For this reason, our current posture is that whenever radioactive seeds are used as a supplement to previous radiation, the skull base should be reconstructed with free tissue transfer to establish a highly vascularized and relatively thick separation between the airway and the intracranial contents.[53] Support for this technique also is reflected in the publication by Vikram.[63]

BENIGN NEOPLASMS

Osteomas and chondromas

Osteomas are most commonly found in the frontal sinus; the ethmoid sinus and maxilla follow, in that order. When located away from the sinus osteum, an osteoma is silent and only discovered incidentally during radiographic examination. In this instance it should be followed with an interval radiograph in 1 to 2 years to assess growth. Osteomas are formed of mature lamellar bone and cause symptoms only when they interfere with sinus drainage or possibly when they impinge on the dura. When the osteoma causes a mucocele, obliterative surgery or wide drainage is recommended (osteoplastic frontal sinus obliteration or external ethmoidectomy).

Chondromas may develop anywhere in the sinonasal tract. Batsakis[2] has emphasized the tendency to underestimate the aggressive nature of these neoplasms. According to him, the histologic differentiation between benign and malignant tumors is "incompletely defined." Because of this histologic uncertainty, resection should be more aggressive than with an osteoma and consideration should be given to "fairly radical treatment."

Schwannomas and neurofibromas

Schwannomas and neurofibromas are indolent tumors arising from peripheral nerve components. A schwannoma is an isolated encapsulated lesion, whereas a neurofibroma is woven into the nerve and is often one of multiple lesions. The tumors cause symptoms by slow progressive growth that may distort tissues by pressure or become symptomatic by obstruction of a sinus osteum. During evaluation a contrast-enhanced CT scan may be performed. Neuromas and neurilemomas demonstrate a characteristic irregular patchy appearance.[40] These lesions are managed by conservative local resection. One should recall that malignant transformation occurs in about one of eight patients with multiple neurofibromatosis (von Recklinghausen's disease).[22]

Ossifying fibromas and cementomas

Although somewhat difficult to differentiate histologically from fibrous dysplasia, ossifying fibromas may be diagnosed by including clinical and radiographic criteria. They occur in an older age group, primarily young adults, and are typified radiographically by a sclerotic bony margin that is evident at surgical resection, when the lesion often "shells out" easily.[22]

Cementomas are described as a variant of ossifying fibromas with a "cementum-like osseous element." These, too, are appropriately managed by local excision, but if any tumor is left, a recurrence is likely.

Odontogenic tumors

Odontogenic tumors are a rare group, accounting for only 1% of all jaw tumors, includes ameloblastoma and the calcifying epithelial tumor of Pindborg.[43] They are locally aggressive, requiring resection with a small margin of normal tissue to prevent recurrence.[22] The vast majority of odontomas are better characterized as hamartomas, emphasizing their benign nature and their evolution from a developmental abnormality in odontogenic material.[43]

INTERMEDIATE NEOPLASMS

Inverted papillomas

Inverted papillomas usually present as polypoid unilateral nasal masses. On occasion they may be found in association with allergic nasal polyps, which accounts for the need to always submit labeled, separate specimens from each side of the nose when performing routine polypectomy. The histology consists of infolded epithelium that may be squamous, transitional, or respiratory. The incidence of frank malignant change approximates 10%.[20,21]

Even when not malignant, these lesions must be treated with respect, because inadequate excision is likely to result in recurrence.[9] A lateral rhinotomy incision combined with medial maxillectomy to allow adequate margins is the classic approach. Recent experience with endoscopic sinus surgery has initiated a new concept. In carefully selected cases inverting papilloma may be removed endoscopically.[44]

Meningiomas

Extracranial meningiomas, which arise from ectopic arachnoid tissue, are very rare tumors. They have a variable histology and may require electron microscopy for identification.[39] Occasionally an intracranial meningioma will invade the sinuses or orbit. In this setting plain skull films may reveal hyperostosis of the ethmoidal region. Further evaluation should consider CT scanning and angiography or MRI.[56] Surgical excision is the only form of definitive management, although radiotherapy may be effectively used to "stabilize" inoperable lesions.

Hemangiomas

On rare occasions a primary hemangioma will occur in the maxilla. Hyams[22] has emphasized the possibility of an erroneous diagnosis when a pyogenic granuloma is mistaken for a true hemangioma. More frequently, the maxilla will become involved with a soft tissue hemangioma of the face or a vascular malformation of the skull. Hemangiomas are typified by rarefaction on radiographs, although they may become sclerotic as they mature. The lesions are typically asymptomatic, and extirpation is indicated only for bleeding or major discomfort. When resection is necessary, it should be preceded by angiography, and selective embolization should be seriously considered as an adjunct to surgical resection.[4]

Hemangiopericytomas

Hemangiopericytomas typically occur in the nose but may involve the sinuses. According to Batsakis,[2] "If there is one common denominator for hemangiopericytomas, it is the lack of uniformity in appearance, growth and biological behavior." Clinical behavior may vary considerably from a slowly enlarging rubbery mass to an infiltrating aggressive neoplasm. It is Batsakis' opinion that these tumors are locally aggressive and must be respected as tumors that are likely to recur and that are associated with delayed recurrence, making 5-year survival an inadequate measure of cure.

MALIGNANT NEOPLASMS

Epidemiology

Numerous environmental agents are considered to have a causal relationship with carcinomas of the paranasal sinuses. The following are all associated with squamous cell carcinomas: aflatoxin found in certain foods and dust; chromium, nickel, mustard gas, polycyclic hydrocarbons, and other organic chemicals, usually from manufacturing processes; and mesothorium (Thorotrast), a radiopaque dye used as a contrast medium within the antrum.[28] Wood dust has a particular association with adenocarcinoma of the ethmoid sinus.[32]

Most series document squamous cell carcinomas to be the most common histologic type, with an incidence of roughly 80%. Adenoid cystic carcinomas and adenocarcinomas are next in frequency (approximately 10%). Numerous other tumors complete the list in small numbers.

Epithelial malignancy

Staging

Staging is appropriately discussed only in the context of carcinomatous tumors because the other lesions are so uncommon that they do not warrant such attention (or such confusion). As Harrison[18] has suggested, the staging system should allow differentiation between distinct stages of disease progression. Unfortunately, most of these tumors present with such advanced disease that the subtle differences

between cases may not be relevant to clinical management or prognosis. Therefore, "one must conclude that attempts at classifying this tumor finitely are both impractical and unrealistic."[18]

Ohngren[45] emphasized the ominous importance of tumor spread in a posterior or superior direction. The imaginary line extending from the medial canthus to the angle of the jaw gives a rough estimate of the dividing line between tumors that may be resected with a good or poor prognosis. He developed a staging system based on personal experience that included topography (tumor location and extent), histology (three grades), and cervical metastases (presence or absence). That the system was effective is borne out by his statistics, which clearly show a difference in 3-year "freedom from symptoms" between groups I (82%), II (63%), and III (25%).

Other systems have been proposed by experienced surgeons. Each represents a personal variation of the generally accepted schemes, but they differ from one another sufficiently to make direct comparison of results impossible, thus negating one of the primary goals of any staging system. The interested reader is referred to Harrison's[18] article for further discussion and references.

In the United States we are probably best served by consistently using the format outlined by the American Joint Committee on Cancer (AJCC) (Box 59-1), although an adjustment based on Harrison's[18] criticism should be seriously considered. In particular, orbital apex involvement and pterygoid muscle involvement should be placed in the T_4 category. It also appears that Ohngren's[45] inclusion of tumor differentiation may be relevant to the staging of these tumors. That this may be a reasonable contention is borne out by Wang's[64] statistics regarding 3-year survival according to cell type: squamous cell, 34% (15 of 44 patients); undifferentiated carcinoma, 29% (4 of 14 patients); transitional cell carcinoma, 40% (2 of 5 patients); and carcinoma with inverted papilloma, 75% (3 of 4 patients). However, Shidnia

---

Box 59-1. Staging criteria: primary tumor (T)

T_x Minimum requirements to assess primary tumor cannot be met

T_0 No evidence of primary tumor

TIS   Carcinoma *in situ*

T_1 Tumor confined to antral mucosa of infrastructure with no bone erosion or destruction

T_2 Tumor confined to suprastructure mucosa without bone destruction, or to infrastructure with destruction of medial or inferior bony walls only

T_3 More extensive tumor invading skin of cheek, orbit, anterior ethmoid sinus, or pterygoid muscle

T_4 Massive tumor with invasion of cribriform plate, posterior ethmoid sinus, sphenoid sinus, nasopharynx, pterygoid plate, or base of skull

and others[58] could not confirm a relationship between histology and survival.

The advent of combined CT and MRI scanning for neoplasms of the paranasal sinuses will allow far more accurate anatomic assessment of individual cases. This improved definition of the tumor boundaries should also allow more precise staging. It is the author's contention that MRI and CT scanning should be required for staging of these neoplasms.

Management

Definitive treatment has included surgery, irradiation, and electrocoagulation in varying combinations. It does not seem that substantial improvements have been achieved in the past 50 years if Ohngren's[45] 3-year statistics are used as a standard of comparison (group I, 82%; group II, 63%; and group III, 25%). More recently, adjunctive chemotherapy has been introduced, but its impact on outcome is still uncertain.

Maxillary sinus. Early (T_1 and T_2) lesions may be treated by surgical resection (maxillectomy) or irradiation. Although Wang[64] has not recommended definitive irradiation, he has reported curing 4 of 4 patients with T_2 maxillary sinus tumors with that modality alone. Bryce[7] has also stated that irradiation alone (5500 rad) is an effective way to manage early tumors, but that 25% to 30% of patients will die of local recurrence.

The majority of patients have advanced (T_3 or T_4) disease when first seen, which most authors agree requires combined therapy for optimal control.[7,54,58,64] Considerable variation exists within each reporting institution regarding the application of surgery and irradiation. All series are retrospective and present a mixture of patient populations, usually receiving the following types of management: surgery for cure, surgery with preoperative or postoperative irradiation, and irradiation with surgical salvage. This hodgepodge of retrospective data leaves one in a muddle, although some trends are becoming apparent.

Surgery alone. Surgery alone is generally accepted as adequate management for tumors isolated to the antral mucosa.[23] As stated previously, most authors agree that T_3 and T_4 lesions require combined therapy. Terz, Young, and Lawrence have taken a more aggressive surgical posture and reported dramatic improvement in survival for patients with T_3 and T_4 lesions when craniofacial resection was performed. According to these authors, craniofacial resection achieved an astonishing 3-year disease-free survival of 72% (15 of 22 patients) among patients who had T_3 or T_4 tumors. The numbers are even more surprising when one realizes that irradiation was not used. However, reporting separately on patients from the same institution and the same time period as that of Terz, Young, and Lawrence,[62] Amendola and others[1] compared the outcome of 19 patients who underwent ''radical craniofacial surgery'' with that of 20 patients treated with megavoltage irradiation and a Caldwell-Luc procedure. Their reported 3-year survival of the group undergoing radical craniofacial surgery was 37%, whereas

the irradiated group had a 3-year survival of 50%. Were the surgical patients reported on by Terz, Young, and Lawrence[62] identical to those reported on by Amendola and others? If so, how do we resolve the dichotomy of reporting, and in what light should we hold any retrospective report concerning an uncommon disorder that is typically managed on an individual basis?

Surgical management should include consideration of immediate rehabilitation. This is usually best achieved with prosthetics that allow immediate restoration of function and yet are removable to allow inspection of the maxillary cavity. Preformed palatal plates may be used to support transoral packing in the postoperative period and may later be modified to occlude the oronasal defect. If one is blessed with a talented prosthetics department, the aftermath of a craniofacial-orbital resection can be reasonably well camouflaged.

Traditionally reconstruction of maxillary sinus defects has been with skin graft and prosthetics. With the advent of free tissue transfer, far more acceptable cosmetic reconstruction including rehabilitation of the bony hard palate for dental rehabilitation is now achievable. In the coming decade, evaluation of the feasibility and appropriateness of this technique will be assessed. Clearly one of the major potential risks is ''covering recurrent disease,'' however since disease recurrence at this site, whether observed or not observed, is essentially untreatable, this may be a moot point.

Combined irradiation and surgery. With T_3 tumors little difference exists between preoperative and postoperative irradiation. Postoperative irradiation will often control microscopically positive resection margins.[58] With the more advanced lesions, especially those where resectability is questionable, preoperative irradiation appears to be the procedure of choice.

A planned preoperative dose of 5500 rad is used in Toronto, followed by radical resection.[7] If no tumor is found, a 5-year survival of 77% occurs; if tumor is found, the survival drops to 23%; overall survival is 50%. Shidnia and others[58] have also noted the favorable effects of a tumor-free specimen. Their group of patients receiving irradiation followed by surgery had an absolute 30-month survival of 28% (9 of 30 patients), whereas their group of patients receiving surgery followed by irradiation had a survival of 45% (11 of 24 patients). Shidnia and others[58] have suggested that the latter group was selected for more favorable lesions because the study was not designed in a prospective manner. For operable lesions (meaning those not extending to the nasopharynx, skull base, or pterygoid fossa), Wang[64] favors radical surgery to remove tumor bulk and establish drainage followed by 5000 to 5500 rad in 6 weeks.

The most emotionally charged decision regarding the management of advanced maxillary sinus tumors is the need for orbital exenteration. The experience of Ketcham and others,[30] which indicates a doubling of survival with removal of the orbital contents for the management of ethmoid neoplasms (57% versus 26%), provides strong encouragement to perform orbital exenteration for advanced operable disease. However, analysis of the benefits of orbital exenteration in two other studies leaves this issue open to question.[49,66]

Radiotherapy. Wang[64] takes special care to shield the eye and the frontal lobe. He has reported a 24% no evidence of disease (NED) for his 34 patients treated with irradiation alone. In contrast, Ellingwood and Million[13] have intentionally included the orbit to include the probable routes of tumor extension within the irradiation field. Their cure rate of 71% suggests a successful regimen. However, all patients treated with this regimen lost vision in the treated eye. Amendola and others[1] have also documented a 3-year absolute survival of 55% using an average of 6600 rad for lesions that were primarily T_4. Then fields were angled posteriorly to avoid the contralateral eye. No complications of irradiation are mentioned in this article, and the authors stress the improved quality of life when irradiation for cure is contrasted with craniofacial resection.

Perhaps the most significant variation from traditional management has been reported by Sakai and others.[54] They have accumulated more than 780 patients since 1957 at Kobe and Osaka Universities in Japan. Their cumulative experience demonstrates impressive support for their current regimen, which consists of 5000 rad, continuous intraarterial 5-fluorouracil (5-FU) infusion, tumor reduction (via the Caldwell-Luc procedure), and immunotherapy. In the reported time period they have seen an increase in 5-year survival from 20% (282 patients treated with 7000 rad and maxillectomy, 1957-1966) to 54% (134 patients treated with the current regimen, 1976-1979). They have simultaneously seen a substantial decrease in the functional disability encountered by their patients. An analogous regimen has been reported from Rotterdam, Holland, with similarly encouraging results in a series of 60 patients (2-year survival, 76%; 5-year survival, 65%).[33]

Inoperable neoplasms. Irradiation may be used to determine operability in tumors that initially appear inoperable. In this situation Wang[64] delivered 6000 rad in 6 weeks, with surgery to follow. He encouraged aggressive surgery if the response to irradiation appeared to make the lesion operable. If margins were subsequently positive, a further boost of local irradiation was considered. Interestingly, Wang had better results with this more advanced group (survival of 58% or 11 of 19 patients) than he did with smaller lesions, in which he favored surgery to be followed by irradiation (survival of 36%, or 5 of 14 patients). The rationale for treating patients with ''curative'' doses of irradiation when their lesions are initially inoperable is borne out by the number of long-term survivors seen in this group of patients.[58,64] This result is probably a manifestation of the heterogeneous nature of the inoperable patients; some are inoperable by virtue of tumor extent, whereas others are medically unsuitable or have refused surgery outright.

Lee and others[38] have documented the potential value of intraarterial infusion chemotherapy (5-FU) and simultaneous irradiation for initially inoperable tumors. They achieved an absolute 2-year survival of 50% in this group with a very poor prognosis. Survival dropped to 28% at 5 years. Unfortunately, optic nerve damage was fairly prevalent and caused bilateral blindness on two occasions. Subsequent to this study Goepfert and others proceeded to develop a technique for ''combined super-selective interarterial and systemic chemotherapy.'' They have reported a 43% complete response rate and a combined complete and partial response rate of 91%. A number of these patients went on to receive radiotherapy and ''extensive cranial facial surgery was avoided in seven of nine patients with CR and one patient with PR (near CR); these eight patients underwent radiotherapy directly after completion of induction chemotherapy.''[38] The utilization of selective chemotherapy and irradiation for advanced tumors of this area has tremendous appeal when contrasted to the horrendous defects created by surgical ablation of lesions in the axial region of the skull. It is hoped that follow-up information on these patients will reveal a sustained result leading to a change in our management.

Ethmoid/sphenoid and frontal sinuses. Ethmoid/sphenoid and frontal sinus tumors are especially likely to present with evidence of advanced disease. Tumor extension to the structures of the skull base can be expected at initial presentation in 50% of patients.[13,31]

Assessment and management of ethmoidal carcinoma should be performed with a specific staging system in mind. The Kadish system[27] is familiar but has some limitations. The author currently favors the four-stage system introduced by Dulgerov and Calcaterra: T_1—tumor involving the nasal cavity or paranasal sinuses (excluding sphenoid), sparing the most superior ethmoidal cells; T_2—tumor involving the nasal cavity or paranasal sinuses (including sphenoid), with extension to or erosion of the cribriform plate; T_3—tumor extending into the orbit or protruding into the anterior cranial fossa; T_4—tumor involving the brain (through dura).[12] Management for esthesioneuroblastoma and adenocarcinoma is generally similar, and based on craniofacial resection and postoperative radiation when surgically feasible. The addition of chemotherapy to the management of advanced esthesioneuroblastoma (T_3 and T_4) is now well established, particularly in light of the experience of Spaulding and others at the University of Virginia.[61]

The argument for craniofacial resection in patients with malignancy extending to or primarily arising from the ethmoid sinus has been presented by Ketcham and others.[29] *En bloc* tumor resection, improved assessment of disease extent, and better cosmesis provide the rationale for applying this technique. The researchers obtained a 5-year survival of 41% in a particularly difficult group of patients, many of whom were referred with advanced disease after failure of previous treatment. Ketcham and others noted a decrease in survival with preservation of the orbital contents (26%) as compared with orbital resection (57%). Further documentation of the techniques and applicability of cranial facial resection and its significant impact on improved local control and survival is provided by Shah,[57] Biller, Krespi, and Som[4] and Panje and others.[47]

Ellingwood and Million[13] have stressed the importance of properly designed fields to include the whole orbit (when necessary) and skull base. Using primary irradiation, they achieved a 5-year actuarial survival of 59% and a 5-year NED of 50%. The incidence of major complications in this series was substantial and included blindness in every eye treated with irradiation of the whole orbit.

In Wang's[64] series, 4 of 12 patients (33%) managed with irradiation alone survived 3 years, whereas 8 of 17 patients (47%) managed with surgery and postoperative irradiation survived 3 years NED.

Primary carcinoma of the frontal sinus is a very uncommon entity. According to a review article by Brownson and Ogura,[6] the survival is 1 of 33 patients. One would anticipate improvement of these statistics as craniofacial resection and appropriately designed irradiation fields are used.

Cervical lymph nodes. Involvement of cervical nodes will occur in about 25% to 35% of cases.[2] Most authors agree that palpable cervical lymph nodes indicate a very poor prognosis.[66] In contrast, the experience of Shidnia and others[58] suggests that if neck disease is discovered at an early stage, it can be successfully managed with neck dissection. These authors advise inclusion of the ipsilateral neck and preauricular area in the initial field of irradiation for T_3 and T_4 tumors.

Adenocarcinomas. Adenocarcinomas have an epidemiologic association with woodworking, furniture making, and leatherwork.[32] They are more commonly found in the upper nasal cavity and ethmoid sinus and are usually lethal by virtue of local progression. In light of its propensity for aggressive local progression, adenocarcinoma should be treated in a surgically aggressive fashion with *en bloc* resection when possible. It is hoped that statistics for this particular disorder will improve as application of craniofacial techniques becomes more frequent.

In contrast to adenoid cystic carcinomas, adenocarcinomas have a relatively low incidence of distant metastasis, but the long-range survival is equally poor.[2] There is a range of histologic differentiation, with patients with the poorly differentiated form having a 5-year survival of no better than 20%,[22] whereas patients with well-differentiated papillary tumors have a better survival.[2]

Adenoid cystic carcinomas. Adenoid cystic carcinomas occur with about the same frequency as adenocarcinomas but most commonly involve the antrum. They have a variable histologic pattern, and substantial biopsy tissue may be necessary before an accurate diagnosis can be established. Also part of the histologic picture is their propensity for invasion along nerve sheath structures. These tumors are more likely to express distant metastases than regional metastasis, although the most likely cause of death is relentless local neoplasm at the skull base.[2] Initially high cure rates (5-year survival of 75%) shrink as time goes on, with the AFIP Registry reporting a 15-year survival of 25%.[22]

Management relies on surgical resection with irradiation added if the margins are in question.[64] Bryce[7] has recommended using only one major modality (surgery or irradiation) at a time because the 5-year survival is good and late recurrence is virtually a certainty. This posture is based on a desire to hold a potentially effective treatment modality in reserve. One wonders whether this is treating the physician or the patient because we do not know if combined treatment decreases the recurrence rate or increases the disease-free interval. A contrasting opinion has been offered by Horree,[19] who has recommended "three-modality therapy," including regional infusion with 5-FU, maxillary resection, and then irradiation. Neoplasms representing the entire spectrum of salivary gland malignancy have been reported to occur in the paranasal sinuses but are not discussed here.

Analysis of experience gained in the few centers that provide neutron irradiation has demonstrated a significant benefit of that form of radiation in the management of salivary gland neoplasms. When confronted with an adenoid cystic carcinoma, and particularly one that is otherwise untreatable, the use of neutron beam irradiation should be seriously considered.[11,34]

Complications. The incidence of complications increases significantly when surgery breaches the intracranial space and also when high doses of irradiation are delivered to the orbit or intracranial contents.

Major complications of surgery are decreased by the use of perioperative antibiotics and by careful attention to dural closure including the use of pericranial flaps. The most significant complications include meningitis, brain abscess, CSF leak, and postoperative wound hemorrhage.

Cataracts are the most common complication of sinus irradiation.[7] Other radiation-induced lesions include osteoradionecrosis, keratitis, optic neuritis, and hypopituitarism. Injury to the optic nerve is made more likely with increased fraction size (250 rad/fraction) and total dose.[64] After high-dose irradiation, which includes the whole orbit, one can expect loss of vision in 100% of cases.[13]

Therapeutic decision making. Taking into consideration the data reviewed previously, some conclusions regarding therapy for advanced disease seem justifiable:

1. Most tumors are at an advanced stage when first recognized and require aggressive multimodality treatment.
2. Survival and local disease control are better when the orbit is included in the therapeutic plan (i.e., exenteration or irradiation).
3. A significant chance of metastasis to the primary (pharyngeal) and secondary (cervical) nodes exists. They should be included in the primary treatment plan.
4. Higher success rates have been reported with primary irradiation, and the associated functional and cosmetic

impairment seems to compare favorably with that of surgery.

5. The best regimen may prove to be a combination of chemotherapy, irradiation, and limited surgical débridement. This, of course, requires the availability of sophisticated equipment and a cooperative effort by a multidisciplinary team.

6. The concept of intraarterial chemotherapy for advanced skull base tumors was advocated by Lee and others[37] and should see continued consideration on the basis of the experience of Robbins and others,[52] who have pioneered the use of intraarterial cisplatinum with thiosulfate rescue and concomitant radiotherapy.

Sarcomas

Osteogenic sarcomas and chondrosarcomas of the facial skeleton are encountered more commonly in the mandible than in the maxilla. They are usually lethal by virtue of relentless local progression. In that light, the most successful therapy is based on wide *en bloc* resection, with 5-year survival being in the 10% to 20% range. Irradiation seems to be an effective adjuvant for both tumors. De Fries and Kornblut[10] have reported a survival of 30% with induction chemotherapy, preoperative irradiation, and widefield ablative surgery. The multiinstitutional analysis of outcome from neutron beam irradiation has identified facial sarcoma as an area in which significant improvement was identified. Neutron beam irradiation, when available, should be considered especially in the management of surgically unapproachable or unresectable lesions.[35]

Hyams[22] has characterized a well-differentiated and a poorly differentiated form of fibrosarcoma. One must consider the diagnosis of aggressive fibromatosis when evaluating a fibrous tumor in young adults.[67] All tumors in this group require *en bloc* excision for cure.[16]

Hematopoietic and lymphoid tumors

The paranasal sinuses are an uncommon primary site for lymphomatous tumors, but any of the multiple subtypes may occur. Because subtyping will determine both the therapy and the prognosis, the most important role of the otolaryngologist is to provide adequate tissue in good condition for histologic processing. If a lymphoma is suspected, the pathology department should be notified before the biopsy is done so that fresh specimens may be properly managed for subtyping.

Treatment is usually chemotherapy, although irradiation alone is adequate for stage I and stage II Hodgkin's disease.[64]

Malignant melanomas

Melanomas of the paranasal sinuses are usually advanced at the time of discovery. In addition to symptoms typical of sinus tumors, the patient may note a black nasal discharge and have a pigmented mass within the nose. Frequently regional or distant metastases exist at the time of initial examination. In the AFIP series,[22] the 5-year survival was 11% and the 20-year survival was 0.5%, with a mean survival of 2.3 years. Although radical surgical removal is the standard of care, it is obviously not very effective. Irradiation has been considered inadequate, but adjustments in fractionation may provide better results, as suggested by Berthelsen,[3] who found local control in three of six patients with nasal melanomas treated with primary irradiation.

PARANASAL SINUS NEOPLASMS IN CHILDREN

Sinus tumors in children are usually benign. The common nasal sinus tumors of children are polyps arising on an allergic basis or in association with cystic fibrosis. The most common true neoplasms are fibroosseous lesions and tumors of dental origin. Mucoceles and hemangiomas are less frequently encountered. The malignant tumors are predominantly embryonal rhabdomyosarcomas, although epithelial malignancies may occur.

Tumors should be assessed radiographically as discussed earlier, and the diagnosis should be established by a transnasal biopsy with a generous tissue sample submitted for pathologic study because special stains and electron microscopy may be necessary.

Tumors are usually managed surgically because (1) most lesions are radioinsensitive, (2) irradiation in excess of 3000 rad will have a substantial effect on growth of the facial skeleton, and (3) there is a significant risk of radiation-induced malignant transformation. Surgery should be designed to respect the developing tooth buds and facial growth centers in the palate, nose, and zygomatic process of the maxilla. The tendency is toward conservative local resection, especially with tumors of dental origin, but some lesions will require *en bloc* resection for a curative effort.

Monostotic fibrous dysplasia is a lesion considered to be a developmental defect of bone.[2,22] As such, it is most common in the pediatric age group and is more common in the maxilla than in the mandible. According to Schramm,[55] in contrast to most bony and odontogenic tumors, fibrous dysplasia sometimes requires wide local removal, including partial maxillectomy, to achieve clear margins. Resection causing a major functional or cosmetic deformity (orbital exenteration, mandibulectomy) is not often warranted.[50] Ossifying fibromas and cementomas, in contrast, are well delineated and may be managed by local excision with a minimal margin.

Rhabdomyosarcomas are the most common malignant neoplasm of the upper respiratory tract in the pediatric age group (age 15 or younger) in the AFIP records.[22] The tumor is aggressive, demonstrating rapid progression and dissemination. According to Hyams,[22] the histologic subcategories of juvenile rhabdomyosarcoma (alveolar, botryoid, and embryonal) have no relevance to the neoplasm's clinical behavior or the prognosis, whereas the Intergroup Rhabdomyosarcoma Study (IRS) had suggested an unfavorable prognosis for cytologic anaplasia or monomorphous round cell patterns.[42] The best survival is obtained with clear surgical margins supplemented by irradiation and chemotherapy.[14] The IRS has evaluated results from 157 nonorbital and 54 orbital rhabdomyosarcoma cases. They have found patients with parameningeal involvement (as indicated by CT evidence of skull base erosion or spinal fluid tests demonstrating pleocytosis as well as elevated protein and decreased glucose levels) to have a poor prognosis. This group of patients has been benefited by a treatment regimen combining intrathecal chemotherapy and craniospinal irradiation.

Patients with a circumscribed local tumor and no evidence of distant metastases have an excellent prognosis when treated with multidrug chemotherapy and adjuvant irradiation. In most instances radical ablative surgery is not considered necessary to achieve a successful outcome.[42]

REFERENCES

1. Amendola BE and others: Carcinoma of the maxillary antrum: surgery of radiotherapy? *Int J Radiat Oncol Biol Phys* 7:743, 1981.
2. Batsakis JG, editor: *Tumors of the head and neck*, ed 2, Baltimore. 1979, Williams & Wilkins.
3. Berthelsen A and others: Melanomas of the mucosa in the oral cavity and the upper respiratory passages, *Cancer* 54:907, 1984.
4. Biller HF, Krespi YP, Som PM: Combined therapy for vascular lesions of the head and neck with intra-arterial embolization and surgical excision, *Otolaryngol Head Neck Surg* 90:37, 1982.
5. Biller HF and others: Superior rhinotomy for en bloc resection of bilateral ethmoid tumors, *Arch Otolaryngol Head Neck Surg* 115:1463, 1989.
6. Brownson RJ, Ogura JH: Primary carcinoma of the frontal sinus, *Laryngoscope* 81:71, 1971.
7. Bryce DP: *Cancer of the antrum*. In Gates GA, editor: *Current therapy in otolaryngology—head and neck surgery 1984-1985*, Philadelphia, 1984, Mosby.
8. Conley J, Price JC: Sublabial approach to the nasal and nasopharyngeal cavities, *Am J Surg* 138:615, 1979.
9. Cummings CW, Goodman ML: Inverted papilloma of the nose and paranasal sinuses, *Arch Otolaryngol* 92:445, 1970.
10. de Fries HO, Kornblut AD: Malignant disease of the osseous adnexae: osteogenic sarcoma of the jaws, *Otolaryngol Clin North Am* 12:129, 1979.
11. Douglas JG and others: *Neutron radiotherapy for adenoid cystic carcinoma of minor salivary glands*. Abstract presented at 37th Annual American Society for Therapeutic Radiation Oncology Meeting, 1995. *Int J Radiat Oncol Biol Phys* 36:87, 1996.
12. Dulguerov P, Calcaterra T: Esthesioneuroblastoma: the UCLA experience 1970-1990, *Laryngoscope* 102(8):843, 1992.
13. Ellingwood KE, Million RR: Cancer of the nasal cavity and ethmoid/sphenoid sinuses, *Cancer* 43:1517, 1979.
14. Feldman BA: Rhabdomyosarcoma of the head and neck, *Laryngoscope* 92:424, 1982.
15. Freeman SB and others: Intraoperative radiotherapy of skull base cancer, *Laryngoscope* 101(5):507, 1991.
16. Fu Y-S, Perzin KH: Nonepithelial tumors of the nasal cavity, paranasal sinuses, and nasopharynx. VI. Fibrous tissue tumors, *Cancer* 37:2912, 1976.
17. Fujii J, Chambers SM, Rhoton AF Jr: Neurovascular relationships of the sphenoid sinus: a microsurgical study, *J Neurosurg* 50:31, 1979.
18. Harrison DFN: Critical look at the classification of maxillary sinus carcinomata, *Ann Otol* 87:3, 1978.
19. Horree WA: Adenoid cystic carcinoma of the maxilla, *Arch Otolaryngol* 100:469, 1974.
20. Hyams VJ: Papillomas of the nasal cavity and paranasal sinuses, *Ann Laryngol* 1, 1970.
21. Hyams VJ: Papillomas of the nasal cavity and paranasal sinuses, *Ann Otol Rhinol Laryngol* 80:192, 1971.
22. Hyams VJ: *Pathology of the nose and paranasal sinuses.* In English GE, editor: *Otolaryngology,* vol 2, New York, 1984, Harper & Row.
23. Jackson RT, Fitz-Hugh GS, Constable WC: Malignant neoplasms of the nasal cavities and paranasal sinuses, *Laryngoscope* 87:726, 1977.
24. Janecka IP and others: Facial translocation: a new approach to the cranial base, *Otolaryngol Head Neck Surg* 103:413, 1990.
25. Jing B-S, Goepfert H, Close LG: Computerized tomography of paranasal sinus neoplasms, *Laryngoscope* 88:1485, 1978.
26. Johns ME and others: Supraorbital rim approach to the anterior skull base, *Laryngoscope* 94:1137, 1984.
27. Kadish S, Goodman M, Wang CC: Olfactory neuroblastoma: a clinical analysis of 17 cases, *Cancer* 37:1571, 1976.
28. Keane WM and others: Epidemiology of head and neck cancer, *Laryngoscope* 91:2037, 1981.
29. Ketcham AS and others: *Surgical treatment of patients with advanced cancer of the paranasal sinuses*. In *Neoplasia of head and neck*, Chicago, 1974, Mosby.
30. Ketcham AS, VanBuren JM: Tumors of the paranasal sinuses: a therapeutic challenge, *Am J Surgery* 150:406, 1985.
31. Kitt VV, Panje WR: Malignancies of the ethmoidal and sphenoidal sinuses: a report of 47 cases, International Conference on Head and Neck Cancer, Baltimore, 1984.
32. Klintenberg C and others: Adenocarcinoma of the ethmoid sinuses, *Cancer* 54:482, 1984.
33. Kneght P, de Jong PC, van Andel JG: Carcinoma of the paranasal sinuses, International Conference on Head and Neck Cancer, Baltimore, 1984.
34. Koh WJ: Fast neutron radiation for inoperable and recurrent salivary gland cancers, *Am J Clin Oncol Cancer Clinical Trials* 12:316, 1989.
35. Laramore GE and others: Fast neutron radiotherapy for sarcomas—soft tissue, bone and cartilage, *Am J Clin Oncol Cancer Clinical Trials* 12: 320, 1989.
36. Larson DL, Christ JE, Jesse RH: Preservation of the orbital contents in cancer of the maxillary sinus, *Arch Otolaryngol* 108:370, 1982.
37. Lee Y-Y and others: Superselective intra-arterial chemotherapy of advanced paranasal sinus tumors, *Arch Otolaryngol Head Neck Surg* 115: 503, 1989.
38. Lee YY and others: Superselective intra-arterial chemotherapy of advanced paranasal sinus tumors, *Arch Otolaryngol Head Neck Surg* 115: 503, 1989.
39. Leipzig B, English J: Sphenoid wing meningioma occurring as a lateral orbital mass, *Laryngoscope* 94:1091, 1984.
40. Mancuso AA, Hanafee WN: *Paranasal sinuses—normal anatomy, methodology, and pathology.* In Mancuso AA, editor: *Computed tomography of the head and neck*, Baltimore, 1982, Williams & Wilkins.
41. Martin H: *Surgery of the head and neck tumors*, New York, 1957, Hoeber-Harper, Inc.
42. Maurer HM, Ragab AH: *Rhabdomyosarcoma.* In Sutow WW, Fernbach DJ, Vietti TJ, editors: *Clinical pediatric oncology*, St Louis, 1984, Mosby.
43. McClatchey KD: *Odontogenic lesions—tumors and cysts.* In Batsakis JG, editor: *Tumors of the head and neck*, ed 2, Baltimore, 1979, Williams & Wilkins.
44. Myers EN, Schramm VL, Barnes EL: Management of inverted papilloma of the nose and sinuses, *Laryngoscope* 91:2071, 1981.
45. Ohngren LG: Malignant tumours of the maxillo-ethmoid region, *Acta Otolaryngol Suppl* 19:1, 1933.
46. Overholt SL and others: Angiography in the diagnosis and management of extracranial vascular lesions of the head and neck, *Laryngoscope* 88:1769, 1978.

47. Panje WR and others: The transfacial approach for combined anterior craniofacial tumor ablation, *Arch Otolaryngol Head Neck Surg* 115: 301, 1989.

48. Perry C and others: Preservation of the eye in paranasal sinus cancer surgery, *Arch Otolaryngol Head Neck Surg* 114:632, 1988.

49. Perry C and others: Preservation of the eye in paranasal sinus cancer surgery, *Arch Otolaryngol Head Neck Surg* 114:632, 1988.

50. Ramsey HE, Strong EW, Frazel EL: Fibrous dysplasia of the craniofacial bones, *Am J Surg* 116:542, 1968.

51. Rate WR and others: Intraoperative radiotherapy for recurrent head and neck cancer, *Cancer* 67:2738, 1991.

52. Robbins KT and others: A targeted supradose cisplatin chemoradiation protocol for advanced head and neck cancer, *Am J Surg* 168:419, 1994.

53. Rostomily TC and others: Personal communication, permanent low-activity ^{125}I seed implants as an adjunct to surgery in the management of advanced adult skull base lesions, *Neurosurgery* 1996.

54. Sakai S and others: Multidisciplinary treatment of maxillary sinus carcinoma, *Cancer* 52:1360, 1983.

55. Schramm VL Jr: Inflammatory and neoplastic masses of the nose and paranasal sinus in children, *Laryngoscope* 89:1887, 1979.

56. Seeger JF: Neuroradiology of the skull base, *Otolaryngol Clin North Am* 17:459, 1984.

57. Shah JP and others: Craniofacial resections for tumors involving the base of the skull, *Am J Surg* 154:352, 1987.

58. Shidnia H and others: The role of radiotherapy in treatment of malignant tumors of the paranasal sinuses, *Laryngoscope* 94:102, 1984.

59. Sisson GA: Symposium—paranasal sinuses, *Laryngoscope* 80:945, 1970.

60. Smith PG and others: Combined pterional-anterolateral approaches to cranial base tumors, *Otolaryngol Head Neck Surg* 103:357, 1990.

61. Spaulding CA and others: Esthesioneuroblastoma: a comparison of two treatment eras, *Int J Radiat Oncol Biol Phys* 15:581, 1988.

62. Terz JJ, Young HF, Lawrence W Jr: Combined craniofacial resection for locally advanced carcinoma of the head and neck, *Am J Surg* 140: 618, 1980.

63. Vikram B, Mishra S: Permanent iodine-125 implants in postoperative radiotherapy for head and neck cancer with positive surgical margins, *Head Neck* 16:155, 1994.

64. Wang CC: *Radiation therapy for head and neck neoplasms*, Boston, 1983, John Wright-PSG, Inc.

65. Weisberger EC, Dedo HH: Cranial neuropathies in sinus disease, *Laryngoscope* 87:357, 1977.

66. Weymuller EA, Reardon EJ, Nash D: A comparison of treatment modalities in carcinoma of the maxillary antrum, *Arch Otolaryngol Head Neck Surg* 106:625, 1980.

67. Wilkins SA and others: Aggressive fibromatosis of the head and neck, *Am J Surg* 130:412, 1975.

Chapter 60

Medical Management of Infectious and Inflammatory Disease

Scott C. Manning

The patient presenting with infrequent episodes of acute sinusitis complicating viral upper respiratory infection usually is easily treated with short courses of antibiotics administered by the primary care physician. Unfortunately, the referral problem of chronic or recurrent rhinitis or sinusitis implies a multifactorial etiology and is not solved by simply making an empiric antibiotic selection. Predisposing factors in chronic disease may include allergic rhinitis, environmental irritants such as cigarette smoke, viral illness (children attending daycare centers), gastroesophageal reflux, anatomic obstruction, immunodeficiency disorder, cystic fibrosis, and ciliary dyskinesia. Antibiotic therapy should be used in conjunction with appropriate measures directed at these factors to achieve resolution of symptoms. The key to breaking a cycle of recurrent or chronic sinusitis is the aggressive combination of antibiotics with therapies directed at predisposing conditions for a time adequate to allow for healing of upper respiratory tract mucosa with return of local immune defense (Table 60-1).

PREDISPOSING FACTORS FOR SINUSITIS

Viral illness

Viruses are probably the most common predisposing factors for sinusitis, especially in children. Children attending daycare centers have double or triple the overall incidence of upper respiratory tract disease, including otitis and sinusitis in those younger than 3 years of age. A multiplicity of viruses has been implicated in the common cold, including influenza, parainfluenza, adenovirus, rhinovirus, and respiratory syncytial virus. Because of the number and antigenic variability of potential causative agents, viral vaccine therapy is not likely to become an effective weapon in the battle against the common cold.

Prevention and therapy

Most viral illness spread occurs through hand-to-hand contact, and studies have shown reduced viral illness among healthcare workers when rigorous hand washing and gloving protocols have been instituted. These measures are particularly important for healthcare workers in pediatric hospitals during seasonal epidemics of respiratory syncytial virus in infants. Parents of children with chronic sinusitis are encouraged to try to find childcare settings with the fewest possible children to reduce viral exposure. Sometimes coordinating vacations or alternative childcare with relatives to remove the patient from the daycare setting for about 1 month allows enough recovery to break a cycle of recurrent sinusitis.

Vitamin C has long been proposed as prevention and therapy for the common cold.[5] Most placebo-controlled trials have shown no benefit for vitamin C as prophylaxis and, at most, a minimal treatment effect, which probably is a result of the mild antihistamine and anticholinergic activity of vitamin C.[3] Similarly, zinc gluconate may have a mild effect in reducing cold symptoms in placebo-controlled trials, but its mechanism of action is not understood.[19] Contrary to prevailing logic, inhalation of heated humidified air has not

Table 60-1. Hierarchy of medical treatment options for patients with chronic rhinosinusitis

Type	Treatment option
Environmental	Reduce exposure to dust, molds, cigarette smoke, pollution, and chemical irritants
Social	Encourage hand washing, reduce time in daycare center or class size
Prophylaxis	Daily nasal saline lavage, topical cromolyn starting before allergy season, management of gastroesophageal reflux
Allergy	Antihistamines, cromolyn, topical corticosteroids, immunotherapy for documented sensitivities
Antimicrobial	Amoxicillin, broad-spectrum for 2 to 3 weeks, prophylaxis, intravenous for threatened suppurative complications
Immunodeficiency	Antibiotic prophylaxis in winter, intravenous gamma-globulin for health-threatening systemic illness

proved beneficial for either viral upper respiratory or allergic rhinitis symptoms in controlled trials.[9]

Antiviral agents currently are being investigated for prevention and management of the common cold. Interferon α-2 may potentially block penetration of viruses through respiratory mucosa.[8] Intranasal interferon α-2, when used as a once-a-day nasal aerosol, has been shown to potentially prevent colds in people exposed to family members with upper respiratory infections. Usage is limited by the cost of interferon and by side effects of nasal drying and congestion. In one placebo study of adults innoculated with rhinovirus, interferon α-2, along with nasal ipratropium and oral naproxen (antimediator therapy), was shown to dramatically reduce cold symptoms.[7]

Several intercellular adhesion molecule (ICAM) receptor antagonist agents currently are under investigation for efficacy in prevention or therapy of colds. Monoclonal antibodies that block or decoy viral binding to ICAM-1 receptors on mucosal cell surfaces may prove to be effective management options when administered at the first onset of cold symptoms.

Environmental irritants

More than one half of the people in the United States are estimated to live in areas where exposure to ozone, sulfur dioxide, nitrogen dioxide, carbon monoxide, lead, and particulates exceed the National Ambient Air Quality Standards. There is increasing evidence that exposure to air pollution may impair respiratory mucociliary protection and potentially increase sensitivities to common aeroallergens.[10] Exposure to outdoor and indoor pollutants is one possible factor

explaining the dramatic increase in immunoglobulin E (IgE)-mediated disease, including asthma and allergic rhinitis, reported from most industrialized areas during the past 20 years.

A careful history of environmental exposures should be a part of the evaluation of every patient with chronic sinusitis. Indoor sources of potentially damaging air pollution include cigarette smoke, smoke from wood burning ovens, formaldehyde, copier fluid, latex, chlorine (pools), paint, and perfumes. At times, medical therapy is consistently ineffective until exposure to offending irritants is reduced or eliminated. People exposed to wood or other particulates may be instructed to wear appropriate masks. Hospital personnel (particularly intensivists) are encouraged to avoid latex if a sensitivity develops (and to follow appropriate hand washing and gloving protocols). Pilots and flight attendants (who are exposed to dry air and increased particulates) are encouraged to use frequent nasal saline lavages. Rarely, patients with severe chemical sensitivities may be encouraged to find other employment to reduce exposure (e.g., persons in the cosmetic industry with severe perfume sensitivity).

Allergic rhinitis

Twenty percent of adults are found to be allergic by skin testing to at least one common aeroallergen, and the percentage probably is much greater among patients presenting with a history of chronic sinusitis. Allergic rhinitis may predispose to recurrent or chronic sinusitis through impairment of mucociliary function, effects on local and systemic immunity, and decreased sinus drainage and ventilation from mucosal congestion within the sinus outflow tracts. Testing for specific IgE antibodies through serologic or skin tests is relatively nonspecific in children 4 years of age or less although an allergic diathesis should be suspected when children have other evidence of atopy such as eczema or when the parents have a strong history of allergic rhinitis. Allergic rhinitis probably is the second most common predisposing condition to chronic sinusitis in children (after viral upper respiratory infection) and perhaps the most common predisposing factor in adults. Therapy aimed at minimizing allergic mucosal inflammation is a vital part of breaking a cycle of recurrent sinusitis in allergic patients. Therapeutic options for allergic rhinitis include environmental control, antihistamines, other antimediator drugs, and immunotherapy.

Environmental control

Sensitivities to dust mite antigen or molds are probably the most common allergies among adult and pediatric sinusitis patients with perennial symptoms of nasal congestion. The dust mite and molds prefer a humid environment, and reducing ambient relative humidity below 50% through dehumidifiers and exhaust fans (in bathrooms) may be beneficial. Cleaning, heating, and cooling systems frequently may reduce mold exposure. In addition, patients with mold allergies are instructed to reduce exposure by not raking leaves in fall. High-efficiency particulate air filters are fairly efficient at reducing light particles, such as pollen (as long as doors and windows are kept closed), but probably do not reduce exposure to heavier dust antigens. Acaricides such as benzyl benzoate powder or tannic acid denature the dust mite antigen and may be beneficial when used to treat carpets and upholstery on a regular basis. Dust mite exposure also may be reduced by using plastic covers around mattresses and pillows, using synthetic linen, minimizing exposure to pets and cockroaches (the dust mite lives on human and animal dander), and by removing old carpet and upholstery.

Antihistamines

Antihistamines work by competitive inhibition of histamine receptor sites on respiratory mucosal target cells. H-1 blockers are relevant to allergic rhinitis and are more likely to be effective for patients with more specific histamine symptoms such as facial itching, watery rhinorrhea, and sneezing. Antihistamines are relatively ineffective in relieving chronic nasal congestion. First generation antihistamines, such as chlorpheniramine, diphenhydramine, and clemastine, demonstrate anticholinergic side effects such as drowsiness (or hyperactivity in children). They work best when used intermittently for brief periods to block specific histamine symptoms. They may be contraindicated when drowsiness could pose a danger such as when driving, operating machinery, or scuba diving. The anticholinergic effect of first generation antihistamines includes drying of secretions, and this may account for their continued popularity as an over-the-counter cold remedy.

Second generation antihistamines have a higher affinity to histamine receptors, affording increased potency and decreased development of tolerance or tachyphylaxis. In addition, they exhibit much less drying and other anticholinergic effects and less or no central sedation. They are safe for use in asthmatic patients.[15] Hepatic metabolism of astemizole and terfenadine may be partially blocked by macrolides, quinolones, and azole drugs, resulting in prolonged Q-T intervals and the potential for ventricular arrhythmias. The risk of conduction abnormalities is increased in patients with hypokalemia or liver disease. The newer second generation antihistamines are less dependent on hepatic metabolism and are safe in combination with other drugs. Loratadine is effective within a few hours, and its efficacy persists for 12 to 24 hours, allowing for once-daily dosing. Cetirizine is effective within 24 hours and also is administered once daily. Cetirizine appears to block other mediator release, such as leukotrienes and kinins, in addition to its antihistamine effect, and it also may inhibit monocyte and lymphocyte chemotaxis. Drugs with leukotriene blockade may prove beneficial in the management of chronic congestion. Cetirizine demonstrated mild sedation in some patients in placebo-controlled trials. Loratadine and cetirizine are approved by the Food and Drug Administration (FDA) for those aged 6 years and older, and both are available in liquid form for children.

Levocabastine is a potent H-1 receptor antagonist with some possible leukotriene inhibition that is being developed for topical nasal use. It is currently available in the United States as a topical ophthalmic preparation. Azelastine recently has been approved as a topical nasal metered dose inhaler, and it also demonstrates leukotriene antagonism.[16] Azelastine is not currently approved for use in children in the United States. All of the second generation antihistamines are relatively expensive compared with the first generation drugs.

Cromolyn

Nasal cromolyn preparations, recently approved for over-the-counter dispensing, work by stabilizing mast cells against degranulation and release of inflammatory mediators. They are safe and have few or no side effects, but they are relatively short-acting, resulting in a need for three to six times daily dosing. Cromolyn preparations work best for patients with specific IgE hypersensitivities when used prophylactically starting before antigen challenge. They are as effective as second generation antihistamines for blocking sneezing and watery rhinorrhea, but they are relatively ineffective for those with chronic nasal congestion from perennial allergic rhinitis. Nedocromil as a 1% nasal solution currently has investigational status, but it appears to have a similar mechanism of action and efficacy.

Glucocorticoids

Corticosteroids stabilize mast cells against mediator release, block formation of inflammatory mediators, and inhibit chemotaxis of inflammatory cells. When used at least 7 days in advance, nasal corticosteroids have been shown to inhibit immediate and late phase reactions to antigenic stimulation in patients with allergic rhinitis.[20] An estimated 90% of patients with allergic rhinitis experience improvement in nasal allergy symptoms, including chronic nasal congestion with topical nasal steroid preparations accounting for a marked increase in popularity of these medications during the past decade. In the United States, the number of prescriptions written for nasal steroids increased from 7 million in 1992 to 9 million in 1994, whereas the number of antihistamine prescriptions decreased.[17]

Except for dexamethasone, intranasal corticosteroids are poorly absorbed through mucosa, allowing for a safe therapeutic ratio when used as directed. With fluticasone and budesonide, some hypothalamic-pituitary-adrenal suppression has been documented at recommended dosing levels in adults.[11] Also, an association between new onset glaucoma and use of an inhaler and nasal glucocorticoids has been reported in older adult patients,[6] and two children have been reported to have experienced disseminated varicella while using nasal beclomethasone spray. Therefore, nasal steroids should be used with caution in young children and older adults, especially if they are using other steroid inhalers. Common side effects of topical nasal steroid use include nasal irritation, mucosal bleeding, and crusting. Septal perforation is a rare complication of nasal steroid use, and the risk may be increased for patients living in dry climates. These side effects appear to be related more to the vehicle than the steroid, and those given preparations using propylene glycol, such as flunisolide, appear to have an increased incidence of nasal burning sensation. Adverse nasal side effects often may be alleviated by switching to a preparation with an aqueous or powder delivery system. Beclomethasone, flunisolide, and triamcinolone acetonide have similar clinical efficacy, whereas budesonide and fluticasone propionate may be slightly more potent.

Short courses of systemic corticosteroids are sometimes used by clinicians to manage severe nasal mucosal congestion in allergic patients so that intranasal steroids preparations subsequently may be inhaled nasally. Contraindications to systemic steroids might include diabetes, peptic ulcer disease, glaucoma, severe hypertension, and advanced osteoporosis.

Immunotherapy

Immunotherapy is indicated for patients with documented IgE-mediated allergies who have failed to achieve sufficient symptom relief from antihistamine and topical nasal glucocorticoid therapy. It generally is not practical for children less than 4 years of age.

Nonspecific rhinitis

Vasomotor or nonallergic rhinitis is a diagnosis of exclusion in patients with symptoms of watery rhinorrhea, congestion, and sneezing but without specific IgE sensitivities. Nasal symptoms may be triggered by emotion, cold air, or other irritants. Patients with vasomotor rhinitis typically do not respond to antihistamine or steroid therapy. Another class of chronic rhinitis sufferers are those patients with aspirin sensitivity sometimes with associated nasal polyps and reactive airway disease. Presumably, aspirin leads to increased lipoxygenase and leukotriene mediator production through blockage of the cyclooxygenase pathway of arachidonic acid metabolism. Patients with nonallergic rhinitis–eosinophilia syndrome (NARES) often respond to nasal corticosteroid therapy for relief of chronic congestion. Chronic rhinitis also may be induced by hormonal changes such as pregnancy or by medications or drugs, including cocaine, birth control pills, β-blockers, ACE inhibitors, and reserpine.

Anticholinergics

Ipratropium is an anticholinergic drug available as a 0.03% or 0.06% nasal spray approved for patients aged 12 years or older. It is a quaternary ammonium molecule with minimal absorption through nasal mucosa, and therefore it exhibits few or no systemic side effects. Potential nasal side effects include excessive drying, epistaxis, and headache. The principal indication for ipratropium nasal spray is for the control of watery rhinorrhea in patients with vasomotor rhinitis. The drug is not effective for control of chronic congestion or sneezing. It is a relatively short-acting drug, and the recommended starting dosage is two sprays each nostril four times a day.

Gastroesophageal reflux

Gastroesophageal reflux is receiving increased attention as a possible etiologic agent behind virtually every respiratory tract ailment but particularly for patients with chronic cough, asthma, or laryngitis. Some clinicians are proposing that reflux may reach the nasopharynx and nasal cavities in some patients, leading to chronic mucosal irritation and sinusitis.[1] The strongest anecdotal evidence for a link between gastroesophageal reflux and chronic sinusitis has been in young children, presumably as a result of the closer proximity of the esophageal inlet and larynx to the soft palate and nasopharynx.

Adult chronic sinusitis patients with a history of heartburn or other reflux symptoms could be started empirically on an antireflux regimen, consisting of antacids and over-the-counter histamine type 2 (H2) antagonists. These patients should be also advised to avoid alcohol and large meals late at night and to try elevating the head of their bed. If symptoms persist, they should be referred to an appropriate medical specialist for further examination.

Gastroesophageal reflux should be suspected in children with chronic congestion and rhinorrhea, particularly if they have a history of excessive spitting up as an infant, low-weight percentile or failure to thrive, chronic stridor, or reactive airway disease. If results of an initial barium swallow evaluation are normal, a pH probe should be considered, ideally with a second channel in the proximal esophagus. Children with documented gastroesophageal reflux are treated by appropriate pediatric specialists in conjunction with head elevation during sleep, thickened feeds, and H2 blockers such as ranitidine. Cisapride is a noncholinergic prokinetic agent that serves to improve gastrointestinal motility and to enhance lower esophageal sphincter pressure, and it often is used in conjunction with ranitidine.

Omeprazole, a hydrogen ion pump inhibitor, is the strongest inhibitor of gastric acid secretion, and it may be indicated for treatment of patients with refractory cases of reflux. It is recommended for short courses of therapy only because of the concern for gastrinoma formation as seen in animal trials. It is not available in liquid form, and no pediatric trials have been published to date.

Immunodeficiency

Many types of primary immunodeficiency have been described over the past 30 years, and considered as a risk factor for those with chronic sinusitis, it is many times more common in the general population than cystic fibrosis or ciliary dysmotility. Recurrent respiratory tract infection is the hallmark of primary immunodeficiency disorders, and therefore the diagnosis should be considered in all patients with sinusitis refractory to medical or surgical therapy. Allergic, autoimmune, and rheumatologic diseases are more common in patients with primary immunodeficiencies, perhaps resulting from T-cell regulatory defects, which potentially up-regulate IgE and down-regulate other immunoglobulins. The clinician should remember that patients with allergies or asthma may have primary immunodeficiencies as an additional predisposing condition for sinusitis.

From the otolaryngologist's perspective, immunodeficiency should be considered in chronic sinusitis patients with unusually severe symptoms, such as facial pain and purulent rhinorrhea, and who fail to respond as expected to appropriate therapy. Examination of these patients usually is done with the help of infectious disease or immunology specialists and often includes total immunoglobulins with immunoglobulin G (IgG) subclasses. Response to polyvalent pneumococcal vaccine measures T-cell independent humoral response to carbohydrate antigens, whereas tetanus toxoid and diphtheria vaccine response provides some measure of T-cell dependent humoral response to protein-dependent antigens. An allergy panel skin test provides some functional measure of cellular immunity.

Patients with common variable immunodeficiency, defined as low total IgG, or other severe immunodeficiency usually have a history of severe infections, such as pneumonia in addition to sinusitis. Patients with decreased functional response to polysaccharide-encapsulated bacteria, so-called vaccine hyporesponse, may present only with a history of refractory severe sinusitis. Patients with vaccine hyporesponse may have associated IgG subclass or immunoglobulin A (IgA) deficiency. Also, clinicians who treat children should remember that children have a physiologic immunodeficiency as quantitative and functional measures of immunity do not reach adult levels until age 12 years. IgG 2 and IgG 4 subclasses, which play a large role in defense against the pyogenic cocci such as *Haemophilus influenzae* and *Moraxella catarrhalis*, develop particularly slowly. Most children achieve near-adult levels of humoral antibodies by age 7 years, and this fact probably accounts for the observation that most chronic rhinitis and sinusitis in children resolve spontaneously by that age.

When primary immunodeficiency is discovered in patients with chronic sinusitis, the principal therapeutic strategy is to aggresively use conventional medical treatments, including prophylactic antibiotics and appropriate allergy management. For young children, the goal is to buy time with conservative therapy (trying to avoid surgery) with the expectation that upper respiratory infections will decrease over time with natural maturation of systemic immunity. Monthly intravenous gamma-globulin therapy is reserved for patients with health-threatening infection as a result of documented humoral antibody deficiencies. It is expensive and carries a small risk of allergic reaction, including anaphylaxis, and of transmission of viruses such as hepatitis C.

Therefore, it should be administered by experts in infectious disease and immunology. In case reports, intravenous gamma-globulin has been used successfully in the treatment of patients with chronic sinusitis, with documented immunodeficiency with unremitting facial pain, mucosal ulcerations, and purulent rhinorrhea with resistant gram-negative bacteria, and who had failed to improve after multiple previous surgical procedures.[12]

BACTERIAL SINUSITIS

Healthy sinuses are a result of adequate ventilation through patent ostia, adequate mucociliary clearance function, and adequate local and systemic immune defense. When conditions allow, opportunistic bacterial flora of the nasal cavities may proliferate and invade sinus mucosa, leading to a cycle of infection with secondary mucosal edema and dysfunction and potentially to more infection.

Acute sinusitis usually is defined as persistent and worsening upper respiratory symptoms for longer than the expected 7-day course of a viral illness but for less than 3 weeks. In placebo studies, the rate of spontaneous resolution for uncomplicated acute sinusitis is at least 40%. As with acute otitis media, the most common cultured pathogens in patients with radiographically documented acute sinusitis are *Streptococcus pneumoniae* in about 30% of patients and nontypeable *H. influenzae* in about 20%. *M. catarrhalis* occasionally is cultured from adults but it is fairly common in children with acute sinusitis, accounting for about 20% of pediatric cases. *Staphylococcus aureus* may be cultured from about 30% of healthy noses, but although it is a common component of normal nasal flora, it is an infrequent isolate in sinus cultures of patients with acute sinusitis. Anaerobes are rarely recovered in significant colony numbers from these patients.

Subacute sinusitis generally is defined as nasal symptoms lasting 3 weeks to 3 months. The profile of cultured pathogens in patients with subacute sinusitis is the same as for those with acute sinusitis. In one prospective study of children with subacute sinusitis defined clinically and radiographically, there were no significant differences in symptom resolution between three groups treated with different antibiotics and one group treated with placebo. All patients received nasal saline and decongestant therapy, and overall symptom resolution was 70% at 3 weeks and 87% at 6 weeks.[4]

Chronic sinusitis usually is defined as symptoms of sinusitis persisting beyond 3 months without improvement. From a practical standpoint, the clinician more commonly hears a story of symptoms waxing and waning with medical therapy over a prolonged period. Culture studies using maxillary sinus taps in patients with chronic sinusitis show similar results to studies of acute sinusitis patients with perhaps an increased overall incidence of nontypeable *H. influenzae*. Patients with refractory chronic sinusitis show an increased incidence of *S. aureus*, anaerobic bacteria, gram-negative organisms, and of polymicrobial infection in general. *Pseudomonas aeruginosa* is commonly cultured from patients who have received multiple courses of antibiotics over a prolonged period. *Pseudomonas* culture also should prompt suspicion of immunodeficiency.

Because of the increased likelihood of polymicrobial infection with resistant organisms, sinus culture is strongly recommended for patients with chronic sinusitis. Maxillary sinus puncture remains the gold standard for obtaining sinus culture material, with many studies in the past showing little correlation between nasal swab and maxillary culture. Careful otoscopic- or endoscopic-guided culturing of obviously purulent secretions in the middle meatus or nasal vestibule is a practical way to obtain rapid guidance in antibiotic selection. When such a culture yields pathogens in high numbers, an assumption may be made that the identified pathogens are playing a role in the infection. Even occasional culturing of office patients with chronic sinusitis may yield valuable information regarding patterns of antibiotic resistance in the community.

Antibiotic therapy

Amoxicillin remains the initial drug of choice for uncomplicated cases of acute sinusitis despite the fact that β-lactamase production is found in up to 40% of isolates of *H. influenzae* and *M. catarrhalis* (Table 60-2). Amoxicillin achieves a high level in sinus fluid at recommended doses, and most β-lactamase resistance is relative and may be overcome by a high enough drug level. Intermediate penicillin resistance of *S. pneumonia* resulting from alterations in penicillin-binding proteins also may be overcome by increasing the dose of amoxicillin. Antibiotic resistance among upper airway bacteria is most prevalent among young children attending daycare centers, and many infectious disease specialists recommend dosing children at 60 mg/kg/day instead of 40 mg/kg/day. Some authors advocate initial therapy with increased doses of penicillin, erythromycin with sulfanilamide, or a second generation cephalosporin in areas with a high incidence of bacterial antibiotic resistance. Amoxicillin is contraindicated in patients with suspected Epstein-Barr virus infection because of a 50% incidence of cutaneous rash. Based on studies showing a 20% incidence of viable bacteria through maxillary sinus tap after 7 days of antibiotic therapy, most authors recommend 10 days of therapy in the manage of acute sinusitis.

The most common empiric initial parenteral antibiotic choices for patients with severe sinusitis with suspected orbital or intracranial extension are cefuroxime, a second generation cephalosporin with good coverage of *Haemophilus* and *Moraxella*, or ceftriaxone, a third generation cephalosporin. Aminoglycosides are considered the first-line drugs for gram-negative serious infections, and vancomycin may come to play an increasing role for patients with severe sinusitis with suppurative complications resulting from resistant *S. aureus* or highly resistant *S. pneumoniae*.

Ideally, antibiotic therapy for patients with chronic sinusitis should be based on culture results. Because of the steady increase in antibiotic resistance, empiric antibiotic selection has less and less likelihood of effectively matching bacterial susceptibilities in the future. Currently, the first-line antibiotics for patients with chronic sinusitis include amoxicillin-clavulanate, second generation cephalosporins, and erythromycin-sulfasoxazole. β-Lactamase-mediated resistance to the early second generation cephalosporins is high among

Table 60-2. Antimicrobial therapy for sinusitis

Type	Organism	Drugs	Comments
Acute	*Streptococcus pneumoniae, Haemophilus influenzae, Moraxella catarrhalis*	Amoxicillin for 10 days	Second-generation cephalosporin or new generation macrolide for penicillin allergic
Subacute	Increased likelihood of resistant *Streptococcus pneumoniae* or β-lactamase positive *Haemophilus influenzae* or *Moraxella catarrhalis*	Back-up drugs for amoxicillin failures	
Chronic	Increased likelihood of resistant organisms and polymicrobial infection including *Pseudomonas* sp. and anerobes	Amoxicillin-clavulanate, second generation cephalosporins, cefixime for *Haemophilus influenzae*, new macrolides, clindamycin for highly resistant *Streptococcus pneumoniae*, 2–3 weeks of therapy	Culture-guided therapy whenever possible, address predisposing conditions
Recurrent chronic	Resistant organisms and polymicrobial infection	Consider 3–4 weeks of prophylaxis after initial therapy	Culture-guided
Suppurative complications	High incidence of gram-negative organisms and *Staphylococcus aureus*	Cefuroxime, ceftriaxone, aminoglycosides	Surgery if no response in 24-48 hours

strains of *H. influenzae* and *M. catarrhalis*. The third generation cephalosporin, cefixime, may be selected for *Haemophilus* or *Moraxella* infections, but it has a poor spectrum of activity against *S. pneumoniae*. The newer generation macrolides, clarithromycin and azithromycin, achieve excellent mucosal levels but should be considered back-up drugs. Azithromycin appears more potent against *H. influenzae* whereas clarithromycin may be slightly better against intermediate resistant *S. pneumoniae*.[14] Clindamycin should be reserved for culture-documented resistant *S. pneumoniae*. Clindamycin has little efficacy against *Haemophilus* infection.

Most clinicians recommend treating patients with chronic sinusitis with a broad spectrum antibiotic for up to 3 weeks. The first outcome measure is improvement in symptoms, which should occur within 3 to 5 days. It is hoped the next outcome will be resolution of symptoms within 7 to 10 days after first improvement. The logic of continuing therapy for another week or so is to allow for further decrease of mucosal edema and mucociliary function to gain resistance against new infection.

Many clinicians will follow the 3-week treatment course of antibiotics with a 3- to 6-week course of once-daily prophylactic antibiotic therapy for patients with a history of rapid recurrence after previous treatment. The goal is to get patients through their window of vulnerability to new infection while mucosal recovery allows for return of normal primary immune defense. Antibiotic prophylaxis probably is worth considering at least once in patients being considered for surgery, but prolonged prophylaxis applies more selection pressure for development of bacterial resistance. Also, prolonged use of antibiotics may promote chronicity of infection by creating β-lactamase–producing normal flora organisms, which can "protect" potentially sensitive pathogens. In addition, normal flora, such as viridans streptococci and nonhemolytic streptococci, may competitively inhibit colonization by pathogenic organisms, and prolonged antibiotics may promote chronic infection by disturbing normal flora.[2] Bacterial interference through management with viridans streptococci has been used in Europe for management of chronic β-hemolytic *Streptococcus* pharyngitis. Overuse of antibiotics also has lead to an increased incidence of pseudomembranous enterocolitis, especially in children. The diagnosis of enterocolitis should be considered in any patient with chronic diarrhea and abdominal discomfort during or after antimicrobial therapy. Cephalosporins probably are the more common cause (more than clindamycin) in most outpatient cases.

Decongestants

Decongestants are α-adrenergic agonists that induce release of norepinephrine from sympathetic nerves, leading to vasoconstriction of dilated mucosal blood vessels (Table 60-3). Decongestants exhibit varying degrees of tachyphylaxis and are best used for short 3- to 5-day courses at the beginning of treatment for patients with sinusitis or allergic rhinitis. The most common oral decongestants are pseudoephedrine and phenylpropanolamine. Common side effects include insomnia, palpitations, and increased blood pressure. Pressor effects are more common in patients with diabetes or thyroid disease and in those patients taking monoamine oxidase inhibitors for management of depression.

Oral decongestants are indicated principally for symptomatic relief of nasal congestion and have not been shown to have therapeutic efficacy for the management of sinusitis. McCormick and others, for example, compared oral brompheniramine and phenylephrine in combination with topical nasal oxymetazoline against topical nasal saline and placebo syrup in children with acute sinusitis.[13] In both groups, symptoms and radiographic findings improved rapidly, and there were no significant differences between the treatment groups.

Topical agents include phenylephrine, oxymetazoline, and naphazoline. Phenylephrine may have a greater tendency to increase blood pressure than oxymetazoline, and all topical decongestants should be used with caution, if at all, in young patients and in the elderly population. All topical agents exhibit rebound vasodilation, which can be demonstrated by rhinometric analysis of nasal resistance as early as 3 days after beginning therapy. Clinical rebound congestion or rhinitis medicamentosa usually requires at least 10 days to 2 weeks of topical decongestant use to become apparent. The management of rebound congestion resulting from prolonged use of topical decongestants consists mainly of administration of topical nasal steroids. Patients also may be instructed to gradually dilute their last bottle of decongestant spray with nasal saline every few days, allowing for gradual weaning.

No controlled studies have shown more rapid resolution of documented sinusitis or otitis with topical decongestants and some studies have increased concern about effects on mucociliary function. Min and others demonstrated a higher incidence of maxillary sinusitis after topical phenylephrine in the rabbit model.[18] Histologic analysis of nasal mucosa after 2 weeks of use showed epithelial ulceration, inflammation, and edema. Similarly, in a trial involving infants with upper respiratory infections, Turner and Darden showed better improvement of middle ear ventilation measured by immitance with placebo nose drops than with topical phenylephrine.[21]

Mucolytics

Guaifenesin is the most commonly used mucolytic agent, and it often is dispensed in combination with a decongestant (see Table 60-3). High doses (up to 2400 mg/day for adults) are required for obtaining an effect on mucous, and at those doses, emesis and abdominal pain are frequently reported mild side effects. Saturated solution of potassium iodide

Table 60-3. Nonantimicrobial pharmacotherapy for rhinosinusitis

Class	Examples	Indications	Comments
Mucolytic	Guaifenisin	Congestion and rhinorrhea symptoms	Symptomatic relief in comparative trial of AIDS patients
Oral decongestant	Phenylpropanolamine, pseudoephedrine	Congestion	Use with caution in children, elderly, and pregnant women; pressor and central nervous system effects
Topical decongestants	Phenylephrine, oxymetazoline	Congestion	Rebound congestion after 1–2 weeks; may damage nasal epithelium; pressor effects especially in elderly or hypertensive patients
Nutritional or "alternative"	Vitamin C, zinc, echinacea, goldenseal	All	Most rhinosinusitis is self-resolving; vitamin C and echinacea may have mild decongestive effect; no evidence of change in "immune function"
Anticholinergics	Ipratropium	Rhinorrhea, vasomotor rhinitis	Short half-life, ineffective for sneezing and congestion
First generation oral antihistamines	Clemastine, diphenhydramine, chlorpheniramine	Sneezing, rhinorrhea, itching	Inexpensive, anticholinergic effects of drying and sedation, ineffective for congestion
Second generation oral antihistamines	Cetirizine, loratadine, fexofenadine, astemizole, terfenadine	Sneezing, rhinorrhea, itching	Expensive, less or no sedation, possibility of drug interactions causing arrhythmia with astemizole and terfenadine
Nasal antihistamines	Azelastine	Sneezing, rhinorrhea, itching, and congestion	Some apparent leukotriene blockade with therapeutic effect for chronic congestion
Nasal antiallergy	Cromolyn, nedocromil	Sneezing, rhinorrhea, itching, congestion	Low incidence of side effects, best given before allergen exposure, nedocromil still investigational for allergic rhinitis
Nasal corticosteroids	Beclomethasone, budesonide triamcinolone, flunisolide, fluticasone	Congestion, general allergy symptoms	Mucosal side effects of drying and bleeding minimized by concurrent use of nasal saline or by aqueous or powder delivery; use with caution in young and elderly patients (varicella, glaucoma)

(SSKI) is another purported mucolytic agent sometimes used in the treatment of patients with sinusitis. There are no placebo-controlled studies demonstrating efficacy of mucolytics in the management of sinusitis, although Wawrose, Tami, and Amoils documented significant improvement in nasal congestion in AIDS patients with low CD4 counts treated with guaifenisin versus placebo.[22]

Nasal saline

Likewise, no comparative studies have documented therapeutic efficacy of nasal saline in the management of sinusitis, but saline has been shown to increase mucociliary flow rates, and it has at least a brief vasoconstrictive effect. Additional goals of nasal saline are to mechanically rinse away predisposing agents such as pollen, mold, dust, and particulate air pollution. Patients with chronic sinusitis are instructed to use saline on at least a twice-daily basis as a preventative measure rather than starting when clinical symptoms manifest. Commercial preparations have the advantage of being sterile and pH neutral, but some brands contain large amounts of benzyl alcohol preservative, which may cause a burning sensation. Nasal saline, when used in conjunction with topical glucocorticoid sprays, may decrease or eliminate side effects, such as burning, drying, crusting, and bleeding, sometimes associated with those

medications. Many clinicians recommend using a dental jet irrigator system to deliver nasal saline in postoperative sinus patients or in those with refractory disease. Advantages of more forceful irrigation may be overshadowed by complications, such as septal irritation and bleeding, and by poor compliance caused by discomfort.

FUNGAL SINUSITIS

Invasive fungal disease, with rare exception, occurs in severely immunodeficient patients. Diabetic patients with ketoacidosis are at risk for developing rhinocerebral infection from fungi in the class Zygomycetes, including the genera *Mucor, Rhizopus*, and *Absidia*. The organisms favor acidic, high glucose environments, and therefore invade vessels, leading to ischemic necrosis. Profoundly neutropenic patients, after receiving a transplant or chemotherapy for malignancy, also are at risk for invasive fungal sinusitis, usually with *Aspergillus* species. The diagnosis of invasive fungal sinusitis depends on a high index of suspicion in patients with signs such as fever, nasal congestion and discharge, paresthetic facial pains, and erythema around nostrils or lower eyelids. Nasal swabs demonstrating fungal forms are highly suggestive, but diagnosis ultimately depends on biopsy results.

The management of invasive fungal sinusitis depends ultimately on reversing the diabetic ketoacidosis or improving the immune status of transplantation or cancer patients. The latter is especially difficult, accounting for the high mortality rates in these patients. Amphotericin B remains the drug of choice for those with confirmed or highly suspected invasive fungal disease with Zygomycetes or *Aspergillus* organisms. The goal in adults is to deliver 2 to 4 over 6 to 8 weeks at 0.25 to 1.0 mg/kg/day as limited by renal toxicity and side effects. Liposomal formulations increase the drug levels at sites of tissue inflammation and may allow for lower total dosing and systemic toxicity. Immunomodulation and hyperbaric oxygen also have been tried with mixed results. Surgery is important for initial diagnosis and for excision of necrotic tissue, allowing for better management efficacy of amphotericin B. It probably is not possible to obtain a true surgical margin in most patients with rhinocerebral invasive fungal diseases as a result of the spread of fungi proximally along vascular pathways (orbit and skull base) well beyond visible mucosal disease. Therefore, some clinicians advocate more conservative endoscopic serial débridement of necrotic tissue more often than radical maxillectomy with orbital exenteration.

SPECIAL CONSIDERATIONS

Acquired immunodeficiency syndrome

Patients with acquired immunodeficiency syndrome (AIDS) appear to have an increased incidence of sinusitis, although most reports are anecdotal. In addition to the usual organisms of sinusitis, AIDS patients have an increased likelihood of culturing pseudomonas and unusual organisms such as *Legionella pneumophila* and *Pneumocystis carinii*. Cases of invasive fungal sinusitis in patients with AIDS are not unusual, but the overall incidence of fungal sinusitis is unknown. Because of the wide spectrum of possible pathogens, antimicrobial therapy for treatment of sinusitis in patients with AIDS should be culture-guided whenever possible. Suspiciously ulcerated or avascular mucosa should have biopsies taken for tissue culture, histology, and fungal stain.

Patients with AIDS who have low CD4 counts may show evidence of hyper-IgE conditions, including allergic rhinitis with severe congestion and thick nasal secretions. In addition to culture-guided antibiotic therapy, management with topical corticosteroids, mucolytics, and decongestants often is helpful for congestion and rhinorrhea symptoms. Most patients respond to medical treatment, with surgery reserved for those with unusual problems such as subperiosteal orbital abscess.

The elderly population

Older patients may have less overall specific sinusitis symptoms, but they complain more of chronic postnasal discharge with congestion, throat clearing, and morning cough. First generation antihistamines are poorly tolerated in older patients because of increased anticholinergic side effects,

such as urinary retention and reduced visual accommodation. Ipratropium nasal spray may be a more appropriate alternative for those with chronic rhinorrhea, and daily saline nose spray and oral gargle may be helpful. Oral decongestants should be used with caution because of the potential for cardiovascular and central nervous system side effects.

Children

Infants are obligate nasal breathers for the first few months of life, and rhinitis of infancy therefore may present with severe respiratory distress when feeding and failure to thrive. Initial management of infantile rhinitis consists of nasal saline drops with topical corticosteroid administration (such as decadron ophthalmic 0.1% drops) reserved for severe cases. Antibiotic therapy should be based on culture; chlamydia is an infrequent but easily missed potential pathogen.

For preschool children, viral exposure is the most common predisposing condition behind a history of chronic rhinosinusitis. A vacation from a daycare center or arrangements for a smaller daycare setting often may break a cycle of recurrent upper respiratory tract disease. In addition, parents should be strongly advised to prevent exposure to cigarette smoke. Gastroesophageal reflux should be suspected in refractory patients, especially in those with a history of lower respiratory tract disease such as asthma, bronchitis, or croup.

If allergic rhinitis is suspected, environmental reduction of dust and mold exposure along with nasal cromolyn are first-line therapies. Although topical nasal corticosteroids are approved by the FDA only in those aged more than 6 years, many clinicians use them in younger patients with careful supervision for defined time intervals, usually at one half the adult dosage.

First generation antihistamines probably are more likely to lead to central nervous system effects in children and are ineffective for those with chronic congestion. Newer second generation antihistamines appear more effective with fewer side effects. In the United States, loratadine and cetirizine are approved for use in children aged 6 years and older (and for younger children in Canada).

The overall strategy in treating children with chronic rhinosinusitis is to address suspected predisposing factors starting with the least costly and invasive therapies. Most children experience spontaneous improvement in symptoms with natural maturation of systemic immunity.

Athletes

For athletes subject to drug testing, the first consideration in managing rhinosinusitis should be to avoid medications proscribed by the relevant testing authority. Commonly proscribed medications include α-agonists such as phenylephrine, ephedrine, pseudoephedrine, and systemic corticosteroids. Topical nasal corticosteroids generally are allowed with a letter from the managing physician.

Pregnancy

Increased nasal congestion caused by hormonal effects is common during pregnancy, usually starting in the second trimester. Conservative measures, such as topical nasal saline or cromolyn, should be tried first, but topical corticosteroids appear to have no teratogenic potential and have a record of safe use in pregnancy. Oral pseudoephedrine at recommended dosages appears to be safe and is widely used. The second generation antihistamines have shown no teratogenic potential in animal studies, but they are relatively new and should be used with caution.

CONCLUSION

Chronic rhinosinusitis is multifactorial, and a balanced approach aimed at likely triggers is necessary to break a cycle of recurrent disease. Patients should be educated about their risk factors to understand the process of treatment and therefore increase compliance with recommended therapies. Logically, therapeutic options should be considered along a hierarchy starting with the least difficult and most risk-free options with more intense therapeutic options added only after initial failure to improve. The therapeutic option of surgery for those with chronic sinusitis is considered last after medical options have been exhausted.

REFERENCES

1. Barbero GJ: Gastroesophageal reflux and upper airway disease, *Otolaryngol Clin North Am* 29:27, 1996.
2. Brook J, Frazier EH: Microbial dynamics of persistent purulent otitis media in children, *J Pediatr* 128:237, 1996.
3. Burns JJ and others, editors: Proceedings of a recent symposium on advances in understanding vitamin C metabolism, *Ann N Y Acad Sci*, 498, 1987.
4. Dohlman AW and others: Subacute sinusitis: are antimicrobials necessary? *J Allergy Clin Immunol* 91:1015, 1993.
5. Dykes MH, Meir P: Ascorbic acid and the common cold: evaluation of its efficacy and toxicity, *JAMA* 213:1073, 1975.
6. Garbe E and others: Inhaled and nasal glucocorticoids and the risks of ocular hypertension or open-angle glaucoma, *JAMA* 227:722, 1997.
7. Gwaltney JM Jr: Combined antiviral and antimediator treatment of rhinovirus colds, *J Infect Dis* 166:776, 1982.
8. Hayden FG, Gwaltney JM Jr: Intranasal interferon alpha-2 for prevention of rhinovirus infection and illness, *J Infect Dis* 148:543, 1983.
9. Hendley JO and others: Effect of inhalation of hot humidified air on experimental rhinovirus infection, *JAMA* 271:1112, 1994.
10. Jorres R, Nowak D, Magnussen H: Effects of ozone on airway responsiveness to inhaled allergens in subjects with allergic asthma or rhinitis, *Am J Respir Crit Care Med* 149:A154, 1994.
11. Knutsson U and others: Effects of intranasal glucocorticoids on endogenous glucocorticoid peripheral and central function, *J Endocrinol* 144:301, 1995.
12. Manning SC and others: Chronic sinusitis as a manifestation of primary immunodeficiency in adults, *Am J Rhinol* 8:29, 1994.
13. McCormick DP and others: A double-blind, placebo-controlled trial of decongestant–antihistamine for the treatment of sinusitis in children, *Clin Pediatr Phila* 35:457, 1996.
14. McCracken G: Microbiologic activity of the newer macrolide antibiotics, *Pediatr Infect Dis J* 16:432, 1997.
15. Meltzer EO: To use or not to use antihistamines in patients with asthma, *Ann Allergy* 64:183, 1990.
16. Meltzer EO and others: Azelastine nasal spray in the management of seasonal allergic rhinitis, *Ann Allergy* 72:354, 1994.
17. Meltzer EO and others: A pharmacologic continuum in the treatment of rhinorrhea: the clinician as economist, *J Allergy Clin Immunol* 95:1147, 1995.
18. Min YG and others: Paranasal sinusitis after long-term use of topical nasal decongestants, *Acta Otolaryngol Stockh* 116:465, 1996.
19. Mossad SB and others: Zinc gluconate lozenges for treating the common cold: a randomized, double-blind, placebo-controlled study, *Ann Intern Med* 125:81, 1996.
20. Pipkorn U and others: Inhibition of mediator release in allergic rhinitis by pretreatment with topical glucocorticoids, *N Engl J Med* 316:1506, 1987.
21. Turner RB, Darden PM: Effect of topical adrenergic decongestants on middle ear pressure in infants with common colds, *Pediatr Infect Dis J* 15:621, 1996.
22. Wawrose SF, Tami TA, Amoils CP: The role of guafenisin in the treatment of sinonasal disease in patients infected with the human immunodeficiency virus (HIV), *Laryngoscope* 102:1225, 1992.

Chapter 61

Primary Sinus Surgery

Jeffrey E. Terrell

Recent advances in understanding the pathophysiology of sinusitis and the importance of the ostiomeatal complex, linked with advances in endoscopic optics, instrumentation, and computed tomography (CT), have led to rapid adoption of endoscopic sinus surgery for chronic sinusitis and other disorders related to the paranasal sinuses. By no means, however, has endoscopic surgery replaced more traditional external or endonasal approaches to sinus disease. In experienced hands, each technique can be successfully performed, and in many ways the more traditional sinus surgery and endoscopic techniques complement each other. Familiarity with both techniques is advantageous.

Although the indications for each procedure may overlap, common to successful surgical outcomes for endoscopic and traditional sinus surgery is the necessity of thoroughly understanding the pathophysiology of nasal and sinus disorders before embarking on a course of medical and surgical management. Interest in the precise anatomy of the lateral nasal wall and paranasal sinuses has been rekindled by the popularization of endoscopic sinus surgery. Intimate familiarity with this anatomy, congenital and acquired variation, and key surgical landmarks is equally essential for all approaches. In this chapter, the majority of the pertinent anatomy will be reviewed in the endoscopic techniques section. Additional anatomic points will be discussed as they apply to the external sinus procedures later in the chapter.

PATHOPHYSIOLOGY OF SINUSITIS: THE OSTIOMEATAL COMPLEX

The pathophysiology of chronic sinusitis is poorly understood at a molecular or biochemical level, but CT imaging, mucociliary flow, and histopathologic studies of chronic sinusitis have shown the importance of a patent ostiomeatal complex for adequate functioning of the sinuses and clearance of infection. Proper sinus function also depends on normal cilia activity, an adequate biphasic mucous blanket, patent ostia, immunoglobin secretions, and other factors. Viral, allergic, bacterial, and other inflammatory processes that affect the sinuses often will lead to inflammation and edema of the mucosa in the region of the ostiomeatal complex. Subsequently, there is obstruction of mucociliary clearance, tissue hypoxia, mucociliary dysfunction, stasis of secretions, bacterial overgrowth, and a cycle of worsening inflammation and obstruction.[80,83,107] Chronic infections often will lead to irreversible changes in the mucosa (including polypoid degeneration) that may require surgical debridement to remove anatomic obstruction, break the inflammatory cycle, allow the mucosa to heal, and thereby enable sinus function to return to normal. Surgical therapy also may need to address underlying anatomic variants or acquired anomalies that may predispose patients to obstruction of the ostiomeatal complex, including septal deviations or spurs, concha bullosa, allergic polyps, fungal debris, or foreign bodies. Surgical therapy alone, without proper pre- and postoperative medical management of underlying comorbidities and mucosal conditions, can lead to troublesome healing and less than optimal results. Therefore, there is great emphasis on management, preoperative evaluation, patient selection, patient education and counseling, and postoperative care, and more technical surgical details.

ENDOSCOPIC SINUS SURGERY

Preoperative assessment

The preoperative evaluation, assessment, medical treatment, and counseling of patients with chronic sinusitis can be as challenging as the surgical management. A systematic method of examining patients for sinus surgery should in-

---

Box 61-1. Preoperative assessment for endoscopic sinus surgery for sinusitis

History

Recurrent acute sinusitis
Chronic sinusitis
Immune status
Comorbid conditions affecting respiratory mucosa (allergy, asthma, aspirin sensitivity, polyps, Wegener's disease, and so on)
Previous surgery, results, and complications
Comorbid medical conditions (i.e., hypertension, bleeding disorders, cardiopulmonary disease)
Eye symptoms, vision, eye surgery

Examination

Anterior rhinoscopy
Nasal endoscopy
   Nasal mucosa status (i.e., allergy, edema, polyp, crusting)
   Vestibule, valve, septum
   Inferior turbinate and meatus
   Middle turbinate and meatus: hiatus semilunaris
   Olfactory groove
   Sphenoethmoid recess, superior turbinate, and sphenoid os
   Nasopharynx
General orbital and ocular examination
Otorhinolaryngologic examination
General examination

Radiologic assessment

Coronal and axial CT scan of sinuses
Consider magnetic resonance imaging (MRI) if potential skull base bony defect or encephalocele

Patient counseling/medical decision-making

Informed consent process

Review of postoperative care

---

clude a "core" of information (Box 61-1). Successful surgery is linked to careful patient examination, selection, education, counseling, participation, and follow-up evaluation.

History

The most important factor in diagnosing chronic or recurrent acute sinusitis is the patient's history. Before surgery is considered for sinusitis, it should be readily apparent that the patient has recurring acute painful infections distinguishable from simple viral infections or chronic infections associated with purulent nasal discharge, nasal congestion, and pressure or pain.[84] Infections also may be associated with maxillary toothache, cough, hyposmia, asthma exacerbations, pharyngitis, or fatigue. Failure to respond to antibiotics

should lead the clinician to question the diagnosis and to reevaluate the patient. It is not uncommon for patients with muscle tension headaches and allergies to be diagnosed with chronic sinusitis and treated with more than one course of antibiotics. A history of nasal congestion associated with clear rhinorrhea, sneezing, itchy eyes, and aggravated by environmental allergens should prompt a more detailed allergic history, examination, workup, and treatment. If possible, allergy management should be instituted before any sinus surgery is contemplated. Patients who complain primarily of postnasal drip also should be evaluated for gastroesophageal reflux or reflux laryngitis. Nasal dryness and crusting leading to chronic bacterial nasal suprainfections with no major sinus pathology are best treated with conservative "nasal toilet," the primary component of which typically is saline sprays or irrigations.

Patients also should be questioned specifically about any asthma or wheezing associated with infections, and any reactive airway disease should be optimized before general anesthesia or surgery during local anesthesia. Patients with asthma or polyps also should be questioned about any sensitivity to aspirin or nonsteroidal antiinflammatory drugs (NSAIDs) that would suggest a diagnosis of Samters triad (asthma, aspirin sensitivity, and nasal polyps) because these patients have severe reactive airway disease and tend to have poorer long-term results with medical or surgical therapy than other patients.[21] These worse outcomes in triad asthma patients may be a result of the extent of mucosal disease at presentation. Kennedy found that when patients with triad asthma or asthma were stratified for the extent of their disease, they did not have a worse outcome than patients without aspirin intolerance or asthma.[41] Pediatric patients with nasal polyps should have a sweat chloride test to rule out cystic fibrosis. Children or young adults with recurring bronchitis, bronchiectasis, polyps, and pseudomonas sinusitis may be candidates for genetic testing for a less severe form of cystic fibrosis, which can occasionally be associated with normal sweat chloride tests.[47]

Patients who have undergone previous sinus surgery in the recent or distant past and who have failed to improve substantially also should be carefully examined to determine, as much as possible, the character of symptoms before the first surgery. Reviewing the history and the first preoperative CT scan will often provide clues of confounding factors and comorbid conditions that need to be addressed before revision surgery. Disorders such as migraine headaches, tension headaches, temporomandibular joint arthritis, dental infections, ozena, reflux, and nasal crusting should be considered because they are common masqueraders of chronic sinusitis. Any previous surgical problem such as hemorrhage, orbital complications, clear rhinorrhea suspicious for cerebrospinal fluid (CSF), infections immediately after surgery, steroid use, recurrence of polyps, or other unusual postoperative events should be recorded and appropriately addressed to avoid similar problems with revision surgery. Previous operative notes are helpful but should always be interpreted with a current CT scan if any major revision surgery is contemplated. May has reviewed several surgical landmarks and techniques that are particularly helpful for revision surgery.[66]

A general history and physical examination also should be performed with the usual emphasis on cardiac and respiratory disorders. Hypertension should be controlled to minimize intraoperative blood loss and postoperative risk of bleeding. A history of cardiac problem may influence whether cocaine or other topical decongestants or anesthetics are used. Aspirin and NSAIDs should be stopped for the appropriate length of time before surgery, and any excessive bleeding history should be investigated. Asthma treatment should be optimized; patients with poorly controlled asthma, reactive airways, steroid-dependent asthma, or other risk factors for postoperative pulmonary exacerbations are potential candidates for perioperative and postoperative steroids. These are usually given in a tapering dose schedule—for the asthma and to improve sinus mucosal healing. These patients often are observed overnight to monitor their pulmonary disease. Patients contemplating surgery on the same side as an only-seeing eye, patients who have occupations that critically depend a sense of smell or taste (e.g., chefs), or patients with other special concerns should be appropriately counseled preoperatively about these special risks.

Anatomy and examination of the nose and paranasal sinuses

The sinus surgeon should understand the endoscopic anatomy of the nose, paranasal sinuses, and surrounding structures to avoid complications, obtain better functional results, and efficiently perform sinus procedures. A review of the literature shows that the rate of complication drops off precipitously with experience.[53,101-103] The "learning curve" is not only a reflection of one's hand–eye coordination but also of one's knowledge of sinus anatomy.

The anatomy of the nose and paranasal sinuses has been well documented by several authors[5,49,86] and is important for accurate diagnostic nasal endoscopy and safe surgical interventions. The middle meatus and the ostiomeatal structures are critical areas to assess, although before the middle meatus is evaluated, the anatomy and any abnormal conditions of the external and internal nasal valves, septum, turbinates, and nasal mucosa should be carefully examined. It is not uncommon for patients to have major nasal obstruction or sinus pathology along with a deviation of the cartilaginous or bony nasal septum. Collapse of the nasal tip, external (alar) valve collapse, and internal valve collapse may be a result of weakness or deformity of the middle or lower third of the nasal structures or may be aggravated by a major septal deformity that may be easily overlooked if routine anterior rhinoscopy with a nasal speculum is not performed.

A systematic evaluation of the nasal cavity should include evaluation of all three turbinates and respective meati, the nasopharynx, the cribriform region, and the sphenoethmoid recess. Limited endoscopy can be performed to evaluate the mucosa in its natural state. Decongestant and anesthetic spray usually is applied to allow full examination of the nasal cavity in most patients with a history of sinusitis.[44] Hypertrophy of the inferior turbinate may be related to allergic rhinitis or may result from a major deviation of the septum. Previous resections of the inferior or middle turbinates should be noted because additional resections may dramatically alter air flow, cause atrophy or dryness of the nasal mucosa, and cause complaints of dryness, crusting, and nasal obstruction or ozena. A concha bullosa often will be noticeable as a wide middle turbinate that may encroach on the middle meatus. Likewise, a septal spur or deviation may obstruct the middle meatus region. Diffuse polypoid changes of the entire nasal and septal mucosa occasionally are seen and usually warrant allergy evaluation. Unilateral nasal polyps, fungiform or papillomatous lesions, and destructive or friable lesions should increase concerns about malignancy, fungal infection, or encephalocele and should trigger appropriate workup before surgical intervention. Endoscopic inspection of the posterior aspect of the nasal cavity with endoscopes should be performed to rule out antrochoanal polyps, to demonstrate any posterior mucopurulent discharge from the middle meatus or sphenoethmoid recess, and to assess the nasopharynx and adenoids for abnormality.

The middle meatus is the final common drainage pathway for the "anterior sinuses," which include the frontal, anterior ethmoid, and maxillary sinuses, and is important from a pathophysiologic standpoint. The uncinate process forms the lateral nasal wall in the middle meatus and the medial wall of the infundibulum in the ostiomeatal complex. Posterior to the uncinate process is the hiatus semilunaris, a crescent-shaped space between the uncinate process and the bulla ethmoidalis (Plate 7, A). The maxillary sinus os lies laterally within the hiatus semilunaris and may sometimes be visible with a 30° endoscope. Abnormality of the middle meatus region is commonly found in patients with chronic sinusitis and may include mucosal edema or polypoid changes of the middle turbinate, uncinate process, or bulla ethmoidalis. These anatomic changes may obstruct the middle meatus. Endoscopy also may show purulent discharge from this region or other abnormal or iatrogenic conditions to be discussed later in this chapter.

The superior turbinate and meatus sometimes are visible on office or surgical endoscopic examination if there are no major mucosal changes or anatomic deformities. The posterior ethmoid cells and sphenoid sinuses drain into the superior meatus and sphenoethmoid recess region. The superior meatus is a good landmark for the os of the sphenoid sinus, which commonly lies medial to or within the superior meatus region. Visualization of the sphenoid sinus os makes sphenoidotomy from the nasal cavity less problematic.

Visualization and palpation of the nose or orbit may show

nasal widening sometimes associated with nasal polyps, mucoceles, or other chronic sinus disease. External erythema, edema, or tenderness to palpation should be noted. A brief orbital and ophthalmologic examination should be performed. A history of unexplained visual loss, blurring, diplopia, or epiphora should prompt a more thorough ophthalmologic evaluation. Any history of serious hyposmia should be recorded. Scratch and sniff objective olfactory testing can be conducted with the University of Pennsylvania Smell Identification test.[19]

Radiographic assessment

Axial and coronal CT scanning has revolutionized the diagnosis of chronic sinusitis and sheds light on the importance of the ethmoid sinus and the ostiomeatal complex. Patients who are candidates for endoscopic sinus surgery may have had previous limited or complete CT scans for diagnostic purposes. For surgical planning, it is preferable to obtain an axial and coronal CT after maximal medical therapy has been completed to estimate the "persistent disease" that has not responded to medical therapy and to guide any surgical intervention.[44] A full sinus CT scan consists of contiguous 3-mm coronal "thin cut" CT images performed perpendicular to the hard palate and extending from the frontal sinuses through the most posterior aspect of the sphenoid sinus.[118] "Bone windows" with edge-enhancing algorithms show the fine bony structures and the overlying mucosal disease. Axial scans, typically taken as 5-mm thick images, help show the relative anatomy of the sinuses, but they are especially important in showing the relationship of the sphenoid sinus to the carotid artery and the relationship of the optic nerve to the posterior ethmoid and sphenoid sinuses.

For patients with "chronic sinusitis," the CT typically is performed after 3 to 6 weeks of adequate antibiotic treatment, steroid sprays, and other appropriate medical therapy to assess "irreversible disease" or that which has not responded to aggressive medical therapy. Any underlying allergies should be evaluated and treated before the CT scan if possible. Patients should be counseled to postpone the CT scan should they develop a condition that might cause mucosal changes on the CT, such as an allergy exacerbation or a common cold.[31] Persistent disease after medical treatment is often found in the ostiomeatal complex region on coronal CT scans and may be as subtle as a few millimeters of mucosal thickening in the infundibulum obstructing the drainage through the ostiomeatal complex, or it may be as severe as pansinus opacification.

Patients with recurrent acute sinusitis may need documentation of an acute infection radiologically if endoscopic documentation is logistically difficult. In such patients, one option is a "screening" or limited sinus CT scan as opposed to a full CT scan. If the treating physician believes the patient is likely experiencing frequent infections that may require surgery, a full CT scan that would be used as an operative guide may be cost effective. If the diagnosis is unclear and

if the CT scan is likely to "rule out" recurrent acute infection, a limited or screening sinus CT scan may be warranted.

Evaluation of the preoperative CT scan should proceed in an orderly fashion with special consideration of the "high-risk" areas for endoscopic sinus surgery, anatomic variants, and unusual findings that might change one's surgical approach.[60] The surgeon should have a systematic way of assessing the CT scans (Box 61-2). The scout film should be evaluated much the same as a lateral sinus film, with special attention to the nasopharynx, which is easily visualized from this view. The remainder of the sinuses are assessed for extent of mucosal disease (ranging from slight mucosal thickening or air fluid levels to complete sinus opacification) and for bony expansion or erosion, anatomic variants, or obstructions to mucociliary flow. Bony expansion or erosion may be caused by chronic osteitis and remodeling as a result of infection or expanding polypoid masses, but these findings also should be concerning for possible tumor, mucocele, encephalocele, or previous surgical procedures or mishaps. Such bony defects often will warrant an external approach to the sinuses to safely dissect diseased tissue from healthy periosteum of the orbit or from dura. Mucoceles may be an exception. Marsupialization of some mucoceles of the frontal, ethmoid, and sphenoid sinuses with erosion of bony barriers can be successfully managed endoscopically with minimal morbidity.[7,43,76] When benign tumors such as inverted papillomas are associated with major sinus opacification, magnetic resonance imaging (MRI) studies should be obtained to differentiate tumor from trapped secretions and to delineate any involvement of periorbita or dura.

The frontal sinus and frontal recess should be evaluated for any "frontal cells" or agger nasi cells that may narrow the nasofrontal recess and predispose the patient to chronic frontal sinus disease.[8] The anterior ethmoid cells are commonly involved with mucosal disease or polyps. Disease in this area obstructs the ostiomeatal complex and often is associated with mucosal disease of the maxillary and frontal sinuses.

The sphenoid sinus may vary considerably in the degree of pneumatization from small cells to large sinuses, with lateral extensions behind the maxillary sinus as far as the foramen lacerum. Sinus septations may be single or multiple and may insert on the posterior wall of the sphenoid sinus directly over the carotid canal rather than in the midline. CT evaluation should include any dehiscence of the walls of the sphenoid sinus, especially over the carotid canals, but also over the optic nerve region, which usually is along the superior lateral aspect of the sphenoid sinus, just posterior to the rostrum of the sphenoid. Although the posterior walls of the sphenoid sinus and the carotid canals are best seen on the axial scans, be aware that these are 5-mm thick cuts averaged to a single image. Small bony dehiscences over the carotid artery, optic nerve, or skull base may not be shown on CT scans. If there is a mass or bony erosion in the region of the sphenoid sinus, contrast should be given to rule out an

Box 61-2. Preoperative assessment of computed
tomography scan for endoscopic sinus
surgery

General

Extent of disease in paranasal sinuses
Ostiomeatal complex disease
Areas of bony expansion
Areas of bony erosion
Areas of bony dehiscence
Extent of previous surgery, status of middle and inferior
   turbinates (concha bullosa)
Septal deviation
Nasal polyposis
Nasopharyngeal disease or masses (scout film)
Foci of hyperintense signal (fungus, inspissated secre-
   tions, tumor)
General abnormalities of orbit and related structures

Maxillary sinuses

Mucosal thickening, air fluid levels
Previous surgical changes (antral windows, Caldwell-
   Luc)
Degree of development
Obstruction of infundibulum
Haller cells
Foreign bodies
Dental abnormalities

Ethmoid sinuses and OMC

Anatomy and height of fovea, cribriform plate and its
   lateral lamella
Bony dehiscences at skull base, lamina papyracea
Mucosal disease in anterior and posterior cells
Proximity of uncinate process to lamina papyracea (risk
   at incision)
Presence of Onodi cell (relative course of optic nerve)
Supraorbital ethmoid cells

Sphenoid sinuses

Extent of mucosal disease in sinus and sphenoethmoidal
   recess
Degree of development
Septations in sinus inserting over carotid artery
Course and dehiscences of optic nerve
Course and dehiscences of carotid artery
Skull base erosion

Frontal sinuses

Extent of frontal sinus aeration and disease
Bony dehiscence of anterior or posterior walls or floor
Anatomy and extent of disease at frontal recess
   Attachment of uncinate process to orbit, skull base, or
      middle turbinate
   Agger nasi cells
   Frontal cells
   Supraorbital ethmoid cells
   Ostiomas or areas of bony sclerosis at frontal recess

angiofibroma, carotid aneurysm, tumor, or encephalocele
and to help delineate the carotid canals. When there is soft
tissue on both sides of a bony defect at the skull base, an
MRI often is indicated to determine preoperatively whether
there may be a meningeoencephalocele or other intracranial
connection and to identify the carotid artery and skull base
anatomy.

The maxillary sinus also should be evaluated for the extent of pneumatization, previous Caldwell-Luc or nasal antral window procedures, dental fragments, apical root abscess, or signs of increased density on the soft tissue
windows. Areas of high attenuation can be seen commonly
when there are inspissated secretions within any sinus (commonly found in patients with pansinusitis), but they also may
be found in those with fungal infections, the most common
of which is the mycetoma or "fungus ball." Occasionally,
areas of calcification are found within tumors, especially
sarcomas. The maxillary sinus commonly has smooth,
round, mucosal retention cysts with no surrounding bony or
mucosal changes. The majority of these are not clinically
significant. It is rare that they expand enough to herniate
into the middle meatus or nasal cavity to form a symptomatic
antrochoanal polyp.

Surgical indications and considerations

Endoscopic techniques have been successfully used to
treat a variety of disorders related to the paranasal sinuses
(Box 61-3). The majority of patients undergoing endoscopic
sinus surgery have chronic sinusitis refractory to maximal
medical treatment, which should consist of antibiotics to
cover *Staphylococcus, Streptococcus, Moraxella catarrhalis,* and *Hemophilus influenza* and anaerobic bacteria.
Nasal steroid sprays are likely to assist in reducing mucosal
edema in an attempt to open the sinus ostia. Guaifenesin is
useful to thin secretions. Underlying disorders such as allergic rhinitis, rhinitis medicamentosa, or atrophic mucosal
changes should be treated as well as possible.

Patients with symptoms of chronic sinusitis generally
should have a fine cut CT scan performed after 4 or more
weeks of appropriate antibiotics. Surgical intervention
would be warranted for patients with (1) CT or endoscopic
evidence of persistent obstruction of the ostiomeatal complex or (2) persistent paranasal sinus mucosal disease after
such treatment. Endoscopic sinus surgery also is indicated
for patients with recurrent acute sinus infections, and although the decision to operate is based on a myriad of factors, a threshold of three to four infections per year is commonly used as a relative indication for surgery. Ideally, at
least one episode of acute sinusitis should be documented
by CT scan or nasal endoscopy. The decision to operate for
patients with chronic or recurrent sinusitis also may depend
on other factors, which include (1) anatomic variants that
may affect resolution of disease, (2) mucosal abnormalities,
allergic rhinitis, or cilia dysfunction, (3) triad asthma or aspirin sensitivity, (4) polypoid disease, (5) comorbidities, such

Box 61-3. Most common indications for endoscopic surgery of sinuses

Inflammatory diseases

    Chronic bacterial sinusitis
    Recurrent acute bacterial sinusitis
    Fungal sinusitis (mycetoma, allergic, fungal)
    Sinonasal polyposis
    Mucoceles of sinuses
    Antrochoanal polyp
    Occasional acute unresolving acute sinusitis

Neoplastic diseases

    Biopsy of nasal masses or tumors
    Resection of limited benign or low grade lesions (i.e., inverted papillomas)
    Tumor debulking

Orbital disorders

    Orbital decompression for Grave's ophthalmopathy
    Endoscopic primary or revision dacrycystorhinostomy
    Endoscopic optic nerve decompression

Other

    Repair of cerebrospinal fluid fistula
    Control of epistaxis
    Choanal atresia repair or revision
    Foreign body removal (nasal or sinus)

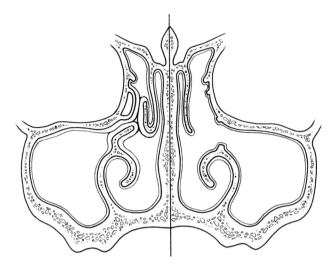

Fig. 61-1. Diseased and inflamed mucosa of the ostiomeatal complex (or anatomic abnormalities) may cause obstruction of the anterior sinuses and predispose patients to sinus infections *(left).* The goal of endoscopic surgery is to widely open the ostiomeatal complex and sinus cavities *(right)* to allow aeration of the sinuses, restoration of normal mucociliary function and proper sinus function, and in this way reduce the frequency and severity of infections.

as immunodeficiency, diabetes or renal failure, (6) unusually resistant bacterial or fungal pathogens, (7) autoimmune disease or Wegener's disease, or other relative contraindications to anesthesia or surgery. The surgical goal for recurrent acute and chronic sinusitis is to remove the anatomic and physiologic obstruction, allow better aeration, and enable the cilia to clear the sinuses (Fig. 61-1). Patients should be counseled that the goal is to lessen the frequency or severity of subsequent sinus infections and not to absolutely prevent infections.

Patients with nasal polyposis may complain of headaches, nasal obstruction, hyposmia, anosmia, recurrent or chronic sinusitis, epiphora, epistaxis, or facial pain. Large polyps may respond partially to control of infection, allergy therapy, systemic steroids, or steroid sprays, but they often will only partially resolve and recur shortly after systemic steroids are stopped. Patients with symptomatic nasal polyps after appropriate treatment are candidates for endoscopic sinus surgery. Patients with polyps not caused by infection, polyps associated with asthma, and polyps associated with aspirin sensitivity (Samter's triad) have a high risk of recurrent polypoid disease[41] and should be counseled as such and monitored closely postoperatively. Patients with aspirin sensitivity and asthma exacerbations caused by sinusitis have dramatic improvement in pulmonary functioning postopera-

tively. There should perhaps be a lower threshold for pursuing surgical therapy in such patients.[23,79]

Endoscopic biopsy of nasal masses or tumors allows for tissue diagnosis with minimal morbidity and without violation of tissue planes, which commonly occurs with external approaches to sinus malignancies. Suspicious nasal or sinus lesions are indications for endoscopic biopsy after appropriate medical and radiologic workup has been performed. Preoperative workup should rule out a distant primary tumor and identify any intracranial communication, excessive vascularity, or related structures that may be "at risk." After treatment of nasal tumors, nasal endoscopy often is an appropriate follow-up modality to survey for recurrence, especially if the sinus has been widely opened to allow for such monitoring.

Endoscopic sinus surgery for curative resection of nasal tumors is limited primarily to benign or low-grade tumors confined to the lateral nasal wall. In these limited instances, complete removal with control of margins should be performed, and the surgeon should routinely inspect one sinus beyond gross tumor to be sure margins are free of tumor. The most common tumor that is sometimes amenable to endoscopic resection is inverted papilloma.[67,106,112] Stankiewicz has recommended that endoscopic surgery only be used for "very limited" inverted papilloma involving the ethmoid sinuses, sphenoid sinuses, lateral wall of the nasal cavity, or medial wall of the maxillary sinus. Papilloma on the lamina should be débrided, and the mucosa should be drilled off to remove any hidden disease. The maxillary sinus almost always should be widely opened to visualize any tumor extending beyond the medial wall. Extension beyond the medial wall or beyond endoscopic visualization or doubt about complete resection should necessitate an external approach. Extensive papillomas should be excised through external approach(es). Patients with multiple resections and recurrence without signs of carcinoma may be candidates for endoscopic monitoring and endoscopic surgical management of local recurrence, reserving radiation therapy for patients who develop carcinoma.[106]

Malignant tumors generally necessitate external procedures for resection. Occasionally, a cancer may originate from the nasal cavity and be pedicalled on a narrow stalk, making it amenable to endoscopic resection, but this is rare.[105]

Endoscopic techniques also may be applied to ophthalmologic procedures, including orbital decompression for Grave's disease[28,71] and dacryocystorhinostomy for patients with lacrimal system obstruction.[28,69] Optic nerve decompression for traumatic indirect optic neuropathy typically is performed through traditional external or microscopic approaches, but it also has been performed endoscopically.

Patients with mucous retention cysts of the maxillary or (less commonly) other sinuses that are asymptomatic and have no suspicious radiologic features are unlikely to benefit from endoscopic surgery. Similarly, other asymptomatic areas of disease on CT scan should, in most instances, not be considered for operative intervention.[84,99]

Perioperative considerations

Before surgery, patients should be assessed for active infection, and attempts should be made to control acute infection, thereby minimizing inflammation and perioperative bleeding. Patients with large nasal polyps may benefit from a short course of steroids for several days preoperatively to shrink the polyps, decrease vascularity of the mucosa and polyps, and reduce bleeding. Patients taking long-term steroids may have more capillary fragility and more bleeding than patients taking shorter courses of steroids. Patients with asthma need to have their medications adjusted to optimize pulmonary function. Severe asthmatics, those with recent steroid use, those with active mild wheezing, and many patients with Samter's triad usually will require a perioperative bolus of steroids and often a postoperative tapering course. Bronchodilators should be used up to the time of surgery. Patients with major coronary artery disease may need special consideration before the use of topical cocaine anesthetic because cocaine may trigger coronary vasospasm. Likewise, these patients may not be good candidates for hypotensive anesthesia. Decongestant sprays, such as oxymetazoline, may be applied to the nasal mucosa preoperatively to improve visualization and vasoconstriction. Preoperative antibiotics to cover *Staphylococcus* and other common pathogens should be considered in most patients and are indicated for any patient with postoperative nasal or sinus packing to reduce the risk of toxic shock syndrome. Broader spectrum antibiotics may be indicated for patients with more severe acute infections or for those with persistent chronic infections.

Anesthesia

There are advantages to local and general anesthesia for endoscopic sinus surgery. Often, the decision depends on the patient's preference, surgeon's training and experience, and the anesthesiologist's experience with monitoring such patients.

Local anesthesia is made difficult by bleeding into the naso- and oropharynx. Once there is much blood in the pharynx, sedated patients are at increased risk of aspiration or bronchospasm. Subsequent administration of narcotics and sedatives must be limited. If patients become more anxious or uncomfortable, bleeding typically increases and may limit the procedure. Pulmonary aspiration of secretions or blood and patient anxiety also may increase the risk of an asthma exacerbation. Attention to hemostasis therefore is critical, and repeated packing of the nose or sinuses with topical anesthetic or decongestant may be necessary during the procedure. If there is extensive sinus disease, large polyps, or concern about blood triggering airway hyperreactivity, local anesthesia may not be optimal. If there are no such considerations and if the patient is likely to tolerate local anesthesia, there are several benefits. Patients can be prepared for surgery and recover from the anesthetic quickly. There is less vasodilation, and therefore there may be less bleeding than with general anesthesia.[26] Additionally, some surgeons believe that local anesthesia may be more safe because trauma to the orbital periosteum or dura is likely to be keenly felt by the patient and serve as a warning signal to the surgeon of impending danger. There have been instances of substantial intracranial and intraorbital complications with local anesthesia, and reliance on the patient's sensation is therefore not warranted. Gittelman, Jacobs, and Skorina showed that complication rates for local and general anesthesia are similar.[26]

During monitored intravenous anesthesia, the patient should be carefully watched for restlessness, confusion, or change in mental status, which may be caused by oversedation and hypoxia, anesthetic toxicity, or drug reaction. Instructing the patient to breathe deeply and delivering supplemental oxygen at 3 to 5 l/min through a nasal cannula taped at the mouth often will prevent transient hypoxia if oversedation occurs. A few deep breaths by the patient often will correct the hypoxia.

The major arguments against general anesthesia are that the patient cannot warn the surgeon of irritation to the dura or orbital periosteum and that vascular dilation caused by the anesthetic agent may be associated with greater amounts of bleeding. Preoperative application of topical decongestants, choice of anesthetic agent, and hypotensive anesthesia (systolic blood pressure < 100 mm Hg) in selected patients may decrease bleeding substantially.[9] At extubation, the surgeon should be aware of the possibility of blood in the airway triggering laryngospasm. This may be averted in most patients by carefully suctioning the hypopharynx and the judicious use of a throat pack intraoperatively and nasal packing postoperatively. If laryngospasm occurs and if positive pressure mask ventilation is attempted, there is a risk of forcing air through any dehiscence of bone into the orbit or into the intracranial cavity. Such a circumstance should be avoided if at all possible.

Local injection of 1% or 2% lidocaine with 1:100,000 or 1:200,000 epinephrine and 4% cocaine solution or crystals (3 mg/kg) can be used safely to provide local anesthesia and vasoconstriction for patients during local or general anesthesia. Cocaine is commonly applied to the middle meatus, septum, anterior ethmoid nerve, and sphenopalatine ganglion to provide anesthesia and vasoconstriction. Local anesthesia is injected at the anterior end of the middle turbinate, the attachment of the middle turbinate superiorly, and the region of the uncinate process with a 25-gauge needle or specialized endoscopic needle. The region of the sphenoethmoid recess or sphenopalatine artery also may be injected with lidocaine with epinephrine using a 25-gauge spinal needle to enhance vasoconstriction, especially if the rostrum of the sphenoid sinus is to be dissected.

Emergence from general anesthesia and extubation are associated with an increased risk of aspiration and bronchospasm. Bleeding should be under control before extubation. Additional nasal packing may be necessary if there is persistent bleeding or increased concern about bleeding. The nasopharynx and hypopharynx should be thoroughly suctioned. If patients are extubated after their airway reflexes have returned, there is less risk of aspiration, laryngospasm, and bronchospasm. In occasional patients with severe reactive airway disease, awake extubation may cause major airway irritation and bronchospasm. These patients may benefit from deep extubation, but care should be taken to assure there is minimal blood in the pharynx to trigger laryngospasm as they transition through the hyperexcitable phase during emergence from anesthesia.

ENDOSCOPIC SINUS SURGERY: ANATOMY AND TECHNIQUE

There are two common approaches to endoscopic sinus surgery: the Messerklinger anterior-to-posterior dissection, and the Wigand posterior-to-anterior dissection. Each has its advantages and disadvantages, and the endoscopic surgeon can benefit from a familiarity with each technique. Key points of the Messerklinger technique have been well described by Kennedy[40] and Stammberger.[98] The following method is primarily modeled after the Messerklinger technique but borrows several concepts from Wigand's dissection. The most important concept incorporated from the Wigand technique is that the roof of the ethmoid is most safely dissected from a posterior to anterior direction. Because the fovea and planum sphenoidale slope at a 15% angle

posteriorly and inferiorly, dissection along the roof of the ethmoid is most safely accomplished working from a posterior to anterior direction, consistently keeping the direction of ''force'' moving away from the skull base, which is ''opening up'' as one proceeds from a posterior to anterior direction. The Wigand technique also allows for opening the larger sphenoid or posterior ethmoid cells first and dissecting anteriorly along the skull base. Identification of the skull base is easier in the sphenoid and posterior ethmoid sinuses, where the cells are larger and the roof is easier to identify and follow. In the technique to be described, the anterior and posterior ethmoid cells are dissected from an anterior to posterior direction, but only along the most inferior aspect of the ethmoid sinus cells. Once the cells have been opened along the most inferior aspects, septations and disease near the roof of the ethmoid are dissected from a posterior to anterior direction as Wigand describes. In all patients, healthy-appearing mucosa is preserved wherever possible to allow faster healing and better mucociliary function.

Uncinate incision

The uncinate process is a crescent-shaped, fine bony wall lying lateral to the middle turbinate. It forms the anterior border of the hiatus semilunaris and the medial wall of the infundibulum.[100] The uncinate may vary in configuration substantially: in most patients, the majority of the uncinate lies in a sagittal plane, but it may occasionally lie in an almost coronal plane and appear like a bulla ethmoidalis cell (Plate 7, B).

The full extent of the uncinate process often can be appreciated by palpating with a curved freer to identify the demarcation between the thin mobile uncinate process and the fixed ascending process of the maxilla lying just anteriorly. The L-shaped bone is then incised with a sickle knife along the anterior edge, which is oriented in a superior to inferior direction, and the posterior limb, which is oriented in a more anterior to posterior direction (see Plate 7, B). The uncinate then is pushed medially so that the most superior aspect of the uncinate can be grasped, twisted, and removed along with any remnant pieces. If the entire uncinate process is removed, the maxillary sinus os usually is visible with a 0° endoscope (Plate 7, C), but almost certainly it can be gently found with a small curved suction or ostium seeker. If the uncinate is not entirely removed, the backbiters are needed to remove the remaining pieces, usually a more time-consuming procedure than a careful initial incision.

Special consideration should be given to related structures in this area. First, the uncinate occasionally may lie close to the medial wall of the orbit. The first cut with the sickle knife, freer, or other instrument should be made after the surgeon has carefully analyzed the CT scan to assess the proximity of the lamina. This cut should be made in such a fashion that the blade engages under the uncinate mucosa and bone, but then is moved tangentially to the uncinate so as not to penetrate the lamina. Should the lamina be penetrated, patients usually will develop mild medial lid ecchymosis and may occasionally experience significant bleeding or orbital complications. The maxillary sinus os often is opened at this point to clarify the relationship of the ethmoid cavities to the orbit and maxillary sinus. Alternatively, it can be opened after the ethmoidectomy.

Maxillary sinus os

There are many different landmarks and techniques used to make identification clear and opening of the maxillary sinus os easier. One of the general landmarks used is the relationship of the os to the middle turbinate. The os is roughly level with the inferior edge of the middle turbinate, about one third the distance from the anterior tip to the posterior end. With the sinus endoscope, the os can be visualized lying deep within the hiatus semilunaris between the uncinate process and the bulla ethmoidalis. The os is most easily identified if the uncinate is completely removed as described previously.[45] If it is not visible after the uncinate resection, a long, narrow, curved suction can be safely placed into the maxillary sinus if the surgeon observes the following caveats. First, the suction should be placed low in the hiatus semilunaris and directed with the curve facing inferiorly and laterally, so as not to penetrate the medial wall of the orbit. Second, one should watch carefully as the maxillary sinus is entered to be sure the suction enters the bony sinus and penetrates the mucosa. If the bone is penetrated but the maxillary sinus mucosa is pushed laterally, there will be a bony opening but no mucosal opening, which predisposes the os to stenosis.

Creation of a wide maxillary antrostomy will allow for easy visualization of the os postoperatively and may prevent stenosis. The "ideal" maxillary sinus os size is not known, but typically it is widened to 5 to 15 mm in diameter. Once the os is identified endoscopically, the posterior edge of the natural os (the posterior fontanelle) may be resected using straight biting forceps, taking care to open bony and mucosal surfaces and to not pull the mucosa off the posterior wall of the maxillary sinus. Once the os is partially opened, the backbiting instruments can be used to remove bone of the anterior fontanelle and any remnants of the uncinate process. Generally, the opening should not extend further forward than the anterior end of the middle turbinate. Opening further anteriorly may injure the nasolacrimal duct and cause infections or stenosis of the duct.

The infundibulum of the maxillary sinus is the funnel-like channel in the antrum leading to the maxillary sinus os. The infundibulum of the maxillary sinus may be obstructed by a large or diseased Haller cell, which is an anterior ethmoid cell lying within the maxillary sinus along the medial floor of the orbit. If this is present, the Haller cell should be removed after the os is widely opened and after the local anatomic landmarks are identified.

Anterior ethmoid cells

The bulla ethmoidalis (Plate 7, *D*) is the most constant and largest anterior ethmoid cell. It forms the posterior border of the hiatus semilunaris and therefore also is a good landmark for the maxillary sinus os. Some surgeons prefer to find the maxillary sinus ostia before removing the bulla ethmoidalis so that they have the bulla as a guide to the maxillary os.

During dissection, the bulla ethmoidalis is entered infero-medially with a suction, curette, or forceps. The anterior and inferior walls are removed carefully and traced superiorly. The superior extent of the bulla ethmoidalis usually is the roof of the ethmoid cells. This is a good landmark for the frontal recess because the bulla usually is at the posterior wall of the frontal recess. As such, it is critical that the entire superior, coronally oriented attachment of the bulla ethmoidalis be resected if there is concern about mucociliary drainage of the frontal sinus or if dissection of the frontal recess is being considered. The bulla attaches laterally to the lamina papyracea. Complete resection of this lateral aspect of the bulla improves visualization of the remainder of the ethmoid cells and facilitates dissection as it proceeds posteriorly. Occasionally, there will be another anterior ethmoid cell, the sinus lateralis, that may be located between the superior aspect of the bulla and the fovea. There may be smaller anterior ethmoid cells posterior to the bulla that need to be exenterated before reaching the basal lamella. Small septations along the roof of the anterior ethmoid cavity may make visualization of the fovea ethmoidalis difficult and complete resection of disease at the roof unsafe at this point. If so, the surgeon can return to the dissection at the fovea after it has been more easily identified in the larger posterior ethmoid cells.

Middle turbinate and basal lamella

To complete the posterior ethmoid sinus dissection, the vertical portion of the basal lamella, which is part of the middle turbinate, should be resected. The middle turbinate and basal lamella are extremely helpful landmarks for endoscopic surgery, particularly revision surgery. It is important to understand the middle turbinate anatomy (and preserve it if possible) to perform endoscopic ethmoidectomy safely and successfully. The middle turbinate and its infrastructure, the basal or ground lamella, is an approximately 4-cm long segment of the ethmoid bone slanting about 15° posteroinferiorly.

There are three main attachments of the middle turbinate and basal lamella, all important clinically in performing endoscopic surgery (Fig. 61-2). The anterior end of the middle turbinate is attached in a sagittal plane to the cribriform plate area. Trauma to this attachment risks damaging the fovea or cribriform plate with possible CSF leak and risks olfactory disturbances or intracranial injury. When the middle turbinate should be resected anteriorly, it is preferable to cut the turbinate sharply rather than to fracture or avulse it. The

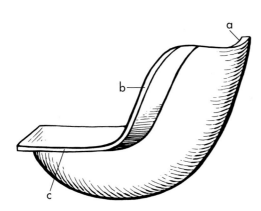

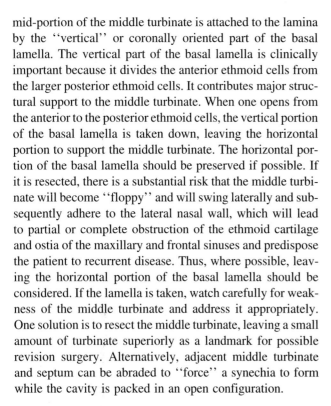

Fig. 61-2. Attachments of the right middle turbinate as viewed from under the lateral aspect of the turbinate. The middle turbinate is attached to the cribriform plate region in a sagittal plane anteriorly *(a)*, to the lamina papyracea in a coronal plane as the vertical portion of the basal lamella *(b)*, and in an axial plane to the lamina papyracea as the horizontal portion of the basal lamella *(c)*. The vertical portion of the basal lamella is taken down when passing from the anterior ethmoid cells to the posterior ethmoid cells during endoscopic ethmoidectomy, but the sagittal and axial attachments are preserved to prevent a weakened turbinate structure and potential lateralization of the turbinate.

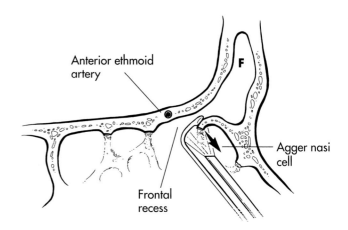

Fig. 61-3. The septations along the roof of the left ethmoid sinus are cleaned in a posterior to anterior direction with a small up-biting forceps and spoon curette until the frontal recess is found. The anterior ethmoid artery often is just posterior to the frontal recess and should not be disturbed if possible. The view of the frontal recess and frontal sinus may be obstructed by an agger nasi cell. Cleaning the roof the ethmoid sinus in a posterior to anterior direction helps to identify the frontal recess. Angled currettes can be used to safely dissect the posterior–superior wall of the agger nasi cell, working with the vector of force away from the skull base as demonstrated.

mid-portion of the middle turbinate is attached to the lamina by the ''vertical'' or coronally oriented part of the basal lamella. The vertical part of the basal lamella is clinically important because it divides the anterior ethmoid cells from the larger posterior ethmoid cells. It contributes major structural support to the middle turbinate. When one opens from the anterior to the posterior ethmoid cells, the vertical portion of the basal lamella is taken down, leaving the horizontal portion to support the middle turbinate. The horizontal portion of the basal lamella should be preserved if possible. If it is resected, there is a substantial risk that the middle turbinate will become ''floppy'' and will swing laterally and subsequently adhere to the lateral nasal wall, which will lead to partial or complete obstruction of the ethmoid cartilage and ostia of the maxillary and frontal sinuses and predispose the patient to recurrent disease. Thus, where possible, leaving the horizontal portion of the basal lamella should be considered. If the lamella is taken, watch carefully for weakness of the middle turbinate and address it appropriately. One solution is to resect the middle turbinate, leaving a small amount of turbinate superiorly as a landmark for possible revision surgery. Alternatively, adjacent middle turbinate and septum can be abraded to ''force'' a synechia to form while the cavity is packed in an open configuration.

Posterior ethmoid cells

The vertical portion of the basal lamella is entered inferomedially, away from the skull base and orbit (Plate 8, *A*). The remainder of the vertical lamella is dissected gently with

a curette, forceps, or suction, with careful attention to the location of the lamina papyracea and skull base at all times. Small septations are taken down to widely open the large posterior ethmoid cells. The possibility that the optic canal or a dehiscent optic nerve may course through the superolateral aspect of the most posterior ethmoid cell (Onodi cell) should be considered. Preoperative evaluation of the CT scan should show if there is an Onodi cell extending posterolaterally to the anterior wall of the sphenoid and whether the optic nerve courses through such a cell. Because these posterior ethmoid cells are much larger than the anterior ethmoid cells, the fovea ethmoidalis is easier to appreciate in the posterior ethmoid region. If a sphenoidotomy is not planned, the entire fovea ethmoidalis then can be cleaned of any septations by following the roof from a posterior to anterior direction, using a small spoon curette and upbiting forceps (Fig. 61-3). As the roof of the ethmoid is cleaned, the posterior or anterior ethmoid arteries may be found coursing laterally to medially across the superior aspect of the ethmoid cavity, sometimes surrounded by a thin bony wall, but occasionally suspended from a small mesentery-like bone or soft mucosal septation as much as 5 mm from the roof.[49] The posterior ethmoid artery generally is just anterior to the rostrum of the sphenoid sinus, and the anterior ethmoid artery courses across the ethmoid cells just posterior to the frontal recess. These arteries should not be traumatized if possible, but they may be cauterized with bipolar cautery if they bleed. If an ethmoid artery should retract into the orbit and continue to bleed, an external ethmoidectomy may be necessary to iden-

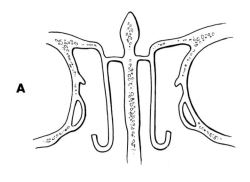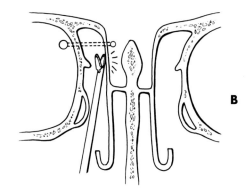

Fig. 61-4. A, The roof of the ethmoid may lie just above the cribriform plate or **B,** as many as 17 mm above the level of the cribriform plate. If this is the case, surgical resection at the roof of the ethmoid can easily result in penetration of the lateral lamella of the cribriform if the surgeon works medial to the plane of the superior attachment of the middle turbinate. Such penetration most commonly occurs where the anterior ethmoid artery crosses through the ethmoid, at which point the bone is very thin and weak.

tify and control the bleeding vessel. It should be noted that the most likely area for penetration of the intracranial cavity is where the anterior ethmoid artery passes through the lateral lamella of the cribriform plate, at which point the bone is only one tenth as thick as other areas of the fovea and cribriform plate.[39] This area also is at increased risk if the olfactory fossa is deep, if the lateral lamella of the cribriform plate is high and thin, and if the discrepancy between the level of the fovea ethmoidalis and cribriform plate is great. When removing disease at the roof of the ethmoid, it is important to stay lateral to the attachment of the middle turbinate and to avoid trauma to the region of the lateral lamella of the cribriform plate (Fig. 61-4).

The lamina papyracea forms the lateral boundary of the ethmoid sinus, dividing the ethmoid sinus from the orbital contents. Clinically, it forms a safety wall for the sinus surgeon, generally protecting the orbital contents from inadvertent trauma. As such, this wall should not be violated or removed during routine sinus procedures without good cause and great care. It is not uncommon that the lamina is naturally dehiscent, with the ethmoid sinus mucoperiosteum adjacent to the orbital periosteum. A dehiscence is of little importance, but if the periorbita is disrupted by the surgeon, there may be damage to the adjacent orbital structures: the medial rectus muscle, the ciliary nerve, the superior oblique muscle, or the optic nerve. The absence of intact lamina bone, the smooth surface of the periorbita, or the yellow glistening appearance of herniated orbital fat should alert the surgeon to the possibility of intraorbital dissection. Gentle palpation of the globe will cause the orbital contents to bulge into the sinus cavity and confirm the finding (Fig. 61-5). If there is only a small amount of fat herniation and no major orbital trauma, the dissection can proceed with care not to traumatize this area further. As the dissection proceeds ante-

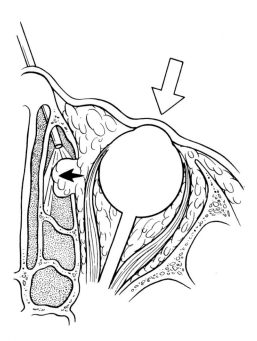

Fig. 61-5. If the surgeon is concerned about orbital penetration or sees tissue suspicious for periosteum or orbital fat, gentle palpation of the globe will cause a pulsation of the tissue in the ethmoid region and alert the surgeon to potential orbital trauma.

riorly, the surgeon may encounter an ethmoid cell in the frontal recess area, the agger nasi cell.

Agger nasi cell

The agger nasi cell is an anterior ethmoid cell lying anterior to the bulla ethmoidalis and pneumatizing the lacrimal bone region. On endoscopic examination, it is evident as a bulging of the lateral nasal wall anterior to the anterior attachment of the middle turbinate. Similarly, on the CT scan, the agger nasi cells are seen on coronal images as ethmoid cells anterior to the leading edge of the middle turbinate. If the agger nasi cells are highly pneumatized, the cells may narrow the frontal recess and predispose patients to frontal sinus disease. When agger nasi cell disease is responsible for frontal sinus disease, the agger nasi cell(s) should be resected if possible.

The posterior–superior wall of the agger nasi cell may be just below the skull base. Straight blunt penetration through this wall may risk penetration of the fovea and intracranial injury. Given this proximity to the skull base, the agger nasi cell often is best removed from a posterior to anterior direction with angled curettes, gently fracturing the wall of the cell with a spoon curette or angled probe (see Fig. 61-3). This is most safely accomplished by always keeping the vector of curettage pointing away from the skull base and orbit, pulling toward the nasal vestibule, to prevent inadvertent penetration of the orbit or cranium. The lateral wall of the agger nasi cell, the lacrimal fossa, is thin and may have dehiscences, which often can be identified by appearance or by gentle palpation of the globe. On occasion, the wall of the agger nasi cell may be so naturally thick or sclerotic from chronic infections that curettes may not be adequate for removal. In such patients, a Hejak punch or small Kerrison-like rongeurs may be used more successfully. Occasionally, such areas of thick bone can be drilled, but care should be taken to avoid trauma to the frontal recess mucosa, which could lead to stenosis and mucocele formation.

During dissection of the agger nasi cell(s) and frontal recess, it is important not to leave free bone fragments loose in the area of the frontal recess; all such pieces should be removed to prevent them from becoming sources of inflammation and obstruction.

Frontal recess and frontal sinus

The frontal recess, or nasofrontal duct as it has been commonly called, is not truly a duct but rather a space that leads to the frontal sinus ostium. Stammberger has aptly described the frontal recess as an hourglass-shaped space defined by the surrounding structures, including the middle turbinate, uncinate process, lamina papyracea, ethmoid bulla, and agger nasi cells.[99] The anatomy of the frontal recess will vary tremendously, depending on the developmental anatomy and abnormal changes of these cells leading to the frontal recess. From an anatomic and technical standpoint, the frontal recess probably is the most challenging aspect of endoscopic procedures.

Successful frontal sinus surgery requires knowledge of the local anatomy and common variants, careful review of the CT images, and precise dissection of the surrounding anatomy. This will remove cells obstructing the view of the recess and clarify landmarks that will be helpful for dissection. Preoperative evaluation of the CT scan, with particular attention to characterize the anatomy of the uncinate process

and agger nasi cells, is helpful. If the uncinate process attaches lateral to the orbit (as it does in 85% of cadavers),[110] the frontal recess will be medial to the attachment of the uncinate. If the uncinate attaches superior to the fovea or medial to the middle turbinate, the frontal recess will be lateral to the uncinate (Fig. 61-6). If the sinus is opacified on CT scan, it often is difficult to define the precise anatomy of the uncinate.

Removing all of the superior attachment of the uncinate aids in dissection of the frontal recess because remnants of the uncinate may obstruct the view of the frontal recess. Generally, the safest technique is to remove as much of the uncinate as possible at the first incision (see Plate 7, B). This can be accomplished by carrying the first sickle knife incision as far superiorly as feasible and by grasping the cut uncinate superiorly to ensure complete removal.[70] At this point in the dissection, the anterior–superior attachment of the bulla ethmoidalis already has been dissected from the roof, but if small remnants are present, they should be removed, leaving a clean smooth fovea ethmoidalis in view. The agger nasi cell, if present, will obstruct the view of the frontal recess if the cell is large. As previously discussed, the presence of an agger nasi cell usually can be anticipated preoperatively based on the CT scans or on its typical appearance as the bulge anterior to the middle turbinate in many patients. Destruction of the posterior and superior wall of the agger nasi cell as described previously often is critical to open the frontal recess. This often will present a technical challenge to the endoscopist because of the ''tight'' anatomy and risk to surrounding orbital and cranial structures. With the uncinate removed, the roof clean, and the agger nasi cells resected, the frontal recess usually is visible if there is good hemostasis. The anterior ethmoid artery typically will traverse the skull base laterally to medially just posterior to the frontal recess. It should be avoided if possible (Plate 8, B). If the recess is not visible, use of a 30° endoscope and gentle palpation of the anterior fovea region with a curved probe may lead to the recess. Failing this, the surgeon is advised to be sure there is still no remnant of agger nasi cell paralleling the fovea and blocking the recess. If present, this can be curetted carefully toward the surgeon and removed to open the recess (see Fig. 61-3). Occasionally, all these techniques fail. If the nature of the disease justifies persistent attempts, a brow incision and an external trephination of the sinus can be performed. Care should be taken to try to avoid trauma to the supratrochlear nerve during soft tissue dissection. A firm or flexible probe then can be passed through the trephination and frontal sinus into the nose to guide endoscopic dissection of the frontal recess.[35,105]

After dissection is complete, the mucosa of the frontal recess should be evaluated. Polypoid disease, postsurgical scar tissue, chronic ethmoid sinusitis, thin bone fragments, and other pathologic changes should be débrided from the recess, but normal-appearing mucosa should not be traumatized. If there is major mucosal trauma, especially circumfer-

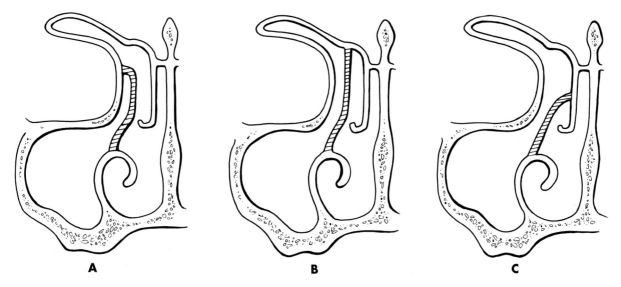

Fig. 61-6. The anatomy of the ostiomeatal complex and uncinate process. **A,** The uncinate process attaches to the lamina papyracea in 85% of cadavers. In such patients, the frontal recess will be found between the uncinate process and the middle turbinate. **B,** However, in 14% of patients the uncinate will attach to the roof of the ethmoid and **C,** in 1% of cadavers to the middle turbinate. If this is the case, the frontal recess and infundibulum are in continuity and the frontal recess will be found between the uncinate process and the lamina papyracea of the orbit.

ential trauma, or concern about stenosis of the frontal recess, a stent may be placed in the frontal recess and sinus and fixed to the septum or lateral nasal wall until the mucosalization is complete and until inflammation has resolved.[33]

In addition to the agger nasi cell, there may be other cells obstructing the view of the frontal recess and sinus. Schaeffer,[90] Van Alyea,[110] and more recently Bent and Kuhn[8] have described the "frontal cell" as one of these potential obstructions. The "frontal cell" originates from the anterior ethmoid sinus above the agger nasi cell and may obstruct the nasofrontal recess or the frontal sinus itself. Bent and Kuhn[8] have classified frontal cells by their relative position as types I to IV (Table 61-1). Type I and II cells lie above the agger nasi cells but below the floor of the frontal sinus. Clinically, these frontal cells may obstruct the frontal recess and cause disease. Type I and II cells often can be managed endonasally with endoscopes, but type III and IV cells are likely to need trephination, an endoscopic approach from above and below, or external procedure, such as an osteoplastic frontal sinus obliteration.[8] Alternatively, chronic frontal sinusitis associated with significant frontal cells may be approached externally with an osteoplastic flap obliteration.[8]

Sphenoid sinus and sphenoid os

Surgery on the sphenoid sinus poses a special problem because of the variable anatomy,[22] sometimes difficult visualization, and associated risk of serious complications from trauma to the nearby carotid artery, optic nerve, and skull base. The sphenoid sinus may vary considerably in the de-

Table 61-1. Types of frontal cells

Type I	Single frontal recess cell above agger nasi cell, but below frontal sinus
Type II	Tier of more than one cell in frontal recess above agger nasi cell, but below frontal sinus
Type III	Large single cell pneumatizing cephalad into frontal sinus
Type IV	Single isolated cell within the frontal sinus

Modified from Bent JP, Cuilty-Siller C, Kuhn FA: The frontal cell as a cause of frontal sinus obstruction, *Am J Rhinol* 8:185, 1994.

gree of pneumatization from small cells to large sinuses, with lateral extensions behind the maxillary sinus as far as the foramen lacerum. As a rough guide, the front wall of the sphenoid sinus in adults is 7 cm posterior to the nasal sill at a 30° angle. It lies just above the choana.

The sphenoid sinus can be entered through the posterior ethmoid cells or from the nasal side; the latter approach is done through the rostrum of the sphenoid or through the natural os. There are several ways to identify the sphenoid sinus os directly through the nose if it is not initially visible or if it is obstructed by disease. The os will lie about one half of the way up the front wall of the sphenoid sinus from the choana—on an average about 8 mm—but this is variable. Also, the os of the sphenoid sinus usually is located in the sphenoethmoidal recess, medial or lateral to the superior or supreme turbinate. The membranous os may be round or elliptical in shape, is less than 4 mm in diameter in more than 70% of patients, and usually is considerably smaller than the actual bony os of the sinus (Plate 8, *C*).[92] Palpation in the area of the sphenoid os with a blunt Cottle elevator often will allow one to gently and safely penetrate through the membranous os into the sinus cavity. If visualization is hampered by a large or polypoid middle turbinate, the posterior inferior aspect of the middle turbinate can be sharply cut to allow better visualization of the sphenoid rostrum. Partial resection of the middle turbinate is especially useful if there is concern that the sphenoid os will not be accessible for postoperative cleaning, is at risk for stenosis or reinfection, or is surrounded by major polypoid disease. If the posterior aspect of the middle turbinate is resected, cautery of the mucosal edges is advisable to coagulate branches of the closely related sphenopalatine artery.

The sphenoid sinuses also can be approached through the posterior medial aspect of the last ethmoid air cell. The sphenoid sinus should be entered as medially as possible, just above the horizontal portion of the basal lamella because the horizontal portion of the basal lamella is the inferior wall of the posterior ethmoid cell. If there is a question whether the surgeon has found a larger posterior ethmoid cell or the sphenoid sinus, the distance can be measured from the cell to the nasal sill and compared with a measure from the rostrum of the sphenoid to the nasal sill. If the dissection probe is in a large cell that is deeper than the distance to the rostrum of the sphenoid, the probe is in the sphenoid sinus. If there is still concern, a cross-table lateral radiograph can confirm the position of the probe. Entering the sphenoid sinus from the posterior ethmoid cells may be more difficult than approaching through the natural os or through the rostrum of the sphenoid.

Once the sphenoid sinus has been entered, the os can be widely opened using a combination of dissection forceps, Hejak forceps, or Kerrison rongeurs (Plate 8, *D*). Care should be taken to remove all small bony fragments that may cause infection or stenosis of the os. Until the sinus is widely opened and easily visualized, one should not penetrate more than a few millimeters past the anterior wall of the sinus, primarily to protect the optic canal and carotid artery from potential injury. The carotid prominence, which may be more or less noticeable with wide angle endoscopes, may have little or no significant bone coverage, and in approximately 25% of patients, there is dehiscence of bone over the artery.[99] This may be detected on axial or coronal CT scans, but the noncontiguous axial scans and the process of volume averaging of images may not show small areas of bony dehiscence. Mucosa within the sinus should be preserved if possible, and diseased mucosa that cannot be removed easily should not be avulsed. The optic canal usually courses superiorly along the lateral aspect of the sphenoid sinus, and there also may be dehiscent bone over it in 6% of patients.[4,49] Instrumentation of the posterior and lateral walls of the sphenoid sinus should be avoided to prevent trauma to the optic nerve and internal carotid artery.[25,37]

The Wigand technique

The Wigand technique[115,116] of a posterior to anterior sphenoethmoidectomy is primarily used for patients with extensive sinus disease and polyposis or for those patients undergoing revision sinus surgery when many of the surgical landmarks are unavailable.[89] In such patients, it is not unusual for the middle turbinate to be markedly distorted by chronic disease or polypoid changes or perhaps be missing as a result of previous surgical procedures. Lacking this and other typical landmarks increases the risk of intracranial and intraorbital trauma. The advantage of the Wigand technique is that the plane of the skull base is identified early in the procedure in the region of the sphenoid and posterior ethmoid cells and may be safely followed anteriorly toward the smaller and more difficult anterior cells. Early identification of the roof with this technique is helpful.

Anesthesia for the Wigand technique is much the same as other techniques and can be local or general. The procedure begins with resection of the posterior–inferior aspect of the middle turbinate to expose the rostrum of the sphenoid and the region of the sphenoid sinus os. The sphenoid sinus is entered and widely opened from the nasal side rather than through the posterior ethmoid cells, as described previously. Once the sphenoid sinus is opened, the plane of the roof of the ethmoid sinuses can be identified, and the posterior ethmoid cells are widely opened. The ethmoid dissection is accomplished with a 0° or 30° endoscope, initially clearing the inferior aspect of each cell and then cleaning small septations at the roof. Care is taken to keep the dissection lateral to the attachment of the middle turbinate to avoid trauma to the lateral lamella of the cribriform plate and potential intracranial trauma. As the dissection proceeds anteriorly, the frontal recess may be opened in the same fashion as described in the Messerklinger technique. The maxillary sinus os is identified and opened.

The disadvantages of the Wigand technique stem from the problem that the surgery cannot be tailored to treat minimal to moderate disease. In many patients, the sphenoid sinus, the posterior ethmoid, and middle turbinate do not need to be resected. Resection of the posterior–inferior portion of the middle turbinate entails resection of the horizontal and vertical portions of the basal lamella and weakens the support to the middle turbinate to the extent that it may easily scar to the lateral nasal wall and obstruct the mucociliary drainage of the frontal, maxillary, and ethmoid regions.

Postoperative care

Successful endoscopic sinus surgery depends on meticulous surgical technique and postoperative care.[72] At the end of the endoscopic sinus procedure, small loose fragments of bone and mucosa should be removed so as not to serve as foci of infection postoperatively. Packing is not necessary in the majority of patients because bleeding is minimal if there is minimal polypoid disease. Otherwise, gentle packing with any of several available materials is reasonable, particularly if the surgeon is concerned about posterior epistaxis. Lateralization of the middle turbinate is a major concern in many patients, and minor preventive measures often are successful. The author prefers to place antibiotic-saturated gelfoam packing in the ethmoid cavity and under the anterior attachment of the middle turbinate, all of which typically is removed after about 1 week.

Antibiotics are typically given postoperatively, and modified as indicated by culture results for patients with chronic active infections. Patients are instructed to avoid strenuous activity, nose blowing, and medications that may affect platelet function for 7 to 10 days. Patients with asthma, excessive intraoperative bleeding, major comorbid conditions, or difficult emergence from anesthesia may require overnight observation.

Patients typically are seen on a weekly basis for débridement of crusts and debris until mucosalization of the cavities is progressing well. If minimal mucosa is removed from the sinus cavities during the procedure, particularly the ethmoid cavities, then remucosalization and improved mucociliary flow tend to occur faster. Areas of early polypoid degeneration may warrant early débridement. Intense postoperative mucosal inflammation or polypoid changes may warrant a course of steroids. Patients with severe polypoid degeneration preoperatively may receive a planned course of postoperative steroids.

Results

Results of endoscopic sinus surgery are difficult to compare because of a lack of a well-accepted staging system to standardize evaluation of the extent of disease, the surgical results, and the patients' subjective symptom complaints. Most studies report retrospective data distinguishing between "improved," "unchanged," or "worse" patient-reported status. Nevertheless, in experienced hands, endoscopic treatment of inflammatory sinus disease is effective with rates of "improvement" at 1- to 2-year follow-up ranging from 83% to 97.5%.* About 10% to 12.5% of patients report symptoms unchanged, and 2% to 5% of patients report worse sinus symptoms after surgery.[41,58,115]

Stammberger[99] and Wigand[115] found that patients with asthma, bronchitis, or aspirin sensitivity had poorer results, with as many as 15.4% of aspirin-triad patients of Wigand's patients reporting a "worse" status after endoscopic sinus surgery. Kennedy found that results were correlated with extent of sinus disease preoperatively rather than presence or absence of asthma or aspirin sensitivity.[41]

The common observation that polypoid disease and patient symptoms can eventually recur was shown by Shaitkin, who found that endoscopic sinus surgery success rates for relieving sinus symptoms decreased over time from 98% at 9 months to 91% at 4 years.[94] Levine and May[53] and also

Lazar[51] have reported revision surgery rates of approximately 10%, typically for polyposis, adhesions, or persistent disease. This only underscores the critical need for meticulous postoperative care to minimize the recurrence of mucosal disease and the need for long-term, detailed symptom and endoscopic follow-up evaluation in reporting of surgical results.

Special problems

Septal deviation

In many patients, there may be a symptomatic or asymptomatic deviation of the nasal septum, which may have predisposed the patient to sinusitis or may make visualization and dissection of the paranasal sinuses difficult. If this is found, a septoplasty may need to be performed along with endoscopic sinus surgery. As a rule of thumb, if the surgeon, with the nasal endoscope in the office, cannot see the entire anterior attachment of the middle turbinate after decongesting the mucosa, the patient is likely to need a septoplasty—for access at the time of surgery and for access during postoperative débridement of the sinus cavities. Occasionally, a septal deviation may only obstruct access to the sphenoid recess and need correction.

The technique of septoplasty is discussed in this text. The surgeon should use the technique with which he or she is most comfortable. As much cartilage or bone as possible should be preserved. Generally, the endoscopist can perform sinus surgery on the most widely patent nasal side before performing the septoplasty. This minimizes edema and blood on the endoscopes, at least on the first side. After the septoplasty has been performed, the opposite sinuses should be easily accessible for dissection. If there is traumatized septal and nasal mucosa that might touch postoperatively and form a synechia, then a septal splint can be applied. Otherwise, a quilting stitch often can adequately approximate the mucoperichondrial flaps of the septum.

Concha bullosa

A concha bullosa (aerated middle turbinate) may be visible as a particularly wide middle turbinate and may, by its size alone, obstruct the middle meatus and ostiomeatal complex, thereby predisposing patients to sinusitis. The concha bullosa, which exists in approximately one third of patients with symptoms of chronic sinusitis, may occasionally become infected itself or form a mucocele.[119] When the concha is not large, it often can be gently crushed in a medial to lateral direction, with care not to traumatize the mucosa severely. A larger concha bullosa can be surgically resected by removing the lateral one half of the concha with a sickle knife, scissors, and forceps. Stenting and compulsive postoperative care may be necessary to prevent scarring of the remaining exposed surface to the lateral nasal wall, especially if the mucosa is taken with the lateral wall of the concha.

* Refs. 36, 41, 52, 85, 96, 99.

Lateralized middle turbinate

Occasionally during endoscopic sinus surgery, the middle turbinate will become ''floppy'' because of disruption of the coronal attachment anteriorly or axial attachment of the turbinate posteriorly. If this occurs, there is a good chance that the middle turbinate may ''lateralize'' and scar to the nasal wall in the early or late postoperative period (Plate 8, *E*). If this is recognized intraoperatively, there are several options. Resection of the middle turbinate can be performed, but the surgeon should consider leaving some superior remnant as a landmark for possible revision surgery. This remnant should be stented away from the lateral nasal wall with absorbable packing for several days postoperatively. If a weakened middle turbinate is not resected, it may be sutured to the septum to allow it to heal fused to the septum. Alternatively, the mucosa of the septum and adjacent middle turbinate can be traumatized with a sickle knife to promote such a synechia and to prevent lateralization. Again, the middle meatus should be packed to prevent tissue contact between the raw turbinate mucosal edges and the cut uncinate edges until the area is mucosalized and the risk decreased.

Mucoceles

Mucoceles of the paranasal sinuses can be managed endoscopically in many patients, but the potential for orbital or intracranial complications may be greater because the mucocele often may be associated with areas of bone dehiscence along the skull base or orbital walls.[43] For the experienced endoscopist, these mucoceles can be marsupialized while avoiding the dehiscence and ''high-risk'' areas. Careful creation of broad exposure, wide opening of the mucocele, drainage, and meticulous postoperative care to keep the mucocele open and cavity visible may obviate the need for an external procedure. Long-term endoscopic or radiologic follow-up evaluation is advisable.

Iatrogenic mucoceles, especially of the frontal sinus, may occur if the frontal recess is obstructed by a lateralized middle turbinate, scar tissue, circumferential stenosis, or bony fragments. Attentive dissection, minimally traumatic handling of the mucosa of the frontal recess, and meticulous postoperative care are critical to prevent this problematic complication.

Extensive polyposis (microdébriders)

Patients with extensive nasal polyposis often have major bony erosion of the middle turbinate, ethmoid septations, lamina papyracea, and potentially of the skull base from the chronic expansive forces or infections. This fact, coupled with the potential for major bleeding intraoperatively and limited visualization, places these patients at increased risk for intraoperative and postoperative complications. Preoperative systemic steroids may help reduce the polypoid mass, degree of inflammation, and bleeding. Polyp removal and hemostasis may be aided by the use of powered microdébrider instruments, several of which are currently available.[30,93]

Isolated sphenoid sinus disease

Isolated sphenoid sinus disease does not require complete ethmoidectomy with complete middle turbinate resection for the surgeon to gain exposure to the rostrum of the sphenoid and sphenoid sinus os. The technique of Wigand, outlined previously, can be used to approach isolated sphenoid sinus disease. The posterior–inferior portion of the middle turbinate can be excised, thereby exposing the rostrum of the sphenoid. The sphenoid sinus os then can be palpated and entered gently to allow wide opening of the front wall of the sphenoid sinus. The sphenoid sinus tends to stenose circumferentially postoperatively, so wide opening usually is indicated. If the middle turbinate lacks adequate support after partial resection, this should be addressed during primary surgery.

Complications of endoscopic sinus surgery

Minor complications of endoscopic sinus surgery occur in 2% to 21% of patients and include periorbital ecchymosis and emphysema, minor epistaxis, adhesions and stenosis of ostia, postoperative sinusitis, asthma exacerbation, and hyposmia (Box 61-4).[16,101-103] In a meta-analysis of rates of minor complications in the literature for groups of 75 or more patients, Levine and May[53] found minor complications occurring in 5.4% of 2583 patients. Major complications, which include intraorbital hemorrhage, visual loss, diplopia, intracranial injury, meningitis, brain abscess, cerebrovascular trauma, epiphora, major epistaxis, and anosmia, have been reported in 0.75% to 8% of patients.* In their meta-analysis, Levine and May[53] reported major complications occurring in 1.1% of 2583 patients undergoing endoscopic sinus surgery. These and other less common complications are listed in Box 61-4.

There is a substantial learning curve when performing endoscopic sinus surgery. Stankiewicz has commented that ''inexperienced sinus surgeons should understand that expertise is attained only through performing many surgical procedures. This includes the need for concurrent multiple cadaver dissections and instructional courses, and limited ethmoidectomy, initially, with gradual progression to extensive ethmoidectomy.''[102,103]

Initially, many surgeons use the endoscope in conjunction with or alternating with an intranasal ethmoidectomy technique using an operative headlight. Prevention of complications during endoscopic sinus surgery depends on thorough preoperative history, examination, medical management, radiologic evaluation, patient counseling, knowledge of the anatomy, surgical training and preparation, and technique.[81] Intraoperatively, complications can be minimized by carefully reviewing the CT scan (which should be available in

---

* Refs. 48, 65, 99, 101, 111, 115.

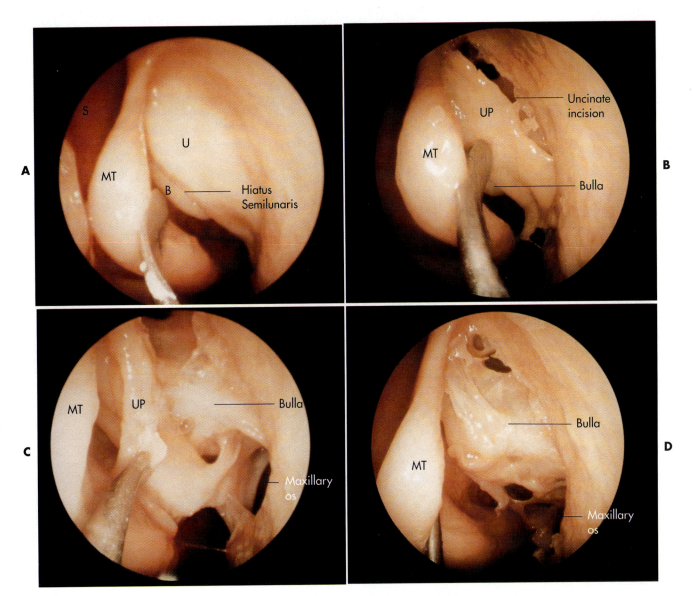

Plate 7. **A,** Endoscopic view of the left middle meatus demonstrating the uncinate process *(U)*, hiatus semilunaris through which the maxillary sinus drains, bulla ethmoidalis cell *(B)*, left middle turbinate *(MT)*, and septum *(S)*. **B,** Uncinate incision. The uncinate incision extends from the attachment of the middle turbinate inferiorly and then curves posteriorly toward the posterior fontanelle. Complete removal of the anterosuperior aspect of the uncinate is critical to provide exposure of the frontal recess. Labeled are the middle turbinate *(MT)*, uncinate process *(UP)*, and bulla ethmoidalis. **C,** The uncinate process *(UP)* has been incised and lifted with a freer to demonstrate the natural maxillary sinus os and to expose the bulla ethmoidalis cell medial to the left middle turbinate *(MT)*. **D,** Left anterior ethmoid cells and maxillary sinus after removal of the uncinate process. The bulla ethmoidalis lies posterior and superior to the maxillary sinus os. It should be opened at its inferomedial region, safely away from the skull base and orbit.

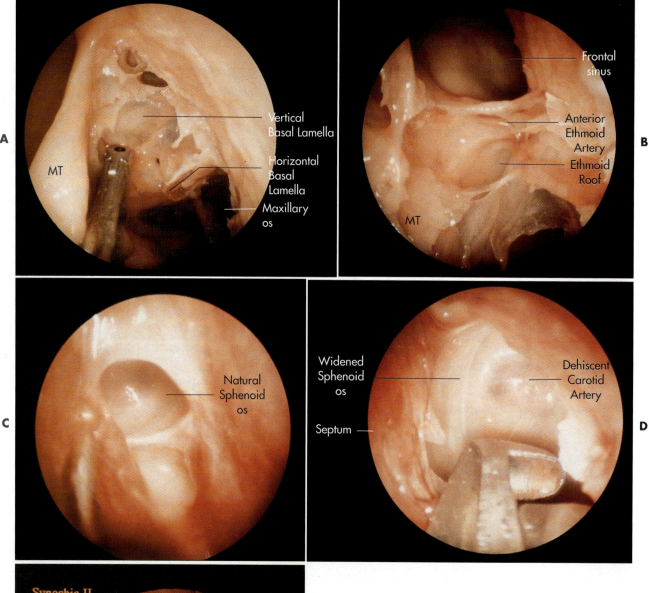

A

Vertical
Basal Lamella

MT

Horizontal
Basal
Lamella

Maxillary
os

B

Frontal
sinus

Anterior
Ethmoid
Artery

Ethmoid
Roof

MT

C

Natural
Sphenoid
os

D

Widened
Sphenoid
os

Septum

Dehiscent
Carotid
Artery

E

Synechia II

MT

S

Plate 8. **A,** The vertical portion of the left basal lamella pictured is opened inferiorly and medially to enter the posterior ethmoid cells distant from the skull base, but the horizontal portion is left intact to support the middle turbinate *(MT)*. **B,** Endoscopic view of the left frontal sinus after complete ethmoidectomy has been performed. Note the anterior ethmoid artery coursing across the skull base just posterior to the frontal sinus opening. MT—Middle turbinate. **C,** Endoscopic view of the left sphenoid os in the spheno-ethmoid recess, just medial to the posterior aspect of the superior turbinate in a cadaver. **D,** The sphenoid os is widened with a Hejak forceps. The posterior and lateral walls are not disturbed in case of a dehiscent carotid artery *(pictured)* or optic nerve. **E,** Synechiae or adhesions from the right middle turbinate to the uncinate process remnants predisposed this patient to recurrent infections postoperatively, and required revision surgery. MT—Middle turbinate; S—Septum.

Box 61-4. Complications of endoscopic sinus
surgery

Minor complications

Periorbital ecchymosis
Periorbital emphysema
Headache
Dental pain
Epistaxis (minor)
Clinically significant adhesions
Postoperative sinusitis
Hyposmia
Asthma exacerbation
Stenosis of ostia

Major complications

Orbital hematoma
Blindness
Diminished visual acuity
Diplopia
CSF leak
Major nasal hemorrhage
Intracranial hemorrhage
Meningitis
Brain abscess
Carotid artery injury
Stroke
Symptomatic epiphora
Anosmia
Focal brain trauma
Tension pneumocephalus

---

the operating room), maintaining a clear unobstructed view of the operative field and eyes and adequate vasoconstriction and hemostasis, frequent reviewing of surgical landmarks, and watching for signs of orbital trauma. Frequent examination and palpation of the orbit intraoperatively will demonstrate any defects of the lamina, in which case the orbital contents will prolapse into the ethmoid sinus cavity with gentle palpation of the globe (see Fig. 61-5).

Early recognition of orbital and intracranial complications is critical. Intraoperative or postoperative ophthalmoplegia, proptosis, ecchymosis, or relative change in pupil size may indicate intraorbital trauma or hemorrhage and warrant immediate evaluation.[15] Early consultation with an ophthalmologist is indicated. Intraorbital hemorrhage discovered *intraoperatively* should be treated by removal of nasal packing, immediate external ethmoidectomy, and orbital decompression with slitting of the periorbita to relieve pressure from the hematoma. If the hemorrhage is noted *postoperatively*, a careful ophthalmologic baseline examination (and subsequent serial examinations) should be obtained, and nasal packing should be removed, which will sometimes suffice. If visual acuity continues to deteriorate despite intravenous decadron (0.1 to 0.5 mg/kg) and Mannitol (0.5 to 1.0 mg/kg), an external ethmoidectomy for orbital decompression is indicated to control the bleeding (usually from the anterior or posterior ethmoid artery). Sudden and rapid hemorrhage into the orbit warrants immediate external ethmoidectomy and orbital decompression. A lateral canthotomy and cantholysis of the lower lid can be performed at the bedside if the patient cannot return to the operating room immediately and if vision is deteriorating.[109] Orbital massage to relieve orbital pressure transiently is controversial and contraindicated in patients with previous eye surgery such as lens implants, retinal detachment repair, or glaucoma surgery.

Postoperative diplopia may be a result of direct or indirect trauma to the extraocular muscles or cranial nerves or caused by the effects of local anesthetic. Anesthetic effects will resolve within a few hours. Nerve injury may recover in 6 to 12 months if the nerve is not severed but otherwise is treated with prisms or strabismus surgery. Muscle injury may be detected by CT scanning and typically will require ophthalmologic surgical repair, which often is difficult.

Blindness in the absence of orbital hemorrhage or increased ocular pressure may indicate direct or indirect trauma to the optic nerve, in which case the patient will have a positive Marcus Gunn pupil or ''afferent pupillary defect'' on the swinging flashlight test. Nasal packing should be removed. If there is no sustained improvement with megadose steroids, an external sphenoethmoidectomy and optic nerve decompression should be considered. The optic nerve sheath may be slit to decompress the nerve further and to drain any perineural hematoma, but this procedure is still controversial.

If there is dehiscence of, or trauma to, the medial wall of the orbit, patients should not have any positive pressure mask ventilation after extubation or surgery and should absolutely avoid nose blowing for several days postoperatively to prevent subcutaneous emphysema of the orbit. If this should occur, it will usually resolve spontaneously in about 1 week.

Obstruction of the lacrimal system resulting in epiphora may occur in the early or late postoperative period and typically is a result of trauma to the nasolacrimal duct from overresection of the anterior edge of the maxillary sinus os.[11] Many of these injuries may be asymptomatic if the tears drain into any part of the nasal cavity. This complication is unusual if the os is not widened past the anterior attachment of the middle turbinate and if any firm bone encountered on widening the os is left alone.[91]

Intracranial injury of the floor of the anterior cranial fossa may be associated with tension pneumocephalus, CSF leak, meningitis, brain hemorrhage, neurologic deficit, brain abscess, or death.[14,15,61,101-103] Penetration of the cribriform plate, lateral lamella of the cribriform plate, or the roof of the ethmoid or sphenoid cavity usually will be associated with a CSF leak, which will wash away the blood around that area of the skull base—coined the ''washout sign'' by May.[65,66] CSF leaks may tamponade themselves intraoperatively and only become evident postoperatively. Patients complaining of intermittent clear rhinorrhea (Fig. 61-7) should be carefully evaluated for CSF leak with high resolution CT scans in the axial and coronal planes to search for bony defects of encephaloceles (Fig. 61-8). Bone defects at the skull base associated with a soft-tissue mass in the sinus region should be investigated using MRI to discern any potential encephalocele herniating through the defect. In patients with rhinorrhea but no obvious site of leakage on endoscopic examination and routine imaging studies, CT cisternography may be helpful, but often such leaks are too small or intermittent to identify. Lumbar puncture and fluorescein injection into the CSF can confirm such leaks and also assist in their identification intraoperatively.[74,99] β-2 Transferrin assays also have been used to confirm CSF rhinorrhea and chloride, protein, and glucose levels, but no chemical test has ideal sensitivity, specificity, and practicality.[6]

Several authors have reported successful endoscopic repair of CSF fistulas.[18,27,32,64,104] Techniques for repair of

CSF leaks and bony defects depend on the size of the defect. Cleaning the mucosa away from a bone defect before repair is helpful to prevent trapping mucosa intracranially. Small cracks in the bone can be repaired with a free mucosal graft or a middle turbinate mucosal flap turned over to cover the defect. Bony defects smaller than 1 cm with minimal leaks can be repaired with similar mucosal grafts and packing. If the dural defect is large or the CSF leak is profuse, inserting a piece of muscle or fascia through the bone defect to plug the leak before ''patching'' with a mucosal graft may be indicated. If the bone defect is larger than 1 cm, a more solid graft should be considered. Composite septal cartilage–mucosal grafts can be fashioned to fit the defect. The dura can be gently lifted inside the bone defect, and the cartilage can be tucked through the defect. Septal or conchal cartilage grafts, turbinate bone and turbinate bone-mucosa grafts are useful. Autologous fibrin glue or single-donor fibrin glue can be used to fix the graft in place. The area then can be packed with several layers of antibiotic-coated gelfoam, followed by a nasal pack to support the graft for 7 to 14

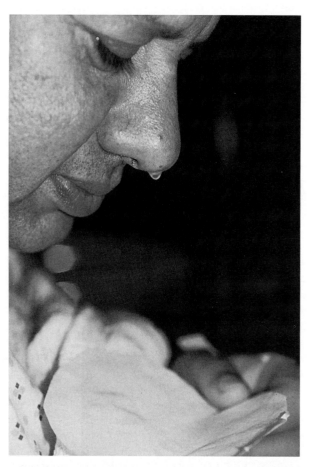

Fig. 61-7. Demonstration of active cerebrospinal fluid rhinorrhea in a patient after fluorescein injection into the intrathecal space (lumbar puncture).

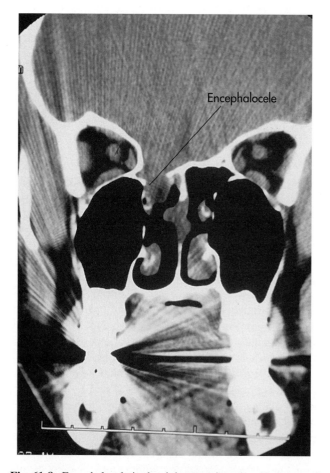

Encephalocele

Fig. 61-8. Encephalocele in the right posterior ethmoid sinus roof in a patient with a history of endoscopic sinus surgery, profuse chronic clear rhinorrhea postoperatively, and meningitis. The skull base defect is apparent.

days. Prophylactic antibiotics are controversial as a meningitis prophylaxis, but they are indicated to lessen the risk of sinusitis or toxic shock syndrome from infected packing.[1] If the patient has a major leak postoperatively, a controlled lumbar drain can be used to remove 8 to 10 ml/hour of CSF to reduce CSF pressures. Such controlled lumbar drains may be placed preoperatively or intraoperatively. Some chronic CSF fistulas may form "tracts," which seem to be more difficult to close with lumbar drainage, but small leaks noted postoperatively may close and stop with conservative management and lumbar drainage for several days. Considering the minimal morbidity of endoscopic techniques versus open or neurosurgical procedures, the success rate of endoscopic repair of CSF leaks is excellent. Dodson[18] reported a success rate of 75.9% with one procedure and 86.2% after a second procedure. He recommended endoscopic approach to CSF rhinorrhea as the preferred initial approach.

Profuse bleeding at the skull base that is difficult to control also should alert one to the possibility of intracranial vascular trauma. Bleeding from the carotid artery should be suspected if the surgeon is working deeper than 7 cm from the nasal spine in adults. The nose and sinus cavities should be promptly packed, the carotid artery compressed in the neck, and hypotensive anesthesia initiated. Neurosurgical consultation should be obtained, arteriography performed, blood transfusions readied, and balloon occlusion of the artery performed if electroencephalographic (EEG) monitoring shows no adverse events associated with a test occlusion.[37,97] Trauma at the roof of the ethmoid may result in major bleeding from the frontopolar branches of the anterior circulation and may require neurosurgical intervention. In patients in whom vascular injury is suspected, there is concern about immediate ischemia, delayed spasm of the vessel, and later aneurysm formation. Trauma near the cribriform plate also is likely to result in hyposmia, parosmia, or anosmia.

EXTERNAL SINUS SURGERY

The Caldwell-Luc procedure

Surgical treatment of chronic maxillary sinus disease has evolved over the past 100 years since the Caldwell-Luc operation was described by George Caldwell[12] in New York in 1893 and Henri Luc[57] in France in 1897. Maxillary antrostomy through the canine fossa already had been described and performed, but Caldwell and Luc developed the concept of combining the canine puncture and stripping the diseased sinus mucosa with the known technique of creating an inferior meatus antrostomy to allow a longer lasting drainage into the nose. This antrostomy also facilitated sinus irrigations and débridement of polypoid or inflammatory tissue from the sinus postoperatively. For decades after the popularization of the Caldwell-Luc procedure, debate continued over whether the antrostomy alone was sufficient and which, if any, patients with chronic inflammatory disease required a

Caldwell-Luc procedure. The inferior meatal antral windows were quick, easy to perform, and associated with minimal complications, but made wide exposure and complete stripping of the sinus mucosa difficult.[20] Yarington[117] reviewed the history of the Caldwell-Luc operation and suggested that inferior antrostomy alone was of minimal benefit and that the Caldwell-Luc procedure was preferred for patients with maxillary sinusitis refractory to medical treatment or complications of the infection. In his series of 271 patients, Yarington found a complication rate of 3% and a success rate of 90%.

Until the popularization of endoscopic sinus surgery, the Caldwell-Luc operation was the standard approach for management of maxillary sinus disease and for access to other regions of the skull base. However, as Blitzer[10] noted, the advent of endoscopic sinus surgery has decreased the frequency of the Caldwell-Luc procedure. The most common indication is still that of irreversible scarring, polypoid mucosal inflammation, and chronic inflammation associated with mucociliary dysfunction. These patients often are poor candidates for endoscopic procedures or have failed such procedures because endoscopic middle meatus antrostomy precludes stripping of the irreversibly diseased mucosa in the antrum. In those with severely diseased sinuses, after middle meatus antrostomy alone, the mucociliary function is not sufficiently improved to allow for ciliary clearance of the sinus cavity: the secretions become stagnant, inspissated, and lead to chronic infection. These patients often require stripping of the diseased mucosa through a Caldwell-Luc approach and a dependent site for drainage and irrigation of the sinus. Similarly, patients with Kartagener's syndrome and other disease of mucociliary function may be candidates for such dependent drainage of the maxillary sinus through an inferior meatus antrostomy because mucociliary function is not expected to develop to assist the sinus in clearing itself through the natural ostia. It also may be possible to accomplish such extensive surgery on the maxillary sinus through a large inferior meatus maxillary antrostomy using endoscopic techniques, but this has not been extensively reported.

In the recent past, the Caldwell-Luc approach also was commonly indicated for those with chronic maxillary sinusitis with or without irreversible mucosal disease, antral choanal polyps, sinusitis of dental etiology, foreign bodies in the maxillary sinuses (e.g., displaced tooth roots), biopsy of maxillary sinus tumors or masses, and localized cellulitis from maxillary sinusitis. Today, to a great degree, these surgical problems have been approached and treated using endoscopic techniques when the surgeon has the training and equipment available. The Caldwell-Luc approach can be used to obtain exposure for the Walsh and Ogura[113] technique of transantral decompression of the orbit for malignant Graves' ophthalmopathy. The Walsh and Ogura technique is indicated in Graves' ophthalmopathy for patients who have loss of visual acuity, corneal exposure, loss of extraocular muscle function, or major cosmetic deformity. The technique involves removal of the anterior wall of the maxilla, the orbital floor, and the lamina papyracea, coupled with serial parallel incisions in the orbital periosteum to allow herniation and decompression of the orbital contents into the maxillary and ethmoid sinuses.

The Caldwell-Luc procedure also is used as an approach for surgical procedures in the ptergomaxillary space, the most common of which are internal maxillary artery ligation for posterior epistaxis,[68,74] vidian neurectomy for severe vasomotor rhinitis,[73,75] and biopsy of lesions in the pterygopalatine fossa. This approach also is used for access to facial fractures such as trimolar fractures, orbital floor fractures, zygomatic arch fractures, and LeForte fractures—often in combination with other approaches (Box 61-5).

Patients with oroantral fistulas failing to respond to conservative medical management and local flap repair often will require a Caldwell-Luc approach to remove foreign bodies, pathologic mucosa, osteitic bone, and granulation tissue from the sinus and to allow proper drainage and ventilation of the sinus.[55] Osteoradionecrosis or osteomyelitis of the maxilla also may need to be resected through a Caldwell-Luc approach.

The Caldwell-Luc procedure can be performed during general or local anesthesia, but it is more commonly done during general anesthesia. Local injection of 1% lidocaine with 1:100,000 epinephrine is infiltrated into the gingivobuccal sulcus for anesthesia and vasoconstriction. Neurosurgical pledgets soaked with 4% cocaine are placed in the inferior meatus, middle meatus, and sphenopalatine artery region to assist with vasoconstriction, hemostasis, and local anesthesia. An incision is made in the gingivobuccal sulcus from the lateral incisor to the first or second molar (Fig. 61-9, *A*). The incision should not be so close to the gingiva that the sulcus is blunted and shallow because patients then will have difficulty wearing dentures. The periosteum is incised sharply and lifted up to and around the infraorbital nerve. The maxillary sinus is opened in the canine fossa in a controlled fashion with a cutting bur or a chisel and mallet, with care not to traumatize the infraorbital nerve, its bony canal, or its foramen with an uncontrolled fracture (Fig. 61-9, *B*). The anterior opening in the sinus then is enlarged only to the extent necessary to assess the abnormality and remove the irreversibly diseased mucosa. Normal mucosa is preserved. Dissection along the roof should be done with con-

---

Box 61-5. Indications for Caldwell-Luc procedure

Chronic maxillary sinusitis
Maxillary sinus disease refractory to endoscopic surgery
Antrochoanal polyp
Maxillary sinus foreign bodies or mycetoma
Approaches to pterygomaxillary space
    Internal maxillary artery ligation
    Vidian neurectomy
    Biopsy of skull base lesions
Trauma
    Tripod, orbital floor, zygomatic arch fractures
    LeForte fractures
Other
    Oroantral fistula
    Ostioradionecrosis or osteomyelitis of maxillary
    Orbital decompression for Grave's ophthalmology

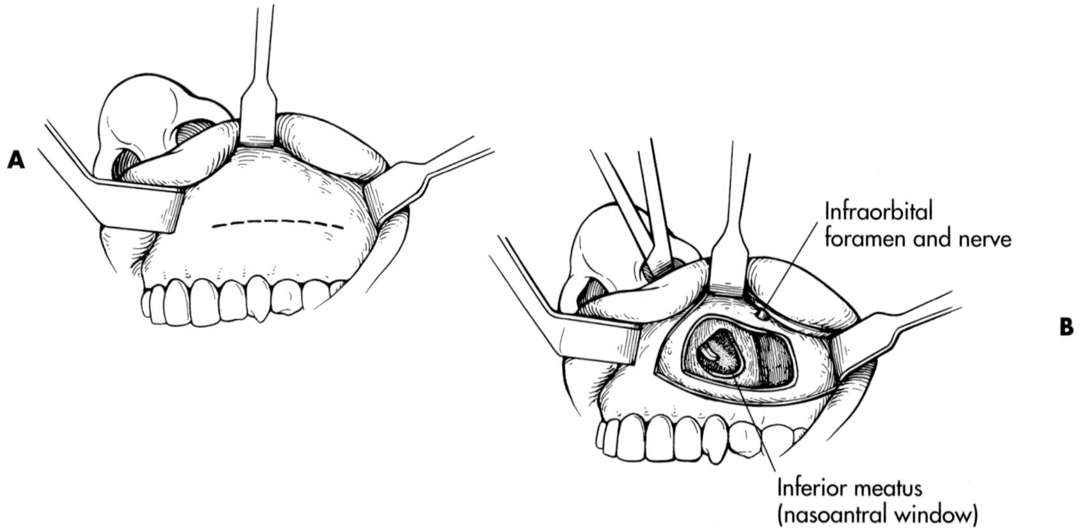

Fig. 61-9. A, The incision for Caldwell-Luc procedure, extending from lateral incisor to first or second molar. **B,** The mucosa, soft tissue, and periosteum have been lifted up to the infraorbital nerve and foramen, which is preserved. The anterior wall is opened in a controlled fashion, mucosal disease removed, and inferior (or natural) antrostomy opened.

sideration that the infraorbital nerve or floor of the orbit may have dehiscent bony coverage. A nasoantral window traditionally has been placed in the inferior meatus because these sinuses are unlikely to have effective mucociliary clearance for several months and therefore will need dependent drainage. This can be done by placing a sharp hemostat under the inferior turbinate in the nose and fracturing the bone. Subsequently, the opening should be enlarged to 1.5 to 2 cm in diameter with a Kerrison forceps. The bone may be drilled from the inferior aspect of the medial wall of the sinus to create such an opening. The preserved nasal mucosa then may be laid into the bony window to decrease the chance of stenosis. As a result of growing recognition of muciliary clearance patterns and the importance of the ostiomeatal complex, Mabry recommends placing an endoscopic middle meatus antrostomy with the Caldwell-Luc approach, a procedure he termed "anterior antrostomy with natural ostium fenestration."[59] Postoperatively, the cavity usually is left unpacked, but if there is substantial bleeding, the antrum can be packed through the inferior window with antibiotic-impregnated 1-inch gauze for 1 to 2 days. The buccal mucosa is closed with interrupted chromic sutures. Ice helps minimize swelling for the first 24 to 48 hours. Antibiotics are indicated if there are any signs of active infection. Irrigations and postoperative removal of clots and crusts are recommended.

Complications of the Caldwell-Luc approach are not insignificant (Box 61-6). DeFreitas and Lucente[17] reviewed their 10-year experience with 670 Caldwell-Luc procedures and found that 53% had complete resolution of their symptoms, 28% had continued symptoms that were responsive to medical management, and 19% had one or more persistent major complications: 12.0% had recurrent sinusitis, 9.1% facial paresthesias, 5.4% recurrent polyps, 2.6% dacryocystitis, 1.5% gingivolabial fistula, 0.7% facial asymmetry, and 0.4% devitalized tooth. Low performed a retrospective study of 185 patients who underwent 216 procedures and found that 17.5% had persistent facial pain or numbness, and 16.7% had tooth or gum pain or numbness.[56] In pediatric patients undergoing Caldwell-Luc procedures, there is concern about dental trauma. Paavolainen, Paavolainen, and

---

Box 61-6. Complications of Caldwell-Luc procedure

Hemorrhage or ecchymosis
Facial paresthesias or numbness
Persistent facial pain
Tooth or gum pain or numbness
Recurrent disease
Oroantral fistula
Dacryocystitis
Devitalized teeth
Facial asymmetry

Tarkkanen[82] found five teeth totally anesthetic as a result of nerve lesions in 3 of 30 children, but there were no instances of developmental disturbances, devitalization, or tooth loss caused by the procedure. They recommended that the "opening into the maxillary sinus should be made as high up as possible to the lateral side of the root of the canine, and the mucosa excised without damaging the bony walls of the sinuses; in addition, the inferior meatus window should not be made too anteriorly, in order to avoid lesion of the first incisor."

INTRANASAL ETHMOIDECTOMY

Indications

The indications for an endonasal ethmoidectomy are similar to those of endoscopic or external ethmoidectomy: primarily, chronic hypertrophic rhinosinusitis and nasal polyposis, sinobronchial syndrome, and recurrent acute pansinusitis. A surgeon's choice of ethmoidectomy techniques greatly depends on his or her training and experience. Although the surgeon has relatively good binocular vision during intranasal ethmoidectomy, one disadvantage of this procedure is the inability to easily visualize and remove disease from the frontal recess. The frontal recess can be more easily identified and cleaned using the angled endoscope and instruments or an external ethmoidectomy approach.

Technique

A septoplasty or submucous resection of the septum, outfracture of inferior turbinate, or in-fracture of the middle turbinate may aid in exposure of the middle meatus and ethmoid region. The nose is decongested and anesthetized in much the same fashion as for endoscopic sinus surgery, frequently using oxymetazalone spray or 4% cocaine pledgets. Middle meatus and nasal polyps are removed with forceps or snares. With the head in minimal extension, the surgeon can visualize the middle meatus, bulla, and hiatus semilunaris with a headlight. The bulla is penetrated and removed with a Takahashi or dissecting forceps. After the anterior ethmoid cells are removed, it is sometimes necessary to remove the anterior one half or two thirds of the middle turbinate to visualize the posterior ethmoid cells and sphenoid os. Removal of the most posterior portion of the middle turbinate may be associated with bleeding from branches of the sphenopalatine vessels and may require vasoconstrictor-soaked packing or gentle cautery. The posterior ethmoid is entered and cleaned with a curette. To complete the ethmoid dissection and clear the frontal recess, the roof of the ethmoid is curetted from a posterior to anterior direction, staying lateral to the attachment of the middle turbinate (to prevent trauma to the cribriform) and avoiding trauma to the fovea or lamina. The sphenoid sinus os can be entered if there is disease present, and a wide opening can be made with Kerrison forceps. Maxillary antrostomies, originally placed in the inferior meatus, are best placed in the middle meatus to widen the natural os and to promote easier physiologic drainage of the maxillary sinus. Some authors propose using the endoscope to assist with maxillary antrostomy.[40] The nasal and ethmoid cavity may be left unpacked or packed with any number of absorbable or nonabsorbable packs, depending on the surgeon's preference and extent of intraoperative bleeding. Again, cleansing of the cavity is performed during the first few postoperative weeks.

Complications of intranasal ethmoidectomy are similar to those of endoscopic or external approaches. Lawson[50] operated on a series of 1077 intranasal ethmoidectomies and reported his results for a subset of 90 patients who had two or more years of follow-up evaluation; he had an overall success rate of 73% for those 90 patients. The success rate was 88% in nonasthmatic patients but decreased to 50% in asthmatic patients. Major complications occurred in 1.1% of the 1077 patients. In this same review, Lawson noted that the complications of intranasal ethmoidectomy seem to be related to many factors, including variation of anatomy, extent of disease, previous surgery, experience of the operator, bleeding, and right-sided surgery. Freedman and Kern[24] reported a complication incidence of 2.8%, the most common of which was hemorrhage (12 of 28 patients), of which only four were orbital hematomas. They reported three exacerbations of asthma, two anxiety reactions, and one case each of meningitis, CSF leak, infraorbital neuralgia, fever, anosmia, nasolacrimal obstruction, and aspirations. Eichel[21] and Taylor[108] noted complication rates of 1.7% to 2.5%, respectively, including among both studies CSF leaks, pneumocephalus, meningitis, retroorbital hemorrhages, nasal hemorrhages requiring transfusions, and orbital injury and minor complications such as orbital ecchymosis, dental paresthesias, nasal synechiae, recurrent headache, and unwitting resection of congenital meningocele. Maniglia[62] described 11 complications of intranasal ethmoidectomy, including four cases of unilateral blindness, two cases of persistent limitations of ocular motility, three cases of CSF fistula and meningitis, one death from anterior cranial fossa cerebral trauma, and one case of carotid cavernous sinus fistula.

EXTERNAL ETHMOIDECTOMY

Technique

The external ethmoidectomy should begin with positioning the patient's head parallel to the floor, protection of the eyes with a Frost stitch or scleral shell, proper decongestant and topical anesthetic application intranasally, and 1% lidocaine with 1:100,000 epinephrine local anesthesia at the incision site. A 3-cm skin incision is made midway between the inner canthus and the dorsum of the nose and may incorporate a Z-plasty or "gull wing" type of extension to prevent webbing of the incision postoperatively (Fig. 61-10, A). The skin incision is followed by blunt dissection of the subcutaneous tissue down to the periosteum, cauterizing or tying

branches of the angular vessels as they are exposed. The periosteum incision may be larger than the skin incision to allow wider exposure of the area. Once incised, the periosteum is lifted anteriorly toward the nasal dorsum and posteriorly over the anterior and posterior lacrimal crests toward the anterior ethmoid artery, which lies in the frontoethmoid suture line approximately 24 mm from the anterior lacrimal crest. The anterior and posterior ethmoid arteries mark the level of the cribriform plate, which is the superior-most aspect of the ethmoid dissection. The anterior ethmoid cells are entered via the thin bone of the lacrimal fossa. The opening is widened anteriorly over the ascending process of the maxilla with a Kerrison rongeur and posteriorly toward the anterior ethmoid artery with a Takahashi forceps (Fig. 61-10, B). The anterior ethmoid artery can be cauterized or clipped and then divided to allow lifting of the periosteum to the posterior ethmoid artery, which lies approximately 12 mm from the anterior ethmoid artery. The posterior ethmoid artery crosses into the posterior ethmoid cells at a point just anterior to the front wall of the sphenoid sinus. It serves as a good landmark for the posterior-most ethmoid cells and the depth of the sphenoid sinus. It may be clipped or cauterized and divided if necessary, but the surgeon should recognize that the optic nerve is approximately 6 mm from this artery and may be susceptible to cautery or traction injury.

The anterior ethmoid air cells are removed with Takahashi forceps. At this point, the lateral nasal wall mucosa, anterior and inferior to the attachment of the middle turbinate, is resected, exposing the septum and middle turbinate. The posterior ethmoid air cells then are entered and removed, exposing the entire middle turbinate, which then can be sharply cut with a scissors. Bleeding from the branches of the sphenopalatine artery can be controlled with cautery or vasoconstrictor-soaked packing. If indicated, the sphenoid sinus can be entered through its natural os, and the front wall can be widely resected. The ethmoid, sphenoid, and nasal cavities usually are packed with antibiotic-impregnated gauze, and the periosteum is closed with 4-0 vicryl sutures, with care not to catch the packing in a suture. The subcutaneous soft tissue is approximated with fine absorbable suture. The skin is closed with permanent sutures or with absorbable sutures and sterile strips. Packing can be removed in stages after 2 to 4 days, and the patient discharged to home on nasal irrigations. Crusts should be gently removed over the next few weeks as healing progresses. Montgomery[74] and Neal[77] reviewed the anatomy, technique, and postoperative care in detail.

Complications

Patients undergoing external ethmoidectomy are subject to the same potential complications as with intranasal or endoscopic techniques, but major complications seem to occur less frequently. Complications more specific to external ethmoidectomy would include diplopia caused by lifting of the periosteal attachment of the trochlea. However, if the

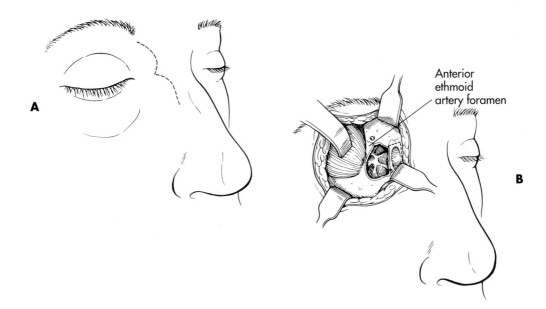

Fig. 61-10. A, The "gull wing" incision for an external ethmoidectomy to prevent webbing in the region of the medial canthus. **B,** The periosteum has been lifted anteriorly over the lateral nasal bones and posteriorly to the ethmoid arteries. The ethmoid cavity has been entered posterior to the lacrimal fossa. Bone of the lacrimal fossa and half of the lateral nasal bone are removed for better exposure of the ethmoid cavity. The anterior ethmoid artery has been cauterized and transected at the foramen. The bone over the lacrimal fossa is removed with some of the lateral nasal bone to provide wide exposure of the ethmoid cavity.

periosteum is well closed, the orbital periosteum gradually reattaches to the orbital roof, and the diplopia gradually resolves. Hypesthesia or neuralgias of the supratrochlear nerve are possible postoperatively if the incision extends too far superiorly and laterally. Webbing or hooding of the incision site near the medial canthus can be prevented by breaking up the incision intraoperatively, as described, or by W-plasty or Z-plasty repair. Penetration of the orbital periosteum with damage to neural, vascular, and muscular structures or stretch injury to the optic nerve is possible but not as likely with external ethmoidectomy, presumably because of the wide exposure and gentle retraction of orbital contents. Intracranial penetration and CSF leak are rare but potential complications that may be managed with rotation of a posteriorly based septal mucosal flap supported by transnasal packing for 5 to 7 days and with broad antibiotic coverage.[74] Minor complications including periorbital edema, supraorbital anesthesia, hemorrhage, or wound infection usually are transient but may occur in as many as 55% of patients as reported by Kimmelman.[46] Synechiae to the septum, stenosis of the sphenoid os, recurrence of disease, and enophthalmos also are potential complications.

TREPHINATION OF THE FRONTAL SINUS

Indications

Trephination of the frontal sinus is indicated for patients with acute frontal sinusitis or acute exacerbation of chronic frontal sinusitis failing to respond to appropriate deconges-

tant therapy and broad spectrum antibiotics systemically. If the patient has persistent pain and upper lid inflammation despite 48 hours of systemic treatment, if there is progression of the infectious process despite such treatment, or if there is an orbital or intracranial complication, a trephination should be considered. Occasionally, a trephination will be performed to obtain culture or biopsy of frontal sinus disease. Some authors advocate that endoscopic approach to the frontal recess be attempted to allow drainage before external incision and trephination, but extensive experience operating at the frontal recess and proper instrumentation are required, whereas the frontal sinus trephination is a relatively simple procedure.

The trephination can be performed during local or general anesthesia. The incision, which is about 2 cm in length, is located just below the medial eyebrow and is injected with lidocaine with epinephrine. After the skin incision is made, it is carried down through the periosteum of the frontal sinus floor, an area of thin bone devoid of marrow and therefore less likely to develop osteomyelitis. A 6- to 10-mm opening is made in the floor using a cutting burr. The sinus is entered, infectious material obtained for pan-cultures and sensitivities, and the sinus irrigated with an antibiotic solution. The sinus cavity can be visualized by insertion of a flexible or rigid endoscope. A singe or preferably double drainage tube system is placed through the incision before wound closure, which allows for antibiotic–saline irrigation of the sinus postoperatively while the patient receives intravenous antibiotics. When the irrigation is clearly and consistently passing through the nasofrontal recess and into the nose, the natural drainage tract is patent and the irrigation catheters or tubes can be removed.

Patients should be aware that anesthesia of the region of the supratrochlear nerve is common but does gradually lessen to some degree with time. The supraorbital nerve should be avoided but occasionally may be traumatized.

EXTERNAL FRONTOETHMOIDECTOMY (LYNCH PROCEDURE)

The external frontoethmoidectomy, popularized by Lynch[46] in 1921, is one of the most commonly performed procedures on the frontal sinus. It can be used to address unilateral isolated frontal sinus disease or can be incorporated with other procedures to treat ipsilateral pansinusitis. Common indications include chronic sinusitis, removal of osteomas and mucoceles, and biopsy or excision of tumors in the region. Because the periosteum and much of the mucosa may be left intact over bone, it is an advantageous approach for those with tumors that will require postoperative radiation therapy. The Lynch procedure is less invasive than the osteoplastic flap operation and allows the surgeon to simultaneously address ethmoid sinus disease that may be more difficult to assess and treat with the osteoplastic operation. Nevertheless, the external frontoethmoidectomy is plagued with the same problem as other external frontal sinus procedures: long-term failure rates of 20% to 30%, primarily resulting from scar tissue closure of the frontal recess with subsequent mucocele formation.

External frontoethmoidectomy is performed during general anesthesia. After a tarsorrhaphy suture has been placed and local lidocaine with epinephrine injected, a curvilinear incision is made, starting just above the caudal margin of the lateral nasal bone midway between the inner canthus and the nasal dorsum (Fig. 61-11, A). The incision is extended superiorly and laterally under the medial portion of the unshaven brow. The angular blood vessels are cauterized, and the periosteum is incised and lifted over the lacrimal fossa, lamina papyracea, and floor of the frontal sinus, thereby exposing the anterior ethmoidal artery in the frontoethmoidal suture line. A complete external ethmoidectomy is performed (see previous). The anterior ethmoidal artery can be clipped or cauterized with a bipolar cautery. The bone across the frontal recess and the medial floor of the frontal sinus is removed until the disease in the sinus can be visualized and removed. The limiting factor for this procedure is the height of the frontal sinuses. The surgeon should preserve as much mucosa as possible, especially along the frontal recess and "duct" area. The key to preventing stenosis is to assure a large drainage area by performing a complete ethmoidectomy. The frontal recess may be stented open with rolled silastic sheeting[3] (Fig. 61-11, B), and which seems to generate the least local reaction. The stent is removed after several weeks when a mucosalized tract has formed, and the patient is followed long-term for stenosis of the tract and recurrent disease.

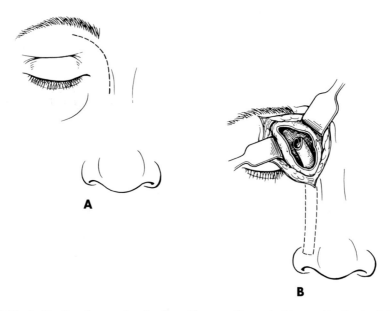

Fig. 61-11. A, The Lynch procedure begins with a curvilinear incision or "gull wing" incision, which extends under the medial brow. The incision is carried down through the periosteum. **B,** The floor of the frontal sinus and "duct" area are opened widely down through the ethmoid sinus to prevent stenosis. The enlarged duct are may be stented open with a rolled silastic sheet, which is sutured within the nasal cavity.

OSTEOPLASTIC FLAP WITH FRONTAL SINUS OBLITERATION

Indications

Open surgical procedures on the frontal sinus typically are performed for patients having chronic sinusitis with persistent symptoms despite maximal medical management, along with neoplasms or fractures. Medical management should include an adequate trial of antibiotics, decongestants, and management of underlying comorbidities and anatomic abnormalities. Conservative surgical management to be considered before frontal sinus obliteration may include frontal sinus trephination, intranasal or external ethmoidectomy, endoscopic ethmoidectomy and frontal recess exploration, and correction of underlying septal deformities or abnormal sinus "cells" in the frontal recess. Patients who have had chronic frontal sinusitis associated with orbital or intracranial complications may require an osteoplastic flap and frontal sinus obliteration after the acute infection has been controlled with systemic antibiotics or surgical drainage of the sinus. Ostiomas of the frontal sinus can be removed through an osteoplastic flap. Savic and Djeric recommended an osteoplastic approach for treatment of frontal ostiomas if they extended beyond the frontal sinus, were enlarging on serial radiologic studies, were encroaching on the region of the nasofrontal duct, or were associated with chronic sinusitis.[88] Less frequent indications include selected cases of frontal sinus fractures or fibrous dysplasia and cholesteatoma of the frontal sinus.[63]

Technique

The osteoplastic frontal sinus procedure can be approached through three potential routes: the coronal approach, a midline forehead approach, or a brow incision.[63] The coronal approach is cosmetically pleasing if the patient is not balding, but it requires more dissection and is associated with more blood loss than the other approaches. The author prefers the mid-forehead approach if the patient has forehead wrinkles that can camouflage the incision. The brow incision is cosmetically poorer than the others, especially if the patient does not wear glasses, and seems to be associated with a higher incidence of forehead pain and paresthesias. For each of these approaches, the incision site is injected with local anesthesia with epinephrine. A skin–soft tissue flap is lifted, leaving the periosteum intact and preserving the supraorbital nerves if possible. The perimeter of the frontal sinus can be identified by creating a template from a preoperative Caldwell-view radiograph of the sinus, taken from a distance of 6 feet. The frontal sinus template is gas-sterilized, and then laid over the frontal sinus with the lower edge lying along the supraorbital rim. The exact margins of the sinuses can be checked using transillumination. The periosteum is incised 0.5 to 1 cm outside the planned bone cuts and lifted just past the edges of the frontal sinuses (Fig. 61-12, *A*). The bone cuts are made with a Stryker saw blade, angling the cut into the sinus. The beveled cut allows for a safety margin to be sure that one enters the sinus rather than the cranial cavity. It also allows the bone

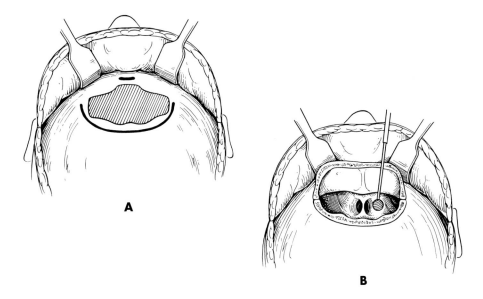

A

B

Fig. 61-12. **A,** The osteoplastic flap procedure. A bicoronal flap has been lifted. The template of the frontal sinus, cut from a 6-foot Caldwell view of the frontal sinuses, is laid over the supraorbital ridge, and periosteal cuts are made outside the template and at the nasion. **B,** The osteoplastic flap has been lifted with a sagittal saw and the mucosa stripped. The bony cavity is then drilled with cutting and diamond burrs to remove all mucosa and to create a more vascular surface area before obliteration of the duct and sinus cavity.

74. Montgomery WW: *Surgery of the upper respiratory system*, vol 1, Philadelphia, 1996, Lea & Febiger.

75. Morgenstein K: *Anatomy and surgery of the pterygopalatine fossa.* In Goldman J, editor: *Principles and practice of rhinology*, New York, 1987, Churchill Livingstone.

76. Moriyama H and others: Mucoceles of ethmoid and sphenoid sinus with visual disturbance, *Arch Otolaryngol Head Neck Surg* 118:142, 1992.

77. Neal GD: External ethmoidectomy, *Otolaryngol Clin North Am* 18: 55, 1985.

78. Neel HB III and others: Modified Lynch procedure for chronic frontal sinus diseases: rationale, technique, and long-term results, *Laryngoscope* 97:1274, 1987.

79. Nishioka GJ and others: Functional endoscopic sinus surgery in patients with chronic sinusitis and asthma, *Otolaryngol Head Neck Surg* 110:494, 1994.

80. Norlander T, Wstrin K, Stierna P: The inflammatory response of the sinus and nasal mucosa during sinusitis: implications for research and therapy, *Acta Otolaryngol (Stockh)* 515:38, 1994.

81. Ohnishi T and others: High-risk areas in endoscopic sinus surgery and prevention of complications, *Laryngoscope* 103:1181, 1993.

82. Paavolainen M, Paavolainen R, Tarkkanen J: Influence of Caldwell-Luc operation on developing permanent teeth, *Laryngoscope* 87:613, 1977.

83. Rachelefsky GS, Katz RM, Siggel SC: Chronic sinusitis in the allergic child, *Pediatr Clin North Am* 35:1091, 1988.

84. Rice D: Endoscopic sinus surgery, *Otolaryngol Head Neck Surg* 111: 100, 1994.

85. Rice DH: Endoscopic sinus surgery: results at 2-year followup, *Otolaryngol Head Neck Surg* 101:476, 1989.

86. Ritter F: *The paranasal sinuses: anatomy and surgical technique*, ed 2, St Louis, 1978, Mosby.

87. Rohrich RJ, Mickel TJ: Frontal sinus obliteration: in search of the ideal autogenous material, *Plast Reconstr Surg* 95:580, 1995 (see comments).

88. Savic DL, Djeric DR: Indications for the surgical treatment of osteomas of the frontal and ethmoid sinuses, *Clin Otolaryngol* 15:397, 1990.

89. Schaefer SD: Endoscopic total sphenoethmoidectomy, *Otolaryngol Clin North Am* 22:727, 1989.

90. Schaeffer J: The genesis, development and adult anatomy of the nasofrontal region in man, *Am J Anat* 20:125, 1916.

91. Serdahl CL, Berris CE, Chole RA: Nasolacrimal duct obstruction after endoscopic sinus surgery, *Arch Ophthalmol* 108:391, 1990.

92. Sethi DS, Stanley RE, Pillay PK: Endoscopic anatomy of the sphenoid sinus and sella turcica, *J Laryngol Otol* 109:951, 1995.

93. Setliff RC, Parsons DS: The ''Hummer'': new instrumentation for functional endoscopic sinus surgery, *Am J Rhinol* 8:275, 1994.

94. Shaitkin B and others: Endoscopic sinus surgery: 4-year follow-up on the first 100 patients, *Laryngoscope* 103:1117, 1993.

95. Shore JW and others: Enophthalmos and upper eyelid retraction following osteoplastic frontal sinusotomy, *Ophthal Plast Reconstr Surg* 3:13, 1987.

96. Smith LF, Brindley PC: Indications, evaluation, complications, and

97. Sofferman R: Complications, prevention and management—carotid artery and optic nerve injury, First International Symposium, Contemporary Sinus Surgery, Pittsburgh, 1990.

98. Stammberger H: Endoscopic endonasal surgery—concepts in treatment of recurring rhinosinusitis. Part II. Surgical technique, *Otolaryngol Head Neck Surg* 94:147, 1986.

99. Stammberger H: *Functional endoscopic sinus surgery*, St Louis, 1991, Mosby.

100. Stammberger HR, Kennedy DW: Paranasal sinuses: anatomic terminology and nomenclature. The Anatomic Terminology Group, *Ann Otol Rhinol Laryngol Suppl* 167:7, 1995.

101. Stankiewicz JA: Complications of endoscopic intranasal ethmoidectomy, *Laryngoscope* 97:1270, 1987.

102. Stankiewicz JA: Complications in endoscopic intranasal ethmoidectomy: an update, *Laryngoscope* 99:686, 1989.

103. Stankiewicz JA: Complications in endoscopic sinus surgery, *Otolaryngol Clin North Am* 22:749, 1989.

104. Stankiewicz JA: Cerebrospinal fluid fistula and endoscopic sinus surgery, *Laryngoscope* 101:250, 1991.

105. Stankiewicz JA: *Advanced endoscopic sinus surgery*, St Louis, 1995, Mosby.

106. Stankiewicz JA, Girgis SJ: Endoscopic surgical treatment of nasal and paranasal sinus inverted papilloma, *Otolaryngol Head Neck Surg* 109:988, 1993 [published erratum appears in *Otolaryngol Head Neck Surg* 110:476, 1994].

107. Sykes DA and others: Relative importance of antibiotic and improved clearance in topical treatment of chronic mucopurulent rhinosinusitis: a controlled study, *Lancet* 2:359, 1986.

108. Taylor JS, Crocker PV, Keebler JS: Intranasal ethmoidectomy and concurrent procedures, *Laryngoscope* 92:739, 1982.

109. Thompson RF and others: Orbital hemorrhage during ethmoid sinus surgery, *Otolaryngol Head Neck Surg* 102:45, 1990.

110. VanAlyea O: Frontal sinus drainage, *Ann Otol Rhinol Laryngol* 55: 267, 1946.

111. Vleming M, Middelweerd RJ, deVries N: Complications of endoscopic sinus surgery, *Arch Otolaryngol Head Neck Surg* 118:617, 1992.

112. Waitz G, Wigand ME: Results of endoscopic sinus surgery for the treatment of inverted papillomas, *Laryngoscope* 102:917, 1992 (see comments).

113. Walsh T, Ogura J: Transantral orbital decompression for malignant exophthalmos, *Laryngoscope* 67:544, 1957.

114. Ward PH, Bauknight S: Proceedings: a serious cosmetic complication of the osteoplastic frontal flap, *Arch Otolaryngol* 98:389, 1973.

115. Wigand M: *Endoscopic surgery of the paranasal sinuses and anterior skull base*, New York, 1990, Thieme.

116. Wigand ME: Transnasal ethmoidectomy under endoscopical control, *Rhinology* 19:7, 1981.

117. Yarington CT: The Caldwell-Luc operation revisited, *Ann Otol Rhinol Laryngol* 83:380, 1984.

118. Zinreich J: Imaging of inflammatory sinus disease, *Otolaryngol Clin North Am* 26:535, 1993.

119. Zinreich SJ, and others: Concha bullosa: CT evaluation, *J Comput Assist Tomogr* 12:778, 1988.

Chapter 62

Revision and Open Sinus Surgery

Neal M. Lofchy
Robert M. Bumsted

REVISION SINUS SURGERY

With the increased popularity of endoscopic sinus surgery comes an increased number of patients undergoing revision procedures. In this chapter, the management of patients requiring revision sinus surgery, including reasons for initial failure, endoscopic approaches, and open and external sinus surgery is discussed (Fig. 62-1). Although rarely done primarily in this age of fiberoptic technology, anyone performing sinus surgery should be well acquainted with nonendoscopic, external approaches to the sinuses. A description of indications, contraindications, technique, complications, and controversies surrounding these different approaches is presented.

Failure of endoscopic sinus surgery

Initially revisions were being done on patients who had undergone external or intranasal (nonendoscopic) sinus surgery, but now many endoscopic failures occur as well.[6] Surgical failures are best defined as patients who have a return or persistence of preoperative symptoms. The most common reasons for failure of endoscopic sinus surgery (ESS) are polyposis, infection, and rhinitis.[7,9,14,16]

Polyps may be diffuse and inadequately removed especially if superior and lateral in the frontal sinus. Even if adequate removal is achieved, polyps may recur in patients with underlying systemic disease. This is common in patients with asthma, acetylsalicylic acid sensitivity, and polyps ("Sampter's Triad") and allergic, cystic fibrosis, and immotile cilia patients. Recurrence of polyps from local disease often is seen when an underlying sinus infection causes inflammatory mucosal changes.

Sinus infections, as with polyps, may occur as a result of inadequate eradication of disease at the time of surgery or recurrence. Superolateral frontal sinus disease, unopened infected ethmoid and agger nasi air cells, and unopened or lateral sphenoid disease are the common reasons for incomplete removal of infection.

It is especially important to ensure complete eradication of infectious foci in patients who are immunocompromised or infected with opportunistic organisms such as tuberculosis or fungi. Infection may recur in these patients as well.

Recurrence of sinus infections may be a direct consequence of surgical technique or postoperative care resulting in poor healing. Adhesions or lateralization of a middle turbinate, stenosis of a maxillary or sphenoid ostium, and scarring of a nasofrontal duct (recess) lead to poor sinus drainage with stasis and subsequent infection. The maxillary antrum may be prone to recurrent infections if the natural ostium has not been correctly identified and cleared of disease. This often is the case when openings are created in the posterior fontanelle or inferior meatus, when an accessory ostium is mistaken for the natural ostium, or when a portion of the uncinate process remains. If this occurs, mucociliary clearance continues to be impeded.[2] Uncontrolled frontal sinus disease also may lead to persistent maxillary sinusitis.

Poorly controlled rhinitis—allergic, vasomotor, or environmental—may lead to recurrence of symptoms postoperatively. Not addressing turbinate hypertrophy with, for example, submucous resection, cryotherapy or laser photocoagulation, or an uncorrected deviated nasal septum causes persistent or recurrent nasal congestion and obstruction.

Avoidance of allergens, immunotherapy, and continued pharmacologic therapy is required in the highly allergic patient. Respiratory irritants such as cigarette smoke, exhaust

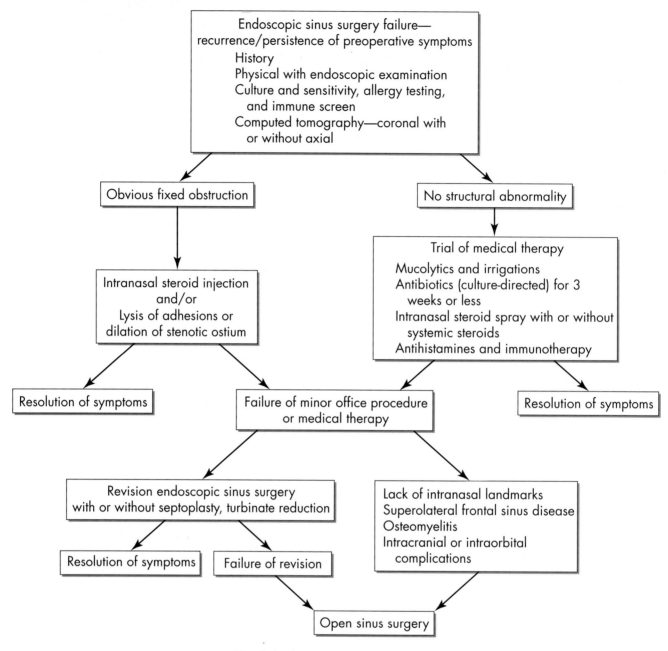

Fig. 62-1. The algorithm of management.

fumes, and chemical vapors may contribute to persistent rhinitis, as will abuse of topical vasoconstrictors.

With proper technique and close follow-up care, persistence or recurrence of symptoms may be prevented.

Management of surgical failures

When initial endoscopic sinus surgery has failed, the underlying cause should be identified. A thorough history is mandatory, and if available, a review of the operative reports, followed by a complete otolaryngologic examination, with special attention to findings on diagnostic nasal endoscopy with and without decongestion. Scarring, stenosis, ad-

hesions, lateralization of the middle turbinate, polyps, turbinate hypertrophy (reversible or fixed), a high septal deviation, and purulent drainage may be identified.

A thorough work-up for an allergic diathesis including skin end-point titration and a radioallergosorbent test (RAST) battery may be necessary if the patient's history suggests allergy and if it has not been performed preoperatively.[1]

A computed tomography (CT) scan—using coronal and possibly axial views—of the paranasal sinuses is the next step. The status of the middle turbinate, lamina papyracea, fovea ethmoidalis, and sphenoid face may be assessed, and a retained ethmoid cell or uncinate process may be discovered.

A stepwise approach to management then is undertaken. Medical treatment is attempted first, including mucolytics, irrigations, systemic antibiotics (culture-directed if possible, for at least 3 or 4 weeks), topical steroid sprays, a systemic oral steroid burst, and immunotherapy if indicated.

Minor office-based procedures

Obvious fixed obstructions noted at endoscopy often may be managed outside the operating room with local anesthetic. Simple lysis of adhesions between a lateralized middle turbinate and the lateral nasal wall may be done with topical cocaine, 4%, and injection of lidocaine, 1%, with epinephrine anesthetic in the office. A stenotic or scarred maxillary ostium or nasofrontal recess may be injected with steroid (triamcinolone 20 mg/ml) under direct endoscopic vision. This technique may be used for those with polyps not responding to topical steroid sprays.

If scarring, stenosis, or polyps do not respond to steroid injections, a minor endoscopic procedure may be performed in the office using conventional endoscopic instruments or laser technology.

Revision endoscopic sinus surgery

Indications. If mucosal disease is extensive, the revision procedure is best performed in the operating room during local anesthesia with sedation or general anesthesia with hypotension. Recurrence or persistence of polyps or sinusitis refractory to medical therapy, with return or even worsening of preoperative symptoms, are the most common indications for revision ESS. Revision often is required in children, with whom a surgeon often errs on the side of conservatism to avoid potential disruption of nasal and sinus growth. In those patients with immotile cilia and cystic fibrosis, one or many revision procedures may be expected when the initial surgery is performed on a young child.[8]

Contraindications. A thorough knowledge of paranasal sinus anatomy and endoscopic techniques and a current CT scan of the sinuses are absolute musts for any surgeon attempting revision ESS. Extensive scarring and obliteration of endoscopic landmarks may make ESS technically more challenging. The technique should be abandoned if the surgeon becomes disoriented or confused. Frontal sinus osteomas or superolateral disease usually are inaccessible endoscopically and should be approached externally. In the presence of osteomyelitis or intracranial or intraorbital complications, endoscopic approaches also should be avoided unless the surgeon has extensive experience.

Surgical technique. The patient is prepped and draped in the supine position in the reverse Trendelenburg position with the eyes left exposed and untaped after the induction of general anesthesia. Intravenous antibiotics (cefazolin, 1 g) and steroid (dexamethasone, 10 mg) are administered. Cocaine, 4%, pledgets are placed intranasally for vasocon-

striction. Intraoral injections of lidocaine, 1%, with 1 : 100,000 epinephrine into the greater palatine canals bilaterally are performed with a control syringe to achieve bilateral sphenopalatine blocks (Fig. 62-2). The same solution then is injected intranasally, under direct endoscopic vision with a 4 mm, 0° endoscope, into the middle meatus areas bilaterally.

If indicated, a septoplasty is performed to alleviate obstruction and to provide easier access to the middle meatus areas.

With careful preoperative examination of the patient endoscopically and of the CT scan, potential pitfalls and "danger areas" to avoid during surgery can be anticipated. These may include dehiscences in the fovea ethmoidalis or in the lamina papyracea with prolapse of orbital contents (seen after external ethmoidectomy).[15] It is crucial that the surgeon locate certain landmarks to keep oriented at all times and to avoid complications. The middle turbinate or its remnant is located; if absent, the anterosuperior attachment site should be identified as an arch at the posterior edge of the lacrimal bone (Fig. 62-3).[11] The maxillary ostium and floor of the orbit along with the lamina papyracea are identified next (Fig. 62-4). Staying inferior to the level of the orbital floor and lateral to the septum above the choana, the sphenoid sinus ostium may be located at a 30° angle above the floor of the nose on the anterior wall of the sinus at 7 to 7.5 cm posterior to the nasal spine of the maxilla (Fig. 62-5). Once the sphenoid is entered, dissection may proceed safely in a posterior to anterior direction using a 4 mm, 30° endoscope. The superior boundary of the dissection is the roof of the sphenoid and the contiguous fovea ethmoidalis, and the lateral boundary is the lateral wall of the sphenoid and the lamina papyracea. Retained ethmoid disease is removed, and if obstructed, the nasofrontal recess is cleared of diseased mucosa. Care is taken not to strip mucosa from the posterior wall of the nasofrontal duct, which could lead to stenosis postoperatively or anterior ethmoid artery hemmorrhage intraoperatively. A ball-tipped frontal sinus seeker may be helpful in locating the duct just behind the anterior middle turbinate attachment. A 70° endoscope may provide a better view of this area. If disease is extensive, further more aggressive frontal sinus surgery may be performed endoscopically, including drilling or curetting bone from the floor of the frontal sinus laterally and medially to the middle turbinate, nasal septum, or even through a created superior septal defect to the contralateral orbit.[5,10] Details of this technique are beyond the scope of this chapter.

If the middle turbinate has not already been resected, a decision should be made as to its fate. A concha bullosa or floppy turbinate that obstructs the middle meatus should be removed, leaving the superior one third as a surgical landmark.

Any inferior turbinate reduction—outfracturing, cryotherapy, submucous resection, cautery, or laser photocoagulation—then is performed if necessary.

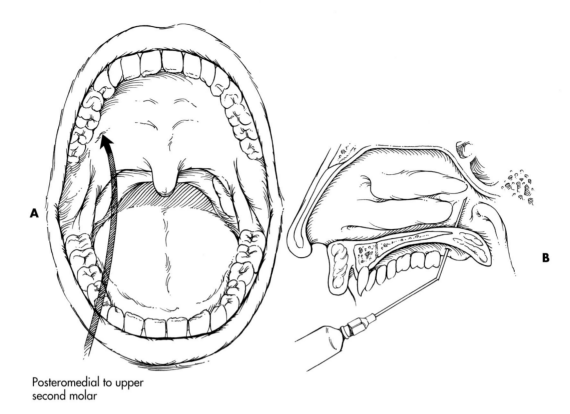

Posteromedial to upper
second molar

Fig. 62-2. The sphenopalatine nerve block. **A,** The injection is made posteromedial to the upper second molar using **B,** a 3.5″ 25-gauge spinal needle bent at a 45° angle to facilitate entry to the greater palatine canal and sphenopalatine ganglion.

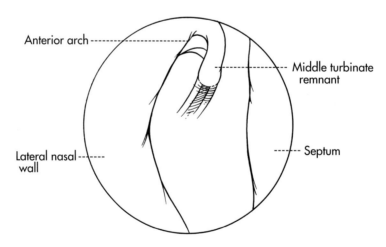

Fig. 62-3. The endoscopic view of the anterosuperior attachment of a right middle turbinate remnant—a key landmark in revision surgery.

Telfa or merocel packs with silk pull-out sutures coated with antibiotic ointment are placed into the ethmoid cavities, if required, for hemostasis. If turbinate or septal work has been done, larger packs may be used to totally occlude the nose. Packing is avoided in small children, other than a rolled Gelfilm stent to the middle meatus if necessary.

Postoperative care. In recovery, the patient is monitored for proptosis or visual changes. The patient may use ice packs on the eyes, and the head of the bed is elevated to at least 30°. Postoperative medications include antibiotics, analgesics, and a tapering dose of methylprednisolone. Nasal packs, if present, are pulled 24 to 48 hours after surgery,

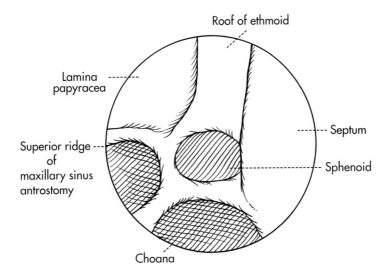

Fig. 62-4. The endoscopic view of the right middle meatus posteriorly, displaying the maxillary ostium and lamina papyracea laterally, the fovea ethmoidalis superiorly, and the sphenoid ostium posteriorly at the level of the orbital floor.

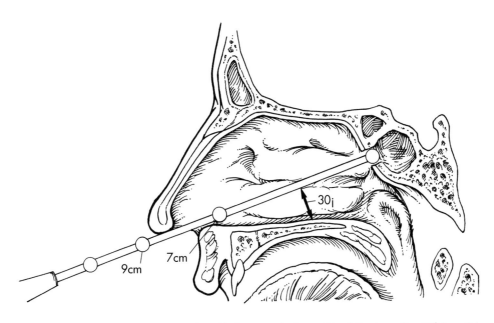

Fig. 62-5. The anterior wall of the sphenoid sinus may be located by following a line 30° from the floor of the nose 7 to 7.5 cm posterior to the maxillary nasal spine.

and any ethmoid cavity packing is removed 1 week later. Patients are given a steroid spray once all the packing has been removed. Frequent postoperative débridement is required for the first 2 or 3 months. Sterile mineral oil drops or saline nasal spray are helpful to soften crusts and make débridement easier. In children, a débridement procedure during general anesthetic is scheduled for 2 weeks after surgery.

Complications. Complications may be orbital, intracranial, vascular, or sinonasal. These complications are listed in Table 62-1. Violation of the lamina papyracea may lead to orbital complications. Intracranial complications result from damage to the fovea ethmoidalis, cribriform plate, or sphenoid sinus roof or lateral wall. A maxillary sinus ostium widened too far anteriorly may lead to nasolacrimal duct damage with resultant epiphora.

Controversies. Surgeons differ in their technique endoscopically; Messerklinger versus Wigand, posterior to anterior versus anterior to posterior, whether or not to do a sphenoidotomy in the absence of sphenoid disease, and

preservation. If floppy, pneumatized, or involved in the disease process (e.g., polypoid), the inferior two thirds should be removed, leaving the superior attachment to the cribriform plate as a future landmark.

External ethmoidectomy

This approach involves a 1- to 2-cm incision anterior to the medial canthus (''Lynch'' incision), which provides access to the ethmoid air cells for eradication of disease and creation of an ethmoid cavity.

Indications. This technique allows for direct visualization of the periorbita throughout the dissection and is excellent for management of orbital complications of suppurative disease. A list of indications can be found in Table 62-4.

Contraindications. Aside from an uncontrolled bleeding disorder or a keloid tendency, there are no absolute contraindications to this procedure.

Technique. The patient is prepped and draped in a supine position with the eyes protected with lubricating ointment and a temporary tarsorrhaphy. Cocaine, 4%, pledgets are placed intranasally within the middle meatus. Lidocaine, 1%, with 1:100,000 epinephrine solution then is infiltrated

Table 62-3. External ethmoidectomy complications

Orbital	Medial canthal ligament damage, telecanthus
	Lacrimal sac or nasolacrimal duct trauma, epiphora
	Trochlea or extraocular muscle injury, diplopia
	Retrobulbar hemorrhage or hematoma
	Optic nerve injury
	Direct globe trauma
	Blindness
Intracranial	Dural tear
	Cerebrospinal fluid leak
	Intracranial hemorrhage
	Meningitis or abscess
Sinonasal	Hemorrhage
	Crusting
	Nasofrontal recess stricture, frontal sinusitis
Facial	Supraorbital or supratrochlear nerve paresthesia
	Webbing or hypertrophic scar

Table 62-4. Indications for external ethmoidectomy

Infection	Persistent or recurrent ethmoid sinusitis, failure of endoscopic sinus surgery
Orbital	Subperiosteal or orbital abscess, hematoma
Intracranial	Cerebrospinal fluid rhinorrhea from cribriform or fovea ethmoidalis
Neoplastic	Benign tumors of ethmoid or orbit, polyps (despite endoscopic sinus surgery)
Trauma	Penetrating wounds, fractures of midface or nasoorbital-ethmoid complex
Surgical access	Frontal sinus (frontoethmoidectomy), sphenoid or pituitary

into the area of incision midway between the medial canthus and the nasal dorsum. The incision is made from the inferomedial border of the eyebrow 2 to 3 cm inferiorly in a curvilinear or W-plasty fashion (Fig. 62-7).

Hemostasis is achieved with bipolar electrocoagulation as dissection proceeds down to the level of the periosteum, which is incised and elevated using a Freer elevator. The lacrimal sac is carefully elevated from its fossa, and the frontoethmoidal suture line is identified and followed posteriorly. The anterior ethmoid artery is identified at the level of the suture line, approximately 24 mm posterior to the anterior lacrimal crest, and then is clipped or electrocoagulated and divided. The periorbita should be retracted gently (avoiding reflex bradycardia and hypotension) with a malleable retractor. If an orbital abscess is present, the periorbita is incised to allow drainage. Further posterior dissection necessitates care at the posterior ethmoid artery located about 12 mm posterior to the anterior ethmoid artery and 6 mm anterior to the optic nerve. Manipulation in this area should be avoided, if possible, to prevent damage to the optic nerve.

The ethmoid cells are entered through the lacrimal fossa or the lamina papyracea posteriorly, staying below the frontoethmoidal suture line that delineates the level of the floor of the anterior cranial fossa. The ethmoid air cells are removed with Blakesley forceps or mastoid curettes within the boundaries of the skull base superiorly, the lamina papyracea laterally, and the middle turbinate medially. The basal lamella marks the location of the large posterior cells. The middle turbinate is spared unless it is involved in the disease process. Intranasal assessment may be done through the external incision, using an endoscope if desired. The nose is packed lightly to the middle meatus, and the incision is closed in layers. In patients with purulent infection or abscess, a drain or catheter may be brought out through the incision. External drainage is rarely necessary because this procedure should provide adequate intranasal drainage of the ethmoid cells.

Postoperative care. Postoperative irrigation with normal saline may be performed through an indwelling catheter, which may be removed when irrigations become clear (nonproductive). Visual acuity and extraocular muscle movements are tested routinely. Wound care with hydrogen peroxide and topical antibiotic ointment is recommended at least three times daily. The packing and sutures may be removed together 5 or 6 days after surgery. Ice packs, head of bed elevation, antibiotics, and intranasal saline spray are routine.

Complications. Complications are listed in Table 62-3. Complications specific to external ethmoidectomy include medial canthal ligament damage resulting in blunting and telecanthus, trochlea injury resulting in diplopia, supraorbital or supratrochlear nerve damage, and hypertrophic scarring or webbing of the incision.

Controversies. Although the classic external ethmoidectomy incision is curvilinear, scar contracture and webbing may be avoided if a W-plasty incision is used. Posterior ethmoid artery ligation or manipulation is rarely indicated and should be avoided. The fate of the middle turbinate is the source of ongoing debates. The authors' philosophy remains the same for all ethmoidal surgery.

Sphenoid sinus

Many open approaches to the sphenoid sinus are described depending on the indication and exposure required (Table 62-5). The following discussion will be confined to external approaches for inflammatory sphenoid sinus disease; the remaining approaches are beyond the scope of this chapter.

Table 62-5. Surgical approaches to the sphenoid sinus

Indication	Route	Incision
Pituitary access	Transseptal	Sublabial
		External rhinoplasty
		Hemitransfixion or Killian
Inflammatory disease	Endoscopic	Sphenoidotomy
	Intranasal	Sphenoidotomy
	Transethmoid	Caldwell-Luc (antral), external ethmoid
Tumor	Transpalatal	Midline, bipedicle, S-shaped

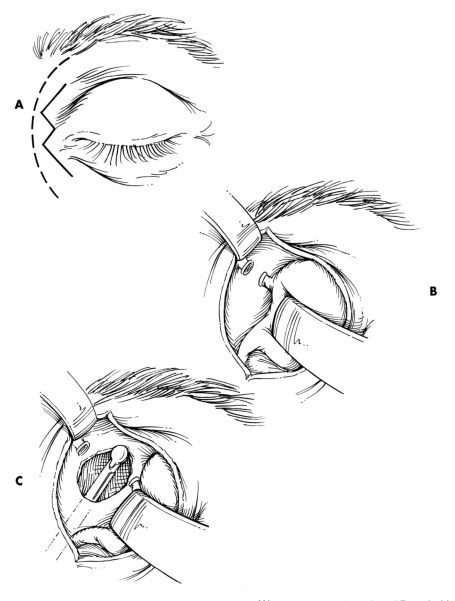

Fig. 62-7. External ethmoidectomy. **A,** A curvilinear or W-plasty incision is made and **B,** periorbita retracted laterally revealing the anterior and posterior ethmoidal arteries at the frontoethmoidal suture line. **C,** Ethmoids are entered via the lacrimal fossa and lamina papyracea and exenterated with a curette or forceps.

External transethmoidal sphenoidotomy

This approach is an extension of the external ethmoidectomy described previously with exenteration of ethmoid and sphenoid sinus contents through an external incision.

Indications. Indications for this procedure are similar to those for external ethmoidectomy with sphenoid sinus involvement in the disease process. A lack of intranasal landmarks from recurrent disease and previous intranasal surgery make this a desirable approach.

Contraindications. See the section on external ethmoidectomy.

Technique. An external ethmoidectomy is performed as detailed previously. The ethmoid cells are removed, exposing the anterior wall of the sphenoid sinus. This wall is fractured with a Blakesley forceps, staying medial and inferior. If the bone is thick, a chisel or drill may be required. The anterior sphenoid sinus wall is enlarged by piecemeal bone removal, and diseased mucosa then is removed carefully, avoiding force superiorly and laterally to safeguard against potential vascular or neurologic complications.

Postoperative care. See the section on external ethmoidectomy.

Complications. Along with potential complications of an external ethmoidectomy, there are those specific to sphenoid manipulation. Knowledge of the anatomy of the sphenoid sinus and its intracranial relationships (Fig. 62-8) allows the surgeon to understand the potential for complications of sphenoid manipulation (Table 62-6). It may be appreciated how mistaking the lateral wall of the sphenoid for an intersinus septum may have dire consequences.

Transantral sphenoethmoidectomy

Transantral sphenoethmoidectomy is a canine fossa approach to expose or remove contents of the maxillary, ethmoid, and sphenoid sinuses.

Indications. The indications are similar to those for a transantral ethmoidectomy, with sphenoid sinus involvement in the disease process.

Contraindications. See the section on transantral ethmoidectomy.

Technique. A transantral ethmoidectomy is performed as described previously. The anterior wall of the sphenoid sinus is exposed after removal of the ethmoid air cells. Entry is achieved in a technique similar to the transethmoidal approach. Another option is to enter the sphenoid sinus prior to ethmoidectomy. A measurement probe is placed intranasally 7 cm from the anterior nasal spine at a 30° angle from the floor of the nose, medial and parallel to the middle turbi-

Table 62-6. Complications of sphenoid sinus surgery

Vascular hemorrhage	Internal carotid artery
	Cavernous sinus
	Retrobulbar
	Intranasal, sphenopalatine
Cranial nerves	Optic chiasm or optic nerve, hemianopsia or blindness
	Occulomotor (III), trochlear (IV), or abducens (VI), diplopia
	Trigeminal (V1, V2), facial numbness
Cerebral	Cerebrospinal fluid leak
	Meningitis or abscess
	Direct brain or brainstem trauma
	Pituitary trauma, hypopituitary

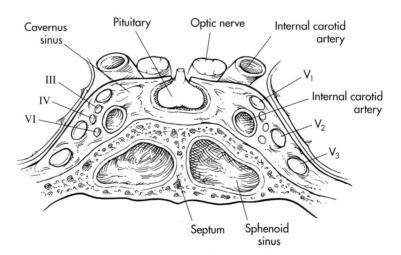

Fig. 62-8. Coronal section of posterior sphenoid sinus displaying anatomic relationships with intracranial structures.

nate. This identifies the natural ostium on the anterior sphenoid wall. Sinus contents are then carefully exenterated from the sphenoid sinus, being certain the bony walls are intact laterally and superiorly.

Postoperative care. See the section on transantral ethmoidectomy.

Complications. Complications include those of the transantral ethmoidectomy approach and those associated with sphenoid sinus surgery (see Tables 62-2, 62-3, and 62-6).

Frontal sinus

Trephination

Frontal sinus trephination involves the creation of an opening into the sinus through the floor (or anterior wall).

Indications. This is a drainage procedure done for patients with symptomatic acute purulent frontal sinusitis refractory to maximal medical therapy. Trephination may be performed as a "first step" with early intracranial complications of frontal sinusitis or frontal bone osteomyelitis to avoid major frontal sinus surgery. Frontal sinoscopy for evaluation of sinus contents or biopsy may be performed through the trephination.

Contraindications. Caldwell and lateral view plain films or axial and coronal CT images should be obtained before trephination. This procedure should not be performed on a patient with an aplastic sinus.

Technique. This procedure may be performed with local anesthetic if the patient is too sick to tolerate a general anesthetic. The patient is prepped and draped in standard fashion, and a superomedial orbital injection of lidocaine, 1%, with 1:100,000 epinephrine is performed to block the supratrochlear and supraorbital nerves. A small incision then is made below the eyebrow and supraorbital rim down through periosteum to bone (Fig. 62-9). The periosteum is elevated with a Freer elevator superiorly and inferiorly to expose the area of the frontal sinus floor. A small drill or chisel is used to enter through the floor of the sinus (anteromedially) slowly to avoid overheating the bone or uncontrolled "popping in." Frontal sinoscopy may be performed using 4 mm, 0° and 30° endoscopes. Cultures of purulent drainage are obtained. A blunt cannula or two plastic or rubber catheters may be inserted to allow further drainage and irrigation with an antibiotic solution or decongestant agents. Dye instillation may be performed to assess nasofrontal duct patency.

Once the infection has cleared and the daily irrigations are completed, the cannula or drainage tubes are removed. The incision heals by secondary intention or, if large, sutures can be placed at the time of surgery, and the wound is closed when the drains are pulled.

Postoperative care. In patients with infection, culture-directed intravenous antibiotics should be administered. Irrigations are performed four times daily with an appropriate antibiotic solution. The drains are left in place for at least 48 hours or until drainage ceases. The drains should not be kept in longer than 14 days to avoid a mucosal foreign body reaction.

Complications. Frontal bone osteomyelitis may occur, or preexisting bone involvement may spread if trephination is performed into an acutely infected area. Trauma to the nasofrontal duct region may lead to stenosis of the duct and chronic frontal sinus infection. Orbital complications may include trauma to the trochlea; injury to the medial canthal ligament, extraocular muscles, or globe; hemorrhage; or blindness. Violation of the posterior table may result in intracranial complications such as dural tear, frontal lobe trauma, meningitis, abscess formation, and hemorrhage.

Controversies. The Kuemmel-Beck technique of trephination advocates going through the anterior wall of the sinus.[12] This procedure is not advised when the area is involved with osteomyelitis because it may promote the spread of the infection.

External frontoethmoidectomy

External frontoethmoidectomy is an open transorbital approach useful for exploring, draining, and removing diseased tissue in the frontal and ethmoid sinuses. A variety of techniques have been described with the classic "Lynch" procedure being the most popular (Fig. 62-10). Other variations include Killian, Reidel, and Lothrop or Chaput-Mayer techniques (Table 62-7).

Indications. This procedure is ideally suited for acute infectious disease of the frontal and ethmoid sinuses with orbital extension. Mucoceles, pyoceles, cutaneous fistulae and cerebrospinal fluid leaks, or intracranial complications from the frontal and ethmoid sinuses may be managed using this approach. Exposure for benign tumors of the frontal or ethmoid sinuses, anterior skull base, or superior nasal cavity may be achieved.

Contraindications. A previous failure of this approach would be a relative contraindication, as would a tendency for hypertrophic scarring or keloid formation.

Technique: the Lynch frontoethmoidectomy. The patient is prepped and draped as if undergoing an external ethmoidectomy, and a similar curvilinear or W incision is made, avoiding damage to the medial canthal ligament and trochlea. The periosteum is elevated to the frontoethmoid suture, and the anterior ethmoid artery is identified and cauterized or clipped and divided. The lamina papyracea is removed, and a complete ethmoidectomy is performed. The middle turbinate is removed if involved in the disease process. The frontal sinus then is opened in the medial part of the floor with a chisel or burr, and then the entire floor is removed with Kerrison rongeurs to provide adequate exposure of the interior. To avoid deformity, the bony defect should not extend beyond the orbital rim anteriorly or superiorly. Diseased tissue from within the sinus is removed, spar-

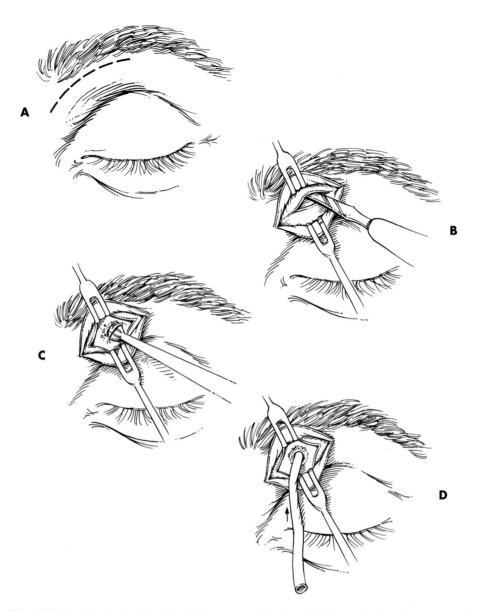

Fig. 62-9. Frontal sinus trephination. **A,** A small incision is made inferomedial to the supraorbital rim and **B,** the periosteum is elevated to expose the frontal sinus floor. **C,** A drill or chisel is used to enter through the floor of the sinus, **D,** which then may be irrigated with a catheter.

ing normal mucosa. This creates a large chute from the frontal sinus through the ethmoid cavity into the nose. Mucosal flaps may be developed from the lateral wall of the nose to line the opening.

The nose is packed with antibiotic-impregnated gauze. The incision then is closed in layers.

Variations

Killian. In very tall frontal sinuses (large, loculated, and so forth) it is difficult to be certain all disease is removed through the floor alone. In the Killian procedure, the floor and much of the anterior wall are removed, leaving a 10-mm bony strut at the supraorbital rim to prevent deformity. This allows excellent exposure to all areas of the frontal sinuses.

Reidel. The entire anterior wall and floor of the frontal sinus are completely removed. The mucosa is removed, and the forehead soft tissue is laid against the posterior table, thereby obliterating the frontal sinus. Because a significant deformity is caused, this technique is rarely used except when the entire anterior wall is diseased.

Lothrop (Chaput-Mayer). In patients with bilateral chronic frontal sinusitis, median drainage is accomplished by taking down the intersinus septum. The nasofrontal ducts then are connected, and a portion of the superior nasal septum with adjoining frontal bone anterior to the duct is removed.

In patients with unilateral disease with a narrow nasofrontal duct and a normally draining contralateral frontal sinus,

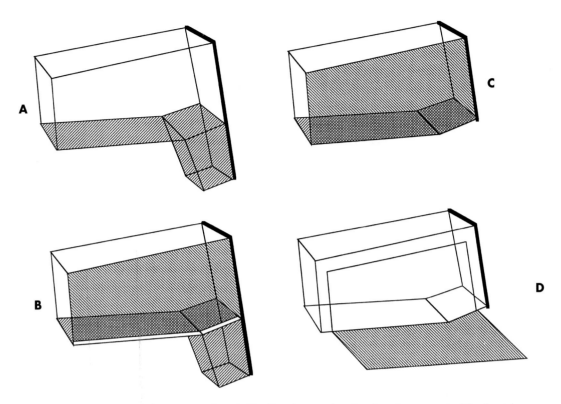

Fig. 62-10. Frontal sinus approaches. **A,** The Lynch procedure involves the removal of the frontal sinus floor and ethmoid air cells. **B,** In the Killian procedure the floor, ethmoids, and a portion of the anterior frontal sinus wall are taken, leaving a supraorbital bony strut. **C,** The Reidel procedure involves the removal of the entire anterior wall and frontal sinus floor. **D,** The osteoplastic flap of the anterior wall is hinged inferiorly; diseased tissue is removed and then replaced.

Table 62-7. Comparison of open frontal sinus approaches

Approach	Resection	Advantages	Disadvantages
Lynch	Ethmoidectomy and removal of the floor of the frontal sinus, with or without middle turbinectomy	Quick and simple, may be good for small malignant lesions	Difficult in tall frontal sinuses, recurrent infection, or mucocele, pyocele
Killian	Anterior ethmoidectomy, with or without middle turbinectomy, floor and anterior wall of frontal sinus (except a supraorbital bony strut)	Good visualization even in large frontal sinuses	Fails to obliterate, there may be a forehead deformity in a large sinus or with bony strut necrosis
Reidel	Complete removal of anterior wall and floor of frontal sinus	Good exposure of entire sinus, easy to obliterate if narrow anterior-posterior diameter	Forehead concavity in larger sinus, fail to obliterate if wide anterior-posterior diameter
Lothrop	Unilateral or bilateral anterior ethmoidectomy, with or without middle turbinectomy, interfrontal septum and superior nasal septum and nasofrontal ducts connected	Good for bilateral disease	Not effective if narrow anterior-posterior diameter of frontal sinus or duct
Osteoplastic	Anterior wall osteoplastic flap based inferiorly, retracted then replaced	Excellent exposure of entire frontal sinus and ducts, minimal cosmetic deformity	Big operation with increased blood loss, not suitable for malignant disease

supplementary drainage may be achieved through the healthy side. This is done simply by removing the intersinus septum down to the floor, avoiding damage to the mucosa and infundibulum of the healthy side.

Postoperative care. Management of nasal packing, wound care, and antibiotic coverage is similar to that for the external ethmoidectomy procedure.

Complications. Complications are all similar to those of the external ethmoidectomy procedure (see Table 62-3). There also are potential risks and complications specific to the method of frontal sinus exposure used. The Lynch procedure is limited in visualization, and therefore patients are prone to recurrent infection. If a complete ethmoidectomy is not done, the drainage port into the nose may scar shut. The Killian technique may lead to forehead deformity with a large frontal sinus or necrosis of the bony strut. The Reidel obliteration results in noticeable forehead concavity in medium- to large-sized sinuses, often necessitating soft-tissue or alloplastic augmentation to reconstruct the defect. A Lothrop or Chaput-Mayer approach carries a risk of cribriform plate damage with resulting anosmia, cerebrospinal fluid (CFE) leak, or meningitis.

Controversies. Although an excellent approach for orbital complications of frontal and ethmoid sinusitis, the external frontoethmoidectomy is not ideally suited for frontal sinus obliteration. The cosmetic deformity resulting from removal of the anterior wall of the sinus is unacceptable when there is a safe, reliable technique that may achieve obliteration without forehead concavity.

Frontal osteoplastic flap and sinus obliteration

The creation of an osteoperiosteal flap of the anterior frontal sinus wall allows for direct access to the entire frontal sinus and nasofrontal ducts. In patients with a chronically diseased frontal sinus, the cavity may be obliterated with an adipose tissue autograft.

Indications. This approach has become the gold standard for chronic frontal sinusitis refractory to conservative therapy or to previous surgical attempts with ESS or frontoethmoidectomy. The exposure achieved with this procedure allows for access to the superior and lateral sinus (inaccessible with ESS) and nasofrontal duct areas. Mucoceles, pyoceles, frontal bone osteomyelitis with bone necrosis, benign frontal sinus tumors, and fractures are indications, as is orbital or intracranial extension of frontal sinus disease.

Contraindications. This procedure is not indicated in patients with small hypoplastic frontal sinuses that do not extend into the frontal bone.

Technique

Unilateral. Frontal sinus disease most often is bilateral, so it is relatively uncommon to perform a unilateral procedure. A unilateral frontal sinus tumor would be the most common indication.

A standard 6 foot Caldwell view radiograph is taken preoperatively, and a template is fashioned by tracing the outline of the frontal sinus on transparent film or just by cutting it directly out of the original film. The template is cut inferiorly above the level of the cribriform, ensuring that the interfrontal septum and supraorbital rim are included. This is autoclaved for the procedure.

The patient is prepped and draped in the supine position with the left abdomen prepped for an adipose autograft. An ipsilateral tarsorrhaphy is performed, or a scleral shield is inserted to protect the eye. Lidocaine, 1%, with 1:100,000 epinephrine is injected into the area of incision along the upper margin of the eyebrow. Beveling the blade to avoid trauma to the eyebrow follicles, the incision is carried down through subcutaneous tissue and frontalis muscle to the periosteum, which is preserved. The anterior wall of the sinus is exposed, and the template is outlined on the periosteum. This then is incised just beyond the outline along the superior, lateral, and medial borders, leaving the inferior portion of periosteum intact. The periosteum is elevated away from the edge of the incision and reflected back to avoid damage during bone cuts. These incisions are made along the outlined area with a Stryker saw or equivalent, beveled inward at about 30° toward the sinus. The supraorbital rim is cut medially and laterally (using chisel cuts if necessary) to allow for a controlled fracture of bone across the floor of the frontal sinus. The bone incision then is completed with an osteotome and mallet, and the flap is pryed away slowly to expose the sinus contents. If diseased mucosa exists, the entire lining is removed with a Freer elevator and Blakesley forceps. The inner cortical bone then is burred away from the sinus walls and inner aspect of the flap to ensure complete removal of mucosa and to provide a viable bed for revascularization of the adipose autograft. If an osteoma is present with normal mucosa and a healthy, patent nasofrontal duct, this step and subsequent obliteration may be avoided.

Subcutaneous fat is harvested from a left lower quadrant abdominal incision. It is done in this location to avoid confusion with an appendectomy scar in the right lower quadrant. Immaculate hemostasis is achieved with electrocoagulation, and a potential dead space is avoided by using a two-layer closure and drain placement if the wound is not perfectly dry. The frontal sinus then is obliterated with the adipose graft, which should fill it completely. The bone flap is returned to its original position, and the periosteal incisions are closed with interrupted 4-0 Vicryl. The wound then is closed in three layers (frontalis, subcutaneous, and skin), and a Penrose drain is placed if necessary. A light pressure dressing is applied.

Bilateral. A template is prepared as described previously. The incision for exposure of the frontal sinuses may be brow, coronal, or midforehead (Table 62-8, Fig. 62-11, A). The coronal incision is preferable if the patient has sufficient hair and is unlikely to develop a receding hairline because the scar will not be visible. This incision is created approximately 2 to 3 cm posterior to the anterior hairline. The hair is prepped at surgery by combing anterior and posterior to the incision line and greasing it down with antibiotic

Table 62-8. Osteoplastic flap incisions

Incision	Indications
Brow	Balding or receding hairline, small frontal sinus
Midforehead	Balding or receding hairline, established forehead rhytids, large sinus
Coronal	Sufficient hair coverage, any size sinus

ointment. Care is taken to remain parallel to the follicles to avoid transecting the roots, which would result in periincisional hair loss.

In patients who are balding, a brow incision or midforehead incision is performed. If the frontal sinus is large, exposure may be difficult through the brow, so a midforehead incision within an established wrinkle is preferred, offering an excellent cosmetic result.

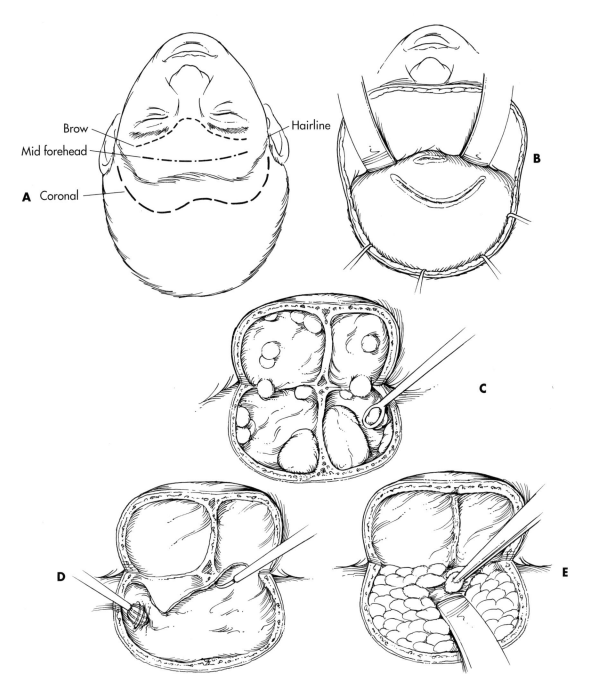

Fig. 62-11. Frontal osteoplastic flap and sinus obliteration. **A,** Depending on the size of the sinus and patient hairline, the incision may be brow, midforehead, or coronal. See text for explanation of parts **B** to **E**.

Regardless of the type of incision used, the skin flap is elevated in the same plane just above the pericranium. Previous infiltration with lidocaine, 1%, with 1:100,000 epinephrine along the incision and the use of hemostatic Raney clips along the wound edge are advised to control blood loss from the well-vascularized scalp.

The sterilized template is placed over the frontal periosteum and positioned to accurately line up with the supraorbital rims bilaterally. The periosteum is incised just beyond the outline of the template as with a unilateral flap; the difference is that a horizontal incision is made across the nasal process (Fig. 62-11, *B*). A beveled bone incision is made around the outline; the supraorbital rims are cut laterally on each side; and the nasal process is transected with an osteotome. The osteotome is used to complete the bone incision, and the intersinus septum is transected from the superior aspect. The flap then may be elevated by prying gently with the osteotome around the bone incision.

Diseased tissue is removed as with the unilateral procedure, and the intersinus septum is burred down (Fig. 62-11 *C, D*). Obliteration is performed with an adipose autograft (Fig. 62-11, *E*) after careful removal of all mucosa. The flap is replaced and fixed with periosteal sutures as described previously. If the flap seems unstable or sinks into the sinus, it should be fixed to surrounding bone with wire sutures or mini- or microplates. Penrose drains are placed, and the wound is closed in three layers. A light pressure dressing is applied.

Postoperative care. The patient is maintained on systemic antibiotics. The pressure dressing and drains may be removed after 24 to 48 hours. Wound care is performed using hydrogen peroxide and antibiotic ointment at least three times daily. Forehead sutures are removed 5 to 7 days after surgery, and scalp staples are left in for at least 1 week to 10 days.

Complications. Fracture or injury to the posterior table of the frontal sinus may result in intracranial complications, including dural tears, CSF leaks, frontal lobe injury, meningitis, or brain abscess. Fracture of the floor of the sinus or orbital roof may result in extraocular muscle injury, globe injury, or hemorrhage causing diplopia or blindness, respectively. Supraorbital nerve injury may be transient as a result of retraction or permanent if transected with subsequent forehead paresthesia, hypoesthesia, or anesthesia. A loss of frontalis function is possible from damage to the muscle or nerve.

Hematoma or seroma formation and possible wound infection or abscess may occur at either the abdominal or frontal wound. Anosmia may result from trauma to the cribriform plate and olfactory nerve.

Controversies. Many would argue that obliteration of the sinus is mandatory with this approach. However, if being performed on a frontal sinus with an osteoma and normal mucosa, the authors believe that obliteration is unnecessary.[17] Management of the nasofrontal duct varies from leaving it alone to occluding it with fascia, muscle, or bone. Either approach should yield excellent results.

References

1. Corey JP, Bumsted RM: Revision endoscopic ethmoidectomy for chronic rhinosinusitis, *Otolaryngol Clin North Am* 22:801, 1989.
2. Duncavage JA: *Maxillary sinus revision surgery.* In Stankiewicz JA, editor: *Advanced endoscopic sinus surgery*, St Louis, 1995, Mosby.
3. Friedman WH, Katsantonis GP: The role of standard techniques in modern sinus surgery, *Otolaryngol Clin North Am* 22:759, 1989.
4. Friedman WH, Katsantonis GP: Transantral revision of recurrent maxillary and ethmoidal disease following functional intranasal surgery, *Otolaryngol Head Neck Surg* 106:367, 1992.
5. Gross WE and others: Modified transnasal endoscopic Lothrop procedure as an alternative to frontal sinus obliteration, *Otolaryngol Head Neck Surg* 113:427, 1995.
6. King JM, Caldarelli DD, Pigato JB: A review of revision functional endoscopic sinus surgery, *Laryngoscope* 104:404, 1994.
7. Lazar RH and others: Revision functional endonasal sinus surgery, *ENT J* 71:131, 1992.
8. Lazar RH, Younis RT, Gross CW: Pediatric functional endonasal sinus surgery: review of 210 cases, *Head Neck* 14:92, 1992.
9. Levine HL: Endoscopic sinus surgery: reasons for failure, *Op Tech Otolaryngol Head Neck Surg* 6:176, 1995.
10. May M, Schaitkin B: Frontal sinus surgery: endonasal drainage instead of an external osteoplastic approach, *Op Tech Otolaryngol Head Neck Surg* 6:184, 1995.
11. May M, Schaitkin B, Kay SL: Revision endoscopic sinus surgery: six friendly surgical landmarks, *Laryngoscope* 104:766, 1994.
12. Messerklinger W, Naumann HH: *Kuemmel-Beck frontal trephine.* In Naumann HH and others, editors: *Head and neck surgery*, ed 2, New York, 1995, Thieme.
13. Montgomery WW, Cheney ML, Turner PA: *External sinus surgery.* In Pillsbury HC, Goldsmith MM, editors: *Operative challenges in otolaryngolgy head and neck surgery*, Chicago, 1990, Mosby.
14. Ng M, Rice DH: Revision sinus surgery, *ENT J* 73:44, 1994.
15. Rice DH, Schaefer SD: *Endoscopic paranasal sinus surgery*, ed 2, New York, 1993, Raven Press.
16. Schaitkin B and others: Endoscopic sinus surgery: 4-year follow-up on the first 100 patients, *Laryngoscope* 103:1117, 1993.
17. Younis RT, Lazar RH: *Osteoplastic frontal sinusectomy procedure and fat obliteration.* In Bailey BJ and others, editors: *Atlas of head and neck surgery—otolaryngology*, Philadelphia, 1996, Lippincott-Raven.

Chapter 63

Cerebrospinal Fluid Leaks

Edward L. Applebaum
James M. Chow

Leakage of cerebrospinal fluid (CSF) from its intracranial location may present difficulties in diagnosis, localization, and management. Physicians may overlook the leakage in a trauma patient with other serious injuries or may confuse the clear fluid discharge with other abnormal conditions. The recognition and the localization of CSF leaks can be challenging, and management varies with etiology and site. The development of skull base surgery has resulted in an increased incidence of CSF leaks, and contemporary diagnostic studies have replaced older techniques of diagnosis and localization. This chapter describes the manifestations of CSF leaks in clinical practice and current methods of diagnosis, localization, and management.

CLASSIFICATION

Cerebrospinal fluid rhinorrhea

CSF rhinorrhea is classified according to a modification of a scheme Ommaya[44] developed (Fig. 63-1). This classification scheme is based on etiology and clinical presentation and has implications for evaluation and management. CSF rhinorrhea may be traumatic or nontraumatic in origin. Traumatic fistulas may be a result of accidental trauma or surgical causes. Accidental trauma is the cause in approximately 80% of patients with CSF rhinorrhea, even though the incidence of CSF rhinorrhea in patients who suffer serious head trauma is only 2% to 3%.[28] Intracranial and extracranial surgical procedures cause approximately 16% of CSF leaks from the nose. The remaining 4% are nontraumatic in origin,[28] and these may be high-pressure or normal-pressure fistulas. High-pressure leaks are more common and result from tumors or hydrocephalus. Tumors account for more than one half of the cases of nontraumatic CSF rhinorrhea and directly

cause the leak by erosion of bone and soft tissue or indirectly through increase of intracranial pressure.[6,44] Hydrocephalus, which may be communicating or obstructive, also increases intracranial pressure. Normal-pressure CSF leaks occur as a result of congenital anomalies or osteomyelitis; occasionally, they may occur without any obvious cause.

Cerebrospinal fluid otorrhea

Although no commonly used classification system exists for CSF otorrhea, this entity also may be traumatic or nontraumatic in origin (Fig. 63-2). Traumatic fistulas may be caused by accidental or surgical trauma. The most common cause of CSF otorrhea is accidental trauma, with CSF leaks occurring in approximately 0.4% to 6.7% of patients with demonstrable skull fractures.[5,20,48] Longitudinal temporal bone fractures result in CSF otorrhea more frequently than transverse fractures do. Longitudinal fractures course from the squama, through the posterior portion of the bony external auditory canal wall, and into the tegmen, where they tear the overlying dura. The tympanic membrane often is torn resulting in a pathway for egress of fluid out of the ear canal. Transverse fractures are less common and usually are associated with an intact tympanic membrane. This fracture line courses perpendicular to the long axis of the temporal bone and may transect the internal auditory canal. When transverse fractures cause CSF leaks into the middle ear, the CSF passes down the eustachian tube into the nasopharynx. If the blow tears the tympanic membrane, CSF leaking from the internal auditory canal will produce otorrhea.

Although a much less frequent etiologic agent than trauma, surgery for chronic suppurative ear disease or malignancy is the second-most common cause of CSF otorrhea. Finally, rare nontraumatic fistulas occur as a result of con-

rhinorrhea tend to occur in adults aged more than 30 years, with a female preponderance of 2:1.[44]

Cerebrospinal fluid otorrhea

When accidental trauma causes CSF otorrhea, the majority of patients develop signs and symptoms immediately. In one report, 94% of those who ultimately developed CSF otorrhea after trauma had an immediate onset.[27] In those patients in whom the tympanic membrane is intact, fluid will be visible behind the tympanic membrane or will drain into the nasopharynx by way of the eustachian tube, causing rhinorrhea or a sensation of postnasal discharge. Additional symptoms may consist of hearing loss, pressure sensation in the ear, or dizziness. When surgical procedures are the cause, CSF otorrhea may present in the same manner as a traumatic CSF otorrhea of accidental origin, although the surgery also may produce CSF leakage from the incision site, a fluctuant mass at the surgical site, or meningitis postoperatively.[39] CSF otorhinorrhea after surgery for acoustic neuroma occurs in approximately 10% to 20% of patients.[17,18,22] Nontraumatic CSF otorrhea of congenital origin usually occurs in children but may develop at any time of life. Children who have this type of otorrhea frequently have a form of Mondini inner ear malformation and have a history of recurring episodes of meningitis. A less common presentation occurs in children who only have hearing loss as a result of middle ear fluid. Myringotomy reveals CSF exuding from the middle ear. These children may have a congenital dehiscence of the fallopian canal or Hyrtl's fissure. Adults who have leakage of CSF into the middle ear may present with hearing loss only, otorrhea, or otorhinorrhea. These patients, who have normal inner ear function, have a CSF fistula as a result of ruptured meningoencephaloceles that present through congenital defects in the tegmen of the temporal bone. Recurrent meningitis is sometimes the only problem in these patients, and its cause may go undetected for years. Although the bone defect in the tegmen probably has been present from birth, CSF leakage may develop years later when the meninges finally are worn through by the constant fluctuations in CSF pressure.[41,47]

Diagnostic studies

Demonstrating extracranial cerebrospinal fluid

The accurate diagnosis of a CSF fistula depends on unequivocal demonstration of extracranial CSF and precise localization of its site of leakage. In many patients with profuse nasal drainage, the diagnosis of extracranial CSF is obvious; it is rarely confused with vasomotor or allergic rhinitis. In patients in whom minimal or intermittent drainage occurs, diagnosis can be difficult. Persistence of a clear, nonsticky, nasal discharge should arouse suspicion of a CSF leak. In a comatose, head injury patient or in anyone suspected of having CSF rhinorrhea, the body should be placed in the lateral position with the face bent downward to increase CSF flow.

Pressure applied to the jugular veins also may make latent CSF leakage apparent.[28] A classic sign of CSF leakage is the presence of a "halo sign," in which a clear fluid area surrounds a blood stain when CSF mixed with blood is absorbed onto paper. In addition, a wet handkerchief that dries without stiffening also is highly suggestive that a clear rhinorrhea is caused by CSF. Usually neither test is sufficient to make the diagnosis. Testing for glucose content in the suspicious fluid also is done sometimes, with a value greater than 30 mg/ml being confirmatory for CSF. Collecting adequate amounts of fluid to analyze for chemical content often is difficult, and the glucose content of tears may be a confounding factor. Glucose oxidase test papers are inaccurate, and their use provides equivocal information. Immunoelectrophoretic identification of B_2 transferrin in fluid suspected to be CSF confirms the diagnosis of a CSF leak.[42,43,51,56] B_2 transferrin, the desialated form of transferrin, almost exclusively is localized to CSF. The only other tissue fluids that contain B_2 transferrin are the aqueous and vitreous humor in the eye and perilymph in the cochlea.[3] This analysis can be done with only a small amount of fluid and recently has become readily available.[42] The radiologic diagnosis of extracranial CSF can be accomplished through the use of computed tomography (CT) cisternography with nonionic contrast (NCTC).[28,46] Metrizamide, which used to be commonly used, is no longer commercially available. Nonionic contrast is injected into the subarachnoid space and visualized by CT (axial, coronal, and sagittal scans). CT readily demonstrates extracranial extravasation of CSF (made radiopaque by the nonionic contrast), thereby not only diagnosing a CSF leak, but also localizing its site (Figs. 63-3 and 63-4). In those with nontraumatic CSF rhinorrhea, plain CT or CT cisternography also is useful as an initial diagnostic test to differentiate between high-pressure leaks and normal pressure leaks. Conventional skull radiographs, noncomputed tomography studies, pneumoencephalography, and subdural pneumography are outdated studies that CT studies have replaced.

Other techniques used to show CSF leakage involve the injection of various colored dyes (methylene blue, indigo carmine, toluidine blue) or radioactive isotopes (radioactive sodium, ^{111}In-DTPA [diethylenetriamine pentaacetic acid] ^{99m}Tc-DTPA) into the subarachnoid space. The former technique has been largely discontinued because of the morbidity it produces.[7,8] The latter technique is currently widely used and involves radionuclide cisternography combined with scintigraphy of pledgets placed intranasally. This technique has a reported overall success rate of 25% to 65% and has been useful in patients with intermittent rhinorrhea not diagnosable by other means.[11,19]

Localizing the site of leakage

Clinical localization of the site of CSF leakage should not be overlooked despite the advances in imaging studies. A leak occurring in only one side of the nose generally corre-

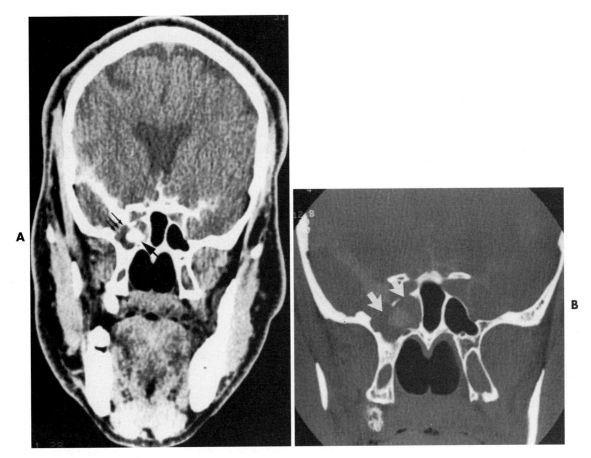

Fig. 63-3. A, The coronal section computed tomography scan (soft-tissue setting) demonstrating metrizamide in the left sphenoid sinus *(large black arrow)* from dehiscence in the roof of the sphenoid sinus *(small black arrow)*. **B,** The same section as in *A* with enhancement of bony detail showing two defects in the roof of the left sphenoid sinus *(white arrows)*.

lates with the side of the defect, although a leak that shifts from one side to the other or occurs bilaterally provides no localizing information. Leakage from the nose when the head is upright or tilted backward suggests that the leak is through the cribriform plate, ethmoid roof, or frontal sinus. Leakage only on tilting the head forward suggests that the leakage is coming from the sphenoid sinus or through the middle ear.[8]

Nasal endoscopic examination can diagnose and localize the site of CFS leak in patients with CFS rhinorrhea. This requires the presence of an active leak at the time of examination. The cribriform plate can be adequately examined in some patients, showing egress of clear fluid from this region or a cephalocele with leakage of clear fluid from this area. Visualization of clear fluid emanating from the middle meatus, superior meatus, or the sphenoethmoid recess indicates the site of leakage to be from the roof of the anterior ethmoid sinus, the posterior ethmoid sinus, or the sphenoid sinus, respectively. CSF also has been visualized emanating from the eustachian tube orifice, indicating the site of leakage to be from the temporal bone.

As previously mentioned, NCTC is useful not only for the diagnosis of extracranial CSF but also for localizing the site. The success rate of this technique depends highly on the presence of an active leak at the time of the study. Manelfe and others[31] have reported a success rate of more than 80% in localizing the site of leakage in active leaks, although the presence of an inactive leak at the time of examination has been reported to result in an identification rate of only 20% to 30%.[30,31] Artificially increasing the CSF pressure to open an inactive CSF leak reportedly has increased the success rate to 100%.[40]

The use of radioactive isotopes injected into the subarachnoid space is not very accurate in localizing the site of leakage. A false-positive result is common because of absorption of radioactivity within the bloodstream and redistribution of this activity through nasal mucosa to the pledgets. Passage of radioactivity to nasal mucosa through the olfactory nerves also may result in false-positive results.[7,21]

Injection of fluorescein into the subarachnoid space also has been used to localize the site of CSF leakage.[7,24] This fluorescent dye is commonly used intraoperatively to local-

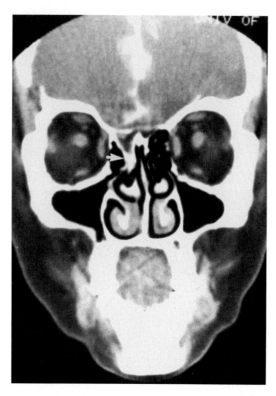

Fig. 63-4. Coronal section computed tomography scan demonstrating metrizamide in the left ethmoid sinus *(white arrow)* from dehiscence in the anterior cranial fossa.

ize exactly the site of CSF leakage. After injection of 0.5 ml of 5% fluorescein diluted by 9.5 ml of CSF[36] into the subarachnoid space and after placing the patient in a head-down position, the investigator can use a microscope or an endoscope to detect yellowish green fluid emanating from the site of the CSF leak. This technique also can be used intraoperatively to diagnose CSF leaks.[50]

Magnetic resonance imaging (MRI) also has been used to localize the site of CSF leakage (Fig. 63-5). Various techniques of MRI have enhanced the ability of MRI to localize the site of the CSF leakage. In one study, the identification and localization of an inactive CSF leak was made in all 11 patients studied.[14] In several other studies, MRI was able to show the site of the CFS leak, whereas NCTC was not able to show the site of the leak.[13,14,38] Further studies directly comparing MRI to NCTC are needed to evaluate the role of MRI in evaluating the patient with a CSF leak. The advantages of MRI (over NCTC) are that MRI is noninvasive (no radiopaque dye is injected), does not involve radiation exposure, and has multiplaner images.

A new imaging technique, positron emission tomography (PET), also has been investigated to determine its ability to localize the site of CSF leakage. This technique is similar to radioactive cisternography and involves intrathecal injection of ^{68}Ga-EDTA. Superimposition of images obtained from PET over images obtained by CT was helpful in locat-

ing sites of CSF leakage.[4] Further studies are needed to compare PET with currently used methods.

MANAGEMENT

The management of patients with CSF rhinorrhea depends on the etiology of the leak, the location of the fistula, and the temporal relationship of the leak to the inciting factor. The majority of traumatic CSF fistulas heal without surgical intervention. Patients who develop CSF rhinorrhea shortly after trauma generally do not need surgery to close the CSF fistula, provided no indication for intracranial exploration coexists. Those patients who show no evidence of resolution of CSF leakage by the end of 1 week probably will require surgical exploration and closure of the leak. Patients who develop CSF rhinorrhea days or weeks after trauma generally do not heal without surgical intervention. Adjacent facial fractures should be reduced early, and reduction may result in cessation of the CSF leakage without further therapy. CSF rhinorrhea resulting from a bullet wound requires exploration. Additional criteria for surgical exploration of patients with CSF rhinorrhea include large defects in the skull base with herniation of brain and evidence of a spicule of bone penetrating the brain.[10] A highly controversial indication for surgery is traumatic CSF rhinorrhea of early onset that is associated with meningitis or a pneumocele. If either of these conditions exists immediately after trauma and resolves with conservative therapy, surgical exploration probably is not required.[6,10] If resolution does not occur, surgical exploration is indicated.

When CSF rhinorrhea results from surgery, the dural injury should be repaired when it occurs. In those patients in whom injury to the dura is not suspected until postoperatively when CSF rhinorrhea occurs, conservative therapy is indicated because the majority of these leaks will close. Massive leaks that occur immediately after surgery usually do not close with conservative measures and require surgical closure.

Several additional points need consideration in the treatment of patients with traumatic CSF rhinorrhea. As mentioned previously, the risk of developing meningitis in the first 3 weeks after trauma has been reported to be approximately 3% to 11%.[28,35] Prophylactic antibiotics have not been shown to be effective in the prevention of meningitis and are not recommended in posttraumatic patients.[25,29] Conservative management of CSF rhinorrhea includes keeping the patient at bed rest in an upright position that minimizes the leak. Coughing, sneezing, nose blowing, and straining are to be avoided. Laxatives are prescribed to reduce straining with bowel movements. If no resolution of the rhinorrhea occurs in 72 hours, repeated or continuous lumbar drainage of CSF may be tried for the next 4 days with removal of 150 ml/day.[10] This therapy is rarely helpful in those with nontraumatic or delayed CSF rhinorrhea.

The first step in the treatment of nontraumatic, high-pressure CSF rhinorrhea is to decrease the high intracranial pres-

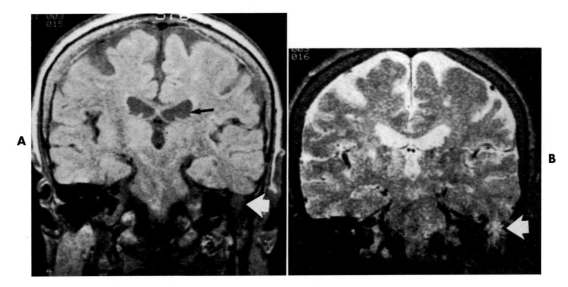

Fig. 63-5. A, Coronal T1-weighted magnetic resonance imaging (MRI) showing cerebrospinal fluid (CSF) in the left mastoid *(white arrow)*, which is of the same intensity as CSF in the lateral ventricle *(black arrow)*. **B,** Coronal T2-weighted MRI of the same section shown in *A*. The *white arrow* indicates CSF in mastoid, which is of the same intensity as CSF in the lateral ventricle.

sure. After this measure, CSF rhinorrhea resolves in most patients. The minority of patients who continue to have CSF rhinorrhea after normalization of intracranial pressure require surgical exploration.[28] Normal-pressure, nontraumatic CSF leaks rarely close with conservative therapy and almost always require surgical exploration and closure.[6]

Operative approaches

The operative management of CSF rhinorrhea can be divided into intracranial and extracranial approaches, each with its advantages and disadvantages. The specific approach selected depends on the site of CSF leakage.

Intracranial approaches require a craniotomy with its attendant morbidity, mortality, and prolonged hospitalization. In addition, anosmia is a frequent complication of craniotomy for CSF rhinorrhea caused by unavoidable trauma to the olfactory nerves.[28] The advantages of intracranial surgery include the ability to achieve a fluid-tight dural closure and to repair multiple areas of leakage. Intracranial approaches can be further subdivided into extradural and intradural repairs. Theoretically, the extradural approach allows the maintenance of intact dura that protects the brain during retraction. From a practical standpoint, the dura tears frequently when it is lifted.[28] Intradural approaches allow a better view of the dura and sometimes a clearer identification of the fistula site, although entering the dura exposes the brain to potential infection. In extradural or intradural approaches, spinal fluid is removed by lumbar drains for several days postoperatively until the edema resolves.

The advantages of an extracranial approach include minimal morbidity and mortality while still achieving excellent visualization of the dural defect. The major requirement for the successful application of this technique is precise, preoperative localization of the leakage site. If the site of leakage is not well defined or if multiple sites of leakage are present, all fistulas may not be closed using an extracranial approach.

In intracranial and extracranial approaches, pedicle flaps should be strongly considered to close areas of leakage that have been irradiated previously. These flaps should be rotated in from sites out of the irradiated field or brought in as free flaps.[33]

Repair of specific sites

Ethmoid roof–cribriform plate

The extracranial route provides the best approach for the repair of a unilateral CSF leak localized to the roof of the ethmoid or the cribriform plate. This surgery can be done through an external approach or through an intranasal approach using an endoscope or a microscope for visualization. The external approach can be done using a naso-orbital incision through which a complete ethmoidectomy is performed. Removal of the middle turbinate aids exposure of the cribriform plate. Using fluorescein enhances accurate visualization of the dural defect. When general anesthesia is administered, 0.5 ml of 5% fluorescein is mixed with 9.5 ml of CSF and slowly injected into the subarachnoid space.[36] On exposure of the site of leakage, egress of fluorescein-stained spinal fluid will be evident by its striking color. Positive-pressure ventilation by the anesthesiologist will increase the rate of CSF flow and may make a leak evident. Although complications from the use of intrathecal fluorescein have been reported, they are rare and reversible. These complications have consisted of lower extremity weakness, numbness, seizures, opisthotonos, and cranial nerve deficits.[37] The dural defect can be sealed with temporalis fascia grafts, fascia lata, or pericranium used alone or bolstered with fat or with mucoperiosteal flaps from the lateral nasal wall or septum.[28,37] If possible, the edges of the fascia are tucked under the bony edges of the dehiscence. If the dura is sealed well, closing a small bony defect at the site of leakage is not necessary.[6] The tissues used to seal the defect are supported by absorbable surgical sponge placed against the graft or flap followed by an intranasally placed antibiotic-impregnated gauze strip. The intranasal packing is removed 1 week after surgery.

The intranasal approach has become the most commonly used approach for the initial closure of CFS leaks in this area as a result of the advent of the rigid endoscope, which allows excellent visualization of the site of leakage, allows easy lifting of the surrounding mucosa, and allows easy placement of the graft over the defect. After localization of the site of leakage with or without use of fluorescein, lifting of mucosa around the defect is accomplished. If a large bony defect is present, septal cartilage or bone can be used to reconstruct the defect before placement of the temporalis fascia graft. A temporalis fascia graft coated with fibrin glue then is placed against the site of CFS leakage. The edges of the graft are subsequently tucked under the mucosal edges. The graft is held in place with a muscle or fat graft coated with fibrin glue and supported by gelfoam. Gauze or a nasal trumpet is used to support the gelfoam.[53] In those patients who have undergone radiotherapy, a septal mucoperichondrial flap additionally may be used.

Encephaloceles that are responsible for a CSF leak can be treated in a similar fashion. The encephalocele can be cauterized with bipolar forceps or excised, and the defect can be reconstructed with bone or cartilage and a graft.[32] The success rate of endoscopic closure of a CFS leak is high and has been reported to range from 76% to 100%.[12,32,53]

An intracranial approach is used if the site of leakage cannot be delinated clearly or if multiple leaks exist. In the extradural and intradural approaches to the repair, fluid-tight closure is accomplished by suturing temporalis fascia, fascia lata, or pericranium to the dural defect. Pedicle pericranium flaps also may be used to provide further support.

Frontal sinus

Leaks of CSF through the frontal sinus are best repaired through an extracranial approach using an osteoplastic flap.[6,46] The advantages and disadvantages of this technique are similar to those of the extracranial repair of CSF leaks of the cribriform plate or roof of the ethmoid. A coronal or brow incision provides access to the frontal sinus, and an inferiorly based osteoplastic flap then is created. Bone fragments and lining mucosa are removed from the sinus, and the leak is identified. Dura then can be sutured directly, which is

usually difficult, or fascia can be inserted through the defect in the posterior wall of the frontal sinus and tucked under the bony edges. To achieve a fluid-tight closure, fascia also can be sutured to the dura, if enough dura is exposed. Fat obliteration of the frontal sinus reinforces the fascia repair and obliterates the nasofrontal ducts, thus eliminating a potential pathway for ascending infection.

Sphenoid sinus

Sphenoid sinus CSF fistulas are best approached through an endoscopic approach. The anterior wall of the sphenoid sinus is exposed and resected, and the site of CFS leak is delineated. The surrounding mucosa then is lifted similar to the technique used in closure of CFS leaks of the roof of the ethmoid sinus. The site of leakage then is grafted with fascia and coated with fibrin glue. This graft is supported by muscle or fat that also is coated with fibrin glue. The sphenoid sinus then is packed with gelfoam, followed by gauze. The nasal cavity also can be packed with gelfoam or gauze. It is not necessary to completely remove mucosa from the sphenoid sinus because the opening to the sphenoid sinus will be maintained. Thus, the risk of developing a mucocele is minimal.

Ear

The precise, preoperative localization of the CSF leak site will determine the surgical approach to the ear. Defects in the tegmen can be exposed by a mastoidectomy or atticotomy. Leaks from the posterior fossa dura into the mastoid are approached through a mastoidectomy. When the defect and leak are confined to the middle ear, a tympanotomy may be all that is required. Craniotomy usually is reserved for those with failures of the various extracranial operations and for patients with large or multiple defects. A small, extradural craniotomy through the temporal squama, in combination with a mastoidectomy, provides the advantages of a limited craniotomy in addition to those of a mastoidectomy.[1] This combined approach facilitates accurate and secure placement of the dural graft.

Many materials have been advocated for dural repair, including, most commonly, temporalis fascia, fascia lata, periosteum, perichondrium, homograft dura, and methyl methacrylate. Composite grafts of conchal cartilage with attached perichondrium have been used to seal the dura and at the same time to provide a covering for the associated defect in the bone. In most patients, direct suture of the graft material to the dura is not possible, so the graft is held in place by abdominal wall adipose tissue or temporalis muscle pedicle flaps.

In mastoidectomy and atticotomy approaches, the leak site is identified, and the bone defect surrounding the dural opening is enlarged. The graft material is inserted through the enlarged opening so that it underlies the dura and is supported circumferentially by bone. The posterior ear canal wall is left intact, if possible, so that the mastoid cavity can be filled with fat or a muscle flap to support the repair site. Also, leaving the canal wall intact eliminates the potential source of infection that would exist from an open mastoid cavity. Small, congenital defects in the tegmen associated with adult-onset CSF leakage have been closed successfully by being packed tightly with bone dust accumulated from the mastoidectomy drilling, rather than through enlargement of the defect to place a soft-tissue graft.

The most frequent locations for middle ear CSF leaks are (1) oval window, (2) round window, and (3) Hyrtl's fissure, in that order.[52] If the explored ear is nonhearing, the site of leakage simply is plugged with the graft. In hearing ears, the CSF leak is sealed with fascia that is packed in place with antibiotic-impregnated ribbon gauze that is removed in 3 to 5 days, at which time the tympanomeatal flap is returned to its original position.[52]

New materials

Lyophilized dura, alcoholic prolamine solution,[26] and fibrin or acrylate glues have been used successfully to close dural defects. Because these substances have only recently been introduced, the long-term success rates with their use compared with those of more conventional methods are unclear. Further studies are needed to define their role in the surgery of CSF leaks.

Results

The failure rate for intracranial repair of CSF rhinorrhea has been reported to be from 6% to 27%.[7,10,27,28] Of these failures, most will require multiple surgical attempts at closure, with a final failure rate ranging from 1% to 10%.[28,49] The failure rate for extracranial repair of CSF rhinorrhea is similar to that reported for intracranial repair, varying from 6% to 33%.[7,23,46] The failure rate for endoscopic repair of a CSF leak has been reported to range from 0% to 24%.[12,32,53] Because of the similar failure rates of extracranial and intracranial procedures, extracranial repair usually is attempted first unless extenuating circumstances require an intracranial procedure, thus avoiding the higher morbidity and mortality of an intracranial approach.

REFERENCES

1. Adkins WY, Osguthrope JD: Mini-craniotomy for management of CSF otorrhea from tegmen defects, *Laryngoscope* 93:1038, 1983.
2. Ahren C, Thulin CA: Lethal intracranial complications following inflation in the external auditory canal in treatment of serous otitis media and due to defects in the petrous bone, *Acta Otolaryngol* 60:407, 1965.
3. Bassiouny M and others: Beta 2 transferrin application in otology, *Am J Otol* 13:552, 1992.
4. Bergstrand G and others: Positron emission tomography with ^{68}Ga-EDTA in the diagnosis and localization of CSF fistulas, *J Comput Assist Tomogr* 6:320, 1982.
5. Besley FA: A contribution to the study of skull fractures, *JAMA* 66:345, 1916.
6. Briant TDR, Bird R: Extracranial repair of cerebrospinal fluid fistulae, *J Otolaryngol* 11:191, 1982.
7. Calcaterra TC: Diagnosis and management of ethmoid cerebrospinal rhinorrhea, *Otolaryngol Clin North Am* 18:99, 1985.
8. Chandler JR: Traumatic cerebrospinal fluid leakage, *Otolaryngol Clin North Am* 16:623, 1983.
9. Ciric IS, Tarkington J: Transphenoidal microsurgery, *Surg Neurol* 2:207, 1974.
10. Cooper PR: *Skull fracture and traumatic cerebro-spinal fluid fistulas in head injury*. In Cooper PR, editor: *Head injury*, Baltimore, 1982, Williams & Wilkins.
11. Curnes JT and others: CSF rhinorrhea: detection and localization using overpressure cisternography with TC-99m-DTPA, *Radiology* 154:795, 1985.
12. Dodson EE and others: Transnasal endoscopic repair of cerebrospinal fluid rhinorrhea and skull base defects: a review of twenty-nine cases, *Otolaryngol Head Neck Surgery* 111:600, 1994.
13. El Gammal T, Brooks BS: MR cisternography: initial experience in 41 cases, *Am J Neuroradiol* 15:1647, 1994.
14. Eljamel MS and others: MRI cisternography, and the localization of CSF fistulae, *Br J Neurosurg* 8:443, 1994.
15. Ferguson BJ and others: Spontaneous CSF otorrhea from tegmen and posterior fossa defects, *Laryngoscope* 96:635, 1986.
16. Gagnon NB, Mohr G, Martinez SN: Unusual dural fistulae, *J Otolaryngol* 13:395, 1984.
17. Gardner G and others: Acoustic tumor management—combined approach surgery with CO_2 laser, *Am J Otol* 5:87, 1983.
18. Glasscock ME, Dickins JRE: Complications of acoustic tumor surgery, *Otolaryngol Clin North Am* 15:883, 1982.
19. Glaubitt D, Haubrich J, Cordoni-Voutsas M: Detection and quantitation of intermittent CSF rhinorrhea during prolonged cisternography with ^{111}In-DTPA, *Am J Neuroradiol* 4:560, 1983.
20. Gurdjian ES: Ear complications in acute craniocerebral injuries, *Radiology* 18:74, 1932.
21. Hasegawa M and others: Transfer of radioisotope from CSF to nasal secretion, *Acta Otolaryngol* 95:359, 1983.
22. House WF, Hitselberger WE: Surgical complications of acoustic tumor surgery, *Arch Otolaryngol* 88:659, 1968.
23. Hubbard JL and others: Spontaneous cerebrospinal fluid rhinorrhea: evolving concepts: diagnosis and surgical management based on the Mayo Clinic experience from 1970 through 1981, *Neurosurgery* 16:314, 1985.
24. Kirchner FR, Proud GO: Method for identification and localization of cerebrospinal fluid rhinorrhea and otorrhea, *Laryngoscope* 70:921, 1960.
25. Klastersky J, Sadeghi M, Brihaye J: Antimicrobial prophylaxis in patients with rhinorrhea or otorrhea: a double blind study, *Surg Neurol* 6:111, 1976.
26. Krahling KH, Konig HJ: A new technique for the sealing of a frontobasal cerebrospinal fluid fistula, *Fortschr Med* 102:1017, 1984.
27. Laun A: Traumatic cerebrospinal fluid fistulas in the anterior and middle cranial fossae, *Acta Neurochir* 60:215, 1982.
28. Loew F and others: Traumatic, spontaneous and postoperative CSF rhinorrhea, *Adv Tech Stand Neurosurg* 11:169, 1984.
29. MacGee EE, Cauthen JC, Brackett CE: Meningitis following acute traumatic cerebrospinal fluid fistula, *J Neurosurg* 33:312, 1970.
30. Mamo L and others: A new radiographic method for the diagnosis of posttraumatic cerebrospinal fistulas, *J Neurosurg* 57:92, 1982.
31. Manelfe C and others: Cerebrospinal fluid rhinorrhea: evaluation with metrizamide cisternography, *Am J Radiol* 138:471, 1982.
32. Mattox DE, Kennedy DW: Endoscopic management of cerebrospinal fluid leaks and cephaloceles, *Laryngoscope* 100:857, 1990.
33. McCarthy JG, Zide BM: The spectrum of calvarial bone grafting: introduction of the vascularized calvarial bone flap, *Plast Reconstr Surg* 74:10, 1984.
34. Messerklinger W: Nasenendoscopie: Nachweis, Lokalisation und Defferential-diagnose der Nasalen Liquorrhoe, *HNO* 20:268, 1972.
35. Mincy JE: Posttraumatic cerebrospinal fluid fistula of the frontal fossa, *J Trauma* 6:618, 1966.
36. Montgomery WW: *Cerebrospinal fistula*. In Montgomery WW, editor:

Surgery of the upper respiratory system, ed 2, Philadelphia, 1979, Lea & Febiger.

37. Mosely JI, Carton CA, Stern WE: Spectrum of complications in the use of intrathecal fluorescein, *J Neurosurg* 48:765, 1979.

38. Murata Y and others: MRI in spontanous cerebrospinal fluid rhinorrhea, *Neuroradiology* 37:453, 1995.

39. Myers DL, Sataloff RT: Spinal fluid leakage after skull base surgical procedures, *Otolaryngol Clin North Am* 17:601, 1984.

40. Naidich TP, Moran CJ: Precise anatomic localization of cerebrospinal fluid rhinorrhea by metrizamide CT cisternography, *J Neurosurg* 53:222, 1980.

41. Neely JG: Classification of spontaneous cerebrospinal fluid middle ear effusion: review of forty-nine cases, *Otolaryngol Head Neck Surg* 93:625, 1985.

42. Normansell DE and others: Detection of beta 2 transferrin in otorrhea and rhinorrhea in a routine clinical laboratory setting, *Clin Diagn Lab Immunol* 1:68, 1994.

43. Oberaschen G, Arrer E: Immunologische Liquordiagnostik mittels B_2—Transferrin—grundlagen und methodik, *Laryngol Rhinol Otol* 65:158, 1986.

44. Ommaya AK: Spinal fluid fistula, *Clin Neurosurg* 23:363, 1976.

45. Papay FA and others: Rigid endoscopic repair of paranasal sinus cerebrospinal fluid fistula, *Laryngoscope* 99:1195, 1989.

46. Park JI, Strelzow VV, Friedman WH: Current management of cerebrospinal fluid rhinorrhea, *Laryngoscope* 93:1294, 1983.

47. Park TS and others: Spontaneous cerebrospinal fluid otorrhea in association with a congenital defect of the cochlear aqueduct and Mondini dysplasia, *Neurosurgery* 11:356, 1982.

48. Raaf J: Posttraumatic cerebrospinal fluid leaks, *Arch Surg* 95:648, 1967.

49. Ray BS, Bergland RM: Cerebrospinal fluid fistula: clinical aspects, techniques of localization, and methods of closure, *J Neurosurg* 30:399, 1969.

50. Reck R, Wissen-Siegert I: Ergebnisse der Fluoreszein-Nasenendoskopie bei der Diagnostik der Rhinoliquorrho, *Laryngol Rhinol Otol* 63:353, 1984.

51. Ryall RG, Peacock MK, Simpson DA: Usefulness of beta 2-transferrin assay in the detection of cerebrospinal fluid leaks following head injury, *J Neurosurg* 77:737, 1992.

52. Schuknecht HF, Zaytoun GM, Moon CN: Adult-onset fluid in the tympanomastoid compartment, *Arch Otolaryngol* 108:759, 1982.

53. Stankiewicz JA: Cerebrospinal fluid fistula and endoscopic sinus surgery, *Laryngoscope* 101:250, 1991.

54. VanGilder JC, Goldenberg IS: Hypophysectomy in metastatic breast cancer, *Arch Surg* 110:293, 1975.

55. von Haacke NP, Croft CB: Cerebrospinal fluid rhinorrhoea and otorrhoea: extracranial repair, *Clin Otolaryngol* 8:317, 1983.

56. Zaret DL and others: Immunofixation to quantify beta 2-transferrin in cerebrospinal fluid to detect leakage of cerebrospinal fluid from skull injury, *Clin Chem* 38:1908, 1992.

PART FIVE

SALIVARY GLANDS

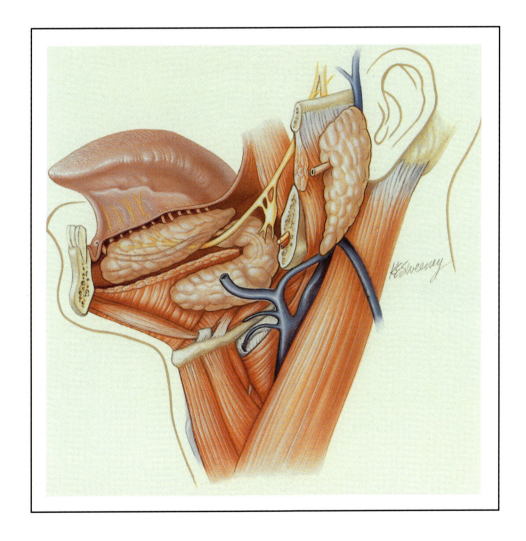

Chapter 64

Anatomy

Daniel O. Graney
John R. Jacobs
Robert C. Kern

PAROTID GLAND

The parotid gland, the largest of the salivary glands, is located on the face and is palpable between the ramus of the mandible and the mastoid process (Fig. 64-1). The lateral surface of the gland is covered only by the skin and dermis of the face, thus the gland is vulnerable to injury even with superficial lacerations of the face. The medial relations of the gland (Fig. 64-2) or deep surface are buttressed by the styloid process and its associated muscles (styloglossus, stylohyoid, and stylopharyngeal) as well as the carotid sheath and its contents (internal carotid artery, internal jugular vein, and cranial nerves [CN] IX, X, and XII). The superior limit of the gland is the zygomatic arch, and the inferior boundary of the gland is the oblique anterior border of the sternocleidomastoid muscle.

The gland is often described as having a superficial and deep lobe, although the exact pattern of the lobulation has been the subject of substantial debate.[1] A simplified view is to think of the gland as an asymmetric dumbbell with the larger end representing the superficial lobe and the smaller end the deep lobe, with the glandular isthmus being the connection between the two. When viewed from above, the groove between the two is filled by the ramus of the mandible and its muscle coverings, the masseter laterally and the medial pterygoid medially. The posterior groove is filled by the mastoid and posterior belly of the digastric muscle. Much of the superficial lobe lies close to the skin and is obvious when the gland is swollen, as happens with parotitis. Because of the close anatomic relationships and the fact that the gland is well encapsulated within a fascial envelope, swelling of the gland during parotitis (as in mumps) can be quite painful,

particularly when the patient opens his or her mouth. The hinge action that occurs when the mandible is depressed compresses the swollen parotid against the mastoid process and the walls of its inelastic capsule and results in a painful masticatory process.

The main portion of the deep lobe lies adjacent to the styloid and carotid sheath structures, as described, but when enlarged by tumor it can contact the lateral pharyngeal wall in the region of the palatine tonsil and appear clinically as a peritonsillar mass.

Clinical considerations

The surgical concept of the parotid gland is of a structure that contains two lobes: superficial and deep. The plane between the two lobes is defined by the facial nerve as it exits the stylomastoid foramen and courses anteriorly through the gland to innervate the fascial muscles of expression. Surgically removing the superficial lobe is often the recommended approach for diagnosis and treatment of tumors of the parotid gland. Crucial to successful removal of the superficial lobe is the accurate identification and preservation of the facial nerve.

The only constant landmark to the location of the facial nerve is the stylomastoid foramen from which the nerve exits the skull base. Although the nerve can and often is displaced by large tumors of the parotid gland, it usually can be identified without dissecting the mastoid tip. The key to identifying the facial nerve successfully is good exposure. The incision starts anteriorly in the pretragal skin creases and extends inferiorly down to the lobule where it is gently curved posteriorly, approximately a centimeter over the mastoid tip be-

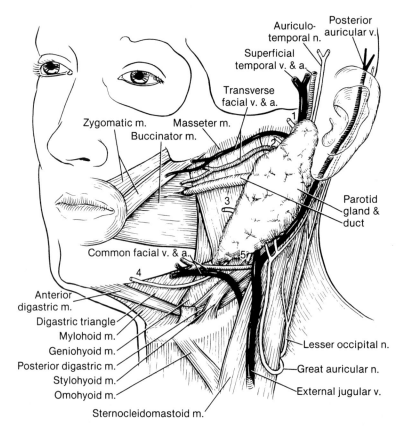

Fig. 64-1. The parotid gland and surrounding structures. Branches of the facial nerve: (1) temporal; (2) zygomatic; (3) buccal; (4) mandibular (marginal); and (5) cervical.

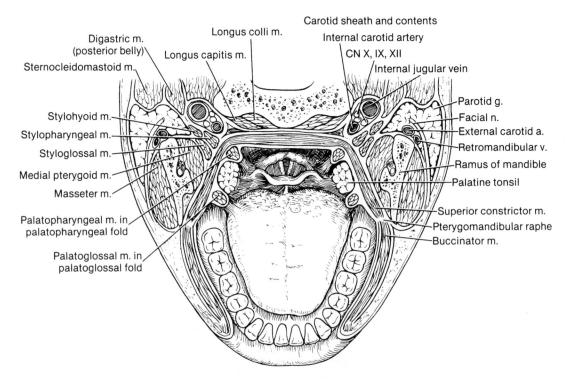

Fig. 64-2. Medial relations of the parotid gland.

fore tracing the anterior border of the sternocleidomastoid muscle. It is then extended anteriorly approximately two fingers' breadths beneath the inferior ramus of the mandible. The skin flap is elevated to expose the entire gland. This usually results in an exposure from the zygomatic arch to the midportion of the posterior belly of the digastric muscle. Careful dissection down the cartilaginous external auditory canal medially is then performed. Care should be taken to avoid dissecting into a "hole." The anterior border of the sternocleidomastoid muscle insertion onto the mastoid tip should be developed to increase exposure. Eventually the cartilaginous pointer will be identified; the facial nerve lies inferior and slightly deeper to the pointer. It is helpful to use an operating headlight and low-power magnifying loops for this portion of the procedure. Once the nerve is identified visually it is important that confirmation be obtained with a single low-power electrical stimulation. The nerve trunk is then traced anteriorly with removal of the so-called superficial lobe. Using a small, pointed hemostat, tunnels are created over the nerve branches and then connected, allowing preservation of the nerve. It is critical that the gland be placed under traction by the surgical assistant.

Occasionally the facial nerve cannot be identified through the pointer. It then becomes necessary to use an alternative method. All of the alternatives with the exception of localization within the mastoid tip through a mastoidectomy require identification of a branch of the facial nerve and retrograde dissection back to the main trunk. Perhaps the most reliable alternative is identifying mandibularis branch as it crosses the facial vein. The ophthalmic and buccal branches also are potential candidates for identification and subsequent retrograde tracing.

Parotid duct

Although the parotid duct usually appears to originate from the superficial lobe, its origin is in fact frequently more complicated. Davis and others[1] have described the formation of the parotid duct as arising from a varied pattern of extraglandular ductules. These ductules may arise from the superficial lobe, the deep lobe, or both, before fusing to form the substance of the parotid duct. The duct traverses the surface of the masseter muscle and crosses the anterior aspect of the mandible approximately a fingers' breadth below the zygomatic process. At this point, the duct abruptly turns medially to pierce the buccinator muscle and the buccal fat pad to enter the oral mucosa, which it penetrates at approximately the level of the second maxillary molar.

Surface relationships of the parotid gland

The lateral surface of the gland or its superficial lobe has a number of important anatomic relationships pertaining to various nerves, arteries, and veins that either emerge or enter the substance of the gland at varying points around its perimeter. If the gland is viewed as a clock face with the superior pole representing the 12 o'clock position and the inferior pole representing the 6 o'clock position, various structures can be seen to enter or leave the gland at these points (see Fig. 64-1). At the 12 o'clock position are three structures: the auriculotemporal nerve and the superficial temporal artery and vein. At the inferior pole, or 6 o'clock position, the structures are the retromandibular vein and its connections with the external and internal jugular veins. Along the anterior margin of the parotid are the various branches of CN VII, which emerge from the substance of the parotid to enter the submuscular plane of the face. These include the temporal, zygomatic, buccal, mandibular, and cervical branches. A transverse facial artery and vein also are related to the anterior aspect of the parotid, located slightly superior to the parotid duct and paralleling the course into the cheek and infraorbital region. At the posterior margin of the gland the posterior auricular and occipital arteries can sometimes be identified, but more often they are buried in the parotid tissue. Superficially located at this posterior aspect of the parotid, however, is the great auricular nerve. This is a peripheral nerve made up of fibers from the roots of cervical nerves C2 and C3 and is one of the major branches of the cervical plexus. This nerve serves to supply cutaneous innervation over the region of the mastoid and the submandibular triangle of the neck.

The contents of the parotid gland include, in addition to CN VII, the external carotid artery, and the retromandibular vein. Each of these structures is discussed.

Origin and course of the intraparotid portion of the seventh cranial nerve

CN VII emerges from the stylomastoid foramen to enter the substance of the parotid gland on its posteromedial surface. The site of entry into the gland is an important surgical landmark and can be found using the "tragal" pointer. If the tip of the index finger is placed at the base of the tragal cartilage and is pushed firmly against the lateral aspect of the skull, the pad of the fingertip lies between the external acoustic meatus and the mastoid process. This in effect represents the site of the stylomastoid foramen and the point at which CN VII emerges from the skull. During parotid surgery, an incision is made along the inferior margin of the external acoustic meatus. The skin is reflected to visualize the cartilage of the meatus and the bone of the mastoid tip.

If one follows the interval between the bone and cartilage medially, that is, deep into the dissection, one eventually reaches the stylomastoid foramen. The depth of the foramen from the level of the skin is approximately 25 mm. As CN VII leaves the stylomastoid foramen, it simultaneously enters the substance of the parotid gland and divides into two major trunks, the temporofacial and the cervicofacial. The branching pattern of these nerves has been studied extensively by Davis and others.[1] Their study describes six types of the facial nerve based on the anastomosis of individual branches. Type I occurs in approximately 13% of cases and represents no anastomosis between the five branches of CN

VII: the temporal, zygomatic, buccal, mandibular, and cervical. The other five types show varying patterns of anastomosis between the individual branches. Although to recognize the potential for variation in anatomic patterns is important for the surgeon, committing the percentages of these to memory seems fruitless because the surgeon cannot select patients on the basis of anatomic variants. For the surgeon, Geraldine's law of anatomy prevails: ''what you see is what you get'' (with apologies to Flip Wilson).

The temporofacial usually is composed of the temporal, zygomatic, and buccal branches, whereas the cervicofacial comprises the mandibular and cervical branches. The trunks divide into their branches within the main body of the gland and then course distally within the superficial lobe to their respective territories on the face and neck. None of the branches traverse the deep lobe.

External carotid artery

Although the external carotid artery can be visualized at the inferior pole of the parotid gland, it may travel superiorly a few millimeters before entering the substance of the gland. The posterior auricular artery is usually given off from its posterior surface before the vessel divides into its two terminal branches, the maxillary artery and the superficial temporal artery. The maxillary artery exits the deep surface of the gland and supplies the various structures of the infratemporal fossa before entering the pterygopalatine fossa. The branches of the terminal part of the maxillary artery supply the maxillary teeth and the palatine and nasal mucosae. Chapter 40 discusses the details of these vessels. Before the superficial temporal artery leaves the superior pole for the parotid, it gives off the transverse facial artery, described previously as following the course of the parotid duct supplying the upper quadrant of the face. Chapter 21 describes the distribution and pattern of anastomosis of the superficial temporal artery in the scalp.

Venous pattern within the parotid gland

The venous structures within the parotid gland fundamentally parallel those of the parotid arteries; they consist of a superficial temporal vein and a series of veins emerging from the infratemporal fossa and the pterygoid venous plexus. The maxillary vein may be somewhat short because it is formed from a series of tributaries rather than a single large vein crossing the infratemporal fossa, as in the case of the maxillary artery. The fusion of the maxillary and superficial temporal veins forms the retromandibular vein within the substance of the parotid. The veins usually occupy the plane between the nerve (superficially located) and the artery (located in the deep lobe). The retromandibular vein exits from the parotid near its inferior pole, where anastomosis with the external jugular vein occurs. Frequently a posterior facial vein connects with the anterior facial vein, the confluence of the two forming a common facial vein that drains into the internal jugular vein (Figs. 64-1 and 64-3). The pattern of venous anastomosis at this point varies in different individuals as well as from side to side in a single individual.

Innervation of the parotid gland

CN IX provides secretomotor function to the parotid gland after a complicated course through the temporal bone and infratemporal fossa (Fig. 64-4). The secretomotor fibers begin in the inferior salivary nucleus of the brainstem and travel with CN IX as it emerges from the jugular foramen. Here a recurrent branch, the tympanic branch (Jacobson's nerve), turns back into the skull by entering a small canal, the inferior tympanic canaliculus, which opens onto the floor of the middle ear or tympanic cavity (see Fig. 64-4). The path of this nerve can be identified on most skulls by the passing of a fine bristle through the tympanic canaliculus, located in the bony septum lying between the jugular and carotid foramina, as the middle ear space through the external acoustic meatus is observed.

From the floor of the tympanic cavity, the nerve fibers enter the mucosa over the promontory and course anterosuperiorly to penetrate the bony roof of the tympanic cavity and enter the subdural space of the middle cranial fossa. It should be noted that the tympanic nerve also contains sensory fibers that are distributed to the mucosa of the middle ear.

After penetrating the roof of the tympanic cavity, the secretomotor fibers descend on the petrous ridge in the middle cranial fossa as a delicate nerve bundle, termed the *lesser petrosal nerve*. The fibers are directed toward the area of the foramen spinosum and the foramen ovale and usually exit from the skull through the latter in proximity to the third division of the trigeminal nerve. Because these fibers are preganglionic parasympathetic secretomotor fibers, they synapse with the cell body of a second neuron before innervating the parotid. The accumulated cell bodies of these second-order neurons form the otic ganglion; they are the source of the postganglionic fibers for innervation of the gland. The ganglion is not always an identifiable structure attached to the mandibular division of the trigeminal nerve, but may be formed by scattered cell bodies trapped within a plexus of trigeminal nerve fibers. Postganglionic fibers from the ganglion do not form a new nerve but join with the auriculotemporal branch of the mandibular division of the trigeminal nerve, which crosses the posterior wall of the infratemporal fossa to the region of the parotid. Most of the secretomotor fibers leave the auriculotemporal nerve and disperse within the parotid substance, so that by the time the nerve crosses the temporomandibular joint it contains only sensor fibers from the scalp.

Frey's syndrome (gustatory sweating, or auriculotemporal nerve syndrome) is familiar to most surgeons who perform parotidectomies. Following parotidectomy the regeneration of these secretomotor fibers becomes misdirected, and the fibers innervate the sweat glands of the skin. The result of these misdirected fibers is facial sweating when CN IX

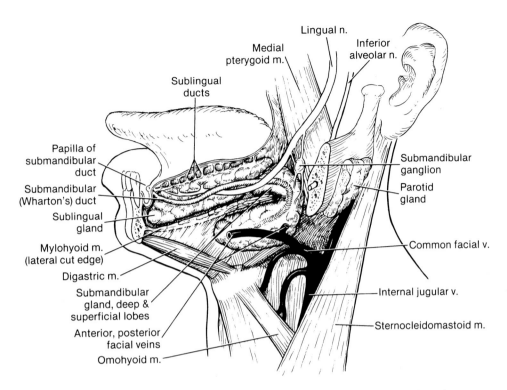

Fig. 64-3. The formation of common facial vein draining into internal jugular vein.

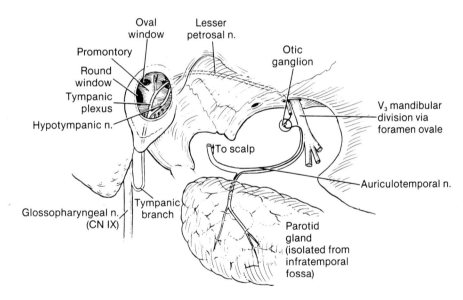

Fig. 64-4. The parotid innervation.

is stimulated during the course of eating. Ross[4] observed increased parotid secretion after electrical stimulation of the tympanic branch of the glossopharyngeal nerve in stapedectomy patients. In a second patient population with Frey's syndrome, Ross resected the tympanic plexus and obtained a mixed result with respect to relief of the patient's symptoms. Although two patients had permanent cures, other patients had a return of symptoms within 30 days. This return resulted from incomplete section of the tympanic plexus with recovery of the remaining nerve fibers several days after surgery. These fibers arise as a hypotympanic nerve from the tympanic plexus near the floor of the tympanic cavity and ascend the anterior aspect of the promontory either within the mucosa or covered by thin bone. A hypotympanic branch has been described in 50% of specimens.[3] Parotid atrophy has been reported in humans[2] and rabbits[5] after interruption of the tympanic plexus.

It appears clear from the current evidence that parasympathetic secretomotor fibers innervate the parotid gland solely through CN IX and that denervation of the gland results in atrophy. The parotid gland, then, contrasts with other salivary glands that appear to be more diffusely innervated.

SUBMANDIBULAR GLAND

The submandibular gland fills the major portion of the digastric or submandibular triangle. The gland rests against the structures forming the floor of the triangle, the mylohyoid and hyoglossus muscles (see Fig. 64-3). The gland has two portions: (1) a superficial lobe lying superficial to the mylohyoid and (2) a deep lobe wrapping around the posterior border of the mylohyoid muscle. The deep lobe cannot be palpated superficially in the neck but can be palpated in the floor of the mouth by a gloved finger while the other hand supports the superficial lobe. The duct of the submandibular gland (Wharton's duct) emerges from the deep lobe and courses anteriorly in the plane between the hyoglossus and mylohyoid muscles. It terminates as an elevated papilla on the floor of the mouth near the frenulum of the tongue, adjacent to the duct from the opposite side. While occupying this plane the duct is crossed twice by the lingual nerve, once on its lateral aspect near its origin and again on the medial aspect of the duct near its termination at the frenulum.

Clinical considerations

The surgical approach to removing the submandibular gland is through an incision placed approximately two fingers' breaths beneath the inferior border of the ramus of the mandible. The incision is carefully dissected down to the level of the platysmal muscle and the fascia lying immediately over the actual gland. At this level, the mandibularis branch of the facial nerve is identified lying on the undersurface of the platysmal muscle and superficial on the fascia overlying the submandibular gland proper. It is usually identified visually without much difficulty. Damage to this nerve will result in drooping of the corner of the lip. The facial vein, which lies beneath the nerve, can be used to raise the nerve out of harm's way by ligation inferior to the nerve and then subsequent dissection of the vein superiorly with the nerve trapped above the vein.

Once the facial nerve is safely out of the operative field, the dissection then can proceed to identification of the posterior border of the mylohyoid muscle. Placement of a Richardson retractor on the posterior border of this muscle along with inferior traction on the gland proper brings into view the important structures that lie on the medial aspect of the gland, the lingual nerve and submandibular gland duct. With the lingual nerve visually identified as it loops into the field, the duct can safely be isolated, divided, and ligated. The facial artery also is in the field and relatively easy to identify by palpation. It is usually ligated twice during the procedure as it arises from the depths of the wound through the undersurface of the gland and over the mandible.

SUBLINGUAL GLAND

The sublingual gland is a flat, oblong structure that accompanies the distal half of the submandibular duct, so the gland occupies the same plane; that is, between the mylohyoid and hyoglossus muscles (see Fig. 64-3). It lies superficially in the floor of the mouth, covered only by the oral mucosa. The gland does not have a single large excretory duct but a series of ductules that open either into the floor of the mouth directly or into the submandibular duct. The submandibular duct thus serves both glands.

INNERVATION OF THE SUBMANDIBULAR AND SUBLINGUAL GLANDS

The submandibular and sublingual glands are innervated by secretomotor fibers of CN VII, which are derived from the superior salivary nucleus. These fibers exit from the brainstem within the intermediary nerve rather than the motor portion of CN VII. The intermediary nerve joins CN VII within the internal acoustic meatus, and its fibers parallel the course of CN VII through the temporal bone (Fig. 64-5). On the posterior wall of the middle ear the chorda tympani branch of CN VII arises from the vertical portion of CN VII and crosses the lateral wall of the middle ear. Its course is constant as it parallels the tympanic membrane, lying between the long process of the incus and the manubrium of the malleus. Anteriorly it pierces the petrotympanic fissure of the middle ear and enters the infratemporal fossa. Here, the nerve has a short independent course before joining the lingual nerve, a branch of the mandibular division of the trigeminal nerve. The fibers follow the course of the lingual nerve until it reaches the floor of the mouth, where the fibers leave the lingual nerve to synapse in the submandibular ganglion, a parasympathetic ganglion. The ganglion is usually a prominent structure attached to the lingual nerve by a plexus of nerve fibers (see Fig. 64-5). Postganglionic secretomotor fibers course directly to the submandibular gland from the ganglion, but some postganglionic fibers return to the lingual nerve and travel anteriorly in the floor of the mouth before supplying the sublingual gland.

Although the innervation of the parotid gland was seen to be quite specific—denervation resulting in glandular atrophy—the same is not true for the submandibular and sublingual glands. Sectioning of the chorda tympani does not produce atrophy of these glands and results in only partial diminution of secretion, even when combined with sectioning of the tympanic branch of the glossopharyngeal nerve.

INNERVATION OF THE TONGUE

Although initially the topic of innervation of the tongue may not seem to fit into the context of this chapter, it is actually quite appropriate when one considers that the tongue

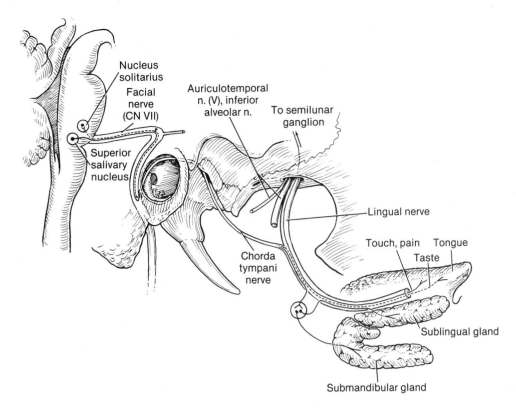

Fig. 64-5. The submandibular innervation.

receives sensory innervation from the chorda tympani branch of the facial nerve, the lingual branch of the trigeminal nerve, and the terminal branch of the glossopharyngeal nerve.

CN XII supplies all of the tongue's musculature by fibers beginning in the hypoglossal nucleus of the medulla. However, the sensory innervation of the tongue is topographically divided into the posterior one third supplied by the glossopharyngeal nerve (CN IX) and the anterior two thirds supplied by the lingual and chorda tympani nerves. In the posterior third the glossopharyngeal nerve supplies both special visceral afferents responsible for taste and general visceral afferents concerned with touch and the gag reflex. The majority of the taste buds in the posterior third of the tongue are located in the epithelium lining the circumvallate papillae, although others can be found in the mucosa of the valleculae and the epiglottis. The peripheral processes of both modalities, taste and touch, have the cell bodies of their neurons in the inferior ganglion of the glossopharyngeal nerve, which is located on the nerve at the level of the jugular foramen. The central processes for both taste and touch project to the nucleus solitarius in the pons.

In the anterior two thirds of the tongue, touch and taste sensations are carried by two different nerves, the lingual and the chorda tympani, respectively. The general sensations of touch, pain, and temperature are carried by fibers through the lingual nerve; the fibers ascend the infratemporal fossa to the foramen ovale, where they join with other fibers of the mandibular division of the trigeminal nerve. The peripheral processes of these neurons have their cell bodies located in the semilunar ganglion of the trigeminal nerve. Central processes project to the nucleus of the spinal tract of CN V in the case of pain and temperature fibers, whereas touch fibers project to the main sensory nucleus of CN V. Taste buds in the anterior two thirds of the tongue are located either in the foliate papillae along the lateral aspect of the tongue or in fungiform papillae, which are more diffusely distributed in the mucosa. Afferent fibers from the taste buds travel posteriorly along the lingual nerve until the junction with the chorda tympani near the roof the infratemporal fossa. The fibers follow the course of the chorda tympani through the middle ear and join the facial nerve on the posterior wall of the tympanic cavity. Following the facial canal, the fibers reach their cell bodies in the geniculate ganglion before projecting centrally through the intermediary nerve to the nucleus solitarius in the pons.

The importance of neuroanatomic pathways is obvious in understanding the various clinical deficits exhibited by patients after either a central pontomedullary lesion or a peripheral trauma affecting the pathways of CN V, VII, or IX.

ANATOMIC PLANES IN THE FLOOR OF THE MOUTH

The surgical approaches to the salivary glands in the floor of the mouth may involve either an intraoral route or an external approach through the submandibular triangle of the neck. Regardless of the approach chosen, the anatomic relationships are fundamentally the same. The surgeon must anticipate anatomic structure during surgical dissection. Memorizing anatomic detail seems tedious, but sometimes simple organizational techniques can facilitate learning. In the floor of the mouth the keys to these relationships are the mylohyoid and the hyoglossus muscles, which form vertical planes for the passage of the neurovascular bundle that is related either superficial or deep to these muscles (Fig. 64-6). In this manner, three planes can be described: the first, superficial to the mylohyoid; the second, superficial to the hyoglossus; and the third, deep to the hyoglossus.

Plane that is superficial to the mylohyoid muscle

The relationships of the mylohyoid muscle are in fact the contents of the submandibular triangle of the neck. Bounded by the two bellies of the digastric and the ramus of the mandible, the triangle forms a three-dimensional space rather than a flat triangle. The skin and platysma close the roof (lateral wall) of the triangle, whereas the mylohyoid and hyoglossus muscles form the floor (medial wall). Superficial to the mylohyoid are the submandibular gland, associated lymph nodes, the facial artery and vein, and the motor nerve to both the mylohyoid muscle and the anterior belly of the digastric muscle. One of the most superficial structures in the space is the mandibular branch of the facial nerve, which after emerging from the parotid usually arcs below the mandible before ascending onto the face again near the anterior part of the triangle. Chapter 21 discusses this nerve's importance to the innervation of the muscle of the lower lip.

Plane that is superficial to the hyoglossus muscle

The structures related to the hyoglossus muscle also might be described as lying deep to the mylohyoid; in effect, they occupy the plane between the two muscles. The deep lobe of the submandibular gland separates these muscles before folding around the posterior border of the mylohyoid before sending the submandibular duct anteriorly to the frenulum of the tongue. The sublingual gland surrounds the duct as it lies against the anterior part of the hyoglossus muscle. In addition to the duct, two nerves occupy this plane, the lingual and CN XII (the hypoglossal nerve). The hypoglossal nerve always courses along the most inferior part of the plane between the two muscles. The lingual nerve enters the floor of the mouth, superior to the submandibular duct and crosses it laterally before ascending on the medial surface of the duct adjacent to the hyoglossus muscle.

Plane that is deep to the hyoglossus muscle

Three structures occupy the plane that is deep to the hyoglossus muscle: the lingual artery, the stylohyoid ligament attaching to the lesser cornu of the hyoid bone, and CN IX (glossopharyngeal nerve) (see Fig. 64-6). The nerve and ligament are not seen in Figure 64-6 because they have terminated posterior to the plane of the section.

The three relationships just described provide an inventory of structures the surgeon should be able to predict during surgical dissection. Whether the challenge is a

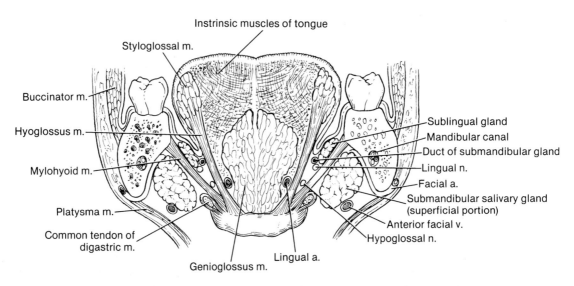

Fig. 64-6. The mylohyoid and hyoglossus muscles form vertical planes for passage of neurovascular bundle.

simple exploration of the floor of the mouth to remove a ductal occlusion or a complicated hemiglossectomy, the anatomy is the same.

REFERENCES

1. Davis RA and others: Surgical anatomy of the facial nerve and parotid gland based upon a study of 350 cervicofacial halves. *Surg Gynecol Obstet* 102:385, 1956.

2. Dishell WD: Tympanic neurectomy in chronic parotitis. *Arch Otolaryngol* 94:471, 1971.

3. Porto AF, Whicker J, Proud GO: An anatomic study of the hypotympanic branch of Jacobson's nerve, *Laryngoscope* 88:56, 1978.

4. Ross JAT: The function of the tympanic plexus as related to Frey's syndrome, *Laryngoscope* 80:1816, 1970.

5. Wallenborn WM and others: Parotid gland atrophy produced by transtympanic destruction of the tympanic plexus, *Laryngoscope* 78:132, 1968.

Chapter 65

Physiology

John G. Batsakis

The study and elucidation of the physiology of salivary tissues have evolved more slowly than those of other tissue/organ systems. Indeed, only since the late 1970s have the misconceptions and misinterpretations of earlier data been corrected; with these corrections has come an appreciation of the physiology's complex nature. The excretory-secretory functions of the salivary duct system rival those of the renal tubules in their metabolic activity, and only recently have the acinar cell processing and delivery of their products been postulated. Saliva, the medium produced by salivary tissue, also remains to be fully characterized despite investigations dating back to Greco-Roman times.

It should also be appreciated that much of the basis of our understanding of salivary physiology is derivative of studies with nonhuman (principally rat) salivary glands.[6] Human data are limited, but those that exist generally conform to the information described in the following pages.

NORMAL PHYSIOLOGY

The salivary glands have a variety of functions. They provide (1) a lubricant to aid in swallowing food, mechanical cleaning, and immunologic defense; (2) digestion by an emulgation of food and enzymatic cleavage (primarily starch by α-amylase); (3) production of hormones or hormone-like products and other metabolically active compounds; (4) excretion of endogenous and exogenous materials, for example, antibodies, blood group–reactive substances, iodine, and viruses; (5) mediation of taste sensations; and (6) defense, which is pertinent only to subhuman species.

For their size the salivary glands produce a large volume of saliva: the maximal rate in humans is about 1 ml/min/g of glandular tissue. The rate of metabolism of salivary glands is also high, accompanied by a high blood flow—both proportional to the rate of saliva formation. The flow of blood to maximally secreting salivary glands is approximately 10 times that of an equal mass of actively contracting skeletal muscle.

Autonomic control

With the exception of the vasodilator action of bradykinin and the stimulation of ductal sodium ion and potassium ion transport by aldosterone, the physiologic control of salivary glands is almost solely affected by the autonomic nervous system.[3,19] Stimulation of sympathetic or parasympathetic nerves produces salivary secretion. The effects of the parasympathetic nerves are predominant; interruption of the sympathetic innervation causes little or no change in function. If interruption of the parasympathetic supply occurs, however, salivary glands undergo atrophy.

Probably there is no truly spontaneous secretion from either the parotid or the submandibular glands. All secretion of saliva results from stimulation of the glands' autonomic innervation or by the action of the substances mimicking the effects of such stimulation.

Functional studies with electrical stimulation of nerves continue to provide new information about the respective roles of the different nerves involved in salivary secretion. Garrett[20] rightly points out that the different nerves and their various transmitters allow a harmonious interplay and the interaction is not ''a contest between two solo performers'' (Table 65-1). The principal stimulus for inducing flow of saliva is parasympathetic. Sympathetic impulses serve more as modulators of the composition of the saliva. There is also some indication that nerve impulses may have an important role in the resynthesis of intracellular secretory material.[20]

The innervation patterns of the major salivary glands differ considerably, not only from species to species but also between glands within the same subject and between differ-

Table 65-1. Salivary gland innervations and functional correlates

Parasympathetic	Sympathetic
Principal stimulus for fluid formation	Weak-to-poor mobilizer of fluid
May be isolated	Additive to parasympathetic; may yield synergistic effect
Causes some exocytosis	Increases exocytosis and modulates composition of saliva
Induces contraction of myoepithelia	Usually induces contraction of myoepithelia
Causes vasodilatation as part of secretory process	Some fibers maintain vascular tone; believed to be anatomically separate from secretory nerves

Modified from Garrett JR: *Innervation of salivary glands: neurohistological and functional aspects.* In LM Sreebny, editor: *The salivary system,* Boca Raton, Fla, 1989, CRC Press.

ent cell types within a gland. The human parotid gland is furnished equally well with both sympathetic and parasympathetic nerve fibers.[12,19] Preganglionic parasympathetic fibers from the ninth cranial nerve (CN IX) travel to the otic ganglion and continue as secretomotor fibers to reach the parotid gland via the auriculotemporal nerve. Sympathetic fibers from the cervical ganglia accompany the blood vessels to the salivary gland. Gangliocytes are not found in the gland itself. Once within the gland, the postganglionic sympathetic and parasympathetic fibers reach myoepithelial cells, intercalated ducts, and acinar cells. Cholinergic and adrenergic terminal axons innervate the same cells, with receptors found on the cell membrane.[19]

Electron-optic study shows two types of neuroeffector arrangements in the glands: epilemmal and hypolemmal.[12,19] In the former the axon lies outside the epithelial basement membrane; in the latter the axon penetrates the basement membrane. Neuroeffector sites occur where a nonmyelinated axon is in intimate relationship with adjacent salivary cells, and neuroactivation takes place where sufficient transmitter is released to activate adjacent cells. This depends on the distances between axon and cells and on the sensitivity of the cell membranes. Most hypolemmal axons are cholinergic. No pattern of order exists, however, and at certain sites hypolemmal axons have been found in the submandibular gland, whereas both adrenergic and cholinergic hypolemmal axons occur in relation to parotid acinar cells.[19]

The parasympathetic nerves are primarily responsible for the flow of saliva during reflex secretion via acetylcholine released from nerves acting on the membranes of effector cells.[12,19] The electrical changes and the movement of ions induced by acetylcholine are associated with permeability changes in activated cell membranes.

Electrophysiology

With a few (nonsalivary) exceptions, all stimulants to secretion cause membrane potential changes in their target cells, and this results at least in part from changes in membrane conductance to certain ions.[38] Two distinct factors contribute to the electrical properties of a cell surface. One is the presence of "fixed" negative charges associated with phospholipids, glycolipids, and glycoproteins that constitute the plasma membrane—the so-called *surface potential*; the other factor is the difference in charge between the inside and the outside of cells—the so-called *transmembrane potential*. The surface potential contributes little to transmembrane potential but it seems to affect the ability of certain stimuli to collapse the transmembrane potential in excitable cells; that is, the ability to generate an action potential. Electrogenic pumps in the plasma membrane, such as the sodium pump, contribute in varying amounts to the setting of membrane potential.[38,46]

Neurotransmitters, hormones, and other regulatory molecules affect the function of salivary cells in a complex manner that is only beginning to be understood.[19,38,46,51] Nearly all of the effects result from a direct regulation of target cells. Receptors, second messengers, and effectors are essential to this regulation of cell function (Table 65-2). With the parotid gland as the prototype, the following is presented to illustrate the interactions of the various modules in the electrophysiologic patterns.

Receptors

The receptors are moieties that interact with ligands involving recognition and transfer of information.[25] The interaction initiates a biologic response or sequence of responses. The quality of the biologic response resides in the receptor-effector and not in the ligand. The binding of a ligand to a specific receptor is the first step in the regulation of cell function by extracellular factors. The majority of regulatory receptors are found in the plasma membrane (proteins or glycoproteins); a few (hormonal) are present within the cell. Once occupied by its specific regulatory molecule, the receptor complex activates an effector process to bring about the cellular response. Activation is either direct or through a second messenger. A receptor may be a single or composite membrane protein and may contain subunits with special functions.

Little is known of the molecular characteristics of salivary gland receptors. Probably, however, adrenergic, muscarinic cholinergic, and other receptors are similar to those found on other cells. Receptors for polypeptide hormones and neurotransmitters are on the plasma membrane, and for exocrine glands they are on the basal or lateral membranes.[50] For some cells, receptor occupancy and biologic effects follow saturation kinetics; for other cells, regulation does not require full occupancy.[25]

Two major classes of receptors are α-adrenergic and β-adrenergic. Lefkowitz and others,[26] have defined two subtypes of each receptor, termed α_1 and α_2 and β_1 and β_2. Table 65-3 outlines their properties. Three of the four subtypes of adrenergic receptors are linked to the same biochem-

Table 65-2. Salivary function and regulatory molecules

Salivary gland	Regulator	Second messenger	Effect
Parotid	Acetylcholine (ACh), α-adrenergic, substance P	Ca^{++}	Production of saliva, limited enzyme secretion, increased cell metabolism
	β-adrenergic, vipadrenergic intestinal peptide (VIP)	AMP	Secretion of enzymes, increased cell metabolism
Submandibular	ACh, α-adrenergic	Ca^{++}	Production of saliva
	β-adrenergic	?cAMP	Production of mucin
	VIP	?cAMP	Potentiates ACh effect, enhances blood flow

Data from Williams JA: Regulatory mechanisms in pancreas and salivary acini, *Ann Rev Physiol* 46:361, 1984.

Table 65-3. Adrenergic receptors

α_1	α_2	β_1	β_2
Physiologic responses			
Smooth muscle contraction in vessels	Smooth muscle contraction in selected vascular bed	Stimulates amylase secretion by salivary glands	Smooth muscle relaxation
	Inhibits release of norepinephrine Stimulates secretion of K and H_2O by salivary glands		Facilitates release of norepinephrine
Location			
After synapse	Before, after, and without synapse	After synapse	Before, after, and without synapse
Mechanism			
Changes of cellular Ca^{++} fluxes	Inhibition of adenylate cyclase	Stimulation of adenylate cyclase	Stimulation of adenylate cyclase

Modified from Lefkowitz RJ, Caron MG, Stiles GL: Mechanisms of membrane-receptor regulation: biochemical, physiological, and clinical insights derived from studies of the adrenergic receptors. *N Engl J Med* 310:1570, 1984.

ical effect on the adenylate cyclase system, which generates the second messenger, adenosine $3':5'$-cyclic phosphate (cAMP). The β_1 and β_2 receptors stimulate the enzyme, whereas the α_2 receptors inhibit it. Rather than being coupled to adenylate cyclase, α_1 receptors appear to be coupled to processes that regulate cellular calcium-ion fluxes.[26]

Second messengers

cAMP and cytosol-free calcium ion have been the most intensively studied second messengers. Others, considered to be messenger-like systems, include guanylic monophosphate (GMP), phospholipids, cytosol pH, and membrane depolarization.[51] In the parotid gland or pancreas, intracellular calcium ion serves as a trigger for acutely stimulating acinar function. The relationship, however, between receptor occupancy, intracellular calcium ion, and the induced response is not known.

Williams[51] has indicated that specific second messengers are not typically linked to specific biologic effects. In the parotid gland, calcium largely mediates stimulation of fluid secretion, whereas in the pancreas, calcium is the major mes-

senger stimulating enzyme release from acinar cells. Conversely, cAMP in salivary glands mediates macromolecular secretion and fluid from the pancreas. Probably the two messengers potentiate each other. The messenger-like systems may be involved in the formation of second messengers, function as transduction mechanisms, or be induced as tertiary phenomena. Not all hormones or neurotransmitters possess known second messengers. They may act as their own second messengers through enzyme activation of their receptors.[51]

Besides the generation of cAMP as a mechanism of neurotransmitter signal transduction, it is likely that a second signal transduction mechanism exists, and this relates to phosphatidylinositol-4, 5-biphosphate turnover.[30]

Effectors

Far less is known about effector systems than about receptors or second messengers. The protein-kinases in salivary tissues are, however, similar to those in the pancreas and other tissues.[51] Both cAMP and calcium-activated kinases exist. All of the kinases phosphorylate different subsets of proteins. Control of exocytotic secretion may involve phosphorylation of granule or plasma membrane or activation of contractility by phosphorylation of the light chain of myosin.[51] A calcium-activated monovalent cation-selective channel is another effector system; that is, ion flux (influx of Na^+ and Ca^{++} and efflux of K^+) leads to a depolarization of the cell.[19,51]

Secretion

Saliva consists of fluid and macromolecules. The fluid component is derived from perfusing blood vessels; the macromolecules are primarily derived from secretory granules of the acinar cells. The fluid is produced at the secretory end-pieces and is currently thought to occur via an osmotic coupling (solute-solvent coupling) of transepithelial fluxes of sodium chloride and water.[22] It is likely that the water and electrolyte fluxes occur transcellularly through acinar cells. Movement of sodium and chloride through the cell and into the acinar lumen provides an osmotic gradient to establish an accompanying water flow across the cell. The currently favored hypothesis to explain how sodium and chloride cross the basal cell membrane is that a cotransport of the two ions occurs with the movement of sodium down its electrochemical gradient, driving the accumulation of chloride against its electrochemical gradient.[22]

For the salivary glands the precise method by which secretion is brought about is still largely unknown. cAMP and calcium-activated phosphorylation of cellular substances are currently believed to be the major effects leading to macromolecular secretion.[51] In the case of electrolyte secretion, attention is directed primarily to ion channels and carriers by which ions enter the cells or to the energy-dependent Na^+-K^+ pump, which carries out ion extrusion. Petersen[38] and Williams[51] postulated a calcium effector system or a channel linking extracellular and intracellular compartments permeable to calcium and capable of different conformations corresponding to different calcium permeabilities. Voltage-sensitive channels permeable to sodium, potassium, or calcium ions open after a depolarization of the plasma membrane.[18,38] The sodium pump exists in all cells, and since more sodium ions are actively pumped out than potassium is taken up, it contributes directly to the membrane potential. The pump is primarily activated by an increase in sodium. Calcium-sensitive ion channels, permeable to sodium, potassium, or chloride ions, open when calcium increases.[38] This is in addition to a calcium-activated channel. Possibly, cyclic nucleotides (e.g., AMP, GMP) activate ion channels or pumps.

Despite the many gaps in our knowledge of the electrophysiology of salivary acinar cells, the action of the major secretagogues can be summarized as follows. In mammalian salivary glands, acetylcholine and epinephrine or norepinephrine act on α-receptors, causing an increase in potassium and sodium ion permeability of the plasma membrane. This results in a pronounced reduction of the surface membrane resistance and a loss of potassium from the cells, balanced by an uptake of sodium. An active electrogenic extrusion of sodium and accumulation of potassium follow. An increase in calcium permeability probably mediates the permeability of sodium and potassium. Epinephrine or norepinephrine, acting on receptors, produce only small potential and resistance changes. The most important effect of β-adrenergic activation is an increase in intracellular cAMP, which stimulates enzyme secretion. Cholinergic or α-adrenergic stimulation causes a marked fluid and some calcium-dependent enzyme secretion.

There is a dissociation of cellular secretory mechanisms underlying protein secretion and fluid/electrolyte secretion in the salivary glands. Of the three major cationic electrolytes—sodium, potassium, and chloride—sodium is the only one with a pattern of very low concentrations at lowest flow rates to high concentrations at the highest rates of flow. Sodium is also the primary contributor to the increasing osmolality of the fluid as the level of secretion increases.[46] In human parotid saliva, sodium is the key in the secretion of fluid because local osmotic effects across the secretory luminal membrane influence the generation of the fluid.[46]

Acinar secretion

Secretory cells, such as the acinar cells of the parotid gland, discharge their products by a process of *exocytosis*, wherein fusion of secretory granules with a delimited portion of the plasmalemma at the apex of the acinar cell occurs. The membrane fusion is the last of a series required for the transfer of export proteins from their synthesis in the rough endoplasmic reticulum (RER) to the extracellular environment. Using the model by Palade,[37] the secretory process can be divided into six successive steps: (1) synthesis, (2) segregation, (3) intracellular transport, (4) concentration, (5) intracellular storage, and (6) discharge.

Synthesis of secretory proteins requires the uptake of amino acids by cells. Much of this synthesis is accomplished by an active transport from the extracellular pool via carrier systems located in the basolateral plasma membrane, with transfer-ribonucleic acid (RNA) molecules delivering the amino acids to the ribosomes of the RER.[37] Production and processing occur in the RER and the Golgi complex, as they do in all eukaryotic cells.[21] Most of the polypeptides produced pass through the Golgi cisternae. Carbohydrate synthesis is also believed to take place in the Golgi complex, but it is more variable than polypeptide synthesis in the RER, which is strictly template controlled.[52]

After synthesis, the secretory proteins are segregated in the cisternal space of the RER. Segregation is regarded as an irreversible step, and the vectorial transportation leading to it is probably obligate for all protein-secreting cells.[37]

From the cisternal space of the RER the secretory proteins are transported to the Golgi complex. The intracellular transport requires energy (adenosine triphosphate synthesis). Condensation and maturation follow the secretory proteins arrival at the condensing vacuoles in a dilute solution. The final result of the concentration step is the conversion of the condensing vacuoles into mature secretion granules. Concentration does not depend on a continuous energy supply but is highly sensitive to pH, with lysis occurring above pH 7.2.[37]

Terminal glycosylation of secretory proteins also occurs in the Golgi complex, and at that level the product is transferred from a high-permeability membrane to a membrane whose lipids approach that of the plasmalemma.

Temporary storage of secreting proteins in the cell is within secretion granules (condensing granules at the end of the concentration step). Their membranes come from the Golgi complex, and their content is an outcome of attached polysomes that have undergone modification.[37,52]

Secretion granules discharge into the glandular lumina by a process of exocytosis (membrane fusion). Such a process is generally accepted for the discharge of macromolecular secretory products. Morphologically the membrane of the secretion granule fuses with the plasmalemma, with a fission of the fused membranes within the area of fusion.[37,52] A continuity is thereby established between the granule and the extracellular lumen, which ensures maintenance of a continuous diffusion barrier between the interior of the cell and the extracellular medium. In exocrine cells the fusion site is limited to the luminal domain, and the consequent exocytosis requires calcium ions and energy (often a cyclic nucleotide–generating system and one or more protein kinases plus a depolarization of plasmalemma).

The procedures the cell uses to recover and redistribute membrane after exocytosis are not known. Recovery of membrane in the form of endocytic vesicles with translocations to Golgi vacuoles and cisternae is most likely. Appreciable amounts of membrane material are probably discharged into the lumen, but as Figure 65-1 suggests, excess apical membrane, removed by interiorization, is then disassembled within the cell to provide new protein molecules via a "cryptic pool."[52]

A Ca^{++} messenger system links surface membrane receptors to the control of epithelial ion fluxes and therefore to the excretion of fluid.[39] The activation of receptors leads to a biphasic Ca^{++} mobilization (composed of an intracellular Ca^{++} release and a component of increased Ca^{++} entry into the extracellular space). The resulting increase in cytosolic Ca^{++} is accompanied by the opening of Ca^{++}-sensitive monovalent ion channels and an efflux of K^+ and entry of Na^+. The increase in cytosolic Na^+ activates the Na^+-K^+ pump.

The role of calcium in amylase secretion is less understood. Although extracellular Ca^{++} does not directly participate in exocytosis, Ca^{++} derived from an intracellular pool is required as a step in amylase secretion after cAMP production. It is believed that cAMP and Ca^{++} function in concert to stimulate exocytosis by unknown mechanisms.[39] It may be that cAMP mobilizes Ca^{++} by phosphorylation of stimulus-affected proteins associated with endoplasmic reticulum (ER). Following this mobilization, the liberated calcium may activate phosphoprotein phosphatases, which dephosphorylate a 24-kDa protein integral to the membrane of secretory granules and cytoplasmic-stimulated proteins. In addition, cAMP would also increase phosphorylation of the 92.5-kDa protein loosely associated with secretory granule membranes.

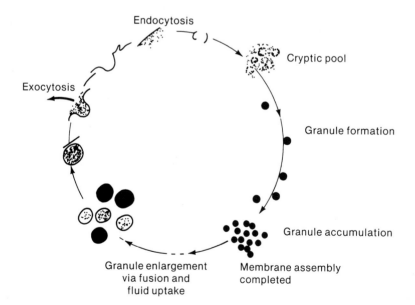

Fig. 65-1. Endo-exocytotic process and granule formation in the acinar cells of salivary tissues. (Modified from Williams MA, Cope GH: Membrane dynamics in the parotid acinar cell during regranulation: a stereological study following isoprenaline-induced secretion, *Anat Rec* 199:389, 1981.)

These changes in phosphorylation of the membrane protein are proposed to lead to exocytosis, perhaps by affecting the interaction of the cytoskeleton or the luminal plasma membrane with the secretory granule.

Saliva

The variability of the composition of saliva can be accounted for by the fact that the several classes of salivary glands contribute different constituents, and because the final product depends on the stimuli evoking the secretion (Table 65-4). The concentration of many of the inorganic constituents further depends on flow rate.

Whole or mixed saliva is composed of approximately 99.5% water and has a specific gravity between 1.002 and 1.012. In humans the amount of saliva secreted in 24 hours is between 1000 and 1500 ml.[3,29] The secretory rate is highest during meals; during sleep or in the absence of stimulation the secretory rate is low or nearly absent.

The pH of saliva depends primarily on the relative concentrations of free and combined CO_2: the ratio of $H_2CO_3/NaHC_3$ and the pH varies directly with the CO_2 content of blood. These bicarbonates (and to a lesser degree, phosphates) buffer saliva. In human mixed saliva the pH varies from 5.75 to 7.05.[3]

If data on flow and composition are to be meaningful, the saliva must be collected under standardized conditions.[3,29] Resting and stimulated secretions should be evaluated, and because many constituents of saliva are circadian, the times of collection should be uniform.

The electrolyte composition of saliva from the parotid and submandibular glands shows differences between each source and is markedly different from plasma. In general, parotid-gland concentrations are higher than those from the submandibular gland.[3,29] Calcium is the main exception, with submandibular calcium nearly twice the concentration of parotid calcium. The electrolytes are relatively independent of plasma concentrations because they reflect an active transport system. Sodium and chloride are directly related to flow rate. Calcium concentrations appear to be flow dependent only at high flow rates.

The organic (nonelectrolyte) analytes are passively diffused from plasma as opposed to actively transported and thereby reflect blood concentrations.[29]

Table 65-5 presents the composition of saliva in adults. The flow-rate data were documented after 2% citric acid was applied to the tongue as the stimulus. After such stimulation, sodium, chloride, bicarbonate, and calcium concentrations increase in the rate of flow, but magnesium, phosphates, urea, ammonia, and uric acid decrease in the rate of flow. Protein is variable in the parotid saliva but increases in saliva from the submandibular gland. The pH increases with flow rate.

The flow rate in nonstimulated parotid glands is about 0.04 ml/min/gland; submandibular saliva has a somewhat higher resting flow rate, 0.05 ml/min/gland.[29] This decreases markedly during sleep; the sleeping flow rate from the parotid gland is nearly nil.

Flow rates after stimulation vary with the stimulus. With usual gustatory stimulation a 0.6 ml/min/gland flow rate is obtained. A range of 0.4 to 1.0 is not uncommon. Discomfort from dryness is usually not a complaint until the rate of flow is below 0.2 ml/min/gland.[29]

Proteins or protein-containing moieties make up the majority of the organic components of saliva. Of the two major salivary glands, the concentration of protein is higher in

Table 65-4. Contribution to saliva and relative viscosities of saliva by salivary glands

Gland	Total saliva (24 hours) (%)	Relative viscosity
Submandibular	71	3.4
Parotid	25	1.5
Sublingual	3 to 4	13.4
Minor (oral, labial)	Trace amounts	—

Data from Mandel ID: Sialochemistry in diseases and clinical situations affecting salivary glands, *Crit Rev Clin Lab Sci* 12:321, 1980.

Table 65-5. Saliva composition in normal adults

Mean values	Parotid gland	Submandibular gland
Flow rate		
(ml/min/gland: stimulated)	0.7	0.6
Inorganic analytes (mEq/l)		
K^+	20	17
Na^+	23	21
Cl^-	23	20
HCO_3	20	18
Ca^{++}	2	3.6
Mg^{++}	0.2	0.3
HPO_4^{-2}	6	4.5
Organic analytes (mg/dl)		
Urea	15	7
Ammonia	0.3	0.2
Uric acid	3	2
Glucose	<1	<1
Cholesterol	<1	?
Fatty acids	1	?
Total lipids	2 to 6	2 to 6
Amino acids	1.5	?
Proteins	250	150

Modified from Mandel ID: Sialochemistry in diseases and clinical situations affecting salivary glands, *Crit Rev Clin Lab Sci* 12:321, 1980.

cholinergic mechanisms. In contrast, release of renal renin is mediated by β-adrenergic receptors and inhibited by α-adrenergic receptors. Plasma angiotensin II concentrations do not have any impact on the release of submandibular gland renin.[8]

The presence of renin in the submandibular glands certainly implies a role in the renin-angiotensin-aldosterone system, despite observations that removal of the gland has no significant effect on plasma concentrations of renin.[8] The findings of other angiotensin-forming enzymes, pseudorenin, and tonin in the submandibular gland are further related implications.[8]

Kallikreins

Kallikreins, which are serine proteases, have been found in and isolated from submandibular glands of many mammalian species including humans, where they exist in many molecular forms (isoenzymes).

The kallikreins are localized in duct cells (secretory granules of the GCT or striated ducts).[4,24,36] No sexual dimorphism exists in kallikrein contents. In the rat the submandibular gland is the richest source of glandular kallikreins, and it may contribute to the blood concentrations of the enzymes.

The glandular kallikreins' physiologic role is poorly understood. They may be involved as mediators of functional vasodilation, and an interrelation between the renin-angiotensin and kallikrein-kinin systems has been suggested.[36]

Peptide hydrolases

The submandibular glands contain a number of peptidases and proteases that are androgen dependent and nearly exclusively found in the GCT cells.[4] These enzymes may also exhibit kininogenase activity and may be related to kallikreins. They may perform important regulatory functions in the submandibular glands by serving as processing enzymes to form stable complexes with biologically active polypeptides. Other suggested biologic functions are vascular effects and stimulation of growth.[4]

Glucagon or glucagon-like substances

Current information about the role of salivary tissues in glucose homeostasis is far from clear despite the presence of glucagon-like immunoreactive substances in the submandibular glands of several species and effective competition with pancreatic glucagon for specific receptors on rat liver cell plasma membrane.[4] There is a reported sexual dimorphism. The substances have not been found in the saliva of humans and do not contribute to plasma levels.

ALTERED PHYSIOLOGY OF SALIVARY TISSUES

Changes in the composition of saliva may occur in various diseases affecting salivary glands or other tissues in the body.[22] In mucoviscidosis, for example, the concentrations of sodium, calcium, phosphorus, urea, and uric acid are in-

creased. The thyroid and salivary glands share a similar iodide-concentrating mechanism, with the inorganic iodide being secreted in saliva because conjugation with proteins does not take place in salivary glands.[13] A decrease in salivary sodium occurs in primary hypertension, and protein alterations are seen in diabetes mellitus and Sjögren's syndrome, among other diseases. Drug-induced alterations are also well known.[45,47]

All or nearly all of the causes of an altered physiologic response by salivary glands have either a defective (increase or decrease) stimulation or obstruction of (change in flow rate) secretion, or physical-chemical changes of product as their underlying bases. Sialadenosis, sialolithiasis, radiation sialadenitis, and Sjögren's syndrome illustrate this.

Sialadenosis

Sialadenosis, or sialosis, is a noninflammatory, parenchymatous disease of the salivary glands whose origins are based in metabolic and secretory disorders of the functional salivary parenchyma and are clinically manifested by recurrent, painless swellings of the salivary glands, principally the parotid.[43,44]

The association of sialadenosis with disorders of endocrine glands, malnutrition, and several neuropathic disorders has led to its classification into three types.[12]

1. *Hormonal.* Parotid enlargement has been described in connection with nearly all endocrine disorders. That accompanying diabetes mellitus is the most common.
2. *Dystrophic-metabolic.* Primarily nutritional in basis, this form is seen in protein deficiency, the malnutrition of alcoholics, and vitamin deficiencies such as beriberi and pellagra.
3. *Neurogenic.* This type of sialadenosis is an outcome of dysfunction of the autonomic nervous system.

Morphologic and biochemical investigations indicate that changes or disorders of the salivary glands' acinar protein secretion are responsible for sialadenosis. Changes in the secretory behavior can be the result of either an excessive stimulation or inhibition of secretion, and both of these probably are aberrations of the autonomic nervous system.[12]

Light and electron-optic study of parotid tissue from patients with sialadenosis demonstrates enlarged acinar cells filled with zymogen granules. The granules, however, are different in different subjects. Donath and Seifert[16] distinguished the following three different types of sialadenosis based on the ultrastructural appearance of the granules:

1. *Dark granule type,* in which densely packed, protein-rich secreting granules are found. No evidence of increased protein synthesis exists.
2. *Light granule type,* in which the acinar cells contain low-optical-density secreting granules. The acinar cells in this form manifest signs of an increased synthesis of proteins.

3. *Mixed granule type*, in which there is a simultaneous presence of light and dark acinar cells.

These types of human sialadenosis can be induced experimentally in the rat by isoproterenol (light granule type) or guanacline (dark and mixed granule type).[12]

Pathogenetically, all of the varied clinical associations, as well as the wide variation in the results of sialochemical and sialometric determinations observed in the sialadenoses, can be explained using peripheral autonomic neuropathology as the fundamental basis.

Sialolithiasis

Sialoliths (calculi) constitute one of the most common causes of salivary gland dysfunction. The composition of salivary calculi has been well studied with methods including histochemical studies, chemical analysis, and electron-optic examinations.[1,48] The calculi consist of a laminated structure of concentric shells of calcareous materials alternating with layers of organic resinous material.[17] Carbohydrates and amino acids compose the organic matrix; the crystalline components consist of calcium phosphate in the form of hydroxyapatite with small amounts of magnesium, carbonate, and ammonium ions. The distribution of the mineral elements varies extensively from one calculus to another: some are lamellar, others are homogeneous.

The process of stone formation is clearly enhanced in the presence of stasis of salivary flow within the duct of the salivary gland. The submandibular gland is the most susceptible for salivary calculi because of the anatomic arrangement of its principal duct and the physiochemical characteristics of its secretion. The nonstimulated saliva from the submandibular gland has a higher pH, higher mucin content, and about twice as much calcium as has parotid saliva. All of these favor mineralization of a mucoid gel formed in the duct system of the submandibular gland.[1] The following, modified from El Deeb,[17] lists physiochemical and anatomic factors predisposing to calculi in the submandibular gland.

1. Submandibular saliva
   a. High mucin content
   b. Alkaline pH
   c. High percentage of organic matter
   d. Concentration of calcium and phosphate salts
   e. Low carbon dioxide level
   f. High phosphatase enzyme content
2. Anatomy
   a. Length and irregular course of Wharton's duct
   b. Dependent position of gland and its duct system
   c. Position of ductal orifice
   d. Size of orifice smaller than duct lumen

Whereas knowledge of salivary calculi in the major salivary glands is relatively well documented, information concerning those in minor salivary glands is limited. Reports indicate that 92% of salivary calculi occur in the submandib-

Table 65-7. Minor salivary gland calculi

Site	Number of cases
Upper lip	71
Buccal mucosa	57
Buccal sulcus	10
Lower lip	9
Palate	3
Alveolar mucosa	3
Tongue	1

Data from Anneroth G, Hansen LS: *Int J Oral Surg* 12:80, 1983; and Jensen JL and others: *Oral Surg* 47:44, 1979.

ular gland, 6% in the parotid gland, and 2% in both the sublingual and minor salivary glands.[17] Probably, however, minor salivary calculi are more common than the literature presents.[2] The principal locations are in the buccal and upper labial mucosa (Table 65-7). The lower lip is seldom involved, and the alveolar and palatal mucosae are even less often afflicted. The preponderant localization of major salivary gland calculi to the submandibular gland and of the minor salivary gland calculi to the buccal mucosa and upper lip suggests that local factors such as trauma and duct morphology may be important. The duct lengths in the labial and buccal mucosal glands are longer than those in the palate and that biochemical and biophysical properties of the secretions are more favorable to stone formation in the lip and buccal mucosa.[23]

Irradiation

Salivary function is extremely responsive to radiation. At least 50% of function is lost after only 1000 cGy (1 week of radiotherapy). In conventional radiotherapy for tumors of the head and neck (6000-7000 cGy over 6 to 7 weeks), the radiation doses cause 80% salivary dysfunction.[33] This dysfunction may exist for years after the radiotherapy. Loss of taste acuity, increased incidence of dental caries, altered nutritional status, and loss of appetite accompany the reduction in salivary function. Damage to the acinar and duct systems is held responsible for the apparent increases in salivary sodium and chloride and for the decrease in bicarbonate during radiotherapy in humans.[34] The principal damage is to the acinar parenchyma.

Sjögren's syndrome

Current evidence indicates that Sjögren's syndrome is the result of a lymphocyte-mediated destruction of exocrine glands, which in turn leads to diminished or absent glandular secretion and mucosal dryness.[28] The syndrome is a consequence of altered immunoregulation in which destruction of the salivary exocrine parenchyma occurs. Pathogenetically, the syndrome and the observed salivary and extrasalivary lesions possibly represent a graft-versus-host disease-like process, in which the histocompatibility antigens of ductal epithelium or lymphoid cells are changed, so that self-recognition does not occur. Patients at risk are those with accompanying genetic abnormalities of T-cell and B-cell cooperation. *In vitro* tests, *in vivo* tests, and the high incidence of non-Hodgkin's lymphomas in patients with the syndrome provide clinical and laboratory support for this reasoning.[5]

Sialochemistry in patients with Sjögren's syndrome also appears to be characteristic and distinguishable from that in patients with parotitis. Stuchell and others[49] indicate that the parotid saliva in patients with the syndrome manifests increased sodium, chloride, IgA, immunoglobin G (IgG), lactoferrin, and albumin. Phosphates are decreased. The increase in IgA is almost all 11S in type—not 7S, which is the major component in patients with parotitis. This finding suggests that the increase in IgA is a result of local synthesis and not a reflection of the serum increase of IgA, as is the case in parotitis.[7]

Cystic fibrosis

Salivary tissue involvement in this recessively inherited disease is preponderantly of the mucous-type glands, especially as manifested by a change in the composition and flow rate of salivary fluid in the labial minor salivary glands. These glands have a disease-related increase in sodium concentration and a decrease in flow rate. According to Izutsu,[22] there are three principal hypotheses for cystic fibrosis–related changes in salivary gland function: (1) alterations in intracellular calcium concentration, (2) autonomic dysregulation of the secretory process, and (3) decreased chloride permeability.

The histomorphologic changes are nonspecific and consist of duct ectasia, inspissation of secretions, and acinar atrophy.

Changes with aging

All salivary glands undergo structural changes with age. With increasing age, the compact lobular structure and uniform appearance of the ducts and acini are altered. The lobules become more loosely structured, acini assume disparate sizes, and intralobular ducts become more prominent. Fibroadipose tissue is found in the glands in all ages, but increases in the elderly as acini atrophy.

The more readily accessible submandibular gland has been studied more than the parotid gland but differences in aging exist between the two glands.[41] Structural changes in the human parotid gland are less manifest, and the overall loss of parenchyma may not be as severe. Parotid glands from patients older than 55 years of age often retain the typical, evenly compact appearance of younger glands.

In comparison with the young adult submandibular gland, the following parenchymal changes are seen: loss of acinar granules with a shrinkage of cells, dilation of intra- and extralobular ducts with a modest hyperplasia of intralobular

ducts, an invariable oncocytic transformation after 70 years of age (infrequent in those younger than 30 years of age), age-related fibrosis around ducts and in septae, an increased glandular adiposity that is independent of the patient's general adiposity, and focal obstructive and chronic inflammatory adenitis with intraductal calculi.[41]

The parotid glands exhibit an age-related fibrosis, but this is usually overshadowed by the increasing glandular adiposity. Because of the wide range of fatty infiltration between patients and across age groups, the mere presence of an extensive intralobular adiposity should not be an indicator of a particular systemic disorder.[42] There is an increasing prevalence of oncocytes with increasing age of the parotid glands, usually commencing in the fifth decade of life. In general, there is no relationship between aging and the amount of lymphoid aggregates, although Scott, Flowers, and Burns[42] indicate the total amount of lymphoid tissue appears to be reduced in those over 75 years of age. Elderly persons have intraductal inspissated secretions and microcalculi, but they are much less numerous than in the submandibular glands.

Most investigators report no change in salivary flow rates in older humans. This is not the case in rodents where significant differences are found in the effects of age on specific glands. We must await data from longitudinal studies on nonmedicated subjects who are also stimulated by the same techniques and free of psychologic aberrations before we can assess the role of aging on salivary flow rate.[15] A similar position should be taken to reconcile the wide range of variability in the concentration of saliva proteins. Animal studies indicate an age-dependent decrease in the production of proteins such as amylase and mucins.[15]

The important calcium-dependent events in salivary cells are functionally defective in the latter half of the lifespan of male Wistar rats. In humans, parotid saliva shows a decrease in electrolyte and osmolality values with aging.[11]

FUTURE DIRECTIONS

Transgenic technology will become essential to understanding salivary gland function and gene expression because of the paucity of salivary gland cell lines that can maintain a differentiated phenotype.[40] The expression of recombinant deoxyribonucleic acid (DNA) constructs can be used to alter normal salivary gland physiology and thus allow examination of salivary function at the molecular level.

Embryonic stem cell–transgenic approaches can be used to investigate the consequences of specific salivary cell deficiencies, and conventional transgenics or adenovirus gene transfer can be used to evaluate dominant transgenes. There have been significant advances in the characterization of salivary-specific promoters, but function definition of these sequences in transgenic animals is necessary to define easily manipulated promoter-enhancers for efficient expression in salivary glands. Adenovirus gene transfer techniques should speed the acquisition of promoter studies in the future.

Table 65-8. Salivary gland promoter/enhancers expressed in transgenic mice

		Site of dominant transgene expression: salivary versus other tissue	
Promoter/enhancer	Kilobase (Kb) pair gene region*	Salivary gland	Other
Human salivary amylase	−1.0 to −0.3	Parotid	Low
Mouse parotid secretory protein	−25-kb gene fragment	High in parotid, also found in sublingual and submandibular	None
Mouse major urine protein	−3.5 to 1.9	Submandibular	None
Rat tissue kallikrein	−1.7 to +2	Submandibular (low)	Several
Mouse renin	16-kb gene fragment	Submandibular	Kidney
Human cystatin	22-kb gene fragment	Parotid, submandibular	Lacrimal

Modified from Samuelson LC: Transgenic approaches to salivary gland research, *Ann Rev Physiol* 58:209, 1996.
* The minimal gene region, in kilobase pairs, sufficient to drive expression in the salivary gland.
The numbering of the gene is relative to the start of transcription, defined as +1.

Table 65-8, modified after Samuelson,[40] presents a number of genes that code for salivary proteins. These include cloned genes that are preponderantly expressed in a single salivary gland (e.g., a α-amylase and parotid secretory protein) as well as genes expressed in extra-salivary tissues (e.g., renin and kallikrein). In most of the examples, the exact nature and positioning of the salivary-specific regulatory sequences have not been fully defined. Amylase is an example. Pancreatic and salivary amylases are encoded by closely related yet distinct genes in both mouse and human subjects.[40] There has also been an independent evolution of the mouse and human salivary amylase genes. Parotid-specific enhancers are found within 1 kb of the human salivary amylase promoter. In the mouse, they lie at a distance from the promoter.[40] Salivary amylase constructs expressed in transgenic mouse salivary glands demonstrate that there has been conservation of salivary transcriptional regulatory mechanisms between mouse and human subjects.

REFERENCES

1. Anneroth G, Eneroth CM, Isacsson G: Morphology of salivary calculi: the distribution of the inorganic component, *J Oral Pathol* 4:257, 1978.
2. Anneroth G, Hansen LS: Minor salivary gland calculi: a clinical and histopathological study of 49 cases, *Int J Oral Surg* 12:80, 1983.
3. Arglebe C: Biochemistry of human saliva, *Adv Otorhinolaryngol* 26:97, 1981.
4. Barka T: Biologically active polypeptides in submandibular glands, *J Histochem Cytochem* 28:836, 1980.
5. Batsakis JG: The pathology of head and neck tumors: the lymphoepithelial lesion and Sjögren's syndrome, part 16, *Head Neck Surg* 5:150, 1982.
6. Baum BJ: Principles of saliva secretion, *Ann N Y Acad Sci* 694:17, 1993.
7. Baum BJ, Fox PC: *Chemistry of saliva*. In Talal N, Moutsopoulos HM, Kassan SS, editors: *Sjögren's syndrome: clinical and immunological aspects*, New York, 1987, Springer-Verlag.
8. Bing J and others: Renin in the submaxillary gland: a review, *J Histochem Cytochem* 28:874, 1980.
9. Bothwell MA, Wilson WH, Shooter EM: The relationship between glandular kallikrein and growth factor-processing proteases of mouse submaxillary gland, *J Biol Chem* 254:7287, 1979.
10. Castle D: *Cell biology of salivary protein secretion*. In Dobrosielski-Vergona K, editor: *Biology of salivary glands*, Boca Raton, Fla, 1993, CRC Press.
11. Chauncey HH, Feller RP, Kapur KK: Longitudinal age-related changes in human parotid saliva composition, *J Dent Res* 66:599, 1987.
12. Chilla R: Sialadenosis of the salivary glands of the head: studies on the physiology and pathophysiology of parotid secretion. *Adv Otorhinolaryngol* 26:1, 1981.
13. Chisholm DM, Mason DK: Salivary gland disease, *Br Med Bull* 31:156, 1975.
14. Cohen RE, Levine MJ: *Salivary glycoproteins*. In Tenovuo J, editor: *Human saliva: clinical chemistry, microbiology, vol I*, Boca Raton, Fla, 1989, CRC Press.
15. Dobrosielski-Vergona K: *Age-related changes in the function of salivary glands*, Boca Raton, Fla, 1993, CRC Press.
16. Donath K, Seifert G: Ultrastructural studies of the parotid gland in sialadenosis, *Virchows Arch* 365:119, 1975 [abstract].
17. El Deeb M, Holte N, Gorlin RJ: Submandibular salivary gland sialoliths perforated through the oral floor, *Oral Surg* 51:134, 1981.
18. Findlay I: A patch-clamp study of potassium channels and whole-cell currents in acinar cells of the mouse lacrimal gland, *J Physiol* 350:179, 1984.
19. Garrett JR: Recent advances in physiology of salivary glands, *Br Med Bull* 31:152, 1975.
20. Garrett JR: *Innervation of salivary glands: neurohistological and functional aspects*. In Sreebny LM, editor: *The salivary system*, Boca Raton, Fla, 1989, CRC Press.
21. Hand AR, Oliver C: Effects of secretory stimulation on the Golgi apparatus and GERL of rat parotid acinar cells, *J Histochem Cytochem* 32:403, 1984.
22. Izutsu KT: *Salivary electrolytes and fluid production in health and disease*. In Sreebny LM, editor: *The salivary system*. Boca Raton, Fla, 1989, CRC Press.
23. Jensen JL and others: Minor salivary gland calculi: a clinicopathologic study of forty-seven new cases, *Oral Surg* 47:44, 1979.
24. Kimura K, Moriya H: Enzyme and immunohistochemical localization of kallikrein. I. The human parotid gland, *Histochemistry* 80:367, 1984.
25. Lefkowitz RJ, Caron MG, Stiles GL: Mechanisms of membrane-receptor regulation: biochemical, physiological, and clinical insights derived from studies of the adrenergic receptors, *N Engl J Med* 310:1570, 1984.
26. Lefkowitz RJ and others: Structure and function of β-adrenergic receptors: regulation at the molecular level, *Adv Cyclic Nucleotide Res* 17:19, 1984.
27. Levine MJ: Salivary macromolecules: a structure/function synopsis, *Ann N Y Acad Sci* 694:11, 1993.

28. Maier J, Bihl H: Effect of radioactive iodine therapy on parotid gland function, *Acta Otolaryngol* 103:318, 1987.

29. Mandel ID: Sialochemistry in diseases and clinical situations affecting salivary glands, *Crit Rev Clin Lab Sci* 12:321, 1980.

30. Michell R: Hormone action at membranes, *Trends Biochem Sci* 9:3, 1984.

31. Minaguchi K, Bennick A: Genetics of human salivary proteins, *J Dent Res* 68:2, 1989.

32. Moro I and others: Immunohistochemical distribution of immunoglobulins, lactoferrin, and lysozyme in human minor salivary glands, *J Oral Pathol* 13:97, 1984.

33. Mossman KL: Quantitative radiation dose-response relationship for normal tissues in man. II. Responses of the salivary glands during radiotherapy, *Radiat Res* 95:392, 1983.

34. Mossman KL, Shatzman AR, Chencharick JD: Effects of radiotherapy on human parotid saliva, *Radiat Res* 88:403, 1981.

35. Murphy RA and others: The mouse submandibular gland: an exocrine organ for growth factors, *J Histochem Cytochem* 28:890, 1980.

36. Orstavik TB: The kallikrein-kinin system in exocrine organs, *J Histochem Cytochem* 28:881, 1980.

37. Palade G: Intracellular aspects of the process of protein synthesis, *Science* 189:347, 1975.

38. Petersen OH: *The electrophysiology of gland cells*, New York, 1980, Academic Press.

39. Putney JW: *Calcium signaling system in salivary glands*. In Schultz SG, Forte JG, Rauner BB, editors: *Handbook of physiology, vol III, section 6: the gastrointestinal system*, Bethesda Md, 1989, American Physiological Society.

40. Samuelson LC: Transgenic approaches to salivary gland research, *Ann Rev Physiol* 58:209, 1996.

41. Scott J: Structure and function in aging human salivary glands, *Gerodontology* 3:149, 1986.

42. Scott J, Flower EA, Burns JA: A quantitative study of histological changes in the human parotid gland occurring with adult age, *J Oral Pathol* 16:505, 1987.

43. Seifert G: Klinische Pathologie der Sialadenitis und Sialadenose. *HNO* 19:1, 1971.

44. Seifert G, Donath K: Die Sialadenose der Parotis, *Deutsche Med Wochenschr* 100:1545, 1975.

45. Setser ME and others: Altered granule discharge and amylase secretion of parotid glands in reserpine-treated rats, *Lab Invest* 41:256, 1979.

46. Shannon IL, Suddick RP, Dowd FJ Jr: *Saliva: composition and secretion: monographs in oral science*, Basel, Switzerland, 1974, S Karger.

47. Simson JAV, Spicer SS, Hall BJ: Morphology and cytochemistry of rat salivary gland acinar secretory granules and their alteration by isoproterenol, *J Ultrastruct Res* 48:465, 1974.

48. Strubel G, Rzekpa-Glinder V: Structure and composition of sialoliths, *J Clin Chem Clin Biochem* 27:244, 1989.

49. Stuchell RN, Mandell ID, Bauermash I: Clinical utilization of sialochemistry in Sjögren's syndrome, *J Oral Pathol* 13:303, 1984.

50. Stumpf WE: Histochemical characteristics and significance of cell receptors in biology and pathology, *Acta Histochem* 29:23, 1984.

51. Williams JA: Regulatory mechanisms in pancreas and salivary acini, *Ann Rev Physiol* 16:361, 1984.

52. Williams MA, Cope GH: Membrane dynamics in the parotid acinar cell during regranulation: a stereological study following isoprenaline-induced secretion, *Anat Rec* 199:389, 1981.

SUGGESTED READINGS

Baum BJ: Neurotransmitter control of secretion, *J Dent Res* 66:628, 1987.

Berne RM, Levy MN: *Physiology*, ed 2, St Louis, 1988, Mosby.

Brandtzaeg P: Immunohistochemical studies on various aspects of glandular immunoglobulin transport in man, *Histochem J* 9:553, 1977.

Crawford JM, Taubman MA, Smith DJ: Minor salivary glands as a major source of secretory immunoglobulin A in the human oral cavity, *Science* 190:1206, 1975.

Foskett JK, Melvin JE: Activation of salivary secretion: coupling of cell volume and (Ca^{++}) in single cells, *Science* 244:1582, 1989.

Fox RI and others: Primary Sjögren syndrome: clinical and immunopathologic features, *Sem Arthritis Rheum* 14:77, 1984.

Hand AR, Oliver C: *Basic mechanisms of cellular secretion: methods in cell biology, vol 23*, New York, 1981, Academic Press.

Johnson LR: *Physiology of the gastrointestinal tract*, ed 2, New York, 1987, Raven Press.

Lefkowitz RJ: Clinical physiology of adrenergic receptor regulation, *Am J Physiol* 243:43, 1982.

Lustmann J, Shteyer A: Salivary calculi: ultrastructural morphology and bacterial etiology, *J Dent Res* 60:1386, 1981.

Mandel ID, Bauermash I: Sialochemistry in Sjögren's syndrome, *Oral Surg* 41:182, 1976.

Mason DK, Chisholm DM: *Salivary glands in health and disease*, Philadelphia, 1975, WB Saunders.

Petersen OH: Mechanisms of action of hormonal and neuronal peptides on exocrine gland cells, *Br Med Bull* 38:297, 1982.

Polak JM, Bloom SR: Neuropeptides in salivary glands, *J Histochem Cytochem* 28:871, 1980.

Putney JW, Weiss SJ: Relationship between receptors, calcium channels, and responses in exocrine gland cells, *Methods Cell Biol* 23:503, 1981.

Rice DH: Advances in diagnosis and management of salivary gland diseases, *West J Med* 140:238, 1984.

Seifert G and others: *Diseases of the salivary glands*, New York, 1986, Georg Thieme Verlag.

Sreebny LM: *The salivary system*, Boca Raton, Fla, 1989, CRC Press.

Tandler B: Salivary gland changes in disease, *J Dent Res* 66:398, 1987.

Tenovuo JT: *Human saliva: clinical chemistry and microbiology, vol 1*, Boca Raton, Fla, 1989, CRC Press.

Thorn NA, Treiman M, Peterson OH: *Molecular mechanisms in secretion*, Copenhagen, 1988, Munksgaard.

Turner RJ: Mechanism of fluid secretion of salivary glands, *Ann N Y Acad Sci* 694:23, 1993.

Vergona K: *The biology of the salivary glands*, Caldwell, NJ, 1992, Telford Press.

Young JA, Van Lennep EW: *The morphology of salivary glands*, New York, 1978, Academic Press.

Chapter 66

Diagnostic Imaging

Dale H. Rice

A variety of diagnostic imaging techniques is available for the investigation of salivary gland disorders. For practical purposes these techniques are of use only for the parotid and submandibular glands. Although sialography of the sublingual glands can be done, it is of little practical value. The techniques in current use are sialography, radionucleotide scanning, ultrasonography, computed tomography (CT) scanning, and magnetic resonance imaging (MRI).

SIALOGRAPHY

Sialography is currently used to evaluate calculi, obstructive disease, inflammatory lesions, penetrating trauma, and mass lesions.

Mercury was used in 1904 for the first sialogram reported.[6] Both water-soluble and oil-soluble contrast media have been used, with water-soluble media currently preferred (Table 66-1). Correct interpretation of the sialogram requires a thorough knowledge of the anatomy of the parotid and submandibular glands. Since Chapter 64 discusses this anatomy, it is not repeated here except for particular points important to the study under discussion.

To perform a sialogram, the following equipment should be available: water-soluble contrast media, such as meglumine diatrizoate 76%, a good light source, a topical anesthetic for the duct orifice, lacrimal dilators, a lacrimal cannula, a syringe, polyethylene tubing, a Rabinov cannula, and a tapered sidehole needle.

First, the ostium is anesthetized. If the precise opening cannot be readily identified, the area should be dried, the gland gently massaged, and the area observed for the flow of saliva. If the duct cannot be easily cannulated, gentle dilation can be performed with lacrimal dilators.

Contrast medium is injected gently until the patient experiences pain. For each gland (parotid or submandibular) an-teroposterior, lateral, and oblique roentgenograms are obtained to eliminate all bony overlapping. A separate injection is done for each exposure to ensure adequate filling of the ductal systems and a good parenchymal phase.

Bilateral studies may be advisable to detect subclinical disease in the contralateral gland. Also, deviations from normal can be better appreciated. Furthermore, displacement of the gland by an extrinsic mass can more readily be seen. Finally, if the diseased side is studied first, radiographs of the contralateral side can serve as drainage views of the diseased side.[33]

In the lateral view the area of the parotid gland varies from 10.1 to 21.2 cm^2 with a variation right to left of 2.5 cm^8. Stensen's duct ranges from 0.8 to 3.2 mm in diameter, with a right-left difference of up to 0.7 mm. The parotid duct is approximately 6 cm long with second- and third-order branching. In the anteroposterior view the duct is approximately 2 cm lateral to the mandible. Accessory lobules are occasionally seen superior to the duct. The submandibular duct is 5 cm long and 2 to 4 cm wide, with branching similar to the parotid. Acinar filling may or may not occur, depending on the pressure of injection, the contrast medium, and the condition of the gland. Retention of water-soluble contrast medium beyond 5 minutes has been established as the norm for secretory ability. In general, if contrast medium is retained, the abnormalities provide the diagnosis.

The most important contraindications to sialography are iodine allergy and acute sialadenitis. If thyroid function tests are to be performed and if iodine interferes with them, they should be completed first.

Several variations in technique have been introduced over the years to improve the capability for diagnosing various lesions. These include simultaneous xeroradiograph,[9] the use of pneumography with tomography,[12] secretory sialography,[24] and CT sialograph.[17] Only secretory sialography is of contemporary interest. It allows a measure of the physiologic function of the gland. CT sialography is excellent for the evaluation of mass lesions, but is unnecessary with contemporary scanners.

Radiopaque calculi can usually be seen on the preliminary radiographs (Fig. 66-1). Twenty percent of submandibular calculi and 80% of parotid calculi are radiolucent. Eighty percent to 90% of all calculi occur in the submandibular gland. Multiple calculi occur in up to 25% of patients who develop calculi.[31] Calculi rarely cause complete obstruction, so contrast medium flows around them, showing a filling defect on sialography. A dilation of the main duct (if the calculus is distal) or of the intraglandular ducts may exist (if the calculus is in the hilum).[20] Occasionally a calculus passes but symptoms persist. This may indicate a ductal stricture that can be demonstrated with sialography. After passage or removal of the calculus, the sialographic appearance of the gland may resemble chronic sialadenitis.

The changes seen in inflammatory diseases depend on the severity and chronicity of the process. These chronic inflammatory lesions are believed to represent a spectrum of diseases from chronic sialadenitis through the benign lymphoepithelial lesion to Sjögren's syndrome. These lesions all involve a lymphoreticular infiltrate combined with acinar atrophy and ductal metaplasia ending in the epimyoepithelial island.[3] The histologic picture is similar, with variations being related only to distribution and severity.

The primary pathogenic event in chronic sialadenitis is believed to be a decreased secretion rate with subsequent stasis. Two theories of initiation are currently espoused. One is that repeated acute episodes or a single severe episode of acute suppurative sialadenitis leads to ductal metaplasia of mucus-secreting glands. This situation leads to an increased mucus content in the saliva, causing stasis. The other is that if the gland is colonized by pyogenic bacteria, an acute suppurative infection occurs, whereas colonization with opportunistic flora leads to chronic, recurrent sialadenitis. This disease is much more common in the parotid gland, presumably because of its longer, narrower duct, making it more susceptible to stasis.[22] Repeated episodes lead to sialectasis, ductal ectasia, and progressive acinar destruction combined with a lymphocytic infiltrate.

As already implied, the sialographic appearance parallels the degree of histologic change, and all chronic inflammatory lesions give similar sialographic changes. The changes that may be seen include saccular dilation of the terminal ducts and acini, segmental strictures and dilation, and pseudocyst formation. Four stages of sialectasis have been described: punctate, globular, cavitary, and destructive. Som and others[29] reported that the punctate and globular forms may actually represent extravasation of contrast media through damaged ducts.

Table 66-1. Comparison of water-soluble and oil-soluble contrast media

	Water soluble	Oil soluble
Miscible with saliva	+ + + +	0
Physiologic solution	+ +	0
Allergic reactions	0	+
Opacification	+ + +	+ + + +
Local reaction	+	+ + + +
Elimination time	Fast	Slow

+ + + +—Most soluble; +—Least soluble.

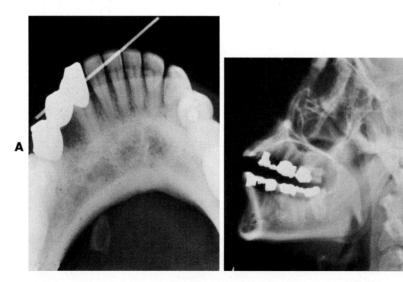

Fig. 66-1. A, plain radiograph showing bullet-shaped calculus in submandibular duct. **B,** A lateral radiograph of the same patient. Calculus can be seen at tooth root level midway between symphysis and third molar.

The benign lymphoepithelial lesion gives a similar sialographic appearance. In fact, some regard this lesion as "end-stage" chronic recurrent parotitis.[2] Similarly, varying degrees of pseudosialectasis characterize the sialographic appearance of either primary or secondary Sjögren's syndrome (Figs. 66-2 to 66-4).

Sialography may be of value in assessing penetrating trauma, especially involving the parotid gland. It may demonstrate occlusion of a duct, a salivary-cutaneous or salivary-oral fistula, or a sialocele (Fig. 66-5). Displacement of the gland by edema or hematoma also can be demonstrated.

Sialography has long been used to evaluate mass lesions. Information can be obtained concerning the size and location of the mass, whether it is intrinsic or extrinsic (Fig. 66-6), and whether it is benign or malignant. Depending on the extent of the lesion and its location, this information can be of variable accuracy. Tumors 1 cm or less are difficult to demonstrate, especially if peripherally located. Masses greater than 1 cm can usually be easily located by their disturbance of the ductal architecture.[33] The mass may drape around or displace the ducts. For benign tumors the margins should be smooth, with no evidence of extravasation of contrast material (Figs. 66-7 and 66-8). Several sialographic changes are characteristic of malignant tumors: (1) destruction of ducts, (2) irregular borders, (3) encasement of major ducts, and (4) cystic cavities that fill with contrast media.

In the deep lobe, the ducts normally can be seen passing around the mandible below the condyle. They are parallel and oblique and course superiorly from lateral to medial. A

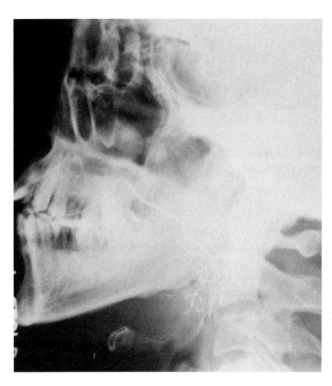

Fig. 66-3. A sialogram showing ductal ectasia common to chronic inflammatory lesions.

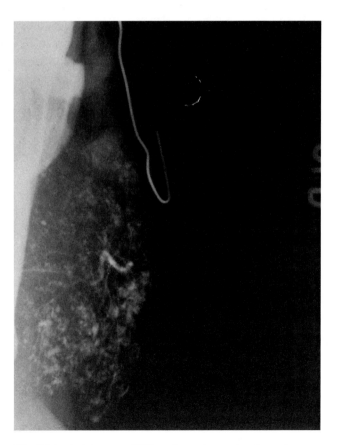

Fig. 66-4. A sialogram of Sjögren's syndrome showing extravasation of contrast media.

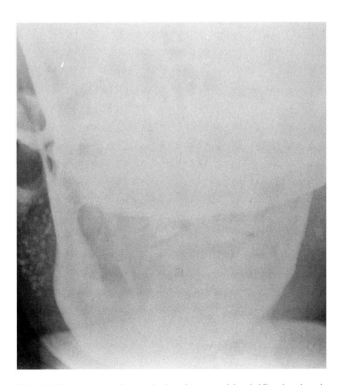

Fig. 66-2. A plain radiograph showing parotid calcification in advanced Sjögren's syndrome.

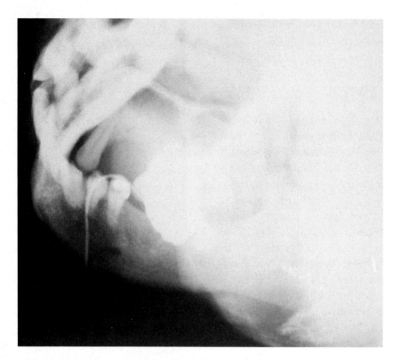

Fig. 66-5. A sialogram showing pseudocyst formation secondary to penetrating injury resulting in lacerated duct.

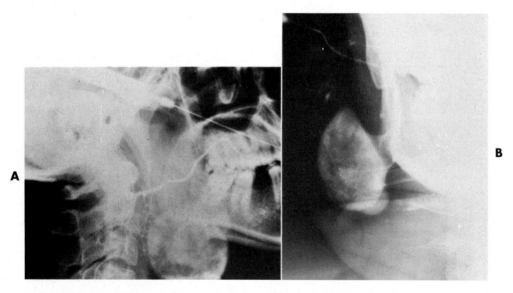

Fig. 66-6. A, A sialogram demonstrating osteochondroma of mandible in patient who presented with "parotid" mass. **B,** A plain radiograph demonstrating the same osteochondroma.

deep-lobe tumor disrupts this and is best seen on the anteroposterior projection.

In one study assessing the accuracy of sialography, five of seven malignant parotid tumors were correctly called. However, 6 of 30 benign tumors were called malignant.[5]

In summary, sialography is currently best for studying the ductal system. No other test supplies useful information about ductal architecture and glandular patterns. On the other hand, sialography has little to offer in the study of mass lesions. The information obtained is severely restricted if the mass is small or extrinsic to the gland.

RADIOSIALOGRAPHY

Salivary glands also can be studied by radioactive scanning. This technique has been used most for the parotid gland. The most popular substance used is technetium. Tech-

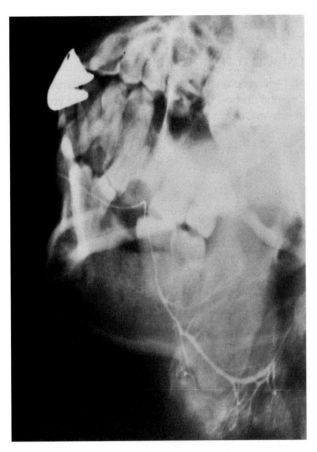

Fig. 66-7. A sialogram demonstrating smooth, curved ductal displacement around pleomorphic adenoma.

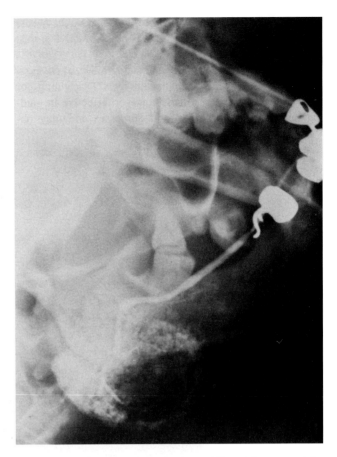

Fig. 66-8. A sialogram demonstrating filling defect caused by pleomorphic adenoma.

netium is an artificially produced element obtained by molybdenum decay (first produced in 1933). The atomic number is 43, and the atomic weight is 99. The half-life of the most stable form is 215,000 years, but in the medical form it is 6 hours. The tetraoxygenated form (pertechtenate) is distributed in body fluids as is iodide, except iodine is not absorbed in the thyroid. It has no β irradiation, but emits γ irradiation at 140 keV energy level.

Radioisotope scanning is used to evaluate parenchymal function and to detect mass lesions. It is of no use in studying the ductal system. Sequential scanning demonstrates uptake of pertechtenate from the vascular system and its subsequent secretion in saliva.[13] In a normal study, uptake in the parotid occurs before uptake in the submandibular gland, and the glands are symmetric. Although uptake occurs in the sublingual and minor glands, this study has little to offer in investigating them. The scan should be performed in the resting state because uptake in the parotid is greater.[30]

Radioisotope scanning was first used to study masses in the parotid. In one study of 106 patients, scanning had a 78% accuracy rate; 22% were incorrect, and all were false-negatives.[10] Warthin's tumor and the rare oncocytoma are radiopositive, but all others are generally radionegative. One case of a radiopositive pleomorphic adenoma has been reported.[14]

The first report of sequential scanning for the assessment of physiologic function was in 1971.[25] In generalized parenchymal disease, such as postradiation or chronic sialadenitis, the abnormality is evident on sequential scanning by the decreased and delayed uptake.

At this time, radioisotope studies have little to offer in the evaluation of salivary gland disease.[7] Sialography provides more information about the ductal system,[26] and CT scanning and MRI are superior in the evaluation of mass lesions.

ULTRASONOGRAPHY

Bozin, Romacheva, and Nakhutine[4] first reported the use of ultrasonography to study the salivary glands. Ultrasound is generally able to distinguish intrinsic from extrinsic masses.[11] One study with histologic follow-up showed that malignant tumors have a low reflectivity with poorly defined borders, whereas pleomorphic adenomas have a variable reflectivity with well-defined borders.[1] Inflammatory lesions have high reflectivity with diffuse borders.

nant parotid neoplasms, and others have confirmed this rate of accuracy.[28] Malignant tumors tend to show irregular outlines, diffuse borders, and nodal metastases.

With the newer generations of CT scanners, equally good results can be obtained using intravenous contrast enhancement rather than sialography. Although CT scans are no substitute for a histologic diagnosis, the general appearance of the mass often gives considerable insight into its histologic type.

The pleomorphic adenoma usually has crisp borders, unless it has become large enough to be lobulated (Figs. 66-13 and 66-14). Similarly, Warthin's tumor is sharply circumscribed.

Malignant neoplasms are often irregular and infiltrative. The low-grade mucoepidermoid carcinoma, when small, is similar in appearance to the pleomorphic adenoma. Larger lesions become lobulated with less regular borders. High-grade mucoepidermoid carcinomas are infiltrative and destructive. Other malignancies are similar to the high-grade mucoepidermoid carcinoma with irregular margins and a density greater than that of normal parotid tissue (Figs. 66-15 and 66-16). All are enhanced by intravenous contrast.

CT is accurate in evaluating deep-lobe and parapharyngeal space lesions.[16] There is a low-density fat plane between the parotid and pharyngeal constrictors that is displaced medially by deep-lobe parotid tumors or laterally by benign parapharyngeal lesions. Deep-lobe tumors may displace the carotid artery medially. Schwannomas and paragangliomas cause a loss of the low-density area around the carotid artery

and may displace the jugular vein, whereas malignant lesions destroy fascial planes.

CT scanning with intravenous contrast enhancement is currently the study of choice for evaluating parotid masses or parapharyngeal masses.

MAGNETIC RESONANCE IMAGING

MRI, which has improved markedly in the past few years, is excellent at separating adjacent soft tissues. It has a further advantage in being able to provide simultaneous coronal, axial, and sagittal views.

Two recent advances have added to its value. The first was the introduction of gadolinium, a paramagnetic compound that enhances vascular lesions. The second was the development of MRI angiography. A general disadvantage of MRI is that it does not show bone. Thus, CT and MRI are often used in a complementary fashion when evaluating lesions in and around the bone.

For salivary gland tumors, gadolinium-enhanced MRI is equal or superior to contrast-enhanced CT (Fig. 66-17).[18]

Both CT and MRI are able to detect a mass within a major salivary gland and determine whether the mass is well circumscribed or infiltrating. They both are able to detect extrinsic and intrinsic masses well, and may even be able to approximate the relative position of the facial nerve in the parotid gland.

With MRI, the variable fat content of the parotid gland gives it an intermediate to bright intensity on the T1-weighted signal. The signal is thus heterogeneous. On T2-

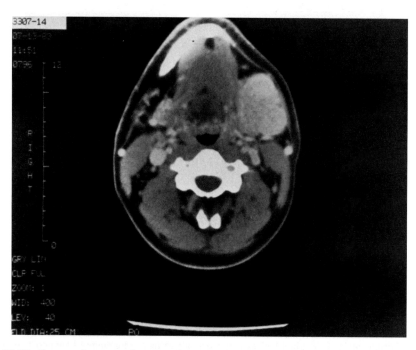

Fig. 66-13. Computed tomography scan of pleomorphic adenoma of the left submandibular gland.

weighted images the gland also is heterogeneous, this time because of the serous secretions and water content of the gland. MRI is quite sensitive to the presence of masses within the gland but less sensitive to subclinical inflammation and not sensitive at all to calcification.[32] In addition, MRI is less sensitive to cystic legions, such as first arch branchial cleft cysts within the parotid gland, than CT. In contrast, however, MRI is often better at outlining the margins of an intraglandular mass than CT.[19] MRI is excellent at detecting infiltrating borders of neoplasms, but like all

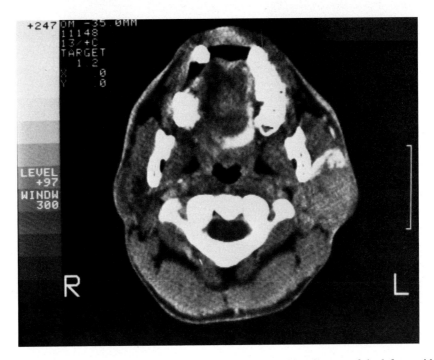

Fig. 66-14. Computed tomography scan of recurrent pleomorphic adenoma of the left parotid.

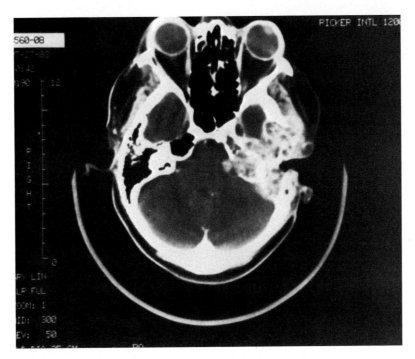

Fig. 66-15. Computed tomography scan of recurrent adenoid cystic carcinoma. Note mass replacing much of left temporal bone.

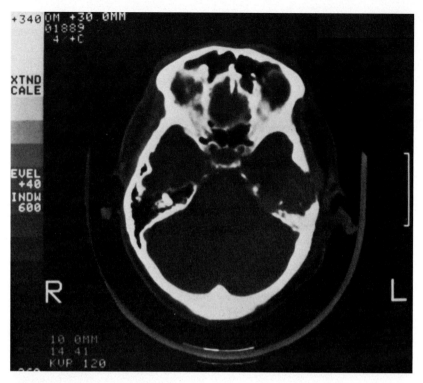

Fig. 66-16. Computed tomography scan of the same patient in Figure 66-15, with scanner set with ''bone windows.'' Note extensive destruction of the left temporal bone.

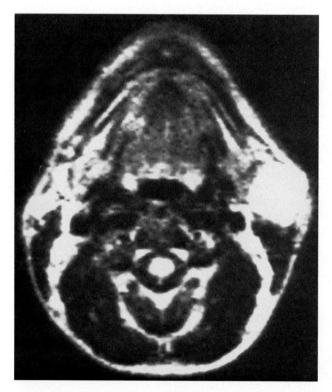

Fig. 66-17. Magnetic resonance imaging scan of patient with large pleomorphic adenoma.

other techniques it does not provide a histologic diagnosis and is never able to tell a benign from a malignant salivary gland legion, except in extreme cases.

REFERENCES

1. Baker S, Ossoinig KD: Ultrasound evaluation of salivary glands, *Trans Am Acad Ophthalmol Otolaryngol* 84:750, 1977.
2. Batsakis JG, Sylvest V: *Pathology of the salivary glands*, Chicago, 1977, American Society of Clinical Pathologists.
3. Batsakis JG and others: Malignancy and the benign lymphoepithelial lesion, *Laryngoscope* 85:389, 1975.
4. Bozin YN, Romacheva IS, Nakhutine EM: Biolocation diagnosis of diseases of parotid and submaxillary salivary glands, *Stomatologia* 50: 27, 1971.
5. Calcaterra TC and others: The value of sialography in diagnosis of parotid tumors, *Arch Otolaryngol* 103:727, 1977.
6. Carpy A, Poirer P: *Traite d'anatomie humane*, Paris, 1904, Masson.
7. Eneroth CM, Ling MG: Radiosialometry. II. The diagnostic accuracy of different evaluation parameters, *Acta Otolaryngol* 81:141, 1976.
8. Ericson S: Sialographic appearances of the normal parotid gland, *Acta Radiol* 14:593, 1973.
9. Ferguson MM and others: Application of xeroradiography in sialography, *Int J Oral Surg* 5:176, 1976.
10. Gates GA: Radiosialographic aspects of salivary gland disorders, *Laryngoscope* 82:115, 1972.
11. Gooding GA: Gray scale ultrasound of the parotid gland, *Am J Roentgenol* 134:469, 1980.
12. Granone FG, Julian G: Submaxillary sialography in combination with pneumoradiography and tomography, *Am J Roentgenol* 104:691, 1968.
13. Greyson ND, Noyak AM: Nuclear medicine in otolaryngological diagnosis, *Otolaryngol Clin North Am* 11:541, 1978.

14. Hendra R, Stebner FC: Evaluation of parotid gland masses by rectilinear scanning, *J Oral Surg* 33:838, 1975.
15. Magaram D, Gooding GA: Ultrasonic guided aspiration of parotid abscess, *Arch Otolaryngol* 107:549, 1981.
16. Mancuso AA, Hanafee WN: *Computed tomography in the head and neck*, Baltimore, 1982, Williams & Wilkins.
17. Mancuso AA, Rice DH, Hanafee WN: Computed tomography of the parotid gland during contrast sialography, *Radiology* 132:211, 1979.
18. Mandelblatt SM and others: Parotid masses: MR imaging, *Radiology* 163:411, 1987.
19. Mirich DR, McArdle CB, Kulkarni MV: Benign pleomorphic adenomas of the salivary glands: surface coil MR imaging versus CT, *J Comput Assist Tomogr* 11:620, 1987.
20. O'Hara AE: Sialography: past, present, and future, *CRC Crit Rev Clin Lab Sci* 4:87, 1973.
21. Pickrell KL, Trought WS, Shearin JC: The use of ultrasound to localize calculi within the parotid gland, *Ann Plast Surg* 1:542, 1978.
22. Rausch S: *Diseases of the salivary glands*. In Gorlin R, editor: *Thoma's oral pathology*, ed 6, vol 2, St Louis, 1974, Mosby.
23. Rice DH, Mancuso AA, Hanafee WN: Computerized tomography with simultaneous sialography in evaluating parotid tumors, *Arch Otolaryngol* 106:472, 1980.
24. Rubin P, Blatt DM: A modification of sialography (preliminary report), *Univ Mich Med Ctr Bull* 21:57, 1955.
25. Schall GE and others: Investigation of major salivary duct obstruction by sequential salivary scintigraphy: report of 3 cases, *Am J Roentgenol Rad Ther Nucl Med* 113:655, 1971.
26. Schmitt G and others: The diagnostic value of sialography and scintigraphy in salivary gland disease, *Br J Radiol* 49:326, 1976.
27. Som PM, Biller HF: The combined computerized tomography-sialogram: a technique to differentiate deep-lobe parotid tumors from extraparotid pharyngomaxillary space tumors, *Ann Otorhinolaryngol* 88:590, 1979.
28. Som PM, Biller HF: The combined CT sialogram, *Radiology* 135:387, 1980.
29. Som PM and others: Manifestations of parotid gland enlargement: radiographic, pathologic, and clinical considerations. Part I. The autoimmune pseudosialectasias, *Radiology* 141:415, 1981.
30. Stephens KW, Robertson JW, Harden RM: Quantitative aspects of pertechnetate concentration in human parotid and submandibular salivary glands, *Br J Radiol* 49:1028, 1976.
31. Suzuki S, Kawashima K: Sialographic study of diseases of the major salivary glands, *Acta Radiol [Diagn]* 8:465, 1969.
32. Teresi LM and others: Parotid masses: MR imaging, *Radiology* 163:405, 1987.
33. Valvassori GE and others: *Radiology of the ear, nose and throat*, Philadelphia, 1982, WB Saunders.

Chapter 67

Infections of the Salivary Glands

Scott M. Gayner
William J. Kane
Thomas V. McCaffrey

Infections of the salivary glands take various forms depending on the etiologic agents involved and the chronicity of the infection. Bacterial infections of the salivary glands are typically the result of mechanical blockage of the salivary ducts or reduced production of saliva, which permits retrograde bacterial contamination of the gland parenchyma. Certain systemic viral infections, such as mumps and acquired immunodeficiency syndrome (AIDS), produce localized salivary gland disease. Many granulomatous infections, through their involvement of the lymphoreticular system in and around the gland parenchyma, can produce pathologic changes in the salivary glands.

PRIMARY INFECTION OF THE SALIVARY GLANDS

Acute suppurative sialoadenitis

Historically, because of the frequency of its postoperative occurrence and the common involvement of the parotid gland, some of the terms associated with acute suppurative parotitis have included *surgical parotitis, surgical "mumps," postoperative parotitis,* and *secondary parotitis.*[8] The incidence of acute suppurative parotitis has been reported to be from 0.01% to 0.02% of all hospital admissions and from 0.002% to 0.04% of all postoperative patients.[43] In acute suppurative sialoadenitis, the initial infection of salivary gland parenchyma is caused by retrograde bacterial migration from the oral cavity.[5] These infections occur in all the major salivary glands, but the parotid gland is most frequently involved, possibly because of the inferior bacteriostatic activity of parotid secretions.[58] In healthy persons, salivary flow constantly flushes contaminants from the ductal

system. Stasis of salivary flow permits retrograde migration of bacteria and contamination of the gland parenchyma. Along with stasis of salivary secretions, compromised host resistance and poor oral hygiene contribute to the pathogenesis of the infection (Fig. 67-1).

Most affected patients are between 50 and 60 years of age; the incidence is equal among men and women. Susceptible patients are frequently debilitated as a result of chronic illness or prolonged recovery from a surgical procedure. Reduction of salivary flow is most frequently the result of dehydration accompanying uncompensated losses of blood and other body fluids following significant hemorrhage, diarrhea, or diaphoresis. Medications with anticholinergic or diuretic side effects further contribute to reduced salivary secretion. Prolonged anorexia reduces the periodic stimulus to salivate and reduces mechanical cleansing associated with mastication. These factors, in addition to the patient's inability to maintain an oral hygiene routine by brushing and flossing, result in an increase in the bacterial count within the oral cavity. Multiple gland involvement is possible, and bilateral involvement occurs in up to 25% of patients with postsurgical parotitis.[31,65]

Local symptoms of suppurative parotitis include a rapid onset of pain, swelling, and induration of the involved gland (Fig. 67-2). Systemic manifestations include fever, chills, malaise, and leukocytosis with neutrophilia. Bimanual manipulation of the gland will frequently result in a suppurative discharge from the duct orifice that should be collected for culture and sensitivity studies before the initiation of empiric antibiotic therapy (Fig. 67-3). The most commonly cultured organism among elderly debilitated patients is penicillin-

rev
of c
acu
tioı
exiı
of p
tis l
pat
pat

Su
ero
chy
inte
spa
bit
and
tis.

St
uli

m

Pa
gl

Pl

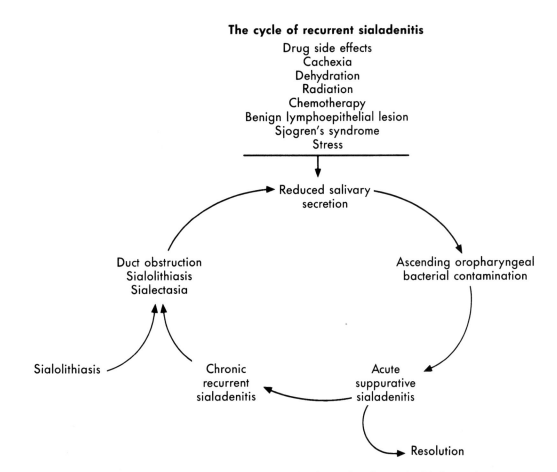

The cycle of recurrent sialadenitis

Drug side effects
Cachexia
Dehydration
Radiation
Chemotherapy
Benign lymphoepithelial lesion
Sjogren's syndrome
Stress

Reduced salivary secretion

Ascending oropharyngeal bacterial contamination

Acute suppurative sialadenitis

Resolution

Chronic recurrent sialadenitis

Sialolithiasis

Duct obstruction
Sialolithiasis
Sialectasia

Fig. 67-1. The detrimental and repetitious cycle of chronic salivary gland inflammation.

Fı
A,
st
si
sp
tr

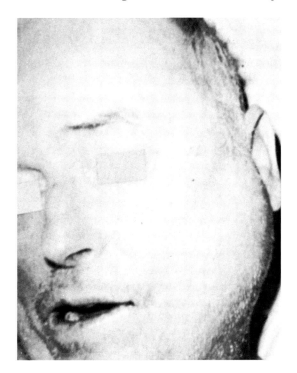

Fig. 67-2. An acutely formed abscess of the parotid gland.

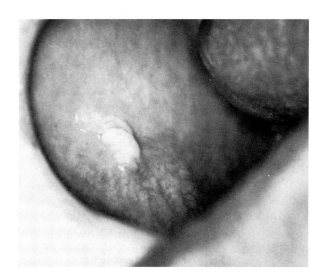

Fig. 67-3. A purulent exudate emerging from the orifice of Stenson's duct.

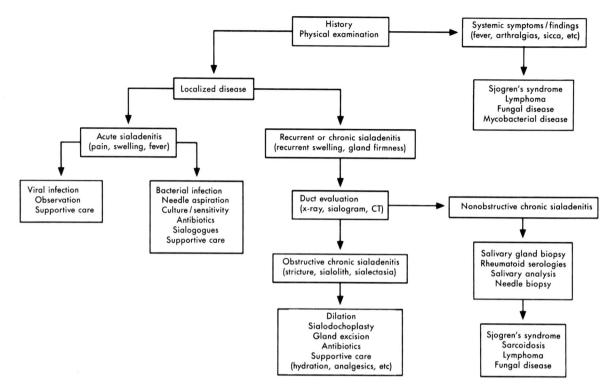

Fig. 67-6. A simplified algorithm for the diagnosis and management of chronic salivary gland inflammation.

episodes of swelling each year, with the swelling lasting from several days to 2 weeks.[22]

Treatment consists of adequate hydration, gland massage, local heat, sialagogues, and appropriate intravenous antibiotics. Empiric therapy prior to culture results should consist of a penicillinase-resistant antistaphylococcal antibiotic. In general, this will lead to rapid resolution of swelling and discomfort.

Biopsy specimens from involved glands show the persistence of chronic infection between symptomatic phases. Infection persists between symptomatic phases, promoting ductal ectasia and abnormal elevation of the viscosity of secretions. Sialochemistry shows an increased protein content of the secretions, and sialography demonstrates the characteristic pattern of sialectasis,[22] which often is bilateral even though the swelling is unilateral. Moreover, the severity of sialographic disturbance does not correlate with the patient's symptoms. The damage can be severe enough to predispose the gland to chronic sialoadenitis persisting into adulthood, which requires surgical removal of the gland. Fortunately, most symptoms abate with adolescence and therefore surgical treatment is rarely required.[35]

Chronic sialoadenitis

Chronic sialoadenitis is a localized condition of the salivary gland characterized by repeated episodes of pain and inflammation, usually culminating in parenchymal degener-

ation and fibrous replacement of the gland substance. Affected patients frequently experience an initial severe episode of acute sialoadenitis. Predisposition to repeated episodes of secondary infection may be attributed to duct obstruction or to duct dilatation and depressed glandular secretion. Asymptomatic intervals can range from a few weeks to several months. As with acute sialoadenitis, the parotid gland is most commonly affected.[53] As the number of inflammatory episodes increases, irreversible alterations to the ductal architecture result in diffuse ductal ectasia with intervening areas of stenosis (Fig. 67-7). Periductal and parenchymal inflammatory infiltration and fibrous replacement progress in proportion to the duration of the disease.

Obstruction of salivary flow is a prominent feature of chronic sialoadenitis. Mechanical impairment of salivary flow is usually caused by an intraductal calculus, stricture, or mucous plug, but lesions of the ductal papilla and extrinsic ductional compression are occasionally responsible. In a review of more than 30 years experience of 92 cases of chronic parotitis (117 parotid glands) the cause of obstruction was determined in one half of the cases.[69] These causes included obstruction due to stones (30%), stricture of the anterior part of Stensen's duct (8%), stricture of the duct orifice (4%), compression by tumor (3%), stenosis secondary to scar in adjacent tissue (2%), congenital dilatation of the main duct (0.8%), and foreign body (0.8%). Typically, the disease is

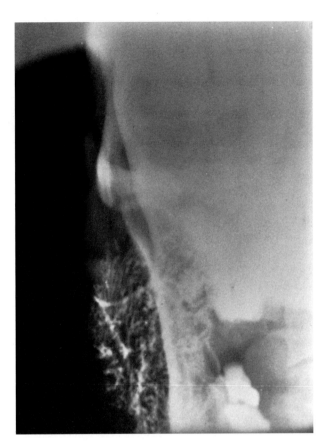

Fig. 67-7. A contrast sialogram demonstrating ductal ectasia.

characterized by recurring painful episodes of swelling accompanied by thickening and diminution of saliva.

Treatment of chronic sialoadenitis can be frustrating and no treatments are consistently successful. Tympanic neurectomy and parotid duct ligation are procedures advocated for chronic parotitis to induce atrophy of the gland, but these have failed to show reliable benefit. Surgical removal of the gland when conservative management has failed to control symptoms has been shown to be safe and effective.[40]

Sialolithiasis

Sialolithiasis refers to the formation of hardened intraluminal deposits in the ductal system of the salivary glands. Salivary calculi are most commonly discovered in association with chronic sialoadenitis, and their development is largely responsible for the recurrent nature of that disease. Approximately 75% of affected patients are between 50 and 80 years of age yet sialolith development in children and infants has been reported.[23] The exact cause of sialolith formation remains unclear, but factors contributing to the development of sialoliths appear to include (1) stagnation of saliva, (2) a focus for sialolith formation resulting from ductal epithelial inflammation and injury, and (3) poorly understood biologic factors favoring precipitation of calcium salts, particularly those associated with chronic inflammation.

Formation of sialoliths at the hilus of the gland is most common, although stones may be distributed throughout the ductal system.

Eighty percent of all salivary duct stones develop in the submandibular (Wharthon's) duct, with 19% occurring in the parotid duct and 1% in the sublingual duct.[7] A predisposition to formation in the submandibular gland may be related to the composition of the secretions, which are more alkaline and viscous; the submandibular gland contains a higher concentration of calcium and phosphate ions than do other major salivary glands.[39] Stagnation of secretions in Wharthon's duct may result from the angulation of the duct as it courses around the mylohyoid muscle and the vertical orientation of the distal duct segment.

Compositional differences between the inner and outer lamellae comprising submandibular and parotid sialoliths suggest a different pattern of evolution at these two anatomic sites.[3] Development of the submandibular sialolith is the primary process that results in impaired salivary flow and ductal inflammation, which secondarily encourages retrograde bacterial migration and resultant sialoadenitis. Conversely, parotid sialoliths may arise because of chronic inflammation that provides the necessary conditions for calculus formation.

Salivary calculi are most frequently composed of calcium phosphate and carbonate, combined with other salts (Mg, Zn, NH_3) and organic material (glycoproteins, mucopolysaccharides, and cellular debris), yet there does not appear to be a relationship between their formation and serum calcium or phosphorous levels.[39]

Symptoms of sialolithiasis consist of colicky postprandial pain and swelling, with variable resolution between attacks. Repeated secondary infection causes ductal strictures and parenchymal atrophy. Erosive luminal trauma can result in extrusion of the stone into the gland parenchyma and fistula formation. Diagnosis is made by history and palpation and imaging techniques, including plain radiography and sialography (Fig. 67-8). Calculi are frequently identified along the course of the involved duct by bimanual palpation of the floor of the mouth. Contrast studies are helpful for the identification of radiolucent stones that are associated with proximal duct dilatation and delayed emptying. Parotid sialoliths are most difficult to diagnose because they are frequently small, palpation is often impeded by the cheek tissues, and in 80% of cases they are radiolucent.[59]

Early management of salivary calculi should be conservative, consisting of measures identical to those outlined for nonobstructive sialoadenitis. Stones palpable near the ductal orifice can frequently be moved manually toward the orifice and removed. Vigorous probing should be avoided because it can initiate an inflammatory episode. If necessary, the ductal orifice can be incisionally enlarged to facilitate stone removal (Fig. 67-9). Sialodochoplasty of Stensen's duct has a high incidence of restricture, so temporary stenting with silastic tubing is necessary. Retained hilar calculi will con-

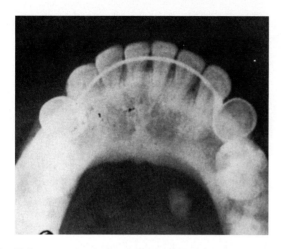

Fig. 67-8. An occlusal-view radiograph demonstrating an opaque calculus in Wharthon's duct.

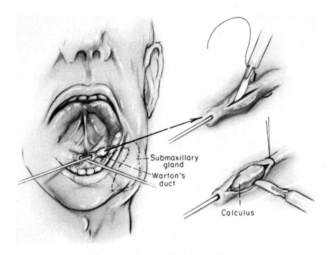

Fig. 67-9. Techniques for localization and retrieval of a submandibular duct calculus.

tinue to predispose the gland to repeated infection and ductal stricture and therefore should be treated by elective surgical removal of the gland. Other treatments, including low-dose irradiation, tympanic neurectomy, and ductal ligation, have proved to be ineffective. Recently, extracorporeal shock wave lithotripsy has been used clinically for the treatment of sialolithiasis.[68]

VIRAL INFECTIONS OF THE SALIVARY GLANDS
Viral diseases

Viral involvement of the salivary glands most commonly occurs through hematogenous dissemination, although infection by retrograde ductal migration does occur. Viral infection of salivary parenchyma is not always locally symptomatic, because transmission from blood to saliva occurs without localizing signs in many systemic viral infections including rabies, hepatitis, influenza, and poliomyelitis.

Mumps

Mumps is the most common cause of nonsuppurative acute sialoadenitis and occurs primarily in children. Bilateral parotid gland swelling occurs in most cases, but submandibular gland swelling occurs in rare cases. Parotid gland inflammation is part of a generalized and highly contagious viral infection caused by a paramyxovirus. The virus is endemic in the community and spreads efficiently by air-borne droplets from salivary, nasal, and urinary excretions. The incubation period averages 18 days, with illness onset signified by pain and swelling in one or both parotid glands. Progression of parotid gland swelling can be rapid and sufficient to cause displacement of the pinna. Pain is usually exacerbated by the physiologic stimulus of eating, which causes contractile ejection of saliva from the inflamed gland. Findings at the orifice of Stensen's duct are usually absent. Infective virus is shed through the saliva for up to a week following gland enlargement. Ductal epithelial desquamation may lead to secondary ductal obstruction and dilatation. Adults are rarely infected due to life-long immunity incurred by childhood exposure or measles, mumps, rubella vaccination.

Proof of diagnosis can be made by hemagglutination inhibition and complement fixation tests, but these are rarely required because of characteristic features present in all but exceptional cases. Routinely obtained laboratory tests are usually unremarkable except for occasional leukopenia. Elevations in serum salivary type isoamylase parallel the pattern and duration of glandular swelling. Histologic examination reveals substantial cytoplasmic vacuolization of acinar cells.

Generally, the symptoms of viremia, including low-grade fever, arthralgia, malaise, and headache, begin to abate within 3 to 7 days. The resolution of gland swelling usually requires several weeks, frequently proceeding symmetrically. As with any viral illness, treatment is directed toward supplemental hydration and rest, with dietary modification to minimize glandular secretory activity. More fulminant infections occasionally progress to include meningoencephalitis, orchitis, pancreatitis, nephritis, and sensorineural hearing loss.

Acute viral parotitis also can arise from other less common endemic organisms including parainfluenza virus, coxsackievirus, echovirus, Epstein-Barr virus (EBV), and choriomeningitis virus.

Acquired immunodeficiency syndrome

Infection with the human immunodeficiency virus (HIV) is frequently associated with lymphoproliferative and cystic enlargement of the major salivary glands, followed by salivary dysfunction.[18] This process, more recently termed *HIV-associated salivary gland disease* (HIV-SGD), has been described among HIV-seropositive patients, and also among high-risk, HIV-seronegative patients. Salivary gland disease in HIV-infected patients is associated with high suppressor

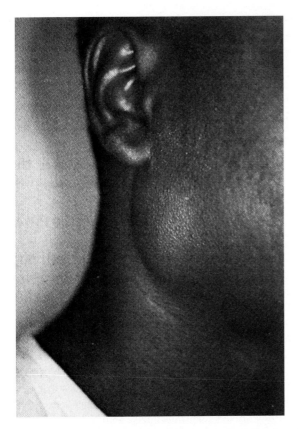

Fig. 67-10. Clinical appearance of human immunodeficiency virus–related enlargement of the parotid gland. (From Debo RF, Davidson M, Petow CA: Pathologic quiz: case 2, *Arch Otolaryngol Head Neck Surg* 116:487, 1990.)

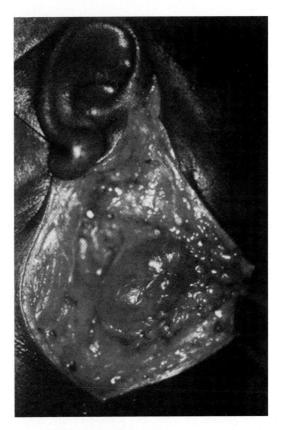

Fig. 67-11. Intraoperative appearance of a parotid gland cyst occurring in a human immunodeficiency virus–seropositive patient. (From Debo RF, Davidson M, Petow CA: Pathologic quiz: case 2, *Arch Otolaryngol Head Neck Surg* 116:487, 1990.)

T-cell counts and lymphocytosis.[56] The age distribution of patients with HIV-SGD falls into two groups: children born of HIV-infected mothers, and adults between 20 and 60 years of age. It is likely that HIV-SGD can occur in all age groups at risk for HIV infection. Salivary gland involvement can be the initial manifestation of HIV infection, with the parotid glands being most frequently affected.[15] Bilateral cystic enlargement of the parotid glands has been observed in 15% to 30% of HIV-infected children,[42] usually in combination with lymphocytic interstitial pneumonitis.[17] HIV is detectable in low concentrations of salivary secretions, but it is presently unknown whether salivary gland involvement is the result of direct infection or is simply a focal manifestation of the progressive generalized lymphadenopathy characteristic of the disease.

The clinical features of HIV-SGD include gradual nontender enlargement of one or more of the salivary glands, most often the parotid, with xerostomia due to compromised glandular secretion,[67] frequently combined with dry eyes and arthralgia (Fig. 67-10). For this reason, the sicca complex symptoms accompanying this disease process have been likened to Sjögren's syndrome and have stimulated investigation of a possible common autoimmune etiology.

Biopsy analysis reveals similar inflammatory infiltrates between Sjögren's syndrome and HIV-SGD, but the serologically detectable antibodies associated with Sjögren's syndrome do not appear in HIV patients with salivary gland abnormalities.[55] This suggests that HIV-SGD is either a separate entity or that the immune reaction is modified because of the nature of the disease. Other opportunistic infections that have been implicated as possible causes include EBV and cytomegaloviruses,[12] but others have disputed these causes.[56] The natural history of HIV-SGD is poorly described. Although glandular swellings may fluctuate, they are generally stable and long standing. The results of some studies would suggest that HIV-SGD is associated with a favorable prognosis.[28]

Histologic examination of excised glands shows numerous adjacent epithelium-lined cysts, up to several centimeters in size, that usually appear to have originated within the substance of a lymph node (Fig. 67-11). These are filled with macrophages and lymphocytes in a watery yellowish fluid containing cholesterol crystals and are surrounded by a dense lymphoid infiltrate with germinal centers.[52]

Appropriate management of these asymptomatic lesions may depend on the patient's status at the time of diagnosis.

Despite a clinical suspicion of HIV, these lesions probably should be treated like any incidental enlargement of the salivary gland, i.e., by surgical removal and pathologic examination. This philosophy is supported by an underlying incidence of lymphoma in up to 10% of patients in one series of HIV-infected patients.[27] Kaposi's sarcoma of the parotid is unusual.[66] However, in the setting of documented HIV infection, other investigators have shown that the findings of needle aspiration and CT or magnetic resonance imaging (MRI) are sufficiently typical to provide a presumptive diagnosis justifying conservative clinical observation of these lesions.[17] Good oral hygiene, sialagogues, and topical fluoride should be maintained. Regression of parotid gland enlargement has been seen with steroids and zidovudine.[56]

GRANULOMATOUS SALIVARY GLAND INFECTIONS

Salivary gland involvement frequently arises as a manifestation of a chronic granulomatous disease involving the lymphatic network in and surrounding the parotid gland. Direct infiltration of the adjacent glandular parenchyma occurs in fulminant cases. Manifestations frequently feature asymptomatic gradual enlargement of a nodule within the gland substance, suggesting a neoplasm. Included among these granulomatous diseases are tuberculous and nontuberculous mycobacterial diseases, actinomycosis, cat-scratch disease (CSD), toxoplasmosis, and tularemia.

Tuberculous mycobacterial disease

Salivary gland involvement is included among the less commonly encountered forms of cervicofacial tuberculosis. However, since the incidence of extrapulmonary tuberculosis at all sites has been increasing steadily since 1985, the diagnosis of *Mycobacterium tuberculosis* must enter into the differential diagnosis. As the number of HIV-positive individuals has increased, so have reports of extrapulmonary infection by *M. tuberculosis*. Gland involvement is characterized by an indolent, painless enlargement mimicking the behavior of a slow-growing neoplasm.[49]

Mycobacterium tuberculosis infection of the major salivary glands can occur more commonly through intraglandular lymph nodes or rarely from parenchymal infiltration. Salivary gland involvement can occur as a primary infection or as a recrudescence of an established pulmonary focus.[16] The parotid gland is more frequently involved in clinically localized tuberculous disease and the submandibular gland is more frequently involved in cases with systemic manifestations of tuberculosis.[4] Isolated salivary gland involvement is most common in the parotid gland, and two pathologic types have been described: (1) diffuse involvement, encompassing the whole gland with irregular nodules in volume and consistency, and (2) localized involvement, with a solid mass corresponding to tuberculosis in the lymph node of the parotid.[41] In most series of extrapulmonary mycobacterial infection, less than 50% of patients had chest-radiograph evidence of previous infection.[6] Constitutional signs including fever, night sweats, and weight loss may be absent. Facial nerve involvement is rare. Even with advances in fine-needle aspiration, most cases of parotid gland mycobacterial infection are not diagnosed preoperatively and diagnosis is made only after operative removal of the gland with its attendant risk of fistula formation.

Nontuberculous mycobacterial disease

Nontuberculous mycobacterial (NTM) infections of the salivary glands are most frequently encountered in children from 16 to 36 months of age. The most common presentation is a rapidly increasing mass,[14] and when the mass occurs in the region of the major salivary glands the diagnosis becomes more difficult. Presentation of a child with a salivary mass rapidly increasing in size without the typical appearance of inflammation raises the possibility of malignancy, granulomatous disease, and other recognized causes of cervical lymphadenopathy.[13] Involvement caused by *Mycobacterium bovis* has become much less common since the widespread pasteurization of milk. NTM infections are widespread in the environment, and the portal of entry is not defined, although the mouth, throat, gingiva, lips, and tonsils have been implicated.[62,64] Lymph nodes in and adjacent to the parotid and submandibular glands are most frequently involved, and sinus tracts can drain to the skin (Fig. 67-12). In NTM infections, skin tests are usually negative unless a higher dose of purified protein derivative is used.[6] Chest radiograph findings and constitutional symptoms are usually absent. Diagnosis is usually based on strong clinical suspicion and exclusion of other causes because tissue staining and microscopic features are nonspecific and culture results require up to 6 weeks. Reports of new tuberculins for

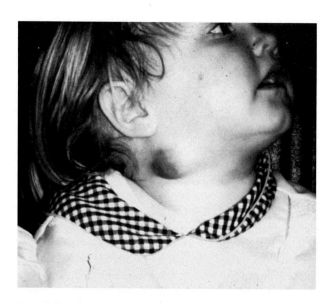

Fig. 67-12. A 4-year-old girl with nontuberculous mycobacterial involvement of periparotid lymph nodes.

skin testing from *Mycobacterium avium, Mycobacterium avium-intracellulare, Mycobacterium malmoense,* and *Mycobacterium scrofulaceum* have shown success.[13] Fine-needle aspiration is preferred to incisional biopsy, which can produce a fistula refractory to healing. Eradication of the disease with antituberculous drugs is usually not successful, and there is no evidence for person-to-person transmission, so excision with preservation of the facial nerve remains the mainstay of treatment.[45,60]

Actinomycosis

Actinomycosis is an infectious disease caused by a gram-positive anaerobic organism. Actinomyces is a normal commensal found in high concentrations in the tonsils[21] and carious teeth, which can rarely infect the major salivary glands. Actinomyces most often infects cervicofacial, ileocecal, and pulmonary sites. *Actinomyces israelii* is the most commonly encountered species, with the balance of cases attributable to *Actinomyces bovis* and *Actinomyces naeslundi.* In most cases, poor oral hygiene combined with trauma to the mucosa permits invasion of the organism, leading to a slowly progressive inflammatory reaction. Diabetes, immune suppression, long-term steroid use, and malnutrition have also been implicated as predisposing factors.[2] Isolated salivary gland involvement probably occurs via retrograde ductal migration and primarily occurs in the parotid gland.[51] Involvement of the salivary glands also can occur as part of direct spread of an invasive cervicofacial infection.

Patients typically have a painless, indurated enlargement of the involved gland that may suggest a neoplasm. Facial nerve involvement has not been described. A history of recent dental disease and manipulation is common. Constitutional symptoms, malaise, leukocytosis, and lymphadenopathy are typically absent. Multiple draining cutaneous fistulas are characteristically the result of lymph node necrosis.

Diagnosis is facilitated by needle aspiration of the mass or a fistula swab with smears and stains to examine for the presence of sulfur granules and the organism. Sulfur granules have also been described for nocardiosis, but their identification in the presence of filamentous gram-positive rods is diagnostic for actinomycosis.[24] Biopsy specimens show firm fibrous encasement of multiloculated abscesses containing whitish-yellow pus. Anaerobic cultures are obtained for species identification and to confirm the diagnosis.

Surgery for cervicofacial actinomycosis, except in the setting of isolated involvement, is mainly of diagnostic use because antibiotics are the mainstay of treatment. The antimicrobial of choice remains penicillin because *Actinomyces* species are not known to be resistant to penicillin. Other acceptable alternatives include clindamycin, doxycycline, or erythromycin. Antimicrobial therapy should consist of a 6-week parenteral course followed by an additional 6 months of oral management to completely eradicate the organism.[26] Response to management is generally favorable, with cure rates approaching 90% despite a delayed diagnosis in most instances.[61]

Cat-scratch disease

CSD is a granulomatous lymphadenitis that most commonly results from cutaneous inoculation caused by scratch trauma from a domestic cat. Roughly 90% of patients who have CSD report a history of exposure to cats, and 75% of these patients have experienced a cat scratch or bite. Dogs have been implicated in 5% of CSD cases. CSD affects approximately 22,000 persons and results in hospitalization of about 2000 persons each year in the United States.[29] Recent evidence suggests that *Rochalimaea henselae*—a rickettsial pathogen that has been isolated from patients with bacillary angiomatosis—is associated with CSD.[50]

Most reported cases occur in the head and neck, frequently involving the skin and lymphatics in and around the parotid and submandibular glands. Lymph node involvement histologically shows reticular cell hyperplasia, granuloma formation, and widening of arteriolar walls. As generalized inflammatory infiltration progresses, stellate areas of necrosis coalesce to form multiple microabscesses.

Usually systemic symptoms are mild or absent, but severe cases can progress to include encephalitis, arthritis, neuroretinitis, osteomyelitis, and hepatitis.[38]

Three of the following criteria are believed to be needed to confirm the diagnosis of CSD: (1) a history of animal contact (usually with a cat or kitten) resulting in a scratch or a primary dermal or eye lesion; (2) regional lymphadenopathy developing about 2 weeks after contact, along with sterile cultures of pus aspirated from the node and laboratory data that exclude other etiologic possibilities; (3) a positive CSD skin test (considered to be at least 5 mm of induration at 48 to 72 hours after the inoculation of 0.1 ml of test material); and (4) a lymph node biopsy revealing histopathology consistent with CSD. Biopsy of lymph nodes in suspected cases may be diagnostic, but biopsy is not without morbidity and should be reserved for cases in which (1) the course of the disease is unusual enough to raise doubts as to the diagnosis, and (2) markedly atypical clinical or laboratory findings are observed. A recently introduced commercially available serologic test to detect antibodies to *R. henselae* may be useful in confirming clinically suspected or atypical cases of CSD.

In the majority of cases no active therapy is required. The patient should be reassured that the lymphadenopathy is self limited and usually will resolve spontaneously in 2 to 4 months. Node aspiration can apparently have diagnostic and therapeutic benefit.[57] If required, judicious use of antipyretics and analgesics is recommended. Case reports and uncontrolled, retrospective reviews of the literature[37] indicate that signs and symptoms of systemic CSD have disappeared promptly in ill patients treated with various antibiotics, but currently antibiotic therapy is not indicated in mild or moderate CSD.

Toxoplasmosis

Toxoplasmosis, an uncommon disease in the United States, is caused by the organism *Toxoplasma gondii*. The usual host for this organism is the domestic cat. Parotid gland disease may involve singular or multiple intraparotid or periparotid lymph nodes. The organism exists in trophozoite, cyst, and oocyst forms, with the latter only existing in the feline vector. Trophozoites and cysts gain entrance to the human host most often through ingestion of infected and undercooked lamb, beef, or chicken, or, less commonly, through cat feces. Digestion of the cyst capsule permits widespread hematogenous dissemination and multiplication of trophozoites in virtually all lymphoreticular organs.

Both disseminated and lymphadenopathic forms of the disease have been described. Immunocompromised individuals are most at risk for the disseminated form of the disease, which features myalgia, lethargy, and anorexia combined with hepatosplenomegaly, pericarditis, and myocarditis. Alternatively, the lymphadenopathic variety occurs much more commonly, with the vast majority of patients presenting with isolated cervical lymphadenopathy.[48]

Definitive diagnosis can only rarely be provided by isolation of the organism. Confirmation of a presumptive histologic diagnosis is made by acute and convalescent serologic testing.[20] Chemotherapy is generally reserved for obviously progressive infections or those involving pregnant or immunocompromised individuals and consists of the combined administration of pyrimethamine and trisulfapyrimidine.

Tularemia

Tularemia is caused by the gram-negative organism *Franciscella tularensis*, which is typically transmitted to humans by insect vectors such as ticks or deer flies, handling of infected animal tissues, or aerosol inhalation.[19] The cottontail rabbit is a principal host in North America, but the organism has been isolated in many animal species throughout the world. In most cutaneously transmitted cases, a reddish papule forms at the site of entry. This may occur in the region of the parotid gland. Following a 2- to 10-day incubation period, neighboring and draining lymph nodes become enlarged, tender, and inflamed. Headache, fever, and other toxic signs can occur. If infectious entry via gastric or pulmonary routes occurs, a skin lesion will not be detected and lymphatic involvement may be more diffuse. Despite phagocytization within the reticuloendothelial organs, the infecting organism can remain viable intracellularly, stimulating a chronic granulomatous disease.

Franciscella tularensis is rarely isolated from human blood[46] and the clinician must rely on serologic tests for diagnosis. Aggressive manipulation of fluctuant nodes during the acute phases of the infection is discouraged because this may disseminate the infectious agent systemically. The organism is resistant to most β-lactam antibiotics, including all penicillins.[54] Successful management has been reported with erythromycin, tetracycline, and ciprofloxacin.[54] Following an interval of antibiotic therapy and the resolution of systemic symptoms, fluctuant cysts, likely to contain sterile fluid, can be safely incised or drained.

SUMMARY

Salivary gland infections manifest differently depending on the agent and the patient population. The acute suppurative infection is bacterial in origin and has quick onset of signs and symptoms usually occurring in elderly, debilitated patients. Chronic sialoadenitis is characterized by repeated episodes of pain and swelling (usually following an episode of acute sialoadenitis) and tends to occur throughout adulthood. Systemic viral infections, such as mumps and AIDS, can produce localized salivary gland disease in any age group but have very different clinical courses. Granulomatous salivary gland infections can occur in children and in elderly patients. They often cause asymptomatic gradual enlargement within a gland nodule suggesting a neoplasm. The differential diagnoses in salivary gland infections are broad but with a careful history and physical examination as well as knowledge of the various etiologic agents that cause disease, the otolaryngologist can make an accurate diagnosis in most cases and recommend appropriate management.

REFERENCES

1. Andrews JC and others: Parotitis and facial nerve dysfunction, *Arch Otolaryngol Head Neck Surg* 115:240, 1989.
2. Bartels LJ, Vrabec DP: Cervicofacial actinomycosis: a variable disorder, *Arch Otolaryngol* 104:705, 1978.
3. Batsakis JG: *Tumors of the head and neck*, ed 2, Baltimore, 1979, Williams & Wilkins.
4. Batsakis JG: *Tumors of the head and neck*, Baltimore, 1974, Williams & Wilkins.
5. Berndt A, Buck R, Buxton R: The pathogenesis of acute suppurative parotitis, *Am J Med Sci* 182:639, 1931.
6. Betts RF, Reese RE: *Lower respiratory tract infections*. In Reese RE, Douglas RG, editors: *A practical approach to infectious diseases*, Boston/Toronto, 1986, Little, Brown.
7. Blatt IM: Studies in sialolithiasis, *South Med J* 57:723, 1964.
8. Branson B and others: The re-emergence of postoperative parotitis, *West J Surg Obstet Gynecol* 67:38, 1959.
9. Brook I: Diagnosis and management of parotitis, *Otolaryngol Head Neck Surg* 118:469, 1992.
10. Brook I, Frazier EH, Thompson DH: Aerobic and anaerobic microbiology of acute suppurative parotitis, *Laryngoscope* 101(2):170, 1991.
11. Coban A and others: Neonatal suppurative parotitis: a vanishing disease? *Eur J Pediatr* 152:1004, 1993.
12. Couderc LJ and others: Sicca complex and infection with human immunodeficiency virus, *Arch Intern Med* 147:898, 1987.
13. Cox HJ, Brightwell AP, Riordan T: Non-tuberculosis mycobacterial infections presenting as salivary gland masses in children: investigation and conservative management, *J Laryngol Otol* 109:525, 1995.
14. Del Beccaro MA, Mendelman PM, Nolan C: Diagnostic usefulness of mycobacterial skin test antigens in childhood lymphadenitis, *Pediatr Infect Dis J* 8:206, 1989.
15. DeVries EJ and others: Salivary gland lymphoproliferative disease in acquired immune disease, *Otolaryngol Head Neck Surg* 99:59, 1988.
16. Donohue W, Bolden T: Tuberculosis of the salivary glands, *Oral Surg* 14:57, 1961.

17. Falloon J and others: Human immunodeficiency virus infection in children, *J Pediatr* 114:1, 1989.

18. Finfer MD and others: Cystic parotid lesions in patients at risk for acquired immunodeficiency syndrome, *Arch Otolaryngol Head Neck Surg* 114:1290, 1988.

19. Foshay L: Tularemia, *Ann Rev Microbiol* 4:313, 1950.

20. Frenkel J: Symposium on parasitic infections: toxoplasmosis, *Pediatr Clin North Am* 32:917, 1985.

21. Gaffney RJ and others: The incidence and role of Actinomyces in recurrent acute tonsillitis, *Clin Otolaryngol* 18:268, 1993.

22. Geterud A, Lindvall AM, Nylen O: Follow-up study of recurrent parotitis in children, *Ann Otol Rhinol Laryngol* 97:341, 1988.

23. Gorlin RJ, Goldman HM, editors: *Thoma's oral pathology*, St Louis, 1970, Mosby.

24. Harris LF, Kakani PR, Selah CE: Actinomycosis: surgical aspects, *Am Surg* 51:262, 1985.

25. Hearth-Holmes M and others: Autoimmune exocrinopathy presenting as recurrent parotitis of childhood, *Arch Otolaryngol Head Neck Surg* 119:347, 1993.

26. Hensher R, Bowerman J: Actinomycosis of the parotid gland, *Br J Oral Maxillofac Surg* 23:128, 1985.

27. Ioachim HL, Ryan JR, Blangrud SM: AIDS-associated lymphadenopathies and lymphomas with primary salivary gland presentation, *Lab Invest* 56:33A, 1987 (abstract).

28. Itescu S, Brancato LJ, Winchester R: A sicca syndrome in HIV infection: association with HLA-DR5 and CD8 lymphocytosis, *Lancet* 2:466, 1989.

29. Jackson LA, Perkins BA, Wenger JD: Cat scratch disease in the United States: an analysis of three national databases, *Am J Public Health* 83(12):1701, 1993.

30. Kaban LB, Donoff RB, Guralnick WC: Acute parotitis: report of a complex and unusual case, *Oral Surg* 31:377, 1973.

31. Lary B: Postoperative suppurative parotitis, *Arch Surg* 89:653, 1963.

32. Leake D, Leake R: Neonatal suppurative parotitis, *Pediatrics* 46:203, 1970.

33. Loughran DH, Smith LG: Infectious disorders of the parotid gland, *N J Med* 85:311, 1988.

34. Lundgren A, Kyle P, Odkvist LM: Nosocomial parotitis, *Acta Otolaryngol (Stockh)* 82:275, 1976.

35. Mandel L: *Inflammatory disorders.* In Rankow RM, Polayes IM, editors: *Diseases of the salivary glands*, Philadelphia, 1976, WB Saunders.

36. Marcy SM, Klein JO: *Focal bacterial infections.* In Remington JS, Klein JO, editors: *Infectious disease of the fetus and newborn infant*, Philadelphia, 1990, WB Saunders.

37. Margileth AM: Antibiotic therapy for cat-scratch disease: clinical study of therapeutic outcome in 268 patients and a review of the literature, *Pediatr Infect Dis J* 11:474, 1992.

38. Margileth AM, Wear DJ, English CK: Systemic cat scratch disease: report of 23 patients with prolonged or recurrent severe bacterial infection, *J Infect Dis* 155:390, 1987.

39. Mason DK, Chisholm DM: *Salivary glands in health and disease*, London, 1975, WB Saunders.

40. O'Brien CJ, Murrant NJ: Surgical management of chronic parotitis, *Head Neck* 15(5):445, 1993.

41. O'Connell JE and others: Mycobacterial infection of the parotid gland: an unusual cause of parotid swelling, *J Laryngol Otol* 107(6):561, 1993.

42. Oleske J and others: Immune deficiency syndrome in children, *JAMA* 249:2345, 1983.

43. Perry RS: Recognition and management of acute suppurative parotitis, *Clin Pharm* 4:566, 1985.

44. Pershall KE, Koopman CF, Coulthard SW: Sialoadenitis in children, *Int J Pediatr Otorhinolaryngol* 11:199, 1986.

45. Pransky SM and others: Cervicofacial mycobacterial adenitis in children: endemic to San Diego? *Laryngoscope* 100:920, 1990.

46. Provenza JM, Klotz SA, Penn RL: Isolation of *Franciscella tularensis* from blood, *J Clin Microbiol* 24:453, 1986.

47. Pruett TL, Simmons RL: Nosocomial gram-negative bacillary parotitis, *JAMA* 256:252, 1984.

48. Rafaty FM: Cervical adenopathy secondary to toxoplasmosis, *Arch Otolaryngol Head Neck Surg* 103:547, 1977.

49. Redon H: *Chirugie des glandes salivaires*, Paris, 1955, Masson.

50. Regnery RL and others: Serologic response of patients with suspected cat scratch disease to "Rochalimaea henselae" antigens, *Lancet* 339:1443, 1992.

51. Roveda S: Cervicofacial actinomycosis: report of two cases involving major salivary glands, *Aust Dent J* 18:7, 1973.

52. Ryan JR and others: Acquired immunodeficiency syndrome (AIDS)-related lymphadenopathies presenting in the salivary gland lymph nodes, *Arch Otolaryngol Head Neck Surg* 111:554, 1985.

53. Saunders JR, Hirata RM, Jacques DA: Salivary glands, *Surg Clin North Am* 66:59, 1986.

54. Scheel O, Reiersen R, Hoel T: Treatment of tularemia with ciprofloxacin, *Eur J Clin Microbiol Infect Dis* 11:447, 1992.

55. Schiedt M and others: Parotid gland enlargement and xerostomia associated with labial sialoadenitis in HIV-infected patients, *J Autoimmun* 2:415, 1989.

56. Schiodt M and others: Natural history of HIV-associated salivary gland disease, *Oral Surg Oral Med Oral Pathol* 74:326, 1992.

57. Spires JR, Smith RH: Cat scratch disease, *Otolaryngol Head Neck Surg* 94:622, 1986.

58. Spratt J: Etiology and therapy of acute pyogenic parotitis, *Surg Gynecol Obstet* 112:391, 1961.

59. Suleiman SI, Hobsley M: Radiographic appearance of parotid duct calculi, *Br J Surg* 67:879, 1980.

60. Waldman RH: Tuberculosis and the atypical mycobacteria, *Otolaryngol Clin North Am* 15:581, 1982.

61. Weese WC, Smith IM: A study of 57 cases of actinomycosis over a 36 year period: a diagnostic "failure" with good prognosis after treatment, *Arch Intern Med* 135:1562, 1972.

62. Wickham K: Clinical significance of nontuberculous mycobacteria, *Scand J Infect Disease* 18:337, 1986.

63. Wittich GR, Scheible WF, Hajek PC: Ultrasonography of the salivary glands, *Radiol Clin North Am* 23:29, 1985.

64. Wolinsky E: Nontuberculosis mycobacteria and associated diseases, *Am Rev Respir Dis* 119:107, 1979.

65. Work WP, Hecht DW: *Inflammatory diseases of the major salivary glands.* In Paparella MM, Shumrick DA, editors: *Otolaryngology*, Philadelphia, 1980, WB Saunders.

66. Yeh CK and others: Kaposi's sarcoma of the parotid gland in acquired immune deficiency syndrome, *Oral Surg Oral Med Oral Pathol* 67:308, 1989.

67. Yeh CK and others: Oral defense mechanisms are impaired early in HIV-1-infected patients, *J Acquir Immun Defic Syndr* 1:361, 1988.

68. Yoshizaki T and others: Clinical evaluation of extracorporeal shock wave lithotripsy for salivary stones, *Ann Otol Rhinol Laryngol* 105:63, 1996.

69. Zhao-ju Z and others: Chronic obstructive parotitis: report of 92 cases, *Oral Surg Oral Med Oral Pathol* 73:434, 1992.

SUGGESTED READINGS

Bartels LJ, Vrabec DP: Cervicofacial actinomycosis: a variable disorder, *Arch Otolaryngol* 104:705, 1978.

Brook I: Diagnosis and management of parotitis, *Otolaryngol Head Neck Surg* 118:469, 1992.

Brook I, Frazier EH, Thompson DH: Aerobic and anaerobic microbiology of acute suppurative parotitis, *Laryngoscope* 101:170, 1991.

Cox HJ, Brightwell AP, Riordan T: Non-tuberculosis mycobacterial infections presenting as salivary gland masses in children: investigation and conservative management, *J Laryngol Otol* 109:525, 1995.

Loughran DH, Smith LG: Infectious disorders of the parotid gland, *New Jersey Med* 85:311, 1988.

Margileth AM: Antibiotic therapy for cat-scratch disease: clinical study of therapeutic outcome in 268 patients and a review of the literature, *Pediatr Infect Dis J* 11:474, 1992.

O'Brien CJ, Murrant NJ: Surgical management of chronic parotitis, *Head Neck* 15(5):445, 1993.

Schiodt M and others: Natural history of HIV-associated salivary gland disease, *Oral Surg Oral Med Oral Pathol Oral Radiol Endod* 74:326, 1992.

Zhao-ju Z and others: Chronic obstructive parotitis: report of 92 cases, *Oral Surg Oral Med Oral Pathol Oral Radiol Endod* 73:434, 1992.

Chapter 68

Trauma

Jeffrey R. Haller

Salivary injuries are relatively uncommon. Earlier experience with treatment of salivary trauma comes from injuries sustained at wartime with one of the largest experiences from World War II.[15] Salivary gland injuries often are associated with multiple trauma victims and can go unnoticed. This is unfortunate because the injuries may be serious with long-term sequelae. The major cause of acute salivary injuries is penetrating trauma. Other acute injuries include blunt trauma or blast injuries. Irradiation (external beam and occasionally radioactive iodine), chronic infection, and chronic obstruction may cause more of a chronic insult to salivary tissue. They are more commonly encountered than acute salivary injuries but are less likely to require or respond to intervention.

Over the years, a number of methods of dealing with salivary injuries have been advocated. Optimal outcomes are the result of early recognition and proper evaluation, leading to proper management (Fig. 68-1). The scope of this chapter focuses primarily on parotid gland and, to a lesser extent, submandibular gland injuries. It emphasizes treatment options and surgical techniques. Chronic injuries are covered, although a more thorough discussion of radiation side effects and sialoadenitis can be found elsewhere in the text.

ANATOMIC CONSIDERATIONS

The parotid gland lays anterior to the ear from the inferior border of the zygoma to just below the angle of the mandible. Anteriorly, it extends 3 to 4 cm over the surface of the masseter muscle, and posteroinferiorly, it extends subcutaneously over the anterior portion of the sternocleidomastoid muscle. Superficial and deep portions of the gland are continuous. The deep portion extends behind the ramus of the mandible lying between the external acoustic meatus and the mastoid process.[13]

The outer surface of the gland is superficial. Only fat and parotid fascia lay between the gland and the skin.

The parotid (Stensen's) duct parallels the zygomatic arch and the buccal branch of the facial nerve. It generally lays inferior to the buccal branch of the facial nerve proximally, but it intersects the nerve as the buccal branch begins to divide. As the parotid duct passes anteriorly across the masseter muscle, it often is accompanied by accessory parotid tissue. Beyond the masseter muscle, the duct turns medially, penetrates the buccinator muscle and opens on the buccal surface of the oral cavity at the level of the upper second molar tooth.[13]

As the facial nerve emerges from the stylomastoid foramen, it almost immediately becomes related to the posterior deep parotid gland. Most commonly, the main trunk is divided into an upper (temporofacial) and a lower (cervicofacial) division. Although describing the next division of the facial nerve as five specific branches is customary (temporal, zygomatic, buccal, marginal mandibular, cervical), a variable number of branches emerge, and the terms indicate regions of distribution rather than individual branches.[13] An extensive cross-anastomotic network exists among nerve branches within the parotid gland. Temporal and marginal mandibular branches have less predictable cross-innervation.[8] These anatomic facts need to be considered when evaluating the location of penetrating injuries to the parotid gland and determining the need for facial nerve repair (Fig. 68-2).

Vascular relationships to the parotid gland are important for deep injuries to the gland. Within the medial portion of the gland lay the external carotid artery and the retromandibular vein. Generally, at the inferior level, the external carotid artery divides into the superficial temporal artery and the internal maxillary artery. Anteriomedial to this deep portion

is required.[25] As other imaging methods for vascular structures evolve, arteriogram may be replaced with less invasive methods, i.e., magnetic resonance angiography (MRA) and Doppler studies. However, arteriogram remains the gold standard against which other methods are tested.

PENETRATING INJURY

Duct injury

Penetrating injuries to the parotid gland not only involve the parenchyma of the gland but may involve Stensen's duct or the facial nerve. Lacerations posterior to the anterior masseter muscle may injure the duct. Although injuries of the parotid duct are uncommon, they are important to recognize to prevent further complications, i.e., infections, posttraumatic fistula, and sialoceles.[22,31] A previous discussion describes methods for identifying the duct through visualization of saliva, cannulating the duct, or sialogram. Everyone suspected of a duct injury also should be checked for facial nerve injury.

Appropriate treatment for parotid duct injury depends on the location of the injury along the duct. If primary anastomosis is not feasible and if the laceration is distal, oral reimplantation may be a reasonable option. Extensive damage of the duct proximally may not allow for primary anastomosis or reimplantation. These injuries need to be treated with proximal ligation in hopes that the gland atrophies.[21]

Many principles of the management of duct injury are controversial, but there is a consensus in the literature that acute parotid injuries should be explored proximally, and all injured structures should be repaired.[23] The proximal end of a divided duct may be identified by massage of the gland and the secretion of clear saliva. Identifying the distal end requires canalization through Stenson's duct in a retrograde fashion. Mobilization of the duct proximally and distally may allow for approximation without tension.

Most authors recommend repairing the duct over a stent. Materials used include 16- to 20-gauge Silastic catheters, No. 9 polyethylene tubing, and large nylon sutures (Fig. 68-3). The stents may prevent inadvertent placement of back wall stitches. Some authors suggest leaving stents in place for up to 2 weeks to help to prevent stricture formation.[1] Many different sutures have been advocated. This author prefers sutures similar to that used in microvascular anastomosis of small vessels. Either 9.0 or 10.0 nylon or proline sutures are acceptable. Under loop magnification or with the assistance of an operating microscope, the injured ends of the duct are adequately débrided. Approximation of the duct ends may be facilitated by placing them in microclamps normally used in microvascular anastomosis (Fig. 68-4). Magnification also allows exact placement of every stitch to ensure inclusion of the mucous membrane lining. Authors differ on suggestions for fixation of the ductal splint. Some favor suturing the splint to the oral mucosa. Abramson[1] describes passing the duct through the parenchyma of the gland proxi-

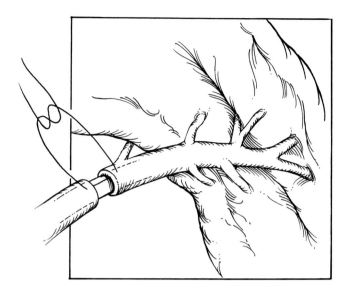

Fig. 68-3. Demonstration of repair of a salivary duct over a polyethylene catheter. (From Olson NR: Traumatic lesions of the salivary glands, *Otolaryngol Clin North Am* 10:345, 1977.)

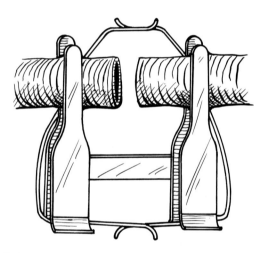

Fig. 68-4. The ends of the salivary gland may be placed in a microvascular framed clamp for ease with an approximation when repairing the duct. (From Julian Mack, University of Utah Medical Illustrations).

mally and then out through the skin.[1] It is fixed externally instead of allowing protrusion of the stent into the mouth (Fig. 68-5).

Injuries to the parenchyma of the major salivary glands that avoid injury to the duct require careful attention. They are treated with meticulous débridement, thorough irrigation, and closed in a layered fashion. A pressure dressing may be applied to prevent the accumulation of saliva and to help to channel it back through the ductal system. The dressing should not be placed too tightly, compromising already devitalized tissue. Additionally, antibiotic coverage should be considered because of the contamination within the

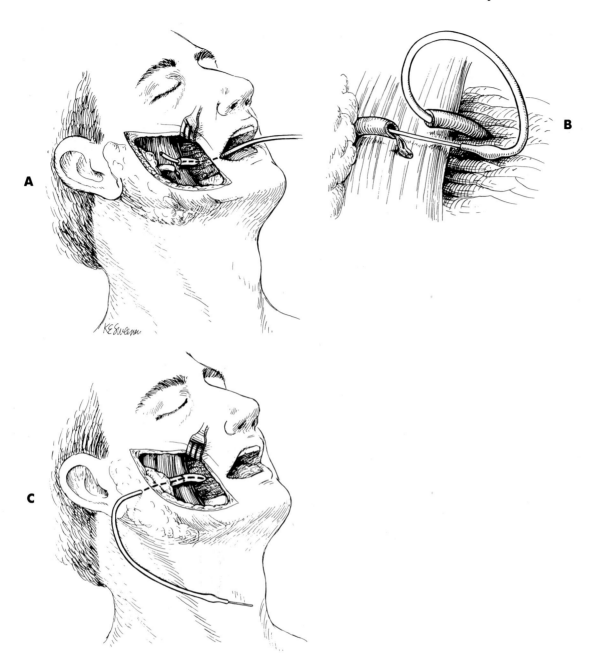

Fig. 68-5. Representation of repair of parotid duct using a polyethylene tube cannulated through the mouth. **A,** The catheter is brought into the wound through the mouth. **B,** A straight needle is placed through the distal end, through the proximal end of the duct threaded through the lateral duct wall at the grand hilum sutured over the skin. **C,** The catheter is advanced posteriorly so the distal end lays within the duct. Therefore, no portion of the catheter lays in the oral cavity so when the catheter is removed it can be done superficially. The catheter is sutured to the overlaying skin. (From Landau R, Stewart M: Conservative management of post traumatic parotid fistula in sialoceles: a prospective study, *Br J Surg* 72:42, 1985.)

wound. This coverage may be tailored to the type of injury sustained.

Posttraumatic parotid fistula or sialoceles

A parotid injury missed at initial presentation may lead to a posttraumatic parotid sialocele or fistula. Many of these present as soft-tissue swelling.[28] Unfortunately, they may go unrecognized as normal edema or a hematoma. Diagnosis at an early stage may allow for primary repair of the injured duct, whereas prolonged waiting allows for granulation tissue formation and great difficulty in primarily repairing the duct. Analysis of the fluid by aspiration may confirm parotid secretion as a result of a high amylase. Additionally, a sialogram may help to confirm a duct injury.[22]

Once beyond the acute development of a salivary fistula or sialocele, the management becomes controversial (Box 68-1). Many can be managed conservatively with repeated aspirations and compression,[16] although injuries to the duct are more resistant to conservative treatment than those originating from the parotid parenchyma.[3] The skin may become irritated, which may result in breakdown and fistula formation. The result may be troublesome as induration and scarring develop.

A variety of surgical methods has been used in the management of a persistent parotid sialocele or fistula. Reexplo-

---

Box 68-1. Management of parotid sialoceles and fistulae classification of reported methods in the literature

Diversion of parotid secretion into the mouth
    Reconstructive methods
        Delayed primary repair of duct
        Reconstruction of duct with vein graft
        Mucosal flaps
        Suture of proximal duct to buccal mucosa
    Formation of a controlled internal fistula
        T-tube or catheter drainage into the mouth
        Drainage of proximal duct by a catheter
Parotidectomy
Local therapy to the fistula
    Excision
    Cauterization
Depression of parotid secretion
    Surgical approaches
        Duct ligation
        Sectioning of the auricotemporal or Jacobsen's nerve
    Conservative approaches
        Administering nothing orally to the patient until the fistula
        Drugs: atropine or Pro-banthine
        Radiotherapy
        Repeated aspiration and pressure dressing

(From Parelch D and others: Posttraumatic parotid fistula in sialocels, *Ann Surg,* 209:105, 1989.)

---

ration of the wound with an attempt to repair or ligate the duct may be difficult because of the scarring and granulation tissue present. One cannot overemphasize the morbidity associated with superficial or total parotidectomy in the presence of such severe fibrosis. The affectiveness of tympanic neurectomy has varied in different reports, which probably is a result of the variations in Jacobson's nerves.[4] Others have attempted inserting a catheter via the intraoral orifice. Their attempt is to create scarring around the lacerated area and allowing saliva to enter into the mouth. This technique has been met with limited success.[11] Radiation with the intention of causing fibrosis is difficult to justify when relatively large doses are needed and long-term risk exists.

Previous work has shown that the amount of saliva excreted by the resting parotid gland is minimal. The major stimulus for parotid secretion appears to be gustatory and mechanical stimulation.[22] Recent work from South Africa has studied these principles and used them in treating chronic salivary fistula and sialoceles.[22,10] They have taken the conservative approach with the addition of probanthine and no oral intake until the injury has healed. Separate authors have been successful with this method and save surgery for the patients who do not respond to an adequate period of conservative therapy.

Traumatic injury to the submandibular gland and sublingual gland is rare because of their protective position by the mandible. Of the few cases reported, the injuries are penetrating trauma.[24,30] Treatment may be similar to that detailed for those with parotid injury, with the exception that the submandibular gland may be removed with minimal risk.

Human and animal bites to the face and salivary gland pose special circumstances. Human bites are associated with more virulent complicating infections and require appropriate antibiotics. Animal bites need an evaluation of the animal as a step to prevent rabies.[5]

Facial nerve injury

Trauma to the parotid region always should be checked for injury to the facial nerve. The facial nerve may be injured by transection, compression, or a crushing injury. A compression injury or crushing injury may cause a functional deficit without anatomic disruption. Electrical testing may be helpful in these patients. In general, the nonpenetrating injuries to the extracranial facial nerve are managed conservatively by expectant observation.[8] If repair is postponed, good results still may be achieved up to 3 weeks or longer.[33] Electromyography may be helpful in establishing recovery potentials of the nerve and in planning exploration.

Lacerated nerves are repaired, depending on their location of injury. If the wound is in front of a vertical line extending from the lateral canthus to mental foramen, repair is not necessary because recovery is likely.[8] Proximal to this line, repair needs to be considered. The timing of repair has been debated in the past. McCabe[18] suggests that the nerve is at its maximal ability to regenerate 21 days after the injury.

He states that metabolically motor neurons from the facial motor nucleus have attained maximum photosynthetic capabilities. Recent data suggest the sooner the integrity of the nerve is reestablished, the better the outcome.[6,9] The timing of nerve repair depends on the condition of the patient, but the author agrees with repairing the nerve as soon as possible after the injury.

Techniques of epineural, perineural, and interfasicular nerve repair exist.[7,26] Despite attempts to define the best method, controversies exist, and the most efficacious method of nerve repair remains clinically unproven. Proponents of perineural and interfasicular repair maintain improved realignment of axons. Opponents believe that this method of repair enhances scarring and decreases blood supply. Terris and Fee[33] believe epineural repair with sutures remains the gold standard against which all other methods should be tested. The author prefers an epineural suture repair. Fine sutures (8-0 or 9-0 nylon) are placed in an interrupted fashion. Magnification is used either with loops or an operating microscope. As few sutures as needed are placed to reduce scarring.

Tissue glues and fine-tuned lasers have theoretical advantages in repairing nerves with less scarring.[14] Although advantages may exist when the nerve is difficult to suture (i.e., when found within the mastoid or at the cerebellopontine angle), no improvement has been seen with these other innovative methods. Fine monofilament suture repair remains the superior method for reconstructing peripheral nerves.

The facial nerve should not be repaired under tension. In patients in whom the cut ends of the facial nerve are separated by more than 1 cm, a nerve graft should be considered. Traditional nerve grafts include the greater auricular and sural nerves. An advantage of the greater auricular nerve is that it is either close or within the operating field. A disadvantage potentially exists of not having adequate length. The greater auricular nerve gives approximately 8 cm. A severe injury with major tissue loss may require more length than the greater auricular nerve allows. Additionally, a numb ear may be bothersome to some patients. The sural nerve has the advantage of an abundant length and an easy two-team approach for harvesting. Recently, the author has used the medial antebrachial cutaneous branch of the median nerve as an alternative donor graft for facial nerve repair. Its advantages include adequate length and a diameter in branching patterns similar to the facial nerve. Additionally, the patient rarely noticed the donor site numbness.[20]

BLUNT TRAUMA

Blunt trauma to the cheek increases concern for skeletal structures. Shetty[29] studied 22 cases of blunt trauma to the cheek. In most patients, there was a fracture of either the mandible, the zygomatic arch, or malar complex. Shetty demonstrated dysfunction in the filling patterns of the parotid gland in patients who sustained these blunt injuries. Therefore, on occasion, salivary complications from blunt injury to the parotid glands may be seen. Otherwise, these injuries can be treated with prudent observation.

RADIATION INJURY TO SALIVARY GLANDS

Radiotherapy impairs function of salivary glands. When salivary glands are included in the radiation field, xerostomia results. If portions of the glands may be protected, the remaining secretory cells have the ability to hypertrophy, and symptoms may decrease after several months.

Additionally, external beam radiation appears to increase the incidence of tumors in salivary tissue. Modan[19] observed a higher frequency of salivary gland tumors in children who had received radiation for other conditions. Also, children who had received radiation to the thymus subsequently developed parotid and submaxillary gland malignancies at a higher rate than expected in the general population.[27] Studies of survivors of the bombing of Hiroshima have a higher incidence of benign and malignant salivary gland tumors.[32]

Acute and chronic sialoadenitis have been found in patients treated with therapeutic doses of I^{131} for thyroid cancer. A cause has been postulated to be a result of radiation injury to the concentration of I^{131} by the glands.[2] Because epithelial cells of the salivary glands divide slowly, it would be expected that the glands would be resistant to radiation, but alteration of the gland has been clearly seen after radiation.[17] Most patients simply experience altered composition of their saliva and have few or no complaints. Occasionally, patients experience severe symptoms, and there are reports of long-term salivary damage.

SIALOADENITIS

Chronic obstruction of the gland leads to obstruction of flow, which may in turn lead to infection. Relieving the gland of the obstruction is the optimal early intervention. If obstruction persists, the gland may become chronically inflamed and edematous, and recurrent infections may occur. Conservative therapy should first be attempted by dilation of the salivary duct and the use of sialagogue and antibiotics. Only after conservative therapy has failed should an attempt be made for surgically removing the glands.

SUMMARY

Although infrequent, salivary gland injuries may be serious and associated with long-term morbidity. Of importance is a thorough evaluation of these injuries because they often are overlooked or underestimated. Surrounding structures also should be thoroughly assessed because injuries severe enough to injure the salivary glands may cause musculoskeletal and neurovascular injuries.

Penetrating injuries to the parotid gland increase attention to duct injuries and facial nerve injuries. Both should be repaired primarily whenever possible. A duct injury missed initially may lead to development of a posttraumatic fistula or sialoceles. Conservative therapy for delayed fistula or sialoceles may be performed with aspiration and compression. Most of these injuries resolve with conservative therapy.

Blunt trauma causes facial nerve injury and glandular duct injury less frequently. Close expectant observation is recommended. Electrical testing may be used to predict the recovery after a facial nerve injury. Salivary injuries, once recognized, are treated similarly to a penetrating injury.

The preferred outcome for the patient stems from an early recognition of injured structures through accurate evaluation followed by appropriate treatment.

REFERENCES

1. Abramson M: Treatment of parotid duct injuries, *Laryngoscope* 83: 1764, 1973.
2. Allweiss P and others: Sialoadenitis following I[131] therapy for thyroid carcinoma: concise communication, *J Nucl Med* 25:755, 1984.
3. Anantha KN, Parkas S: Parotid fistula, *Surgery* 69:641, 1982.
4. Arulpragasam AC: Treatment of parotid fistula, *J Laryngol Otolaryngol* 81:329, 1967.
5. Bailey BJ: *Salivary trauma.* In Cummings CW, editor: *Otolaryngology—head and neck Surgery*, ed. 2, St Louis, 1993, Mosby.
6. Barrs DM: Facial nerve trauma. Optimal timing of repair, *Laryngoscope* 101:835, 1991.
7. Bora FW: Peripheral nerve repair in cats, *J Bone Joints Surg Am* 49: 659, 1967.
8. Coker NJ: Management of traumatic injuries to the facial nerve, *Otolaryngol Clin North Am* 4:215, 1991.
9. DeMedinacilli L, Seaber AV: Experimental nerve reconnection. Importance of initial repair, *Microsurg* 10:56, 1989.
10. Demetriades D: Surgical management of post traumatic parotid sialoceles and fistula, *Injury* 22:183, 1991.
11. Epker B, Burnette J: Trauma to the parotid gland and duct: primary treatment and management of complications, *J Oral Surg* 28:657, 1970.
12. Harnsberger HR: *Handbook of head and neck imaging*, ed 2, St Louis, 1995, Mosby.
13. Hollingshead: *Head and neck anatomy*.
14. Huang TC and others: Laser vs. suture nerve anastomosis, *Otolaryngol Head Neck Surg* 107:14, 1992.
15. Landau R, Stewart M: Conservative management of post traumatic parotid fistula in sialoceles: a prospective study, *Br J Surg* 72:42, 1985.
16. Langenbrunner DJ: Treatment of sialocele and experimental study in dogs, *Trans Am Acad Ophthalmol Otolaryngol* 80:375, 1975.
17. Maier H, Bihl H: Effect of radioactive iodine therapy on parotid gland function, *Acta Otolaryngol (Stockh)* 103:318, 1987.
18. McCabe BF: Facial nerve grafting, *Plast Reconst Surg* 45:70, 1970.
19. Modan B: Radiation-induced head and neck tumors, *Lancet* 1:277, 1974.
20. Newley JA and others: Use of the anterior branch of the medial antebrachial cutaneous nerve graft as a repair of defects of the digital nerve, *J Bone Joints Surg* 4:563, 1989.
21. Olson NR: Traumatic lesions of the salivary glands, *Otolaryngol Clin North Am* 10:345, 1977.
22. Parekh D and others: Post traumatic parotid fistula in sialoceles, *Ann Surg* 209:105, 1989.
23. Parekh D, Stewart M, Demetriades D: *Parotid Injury.* In Pantanowitz D, editor: *Modern surgery in Africa*, Johannesburg, 1988, Southern Publishers.
24. Roebker JJ, Hall LC, Lukin RR: Fractured submandibular gland: CT findings, *J Comput Assist Tomogr* 15:1068, 1991.
25. Roon AJ, Christensen N: Evaluation and treatment of penetrating cervical injuries, *J Trauma* 19:391, 1979.
26. Rosen JM, Hentz BR, Kaplan N: Fascicular sutureless and suture repair of peripheral nerves: a comparison study in laboratory animals, *Orthop Rev* 8:85, 1979.
27. Saenger EL: Neoplasia following therapeutic radiation for benign conditions in childhood, *Radiology* 74:889, 1960.
28. Shapiro DN, Gallo J, Moss M: Subcutaneous parotid infusion after mandibular osteotomy, *J Oral Surg* 36:397, 1978.
29. Shetty DK: Effects of direct blunt trauma on the parotid gland, *Deutsche Zahn Mund Kieferheilk* 62:148, 1974.
30. Singh B, Shaha A: Traumatics of submandibular salivary gland fistula, *J Oral Maxill Facial Surg* 53:338, 1995.
31. Tachmes L and others: Parotid gland in facial nerve trauma: a retrospective review, *J Trauma* 30:1395, 1990.
32. Takeichi N: Salivary gland tumors in atomic bomb survivors of Hiroshima, Japan, *Cancer* 52:377, 1983.
33. Terris DJ, Fee WE: Current issues in nerve repair, *Arch Otolaryngol Head Neck Surg* 119:725, 1993.

Chapter 69

Neoplasms of the Salivary Glands

Ehab Y. Hanna
James Y. Suen

Salivary gland neoplasms are challenging because of their relative infrequency, inconsistent classification, and highly variable biologic behavior. These factors present some difficulty when attempting to compare data from various institutions describing their experience with salivary gland tumors. There are some general features that could be drawn from the literature regarding the incidence, etiology, pathology, and patterns of behavior of the various benign and malignant tumors of the salivary glands. These salient features and guidelines for treatment of these challenging tumors are discussed herein.

HISTOPATHOLOGIC CLASSIFICATION

Tumors of the salivary glands display a variety of histologic appearances and vary in behavior from totally benign to high grade and usually fatal malignancies. During the past 40 years, several classification schemes have been proposed, of which the most comprehensive are those of the Armed Forces Institute of Pathology (AFIP) and the World Health Organization (WHO), which were revised in 1991.[126] The WHO is more concise, but both are readily applicable by practicing surgical pathologists and encompass most of the range of tumors likely to be encountered. The second edition of the *World Health Organization's Histologic Classification* of salivary gland tumors is more extensive and detailed than the previous edition published 20 years ago. The new edition is based on data regarding newly described tumor entities and the behavior and prognosis of previously classified tumors.[122]

Tumors of the salivary glands may be broadly divided into benign neoplasms, tumor-like conditions, and malignant neoplasms. These tumor-like conditions may be confused with benign or malignant tumors of the salivary glands and are included in this chapter. Benign tumors of the salivary glands may be of an epithelial or nonepithelial origin. Epithelial benign neoplasms include the various adenomas, papillomas, and cystadenomas (Box 69-1).

The group of malignant salivary gland tumors contains carcinomas, malignant nonepithelial tumors, malignant lymphomas, and secondary tumors (see Box 69-1). New entities in this classification are polymorphous low-grade adenocarcinoma, basal cell adenocarcinoma, salivary duct carcinoma, and malignant myoepithelioma. Carcinoma arising in a pleomorphic adenoma may be distinguished as noninvasive and invasive carcinoma and carcinosarcoma.[121]

Malignant nonepithelial tumors are mostly malignant fibrous histiocytoma, malignant schwannoma, and rhabdomyosarcoma. The majority of malignant lymphomas are non-Hodgkin's lymphomas with high differentiation. Many lymphomas are associated with chronic immunosialadenitis (Sjögren's syndrome). Secondary tumors are mostly metastases from primary squamous cell carcinomas or from melanomas of the skin of the head and neck. Hematogeneous metastases are rare and originate mainly from the lungs, kidneys, or breasts.[121]

HISTOGENESIS

Understanding the origin of benign salivary gland tumors requires knowledge of the embryology and ultrastructure of the normal salivary gland. The major salivary glands origi-

Box 69-1. The world health organization's histologic classification of salivary gland tumors (1992)

1 Adenomas
  1.1 Pleomorphic adenoma
  1.2 Myoepithelioma (myoepithelial adenoma)
  1.3 Basal cell adenoma
  1.4 Warthin's tumor (adenolymphoma)
  1.5 Oncocytoma (oncocytic adenoma)
  1.6 Canalicular adenoma
  1.7 Sebaceous adenoma
  1.8 Ductal papilloma
    1.8.1 Inverted ductal papilloma
    1.8.2 Intraductal papilloma
    1.8.3 Sialadenoma papilliferum
  1.9 Cystadenoma
    1.9.1 Papillary cystadenoma
    1.9.2 Mucinous cystadenoma
2 Carcinomas
  2.1 Acinic cell carcinoma
  2.2 Mucoepidermoid carcinoma
  2.3 Adenoid cystic carcinoma
  2.4 Polymorphous low-grade adenocarcinoma (terminal duct adenocarcinoma)
  2.5 Epithelial-myoepithelial carcinoma
  2.6 Basal cell adenocarcinoma
  2.7 Sebaceous carcinoma
  2.8 Papillary cystadenocarcinoma
  2.9 Mucinous adenocarcinoma
  2.10 Oncocytic carcinoma
  2.11 Salivary duct carcinoma
  2.12 Adenocarcinoma
  2.13 Malignant myoepithelioma (myoepithelial carcinoma)
  2.15 Squamous cell carcinoma
  2.16 Small cell carcinoma
  2.17 Undifferentiated carcinoma
  2.18 Other carcinomas
3 Nonepithelial tumors
4 Malignant lymphomas
5 Secondary tumors
6 Unclassified tumors
7 Tumor-like lesions
  7.1 Sialadenosis
  7.2 Oncocytosis
  7.3 Necrotizing sialometaplasia (salivary gland infarction)
  7.4 Benign lymphoepithelial lesion
  7.5 Salivary gland cysts
  7.6 Chronic sclerosing sialedenitis of submandibular gland (Kuttner tumor)
  7.7 Cystic lymphoid hyperplasia in patients with acquired immunodeficiency syndrome

nate from ectoderm and begin their development as solid ingrowths from the oral epithelium. These ingrowths continue to develop into tubules that later become the ductal system of the salivary glands. In the major salivary glands, serous and mucous cells are arranged into acini, which are drained by a series of ducts: an intercalated duct that drains into a striated duct, which empties into an excretory duct. Contractile myoepithelial cells surround the acini and intercalated ducts and help drain saliva through the ductal system (Fig. 69-1). Serous acini predominate the parotid gland; mucinous acini are more abundant in the submandibular gland, and in the minor salivary glands which are scattered throughout the upper aerodigestive tract.

The differentiated epithelium lining the acini and each portion of the ductal system is unique and is distinctively different in various portions of the salivary unit. The histologic differences found in benign and malignant neoplasms of the salivary glands could be explained, at least in part, by their origin from different cells along this acinar–ductal subunit (the multicellular theory). For example, pleomorphic adenomas originate from the intercalated duct cells and myoepithelial cells; oncocytic tumors originate from the striated duct cells; acinous cell tumors originate from the acinar cells, and mucoepidermoid tumors and squamous cell carcinomas develop in the excretory duct cells. An alternative theory, the reserve cell theory, assumes that the origin of salivary neoplasms may be traced to the basal cells of either the excretory or the intercalated duct.

Either of these two types of cells may act as a reserve cell with the potential for differentiation into a variety of epithelial cells.[16] According to this theory, squamous cell carcinoma and mucoepidermoid carcinoma originate from the reserve cell of the excretory duct, whereas mixed tumors, Warthin's tumor, oncocytic tumors, adenoid cystic carcinoma, and acinous tumors originate from the reserve cell of the intercalated duct. Recently, there have been several studies that provide some molecular evidence to support the reserve cell theory of salivary gland tumorigenesis.[37,86,101]

ETIOLOGY

The etiology of salivary gland neoplasms, like that of most other types of tumors, remains unknown, although there is growing evidence that some environmental factors and certain genetic abberations may be involved in the development of salivary gland neoplasia.

Environmental factors

Radiation

In 1996, the Radiation Epidemiology Branch of the National Cancer Institute published a study on the risk of developing salivary gland tumors among atomic bomb survivors.[77] The study indicated that these survivors had a higher radiation-related risk of developing benign and malignant salivary gland tumors compared with the general population.

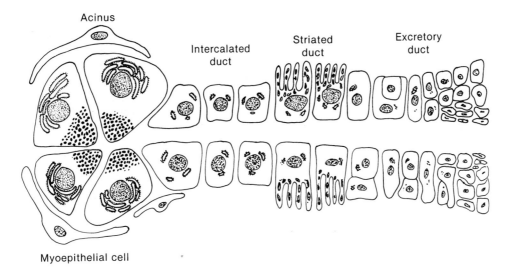

Fig. 69-1. Structural elements of the salivary gland unit.

Dose–response analyses found statistically significant increases in risk with increasing atomic bomb exposure for malignant and benign tumors. The risk was higher for occurrence of malignant tumors, especially mucoepidermoid carcinoma. Among those with benign neoplasms, Warthin's tumor showed the highest dose–response-related risk. Spitz and Batsakis[137] conducted a study of 498 patients with histopathologically confirmed carcinoma of the major salivary glands to ascertain the role of radiotherapy as a possible risk factor in the development of salivary gland cancer. Of the 57 patients who had a history of radiation exposure, 49 patients had been irradiated in a field encompassing the salivary gland area.

Epstein-Barr virus

There is some evidence to indicate that Epstein-Barr virus (EBV) may be implicated in the development of certain types of salivary gland neoplasms. A recent study from Greenland found a relatively high incidence of familial clusters of nasopharyngeal carcinoma and anaplastic salivary gland carcinoma.[5] This may be a result of an enhanced oncogenic potential of an EBV strain that apparently occurs more frequently in Greenland than in other parts of the world.[5] Similarly, there is a relatively high geographic concentration of lymphoepithelial carcinoma originating in the salivary glands among Eskimo and southern Chinese populations.[96] Several other recent studies from the Far East have shown a consistent association between EBV and lymphoepithelial carcinoma of the salivary gland. The presence of the virus in a clonal form and the expression of its viral oncoprotein provide further evidence of the role of EBV in the oncogenesis of this tumor.[84] These findings suggest that lymphoepithelial carcinoma of the salivary gland in the Taiwanese Chinese population may share a similar EBV-related pathogenesis with that of nasopharyngeal carcinoma.[146] The consistent association of EBV with lymphoepithelial carcinoma of the salivary gland suggests that the virus probably plays a causal role in this tumor, at least in the Asian population, whereas there is no evidence of a causal role of EBV in other primary tumors of the salivary gland.[30]

Other factors

In addition to radiation exposure and the possible role of oncogenic viruses, other environmental and dietary factors may contribute to the development of salivary gland malignancy. Occupational exposure to silica dust was linked to a 2.5-fold increased risk of salivary gland cancer.[161] The risk also was significantly increased among patients who reported using kerosene as cooking fuel or having a previous history of head radiographic examinations. Dietary analyses revealed a significant protective effect of consumption of dark-yellow vegetables or liver, with about 70% reduced risk of salivary gland cancer among people in the highest intake group of these foods.[161] Although tobacco use was not associated with a higher incidence of malignant salivary neoplasms, Warthin's tumor is strongly associated with cigarette smoking.[107]

Genetic factors

Certain genetic aberrations may be responsible for an increased likelihood of developing salivary gland neoplasms. Several such aberrations recently have been described in the literature. These genetic alterations may include allelic loss, structural rearrangement of chromosomal units (most commonly translocations), the absence of one chromosome (monosomy), and the presence of an extra chromosome (polysomy). Any of these factors may be the sole karyotypic abnormality, which usually indicates that it is an early genetic aberration in the development of neoplasia, or several genetic alterations may coexist.

Allelic loss

Johns and others found that pleomorphic adenomas showed few areas of allelic loss; the most prominent chromosomal arm involved was 12q, which was lost in more than 35% of patients.[69] The most significant allelic losses in those with adenoid cystic carcinoma were 1p, 2p, 6q, 17p, 19q, and 20p. Mucoepidermoid carcinoma showed 50% or greater loss at 2q, 5p, 12p, and 16q. Although losses at 9p, 3p, and 17p are common in patients with squamous cell carcinoma of the head and neck, only the carcinoma ex-mixed tumors showed loss at these loci, consistent with progression to a more aggressive phenotype. It seems that salivary gland tumors display allelic loss patterns differently from other tumor types, suggesting distinct genetic pathways in the progression of these tumors.[69]

Monosomy and polysomy

In 1994, El Naggar and others described trisomy 5 as the only karyotypic abnormality in a moderately differentiated primary mucoepidermoid carcinoma of the base of the tongue.[40] This finding was remarkably different from previous cytogenetic studies of mucoepidermoid carcinomas, which have shown heterogeneous and unrelated chromosomal aberrations. Their results suggest that trisomy 5 may be an early aberration in the development of this neoplasm. Other studies suggest that polysomy of chromosomes 3 and 17 occurs during the development of salivary gland tumors, and its frequency is higher in adenoid cystic carcinoma compared with pleomorphic adenoma. In addition, monosomy of chromosome 17 could possibly be significant in salivary gland tumors.[88]

Structural rearrangement

The most common genetic structural rearrangement in salivary gland malignancy is translocation of genetic material involving chromosome 11.[97] This finding was most commonly reported in cases of mucoepidermoid carcinoma. In 1996, El-Naggar and others described the cytogenetic analysis of a mucoepidermoid carcinoma of the minor salivary gland with t(11,19) (q21; p3.1) as the sole karyotypic abnormality.[40] Their findings indicated that this translocation is an early and most likely a primary event in the development of at least a subset of these neoplasms.

INCIDENCE

Salivary gland tumors are relatively rare and constitute 3% to 4% of all head and neck neoplasms. The majority (70%) of salivary gland tumors originate in the parotid gland (Fig. 69-2). Although the majority of minor salivary gland tumors are malignant, three fourths of parotid tumors are benign (Fig. 69-3). Spiro and others reviewed the Memorial Sloan Kettering experience with salivary neoplasms during a 35-year period.[131] The distribution of these 2807 patients is shown in Table 69-1. Benign neoplasms constituted 54% (1529 patients) of all tumors. Pleomorphic adenoma (1280 patients) constituted 84% of benign tumors and 45% of all salivary gland neoplasms. Warthin's tumor was the second-most common benign tumor and comprised 12% (183 pa-

Table 69-1. The distribution of 2807 salivary neoplasms

Histology	Number of patients	Percent
Pleomorphic adenoma	1274	45.4
Warthin's tumor	183	6.5
Benign cyst	29	1.0
Lymphoepithelial lesion	17	0.6
Oncocytoma	20	0.7
Monomorphic adenoma	6	0.2
Mucoepidermoid carcinoma	439	15.7
Adenoidcystic carcinoma	282	10.0
Adenocarcinoma	225	8.0
Malignant mixed tumor	161	5.7
Acinic cell carcinoma	84	3.0
Epidermoid carcinoma	53	1.9
Other (anaplastic)	35	1.3
Total	2807	100

Spiro RH: Salivary neoplasms: overview of a 35-year experience with 2,807 patients, *Head Neck Surg* 8:177, 1986.

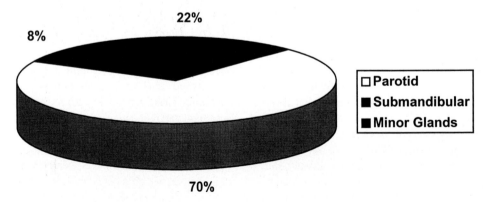

Fig. 69-2. The site of origin of salivary neoplasms.

tients) of all benign tumors. Malignant neoplasms consti-tuted 46% (1278 patients) of all tumors, of which mucoepi-dermoid carcinoma and adenoid cystic carcinoma were the most common (Fig. 69-4).

PATIENT EVALUATION

Clinical features

A careful history and physical examination is the first step in trying to differentiate between a benign and a malig-nant lesion in the parotid gland. Classically, benign neo-plasms of the salivary glands are painless, slow-growing masses. A sudden increase in size usually may be traced to infection, cystic degeneration, hemorrhage inside the mass, or malignant transformation. When this occurs, a patient may complain that the previously painless mass is now tender. As a rule, benign lesions of the parotid gland are freely mobile and have no associated nerve paralysis or overlying ulceration. Seventeen cases of facial nerve dysfunction have been reported in patients with histologically benign, non-neurogenic masses of the parotid gland in the English lan-guage literature.[127] Because this condition is so rare, a facial nerve paralysis generally is associated with a malignant tumor.

Similar to benign neoplasms, malignant tumors of the parotid gland usually present as a painless swelling, although certain clinical features associated with a parotid mass usu-ally indicate malignancy, albeit advanced. These features include facial nerve paresis or paralysis, pain, fixation of the mass to the overlying skin or underlying structures, and associated cervical adenopathy. It should be noted that these findings usually indicate local or regional extension of the tumor, and the diagnosis of parotid malignancy should not await the development of these signs and symptoms. The possibility of malignancy should be ruled out in patients presenting with any mass in the parotid gland. This usually requires histologic evaluation with a fine-needle biopsy or parotidectomy.

Metastatic disease to the parotid gland from skin malig-nancy may be unveiled by a careful history of present or previously excised skin cancer of the scalp or face. A careful examination of these areas for evidence of a coexisting skin cancer or a scar of previous excision also should be done. The oropharynx also should be examined carefully to rule out deep-lobe parotid involvement. A mass in the deep lobe of the parotid gland or a tumor originating from the minor salivary glands in the parapharyngeal space may displace

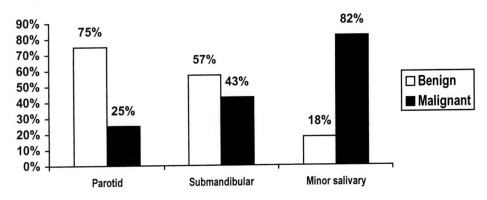

Fig. 69-3. The incidence of benign and malignant salivary neoplasms according to the site of origin.

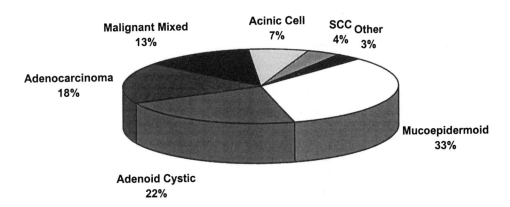

Fig. 69-4. Malignant salivary neoplasms.

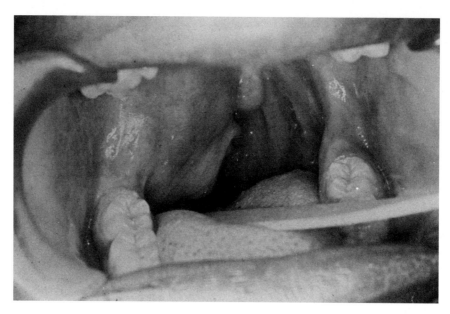

Fig. 69-5. Pleomorphic adenoma of the deep lobe of a parotid gland, causing medial displacement of the palate and tonsil.

the soft palate or tonsils medially (Fig. 69-5). This could be mistaken for tonsillar enlargement and lead to an attempt at intraoral biopsy or excision, resulting in tumor seeding or mucosal scarring and making definitive resection through a transparotid and/or transcervical approach more difficult.

Benign and malignant tumors of the submandibular gland usually present as painless swelling or a mass in the submandibular triangle. In patients with malignant tumors, involvement of the skin or fixation to the mandible indicates local extension. Ipsilateral weakness or numbness of the tongue indicates perineural spread of malignancy along the hypoglossal or lingual nerves, respectively. Enlargement of the submandibular or upper cervical lymph nodes may be a result of reactive lymphadenopathy associated with submandibular sialadenitis or may indicate regional metastasis of malignancy in the submandibular gland.

Benign tumors of the minor salivary gland are rare and usually present as a painless, submucosal mass. The overlying mucosa usually is normal, and the tumors rarely ulcerate. The clinical presentation of malignant tumors of the minor salivary glands depends on the site of origin and does not differ from the presentation of other malignant tumors in these sites. The palate is the most common site of involvement, and adenoid cystic carcinoma is the most common histology encountered. Palatal tumors usually present as ulcerative lesions or submucosal masses (Fig. 69-6). The second-most common site is the sinonasal tract, and these patients usually present with nasal obstruction, epistaxis, or a nasal mass. Numbness or tingling in the distribution of the branches of the trigeminal nerve may indicate perineural spread, which occurs most frequently in patients with adenoid cystic carcinoma. Careful evaluation of the dermatomal

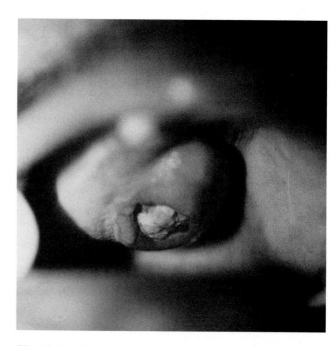

Fig. 69-6. Adenoid cystic carcinoma of the palate presenting as an ulcerative mass.

distribution of the three divisions of the trigeminal nerve should be done, and any hyposthesia or anesthesia should be considered evidence of perineural involvement.

Fine-needle aspiration biopsy

The accuracy of fine-needle aspiration biopsy (FNAB) in the diagnosis of salivary tumors has been well established. In the past 5 years, several studies from various countries

Table 69-2. Sensitivity and specificity of fine-needle aspiration biopsy

Study/Year	Country	Total patients	Patients with malignancy	Sensitivity, %	Specificity, %
Orell,[100] 1995	Australia	325	—	85.5	99.5
Candel,[27] 1993	USA	163	15	95.7	100
Roland,[114] 1993	United Kingdom	92	—	90.9	100
Bhatia,[20] 1993	India	101	34	99	100
Chan,[29] 1992	Hong Kong	112	36	86	99
Abad,[1] 1992	Spain	97	18	90	96.3

have reported an exceptionally high degree of sensitivity and specificity of FNAB. Examples of such studies are summarized in Table 69-2. The overall sensitivity ranges from 85.5% to 99%, and the overall specificity ranges from 96.3% to 100%.* Diagnostic accuracy depends on the experience of the cytopathologist, which in turn depends on the volume of patients with salivary neoplasms evaluated in any given institution. The reported sensitivity and specificity of FNAB were slightly lower in a community hospital setting compared with large academic centers.[109] The most common source of diagnostic error is inadequate sampling. Among 582 FNABs of major and minor salivary glands, lack of cytologic and histologic correlation was noted in 21 cases. Of these, the cause in 10 FNABs was inadequate cytologic sampling of the lesion.[90]

In addition to being accurate, FNAB is safe, simple to perform, and relatively inexpensive, although one essential question is worth asking. Is FNAB necessary in the evaluation of salivary gland masses? Would its results change the course of management based on clinical assessment? In an attempt to answer this question, Heller and others performed a study to determine the impact of FNAB on patient treatment.[61] One hundred one patients underwent FNAB of major salivary gland masses. The physician's initial clinical impression was compared with the FNAB diagnosis and the final diagnosis in each case. Overall, results of FNAB resulted in a change in the clinical approach to 35% of the patients. Examples of such changes in planned management included avoiding a relatively large resection for lymphomas and sialadenitis. FNAB also allows better preoperative counseling of patients, which helps alleviate an already high level of anxiety to them and their families.[27] Based on these findings, the performance of FNAB may be helpful in treatment planning for patients presenting with salivary gland masses.[61]

Imaging

The routine use of imaging in patients with small well-defined masses of the superficial lobe of the parotid gland probably is not warranted because imaging results in such

instances rarely change the planned treatment. Tumors that present with clinical findings suggestive of malignancy, tumors originating from the deep lobe of the parotid gland or the parapharyngeal space, and submandibular and minor salivary gland tumors should be evaluated with high resolution imaging. Computed tomography (CT) and magnetic resonance imaging (MRI) give a better understanding of the location and extent of the tumor, its relation to major neurovascular structures, perineural spread of malignancy, skull base invasion, and intracranial extension. Conventional radiography and sialography are rarely used because they provide little useful information. Nuclear imaging using technetium 99m pertechnetate is helpful only in patients with oncocytic and Warthin's tumors.[66] Because FNAB may provide better information, nuclear imaging is rarely obtained. High resolution ultrasound evaluation is useful to experienced radiologists and may detect calculi, abscesses, and cysts and has been reported to correctly assess up to 90% of benign versus malignant tumors.[56]

Computed tomography and magnetic resonance imaging

CT and MRI provide information that is superior to that provided by other imaging techniques or by physical examination.[60] To obtain the maximum amount of information possible, CT scanning should be performed with intravenous injection of contrast material. The normal parotid gland has a high fat content and is easily visualized on CT and MRI, and therefore both techniques may show whether a mass in that region is intraglandular or extraglandular (Fig. 69-7). Generally, CT and MRI do not provide information regarding the specific histologic diagnosis, except in rare cases. An example of such a rare scenario is in patients with lipoma of the parotid gland (Fig. 69-8). CT and MRI may give useful information that may differentiate benign from malignant tumors. In contrast to benign tumors, which invariably have well-defined margins, malignant tumors usually exhibit irregular margins (Fig. 69-9). Extension of the tumor beyond the confines of the gland may be seen adequately on CT and MRI. Bony destruction of the mandible or skull base is best visualized on CT, whereas bone marrow involvement is better demonstrated on MRI. Both studies may adequately evaluate the neck for metastatic adenopathy. CT has the ad-

*Refs. 1, 20, 27, 29, 100, 114.

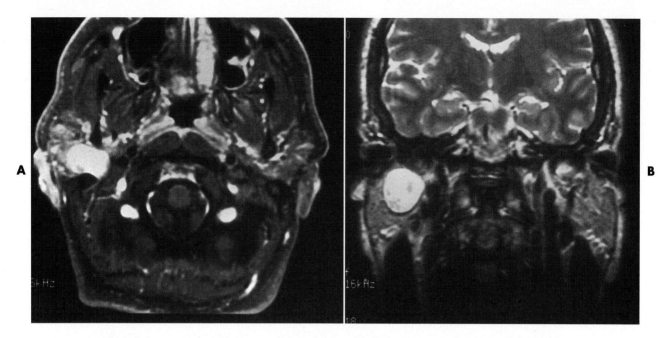

Fig. 69-7. A 35-year-old patient presented with gradually progressive facial palsy. The ipsilateral parotid gland was slightly more prominent, but no distinct masses were palapable. **A,** An axial and **B,** a coronal magnetic resonance imaging scan showed a mass within the deep lobe of the parotid gland. This well-defined mass had smooth borders and enhanced brightly in **A,** the T1-weighted (with gadolinium); and **B,** the T2-weighted images. Surgical exploration revealed a facial nerve neuroma. The tumor was resected with reconstruction of the facial nerve with a cable graft. At 3-year follow-up evaluation, the patient has a House-Brackman grade III facial function and no evidence of recurrence.

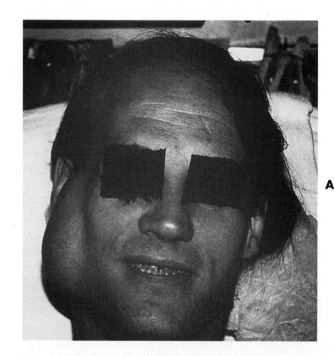

Fig. 69-8. A, A 40-year-old man with a large, painless parotid mass, which has been slow-growing. The fine-needle aspiration biopsy was indeterminate.

Continued

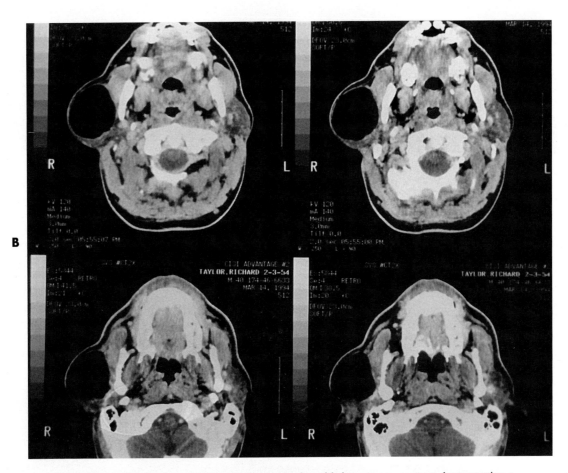

Fig. 69-8, cont'd. B, An axial computed tomography with intravenous contrast demonstrating a large, rounded, well-defined mass, with smooth borders in the parotid gland. The mass was nonenhancing and had the same density as the subcutaneous fat. These findings were pathognomonic of parotid lipoma. A superficial parotidectomy was performed, and the diagnosis was confirmed.

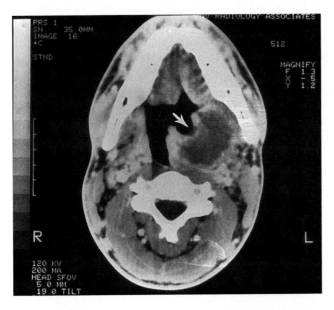

Fig. 69-9. Axial computed tomography with intravenous contrast showing a mass in the oral cavity, which exhibits an enhancing irregular border, with surface ulceration (*arrow*). The low density center is consistent with necrosis. These findings are highly suggestive of a malignant neoplasm. There is no evidence of gross invasion of the mandible. The biopsy confirmed a malignant mixed tumor.

vantage of being less expensive and more available than MRI, although CT images are more susceptible to degradation by dental artifact.[60] MRI is superior to CT in demonstrating the internal architecture of salivary gland tumors in a multiplanar fashion and in delineating the interface between the tumor and normal salivary gland.[13]

Perineural spread is common in patients with salivary gland malignancy, especially in those with adenoid cystic carcinoma. Perineural spread is a precursor of skull base invasion, facial nerve and trigeminal ganglion infiltration, and cavernous sinus involvement. These findings have a profound negative impact on survival rate and may drastically change the therapeutic plan, including the surgical approach and adjuvant therapy.[58] Although patients with perineural spread may present with sensory or motor manifestations of abnormal nerve function, they often are asymptomatic. High resolution imaging is of paramount importance in such patients to detect perineural involvement. The criteria of nerve involvement on CT rely on bony changes in the foramina, fissures, or canals wherein nerves normally traverse the skull base. These changes include bone erosion, sclerotic margins, and widening of the normal diameter of these cranial base

channels (Fig. 69-10), although these findings are late indicators of perineural spread. Perineural spread may be detected earlier on MRI because of the better soft-tissue delineation. The capability of MRI to detect the different signal intensity of tumor, fat, nerve, cerebrospinal fluid, meninges, and brain allows for better assessment of perineural spread. The criteria of nerve involvement on MRI include replacement of normal perineural fat with tumor, enhancement with gadolinium (regardless of size), and increased size of the nerve in question (regardless of enhancement). Using these criteria, MRI is more sensitive and specific in evaluating perineural spread than CT.[58] MRI also is superior to CT in evaluating intracranial extension of tumor, especially in delineating the relationship of tumor to the cavernous carotid artery and the brain parenchyma (Fig. 69-11).

Although parapharyngeal space masses are well visualized by both techniques, they are better delineated with MRI than CT (Fig. 69-12). This is because of the different signal intensity of tumor, fat, and muscle on MRI. Most salivary tumors have low-to-intermediate T1 signal intensities and intermediate-to-high T2 signal intensities. The differential diagnosis of parapharyngeal masses include deep lobe par-

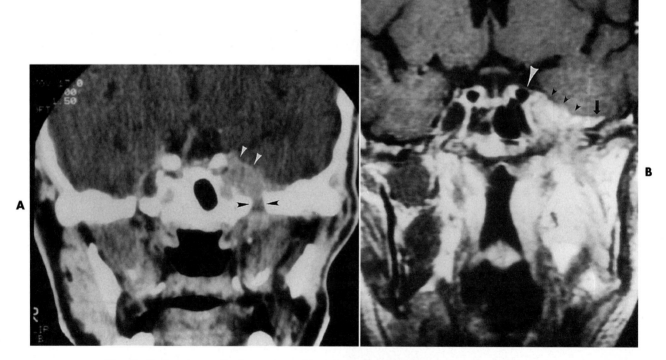

Fig. 69-10. Imaging studies in a patient with perineural spread of adenoid cystic carcinoma along the third division of the trigeminal nerve (V3), involving the cavernous sinus and the dura of the middle cranial fossa. **A,** A coronal computed tomography with intravenous contrast showing widening of the left foramen ovale (*black arrowheads*) compared with the one on the right. There also is enhancement and thickening along the left Meckel's cave (*white arrowheads*). **B,** A coronary T1-weighted magnetic resonance imaging scan with gadolinium showing marked thickening and enhancement of V3, trigeminal ganglion, and the lateral cavernous sinus (*black arrowheads*). The tumor abuts the cavernous carotid artery (*white arrowhead*). There is enhancement of the dura along the floor of the middle cranial fossa (dural tail) (*black arrow*). This usually is a sign of dural involvement.

otid tumors, minor salivary gland tumors, and neurogenic and vascular tumors. Deep lobe parotid tumors and minor salivary gland tumors of the parapharyngeal space lie in the prestyloid compartment, anterior to the carotid artery, and displace the parapharyngeal fat medially (see Fig. 69-12). Deep lobe tumors are connected to the parotid gland in at least one imaging section. Minor salivary gland tumors are completely surrounded by fat.[60] By contrast, neurogenic tumors and glomus tumors lie in the poststyloid compartment, posterior to the carotid artery, which is displaced anteriorly. Neurogenic tumors usually enhance intensely with gadolinium, whereas glomus tumors have a characteristic serpiginous flow void (salt and pepper appearance) on MRI.

Other imaging studies

Ultrasonography. Ultrasonography has the advantage of being inexpensive, noninvasive, simple to perform, and virtually free of complications. It can be used to differentiate solid from cystic masses in the salivary glands. Its use is limited by its ability to visualize only relatively superficial

masses.[60] It has been supplanted by CT and MRI in the evaluation of salivary gland tumors.

Color Doppler sonography. Color duplex scanning is a noninvasive procedure that may be helpful in the preoperative assessment of salivary gland tumors.[4] Color Doppler sonography has been recently used to evaluate the vascular anatomy of the salivary glands. It can distinguish between the physiologic changes that occur during salivary stimulation in healthy subjects and the flow alterations that occur in diseased glands. Specific patterns of peak systolic vascular shifts were described in various abnormal processes, including Sjögren's syndrome, pleomorphic adenoma, and malignant tumors.[92]

Positron emission tomography. A recent study evaluated the ability of positron emission tomography (PET) to differentiate benign from malignant lesions of the salivary glands before surgery.[75] Salivary gland masses were evaluated in 26 patients using PET scans after the administration of fluorine-18 fluorodeoxyglucose (FDG). PET findings helped correctly differentiate benign from malignant masses

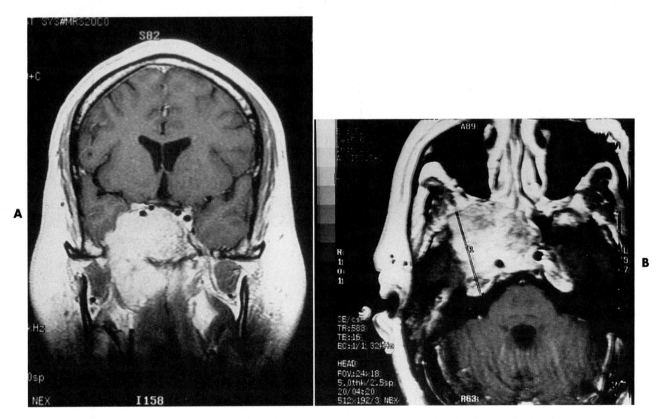

Fig. 69-11. A 47-year-old patient who presented with headache and diplopia. On examination, he was found to have a right abducent palsy, and a polypoid mass in the right fossa of Rusenmuller. The biopsy showed adenoid cystic carcinoma. **A,** Coronal and **B,** axial T1-weighted magnetic resonance imaging scan showing the origin of the mass in the right nasopharynx, with extension in the infratemporal and pterygopalatine fossae. There is destruction of the skull base with intracranial extension elevating the temporal lobe. There is evidence of involvement of the cavernous carotid artery bilaterally. Surgical resection was done through a temporal–infratemporal fossa combined approach with gross total removal of tumor. The patient received 70 cGy of radiation postoperatively. At a 3-year follow-up, there is no progression of residual disease.

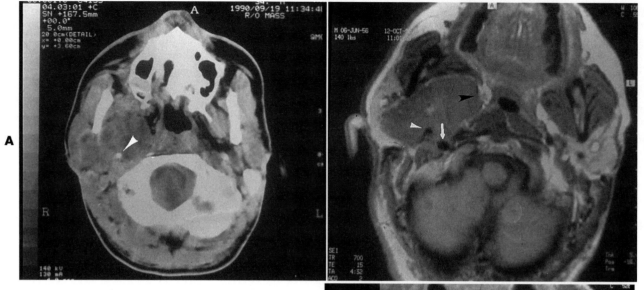

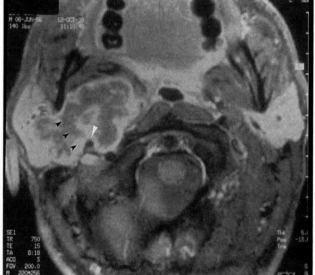

Fig. 69-12. Large pleomorphic adenoma of the parotid gland. **A,** Axial computed tomography with contrast, and **B,** T1-weighted without and **C,** with gadolinium. The tumor involves the superficial and deep lobe of the parotid gland and lies anterior to the styloid process (prestyloid) (*white arrowhead* in **A, B,** and **C**). The fat of the parapharyngeal space is displaced medially (*black arrowhead* in **B**), and the carotid artery displaced posteriorly (*white arrow* in **B**). The isthmus of tumor between the superficial and deep components passes through the stylomandibular space, and therefore, is relatively narrow giving the appearance of a "dumbbell" (*black arrowheads* in **C**).

in 69% of patients, but false-positive results for malignancy occurred in 31% of patients. The investigators concluded that FDG PET is not useful in classifying salivary gland tumors as benign or malignant.[75]

Benign Tumors

ADENOMAS

Pleomorphic Adenomas

Pleomorphic adenomas (benign mixed tumors) are the most common tumors of the salivary gland. The majority originate in the parotid gland (Fig. 69-13). The term *pleomorphic* was chosen to describe the these tumors because they contain epithelial and connective tissue elements. Although the histogenesis of this type of tumor has been de-

bated, the current theory is that pleomorphic adenomas originate from intercalated and myoepithelial cells.

Pleomorphic adenomas are painless, slow growing, and usually found as incidental masses in the cheek or near the angle of the mandible. About 90% of these tumors originate superficial to the plane of the facial nerve. The 10% that originate in the deep lobe may extend through the space between the angle of the mandible and the styloid process and present as a parapharyngeal space mass. They also may present with intraoral swelling and medial displacement of the tonsil and lateral pharyngeal wall.

Pleomorphic adenomas of the submandibular and minor salivary glands also present as swelling in those glands. When they originate in the minor salivary glands, they mostly occur in the hard and soft palate. The second-most common place of origin is the upper lip. Unlike most mixed

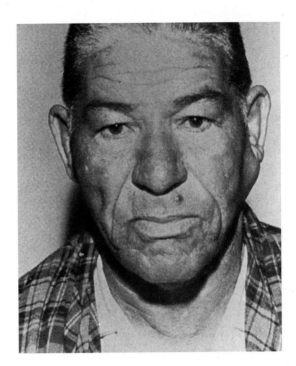

Fig. 69-13. A 60-year-old man with pleomorphic adenoma of the parotid gland.

tumors, those in the palate and lip frequently lack a capsule. Commonly, pleomorphic adenomas of the parapharyngeal space present as asymptomatic masses. Although the parapharyngeal space contains the great vessels and cranial nerves (CN) IX to XII, involvement of these structures is rare. Most of the tumors represent medial extension from a tumor of the deep lobe of the parotid gland but they also may originate from the minor salivary gland tissue that naturally occurs in the parapharyngeal space.

On gross pathologic examination, pleomorphic adenomas are solitary, firm, round tumors with a thin, delicate, incomplete capsule (Fig. 69-14). The cut surface is characteristically solid and is either hard, rubbery, or soft in consistency. The color varies from whitish gray to pale yellow. Microscopically, the tumors have islands of stellate and spindle cells that are interspersed with a mixoid background. Glandular areas of tubular epithelium also have been reported. Commonly, microscopic extensions of tumor extend through the capsule. Variations of this tumor type are common and may include squamous metaplasia, calcification, cartilage-appearing tissue, oxyphilic cells, and a palisading appearance of the underlying stroma. Malignant transformation of pleomorphic adenomas is rare and occurs most frequently in patients with long-standing tumors. Case reports of clinically metastatic disease with histologically benign tumors also have been reported.

Pleomorphic adenoma should not recur after adequate surgical excision. Most recurrences may be traced to enucleation of the mass with no appreciation of the pseudopod-

like extensions of tumor. Although it appears encapsulated, if a surrounding cuff of normal tissue is not removed along with the tumor, the risk of recurrence is high. Recurrences frequently occur in multiple sites. Consequently, the treatment of choice for patients with pleomorphic adenomas of the parotid gland, submandibular gland, or minor salivary gland is excision of tumor with a surrounding cuff of normal tissue.

In patients with tumors of the parotid gland, treatment usually is removal of the tumor with an adequate margin and facial nerve preservation. Because most of the tumors originate in the superficial lobe, superficial parotidectomy often is required. Large pleomorphic adenomas may be intimately related to the facial nerve, and unless the tumor is dissected meticulously, damage to the facial nerve may occur.

Recurrent pleomorphic adenomas may present a more complex problem. There frequently are multiple foci of recurrence, and they may continue to manifest over several years. Provided that a recurrence is nonprogressive and asymptomatic, it may be prudent to observe stable recurrent disease for some time. During this observation time, other recurrences may manifest, and in such cases, multiple surgeries may be avoided. Another reason for observing patients with small asymptomatic recurrent pleomorphic adenomas is the increased risk to the facial nerve during revision surgery. The scarring and altered anatomy puts the nerve at greater risk for surgical injury during the dissection. Under such circumstances, facial nerve monitoring during surgery may be helpful in reducing the risk of damage to the facial nerve.

Radiotherapy may be considered in the treatment of recurrent pleomorphic adenoma when surgery is no longer a feasible option.

Monomorphic adenomas

Monomorphic adenomas are benign tumors of the salivary glands that also originate from ductal epithelium. These tumors usually occur in the parotid gland and in the minor salivary glands of the upper lip. They also have been described in other areas wherein minor salivary glands are found, like the hard and soft palate and buccal mucosa; these tumors represent 1% to 3% of all salivary gland neoplasms.[9] There is no gender predilection, and the average age of patients is more than 60 years. As with most benign tumors, monomorphic adenomas classically appear as asymptomatic, slow-growing masses. Facial nerve involvement is rare. Histologically, these tumors are distinguished from pleomorphic adenomas by their absence of chondromyxoid stroma and the presence of a uniform epithelial pattern.

Basal cell adenomas

Basal cell adenomas are the predominant tissue type of monomorphic adenomas. Most of these tumors also occur in the parotid gland or in the minor salivary glands of the

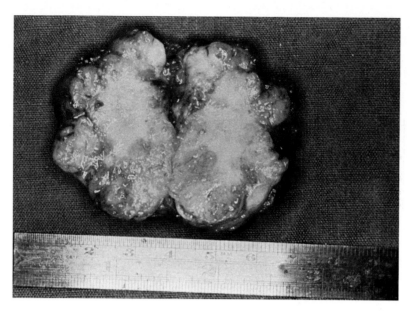

Fig. 69-14. Gross section of pleomorphic adenoma.

upper lip. The tumors are solid and well circumscribed. The cut surface is gray-white, gray-red, or pink-brown. Tumors originating in the parotid gland usually have a capsule, whereas those originating in the lip do not. Histologically, a solid growth pattern is more common in parotid tumors, consisting of isomorphic cells with dark nuclei and rare mitoses. The epithelium is demarcated from surrounding stroma by a row of peripheral cells that show prominent nuclear palisading. This effect is a result of the presence of an intact basement membrane and helps to differentiate this tumor from a pleomorphic adenoma. Adenomas originating in the upper lip usually have a tubular or canalicular pattern.

Clinically, basal cell adenomas may be confused with enlarged lymph nodes, sebaceous cysts, mucoceles, lipomas, nasolabial cysts, or pleomorphic adenomas. On FNAB, they may be confused with the solid variety of adenoid cystic carcinoma.[138] Cytologic features of the cell–stroma interface are useful to distinguish between monomorphic adenomas of the basal cell type and adenoid cystic carcinoma. In patients with basal cell adenomas, the collagenous stroma interdigitates with adjacent cells, whereas in those with adenoid cystic carcinoma, the two are separated by a sharp smooth border. Further, the stroma of basal cell adenomas may contain rare spindle cells or capillaries, but the cylinders of adenoid cystic carcinoma are acellular. On histopathologic examination, distinction between these two tumor types usually is evident, although basal cell adenomas are not always encapsulated. Instead of invading surrounding tissue, they usually show a pattern of circumscription. The stroma also is more vascular. Because basal cell adenomas are benign, treatment is excision with a cuff of normal surrounding tissue.

Clear cell adenomas

Clear cell adenomas also have a propensity to occur in the parotid gland. They are slow growing, asymptomatic, solid, and well circumscribed. Their cut surface is gray-white or yellow. Histologically, these tumors are made up of two uniform cell types: a dark eosinophilic layer representing the epithelium of the intercalated duct, and an outer layer of clear cells that are glycogen-rich. These tumors should be differentiated from acinic cell carcinomas and mucoepidermoid carcinomas. Both of these malignancies may have large numbers of relatively benign-appearing clear cells, although they lack the orderly cytoplasmic architecture and the abundance of glycogen. Reports have been conflicting as to the behavior of clear cell adenomas. Because of the accounts of isolated infiltration, recurrence, and possible metastases, some regard these tumors as low-grade carcinomas. Treatment is surgical excision.

Sebaceous lymphadenomas

Sebaceous lymphadenomas are rare benign tumors of the salivary glands. They are found in normal sebaceous glands that originate from the blind ends of intralobular ducts in otherwise normal salivary glands. Rarely, a sebaceous lymphadenoma originates from minor salivary gland tissue. No cases of malignant counterparts have been reported. These tumors are slow growing, asymptomatic, and usually occur in the parotid gland. Ectopic sebaceous glands in the lips and oropharynx are thought to be present in about 80%

of the population. They usually are found in middle-aged and elderly people. Microscopically, these tumors are composed of cysts lined with squamous epithelium and sebaceous cells. The surrounding lymphoid stroma may contain germinal centers. Surgical excision is the treatment of choice.

Warthin's tumor

Warthin's tumor also is known as *papillary cystadenoma lymphomatosum* or *adenolymphoma*. This type of tumor occurs almost exclusively in the parotid gland and accounts for 10% to 15% of all parotid tumors. After pleomorphic adenoma, it is the second-most common benign salivary tumor. Warthin's tumor is unique in several ways. It contains lymphoid tissue, has a striking male predominance, is bilateral in 10% of patients, commonly has unilateral multifocal involvement, and is rare in blacks.

Although patients with Warthin's tumor typically are asymptomatic, a few patients will present with swelling, pain, and other inflammatory changes. These changes may be a result of reactive changes in the associated rich lymphoid stroma. A Warthin's tumor commonly is found in the superficial lobe of the parotid gland near the angle of the mandible. This type of tumor also has been reported to be found in the parapharyngeal space and less commonly in the submandibular gland and the minor salivary glands of the lower lip and palate.

Embryologically, the parotid gland is the first salivary gland to develop and the last to become encapsulated. One hypothesis concerning the histogenesis of Warthin's tumor is the incorporation of salivary ducts and lymphatic tissue during this late encapsulation. The identification of normal nodal structures, such as subcapsular sinuses, and the occurrence of these tumors in lymph nodes outside the parotid gland support this hypothesis. Further support is derived from T- and B-cell markers that represent normal lymph nodes that have been identified in Warthin's tumors.

On gross pathologic examination, Warthin's tumors are encapsulated with a smooth or lobulated surface. Papillary cysts are commonly found on sectioning and may contain mucoid brown fluid. Solid gray tissue encapsulates white nodules of lymphoid tissue. Lymph node architecture may be distorted by epithelial components compressing the lymphatic sinuses. Electron microscopy shows a tremendous number of mitochondria in the epithelial cells, which are responsible for its granular eosinophilic appearance. Mitochondria-rich oncocytes are found in Warthin's tumors and oncocytomas—the only other tumor type with frequent bilateral presentation. Oncocytes selectively incorporate technetium Tc 99m and appear as hot spots on a radionucleotide scan. Most other neoplasms show either normal uptake or appear as cold nodules. The treatment is surgical excision, usually a parotidectomy with preservation of the facial nerve. Inadequate excision or tumor multicentricity may explain tumor recurrence.

Oncocytomas

Oncocytomas or oncocytic adenomas account for less than 1% of all salivary gland tumors. They usually are benign and originate from oncocytes. These cells are epithelial in origin and may be found individually or in groups in otherwise normal major or minor salivary glands. They also are found in the pancreas; respiratory tract; thyroid, parathyroid, pituitary, and adrenal glands; and the kidney, although the majority of tumors occur in the superficial lobe of the parotid gland. Most patients with oncocytomas are 55 to 70 years of age at diagnosis. The gender distribution is almost equal. These tumors are painless, slow growing, and show a predilection for technetium Tc 99m and appear as hot spots on radionucleotide scan.

On gross pathologic examination, oncocytomas of the major salivary glands are well circumscribed and encapsulated. Those originating from minor salivary glands have less well-defined borders and are not encapsulated. The surface is pink-to-rust in color. Microscopically, the tumor has a granular appearance as a result of abundant mitochondria. The concentration of mitochondria differentiates oncocytomas from other tumors. A true oncocytoma contains no lymphoid tissue. The extensive lymphoid component that is typical of a Warthin's tumor never is encountered. Histologically, these tumors should be differentiated from other salivary gland neoplasms that have an oncocytic component, including adenoid cystic carcinoma, pleomorphic adenoma, mucoepidermoid carcinoma, and adenocarcinoma. Metastatic thyroid carcinoma or renal cell carcinoma with a large number of oncocytes should be differentiated from oncocytomas.

Oncocytomas originating from minor salivary glands tend to grow in an irregular and locally invasive pattern. They are less predictable than those originating in the parotid glands. Those originating from minor salivary glands in the respiratory tract may invade surrounding cartilage or bone. Although histologically benign, they have a destructive potential. Rarely do they demonstrate histologic criteria for malignancy, and their treatment requires surgical excision.

Oncocytic papillary cystadenoma

Oncocytic papillary cystadenoma is an uncommon tumor type originating in the parotid gland. Most of these tumors have originated in the larynx, although they also have been noted in the nasopharynx, palate, buccal mucosa, and the accessory tear ducts. These tumors have no gender predilection and usually are found in those aged 50 years or more. Patients usually present with a painless mass. Those with laryngeal lesions may present with hoarseness or coughing. The minor salivary glands of the false cords and ventricles are common sites of presentation, but this tumor type also may originate from any site in the laryngeal mucosa. Although they are usually solitary tumors, there have been reports of multiple tumors.

On gross pathologic examination oncocytic papillary cytadenoma are smooth and round cysts that may be pedunculated. Microscopically, these tumors look like a Warthin's tumor, although the lymphoid stroma is absent. Whether these are true tumors has been debated. They may reflect metaplasia or hyperplasia of preexisting salivary gland ducts, but nonetheless, they are treated with surgical excision.

Myoepithelioma

Myoepithelioma originates from myoepithelial cells that lie beneath the ductal and acinar epithelium in the salivary glands. These cells also have been identified in sweat glands and mammary glands. They have the ability to contract, and their pumping action helps to express secretions from the salivary glands. Myoepitheliomas are well demarcated, and the external surface is smooth. The cut surface is homogenous and white. Microscopically, these tumors have a thin capsule, except when they occur in the palate, wherein they lack encapsulation. The cells are benign-appearing and spindle- or polygonal-shaped, and mitoses are rare. Clinically, these tumors are difficult to distinguish from pleomorphic adenomas. They are painless, slow-growing masses. There is no gender predilection, and they occur in the major and minor salivary glands. Histologically, they should be differentiated from plasmacytomas and any tumors with spindle cells, including neurilemoma, fibroma, meningioma, and leiomyoma. The majority of these tumors behave in a benign manner, although there have been reports of local aggressiveness. They are treated by surgical excision.

Sialoadenoma papilliferum

Sialoadenoma papilliferum is a rare, benign salivary gland tumor that gets its name from the skin tumor *syringocystadenoma papilliferum*, which it resembles on gross pathologic and microscopic examination. This tumor is painless and exhibits slow-to-moderate growth. It originates in the major and minor salivary glands, most commonly in men aged about 60 years. Microscopically, the tumor originates from the superficial extralobular salivary gland ducts. The cell of origin is thought to be the pluripotential myoepithelial cell.

Clinically, the differential diagnosis includes other papillary lesions like a squamous papilloma, verrucous hyperplasia, or carcinoma. It usually can be distinguished from other intraoral minor salivary gland tumors because it is exophytic and not a smooth, mucosa-covered mass. They are treated with surgical excision.

Inverted ductal papilloma

Inverted ductal papilloma is an inverted papilloma that originates from the excretory ducts of the minor salivary glands. This tumor is a different entity from the inverted oral papilloma, which is endophytic and does not bear any clinical resemblance to inverted ductal papilloma. The few cases that have been reported occur equally in men and women. The lesions are raised but not ulcerated. The preoperative differential diagnosis includes a salivary gland tumor, fibroma, and lipoma. Treatment should be conservative, but excision should be complete.

Hemangiomas

Hemangiomas are the most common salivary gland tumors found in children and usually involve the parotid gland. Less often, they are found in the submandibular gland or surrounding tissues. Considerable confusion about the terminology of vascular lesions existed until Mulliken[94] offered a classification that is rational, simple, and based on clinical and biologic behavior. He divided congenital vascular lesions into two groups: hemangiomas and vascular malformations. Hemangiomas usually are seen in infants. They may be present at birth but commonly appear several days to weeks later. A rapid growth phase occurs around the age of 1 to 6 months, followed by gradual involution over 1 to 12 years. During the growth phase, endothelial cells proliferate rapidly and become flat during involution.

Hemangiomas of the parotid area more often are seen in female patients and usually are asymptomatic, unilateral, and compressible masses. The overlying skin may be normal or may be involved. It is not uncommon to see other skin lesions present (Fig. 69-15). On gross pathologic examination, this tumor is dark red, lobulated, and nonencapsulated. Microscopically, these tumors are comprised of capillaries lined by proliferative endothelial cells. Blood vessels are uniform in size. Mitoses occur frequently but are not indicators of behavior.

Hemangiomas may become extremely large with complications such as bleeding, heart failure, and even death (Fig. 69-16). Treatment initially should consist of steroids administered 2 to 4 mg/kg per day. If the hemangioma is responsive to steroids, the result usually is immediate and often dramatic. Unfortunately, the response rate to steroids is only 40% to 60%. In such patients, interferon may be helpful, but it should be reserved for life-threatening situations because of its toxicity and the necessity to continue the drug for prolonged periods. Surgical excision or various types of laser treatments may be performed for select circumstances.[151] Hemangiomas usually involute completely, but they may take years and may result in medical or psychologic problems for children.

Tumor-Like Conditions

Certain conditions affect the salivary glands and may be difficult to differentiate from benign and malignant neoplasms. It is important to understand these tumor-like conditions and be able to differentiate them from tumors of the salivary glands. The following should be considered in the differential diagnosis of salivary gland abnormalities.

NECROTIZING SIALOMETAPLASIA

Necrotizing sialometaplasia is not a tumor, but it may be mistaken for one because it usually presents as a single

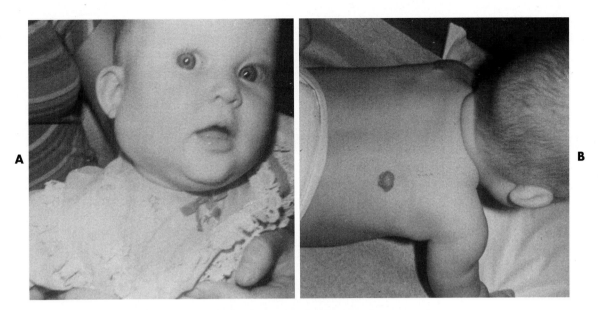

Fig. 69-15. An infant with hemangioma of, **A,** parotid gland and **B,** skin.

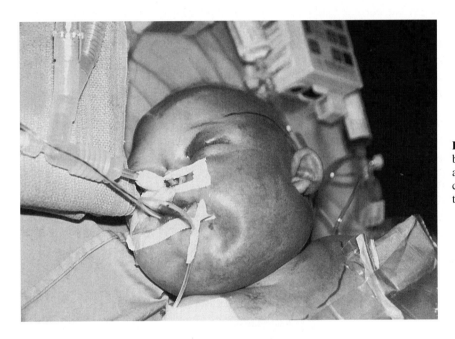

Fig. 69-16. Three-month-old child with Kasabach-Merritt syndrome who had massive hemangioma of the entire face, neck, and upper chest. The child also had lesions throughout the intestine and died of this disease.

unilateral, painless, or slightly painful ulcer on the hard palate. It normally involves the mucoserous glands of the hard palate and is a benign self-healing lesion of the salivary glands. First described by Abrams[2] in 1973, it usually is seen in patients aged more than 40 years and is two to three times more common in men than women. Clinically, the ulcer usually is round, sharply circumscribed with an erythematous halo and usually is between 1 to 3 cm in diameter. In a few cases, necrotizing sialometaplasia presented as a nonulcerated swelling with the clinical appearance of an infectious process.[118] It frequently is misdiagnosed as squa-

mous cell carcinoma or mucoepidermoid carcinoma, although microscopically, necrotizing sialometaplasia has several characteristics[108]:

1. Lobular infarction with or without extravasation of mucous;
2. Pseudoepitheliomatous hyperplasia at the periphery of the ulcer;
3. Squamous metaplasia of ducts and acini;
4. Inflammation as a result of extravasated mucous; and
5. Preservation of lobular architecture

The cause of necrotizing sialometaplasia is unknown, although its histology and clinical course suggest that it may represent a reparative process that occurs in response to ischemic necrosis of salivary gland tissue.[103] A biopsy is necessary to confirm this lesion. Necrotizing sialometaplasia undergoes spontaneous, albeit slow, healing over a period of 6 to 10 weeks. After it heals, recurrence is uncommon.

BENIGN LYMPHOEPITHELIAL LESIONS

In 1952, Godwin proposed the term *benign lymphoepithelial lesion* (BLL) to cover a group of diseases such as Mikulicz's disease, sicca complex, Sjögren's syndrome, and chronic punctate sialadenitis.[53] This term stresses the benign nature and the histologic features of this type of lesion. The etiology is unknown, but it is thought to be reactive rather than neoplastic. The histologic pattern may be confused with malignant lymphoma, metastatic carcinoma, chronic sialoadenitis, or sarcoidosis.

BLLs usually present in women aged 40 to 59 years, but they may be seen in children and in adults of either gender. BLLs usually present as unilateral, bilateral, or even successive enlargements of the salivary or lacrimal glands. They usually are asymptomatic but may present with mild pain. The glands usually are diffusely enlarged but may have circumscribed discrete nodules. On gross pathologic examination, the capsule and overall architecture of the glands remain intact. The cut surface usually is smooth, rubbery, homogeneous, and pink, tan, or white. Sialograms characteristically show sialectasia, which may be punctate, globular, or cavitary. Patients with BLL may develop malignant lymphoma or anaplastic carcinomas.* For some unknown reason, anaplastic carcinomas are seen more commonly in Eskimos who have BLL.[7,150] Treatment of BLL is primarily symptomatic, unless there is a suspicion of lymphoma or anaplastic carcinoma, and if found, these should be treated as such. BLL in children may resolve spontaneously around the age of puberty.[108] BLL occurs in several clinical syndrome settings.

Mikulicz's disease

The term *Mikulicz's disease* has been used for many years to describe patients who have asymptomatic enlargement of the salivary or lacrimal glands without an underlying or associated local disease.[72]

Sjögren's syndrome

Sjögren's syndrome is considered a chronic autoimmune disease and is characterized by a triad consisting of keratojunctivitis sicca, xerostomia, and a collagen vascular disease, usually rheumatoid arthritis. In the absence of a connective tissue disease, the term *sicca complex* has been used. Sjögren's syndrome is seen primarily in women aged about 50 years, and it rarely occurs in children. Salivary

gland enlargement is seen in only 50% of the patients.[142,143] The enlargement is more commonly diffuse rather than nodular (Fig. 69-17). Xerostomia usually is caused more by the involvement of minor rather than major salivary glands. Because the minor salivary glands usually are involved, a diagnosis may be made by performing a biopsy on the minor salivary glands on the inner aspect of the lip.[149]

Histologically, myoepithelial cells are integral components of this lesion type. Periductal inflammation and progressive atrophy of acinar parenchyma accompany replacement by increased amounts of inflammatory tissue. As the ductal lumens disappear, the myoepithelial component becomes more prominent. The association of Sjögren's syndrome with lymphomas of the parotid gland will be discussed in the section on malignant neoplasms.

Sialoadenosis

Sialoadenosis is a noninflammatory, non-neoplastic enlargement of salivary glands. Its etiology is unknown, but it is believed to be associated primarily with malnutrition. It also is referred to as *sialosis* or *nutritional mumps*.[45,123] The parotid glands usually are affected, and the enlargement is gradual and asymptomatic. This enlargement usually is bilateral but not necessarily symmetric. A number of conditions have been associated with sialoadenosis, primarily those that contribute to poor nutritional status. These conditions include alcoholism, malnutrition, diabetes, or kwashiorkor.[22,62] Alcoholism, with or without cirrhosis, and malnutrition are the most common conditions associated with sialoadenosis.

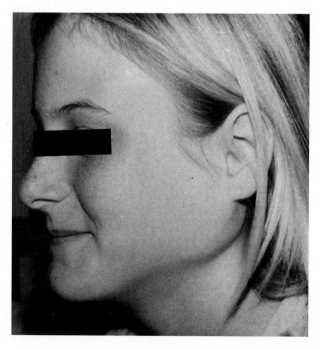

Fig. 69-17. A 14-year-old girl with sarcoidosis.

---

* Refs. 7, 12, 53, 54, 108, 150.

Histologically, the glands show acinar cells hypertrophy, fatty infiltration, or a combination of the two. There rarely is a chronic inflammatory infiltrate. There may be mild-to-moderate fibrosis of the interlobularly septae. The salivary gland function usually is normal, although the amylase level in the saliva may be increased.[24,91] Treatment is rarely necessary, except for managing the malnutrition. As the nutritional status improves, the enlargement of the gland usually decreases. Sialadenosis may be confused with a tumor, but a careful history frequently is all that is necessary to diagnose it. Biopsy may be diagnostic.

TRUE CYSTS OF MAJOR SALIVARY GLANDS

A pseudocyst is the result of extravasation of mucin into a gland. A true cyst may be distinguished from a pseudocyst by the presence of an epithelial lining. Neoplasms, especially Warthin's tumors, also may be cystic. True cysts involving the major salivary glands, originate primarily in the parotid gland.[11,157] There are two categories: congenital and acquired.

Congenital cysts

Congenital cysts also are known as *branchial cleft cysts* and *lymphoepithelial cysts*. They usually are present at birth, but they may not become obvious until adulthood.[50,128,154,159,160] They present as painless, unilateral swelling and may become infected and cause pain related to the infection. There are two types of congenital cysts. The first type usually is just adjacent to the ear, either medial, inferior, or posterior. The second type usually is more intimately associated with the substance of the parotid gland. Sinuses and fistulas may be present and may extend to the external auditory canal or to the skin surface.[99,158] Histologically, they are filled with a fluid and have a lining of squamous epithelium or ciliated columnar epithelium. The wall may contain lymphoid tissue and even skin appendages or cartilage. The cysts may be confused with benign tumors. They are treated with surgical excision that should include the sinus and fistula tract. Recurrence is almost certain if the cyst is not removed completely.

Acquired cysts

These cysts usually originate in the major salivary glands and are a result of obstruction. They may occur from trauma to the salivary gland, although trauma usually results in a pseudocyst.[106] They also are known as retention cysts, and when they are associated with sublingual ducts, they form ranulas. Ranulas occur in the floor of mouth and commonly "plunge" into the submandibular triangle and may be extensive. They should be excised completely to avoid recurrence.

Microscopically, the cyst lining consists of a layer of cuboidal or columnar or squamous epithelium. Lymphoid tissue is not present in the acquired cysts. These cysts also may be confused with benign neoplasms. Complete excision is required for treatment.

VASCULAR MALFORMATIONS

Vascular malformations are different from hemangiomas of the parotid gland. These vascular malformations are not true neoplasms and are divided into different categories, which will be discussed briefly.

Venous malformations

Venous malformations usually are noted at the time of birth and continue to grow as the patient ages. They may become extremely large by the time the child is fully grown. Unlike hemangiomas, which grow by cellular proliferation, enlargement of venous malformations is primarily a result of dilation of the existing vessels and does not represent cellular division. These may or may not need treatment, depending on the size and complications. These malformations can be seen involving the parotid gland (Fig. 69-18) and may be difficult to remove. If the venous malformations are small, they may be surgically removed with or without removing the adjacent salivary glands. An MRI scan is the best imaging modality to determine the extent of disease. Arteriograms are not helpful.

Arteriovenous malformations

Arteriovenous malformations differ from arteriovenous fistulas as the malformations are congenital (but may not manifest for several years), whereas the fistulas are acquired, usually as a result of trauma. Arteriovenous malformations involve shunting of blood from the arterial vessels directly into the venous system, causing major enlargement of the vascular lesion. Generally, these malformations should be removed completely to stop their progress. They may involve the parotid gland and may appear as a parotid mass. An arteriogram is essential to diagnose the presence and extent of the malformation, and surgical resection is the best treatment.

Lymphatic malformations

Lymphatic malformations usually are present at birth and gradually grow. They may involve the salivary glands, causing enlargement. In some patients, the lymphatic aggregates may be nodular, simulating a mass. They usually are diffuse and infiltrate locally in the tissue planes of the adjacent structures. These malformations are treated by surgical resection, which may be tedious.

HUMAN IMMUNODEFICIENCY VIRUS INVOLVEMENT

The parotid gland may enlarge in patients with the human immunodeficiency virus (HIV). Multiple lymphoepithelial cysts may be seen in the parotid gland in these patients. MRI scans can be diagnostic when multiple cysts are noted in the

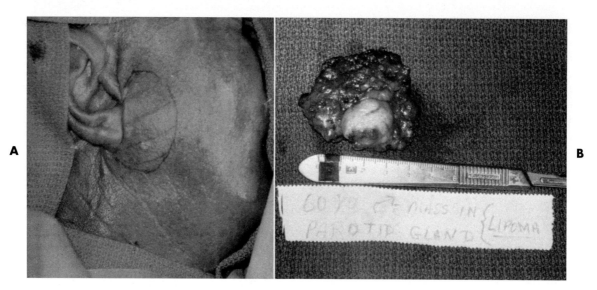

Fig. 69-18. A, A 61-year-old man with a lipoma in the parotid gland; **B,** lipoma in the superficial lobe of the parotid.

parotid gland.[115,68] Surgery is not indicated unless there is suspicion of malignancy.

PRINCIPLES OF MANAGEMENT OF BENIGN NEOPLASM

Management of benign salivary gland tumors has not changed dramatically for years. Benign salivary gland tumors should be excised completely with an adequate margin to avoid local recurrences. Generally, tumors in the parotid gland are removed with an adequate cuff of surrounding normal tissue, and the facial nerve is dissected and carefully preserved. The extent of dissection of the facial nerve and the amount of parotid tissue resection depend on the size, location, and histology of the tumor.

Small adenomas located in the tail of the parotid gland may require only dissection of the lower division of the facial nerve with removal of the tumor and the surrounding parotid tissue, avoiding unnecessary dissection of the upper division. Larger tumors of the superficial lobe usually require a complete superficial parotidectomy. Deep lobe tumors require a total parotidectomy, with facial nerve preservation. Parapharyngeal tumors are excised through a cervical–parotid approach (*vide infra*).

A tumor of the submandibular gland requires submandibular gland resection. If the tumor originates from a minor salivary gland, the tumor and a cuff of normal tissue should be excised. Simple enucleation should be discouraged because of the increased risk of recurrence. Pediatric hemangiomas will involute but may be resected in special cases. Vascular malformations of salivary glands in the elderly population may be excised or managed with lasers. Lymphangiomas may require surgical excision.

Malignant Neoplasms
PATHOLOGY

Adenoid cystic carcinoma

Understanding the pathology and biologic features of adenoid cystic carcinoma has evolved over many decades, mainly as a result of its highly variable natural history and relatively infrequent occurrence. It took almost 100 years to fully appreciate the capricious nature of adenoid cystic carcinoma (ACC). In 1854, Lorain and Robin described an "unusual sinus tumor" that may have been the first description of ACC in the literature.[89] In 1856, Billroth coined the term *Cylindroma* to describe the pathologic features of this rare salivary gland tumor,[21] but it was not until 1942 that the malignant nature of this disease was identified when Dockery and Mayo described it as *Adenocarcinoma, cylindroma type.*[38] In 1953, Foote and Frazell coined the term *adenoid cystic carcinoma,* which best describes the histologic characteristics of this type of tumor.[48]

Adenoid cystic carcinoma constitutes 10% of all salivary neoplasms. It is the second-most common malignant tumor of the salivary glands; mucoepidermoid carcinoma is the most common. ACC is the most common malignant tumor found in the submandibular, sublingual, and minor salivary glands.[134] It is slightly more common in female patients, and approximately 90% of patients are aged 30 to 70 years with a peak incidence in those aged 40 to 59 years. In a review of 242 cases, Spiro, Huvos, and Strong[134] found that more than two thirds of ACCs occurred in the minor salivary glands (Fig. 69-19). The incidence of ACC relative to other salivary neoplasms varies by site of origin (Table 69-3). The

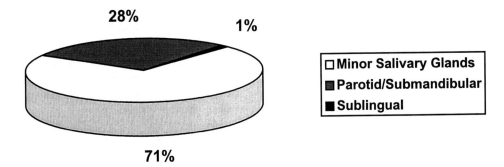

28%

1%

☐ **Minor Salivary Glands**
■ **Parotid/Submandibular**
■ **Sublingual**

71%

Fig. 69-19. Distribution of adenoid cystic carcinoma among minor and major salivary glands.

Table 69-3. The incidence of adenoid cystic carcinoma relative to other salivary neoplasms according to site

Salivary neoplasms	Total	ACC	%
Parotid gland	1674	35	2
Submandibular gland	239	33	14
Minor salivary glands	564	174	31
Total	2477	242	10

Spiro R, Huvos A, Strong E: Adenoid cystic carcinoma of salivary origin: a clinicopathologic study of 242 cases, *Am J Surg* 128:512, 1974.

Table 69-4. The distribution of adenoid cystic carcinoma by site in 242 cases

Site	Number of patients	Percent of total
Palate	64	26
Parotid	35	15
Submandibular	33	14
Antrum	30	12
Tongue	26	11
Nasal cavity	14	6
Cheek/lips	13	5
Gingiva	10	4
FOM/sublingual	9	4
Larynx	3	1
Pharynx	3	1
Tonsil	2	1
Total	242	100

Spiro R, Huvos A, Strong E: Adenoid cystic carcinoma of salivary origin: a clinicopathologic study of 242 cases, *Am J Surg* 128:512, 1974.

most common site of origin is the oral cavity (50%), followed by the sinonasal tract (18%; Table 69-4).

ACC is described in three histologic subtypes based on tumor architecture: cribriform, tubular, and solid. The cribriform pattern has the classic "Swiss cheese appearance," wherein the cells are arranged in nests separated by round or oval spaces. It is suggested that this characteristic stromal architecture of ACC, represented by stromal pseudocysts, results from their own secretion of basement membrane molecules and fibronectin.[31] The tubular (or trabecular) pattern has a more glandular architecture, whereas the solid (or basaloid) pattern shows sheets of cells with little or no luminal spaces. The tubular variety has the best prognosis; the solid variety has the worst, and the cribriform pattern has an intermediate prognosis. Eneroth, Hjertman, and Moberger[43] reported that the 5-year and 10-year survival rates for the solid variety are 17% and 0%, respectively. Conversely, patients with the cribriform pattern had 5-year and 10-year survival rates of 100% and 62%, respectively. Most ACCs usually exhibit a mixed architecture of more than one pattern, and their classification in such cases depends on the predominant histologic subtype. Using these criteria, Perzin, Gullane, and Clairmont[104] found that the cribriform pattern is the most common variety of ACC (Fig. 69-20).

Adenoid cystic carcinoma usually exhibits a protracted course characterized by an indolent growth pattern and a relentless tendency for local and perineural invasion. This neurotropic tendency is characteristic of ACC and has been

reported to occur in 20% to 80% of patients.[58] The description and reporting of perineural spread in ACCs depends largely on the diligence of histopathologic examination of tumor specimens, which explains, at least in part, the wide range in the incidence of perineural spread reported in the literature.

The pathogenesis of perineural involvement is poorly understood and was thought to be caused by spread of tumor through perineural lymphatics. According to this theory, spread occurs by emboli along the nerve lymphatics, and therefore skip lesions may occur with no direct continuity with the main tumor mass. If this mechanism was true, the achievement of negative surgical margins through *en bloc* resection of ACC would be not only impossible to guarantee but also meaningless. This notion of perineural lymphatic emboli was dispelled by well-executed studies, which showed that neural spread occurs by direct invasion of malignant cells through the path of least resistance either in the perineural or endoneural spaces (Fig. 69-21).[10,80] This theory assumes microscopic continuity of perineural tumor with the site of origin of the primary tumor and provides the

rence, distant metastasis, and shorter survival rate compared with low-grade MECs. Hickman, Cawson, and Duffy found that the overall 5- and 10-year survival rates for MEC are 71% and 50%, respectively.[64] Clode and others reported a 5-year cumulative survival rate of 70% for patients with low-grade MEC and 47% for those with high-grade MEC.[33]

Acinic cell carcinoma

Acinic cell carcinoma represents 3% of all salivary gland neoplasms. The majority of these tumors occur in the parotid gland (80% to 90%), wherein they constitute approximately 15% of its malignant neoplasms.[34,120] Although the mean age of presentation is 40 to 49 years, acinic cell carcinoma may occur at any age. Two thirds of cases occur in female patients.[34] Bilateral involvement occurs in 3% of patients, making acinic cell carcinoma the second-most common neoplasm, after Warthin's tumor, to exhibit bilateral presentation.[85]

On gross pathologic examination, acinic cell carcinoma appears fairly well circumscribed by a layer of surrounding dense fibrous tissue. Microscopic examination reveals nests of cells with basophilic cytoplasm and frequently an associated lymphoid infiltrate in the supporting stroma. Four histologic patterns are described: solid, microcystic, papillary-cystic, and follicular.[121,122] It is not uncommon for these patterns to coexist in the same tumor. Unlike ACC or MEC, these histologic patterns do not correlate with the biologic behavior or prognosis. Acinic cell carcinoma generally is regarded as a relatively low-grade malignancy. Compared with ACC or MECs, acinic cell carcinoma has a more favorable prognosis.[121,122] Although acinic cell carcinomas seldom metastasize, they have a high tendency to recur locally if they are incompletely excised. Adequate surgical resection results in cure rates at 5, 10, and 15 years of 76%, 63%, and 55%, respectively.[133] The 5-, 10-, and 15-year survival rates for acinic cell carcinoma are 78%, 63%, and 44%, respectively.[105]

Malignant mixed tumor

As their name implies, malignant mixed tumors represent a malignancy with epithelial and mesenchymal elements. They constitute 3% to 12% of salivary gland cancer, and about three fourths of them originate in the parotid gland. When they originate from a preexisting pleomorphic adenoma, they are called *carcinoma ex-pleomorphic adenoma.* The malignant components and metastasis of this variety are purely epithelial in origin. By contrast, *de novo* malignant mixed tumor is a true carcinosarcoma with malignant features of the epithelial and mesenchymal elements that are present in the primary tumor and its metastasis. The mesenchymal component shows mostly a chondrosarcomatous pattern. This rare true malignant mixed tumor is highly lethal, with a 5-year survival rate of 0%.[122]

Carcinoma ex-pleomorphic adenoma is the more common variety, and it occurs in 3% to 4% of all benign mixed

tumors. The risk of malignant transformation of a pleomorphic adenoma increases with the duration of disease. This risk within the first 5 years is 1.5%, but it increases to 9.5% after a pleomorphic adenoma has been present for more than 15 years.[121,122] Patients with malignant mixed tumors typically are 10 to 20 years older than those with benign mixed tumors. There also is an approximately 7% risk of associated carcinoma with recurrent pleomorphic adenoma. Findings suggesting malignant changes in a pleomorphic adenoma include microscopic foci of necrosis, hemorrhage, calcification, or excessive hyalinization.[121,122] The presence, absence, and degree of local invasion and the histologic differentiation allow the pathologist to distinguish between a noninvasive and an invasive variety of carcinoma in a pleomorphic adenoma. Noninvasive carcinoma consists of circumscribed malignant areas in a pleomorphic adenoma without infiltration of the surrounding tissue. Other terms used to describe this entity are *intracapsular carcinoma* or *carcinoma in situ.*[122] Complete surgical excision in such patients results in an excellent prognosis. The prognosis for invasive carcinoma depends on the degree of local infiltration. Patients with lesions with less than 8-mm invasion have a 5-year survival rate of 100%. By contrast, those with carcinomas that invade more than 8 mm have a 5-year survival rate of less than 50%.[121,122] Invasive malignant mixed tumors have a relatively high rate of regional (25%) and distant (33%) metastasis. This may account, at least in part, for their poor prognosis. Spiro reported 5-, 10-, and 15-year survival rates of 40%, 24%, and 19%, respectively.[131]

Epithelial–myoepithelial carcinoma

Epithelial–myoepithelial carcinomas comprise approximately 1% of all salivary gland neoplasms.[14] Histopathologically, they are characterized by a dual cell population of epithelial (ductal) cells and myoepithelial cells.[32,47] These cells vary in their dominance and phenotypic expression.[14] Like ACC, this type of tumor may exhibit a solid, tubular, or cribriform pattern. It most commonly involves the parotid gland and mainly affects patients aged 50 to 79 years. There is definite female preponderance.[47] The clinical course is characterized by a high incidence of local recurrence (50%) and not infrequent distant metastasis (25%). The rate of recurrence and the development of metastasis may be related to the presence of deoxyribonucleic acid (DNA) aneuploidy and a predominantly solid histologic pattern.[32,47] In a recent report by Fonseca and Soares on 22 cases of epithelial–myoepithelial carcinoma, 40% of patients died of their disease.[47]

Salivary duct carcinoma

Salivary duct carcinoma (SDC) is a high-grade aggressive malignancy of the major salivary glands. Initially named after its resemblance to intraductal carcinoma of the breast, this entity derives its histogenesis from the excretory duct reserve cells, which also are the source of origin of other biologically high-grade neoplasms. The prognosis of this disease is dismal, and therefore it is important for the pathologist to clearly make the distinction between this malignancy and more indolent neoplasms, such as terminal duct adenocarcinoma (polymorphous low-grade adenocarcinoma).[95]

The microscopic features of SDC are remarkably similar to those of mammary ductal carcinoma, raising the question of whether these tumors share antigenic or hormonal features. In a recent study by Lewis and others, such hormonal concordance was not found.[87] In their report of 26 patients with SDC of the major salivary glands treated at the Mayo Clinic from 1960 to 1989, 35% recurred locally, 62% showed distant metastasis, and 77% died of disease at a mean interval of 3 years after diagnosis.[87] A similarly dismal prognosis recently was reported for SDC of the minor salivary glands.[44]

Polymorphous low-grade adenocarcinoma

Polymorphous low-grade adenocarcinoma (PLGA), also known as *terminal duct* or *lobular carcinoma*, first was described in 1983.[17] Before that time, most of these neoplasms were diagnosed as pleomorphic adenomas, variants of monomorphic adenomas, malignant mixed tumors, ACCs, or adenocarcinoma not otherwise specified.[148] This may have been a result of its highly varied histologic pattern—hence the name "polymorphous"—including cords, tubules, papillae, glandular structures, and solid aggregates.[121,122] Despite this varied histologic pattern, the tumor is characterized by cytologic uniformity, mostly myoepithelial or luminal ductal cells.

The overwhelming majority of PLGAs originate in the oral cavity, mostly the palate or buccal mucosa. PLGA's clinical course is that of slow growth, and the tumor may be present for many years before diagnosis. Recently, Vincent, Hammond, and Finkelstein[148] described 204 cases in the literature (including 15 of their own). In their report, PLGA was twice as common in female patients than male patients. Forty-nine percent of tumors originated in palatal mucosa. Lymph node metastasis occurred in 9% of patients, either at the time of presentation or during the course of their disease. The local recurrence rate was 17%. Five patients had multiple recurrences, and 13 recurrences were at or beyond 5 years after the initial diagnosis. None of the 15 patients in their own series developed distant metastasis.

Hyalinizing clear cell carcinoma

Milchgrub and others[93] coined the term *hyalinizing clear cell carcinoma* to distinguish this neoplasm from other clinicopathologic entities formerly described as "clear cell neoplasms." In their series of 11 patients, the majority were women who presented with a painless mass. Nine tumors originated in minor salivary glands of the oral cavity (82%). Microscopically, tumors were characterized by the formation of trabeculae, cords, islands, or nests of monomorphic clear cells that were glycogen-rich and mucin-negative and were surrounded by hyalinized bands with foci of myxohya-

line stroma. Cells with eosinophilic and granular cytoplasm also were noted. Both cell types showed minimal nuclear pleomorphism and a low mitotic index. All of the neoplasms had infiltrative borders.[93] The clinical course of these neoplasms is that of a low-grade malignancy.[15] Fewer than 20% of patients show regional metastasis. None of the 11 patients reported by Milchgrub died of their disease, with a mean follow-up period of 3.6 years.[93]

Adenocarcinoma

The term *adenocarcinoma* implies an epithelial malignancy that originates from a glandular unit and in its most differentiated form maintains a glandular cytoarchitecture. Previously, a variety of heterogeneous tumors originating from salivary glandular subunits were collectively described as "adenocarcinomas." With refinements in histopathologic evaluation, these tumors now are classified in more homogeneous subgroups that have specific histopathologic characteristics and share similar biologic behavior. Clinicopathologic entities, such as SDC, terminal duct carcinoma, and epimyoepithelial carcinoma (formerly classified as adenocarcinoma), are examples of this refinement in classification.[13]

There remain adenocarcinomas of salivary tissues that cannot be accommodated in conventional classifications and are collectively given the term *adenocarcinoma; not otherwise specified (NOS)*. The exact incidence of this subgroup of tumors is difficult to determine. As refinements in classification with clinicopathologic correlations proceed, the number of cases of "adenocarcinomas; (NOS)" of salivary tissue decrease. They are the least common of salivary carcinomas and manifest a cytoarchitecture ranging from a well-differentiated, low-grade appearance to high-grade, invasive lesions.[13] They share some common salient features. They are more common in the major salivary glands and originate from the excretory or striated duct. They may exhibit a solid or cystic pattern, which may be papillary or nonpapillary. Some tumors are mucin-producing, whereas others are not.[13] Poor prognostic indicators include advanced stage, high histologic grade, infiltrative growth pattern, and maybe abnormal DNA content.

Squamous cell carcinoma

Primary squamous cell carcinoma (SCC) of the parotid gland is rare. It should be distinguished from the more common metastatic SCC to the intraparotid lymph nodes from cutaneous malignancy of the face and scalp. It also should be distinguished from direct parotid involvement with cancer of the external ear or preauricular region. Another differential diagnosis that should be ruled out is high-grade undifferentiated MEC, with little or no evidence of mucin-producing elements on light microscopy. Under such circumstances, the use of electron microscopy and special stains for mucin may help establish the diagnosis. Recently, immunohistochemical testing for markers of glandular differentiation in salivary gland tumors have been described.[46,145] Such antigenic markers may be useful in distinguishing undifferentiated MEC from SCC of the salivary glands.

The exact incidence of primary SCC of the salivary glands is difficult to determine from published data. The reported incidence of SCC of the salivary glands varies from 0.5% to 9% in the parotid gland, and from 2% to 11% in the submandibular glands. Batsakis and others[18] indicated that the true incidence of primary SCC of the salivary glands is only 0.3% to 1.5%. Most patients present with advanced stage disease, and nodal metastasis occurs in about one half the patients.[124] This may explain, at least in part, the poor prognosis associated with primary SCC of the salivary glands. In a series of 50 patients reported by Shemen, Huvos, and Spiro,[124] the incidence of locoregional failure was 51% for those with SCC of the parotid gland and 67% in patients with SCC of the submandibular gland.

Undifferentiated carcinoma

The term *undifferentiated carcinoma* describes an epithelial malignancy that, because of lack of distinguishing histologic characteristics, could not be otherwise classified. The diagnosis of undifferentiated carcinoma undoubtedly will be less used as refinements in histopathologic diagnosis continue with the use of electron microscopy, special stains, and immunohistochemistry. A special subtype is the undifferentiated carcinoma with lymphoid stroma, which previously was described as malignant lymphoepithelial of the salivary gland.[122] This tumor has a relatively high incidence in Inuit and Chinese populations and is indistinguishable histologically from the lymphoepithelial undifferentiated carcinoma of the nasopharynx. The etiology of this tumor type also has been linked to EBV.

Lymphoma

Lymphomas of the salivary glands may originate either from intraglandular lymph nodes (nodal) or from the lymphoid tissue dispersed within the salivary gland parenchyma (extranodal), which is considered a part of the mucosa-associated lymphoid tissue (MALT) system.[141] Lymphoma of the salivary gland may involve the salivary glands as the only manifestation of the disease (primary) or as a part of disseminated lymphoma.[122] Primary lymphomas of the salivary glands usually are associated with chronic immunosialadenitis (benign lymphoepithelial lesion or Sjögren's syndrome). The risk of malignant lymphoma in patients with Sjögren's syndrome is forty-fourfold higher than that in the healthy population.[71]

Approximately 5% of all extranodal lymphomas affect the salivary glands, and more than 90% of salivary gland lymphomas occur in the parotid gland.[122] This predilection for origin in the parotid gland undoubtedly is a result of the abundance of lymphoid aggregates within its salivary parenchyma. Most salivary gland lymphomas are of the non-Hodgkin's variety (85%). Salivary gland lymphomas associated with Sjögren's syndrome have a significantly worse prognosis than those originating in healthy glands or in glands with benign lymphoepithelial lesions without the manifestations of Sjögren's syndrome.

Secondary (metastatic) tumors

Hematogenous metastases to the salivary glands from infraclavicular primaries are rare. These metastases are mainly from the lungs, kidneys, and breasts. The majority of metastases to the salivary glands are caused by lymphatic spread from cutaneous malignancy of the head and neck. The parotid gland is the most common site of involvement because of the presence of intraparotid lymph nodes, which reflects the lymphatic drainage pattern of the skin of the ear, face, and scalp. The area of skin that has the highest predilection of metastasis to the parotid gland is located anterior to the midcoronal plane and extends anteriorly to the oblique line corresponding to the course of the facial vessels. This underscores the importance of careful examination of the skin of the head and neck, particularly the ears, cheeks, forehead, temples, and scalp for evidence of cutaneous malignancy in any patient presenting with a parotid mass.

Metastatic tumors account for less than 10% of malignant parotid gland tumors, and of these, 40% are SCCs, and 40% are melanomas. The incidence of metastasis to the parotid gland from SCC[82] or melanoma[81] is about 1.5%. About two thirds of metastatic SCCs to the parotid gland occur within the first year after treatment of the primary skin cancer.[82] The incidence of parotid metastasis from cutaneous melanoma of the head and neck correlates with the thickness of the primary tumor.

STAGING

The American Joint Commission on Cancer describes a staging system for major salivary gland cancer that follows the TNM system of staging.[59] Primary tumor (T) stage primarily depends on the size of the primary tumor, with two subcategories for each stage reflecting the presence or absence of local extension (Table 69-5). Minor salivary gland

Table 69-5. Staging system for major salivary gland cancer

T Stage	Extent of tumor
Tx	Primary tumor cannot be assessed
T0	No evidence of primary tumor
T1	Tumor < 2cm in greatest dimension
T2	Tumor 2-4 cm in greatest dimension
T3	Tumor 4-6 cm in greatest dimension
T4	Tumor > 6 cm in greatest dimension

All categories are subdivided: (a) no local extension; (b) local extension. Local extension is clinical or macroscopic invasion of skin, soft tissue, bone, or nerve.

Microscopic evidence alone is not a local extension for classification purposes.

cancer is staged according to the staging system used to classify primary tumors in their particular site of origin (e.g., oral cavity, oropharynx, and so on).

TREATMENT

Surgery

The principal treatment of salivary gland cancer is surgical resection, used either as a single modality or, in most patients, in conjunction with adjuvant radiotherapy.[102,110,144] The goals of surgical treatment are complete excision of the tumor, while avoiding unnecessary morbidity. The surgical approach and the scope of resection depend on the location and extent of the tumor.

Parotid gland

Small, localized tumors of the superficial lobe of the parotid gland, which are located lateral to the plane of the facial nerve, may be adequately treated with a superficial parotidectomy. Larger tumors and tumors involving the deep lobe of the parotid gland usually require a total parotidectomy. The facial nerve is dissected and preserved, unless it is directly involved by the tumor.[57,155] Preoperative weakness or paralysis of the facial nerve usually indicates tumor involvement, and in these patients the nerve should be sacrificed.[156] The nerve also should be sacrificed if there is intraoperative evidence of gross invasion or microscopic infiltration of the nerve by tumor, even in the presence of normal preoperative facial nerve function. This need to sacrifice the facial nerve is more likely to occur in patients with larger and high-grade tumors and in those with tumors that extend from the superficial to the deep lobe transgressing the plane of the facial nerve. Surgical margins on the distal and proximal nerve stumps should be checked because of the possibility of perineural spread for some distance from the area of the primary tumor. In certain patients, achieving negative surgical margins on the proximal stump of the facial nerve may require a mastoidectomy and facial nerve dissection along its course in the temporal bone. If the facial nerve is sacrificed, nerve repair may be done by using either direct neurorrhaphy of the cut edges or a cable graft, depending on the length of the resected segment. Tumors extending beyond the confines of the parotid gland may require resection of surrounding structures, including the skin, mandibular ramus, masseter muscle, infratemporal fossa dissection, or subtotal petrosectomy.[83]

Submandibular gland

Surgical management of submandibular salivary gland malignancy depends on the extent of the tumor. Small tumors confined to the gland itself are treated with resection of the submandibular gland. Tumors transgressing the confines of the gland to invade surrounding structures are treated with a wider *en bloc* excision.[26] This excision may require removal of the contents of the submandibular triangle, resec-

tion of the floor or mouth, or marginal or segmental mandibulectomy, depending on the extent of the tumor.[153] Special attention should be given to the lingual, hypoglossal, mylohyoid, and marginal mandibular nerves because they may be involved by perineural spread of tumor. Thickening and nodularity of these nerves may indicate perineural involvement, and in such patients, histologic confirmation by frozen-section may be useful in establishing nerve invasion and in obtaining negative surgical margins.

Minor salivary glands

Surgical resection of minor salivary gland cancers depends on their site of origin and extent of disease. In the oral cavity, this may only require a wide local excision of localized low-grade tumors. Larger or high-grade tumors may require wider excisions, including marginal or segmental mandibulectomy or partial or total resection of the hard or soft palate.[102,116] Sinonasal salivary gland malignancies usually are high grade and present at an advanced stage. Surgical resection may require partial or total maxillectomy, infratemporal fossa dissection, or anterior craniofacial resection. Palatal defects resulting from these resections are best managed by prosthetic rehabilitation. The branches of the second (V2) and third (V3) divisions of the trigeminal nerve are at high risk for perineural spread of minor salivary gland malignancy. These nerves may provide an avenue for early skull base invasion. Cranial base resections may be required in some patients to eradicate the tumor and to obtain negative surgical margins.

Neck dissection

There is universal agreement in the literature that a neck dissection is indicated when there is clinical evidence of metastatic disease in the cervical lymph nodes. This dissection usually involves a comprehensive cervical lymphadenectomy and either a modified radical or radical neck dissection, depending on the extent of disease. Controversy still exists regarding the surgical management of the clinically negative neck. The indications and type of elective neck dissection are not well defined in the literature.

To better define the indications for elective neck treatment, Armstrong and others studied the incidence of clinical and occult nodal disease in 474 patients with salivary gland cancer.[6] Clinically positive nodes were present in 14% (67 of 474) of patients. Overall, clinically occult, pathologically positive nodes occurred in 12% (47 of 407) of patients. Considering the low frequency of occult metastases in the entire group, routine elective treatment of the neck was not recommended, although the incidence of occult metastatic disease was dramatically influenced by tumor size and histologic grade. Tumors 4 cm or larger had a 20% (32 of 164) risk of occult metastases compared with a 4% (9 of 220) risk for smaller tumors ($P < 0.00001$). High-grade tumors (regardless of histologic type) had a 49% (29 of 59) risk of occult metastases compared with a 7% (15 of 221) risk for intermediate-grade or low-grade tumors ($P < 0.00001$). Rodriguez-Cuevas and others[113] also found an increased risk (50%) of occult node metastases in patients with high-grade carcinomas, whereas no cases were found in those with low-grade carcinomas ($P < 0.05$). These findings demonstrate that the incidence of occult regional disease in patients with large or high-grade tumors is relatively high, and therefore an elective neck dissection should be considered in these patients. A selective (supraomohyoid) neck dissection may be used as a staging procedure in such patients. Suspicious nodes should be sent for frozen-section diagnosis, and if results are positive for metastatic carcinoma, a comprehensive neck dissection is performed. Elective neck dissection is not recommended for those with low-grade malignancy of the salivary glands.[6,113]

Surgical technique

Parotidectomy. The patient is placed in the supine position, and the head is turned to the opposite side. The skin incision is placed in a preauricular crease and extends superiorly to the level of the root of the helix. The incision extends inferiorly around the lobule of ear over the mastoid tip. It then gently curves down along the sternocleidomastoid muscle and then slightly forward in a natural skin crease in the upper neck. Skin flaps are elevated in the plane superficial to the parotid fascia in the preauricular region and in the subplatysmal plane in the cervical portion of the incision. The greater auricular nerve and the external jugular vein are identified over the sternocleidomastoid muscle and are divided to free the tail of the parotid gland (Fig. 69-23). The posterior belly of the digastric muscle is exposed until the point of its attachment to the mastoid bone. The fascia between the parotid gland and the cartilaginous external auditory canal is dissected, and the parotid gland is retracted anteriorly, which exposes the tragal pointer. The most common way of identifying the main trunk of the facial nerve is in its course in the region located between the tragal pointer and the attachment of the posterior belly of the digastric muscle (Fig. 69-24). Unless displaced by tumor, the nerve usually is located approximately 1.0 to 1.5 cm deep and inferior to the tragal pointer. Another reliable, and perhaps a more constant landmark to identify the facial nerve is the tympanomastoid suture line, which could be followed medially to the main trunk of the nerve. The nerve usually is 6 to 8 mm deep to the tympanomastoid suture line. In certain patients in whom the tumor is directly overlying the region of the main trunk of the facial nerve, one or more of the peripheral branches of the nerve are identified distally and traced proximally toward the main trunk. The marginal mandibular branch may be identified below the lower border of the mandible as it crosses superficial to the facial vessels in the plane immediately underneath the deep cervical fascia (Fig. 69-25). Alternatively, the buccal branch may be identified underneath the parotidomasseteric fascia, coursing parallel to the parotid duct.

Once the facial nerve is identified, the overlying parotid

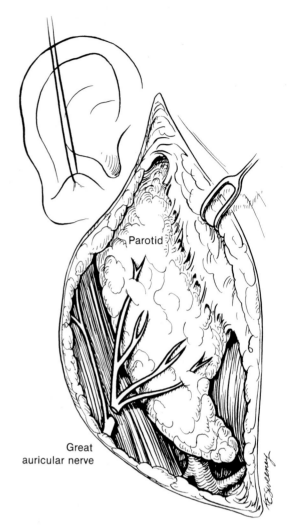

Fig. 69-23. Separation of tail of parotid from sternocleidomastoid, usually requiring sectioning of greater auricular nerve.

tissue is meticulously elevated from the nerve with a fine clamp, and the bridge of tissue between the blades of the clamp are carefully divided (Fig. 69-26). If the main trunk of the nerve is identified first, then the overlying parotid tissue is progressively dissected free of the nerve to the first branching of the nerve, usually into an upper and a lower division. Subsequent branching of the nerve (*pes anserinus*) is sequentially dissected in a similar fashion until the entire superficial lobe of the parotid gland lying lateral to the facial nerve is delivered (Fig. 69-27). This completes a superficial or lateral parotidectomy.

If a total parotidectomy is indicated, the procedure is extended by meticulous dissection of the main trunk and the branches of the facial nerve from the underlying parotid tissue in a gentle and atraumatic fashion, which allows the salivary tissue lying deep to the facial nerve to be delivered while preserving the nerve and its function.

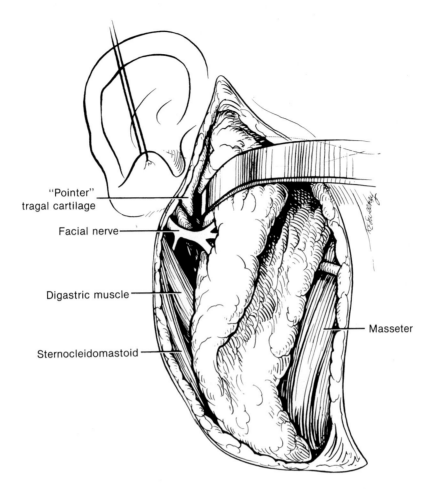

"Pointer"
tragal cartilage

Facial nerve

Digastric muscle

Sternocleidomastoid

Masseter

Fig. 69-24. Blunt dissection of parotid gland from external auditory canal cartilage exposes tragal pointer. The facial nerve lies approximately 1 cm deep and slightly anteroinferior to pointer, and 6 to 8 mm deep to tympanomastoid suture line.

Complications

Facial nerve paresis or paralysis. Facial nerve dysfunction may result from traction injury to the facial nerve during its dissection. As long as the anatomic integrity of the nerve is preserved, this type of injury usually results in neuropraxia, and complete recovery is anticipated. The degree of weakness or paralysis may range from minimal partial weakness of one or more branches of the facial nerve to complete paralysis of all branches of the nerve. Recovery of facial nerve function may be prompt and complete within days, or it may be delayed for several months.

If the facial nerve is sacrificed, nerve repair may be done by using either direct neurorrhaphy of the cut edges or a cable graft, depending on the length of the resected segment. Immediate rehabilitation of the paralyzed face requires diligent eye care to prevent exposure keratitis. This care involves liberal use of artificial tears, lubricating ointment, and protection with an appropriate eye dressing and eyewear. A temporary tarsorrhaphy may be needed for patients with lower eyelid ectropion. A gold weight implant may be needed in patients with corneal exposure. If the facial nerve is not repaired or grafted, one or more of the various surgical procedures for facial rehabilitation of the paralyzed face may be indicated.

Gustatory sweating "Frey's syndrome". Patients with Frey's syndrome experience flushing and sweating of the ipsilateral facial skin during mastication (gustatory sweating). The symptoms may vary in severity from barely noticeable to severe and bothersome. The true incidence of postoperative Frey's syndrome is unknown, but it is estimated to be between 35% and 60%. The incidence probably would be higher if the syndrome is searched for by directed symptom-specific questions. The presumed pathophysiology of Frey's syndrome involves aberrant cross-reinnervation between the postganglionic secretomotor parasympathetic fibers to the parotid gland and the postganglionic sympathetic fibers supplying the sweat glands of the skin.

The diagnosis of Frey's syndrome depends largely on the patient's symptoms. An objective method of confirming the

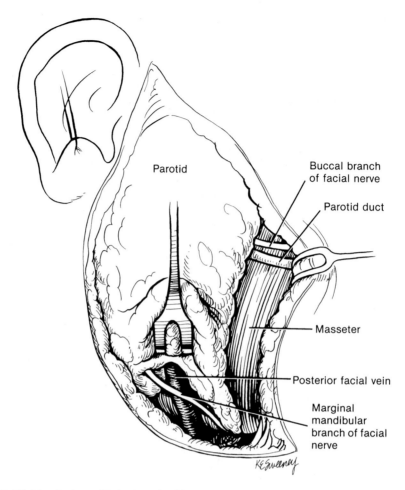

Fig. 69-25. Marginal mandibular branch of facial nerve, which can reliably be found by tracing of posterior facial vein superiorly. Marginal division almost always crosses superficial to vein. Also diagrammed is relationship of buccal branch to parotid duct.

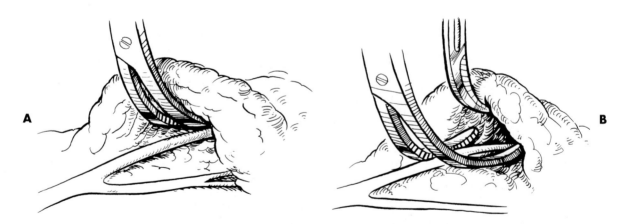

Fig. 69-26. Demonstration of technique of following each branch of facial nerve. **A,** Tunnels are created in plane of nerve. **B,** Overlying parotid tissue is cut with No. 12 blade.

Continued

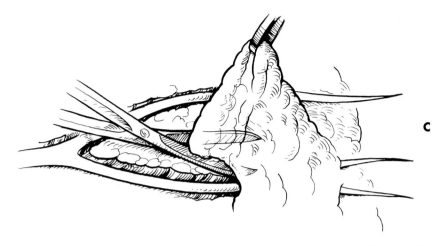

Fig. 69-26, cont'd. C, Each successive tunnel is serially connected to previous tunnel.

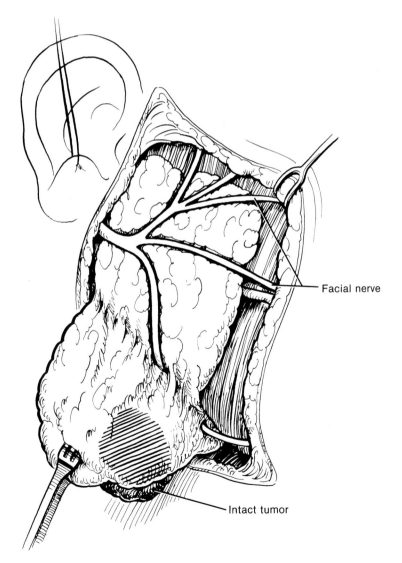

Facial nerve

Intact tumor

Fig. 69-27. Nearly completed process, with tumor within intact superficial parotidectomy specimen.

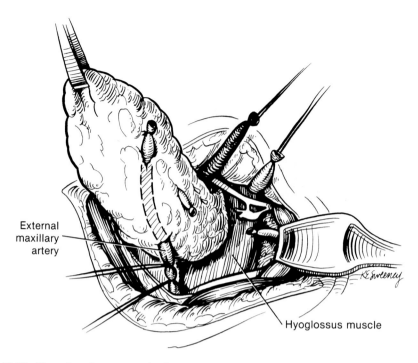

Fig. 69-31. Hypoglossal nerve, running between the hypoglossus and myelohyoid muscles. External maxillary artery must be divided the second time.

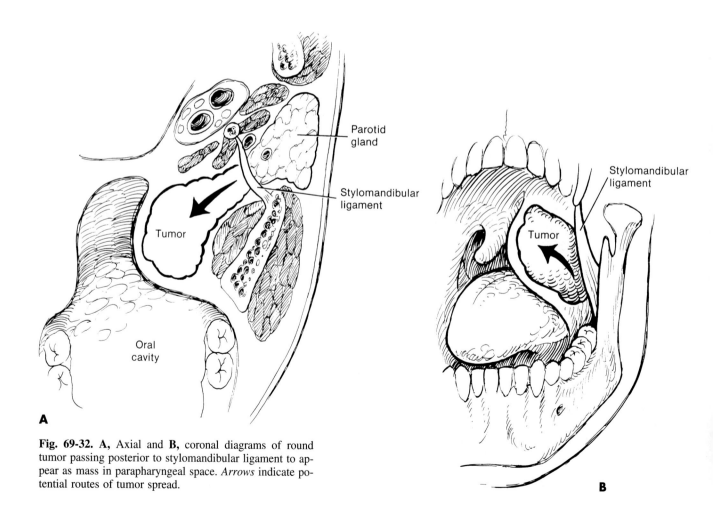

Fig. 69-32. A, Axial and **B,** coronal diagrams of round tumor passing posterior to stylomandibular ligament to appear as mass in parapharyngeal space. *Arrows* indicate potential routes of tumor spread.

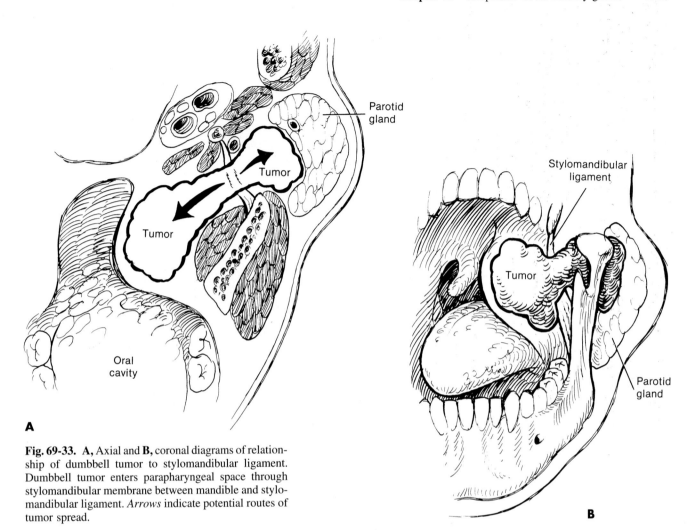

Fig. 69-33. A, Axial and **B,** coronal diagrams of relationship of dumbbell tumor to stylomandibular ligament. Dumbbell tumor enters parapharyngeal space through stylomandibular membrane between mandible and stylomandibular ligament. *Arrows* indicate potential routes of tumor spread.

palpable in the pretragal region, and the deep component, if it is large enough, may displace the palate and tonsil medially. Tumors originating from the minor salivary glands within the parapharyngeal space have no connection to the parotid gland. Whatever their site of origin, parapharyngeal salivary gland tumors are located in the prestyloid compartment of the parapharyngeal space (see Fig. 69-12).

Surgical excision of salivary gland tumors within the parapharyngeal space is best done through an external approach. Olsen[98] used two surgical approaches to treat 44 patients with tumors in the parapharyngeal space. A cervical–parotid approach was used in 35 patients, and the cervical–parotid approach with midline mandibulotomy was used in nine patients. Of the 44 tumors, 32 were benign lesions, and 12 were malignant neoplasms. The use of these two approaches resulted in a low morbidity rate and provided a safe, efficacious method to excise parapharyngeal space neoplasms.

The cervical–parotid approach. The incision of the cervical–parotid approach is that of a parotidectomy with a cervial extension. If the tumor involves the deep lobe of the parotid gland, a superficial parotidectomy is done first. If

the tumor originates from the minor salivary glands of the parapharyngeal space, the inferior division of the facial nerve is identified and carefully preserved (Fig. 69-34). The sternocleidomastoid next is retracted laterally, and the upper jugular lymph nodes are removed to allow identification of the internal jugular vein, external and internal carotid arteries, and the last four CNs (IX, X, XI, and XII) (Fig. 69-35). The posterior belly of a diagastric and the stylohyoid muscle are identified, divided near their mastoid and styloid attachments, respectively, and are retracted medially, which allows further superior exposure of the internal carotid artery, internal jugular vein, and adjacent nerves.[98] The external carotid artery then is divided near its entrance into the parotid tissue, which allows adequate visualization of the stylomandibular ligament and the styloid process. The stylomandibular ligament is divided, which allows further anterior retraction of the mandible and provides a wide opening into the parapharyngeal space (Fig. 69-36). The styloid process may be resected for further exposure and to facilitate delivery of larger tumors. Through this exposure, the tumor may be easily visualized and safely excised (Fig. 69-37).

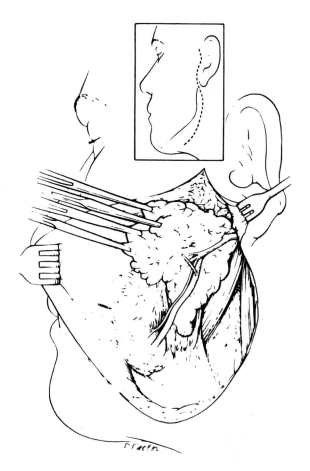

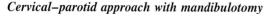

Fig. 69-34. Exposure of the facial nerve and its inferior division: cervical–parotid approach.

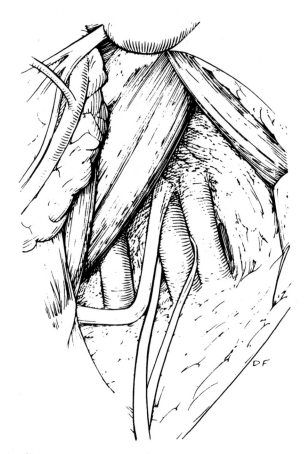

Fig. 69-35. Exposure of vessels and nerves in the upper neck: cervical–parotid approach.

Cervical–parotid approach with mandibulotomy

This approach is more likely to be used in patients with malignant lesions, particularly those with lesions located in the superior aspect of the parapharyngeal space approaching the eustachian tube and skull base.[98] The enhanced exposure offered by the mandibulotomy allows the visualization necessary for resection of the tumor with adequate margins. First, a cervical–parotid approach is performed as described in the previous section. If a mandibulotomy is indicated, a preliminary tracheostomy is performed. Next, the cervical portion of the incision is extended through the chin to split the lower lip in the midline. The mandible is exposed, and a stair-step osteotomy is placed either in the midline (median mandibulotomy) or just anterior to the mental foramen (a paramedian mandibulotomy; Fig. 69-38). A paralingual incision then is made along the floor of mouth and extends back to the anterior tonsillar pillar and up to the level of the hard palate (Fig. 69-39). The myelohyoid muscle is divided while carefully preserving the hypoglossal and lingual nerves. The tongue is retracted medially, and the parapharyngeal and retropharyngeal spaces are opened widely (Fig. 69-40). The tumor now may be excised safely and adequately while pro-

tecting the critical neurovascular structures of the parapharyngeal space. Closure involves a water-tight intraoral suture line and rigid fixation of the mandibulotomy. For mandibular fixation, it is preferable to use plates that have been contoured, applied to the mandible, and then removed before the osteotomy, which minimizes any malocclusion caused by the osteotomy. A nasogastric tube is inserted for feeding. Within 7 to 10 days, most patients will have their tracheostomy decannulated and are able to resume oral feeding.

Radiotherapy

Adjuvant (postoperative) radiotherapy

Several reports suggest that the use of adjuvant radiotherapy in conjunction with surgery is superior to surgery alone in the treatment of high-grade or advanced cancers of the major and minor salivary glands. Theriault and Fitzpatrick reported the outcome of 271 patients with parotid carcinomas.[144] Among these were 64 patients with MECs (24%) (all degrees of differentiation), 50 (18%) with adenocarcinomas, 40 (15%) with malignant mixed tumors, 39 (14%) with ACCs, 37 (14%) with undifferentiated tumors, 21 (8%) with acinic carcinomas, and 20 (7%) with SCCs. The prognostic

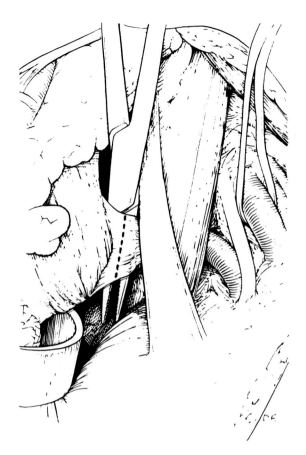

Fig. 69-36. Division of stylomandibular ligament: cervical–parotid approach.

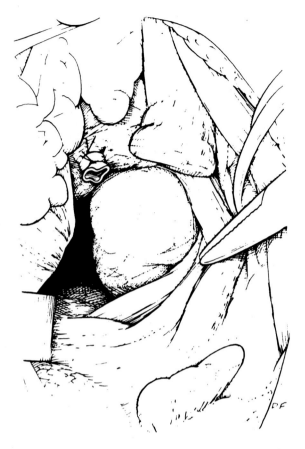

Fig. 69-37. Tumor exposure: cervical–parotid approach.

characteristics were similar for the 67 (25%) patients treated by surgery and for the 169 (62%) patients treated with surgery and postoperative radiotherapy. Patients treated with combined therapy had a 10-year relapse-free rate of 62% compared with 22% for those treated by surgery alone ($P = 0.0005$).

Borthne and others demonstrated that radiotherapy lowered the recurrence rates after surgery and controlled approximately one third of the inoperable tumors.[23] Their data suggested that a dose–response relationship exists for those with salivary gland cancers and that the radiation dose should not be less than 70 Gy/7 weeks.

Recently, Garden and others reported the MD Anderson Cancer Center experience with adjuvant radiotherapy in the treatment of 160 patients with minor salivary gland cancers.[51] Microscopic positive margins were present in 64 (40%) patients. One half of the patients had pathologic evidence of perineural invasion. Radiation doses ranged from 50 to 75 Gy (median, 60 Gy). With a median follow-up period of 110 months, 57 (36%) patients experienced disease relapse. Nineteen (12%) patients had a local recurrence. Regional failures occurred in 3 of 13 patients with initially node-positive disease but were uncommon (< 5%) in pa-

tients with node-negative disease, regardless of elective neck treatments. Distant metastases developed in 43 patients, mostly (79%) within 5 years of treatment. Actuarial overall survival rates at 5, 10, and 15 years were 81%, 65%, and 43%, respectively. Complications from radiotherapy occurred in 51 patients and were of three predominate types: hearing loss (26 patients), ocular injury (15 patients), and bone exposure and necrosis (12 patients). However, their data suggested that improved radiotherapeutic techniques, including better immobilization, customized beam shaping, and treating multiple fields per day, have substantially reduced the risk of serious complications during the past decade. They concluded that postoperative radiotherapy is effective in preventing local recurrence in most patients with minor salivary gland tumors after gross total excision. When local failure occurs, it tends to be a late event. For most patients, a postoperative dose of 60 Gy in 30 fractions to the operative bed is adequate; if there is named nerve invasion, the path of the nerve is treated electively to its ganglion.

Although the addition of adjuvant radiotherapy should not be considered as an adequate substitute for clear surgical margins, in many patients, it is not possible to obtain negative margins of resection. In such patients, the use of postoperative radiation may enhance local control. In 1994, Sakata and others described 17 patients with positive surgical margins after resection of cancer of the major salivary glands.[117] All patients received postoperative radiotherapy. Overall local control at 5 years was 65%.

Recently, Shingaki and others compared 22 patients with salivary gland malignancy treated with surgery alone, with 22 patients treated with combination surgery and radiotherapy.[125] In the surgery group, local recurrence developed in 8 patients with evidence of residual disease at the surgical margins, whereas local control was achieved in 7 of 15 patients with positive surgical margins in the combination group, and the control rate was related to the amount of residual disease. Neck metastasis, which developed in 13 patients (30%), was not affected by the status of surgical margins or by the treatment modality. On the other hand, the incidence of distant metastasis seen in 19 patients (43%) was much higher in patients with positive surgical margins, and the development of distant metastasis in these patients was not prevented by postoperative irradiation. These findings underscore the importance of investigating other therapeutic modalities, such as chemotherapy, to reduce the occurrence of distant disease in such a high-risk patient population.

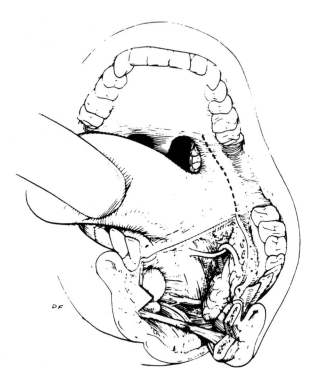

Fig. 69-39. Intraoral incision and identification and preservation of lingual and hypoglossal nerves.

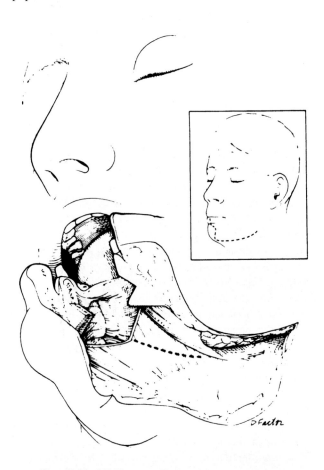

Fig. 69-38. Midline mandibular stair-step osteotomy.

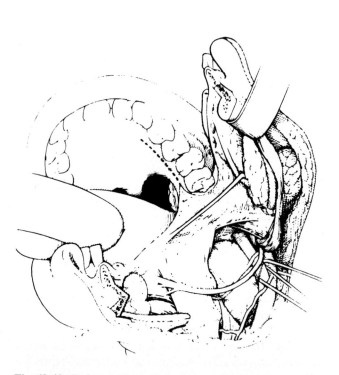

Fig. 69-40. Defect and operative exposure after tumor removal by cervical–parotid approach with midline mandibulotomy.

In conclusion, postoperative radiotherapy generally is recommended for patients with poor prognostic indicators, including high-grade tumors, large primary lesions, perineural invasion, bone invasion, cervical lymph node metastasis, and positive margins. Although a clear-cut survival advantage has not been proven, the addition of postoperative radiotherapy improves locoregional control for patients with such adverse prognostic parameters.[19]

Radiotherapy as a single modality

To compare the effectiveness of radiotherapy used alone or combined with surgery in the treatment of those with minor salivary gland malignancy, Parsons and others reported the results of treatment of 95 patients with minor salivary gland cancer.[102] Fifty-one patients were treated with radiotherapy alone, and 44 were treated by surgical resection plus radiotherapy. Although the tumor was locally controlled in 20 patients with previously untreated primary lesions after radiotherapy alone, freedom-from-relapse rates were higher for patients who received combined treatment ($P = 0.068$). Hosokawa and others achieved 72.3% local control in 41 patients with ACC treated with radiotherapy alone.[67] Despite the high local control rate, the disease-free survival rate of the patients at 10 years was only 20.8%. These findings indicate that in those with resectable tumors, complete surgical excision followed by radiotherapy is the preferred treatment for high-grade and advanced tumors.

Radiotherapy for inoperable tumors

During the past decade, there has been substantial evidence that fast-neutron radiotherapy provides higher rates of locoregional control of unresectable salivary gland cancer compared with photon or electron radiotherapy,[28,63,76,119,139] and perhaps should be considered the initial treatment of choice in such patients.[79] Buchholz and others reported the outcome of 53 patients with locally advanced salivary gland malignant neoplasm treated with fast-neutron radiotherapy.[25] All patients received treatment for gross inoperable, residual unresectable, or recurrent disease. With a median follow-up period of 42 months and a minimum follow-up period of 1 year, the overall locoregional tumor control rate was 77% (40 of 52 patients). The 5-year actuarial overall locoregional control rate was 65%. Grouping patients according to previous treatment status, actuarial 5-year locoregional control rates were 92% for patients treated definitively (without a previous surgical procedure), 63% for those treated postoperatively for gross residual disease, and 51% for those treated for recurrent disease after a surgical procedure. This study suggested that neutron irradiation alone should be the therapy of choice in the treatment of patients with advanced-stage salivary gland tumors and that surgery should be limited to those in whom disease-free margins may be obtained. The potential morbidity of a debunking surgical procedure before neutron irradiation is not warranted by an improvement in locoregional control over that

achievable with neutron therapy alone.[25] These impressive results are encouraging, although the use of fast-neutron radiotherapy is hampered by its lack of wide-spread availability. Currently, only few facilities are equipped with the technology and expertise of delivering fast-neutron radiotherapy.

Other investigators described their experience with photon beam radiotherapy for the treatment of patients with unresectable salivary gland cancer and reported comparable results to those obtained by fast-neutron therapy. Wang and Goodman[152] presented their experience with 24 patients with inoperable or unresectable cancer of the parotid gland (9 patients) or the minor salivary glands (15 patients) treated by photon irradiation. The 5-year actuarial local control of parotid gland lesions after photon irradiation was 100%, and the survival rate was 65%. For those with the minor salivary gland lesions, the 5-year actuarial local control was 78%, and the survival rate with or without disease was 93%. All lesions were irradiated by accelerated hyperfractionated photons (twice daily) with 1.6 Gy per fraction and intermixed with various boost techniques, including electron beam, intraoral cone, interstitial implant, or submental photons for a total of 65 to 70 Gy.

The Radiation Therapy Oncology Group (RTOG) in the United States and the Medical Research Council (MRC) in Great Britain sponsored a study comparing the efficacy of fast-neutron radiotherapy versus conventional photon or electron radiotherapy for unresectable, malignant salivary gland tumors. Thirty-two patients with inoperable, recurrent, or unresectable malignant salivary gland tumors were entered; 17 patients were randomized to receive neutrons, and 15 patients were randomized to receive photons. In 1988, the initial report on the outcome of 25 analyzable patients with minimum follow-up time of 2 years was published (Table 69-6).[55]

After 32 patients were entered into this study, it appeared that the group receiving fast-neutron radiotherapy had a significantly improved locoregional control rate and also a borderline improvement in survival rate, and the study was stopped earlier than planned for ethical reasons. In 1993, Laramore and others published the final report on this study.[79] At 10-year follow-up evaluation, although there was

Table 69-6. Neutron versus photon therapy for inoperable salivary gland cancers

2-year follow-up	Neutron therapy, %	Photon therapy, %	P value
Initial complete response	85	33	
Locoregional control	67	17	$P < 0.005$
2-year survival rate	62	25	$P = 0.10$

Griffin TW and others: Neutron vs photon irradiation of inoperable salivary gland tumors: results of an RTOG-MRC cooperative randomized study, *Int J Rad Oncol Biol Phys* 15:1085, 1988.

a statistically significant improvement in locoregional control for the neutron group (56% versus 25%; $P = 0.009$), there was no improvement in survival rate (15% versus 25%; $P =$ not significant). Distant metastases accounted for the majority of failures on the neutron arm, and locoregional failures accounted for the majority of failures on the photon arm. Although the incidence of morbidity graded ''severe'' was greater on the neutron arm, there was no significant difference in ''life-threatening'' complications. This well-executed study showed that fast-neutron radiotherapy appears to be the treatment of choice for patients with inoperable primary or recurrent malignant salivary gland tumors. It is hoped that fast-neutron therapy will be more widely available for patients with unresectable salivary gland malignancy.

Chemotherapy

The poor outcome of patients with advanced, recurrent, or high-grade salivary gland cancers prompted several investigators to explore the effectiveness of adjuvant chemotherapy. Because a high percentage of patients with poor prognostic criteria succumb to their disease as a result of systemic metastasis, it was hoped that the addition of adjuvant chemotherapy to standard treatment modalities would improve patients' survival rates. The data in the literature regarding the effectiveness of chemotherapy against salivary gland cancers are difficult to interpret. Most studies report few patients, treated for different histologic types with various drug combinations, and include previously untreated patients with those with recurrent disease.[111,112,147]

In an effort to arrive at a rational basis for recommending specific drug regimens for specific histologic types of salivary gland cancers, Suen and Johns[140] conducted a review of the literature and surveyed the experience of numerous institutions with chemotherapy for salivary gland malignancy. Eighty-five patients with salivary gland cancers treated with chemotherapy were evaluated, and the overall response rate (complete and partial) was 42%. Although disease responded whether it was local, regional, or distant disease, there was a higher response rate in locoregional disease compared with distant metastases.

Similarly, Kaplan, Johns, and Cantrell[74] reviewed 116 patients and found that adenocarcinomas responded best to a combination of cisplatinum, adriamycin, and 5-fluorouracil. High-grade MEC may respond best to chemotherapeutic regimens effective against SCC. Similar findings were reported by Venook and others.[147] Airoldi and others[3] found that combination therapy (9% complete response [CR], 36% partial response [PR]) is more effective than single-drug treatment (no CR, 23% PR). The median response duration was 7.5 months after combination chemotherapy, and 4 months after single-agent chemotherapy. Median overall survival time was 8 months in the combination chemotherapy group and 5.5 months in the single-agent chemotherapy group. The

most effective drug regimens included cisplatinum, adriamycin, 5-fluorouracil, and epirubicin in different combinations.

Although there is evidence that salivary gland cancers show some response to various chemotherapeutic agents,[39] these responses are rarely complete, usually are short-lived, and have not resulted in significant improvement in long-term survival rates.[70] New drug combination and high-dose chemotherapy with autologous bone marrow transplantation are being explored in the treatment of patients with advanced salivary gland cancer.[129] Before any conclusions could be made about the efficacy of chemotherapy in those with salivary gland malignancy, well-executed, multiinstitutional, prospective, randomized clinical trials of specific drug regimens for specific histologic types are needed.

FACTORS INFLUENCING SURVIVAL

Stage

The stage of disease probably is the most significant factor in determining the outcome of cancers originating in the major[49,135] or the minor[132,134,136] salivary glands. Using a multivariate analysis of the outcome of 353 patients with minor salivary gland malignancy, Spiro and others[136] found that survival was significantly influenced by the clinical stage and the histologic grade, but the applicability of grading was limited to patients with MEC or adenocarcinoma. Ten-year overall survival rate was 83%, 53%, 35%, and 24% for patients with stage I through stage IV tumors, respectively.

With regards to ACC, Spiro and Huvos[132] found that the stage of disease was much more significant than grade in predicting the outcome of management. Cumulative 10-year survival rate was 75%, 43%, and 15% for stage I, stage II, and stage III and IV patients, respectively. Cause-specific survival at 10, 15, and 20 years is shown in Figure 69-41. The incidence of local recurrence after treatment was lowest in those with stage I (23%) versus other stages (60%) of tumors. Similarly, the incidence of regional metastasis was lowest in patients with stage I (19%) versus other stages (43%).[132,134] Neither survival, regional metastases, nor distant dissemination was predictable on the basis of tumor grade alone.

Histology and grade

The biologic behavior of malignant tumors of the salivary glands depends largely on the histologic type of malignancy.[49] SCC, malignant mixed tumors, undifferentiated carcinoma, and salivary duct carcinoma generally are considered high-grade tumors and usually exhibit an aggressive biologic course, resulting in a poor outcome. By contrast, acinic cell carcinoma and polymorphous low-grade adenocarcinoma are considered low-grade tumors with more favorable prognosis.

ACC generally is considered a high-grade malignancy with a relentless tendency for local recurrence and ultimately

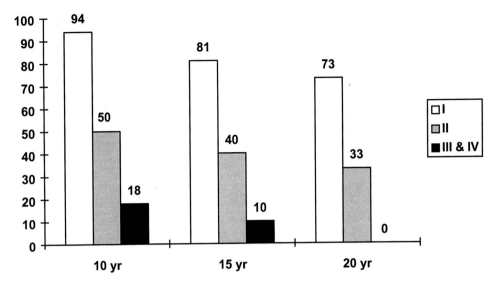

Fig. 69-41. Effect of stage on survival in adenoid cystic carcinoma.

Table 69-7. Effect of histologic pattern on the clinical course of adenoid cystic carcinoma

Pattern	Total	NER	NED-RC	AWD	DOD
Tubular	22	9 (41%)	2 (9%)	2 (9%)	9 (41%)
Cribriform	27	3 (11%)	4 (15%)	5 (19%)	15 (55%)
Solid	13	0	0	6 (46%)	7 (54%)
Total	62	12 (19%)	6 (10%)	13 (21%)	31 (50%)

Perzin KH, Gullane P, Clairmont AC: Adenoid cystic carcinoma in the salivary glands: a correlation of histologic features and clinical course, *Cancer* 42: 265, 1978.
NER—No evidence of recurrence; NED-RC—No evidence of disease-recurrence controlled; AWD—Alive with disease; DOD—Dead of disease.

a poor prognosis, although the three histologic patterns of ACC may have different biologic behavior and therefore different outcome. Generally, patients with the tubular pattern of ACC have a significantly better prognosis than patients with the solid pattern. Perzin and others[104] reported the outcome of 62 patients with ACC and found that of the 12 patients with no evidence of recurrence (NER), 9 (75%) had the tubular pattern. By contrast, all of the patients with the solid pattern experienced recurrent disease, and more than half of them died of disease (Table 69-7). This tendency for a high incidence of local recurrence of patients with the solid pattern of ACC may have been related to the difficulty of achieving clear surgical margins in these patients. None of the 13 patients with solid pattern ACC had negative margins (0%), whereas 3 of 24 patients (13%) with the cribriform pattern and 9 of 21 patients (43%) with the tubular pattern had clear surgical margins.[104] As previously mentioned, Spiro and Huvos[132] found that the stage of disease had a much more significant impact on prognosis than the histologic pattern of ACC.

Most authors agree that the outcome of those with MEC correlates highly with the tumor's grade, although the histo-

pathologic criteria most useful for grading MECs are still controversial. Auclair, Goode, and Ellis[8] proposed a grading system using specific histopathologic features and correlated them with clinical parameters and outcome in patients with intraoral MEC. Histopathologic criteria that indicated high-grade behavior were an intracystic component of less than 20%, four or more mitotic figures per 10 high-power fields, neural invasion, necrosis, and cellular anaplasia. The simultaneous assessment of these features showed improved prognostic correlation over individual parameters, and a quantitative grading system was devised using these features. Tumors with a point score of zero to four were considered low grade, and none of 122 patients with scores in this range died of their tumor, although nine had recurrences only, and three had regional metastases. Point scores of seven or above indicated highly aggressive behavior. Six of 10 patients with these high scores died of their disease. Most of these six patients had recurrences and regional metastases, and all had distant metastases. Two other patients had regional metastases only. Scores of five to six were considered intermediate between low-grade and high-grade scores because only 1 of 13 patients with these scores died of disease. Similarly,

Hicks and others[65] described a three-tiered grading system for MEC of the major salivary glands. Tumor size increased from 2.1 cm for low-grade tumors to 3.8 cm for high-grade tumors ($P = 0.01$). This histologic grading of MEC of the major salivary glands correlated well with clinical, pathologic, and flow cytometric factors that influenced the prognosis and overall survival (Table 69-8).

Site

The primary site of origin of salivary gland cancer has a definite correlation with prognosis and outcome. Generally, patients with cancers of the major salivary glands have a better prognosis than those with cancers originating in the minor salivary glands. Of all cancers originating from the minor salivary glands, those originating from the sinonasal tract tend to have the worst outcome. Spiro, Huvos, and Strong[134] reported a 10-year cure rate of 29% for patients with ACC of the parotid gland, but it was only 7% for those patients whose tumors originated from the sinonasal tract.

The poor outcome of patients with minor salivary gland cancers, particularly those of sinonasal origin, may be explained by several factors that have a detrimental impact on prognosis. First, cancers of the minor salivary glands tend to present at a more advanced stage of disease. Approximately 90% of patients with ACC of the nose and sinuses presented with advanced stage (III and IV) disease (Fig. 69-42). Second, carcinomas of the minor salivary glands have

a higher incidence of extension and fixation to contiguous structures compared with tumors originating in the major salivary glands (Table 69-9). This poses greater difficulty in achieving complete surgical resection with negative margins. Consequently, the incidence of local recurrence after management of salivary gland cancers is highest for those with sinonasal tumors (63%) than for patients with other minor salivary gland tumors (54%) or major salivary gland tumors (32%).[132,134] Third, tumors in the minor salivary glands of the oral cavity and paranasal sinuses tend to have a relatively high incidence of bone involvement, which probably is because of the immediate proximity of the mucoperiosteum of the palate and the sinonasal tract to the underlying bone. Spiro, Huvos, and Strong[134] reported that bony involvement occurred in 87 of 171 patients (51%) with ACC of the minor salivary glands. Bony involvement had a significant negative impact on prognosis. The 10-year "cure" rate for patients without evidence of bony involvement was 32% compared with 7% for patients with evidence of bone invasion.[134]

Nodal metastasis

The presence of metastatic disease in the regional lymph nodes generally is considered a predictor of poor prognosis in patients with salivary gland malignancy.[49,144] The 10- and 20-year survival rates of patients with nodal metastasis from ACC was only 38% and 8%, respectively, compared with

Table 69-8. Effect of histologic grade of mucoepidermoid carcinoma on clinical outcome

Grade	Positive margins, %	LN metastasis, %	Deoxynucleic acid aneuploidy, %	Proliferative fraction, %	Radiotherapy, %	Recurrence, %	Survival, %
Low	0	0	0	5	14	0	100
Intermediate	44	22	13	7	35	39	70
High	61	72	28	13	61	61	22

Adapted from Hicks MJ and others: Histocytologic grading of mucoepidermoid carcinoma of major salivary glands in prognosis and survival: a clinicopathologic and flow cytometric investigation, *Head Neck* 17:89, 1995.

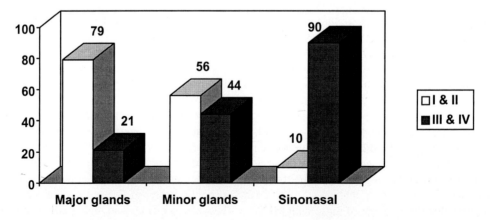

Fig. 69-42. Stage of disease by site of the origin in adenoid cystic carcinoma.

62% and 50%, respectively, in patients without evidence of regional disease in the lymph nodes.[132]

Similarly, Perzin, Gullane, and Clairmont[104] found that nodal metastasis had a significant negative impact on the outcome of patients with ACC. Of the seven patients with nodal disease in their series, five patients died of disease, one patient was alive with disease, and only one patient was without evidence of disease. By contrast, 8 of the 18 patients without evidence of lymph node metastasis were alive with no evidence of disease.

Surgical margins

Some authors consider that the presence or absence of tumor at the lines of surgical resection is the most important factor influencing prognosis. For instance, Perzin, Gullane, and Clairmont[104] found only 12 of 58 patients (20%) with ACC who had negative margins of resection. The outcome of this group of patients was significantly better than the 46 patients with evidence of tumor at the margins of surgical resection (Fig. 69-43).

Although Garden and others[52] agree that microscopic positive margins constitute an adverse prognostic factor,

Table 69-9. Incidence of local extension/fixation by site of origin in adenoid cystic carcinoma

Fixation or extension to contiguous structures	
Sinonasal, larynx, pharynx	39/49 (80%)
Mouth	63/125 (50%)
Parotid/submandibular	23/68 (34%)

Spiro R, Huvos A, Strong E: Adenoid cystic carcinoma of salivary origin: a clinicopathologic study of 242 cases, *Am J Surg* 128:512, 1974.

they contend that even when present, local control was possible in more than 80% of their patients with ACC treated with aggressive surgery and postoperative radiotherapy (see Fig. 69-11). Using this approach and with a minimum follow-up period of 2 years, 15 of the 83 patients (18%) with positive margins developed local recurrences compared with 5 of 55 patients (9%) with close or uncertain margins and with 3 of 60 patients (5%) with negative margins (P = 0.02). There was a trend toward better local control with increasing radiation dose in patients with positive margins. Crude control rates were 40% and 88% for doses of less than 56 Gy and 56 Gy or higher, respectively (P = 0.006). They concluded that excellent local control rates were obtained in this population using surgery and postoperative radiotherapy and recommended a radiation dose of 66 Gy for patients with positive margins. Despite effective local therapy, failure as a result of distant metastatic disease remains a major problem in these patients, and effective management to address this problem is lacking.[52]

Perineural spread

Perineural spread (PNS) carries with it a poor prognosis in patients with SCC of the head and neck.[130] Whether this is because of an inherently aggressive behavior of tumors with neurotropic tendency or because of the difficulty of obtaining tumor-free margins of resection in these patients is still unclear.[58] There is still considerable controversy about the prognostic importance of PNS in patients with ACC. The incidence of PNS in patients with ACC is overwhelmingly high and, as previously mentioned, depends on the diligence of the pathologist in searching for and reporting this peculiar and almost universal neurotropism of ACC. There have been conflicting reports in the literature regarding the prognostic importance of finding perineural spread

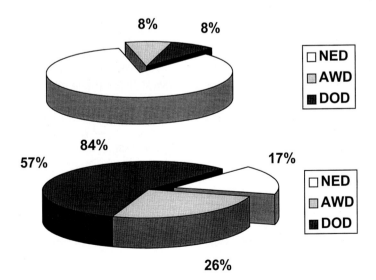

Fig. 69-43. The effect of surgical margins on the outcome of 62 patients with adenoid cystic carcinoma.

Table 69-10. Chapter highlights

Summary	Highlights
General	70% of salivary tumors occur in the parotid gland, three fourths of which are benign, mostly pleomorphic adenomas.
	Most minor salivary gland tumors are malignant. The palate is the most common site, and the most common histology is adenoid cystic carcinoma, followed by mucoepidermoid carcinoma.
Clinical presentation	Salivary gland tumors present mostly as painless swellings.
	Signs of malignancy include:
	Nerve paralysis
	Ulceration
	Pain
	Rapid growth
	Fixation
	Nodal metastasis
Fine-needle biopsy	Safe, inexpensive, accurate
	Helps establish the diagnosis and plan management
Imaging	Computed tomography/magnetic resonance imaging are the studies of choice.
	Indications:
	Large tumors of the parotid
	Deep-lobe parotid tumors
	Parapharyngeal tumors
	Malignant tumors
	Minor salivary gland tumors
	Most submandibular gland tumors
Treatment	Benign: Complete surgical excision.
	Malignant:
	En bloc surgical excision of the primary tumor
	Therapeutic neck dissection for N+ patients
	Elective neck dissection for N0 patients with advanced or high-grade tumors
Radiation therapy	Postoperative radiation for malignant tumors with any of the following poor prognostic indicators:
	Advanced stage
	High grade
	Nodal metastasis
	Facial nerve paralysis
	Perineural spread
	Positive margins
	Neutron therapy for inoperable malignant tumors

in ACC, although there is considerable evidence to suggest that involvement of "major" or "named" nerves is a poor prognostic indicator.

Recently, Garden and others[52] found evidence of PNS in 136 of 198 patients (69%) with ACC and in whom 55 patients (28%) had invasion in a major (named) nerve. Perineural invasion was an adverse prognostic factor only when a major (named) nerve was involved. The crude failure rates in patients with and without a major (named) nerve involved were 18% (10 out of 55) and 9% (13 out of 143), respectively ($P = 0.02$).

Facial nerve paralysis

Eneroth[42] reported facial nerve paralysis in 46 of 378 patients (12%) with cancer of the parotid gland. All of the patients with facial nerve paralysis eventually died of their disease, and the average survival time after the onset of paralysis was 2.7 years. The incidence of systemic metastasis in these patients was 77%. Similarly, Spiro, Huvos, and

Strong[135] found evidence of facial nerve dysfunction in 43 of 288 patients (15%) with carcinoma of the parotid gland. Their study did not support Eneroth's assertion that the presence of facial nerve paralysis is invariably a sign of incurable cancer of the parotid gland, and they reported a 5-year survival rate of 14% in such patients. Conley and Hamaker reported that 9 of 34 patients (27%) with facial paralysis were free of disease at 5 years.[36] It is clear from these studies that although facial nerve paralysis may not be associated with a 100% mortality rate, it is an indicator of a poor prognosis.

Pain

Patients with ACC who present with pain appear to have a less favorable outcome compared with patients presenting with an asymptomatic swelling. The 10-year "cure" rate was only 13% for patients presenting with pain compared with 29% for patients presenting with a painless swelling.[134] This finding may be as result of an increased likelihood of pain in the presence of local invasion of bone or sensory nerves.

REFERENCES

1. Abad MM and others: Statistical evaluation of the predictive power of fine needle aspiration (FNA) of salivary glands. Results and cyto-histological correlation, *Pathol Res Pract* 188:340, 1992.
2. Abrams AM, Melrose RJ, Howell FV: Necrotizing sialometaplasia, *Cancer* 32:130, 1973.
3. Airoldi M and others: Chemotherapy for recurrent salivary gland malignancies: experience of the ENT Department of Turin University, *ORL J Otorhinolaryngol Relat Spec* 56:105, 1994.
4. Ajayi BA and others: Salivary gland tumours: is colour Doppler imaging of added value in their preoperative assessment? *Eur J Surg Oncol* 18:463, 1992.
5. Albeck H and others: Familial clusters of nasopharyngeal carcinoma and salivary gland carcinomas in Greenland natives, *Cancer* 72:196, 1993.
6. Armstrong JG and others: The indications for elective treatment of the neck in cancer of the major salivary glands, *Cancer* 69:615, 1992.
7. Arthaud JB: Anaplastic parotid carcinoma (''malignant lymphoepithelial lesions'') in seven Alaskan natives, *Am J Clin Pathol* 57:275, 1972.
8. Auclair PL, Goode RK, Ellis GL: Mucoepidermoid carcinoma of intraoral salivary glands: evaluation and application of grading criteria in 143 cases, *Cancer* 69:2021, 1992.
9. Batsakis JG: Oral monomorphic adenomas, *Ann Otol Rhinol Laryngol* 100:348, 1991.
10. Batsakis JG: Nerves and neurotropic carcinomas, *Ann Otol Rhinol Laryngol* 94:426, 1985.
11. Batsakis JG: *Tumors of the head and neck*, Baltimore, 1979, Williams & Wilkins.
12. Batsakis JG and others: Malignancy and the benign lymphoepithelial lesion, *Laryngoscope* 85:389, 1975.
13. Batsakis JG, el-Naggar AK, Luna MA: ''Adenocarcinoma, not otherwise specified'': a diminishing group of salivary carcinomas, *Ann Otol Rhinol Laryngol* 101:102, 1992.
14. Batsakis JG, el-Naggar AK, Luna MA: Epithelial-myoepithelial carcinoma of salivary glands, *Ann Otol Rhinol Laryngol* 101:540, 1992.
15. Batsakis JG, el-Naggar AK, Luna MA: Hyalinizing clear cell carcinoma of salivary origin, *Ann Otol Rhinol Laryngol* 103:746, 1994.
16. Batsakis JG, Regezi JA: The pathology of head and neck tumors: salivary glands. Part 1, *Head Neck Surg* 1:59, 1978.
17. Batsakis JG and others: Adenocarcinoma of the oral cavity: a clinicopathologic study of terminal duct carcinoma, *J Laryngol Otol* 97:825, 1983.
18. Batsakis JG and others: Primary squamous cell carcinoma of the parotid gland, *Arch Otolaryngol* 102:355, 1976.
19. Beckhardt RN and others: Minor salivary gland tumors of the palate: clinical and pathologic correlates of outcome, *Laryngoscope* 105:1155, 1995.
20. Bhatia A: Fine needle aspiration cytology in the diagnosis of mass lesions of the salivary gland, *Indian J Cancer* 30:26, 1993.
21. Billroth T: Die Cylindergeschwulst (cylindroma) in Untersuchungen uber die Entwicklung der Blutgerfarse, nebst Beobachtungen aus der Koniglichen chirurgischen Universitats-Kilinik zu Berlin, Berlin, 1856, G Reimer.
22. Borsanyi SJ, Blanchard CL: Asymptomatic enlargement of the parotid glands in alcoholic cirrhosis, *South Med J* 54:678, 1961.
23. Borthne A and others: Salivary gland malignant neoplasms: treatment and prognosis, *Int J Radiat Oncol Biol Physics* 12:747, 1986.
24. Brick IB: Parotid enlargement in cirrhosis of the liver, *Ann Intern Med* 49:438, 1958.
25. Buchholz TA and others: The role of fast neutron radiation therapy in the management of advanced salivary gland malignant neoplasms, *Cancer* 69:2779, 1992.
26. Byers RM, Jesse RH, Guillamondequi OM: Malignant tumors of the submaxillary gland, *Am J Surg* 126:458, 1973.
27. Candel A and others: Is fine needle aspiration biopsy of salivary gland masses really necessary? *Ear Nose Throat J* 72:485, 1993.
28. Catterall M, Errington RD: The implications of improved treatment of malignant salivary gland tumors by fast neutron radiotherapy, *Int J Rad Oncol Biol Physics* 13:1313, 1987.
29. Chan MK and others: Cytodiagnosis of 112 salivary gland lesions. Correlation with histologic and frozen section diagnosis, *Acta Cytol* 36:353, 1992.
30. Chan JK and others: Specific association of Epstein-Barr virus with lymphoepithelial carcinoma among tumors and tumorlike lesions of the salivary gland, *Arch Pathol Lab Med* 118:994, 1994.
31. Cheng J and others: Biosynthesis of basement membrane molecules by salivary adenoid cystic carcinoma cells: an immunofluorescence and confocal microscopic study, *Virchows Arch* 426:577, 1995.
32. Cho KJ and others: Epithelial-myoepithelial carcinoma of salivary glands. A clinicopathologic, DNA flow cytometric, and immunohistochemical study of Ki-67 and HER-2/neu oncogene, *Am J Clin Pathol* 103:432, 1995.
33. Clode and others: Mucoepidermoid carcinoma of the salivary glands: a reprisal of the influence of tumor differentiation on prognosis, *J Surg Oncol* 46:100, 1991.
34. Colmenero C, Patron M, Sierra I: Acinic cell carcinoma of the salivary glands, *J Craniomaxillofac Surg* 19:260, 1991.
35. Conley J, Casler J: *Data and statistics*. In Conley J, Casler J, editors: *Adenoid cystic cancer of the head and neck*, New York, 1991, Thieme.
36. Conley J, Hamaker RC: Prognosis of malignant tumors of the parotid gland with facial paralysis, *Arch Otol* 101:39, 1975.
37. Dardick I, Burford-Mason AP: Current status of histogenetic and morphogenetic concepts of salivary gland tumorigenesis, *Crit Rev Oral Biol Med* 4:639, 1993.
38. Dockerty MB, Mayo CW: Tumors of the submaxillary gland with special reference to mixed tumors, *Surg Gynecol Obstet* 74:1033, 1942.
39. Eisenberger MA: Supporting evidence for an active treatment program for advanced salivary gland carcinomas, *Cancer Treatment Reports* 69:319, 1985.
40. El-Naggar AK and others: A mucoepidermoid carcinoma of minor salivary gland with t(11;19) (q21; p3.1) as the only karyotypic abnormality, *Cancer Gen Cytogen* 87:29, 1996.
41. El-Naggar A and others: Trisomy 5 as the sole chromosomal abnormality in a primary mucoepidermoid carcinoma of the minor salivary gland, *Cancer Gen Cytogen* 76:96, 1994.
42. Eneroth CM: Facial paralysis: a criterion of malignancy in parotid tumors, *Arch Otol* 95:300, 1972.
43. Eneroth CM, Hjertman L, Moberger G: Adenoid cystic carcinoma of the palate, *Acta Otolaryngol* 66:248, 1968.
44. Epivatianos A, Dimitrakopoulos J, Trigonidis G: Intraoral salivary duct carcinoma: a clinicopathological study of four cases and review of the literature, *Ann Dentist* 54:36, 1995.
45. Evans RW, Cruickshank AH: *Epithelial tumors of the salivary glands*, Philadelphia, 1970, WB Saunders.
46. Fonseca I and others: Simple mucin-type carbohydrate antigens (T, Tn and sialosyl-Tn) in mucoepidermoid carcinoma of the salivary glands, *Histopathology* 25:537, 1994.
47. Fonseca I, Soares J: Epithelial-myoepithelial carcinoma of the salivary glands. A study of 22 cases, *Virchows Arch A Pathol Anat Histopathol* 422:389, 1993.
48. Foote FW, Frazell EL: *Tumors of the major salivary glands*, Cancer 6:1065, 1953.
49. Fu KK and others: Carcinoma of the major and minor salivary glands: analysis and treatment results and sites and causes of failures, *Cancer* 40:2882, 1977.

50. Gaisford JC, Anderson VS: First branchial cleft cysts and sinuses, *Plast Reconstr Surg* 55:299, 1975.

51. Garden AS and others: Postoperative radiation therapy for malignant tumors of minor salivary glands. Outcome and patterns of failure, *Cancer* 73:2563, 1994.

52. Garden AS and others: The influence of positive margins and nerve invasion in adenoid cystic carcinoma of the head and neck treated with surgery and radiation, *Int J Rad Oncol Biol Physics* 32:619, 1995.

53. Godwin JT: Benign lymphoepithelial lesion of the parotid gland, *Cancer* 5:1089, 1952.

54. Gravanis MB, Giansanti JS: Malignant histopathologic counterpart of the benign lymphoepithelial lesion, *Cancer* 26:1332, 1970.

55. Griffin TW and others: Neutron vs photon irradiation of inoperable salivary gland tumors: results of an RTOG-MRC cooperative randomized study, *Int J Rad Oncol Biol Physics* 15:1085, 1988.

56. Gritzman N: Sonography of the salivary glands, *Am J Roentgenol* 153:161, 1989.

57. Guillamondequi OM and others: Aggressive surgery in treatment for parotid cancer: the role of adjunctive postoperative radiotherapy, *AJR Am J Roentgenol* 123:49, 1975.

58. Hanna E, Janecka I: Perineural spread in head and neck and skull base cancer, *Crit Rev Neurosurg* 4:109, 1994.

59. Hehrs OH and others, editors: *Salivary glands (including parotid, submaxillary and sublingual). In American Joint Committee on Cancer: manual for staging of cancer,* eds, Philadelphia, 1988, JB Lippincott.

60. Heller KS: *Salivary gland cancer–diagnostic evaluation. In* Johnson JT, Didolkar, editors: *Head and neck cancer,* vol 3, 1993, Elsevier Science Publishing.

61. Heller KS and others: Value of the fine needle aspiration biopsy of salivary gland masses in clinical decision-making, *Am J Surg* 164:667, 1992.

62. Hemenway WG, Allen GW: Chronic enlargement of the parotid gland: hypertrophy and fatty infiltration, *Laryngoscope* 69:1508, 1959.

63. Henry LW and others: Evolution of fast neutron teletherapy for advanced carcinomas of the major salivary glands, *Cancer* 44:814, 1979.

64. Hickman RE, Cawson RA, Duffy SW: The prognosis of specific types of salivary gland tumors, *Cancer* 54:1620, 1984.

65. Hicks MJ and others: Histocytologic grading of mucoepidermoid carcinoma of major salivary glands in prognosis and survival: a clinicopathologic and flow cytometric investigation, *Head Neck* 17:89, 1995.

66. Higashi T and others: Technetium-99m pertechnetate and gallium-67 imaging in salivary gland disease, *Clin Nucl Med* 14:504, 1989.

67. Hosokawa Y and others: Analysis of adenoid cystic carcinoma treated by radiotherapy, *Oral Surg Oral Med Oral Pathol* 74:251, 1992.

68. Huang RD and others: Benign cystic vs. solid lesions of the parotid gland in HIV patients, *Head Neck* 13:522, 1991.

69. Johns MM III and others: Allelotype of salivary gland tumors, *Cancer Res* 56:1151, 1996.

70. Jones AS and others: A randomized phase II trial of epirubicin and 5-fluorouracil versus cisplatinum in the palliation of advanced and recurrent malignant tumour of the salivary glands, *Br J Cancer* 67:112, 1993.

71. Jordan RC, Speight PM: Lymphoma in Sjögren's syndrome. From histopathology to molecular pathology, *Oral Surg Oral Med Oral Path Oral Radiol Endodont* 81:308, 1996.

72. Kahn LB: Benign lymphoepithelial lesion (Mikulicz' disease) of the salivary gland: an ultrastructural study, *Human Pathol* 10:99, 1979.

73. Kaneda T and others: Imaging tumors of the minor salivary glands, *Oral Surg Oral Med Oral Pathol* 78:385, 1994.

74. Kaplan MJ, Johns ME, Cantrell RW: Chemotherapy for salivary gland cancer, *Otolaryngol Head Neck Surg* 95:165, 1986.

75. Keyes JW Jr and others: Salivary gland tumors: pretherapy evaluation with PET, *Radiology* 192:99, 1994.

76. Koh W and others: Fast neutron radiation for inoperable and recurrent salivary gland cancers, *Am J Clin Oncol* 12:316, 1989.

77. Land CE and others: Incidence of salivary gland tumors among atomic bomb survivors, 1950–1987. Evaluation of radiation-related risk, *Radiat Res* 146:28, 1996.

78. Laramore GE: Fast neutron radiotherapy for inoperable salivary gland tumors: is it the treatment of choice? *Int J Rad Oncol Biol Phys* 13:1421, 1987.

79. Laramore GE and others: Neutron versus photon irradiation for unresectable salivary gland tumors: final report of an RTOG-MRC randomized clinical trial, *Int J Rad Oncol Biol Phys* 27:235, 1993.

80. Larson and others: Perineural lymphatics: myth or fact, *Am J Surg* 112:488, 1966.

81. Laudadio P, Leroni AR, Cerasoli PT: Metastatic malignant melanoma in the parotid gland, *ORL J Otorhinolaryngol Relat Spec* 46:42, 1984.

82. Lee K, McKean ME, McGregor IA: Metastatic patterns of squamous carcinoma in the parotid lymph nodes, *Br J Plast Surg* 38:6, 1985.

83. Leonetti and others: Subtotal petrosectomy in the management of advanced parotid neoplasms, *Otolaryngol Head Neck Surg* 108:270, 1993.

84. Leung SY and others: Lymphoepithelial carcinoma of the salivary gland: in situ detection of Epstein-Barr virus, *J Clin Pathol* 48:1022, 1995.

85. Levin JM, Robinson DW, Lin F: Acinic cell carcinoma: collective review including bilateral cases, *Arch Surg* 110:64, 1975.

86. Levin RJ, Bradley MK: Neuroectodermal antigens persist in benign and malignant salivary gland tumor cultures, *Arch Otolaryngol Head Neck Surg* 122:551, 1996.

87. Lewis JE and others: Salivary duct carcinoma. Clinicopathologic and immunohistochemical review of 26 cases, *Cancer* 77:223, 1996.

88. Li X and others: A fluorescence in situ hybridization (FISH) analysis with centromere-specific DNA probes of chromosomes 3 and 17 in pleomorphic adenomas and adenoid cystic carcinomas, *J Oral Pathol Med* 24:398, 1995.

89. Lorain P, Robin C: Memoire sur deux nouvelles observations de tumeurs heteradeniques et sur la nature du tissu qui les compose, *CR Soc Biol* 6:209, 1854.

90. MacLeod CB, Frable WJ: Fine-needle aspiration biopsy of the salivary gland: problem cases, *Diagn Cytopathol* 9:216, 1993.

91. Mandel L, Baurmash H: Parotid enlargement due to alcoholism, *J Am Dent Assoc* 82:369, 1971.

92. Martinoli C and others: Color Doppler sonography of salivary glands, *AJR Am J Roentgenol* 163:933, 1994.

93. Milchgrub S and others: Hyalinizing clear cell carcinoma of salivary gland, *Am J Surg Pathol* 18:74, 1994.

94. Mulliken JB, Young AE: *Vascular birthmarks,* Philadelphia, 1988, WB Saunders.

95. Murrah VA, Batsakis JG: Salivary duct carcinoma, *Ann Otol Rhinol Laryngol* 103:244, 1994.

96. Nagao T and others: Epstein-Barr virus-associated undifferentiated carcinoma with lymphoid stroma of the salivary gland in Japanese patients. Comparison with benign lymphoepithelial lesion, *Cancer* 78:695, 1996.

97. Nordkvist A and others: Recurrent rearrangements of 11q14-22 in mucoepidermoid carcinoma, *Cancer Gen Cytogen* 74:77, 1994.

98. Olsen KD: Tumors and surgery of the parapharyngeal space, *Laryngoscope* 104(suppl 63):1, 1994.

99. Olsen KD, Maragos NF, Weiland LH: First branchial cleft abnormalities, *Laryngoscope* 90:423, 1980.

100. Orell SR: Diagnostic difficulties in the interpretation of fine needle aspirates of salivary gland lesions: the problem revisited, *Cytopathology* 6:285, 1995.

101. Pammer J and others: Expression of bcl-2 in salivary glands and salivary gland adenomas. A contribution to the reserve cell theory, *Pathol Res Pract* 191:35, 1995.

102. Parsons JT and others: Management of minor salivary gland carcinomas, *Int J Radiat Oncol Biol Phys* 35:443, 1996.

103. Peel RL, Gnepp DR: *Disease of the salivary glands.* In Barnes L, editor: *Surgical pathology of the head and neck,* New York, 1985, Marcel Dekker.

104. Perzin KH, Gullane P, Clairmont AC: Adenoid cystic carcinoma in the salivary glands: a correlation of histologic features and clinical course, *Cancer* 42:265, 1978.

105. Perzin KH, LiVolsi VA: Acinic cell carcinoma arising in the salivary glands: a clinicopathologic study, *Cancer* 44:1434, 1979.

106. Pieterse AS, Seymour AE: Parotid cysts. An analysis of 16 cases and suggested classification, *Pathology* 13:225, 1981.

107. Pinkston JA, Cole P: Cigarette smoking and Warthin's tumor, *Am J Epidemiol* 144:183, 1996.

108. Pinkus GS, Dekker A: Benign lymphoepithelial lesion of parotid glands associated with reticulum cell sarcoma, *Cancer* 25:121, 1970.

109. Pitts DB and others: Fine-needle aspiration in the diagnosis of salivary gland disorders in the community hospital setting, *Arch Otolaryngol Head Neck Surg* 118:479, 1992.

110. Plambeck K and others: Mucoepidermoid carcinoma of the salivary glands, clinical data and follow-up of 52 cases, *J Cancer Res Clin Oncol* 122:177, 1996.

111. Posner MR and others: Chemotherapy of advanced salivary gland neoplasms, *Cancer* 50:2261, 1982.

112. Rentschler R, Burgess MA, Byers R: Chemotherapy of malignant major salivary gland neoplasms. A 25-year review of M.D. Anderson Hospital experience, *Cancer* 40:619, 1977.

113. Rodriguez-Cuevas S and others: Risk of nodal metastases from malignant salivary gland tumors related to tumor size and grade of malignancy, *Eur Arch Otorhinolaryngol* 252:139, 1995.

114. Roland NJ and others: Fine needle aspiration cytology of salivary gland lesions reported immediately in a head and neck clinic, *J Laryngol Otol* 107:1025, 1993.

115. Ryan Jr and others: Acquired immunodeficiency syndrome-related lymphadenopathies presenting in the salivary lymph nodes, *Arch Otolaryngol Head Neck Surg* 3:554, 1985.

116. Sadeghi A and others: Minor salivary gland tumors of the head and neck: treatment strategies and prognosis, *Am J Clin Oncol* 16:3, 1993.

117. Sakata K and others: Radiation therapy for patients of malignant salivary gland tumors with positive surgical margins, *Strahlentherapie und Onkologie* 170:342, 1994.

118. Santis HR and others: Necrotizing sialometaplasia: an early, nonulcerative presentation, *Oral Surg* 53:387, 1982.

119. Saroja KR and others: An update on malignant salivary gland tumors treated with neutrons at Fermilab, *Int J Rad Oncol Biol Physics* 13:1319, 1987.

120. Sato S, Kawamura H: Acinic cell tumor of the hard palate, *Int J Oral Maxillofac Surg* 20:271, 1991.

121. Seifert G: Histopathology of malignant salivary gland tumours, *Eur J Cancer B Oral Oncol* 28B:49, 1992.

122. Seifert G, Sobin LH: The World Health Organization's histological classification of salivary gland tumors: a commentary on the second edition, *Cancer* 70:379, 1992.

123. Shafer WG, Hine MK, Levy BM: *Oral pathology,* Philadelphia, 1974, WB Saunders.

124. Shemen LJ, Huvos AG, Spiro RH: Squamous cell carcinoma of salivary gland origin, *Head Neck Surg* 9:235, 1987.

125. Shingaki S and others: The role of radiotherapy in the management of salivary gland carcinomas, *J Cranio Maxillo Facial Surg* 20:220, 1992.

126. Simpson RH: Classification of salivary gland tumours—a brief histopathological review, *Histopathology* 10:737, 1995.

127. Sismanis A and others: Diagnosis of salivary gland tumors by fine-needle aspiration biopsy, *Head Neck Surg* 3:482, 1981.

128. Sisson GA, Summers GW: Branchiogenic cysts within the parotid gland, *Arch Otolaryngol* 96:165, 1972.

129. Slichenmyer WJ, LeMaistre CF, Von Hoff DD: Response of metastatic adenoid cystic carcinoma and Merkel cell tumor to high-dose melphalan with autologous bone marrow transplantation, *Invest N Drugs* 10:45, 1992.

130. Soo KC and others: Prognostic implications of perineural spread in squamous cell carcinomas of the head and neck, *Laryngoscope* 96:1145, 1986.

131. Spiro RH: Salivary neoplasms: overview of a 35-year experience with 2,807 patients, *Head Neck Surg* 8:177, 1986.

132. Spiro RH, Huvos AG: Stage means more than grade in adenoid cystic carcinoma, *Am J Surg* 164:623, 1992.

133. Spiro RH, Huvos AG, Strong EW: Acinic cell carcinoma of salivary origin: a clinicopathologic study of 67 cases, *Cancer* 41:924, 1978.

134. Spiro R, Huvos A, Strong E: Adenoid cystic carcinoma of salivary origin: a clinicopathologic study of 242 cases, *Am J Surg* 128:512, 1974.

135. Spiro RH, Huvos AG, Strong EW: Cancer of the parotid gland: a clinicopathologic study of 288 primary cases, *Am J Surg* 130:452, 1975.

136. Spiro RH and others: The importance of clinical staging of minor salivary gland carcinoma, *Am J Surg* 162:330, 1991.

137. Spitz MR, Batsakis JG: Major salivary gland carcinoma: descriptive epidemiology and survival of 498 patients, *Arch Otolaryngol Head Neck Surg* 110:45, 1984.

138. Stanley MW and others: Basal cell (monomorphic) and minimally pleomorphic adenomas of the salivary glands. Distinction from the solid (anaplastic) type of adenoid cystic carcinoma in fine-needle aspiration, *Am J Clin Pathol* 106:35, 1996.

139. Stelzer KJ and others: Fast neutron radiotherapy. The University of Washington experience, *Acta Oncol* 33:275, 1994.

140. Suen JY, Johns ME: Chemotherapy for salivary gland cancer, *Laryngoscope* 92:235, 1982.

141. Takahashi H and others: Primary malignant lymphoma of the salivary gland: a tumor of mucosa-associated lymphoid tissue, *J Oral Pathol Med* 21:318, 1992.

142. Talal N: *Sjögren's syndrome and connective tissue disease with other immunologic disorders.* In McCarty DJ, editor: *Arthritis and allied conditions,* ed 9, Philadelphia, 1979, Lea & Febiger.

143. Thackray AC, Lucas RB: *Tumors of the major salivary glands, atlas of pathology,* series II, fascicle 10, Washington DC, 1974, Armed Forces Institute of Pathology.

144. Theriault C, Fitzpatrick PJ: Malignant parotid tumors: prognostic factors and optimum treatment, *Am J Clin Oncol* 9:510, 1986.

145. Therkildsen MH and others: Simple mucin-type Tn and sialosyl-Tn carbohydrate antigens in salivary gland carcinomas, *Cancer* 72:1147, 1993.

146. Tsai CC, Chen CL, Hsu HC: Expression of Epstein-Barr virus in carcinomas of major salivary glands: a strong association with lymphoepithelioma-like carcinoma, *Human Pathol* 27:258, 1996.

147. Venook AP and others: Cisplatin, doxorubicin, and 5-fluorouracil chemotherapy for salivary gland malignancies: a pilot study of the Northern California Oncology Group, *J Clin Oncol* 5:951, 1987.

148. Vincent SD, Hammond HL, Finkelstein MW: Clinical and therapeutic features of polymorphous low-grade adenocarcinoma, *Oral Surg Oral Med Oral Pathol* 77:41, 1994.

149. Waldron CA: The histopathology of Sjögren's syndrome in labial salivary gland biopsies, *Oral Surg* 37:217, 1974.

150. Wallace AC and others: Salivary gland tumors in Canadian Eskimos, *Cancer* 16:1338, 1963.

151. Waner M, Suen JY: The treatment of hemangiomas of the head and neck, *Laryngoscope* 102:1123, 1991.

152. Wang CC, Goodman M: Photon irradiation of unresectable car-

cinomas of salivary glands, *Int J Rad Oncol Biol Phys* 21:569, 1991.

153. Weber RS and others: Submandibular gland tumors: Adverse histologic factors and therapeutic implications, *Arch Otolaryngol Head Neck Surg* 116:1055, 1990.

154. Weitzner S: Lymphoepithelial (branchial) cyst of parotid gland, *Oral Surg* 35:85, 1973.

155. Woods JE: The facial nerve in parotid malignancy, *Am J Surg* 146:493, 1983.

156. Woods JE, Chong GC, Beahrs OH: Experience with 1,360 primary parotid tumors, *Am J Surg* 130:460, 1975.

157. Work WP: Cysts and congenital lesions of the parotid gland, *Otolaryngol Clin North Am* 10:339, 1977.

158. Work WP: Newer concepts of first branchial cleft defects, *Laryngoscope* 82:1581, 1972.

159. Work WP, Hecht DW: Non-neoplastic lesions of the parotid gland, *Ann Otol Rhinol Laryngol* 77:462, 1968.

160. Work WP, Proctor CA: The otologist and first branchial cleft anomalies, *Ann Otol Rhinol Laryngol* 72:548, 1963.

161. Zheng W and others: Diet and other risk factors for cancer of the salivary glands: a population-based case-control study, *Int J Cancer* 67:194, 1996.

Chapter 70

Rehabilitation of Facial Paralysis

Roger L. Crumley
Timothy A. Scott
William B. Armstrong

Unilateral facial paralysis is usually a devastating emotional ordeal. The ability to restore symmetry and motion to patients afflicted with facial paralysis is one of the most rewarding skills of the well-trained reconstructive surgeon. This chapter discusses rehabilitation of facial nerve injuries. Many of the diagnostic considerations and surgical techniques described are applicable to otogenic paralyses (intratemporal), as well as injuries and diseases that affect the parotid and facial portions of the facial nerve.

The facial nerve, once damaged, rarely attains full recovery of function. The slightest injury to one branch, even if the nerve is not divided, may produce permanent weakness or an other dysfunction, such as spasm or synkinesis. Any patient sustaining facial nerve injuries or contemplating parotidectomy, and any preoperative patient with the slightest chance of sustaining surgical facial nerve injury should be told that his or her face will never regain *normal* movements. It is worthwhile for the surgeon to take an extra moment to confirm that the patient understands this concept. Videotapes, photographs, or movies of other patients are often necessary before the true meaning of facial paralysis is conveyed to the patient.

Many patients listen to the physician's words, yet are unable to fully understand the visual impact of facial paralysis or synkinesis. Therefore, it is unwise and unfair to describe hypoglossal-facial anastomosis or muscle transposition in such a way that the patient may believe that the facial nerve and movements will be restored. A realistic approach yields the rewards of patient compliance, understanding, satisfaction, and acceptance of reality.

CAUSES OF FACIAL PARALYSIS

The pathogenesis and eventual course of facial paralysis vary depending on the causative injury or disease. Bell's palsy, for example, rarely requires facial reanimation surgery. This chapter focuses on clinical situations requiring surgical reanimation.

REANIMATION MODALITIES

In clinical situations requiring facial reanimation, the technique used often depends on the availability of a viable proximal facial nerve. Tumor ablation with facial nerve sacrifice (as in radical parotidectomy for parotid malignancy) dictates immediate facial nerve restitution, usually by cable grafting. When the nerve's continuity and viability are in question, however, as may be seen during and following cerebellopontine angle surgery, it is wise to wait 9 to 12 months before an extratemporal facial nerve operative procedure is undertaken. Hence, no modality is universally appropriate for all afflictions of facial nerve function. As a general rule, however, the order of preference is as follows:

1. Spontaneous facial nerve regeneration (observation)
2. Facial nerve neurorrhaphy
3. Facial nerve cable graft
4. Nerve transposition
5. Muscle transposition

FACTORS DETERMINING REHABILITATION

A wide array of facial reanimation operations are available to the surgeon. Many of these procedures provide dramatic corrective results when appropriately applied, but their use may be injudicious in other patients.

Any single protocol is ill advised for the management of facial paralysis because patients' needs vary. The high school student with a parotid malignancy deserves the best long-term reanimation result possible; the ipsilateral nerve should be used in such cases. A nerve graft or substitution in an elderly person with a malignancy would be ill advised because the immediate result gained from a fascia or muscle sling would be preferable. Cosmetic results are not as important for this latter patient, so the most expeditious procedure to restore function should be selected. All the factors determining the outcome of rehabilitation should be considered before any facial reanimation procedure is undertaken. Many of these procedures depend on the status of the existing muscles and nerves; other procedures depend on the patient's ability to achieve animation following the procedures and factors such as age, radiation exposure, and any preexisting disease, such as diabetes, and so forth.

Needs of the patient

The patient's needs should be paramount in surgical planning for facial paralysis. Naturally, if the patient demands that normal function be restored, no operation will prove satisfactory because normal function is generally irretrievable.

Factors influencing the timing and performance of facial reanimation procedures follow:

1. Eye protection
2. Presence of partial regeneration
3. Donor site morbidity
4. Proximal and distal nerve integrity
5. Viability of facial muscles (no denervation atrophy)
6. Status of donor nerves
7. Time elapsed since last injury
8. Age
9. Radiation injury
10. Diabetes and other metabolic and/or vascular disorders
11. Nutrition

Eye protection

Evaluation and treatment of eyelid paralysis

Ocular symptoms in facial palsy arise from several mechanisms. The ability to prevent, diagnose, and treat paralytic eyelid sequelae before major complications occur is essential in treating any patient with facial paralysis. In most patients the outcome of the paralyzed eyelid is directly related to patient education and compliance. It is therefore the physician's responsibility to work closely with the patient to ensure understanding of the goals of eye care as well as the potential for serious ocular complications.

Paralysis of the orbicularis oculi results in drying and exposure of the cornea. Inability to protect the cornea occurs secondary to ectropion because the atonic lower lid and lacri-mal punctum fail to appose the globe and bulbar conjunctiva. This causes faulty eyelid closure and improper distribution of tears across the cornea.

Epiphora may result from failure of tears to enter the lacrimal punctum, secondary to the loss of the orbicularis oculi tear-pumping mechanism. The response to abnormal corneal sensation may be reflex tear hypersecretion, which further increases the epiphora.

Any facial paralysis patient with a poor Bell's phenomenon is at risk for developing exposure keratitis. Eye pain may herald the onset of keratitis. However in patients with diminished corneal sensation, exposure keratitis may asymptomatically progress to corneal ulceration. Thus, all patients with diminished orbicularis oculi function should have ophthalmologic consultation.

Nonsurgical methods of treatment

Initial efforts in eye care should be directed toward moisturizing the dry eye and preventing exposure. If the eyelid paralysis is temporary or partial, these local measures may be all that are necessary to protect the eye adequately. Artificial tears are commonly the first method used to keep the eye moist. Ointments also may be used, but they are less practical in the daytime because they tend to blur vision.

Lacriserts, contact lenses, and occlusive bubbles are commonly used, although patient compliance may be problematic[22] (Fig. 70-1). The eyelids are frequently patched or taped, but if incorrectly used, these methods may result in corneal injuries. Tape should not be placed vertically across the eyelashes, but applied horizontally above the eyelashes on the upper eyelid, or supporting the lateral canthal portions of the lower eyelid.[64] When an eye patch is used, care must be taken that the eye cannot open because this allows contact between the patch and the cornea.

Surgical methods

Procedures to treat the paralyzed lower lid (ectropion)

Tarsorrhaphy. The temporary lateral tarsorrhaphy is an expeditious and effective method for protecting the eye in patients with mild lagophthalmos and mild corneal exposure. A horizontal mattress suture of 7-0 silk or nylon is placed laterally so as to approximate the gray line (mucocutaneous junction) of the upper and lower lids. Tarsorraphy sutures will remain effective longer if they are placed through bolsters made of rubber (Robinson) catheters.

For longer lasting protection, the lid adhesion tarsorraphy is preferred. The lid margin (gray line) of each lid is denuded 4 to 6 mm from the lateral canthus, and a similar suture technique is used to approximate the denuded mucocutaneous junctions of upper and lower lids (Fig. 70-2). Like the temporary lateral tarsorraphy, this procedure can be reversed if function returns.

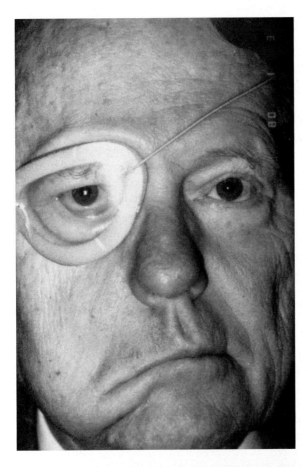

Fig. 70-1. Occlusive bubble worn by a patient following acoustic neuroma surgery. The appliance has a foam rubber skin contact surface that is firmly attached to a thin plexiglass lens. The authors have found that patient compliance is relatively high with this type of device. (Courtesy of Moisture Chamber, Pro-optics, Palatine, Ill.)

Fig. 70-2. A, Tiny single skin hook being used to avert the lower lid for denuding of ''gray line'' (mucocutaneous junction). Note that gray line of upper lid has been denuded. **B,** Healed tarsorraphy at 4 months. Increased eye closure may be achieved by extending the denudation and sutures medially.

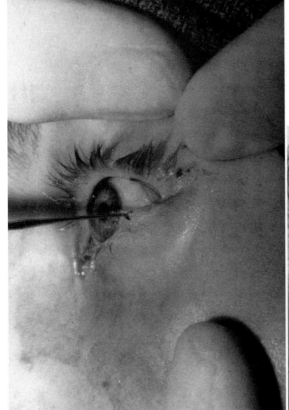

A

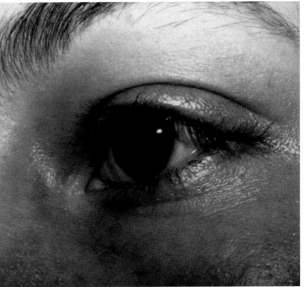

B

Wedge resection and canthoplasty. Wedge resection and canthoplasty are highly effective methods in the repair of paralytic ectropion. Wedge resection of all layers of the lower lid is simple and expeditious, but when lower lid laxity is moderate to severe, lateral canthoplasty is more reliable. In cases of severe ectropion, the lower lid punctum may be everted. In these instances a medial canthoplasty is used to restore the physiologic relationship of the punctum to the globe.[30,31]

Procedures to treat the paralyzed upper lid (lagophthalmos)

Weights, springs, and slings. Eyelid closure in patients exhibiting lagophthalmos can be obtained in several ways. Perhaps the most popular and effective technique is gold weight insertion into the upper lid. Preoperative assessment determines the amount of weight to be used by taping weights to the upper eyelid until the distance between the eyelids is 1 mm or less. An additional 0.2 g is added to the gold weight to counteract the strengthened levator muscle function that usually develops.

Under local anesthesia an incision is made extending equally between the medial third and middle third of the supratarsal crease and the skin is elevated to the superior border of the tarsus. A pocket is formed immediately superficial to the tarsus to accommodate the dimensions of the weight. The weight is placed so that its inferior border is parallel to and 3 mm from the eyelash line, with the weight's fenestrations positioned superiorly. It is secured with sutures to the tarsus, and the orbicularis-levator complex is reapproximated. The position of the weight is evaluated for proper size and orientation and the skin is closed.[22]

Gold weights have some disadvantages; a slight incidence of extrusion is associated with their use. In addition, weights depend on gravity and therefore do not protect the cornea when the patient is supine, so a nighttime ointment is often required. Finally, the gold weight can occasionally be noticed by the casual observer as a bump in the eyelid.

Palpebral springs and silastic slings as described by Morel-Fatio and Arion, respectively, also have been used for lagophthalmos.[4,45] The palpebral spring technique has undergone several modifications since it was originally described, yet remains the procedure of choice in some surgeons' hands for severe lagophthalmos. Silastic slings are used less frequently and are complicated by lateral ectropion.[32] Both procedures share the disadvantage of extrusion, and they are more difficult to place than eyelid weights.

Presence of partial regeneration

Partial regeneration is often overlooked, but it is extremely important in understanding which operation to perform. If the facial nerve has undergone enough regeneration to permit a few axons to reach the facial muscles, this partial innervation may be sufficient to preserve the muscles for many years, even though they may be totally paralyzed. This situation will optimize results from hypoglossal-facial anastomosis, which is generally preferable to muscle transfer.

Donor consequences

Many surgical procedures designed for facial reanimation borrow neural elements or signals from other systems, i.e., the hypoglossal and trigeminal systems. The consequences of sacrificing the donor nerve ("donor deficit") are most important in planning for the overall needs of the patient. Certainly, the surgeon must assess the donor nerve preoperatively in all cases. The hypoglossal nerve must be tested for strength and vitality before it is transected and anastomosed to the distal facial nerve. Similarly, the trigeminal nerve must be intact and functional when its muscles, either masseter or temporalis, are considered for transposition into the facial muscle system.

The donor effects of facial reanimation surgery may be quite detrimental to the patient's welfare. For example, a patient with prior hypoglossal nerve injury on the opposite side could become an "oral cripple" if the remaining hypoglossal nerve were transected for use in a XII-VII anastomosis.

The ideal reanimation procedure is one with the following characteristics: (1) no donor deficit, (2) immediate restitution of facial movement, (3) appropriate involuntary emotional response, (4) normal voluntary motion, and (5) facial symmetry.

No currently available operative procedure satisfies all parameters. In fact, even a bacteriologically sterile and precise surgical transection and immediate microsurgical repair of the facial nerve will not allow a normal result. Therefore, the surgeon must clearly understand all operations available as well as his or her potential results and sequelae.

Status of the proximal facial nerve

As a general rule, the most desired neural source for rejuvenation of the paralyzed face is the ipsilateral facial nerve. Anastomosis or grafting to the ipsilateral nerve has no donor consequence (other than the minor hypesthesia or anesthesia from harvesting of a nerve graft) and allows at least some degree of voluntary and involuntary control of facial movement. Exceptions to this general rule are those situations in which the patient needs prompt relief from corneal exposure or drooling, and a tissue transfer/sling technique may be preferred because its effects are immediate.

For these reasons, the integrity of the proximal facial nerve is most important. As with other motor nerves, no reliable electrical tests exist to confirm the viability of the proximal nerve when it is discontinuous with its distal portion. The following are factors that affect proximal nerve viability, thereby enabling the clinician to make a qualified assessment.[19] (1) Nature of nerve injury, clean transection, crush, and so forth, (2) location of injury (proximal versus distal), (3) age (younger nerves tend to regenerate more quickly and fully), (4) nutritional status (directly affects nerve regeneration), and (5) history of radiation (impedes neural regeneration).

Status of the distal nerve

The facial nerve distal to the injury serves as a conduit for neural regeneration to the facial muscles following neurorraphy, grafting, or hypoglossal-facial anastomosis. Consequently, the anatomic integrity and continuity of the distal nerve to the facial muscles is critical.

When the surgeon is dealing with acute injuries (<72 hours old), the electrical stimulator may be used to identify the distal nerve and the muscular innervation of distal branches. After this "golden period," however, the surgeon must rely on visual identification of the divisions and branches of the distal nerve because the ability to be stimulated electrically is generally lost after approximately 72 hours. For this reason, transected nerve branches in trauma or tumor cases should be tagged for identification by placing a small colored suture around or adjacent to each nerve branch. Any anatomic or surgical landmarks should be precisely dictated in the operative note. If no suture markers are available, and the "golden period" has elapsed, careful surgical searching (preferably with loupes or an operating microscope) may reveal each of the divisions or branches of the facial nerve. A topographic map is essential in guiding the dissection. A review by Bernstein describes the variability with which these branches are placed.[6] The following landmarks are helpful (Fig. 70-3).

1. The pes anserinus can be found 1.5-cm deep to a point 1-cm anterior and 2-cm inferior to the tragal cartilage.
2. The superior division courses from the pes anserinus to the lateral corner of the eyebrow, convex postero-

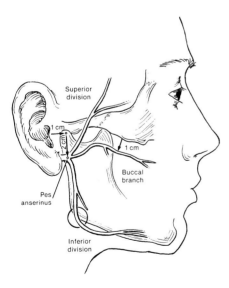

Fig. 70-3. Topographic map of distal facial nerve anatomy, useful as a guide in finding nonstimulatable nerve branches for grafting. Pes anserinus is 2 cm inferior to a point 1 cm anterior to tragus. Marginal mandibular branch courses from the pes anserinus to the angle of the mandible: buccal branch parallels the zygomatic arch 1 cm below its inferior border. Superior division arcs from pes anserinus toward lateral end of the eyebrow, under line that is convex superiorly.

superiorly (see Fig. 70-3). Bernstein[6] stressed that these temporal branches may be multiple, and as far posterior as the superficial temporal vessels.

3. The buccal branch courses superiorly then anteromedially, passing 1-cm inferior to the inferior border of the zygomatic arch (see Fig. 70-3).
4. The marginal mandibular branch passes from the pes anserinus directly over the angle of the mandible and then under the inferior border of the mandible for approximately 3 cm. It then crosses above the mandible at the level of the facial vessels.

Several anatomic variations may exist, requiring ingenuity in nerve grafting. When the facial nerve trunk and pes anserinus are intact, a cable graft (or hypoglossal nerve) should be sutured to that portion of the main nerve trunk. However, certain injuries and surgical procedures may sacrifice important individual portions of the nerve, requiring selective routing of reinnervation to specific divisions. The order of priority for reinnervation of facial nerve branches is as follows: (1) buccal and zygomatic branches (equal), (2) marginal mandibular, (3) frontal, and (4) cervical (the latter may be disregarded or excluded).

As an example of selective routing, when a parotid tumor operation results in excision of the pes anserinus and the proximal facial branches, a branched nerve graft may be placed to reinnervate the zygomatic and the buccal branches, excluding the less important branches.

When nerve grafts are sutured to the entire facial nerve trunk, the relatively unimportant cervical branch appears to be the most easily innervated, and may steal reinnervation axons needed for more important facial muscles. Fisch[21] advises clipping this branch to route innervation to the more important portions of the face. Minimal data exists, however, to confirm the efficacy of this technique.

If no nerve branches are found, and electromyography (EMG) shows that denervated facial muscles are present, the nerve graft may be sutured directly to the muscles that the surgeon wants to reinnervate. This technique is known as *muscular neurotization.* In these instances, the most important muscles are those of the midface (zygomaticus major and minor, levator labii superioris) and orbicularis oculi muscles. Reinnervation will not be as complete as in routine nerve grafting, because the regenerating axons must form new connections to the old motor endplates, or create their own.[1]

Viability of facial muscles

Several variables affect the facial muscles and the results of nerve grafting and transfer procedures. Variables that may limit the results of the most precisely performed operation are: (1) scar tissue, (2) congenital absence, (3) denervation atrophy, and (4) subclinical innervation.

Electromyography is an indispensable tool in determining whether denervation atrophy or subclinical innervation exists. EMG is the single most important test in determining the type of operative procedure to be performed. It is impor-

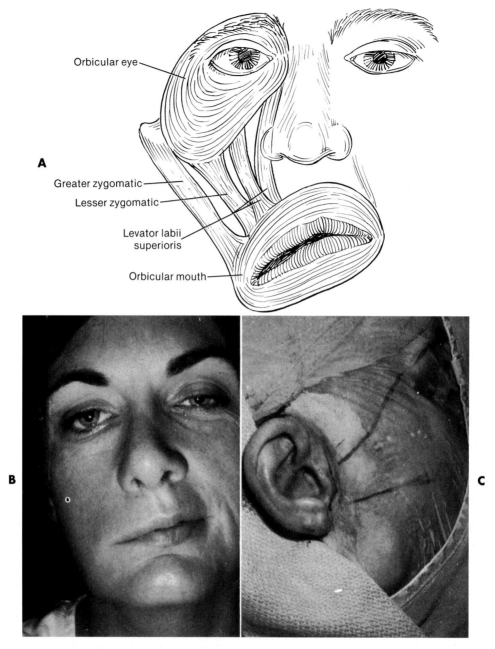

Fig. 70-4. Facial muscles. **A,** The most important muscles for reanimation. Levator labii superioris, along with lesser zygomatic muscle, is probably the most significant muscle for elevation of upper lip. Greater zygomatic muscle is also critical as the strongest elevator of oral commissura. **B,** Example of a delayed nerve graft. A patient with parotid malignancy removed without immediate reconstruction (because of intraoperative anesthesia considerations). Patient was referred for nerve grafting after 9 months elapsed. Note elongation of buccal-smile complex of muscles (greater and lesser zygomatic, levator labii superioris) and paralysis of orbicular eye muscle. **C,** Preoperative surface markings for nerve branches. Nerve stimulator cannot be used to locate distal branches after 9-month time lapse. Markings are for superior division and buccal branch, based on landmarks described in Figure 70-3 and prior operative report.

Continued

making this portion difficult to dissect free for suture. This difficult region exists roughly from 1 cm above to 1 cm below the stylomastoid foramen. Use of the mastoid portion of the facial nerve may require use of the longer sural or medial antebrachial cutaneous nerve rather than the greater auricular nerve as a cable graft.

Distally, several situations may be encountered that require some ingenuity in effecting reanimation. When the distal anastomotic site is at or proximal to the pes anserinus, a simple nerve-to-nerve suture will suffice. More frequently, however, after resection for parotid malignancy, several branches or divisions may present for anastomosis. In these cases, priority must be given to the zygomatic and buccal branches, sometimes to the exclusion of other less important facial nerve branches, because of the branching pattern of the nerve graft. Frequently, a two-branch graft can be prepared from the greater auricular or the sural nerve. This situation favors suturing of one branch of the nerve graft to the buccal branch and the other graft branch to the zygomatic branch or superior division. This technique will direct innervation to the important orbicularis oculi muscle and the muscles of the buccal-smile complex (Fig. 70-4).

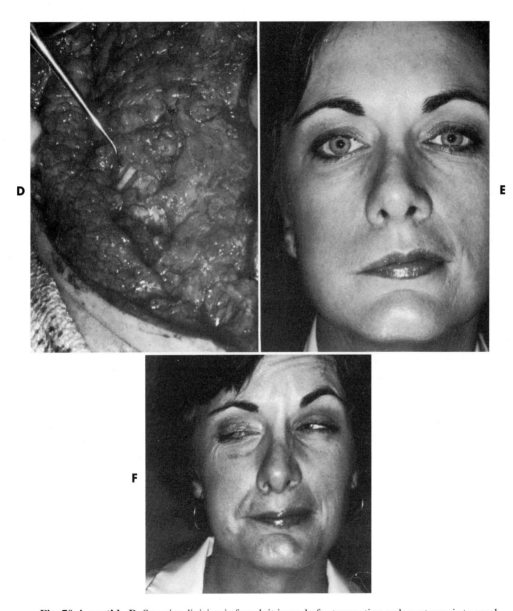

Fig. 70-4, cont'd. D, Superior division is found; it is ready for transection and anastomosis to sural graft (from midmastoid nerve segment). **E,** One year after operation. This is typical result of nerve graft when *delayed*. Orbicular eye and buccal branch muscles are improved but not normally or completely reinnervated. **F,** Voluntary motion in both zygomatic and buccal branches, with synkinesia. This result also is typical of most nerve grafts in that temporal branch (to occipitofrontal muscle) shows no reinnervation. Note hairstyle designed to camouflage occipitofrontal muscle paralysis.

In the rare instance when time has elapsed and distal nerve branches cannot be found, it is acceptable to route the necessarily longer nerve grafts directly to the important muscles cited, usually the orbicularis oculi and the zygomaticus major. Attachment of the graft into a denuded portion of muscle will allow neurotization to occur.

Choosing a donor nerve

Several donor nerves are available for facial nerve grafting. Three of the most common nerves used are the greater auricular nerve, the sural nerve, and the medial antebrachial cutaneous nerve. Since each has distinctive advantages and limitations, the reconstructive surgeon should be familiar with each of these donor nerves to allow greater flexibility in graft reconstructions.

When harvesting the greater auricular nerve, tumor considerations mandate that the ipsilateral nerve not be used. Consequently, the opposite neck should always be prepped and draped for harvesting the contralateral nerve in parotid tumor cases. The nerve is easily identified, arising from the posterior surface of the sternocleidomastoid muscle at Erb's point and traveling obliquely along the sternocleidomastoid muscle toward the ear. The surgical landmarks are well defined: a line drawn from the mastoid tip to the angle of the mandible is then bisected by a perpendicular line that crosses the sternocleidomastoid muscle from inferoposterior to anterosuperior, passing toward the parotid gland. A small horizontal incision in an upper neck skin crease is made along the path of the nerve. The nerve is identified in the subcutaneous tissues and followed superiorly to the parotid gland dissecting each of the three branches, and inferiorly to the posterior border of the sternocleidomastoid muscle. Up to 10 cm of nerve can be harvested. The greater auricular nerve has several advantages: the size and fascicular pattern are similar to the facial nerve, it is easily harvested in familiar anatomy, and it has a favorable distal branching pattern for facial nerve grafting. The main limitation of this graft is the maximum of 10 cm available for grafting.

The sural nerve also is commonly used for facial nerve grafting. In contrast to the greater auricular nerve, the sural nerve is the longest donor nerve available, with up to 70 cm of graft available when all branches are dissected into the popliteal fossa. The donor site is located distant from the surgical resection, allowing a second team to simultaneously harvest nerve tissue. Donor site morbidity is low. However, caution should be used when working with people with diabetes or other patients with peripheral vascular disease, because ischemic pressure necrosis could result in the area of sensory deficit along the lateral aspect of the foot. The sural nerve is of larger diameter than the greater auricular nerve or the facial nerve, and has more prominent connective tissue than the greater auricular nerve or medial antebrachial cutaneous nerve.

The sural nerve is formed by the junction of the medial sural cutaneous nerve and the peroneal communicating branch of the lateral sural cutaneous nerve between the two heads of the gastrocnemius muscle. The nerve lies immediately deep and behind the lesser saphenous vein. Multiple nerve branches arise near the lateral malleolus. A pneumatic tourniquet should be applied to the thigh and a transverse incision made immediately behind the lateral malleolus. As many "stair-step" horizontal incisions as necessary should be used, coursing over the length of the nerve during the harvesting procedure. It is important to avoid tugging on the nerve while harvesting. The nerve should be harvested immediately prior to grafting and placed in lactated Ringer's solution after débriding away any small pieces of fat or other soft tissue that might interfere with vascularization of the graft.

The medial antebrachial cutaneous nerve has been described in the orthopedic literature for peripheral nerve repairs, and is used in situ with forearm microvascular flaps for sensory innervation in head and neck cancer reconstruction. This nerve has several properties that warrant consideration for use in facial nerve reconstruction.[9] The medial antebrachial cutaneous nerve arises from the medial cord of the brachial plexus, contains fibers from C-8 and T-1, and supplies sensation to the medial aspect of the forearm. This nerve has a consistent anatomy traveling in the bicipital groove immediately adjacent to the basilic vein. Nerve diameter and branching pattern are similar to the facial nerve, and there is minimal donor site morbidity with nerve harvest.

The entire arm is prepped and placed in a stockinet. The use of a tourniquet aids dissection. A linear incision is made in the bicipital furrow of the medial aspect of the arm. The nerve is located in the subcutaneous tissue immediately adjacent to the basilic vein. The median nerve lies medial to the basilic vein, and is readily identified and preserved. The medial antebrachial cutaneous nerve divides into anterior and posterior branches in the distal third of the arm. These can be dissected into the forearm to obtain adequate length. More than 20 cm of nerve can be harvested without difficulty. See Cheney[9] for further anatomic details.

Surgical technique

For the surgical technique of neurorrhaphy, interrupted sutures of 9-0 or 10-0 monofilament nylon are preferred. A 75- or 100-micron needle is appropriate. A straight and a curved pair of jeweler's forceps as well as a Castroviejo needle holder are satisfactory instruments for performing the anastomosis. Both ends of the nerve graft and the proximal and distal stumps should be transected cleanly with a fresh sterile razor blade.[38] Some oozing of axoplasm will usually be seen at the proximal stump following preparation, but this generally can be ignored. For nerve trunk anastomosis, four simple epineural sutures will usually coapt the nerve ends accurately. However, obvious discrepancies in size or other epineural gaps should be closed with additional sutures. The needle should pass through epineurium only to avoid injury to the fascicular neural contents. The nerve graft should lie in the healthiest possible bed of supporting tissue, with approximately 8 to 10 mm of extra length for each anastomosis. Thus, the graft should lie in a somewhat ''lazy S'' configuration (see Fig. 70-4), which appears to minimize tension during healing. Hemovac and other suction drainage systems should be placed away from any portions of the nerve graft. When adequate nerve stumps exist, securing them with a special microneural nerve clamp is helpful. This facilitates the anastomosis in a manner similar to a microvascular anastomosis.

When one division is excised or injured and other portions of the nerve remain intact, it may be desirable to graft from a fascicle within the pes anserinus to a distal branch. It is possible to dissect the nerves and divisions proximally into the pes anserinus and perform fascicular dissection at this point. Curved jeweler's forceps used for dissecting in the plane and in a direction parallel to the nerve fascicles will allow this dissection (Fig. 70-5). The distal buccal branch

often has several small filaments, so it may be necessary to select the larger of these for distal anastomosis.

Approximation of the nerve ends using an acrylic glue has been described (Histacryl or cyano-butyl-acrylate).[42] Subsequent investigators have shown that neural anastomosis with this tissue adhesive yields results similar to nerve suture. The technique is most helpful in tight temporal bone anatomic surgical situations rather than in distal facial anastomosis.[54]

Following temporal bone resection, the nerve may be routed from the tympanic or the labyrinthine portions directly to the face through a bony window near the posterior root of the zygomatic arch. This will shorten the necessary length of the nerve graft. However, when using this technique it is important to ensure the nerve graft's protection from trauma at the temporomandibular joint if the joint is preserved. Conley and Baker have reported excellent results using similar techniques.[11,12]

Millesi[44] introduced interfascicular nerve repair, reason-

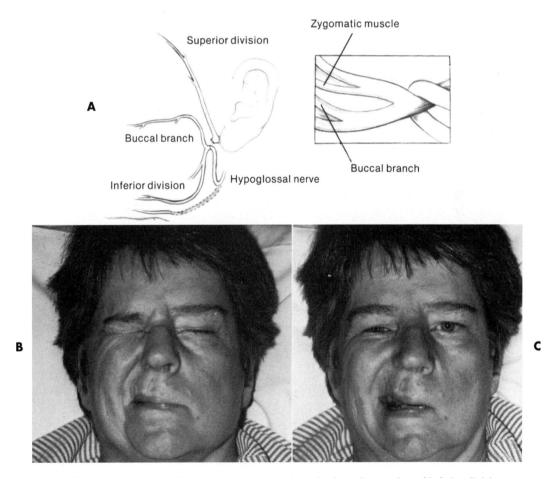

Fig. 70-5. A, Hypoglossal-facial anastomosis showing selective reinnervation of inferior division, leaving superior division innervation intact. *Inset* shows fascicular dissection before anastomosis (see **E** and **D**). **B** and **C,** Preoperative view of patient with long standing segmental paralysis of inferior division of facial nerve. Zygomatic branch to orbicular eye muscle shows preservation of innervation.

Continued

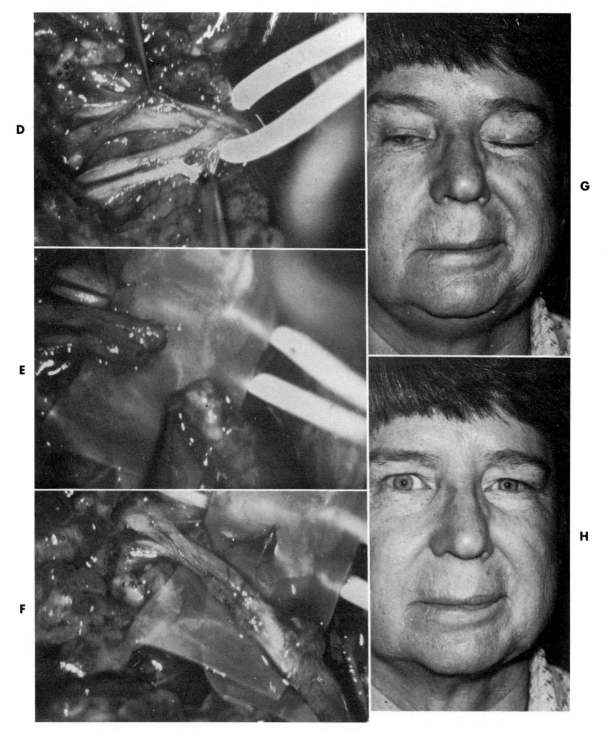

Fig. 70-5, cont'd. D, Perineural dissection of pes anserinus reveals fascicles destined for zygomatic and buccal branches (see *A*). **E,** Buccal branch and inferior division transected. Neurosurgical loop protects intact superior division underneath background piece of polymeric silicone (Silastic). Hypoglossal nerve *(lower right)* is ready for anastomosis. **F,** Completed anastomosis of hypoglossal nerve to buccal branch and inferior division of facial nerve. Superior division intact in continuity with proximal facial nerve. **G,** Strong reinnervation to entire face, 1 year after operation. Patient uses hypoglossal innervation to buccal branch muscles to enhance eye closure. **H,** Upward movement of oral commissura mediated by hypoglossal nerve, without associated or synkinetic eye closure.

ing that the exact microsurgical approximation of nerve fascicles or fascicle groups might minimize synkinesis or mass movement. It is well known that this type of repair is preferred in nerve injuries in the extremities; however, such repairs have not been universally accepted for use in the facial nerve. Several reasons exist for this limited acceptance. The tympanic, and in many cases, the mastoid portions of the nerve have only one or two fascicles, and the intraneural topography is questionable. There are few, if any, sensory fibers in the facial nerve in its extratemporal portion, so performing sensory-to-sensory fascicular repair is not of value.

The authors, as well as May and Miehlke (in independent reports), have reported that discrete, spatially oriented fascicles are present in the nerve near the stylomastoid foramen.[16,35,41] Other authors, notably Sir Sidney Sunderland[58] and Tomander and others,[61] have reported conflicting data demonstrating that various portions of the face are represented in a random fashion in the proximal nerve. Presently, it is probably best to perform fascicular repair when the injury obviously lends itself to the technique (i.e., clean lacerations through the pes anserinus, branch nerve grafts that require fascicular dissection in the pes, and so on). Basic research has yet to reveal the exact neural topography of the more proximal portions of the nerve.

Cross-face nerve grafting

The creative and physiologic method of cross-face nerve grafting provides the possibility for facial nerve control of previously paralyzed facial muscles. It is the only procedure that has the theoretic ability of specific divisional control of facial muscle groups (e.g., the buccal branch controlling the buccal branch distribution, the zygomatic branch innervating the orbicularis oculi). Originally described by Scaramella[53] and Smith[56] in independent reports in 1971, the technique has not proven as advantageous as first thought. Anderl[2] subsequently described his own results as good in 9 of 23 patients, whereas Samii[52] reported that only 1 of 10 patients had good movement as a result of this technique. A more recent update by Ferreira[20] indicates that those patients operated on in the first 6 months of the paralysis did better than those operated on at a later date; however, some of these patients may have undergone partial spontaneous reinnervation because they appeared to have had lesions without total palsy, and the traditional waiting period of 1 year was not allowed to elapse.

The cross-face technique suffers from a lack of sufficient axon population and neural excitatory vitality. It is of marginal value at the time of this writing, although it may be useful with free muscle transfers. Conley has discussed the shortcomings and unproven status of cross-face grafting.[10,12]

Surgical technique

The operative technique of cross-face grafting consists of transection of several fascicles, usually of the buccal branch, on the nonparalyzed side through a nasolabial fold incision. One to three sural nerve grafts are approximated to these normal contralateral branches. The nerve grafts are then passed through subcutaneous tunnels, usually in the upper lip. Cross-face grafts for the eye region are often passed above the eyebrow.

The anastomosis with the paralyzed facial nerve branches is done by most surgeons at a second stage, 6 to 12 months after the first. As described by most authors, the first stage is performed in the first 6 months of paralysis. This is not advisable unless the paralysis is of known permanence; for example, if spontaneous ipsilateral facial nerve regeneration may induce reanimation, then the surgeon should wait. Tinel's sign may often be elicited on the paralyzed side after several months because of sensory fibers accompanying the motor fibers through the cross-face graft. At this time, the cross-face graft is explored and sutured to the appropriate branches on the paralyzed side. This is approached through a parotidectomy/rhytidectomy approach, and is usually performed within the parotid portion of the paralyzed side.

Cross-face grafting currently is only used in conjunction with free muscle transfers. Reinnervation of paralyzed facial muscles has not proven sufficient to justify use of this procedure without muscle transfer.

NERVE TRANSPOSITION

Reinnervation by connecting an intact proximal facial nerve to the distal ipsilateral facial nerve is generally the preferred method for facial paralysis rehabilitation. Only when a proximal facial nerve stump is not viable or available should attention be turned to other systems, for example, muscle or nerve transfer.

Hypoglossal nerve transfer

Of the various nerves available for anastomosis with the facial nerve the hypoglossal nerve is preferred because an anatomic and a functional relationship exists between the facial and hypoglossal nerves. They both arise from a similar collection of neurons in the brainstem, and they also share similar reflex responses following trigeminal nerve stimulation.[57] In addition, the hypoglossal nerve is in close anatomic proximity, and is readily available during other operations on the facial nerve. Hypoglossal nerve transection results in less donor disability than sacrifice of the spinal accessory, phrenic, or other regional nerves that have been used for facial reanimation. The most common criticism of hypoglossal nerve transfer is that it results in lack of voluntary emotional control. Although this is true, it also is usually true of ipsilateral facial nerve anastomosis as well, in that mass movements and spasms preclude any voluntary control of eye closure, smiling, or other emotional movements.

Surgical technique

A parotidectomy incision with an extension inferiorly toward the hyoid bone is usually used in hypoglossal nerve transfer. The procedure also may be performed with some-

cle must be delivered into the face. A large group of patients who fit into this category are those whose complete paralysis has lasted 2 years or more. These patients are usually characterized by severe denervation atrophy as noted on EMG. In these situations, muscle transfer is the preferred technique of reanimation.

Since the masseter was first used for facial reanimation in 1908, many modifications have been described.[33] Many authors, notably Conley, prefer the masseter muscle for rehabilitation of the lower and mid-face.[14]

The masseter transfer procedure is generally performed for rehabilitation of the sagging paralyzed oral commissure and the buccal-smile complex of muscles. The masseter's upper origin from the zygomatic arch allows a predominantly posterior pull on the lower mid-face. Transfer of the muscle can be accomplished externally through a rhytidectomy/parotidectomy incision, or intraorally using a mucosal incision in the gingivobuccal sulcus lateral to the ascending ramus of the mandible (Fig. 70-7). The masseter's blood supply is medial and deep, and its nerve supply passes through the sigmoid notch between the condylar and coronoid processes of the mandible to reach the upper deep surface of the muscle. The nerve supply then ramifies and courses distally and inferiorly, terminating near the periosteal attachments on the lateral aspect of the mandibular angle and body. In general, the external approach is preferred, insofar as the intraoral approach is associated with somewhat limited access, poorer muscle mobilization, and less vascular control. The troublesome facial artery branches may be difficult to secure when using this limited exposure, thus the external approach is preferred.

A generous parotidectomy incision is made and extended inferiorly below the mastoid tip. The parotid gland and masseteric fascia is exposed. The posterior border of the muscle is freed from the mandible's ascending ramus, and the inferior attachments at the lower border of the mandible also are detached with electrosurgical cutting current. The nerve supply courses along the deep surface approximately midway between the anterior and the posterior borders of the muscle (see Fig. 70-7). It is advisable to transfer the entire anterior-posterior diameter of the muscle and preserve the deep fascial layer when dissecting the muscle free from the mandible. Mobilization of the periosteal attachments along the inferior border will allow secure tissue for anchoring sutures and promote more length of the transposed muscle.

Continued dissection is then carried forward to the nasolabial fold in the subcutaneous plane using large Metzenbaum or rhytidectomy scissors. The external incisions are made at or just medial to the nasolabial fold, the lateral oral commissure, and at the vermilion cutaneous junction of the lower lip. Each of these incisions is connected to the cheek tunnel, allowing transfer of slips of the masseter muscle. The muscle may be divided into three slips for attachment at these three sites, or the entire periosteal end of the muscle may be used to suture the remnants of the orbicularis oris muscle from the lateral upper lip to the commissure and

below. These muscle slips are sutured to the dermis and the orbicularis oris muscle using 4-0 clear nylon sutures. May[36] reported that suturing to the mucocutaneous line deep to the orbicularis muscle promotes a more healthy nasolabial fold and overall results, compared with suturing to the dermis. The best results depend on the following:

1. Gross overcorrection: no matter how this procedure is performed, gravity and natural laxity of the tissues will allow for sagging of the oral commissure, so that the intraoperative result should be a contorted hyperelevation of the oral commissure.
2. Preservation of masseteric nerve supply.
3. Placement of many sutures in the transposed muscle: the surgical assistant should hold the oral commissure at the exaggerated overcorrected level during attachment of the muscle.
4. Following skin closure (the commissure should continue to be held upward), the skin of the perioral and cheek region should be painted with benzoin or Mastisol, and a tape dressing (which maintains overcorrection) left in place for 7 days to retain overcorrection.

Perioperative antibiotics are recommended. The patient should not be given anything orally; nasogastric feedings should be administered for the first 5 days to minimize masseter movement.

Results from the masseteric procedure are quite gratifying and usually yield a high degree of facial symmetry. However, the masseter's arc of rotation will not allow for rehabilitation around the orbit. For this reason, the temporalis may be combined with masseter transfer, or the orbital region treated separately with such procedures as canthoplasty and gold weights.

Temporalis transfer

Although Gillies[23] is usually given credit for introducing the temporalis procedure, Rubin[49,50] deserves much credit for refining the goals of the procedure and the operative technique in the United States. Like the masseter transfer, the temporalis transfer procedure requires an intact ipsilateral trigeminal nerve. The nerve supply to the temporalis lies along the deep surface of the muscle. The upper origin of the temporalis muscle is fan-shaped and arises from the periosteum of the entire temporal fossa. The muscle belly converges on a short tendinous portion deep to the zygomatic arch and inserts on the coronoid process and a portion of the ascending ramus of the mandible. The muscle is best exposed through an incision that passes above the ear, slightly posteriorly, and then in an anteromedial arc. This will expose the entire upper portion of the muscle (Fig. 70-8). A convenient aponeurotic dissection plane exists lateral to the temporalis fascia.

In Rubin's technique, the muscle is dissected free from the periosteum and attached to fascial strips, which are turned down inferiorly to reach the oral commissure and

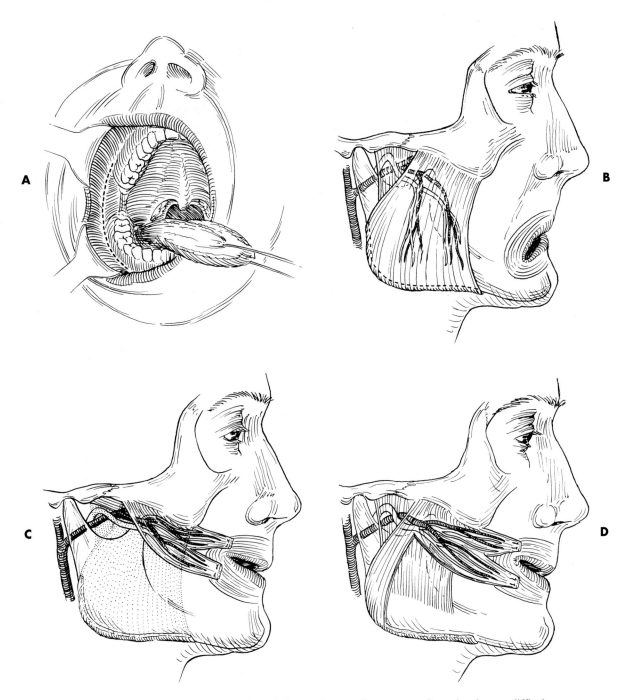

Fig. 70-7. Masseter transfer procedure. **A,** Intraoral approach to masseter. Procedure is more difficult when performed in this manner; external approach is preferred. **B,** Correct incisions in muscle and periosteum. Periosteum must be incorporated in lower portion of muscle flap to leave tissue secure for suturing to lip region. **C** and **D,** Entire muscle, rather than only anterior elements, is transposed, so that masseteric nerve supply is transferred intact with muscle belly.

Continued

E
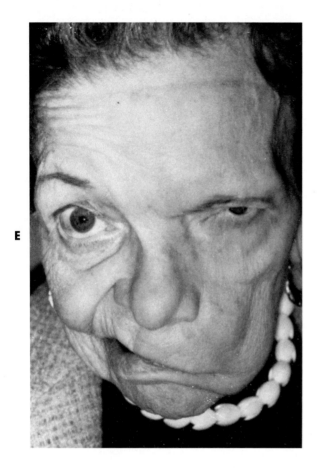

F
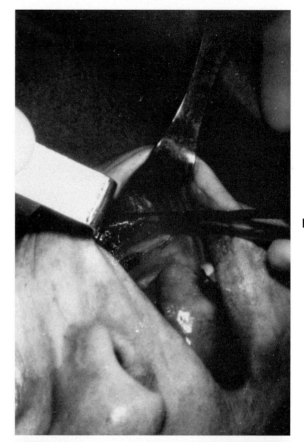

Fig. 70-7, cont'd. E, Elderly woman with complete peripheral facial paralysis. Note severe brow ptosis, medial tarsorraphy, and severe redundancy of cheek, paranasal, and lateral lip tissues on the left. **F,** Intraoperative photograph showing intraoral masseter transfer. Large Kelly clamp is used to grasp the inferior portion of the masseter, which will be passed through the cheek tissues to a nasolabial fold incision. (see **A** through **D**). **G,** Photograph taken after brow-lifting procedure (tarsorraphy has been left for eye safety). Masseter transfer has successfully raised the corner of the mouth and the nasolabial fold. The patient declined further excision of the nasolabial fold for improved cosmesis.

G
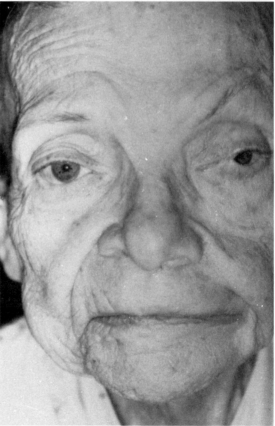

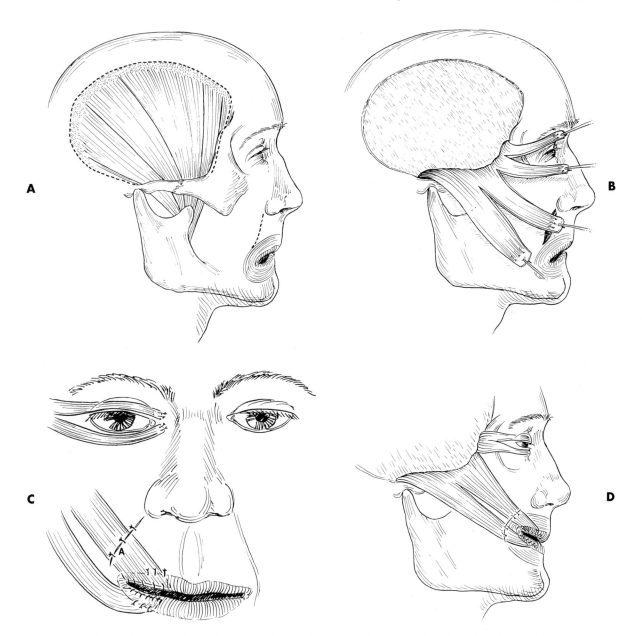

Fig. 70-8. Temporal muscle transposition. **A,** *Dotted line* illustrates incision in pericranium peripheral to edge of muscle. This results in strong periosteum to hold sutures in transposed position. Nerve supply on deep side of muscle is not shown. **B,** Temporal muscle divided into four slips. Note pericranium at end of slips sutured to muscle to reinforce suture site. Temporal fascia superficial to muscle can be used in same way. **C,** Transposed slips sutured to perioral muscles. Creativity and compulsivity must be used during this portion of procedure. Overcorrection is mandatory. Sutures *(A)* must be placed in subdermis inferior to incision or in submucosal portion of wound deep to orbicularis oris muscle.[36] **D,** Completed procedure. Wide tunnel over zygomatic arch precludes unsightly bulge of muscle, which would otherwise be produced. Superior pull of temporal muscle is somewhat preferred to the posterolateral pull of masseter muscle (see Fig. 70-7).

eyelid area. If these fascial strips are omitted, the transposed muscle's length is insufficient to reach the lateral oral commissure.

More recently, Rubin[50] refined his temporalis transfer technique by including a slip of masseter muscle that is sutured to the oral commissure and lower lip. The resulting masseteric pull improves results by providing more posterior and lateral vectors to the oral commissure.

The authors prefer to use the technique described by Baker and Conley,[13] who describe retaining the integrity of the upper muscle and its overlying fascia. The latter is dissected free, then turned inferiorly for suturing to the oral commissure.

A tunnel at least 1 to 1.5 inches wide must be made over the zygomatic arch to allow the muscle to turn inferiorly and eliminate an unsightly bulge. The attachment of the strip should be just medial to the nasolabial fold so that the natural crease is reproduced by the muscle pull. As with the masseteric procedure, a marked overcorrection is necessary on the operating table. A soft silicone block may be used to fill the depression in the donor defect; hairstyling may obviate the necessity for this step.

Although the gold weight–canthoplasty technique is often preferred, the temporalis muscle can be used for orbital rehabilitation. The anterior third of the temporalis muscle is turned laterally into the eyelids (see Fig. 70-8). Subcutaneous tunnel dissection between the paralyzed orbicularis oculi and the eyelid skin allows passage of the fascial strips medially through both eyelids to the medial canthus, where they are sutured. As with any reconstructive procedure, adjustments and suture revisions should be checked carefully on the operating table to ensure proper eyelid contour.

With both masseter and temporalis transfer, facial muscle activation originates from the trigeminal nerve. Patients need to learn through videotape, biofeedback, or similar methods the proper way to contract the muscles by chewing or biting. Some younger patients may actually learn how to incorporate these movements into their own facial expressions, e.g., smiles, grimaces, and so forth. However, patients should be told preoperatively that muscle transfer procedures will not allow any emotional or involuntary reanimation. In the best hands, these techniques provide symmetry and tone in repose, with some learned and induced movements on attempted chewing.

The surgeon must not forget the importance of corneal protection while planning and executing any of the described reanimation surgical procedures. To allow corneal desiccation and loss of the eye would be a tragic accompaniment to an otherwise successful reanimation result. Simple suture tarsorrhaphy provides eyelid closure during the healing period before eyelid function returns, following temporalis transposition, XII-VII anastomosis, facial nerve neurorraphy, or grafting.

SUMMARY

A variety of techniques are available for facial nerve rehabilitation following paralysis. The surgeon should know the advantages and disadvantages of the various techniques in order to apply them properly in each clinical situation. Thorough knowledge of neuromuscular pathophysiology also is important in understanding how time affects the choice of rehabilitative procedures. When properly informed of the limitations of these operative procedures, most patients can be rehabilitated and many of their symptoms alleviated.

REFERENCES

1. Aitken JT: Growth of nerve implants in voluntary muscle, *J Anat* 84: 38, 1950.
2. Anderl H: Cross-face nerve transplant, *Clin Plast Surg* 6:433, 1973.
3. Anonsen CK and others: Reinnervation of skeletal muscle with a neuromuscular pedicle, *Otolaryngol Head Neck Surg* 93:48, 1985.
4. Arion HG: Dynamic closure of the lids in paralysis of the orbicularis muscle, *Int J Surg* 57:48, 1972.
5. Barrs DM: Facial nerve trauma: optimal timing for repair, *Laryngoscope* 101:835, 1991.
6. Bernstein L: Surgical anatomy of the extraparotid distribution of the facial nerve, *Arch Otolaryngol* 110:177, 1984.
7. Borodic GE and others: Botulinum A toxin for treatment of aberrant facial nerve regeneration, *Plast Reconstr Surg* 91:1042, 1993.
8. Buncke HJ, Alpert BS, Gordon I: Free serratus anterior muscle transfer of unilateral facial paralysis, Paper presented at the annual meeting of the American Association of Plastic Surgeons, Chicago, May, 1984.
9. Cheney, ML: *Medial antebrachial cutaneous nerve graft.* In Urken ML and others, editors: *Atlas of regional and free flaps for head and neck reconstruction,* New York, 1995, Raven Press.
10. Conley J: *Facial rehabilitation: new potentials.* In Baker CD, editor: *Clinical plastic surgery,* Philadelphia, 1979, WB Saunders.
11. Conley J, Baker CD: Hypoglossal-facial nerve anastomosis for reinnervation of the paralyzed face, *Plast Reconstr Surg* 63:63, 1979.
12. Conley J, Baker CD: Myths and misconceptions in the rehabilitation of facial paralysis, *Plast Reconstr Surg* 71:538, 1983.
13. Conley J, Baker CD: Regional muscle transposition for rehabilitation of the paralyzed face, *Clin Plast Surg* 6:317, 1979.
14. Conley J, Baker CD: The surgical treatment of extratemporal facial paralysis, *Head Neck Surg* 1:12, 1978.
15. Conley J, Miehlke A: *Factors influencing results in extratemporal facial nerve repair.* In Fisch U, editor: *Facial nerve surgery,* Birmingham, Ala, 1977, Aesculapius Publishing.
16. Crumley R: Spatial anatomy of facial nerve fibers: a preliminary report, *Laryngoscope* 90:274, 1980.
17. Dellon AL, Mackinnon SE: Segmentally innervated latissimus dorsi muscle: microsurgical transfer for facial reanimation, *J Reconstr Microsurg* 2:7, 1985.
18. Dressler D, Schonle PW: Botulinum toxin to suppress hyperkinesias after hypoglossal-facial nerve anastomosis, *Eur Arch OtoRhinolaryngol,* 247:391, 1990.
19. Ducker TB, Kempe LG, Hayes GJ: The metabolic background for peripheral nerve surgery, *J Neurosurg* 30:270, 1969.
20. Ferreira M: Cross-facial nerve grafting, *Clin Plast Surg* 11:211, 1984.
21. Fisch U: *Facial nerve surgery,* Birmingham, Ala, 1977, Aesculapius Publishing.
22. Freeman MS and others: Surgical therapy of the eyelids in patients with facial paralysis, *Laryngoscope* 100:1086, 1990.
23. Gillies H: Facial paralysis, *Proc R Soc Med* 27:1372, 1934.
24. Gutman E, Young J: The reinnervation of muscle after various periods of atrophy, *J Anat* 78:15, 1944.
25. Hakelius L: Free muscle grafting, *Clin Plast Surg* 6:301, 1979.

26. Hardy R, Perret G, Myers RD: Phrenicofacial anastomosis for facial paralysis, *J Neurosurg* 14:400, 1957.

27. Harii K: Microneurovascular free muscle transplantation for reanimation of facial paralysis, *Clin Plast Surg* 6:361, 1979.

28. Harii K, Ohmori K, Torii S: Free gracilis transplantation with microneurovascular anastomosis for the treatment of facial paralysis, *Plast Reconstr Surg* 57:133, 1976.

29. Harrison DH: The pectoralis minor vascularized muscle graft for the treatment of unilateral facial palsy, *Plast Reconstr Surg* 75:206, 1985.

30. Jelks GW, Smith B, Bosniak S: The evaluation and management of the eye in facial palsy, *Clin Plast Surg* 6:397, 1979.

31. Kazanjian VH, Converse JM: *Facial palsy.* In Converse JM, editor: *Surgical treatment of facial injuries,* ed 3, Baltimore, 1974, Williams & Wilkins.

32. Levine R: *Eyelid reanimation surgery.* In May M, editor: *The facial nerve,* New York, 1986, Thieme.

33. Lexer E, Eden R: Uber die Chirurgische Behandlung der Peripheren Facialislahmung, *Beitr Klin* 73:116, 1911.

34. Maas CS and others: Primary surgical management for rehabilitation of the paralyzed eye, *Otolaryngol Head Neck Surg* 110:288, 1994.

35. May M: Anatomy of the facial nerve, *Laryngoscope* 83:1311, 1973.

36. May M: Muscle transposition for facial reanimation, *Arch Otolaryngol* 110:184, 1984.

37. May M, Sobol SM, Mester SJ: Hypoglossal-facial nerve interpositional-jump graft for facial reanimation without tongue atrophy, *Otolaryngol Head Neck Surg* 104:818, 1991.

38. McCabe B: Facial nerve grafting, *Plast Reconstr Surg* 45:70, 1970.

39. McGuirt WF, McCabe BF: Effect of radiation therapy on facial nerve cable autografts, *Laryngoscope* 87:415, 1977.

40. McKee NH, Kuzon WM: Functioning free muscle transplantation: making it work. What is known? *Ann Plast Surg* 23:249, 1989.

41. Miehlke A: Topography of the course of fibers in the fascialis stem, *Arch Klin Exp Ohren Nasen Kehlkopfkunde (Berlin)* 171, 1958.

42. Miehlke A: Probleme Beider Naht der Feinstenperipheren Neruen im Bereich der Otolaryngologie, *Melsunger Med Mitteilungen* 42:71, 1968.

43. Miehlke A, Stennart E, Chilla R: New aspects in facial nerve surgery, *Clin Plast Surg* 6:3, 1979.

44. Millesi H: *Facial nerve suture.* In Fisch U, editor: *Facial nerve surgery,* Birmingham, Ala, 1977, Aesculapius Publishing.

45. Morel-Fatio D, Lalardrie JP: Palliative surgical treatment of facial paralysis: the palpepral spring, *Plast Reconstr Surg* 33:446, 1964.

46. O'Brien BMC, Franklin JD, Morrison WA: Cross-facial nerve grafts and microneurovascular free muscle transfers for long established facial palsy, *Br J Plast Surg* 33:202, 1980.

47. Pillsbury HC, Fisch U: Extratemporal facial nerve grafting and radiotherapy, *Arch Otolaryngol* 105:441, 1979.

48. Rubin LR: The anatomy of a smile: its importance in the treatment of facial paralysis, *Plast Reconstr Surg* 53:384, 1974.

49. Rubin LR: *Reanimation of the paralyzed face: new approaches,* St Louis, 1977, Mosby.

50. Rubin LR: *Reanimation of total unilateral facial paralysis by the contiguous facial muscle technique.* In Rubin LR, editor: *The paralyzed face,* St Louis, 1991, Mosby.

51. Sachs M, Conley J: Dual simultaneous systems for facial reanimation, *Arch Otolaryngol* 109:137, 1983.

52. Samii M: *Nerves of the head and neck: management of peripheral nerve problems.* In Omer G, Spinner M, editors: *Management of peripheral nerve problems,* Philadelphia, 1979, WB Saunders.

53. Scaramella LL: L'anastomosi tradue nervi facciali, *Arch Otologia* 82:208, 1971.

54. Siedentop KH, Loewy A: Facial nerve repair with tissue adhesive, *Arch Otolaryngol* 105:423, 1979.

55. Smith JD, Crumley RL, Harker JD: Facial paralysis in the newborn, *Otolaryngol Head Neck Surg* 89:1021, 1981.

56. Smith JW: *A new technique of facial animation: transactions of fifth international congress of plastic and reconstructive surgery,* Chatswood, MSW, Australia, 1971, Butterworths.

57. Stennart E: Hypoglossal-facial anastomosis: its significance for modern facial surgery, *Clin Plast Surg* 6:471, 1979.

58. Sunderland S: *Mass movements after facial nerve injury.* In Fisch U, editor: *Facial surgery,* Birmingham, Ala, 1977, Aesculapius Publishing.

59. Terzis JK: Pectoralis minor: a unique muscle for correction of facial palsy, *Plast Reconstr Surg* 83:767, 1989.

60. Thompson N: Autogenous free grafts of skeletal muscle, *Plast Reconstr Surg* 48:11, 1971.

61. Tomander L, Aldshogius H, Grant G: *Motor fiber organization of the facial nerve in the rat.* In House W, editor: *Disorders of the facial nerve,* New York, 1980, Raven Press.

62. Tucker H: The management of facial paralysis due to extracranial injuries, *Laryngoscope* 88:348, 1978.

63. Wells MD, Manktelow RT: Surgical management of facial palsy, *Clin Plast Surg* 17:645, 1990.

64. Wesley RE, Jackson CG: *Facial palsy.* In Hornblass A, editor: *Oculoplastic, orbital and reconstructive surgery, vol I, Eyelids,* Baltimore, 1988, Williams & Wilkins.

PART SIX

ORAL CAVITY/ OROPHARYNX/ NASOPHARYNX

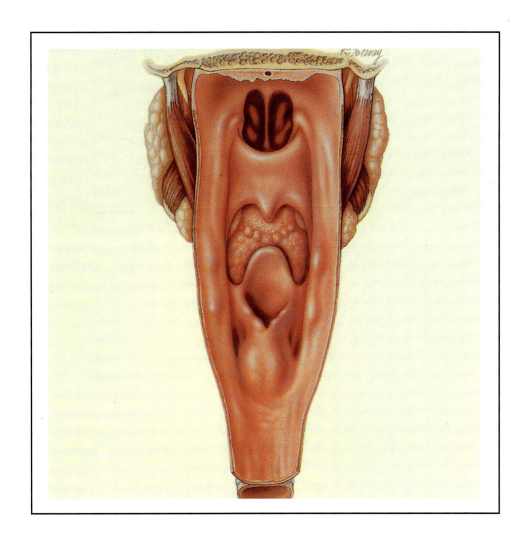

Chapter 71

Anatomy

Daniel O. Graney
Guy J. Petruzzelli
Eugene N. Myers

PHARYNX

The pharynx (Fig. 71-1) is a common aerodigestive tract, which is subdivided anatomically into the nasopharynx, oropharynx, and laryngopharynx (hypopharynx). At approximately the level of the sixth cervical vertebra the pharynx becomes the esophagus, and anterior to the pharynx the larynx becomes the trachea. Although the pharynx in toto is not usually a site or target of surgery, areas of the lateral pharynx are often approached during total parotidectomies or surgical treatment of neoplasms. An alternate approach, for example, from the mucosal or interior surface of the pharynx, may be necessary, as in the case of a peritonsilar mass or laryngeal polyp. Thus, it is important for the surgeon to understand both the medial and lateral anatomic relationships of the pharynx.

The anatomic perspective may cause disorientation and confuse surgical relationships. This chapter approaches the anatomic relationships of the entire pharynx as viewed from its lateral surface, from the skull base to the level of the cricoid cartilage. The pharynx is then rotated 90° for viewing from the posterior aspect; finally it is rotated another 90° for viewing the relationships from the medial surface. The key point is the constancy of anatomic relationships in a changing perspective.

Because the pharynx is constructed from three U-shaped constrictor muscles that are more narrow anteriorly than they are posteriorly, a series of four intervals occurs between the muscles, from the skull base to the esophagus. In the following discussion, the strategy is to describe, first, the musculoskeletal framework of the pharynx and the respective intervals between the parts of the pharynx and, second, the

appropriate muscles, ligaments, and accompanying neurovascular bundles filling these interspaces.

Musculoskeletal framework

The pharyngeal wall is composed of stratified squamous epithelium covering a myofascial layer extending from the skull base to the esophagus. The muscles of the pharyngeal wall are the paired superior, middle, and inferior constrictors. The fasciae of the pharyngeal wall are the well-developed dense pharyngobasilar fascia and the thinner buccopharyngeal fascia.

The pharyngobasilar fascia has its origin at the basiocciput and extends horizontally along the petrous portion of the temporal bone to the carotid canal, at which point it turns anteriorly and attaches to the medial pterygoid lamina and pterygomandibular raphe. The buccopharyngeal fascia is a reflection of the middle layer of the deep cervical fascia and comprises the external investing layer of the superior pharyngeal constrictor and buccinator muscles. It originates at the skull base and extends into the neck to eventually fuse with the pretracheal and visceral fasciae.

The paired superior pharyngeal constrictor muscles arise from the inferior one third of the posterior border of the medial pterygoid plate and the hamulus and the pterygomandibular raphe. The fibers radiate posteriorly, inferiorly, and superiorly, condensing in the posterior midline pharyngeal raphe, which attaches superiorly at the pharyngeal tubercle. The superior constrictor is attached to the skull base at three points, the two pterygoid hamuli and the pharyngeal tubercle, thus leaving a bean-shaped interval in the posterior pharyngeal wall composed only of pharyngobasilar fascia.

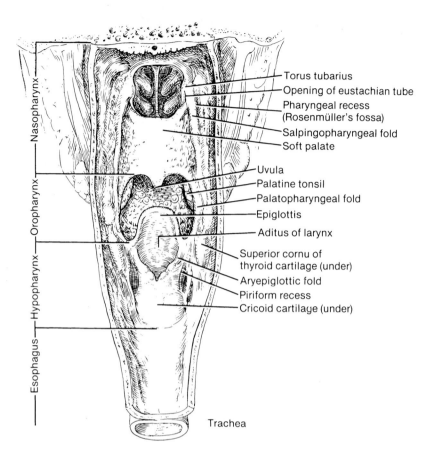

Fig. 71-1. The posterior view of the pharynx.

Fibers of the middle pharyngeal constrictor arise from the greater and lesser cornua of the hyoid bone and the stylohyoid ligament. In an analogous fashion to the superior constrictor, the fibers of the middle constrictor radiate posteriorly, inferiorly, and superiorly, condensing in the posterior midline pharyngeal raphe, which overlaps the superior constrictor.

The inferior pharyngeal constrictor is the thickest and most well developed of the three muscles. These fibers arise from the oblique line of the thyroid cartilage and the posterior aspect of the cricoid cartilage. The fibers of the inferior constrictor radiate posteriorly, inferiorly, and superiorly, condensing in the posterior midline pharyngeal raphe, which overlaps the middle constrictor.

Inferiorly, at the level of the cricoid cartilage, the lowermost (horizontal) fibers of the inferior constrictor interdigitate with the transverse muscle layer of the esophagus and thicken to form the specialized cricopharyngeus muscle. The cricopharyngeus muscle is innervated by the pharyngeal plexus (cranial nerve [CN] X) and is involved in the coordinated series of events associated with deglutition. Cricopharyngeal dysfunction has many causes. Idiopathic cricopharyngeal hypertonicity and cricopharyngeal achalasia result

in difficulty in swallowing or dysphagia. Systemic neuromuscular diseases, such as amyotrophic lateral sclerosis, myasthenia gravis, polymyositis, myotonic dystrophy, or muscular dystrophy, may cause cricopharyngeal dysfunction and result in uncoordinated swallowing with aspiration.[11] Similar symptoms may be present in patients with central nervous system pathologic conditions such as multiple sclerosis, Parkinson's disease, Huntington's disease or following cerebrovascular accidents.[3] Congenital weakness of this muscle may result in herniation of the pharyngoesophageal mucosa and development of a diverticulum. In many cases, vertical sectioning of the cricopharyngeus muscle fibers (cricopharyngeal myotomy) may provide symptomatic relief.

As a unit, the pharyngeal constrictors can be seen as a series of telescoping muscles with the lower fibers overlapping those above. They share a common insertion, that being the posterior pharyngeal raphe attaching at the pharyngeal tubercle. The motor innervation of the constrictors is from the external branch of the superior laryngeal nerve and the recurrent laryngeal nerve (CN X). It is uncertain whether CN IX contributes to the motor innervation of the constrictors. The blood supply to the constrictors is through the pharyngeal branches of the superior and inferior laryngeal arter-

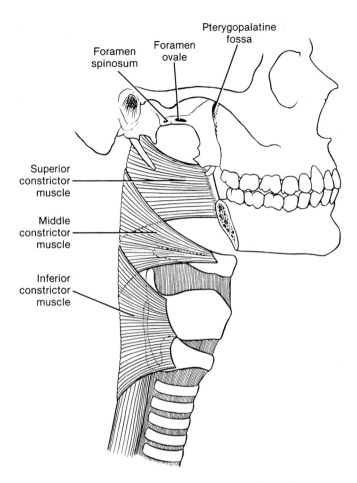

Fig. 71-2. The lateral view of the pharyngeal muscles.

ies, and branches of the external carotid and subclavian arteries, respectively.

When viewed from the lateral aspect, an interval is seen above or below each constrictor muscle (Fig. 71-2). The first of these intervals is between the superior constrictor and the skull base; the second interval is between the superior and middle constrictor muscles; the third interval is between the middle and inferior constrictor muscles, although it is mostly filled in by the thyrohyoid membrane; and the fourth interval is between the fibers of the inferior constrictor and the esophagus. As noted previously, each of these spaces contains certain structures and is invested as well by buccopharyngeal (visceral) fascia, which is part of the internal layer of deep cervical fascia.

INTERVAL BETWEEN SKULL BASE AND SUPERIOR CONSTRICTOR MUSCLE

The interval between the skull base and the superior constrictor muscle is closed by a fascial membrane (the pharyngobasilar fascia, between the pharynx and the skull base), which is part of the buccopharyngeal fascia. In addition, two small muscles are located in the interval: the tensor veli palatini (TVP) and levator veli palatini muscles (Fig. 71-3). These muscles arise from the pterygoid fossa between the lateral and medial pterygoid plates and insert into the soft palate. The TVP is a broad, flat band of muscle, compared with the more cylindric form of the levator veli palatini.

As the TVP fibers descend from the sphenoid bone they cross laterally to the superior constrictor muscle and course anteriorly to the hamulus and pterygomandibular raphe. At this point, the hamulus serves as a fulcrum for the aponeurotic part of the TVP as its fibers condense and twist into a relatively narrow band before inserting on the anterior aspect of the soft palate (see Fig. 71-5). This portion of the soft palate is tensed by the action of the TVP muscle. In contrast, the levator veli palatini muscle crosses the superior border of the superior constrictor and enters the nasopharyngeal mucosa and the lateral border of the soft palate.

The fibers remain as a cylindric mass until they reach the tip of the uvula. Contraction of the levator veli palatini muscle fibers elevates the soft palate and assists in sealing the oral cavity from the nasopharynx. Most authors state that the TVP also has an important role in opening the eustachian tube,[6,12,14,16] but others attribute this function to the levator veli palatini.[18]

TVP dysfunction produced congenitally, experimentally, or by extirpative tumor surgery leads to middle ear dysfunction and conductive hearing loss. Congenital TVP dysfunction and resultant middle ear disease in children with cleft palates has been well described.[7] Recently, Casselbrant and others[4] have demonstrated transient eustachian tube dysfunction, negative middle ear pressure, and serous middle ear effusion in monkeys after intramuscular injection of *Clostridium botulinum* toxin into the TVP.

In a review by Myers and others,[13] approximately one fourth of patients presenting with nasopharyngeal, oropharyngeal, or maxillary antral cancers had middle ear–eustachian tube dysfunction. Tubal dysfunction was associated with large tumors (T_3 or T_4). In these cases middle ear–tubal dysfunction was caused by (1) mechanical obstruction of the torus by tumor, or (2) tumor infiltration into the TVP resulting in muscle dysfunction and functional tubal obstruction. Eighty-one percent of patients with surgical resection of the TVP developed middle ear–eustachian tube dysfunction.

Also traversing the interval above the superior constrictor muscle are two arteries: the ascending pharyngeal, which arises from the bifurcation of the internal and external carotid arteries, and the ascending palatine, a branch of the facial artery. These arteries contribute to the blood supply of the palatine tonsil and adjacent mucosa.

Other important landmarks in this region are the foramen spinosum and foramen ovale, which provide passage for the middle meningeal artery and mandibular branch of the trigeminal nerve, respectively (see Fig. 71-3). At this point, the mandibular division branches into the buccal, lingual, inferior alveolar, and auriculotemporal nerves and is the site of the otic ganglion.

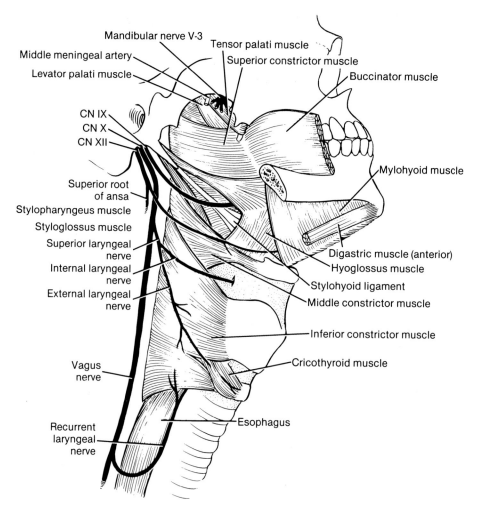

Fig. 71-3. The lateral view of the pharynx with adjacent nerves.

INTERVAL BETWEEN SUPERIOR AND MIDDLE CONSTRICTOR MUSCLES

The gap between the superior and middle constrictor muscles is filled by the prominent stylopharyngeus muscle, which originates from the styloid process. It traverses the interspace between the two constrictors and is directed inferiorly along the lateral pharyngeal wall, where its fibers insert into the fascia overlying the medial aspect of the middle constrictor. Accompanying the stylopharyngeus muscle is CN IX, the glossopharyngeal, which supplies motor innervation to the muscle. After penetrating the interval between the two muscles, the glossopharyngeal nerve courses deep to the hyoglossus and enters the posterior third of the tongue, where it supplies the tongue with afferent fibers for pain, temperature, and taste. Sensory fibers also are distributed to the palatine tonsil and mucosal wall as far superiorly as the eustachian tube and to the middle ear mucosa. Because it can be confused with CN IX in the surgical field, it should be noted that the stylohyoid ligament also traverses this interval

before inserting into the lesser cornu of the hyoid bone (see Fig. 71-3).

Finally, the lingual artery, after arising from the external carotid artery, enters the pharynx above the superior border of the middle constrictor and parallels the course of CN IX on the medial aspect of the hyoglossus muscle. En route to the tongue it sends branches to the inferior pole of the palatine tonsil.

INTERVAL BETWEEN MIDDLE AND INFERIOR CONSTRICTOR MUSCLES

Although the muscles do not form a continuous sheet in the interval between the middle and inferior constrictor muscles, there is no real gap between them because the space is closed by the thyrohyoid membrane. In this region, the structures are more accurately said to pierce the thyrohyoid membrane rather than to traverse an interval. Thus, the structures piercing the thyrohyoid membrane are the superior laryngeal artery and vein and the internal laryngeal nerve. The artery arises from the superior thyroid artery as it loops onto the superior lobe of the thyroid gland. Entering the submucosa of the larynx, it supplies the mucosal wall of the piriform recess and the mucosa of the larynx. Venous drainage of this area follows the superior laryngeal vein to the superior thyroid vein, a tributary of the internal jugular.

Accompanying these vessels is the internal laryngeal nerve, which is strictly a sensory nerve from the mucosa of the piriform sinus and larynx inferiorly as far as the false vocal folds. The internal laryngeal nerve is formed when the superior laryngeal nerve divides into internal and external branches (see Fig. 71-3). The superior laryngeal nerve arises as a branch of the vagus in the upper cervical area. It descends in the carotid sheath for 2 to 4 cm before dividing into the internal and external laryngeal nerves. During various laryngeal procedures the internal laryngeal nerve can be anesthetized by application of a topical cocaine solution in the piriform sinus or by cutaneous injection with a local anesthetic through the thyrohyoid membrane and infiltrating the submucosa. The external laryngeal nerve does not enter the larynx but parallels the superior thyroid artery and the fibers of the inferior constrictor muscle, which it supplies before innervating the cricothyroid muscle. During thyroid surgery this nerve is in jeopardy when the superior thyroid artery is ligated.

INTERVAL BETWEEN INFERIOR CONSTRICTOR AND ESOPHAGUS

The space between the inferior constrictor muscle and the esophagus is traversed only by a neurovascular bundle, composed of the inferior laryngeal artery and vein and the recurrent laryngeal nerve. The inferior thyroid artery is one of the branches of the thyrocervical trunk from the first part of the subclavian artery. The origins of the recurrent laryngeal nerve branches of the vagus differ on the right and left sides. On the left side, the branch begins at the aortic arch in the mediastinum, takes a recurrent course around the arterial ligament, and enters the tracheoesophageal groove. Ascending in the groove to the junction of the esophagus and inferior constrictor muscle, it enters the larynx and supplies motor innervation to the intrinsic laryngeal muscles. In addition, the nerve supplies sensory innervation to the mucosa of the larynx as far superiorly as the true vocal cords.

On the right side, the recurrent nerve is given off at the subclavian artery and, after looping posterior to the artery, enters the tracheoesophageal groove and ascends in a manner similar to the left.

POSTERIOR VIEW OF PHARYNX

When the pharynx is viewed posteriorly, the muscular wall appears to be a continuous structure until it is cleared of fascia, which reveals the overlapping of the three individual pharyngeal constrictors' muscle fibers.

After the pharynx is opened by a vertical midline incision (admittedly, this is not a routine surgical approach), a unique view of the three subdivisions of the pharynx can be obtained (see Fig. 71-1). The nasopharynx begins as far as the tip of the uvula. The oropharynx is outlined by a line drawn from the tip of the uvula following along the palatopharyngeal fold to the level of the epiglottis. Finally, the laryngopharynx extends from the epiglottis to the level of the cricoid cartilage.

Each of these three regions has special mucosal landmarks as well as important anatomic relationships that underlie the mucosa. For better viewing of these features the orientation is rotated another 90°, which looks laterally on the mucosal regions from their medial surface (Fig. 71-4). This is in effect the "other side," or mucosal view of the pharynx.

MUCOSAL VIEW OF NASOPHARYNX

There are several important landmarks on the nasopharyngeal mucosa, which can be seen either on an anatomic specimen or during nasopharyngoscopy. These include the opening of the eustachian tube with its prominent ridge, the torus. The torus is the slightly enlarged cartilaginous portion of the pharyngeal end of the eustachian tube that produces a raised area of mucosa over the opening of the eustachian tube. From the posterior part of the torus the salpingopharyngeus muscle sweeps posteriorly and inferiorly, raising a mucosal fold (the salpingopharyngeal fold). The pharyngeal recess (Rosenmüller's fossa) is formed between the salpingopharyngeal fold and the wall of the pharynx by the elevation of this fold. Diffuse lymphatic nodules in the mucosa underlying the fold and pharyngeal recess form the tubal tonsil (Gerlach's tonsil). In the center of the eustachian tube opening there is usually a slight elevation of mucosa because of the underlying levator veli palatini muscle.

The roof of the nasopharynx at this point is formed by the inferior surface of the sphenoid bone and the floor of the sphenoid sinus. There is frequently a depression in the midline of the bony roof, producing a concavity of the mucosa at this point (the pharyngeal bursa). The mucosa is infiltrated with lymphatic nodules at the periphery of the pharyngeal bursa, which may be sufficiently elevated to form the pharyngeal tonsil or adenoids. Occasionally, a cystic mass (Thornwaldt's cyst) may be found in the depth of the pharyngeal bursa. This is derived from a persisting remnant of the cranial end of the embryonic notochord, which can become cystic later in life.

Slightly superior to the bursa but still in the midline of the nasopharynx is the potential site of a craniopharyngioma. This tumor is formed from residual epithelial elements of Rathke's pouch, an evagination of the stomodeal roof that contributes to the formation of the anterior lobe of the pituitary gland during embryonic development. Besides presenting as a mass in the nasopharynx, epithelial rests from the epithelium of Rathke's pouch also can be found within the sphenoid bone or as suprasellar cysts. Entrapment within the

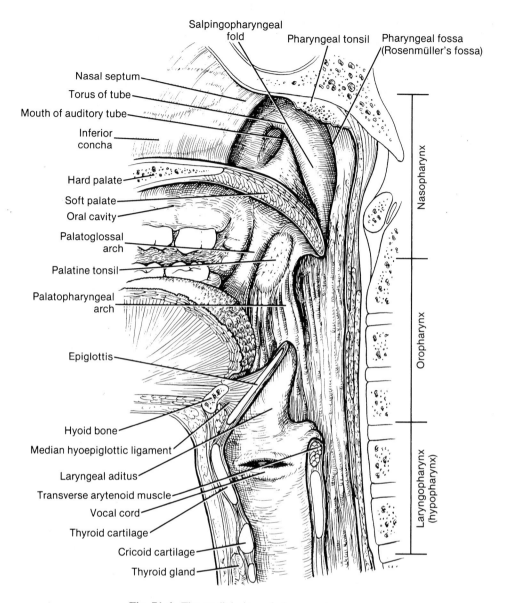

Salpingopharyngeal fold

Pharyngeal tonsil

Pharyngeal fossa (Rosenmüller's fossa)

Nasal septum

Torus of tube

Mouth of auditory tube

Inferior concha

Hard palate

Soft palate

Oral cavity

Palatoglossal arch

Palatine tonsil

Palatopharyngeal arch

Epiglottis

Hyoid bone

Median hyoepiglottic ligament

Laryngeal aditus

Transverse arytenoid muscle

Vocal cord

Thyroid cartilage

Cricoid cartilage

Thyroid gland

Nasopharynx

Oropharynx

Laryngopharynx (hypopharynx)

Fig. 71-4. The medial view of pharyngeal mucosa.

sphenoid bone occurs because the course of Rathke's pouch is through the mesenchymal anlage of the sphenoid bone before it is ossified. A parallel phenomenon, perhaps more familiar to the physician, is the entrapment of remnants of the thyroglossal duct in the hyoid bone after it is transformed from a mesenchymal mass to bone.

In addition to these midline structures, important clinical relationships exist laterally along the basisphenoid. Medial to the bony orifice of the eustachian tube lies the foramen lacerum, its fibrocartilage, and the carotid canal. Anterior to the bony orifice lies the foramen spinosum and more medially, the foramen ovale. These foramina provide direct preformed pathways for nasopharyngeal carcinoma to extend intracranially from the fossa of Rosenmüller.

When the mucosa is removed from the medial aspect of

the pharyngeal wall, many of the structures that traverse the interval between the skull base and the superior constrictor muscle can be seen (Fig. 71-5). As described from the lateral aspect, these are the TVP, levator veli palatini, ascending palatine artery, and ascending pharyngeal artery. This particular view also illustrates the salpingopharyngeus muscle, which underlies the fold.

MUCOSAL VIEW OF OROPHARYNX

The oropharynx is defined superiorly by the soft palate and inferiorly by the epiglottis; it includes the tonsillar crypt and the palatine tonsil. It is limited anteriorly by the posterior third of the tongue and posteriorly by the midline wall of the pharyngeal constrictor muscles. Other landmarks of this area are the terminal sulcus and the foramen cecum.

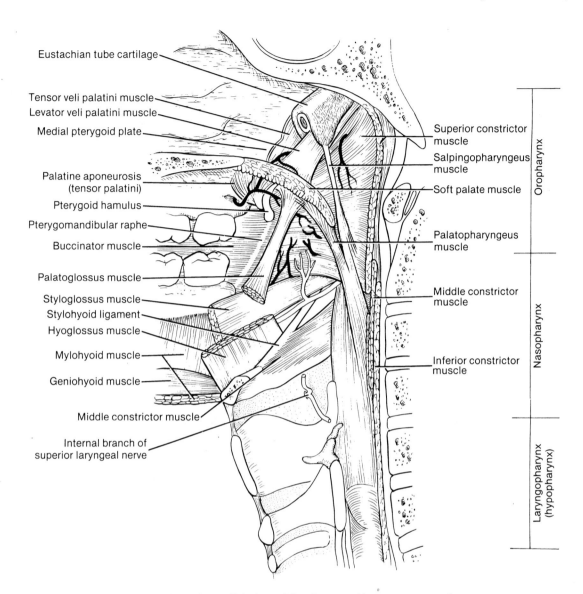

Fig. 71-5. The medial view of the pharynx with mucosa removed.

The sulcus is the boundary between the anterior two thirds of the tongue and the posterior one third. It marks the position of the circumvallate papillae lying anterior to it. At the apex of the V-shaped sulcus is the foramen cecum, representing the site at which the thyroglossal duct pouches out from the floor of the pharynx during development of the thyroid gland. Since the anterior two thirds of the tongue lies in the oral cavity, and the posterior third of the tongue is in the oral pharynx, the terminal sulcus also divides somatic (anterior) and visceral (posterior) innervations of the tongue.

At the base of the posterior part of the tongue are two small fossae, the lingual valleculae. These are bounded by the median glossoepiglottic fold (between the tongue base and the apex of the epiglottis) and paired lateral glossoepiglottic folds (from the lateral surface of the tongue to the lateral and inferior margins of the epiglottis).

The bed of the tonsil crypt is the lateral pharyngeal wall, which at this point is formed by the middle constrictor muscle of the pharynx. The anterior and posterior pillars of this region are formed by the palatoglossal and palatopharyngeal folds (Fig. 71-6). These folds are elevations of the mucosa created by the underlying muscles, the palatoglossus and palatopharyngeus. The superior pole of the tonsil rests against the soft palate, whereas the inferior pole is at the inferior border of the middle constrictor muscle. During a tonsillectomy, if the lateral wall or bed of the tonsil is penetrated, the adjacent lateral space or parapharyngeal space is entered.

The inferior pole of the palatine tonsil is of interest because of its relationship to the interval between the middle and inferior constrictor muscles. As already described, the important relationships of this space are the stylopharyngeus muscle, the glossopharyngeal nerve (CN IX), the lingual artery, and the stylohyoid ligament. Attempts to clamp ton-

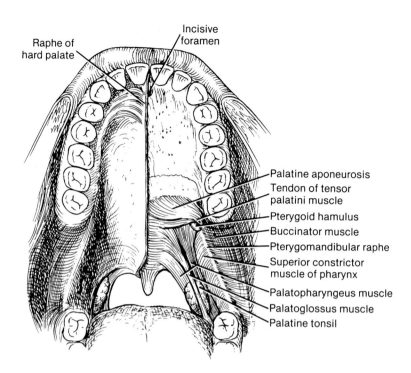

Fig. 71-6. Landmarks of the oropharynx and tonsillar bed.

sillar branches of the lingual or facial arteries supplying the inferior pole of the tonsil can jeopardize CN IX because of its relationship to the inferior pole of the tonsil. The sensory (touch, pain, and taste) distribution of CN IX is to the posterior portion of the tongue, lateral wall of the oropharynx, and upper portion of the laryngopharynx. Paralysis of CN IX may produce sufficient loss of sensation to cause the patient to choke during swallowing, since proper reflex control of the upper airway is lost.

MUSCULATURE OF SOFT PALATE

The muscles of the soft palate should be considered as part of the pharyngeal muscle group, not only because of their importance in swallowing but also because of the similarity in their innervation and development. With the exception of the TVP, which is derived from the mesoderm of the first branchial arch, all other muscles of the soft palate are derived from the fourth through the sixth branchial arch mesoderm.

The soft palate is composed of five muscles: the TVP, levator veli palatini, palatoglossus, palatopharyngeus, and uvular. The primary role of the soft palate is closure of the nasopharynx during the second phase of deglutition. It also has an important role in speech.

DEGLUTITION

In 1813 the act of swallowing was divided into three phases by Magendie, a French physiologist.[17] These stages are still used to describe the basic events of deglutition. Other reviews of this subject include those of Bosma,[2] Ramsey and others,[15] and Warwick and Williams.[19]

Stage 1

Stage 1 is primarily the movement of the anterior tongue, pressing the bolus of food against the hard palate and initiating the movement of the mass to the posterior part of the tongue and oral cavity. Although the intrinsic tongue muscles are important in this regard, the suprahyoid muscles (digastric, stylohyoid, geniohyoid, and mylohyoid) are particularly required in the movement of solid, as compared with liquid, masses. As the suprahyoid muscles contract, they elevate the hyoid bone directly and the laryngeal apparatus indirectly.

Patients undergoing resection of oral cavity/oropharyngeal neoplasms and reconstruction of the resulting defects frequently experience difficulties with the oral phase of swallowing. Logemann[10] has shown increased oral transit times for solids and liquids in patients undergoing resections of neoplasms of the anterior and lateral floor of the mouth. Transit times were increased significantly when reconstruction was done with local tissue flaps that tethered the tongue and impaired retropulsion of the bolus.

Komisar[9] has demonstrated that patients who have undergone mandibular reconstruction have more problems with deglutition and mastication than those patients whose mandibular defects have not been reconstructed. Postoperative scarring, fibrosis, and the loss of masticator muscle mass are all factors that cause impaired swallowing postoperatively. The restoration of anatomic continuity of the mandible, although providing acceptable cosmesis, does not appear to restore normal or, in some cases, even serviceable oral function in deglutition.

Stage 2

Stage 1 is sometimes called the voluntary stage, and stage 2 is called the involuntary stage. As the tongue presses the bolus of food against the soft palate, it is somewhat elevated and tensed by the levator and TVP muscles, respectively. At the same time the nasopharynx is effectively sealed, preventing the regurgitation of the food superiorly into the nasopharynx, and the bolus is forced into the oropharynx. A simultaneous narrowing of the fauces or oropharyngeal isthmus is accomplished by the contraction of the palatoglossus and palatopharyngeus muscles. The styloglossus also assists in the complete elevation of the tongue, whereas the stylopharyngeus muscle assists in elevating the pharynx. After entry into the oropharynx, the bolus is propelled downward into the esophagus by the synchronous contraction of the pharyngeal constrictors.[2] An important element of stage 2 is the sealing of the aditus of the larynx. Although this is an active event caused by the action of the muscles associated with the quadrangular membrane (aryepiglotticus, thyroepiglotticus, and thyroarytenoideus), there is some question as to whether the role of the epiglottis is active or passive. Fink[8] has suggested that the primary mechanism of laryngeal closure by the epiglottis is related to biomechanical forces on the epiglottic cartilage caused by the elevation and abutment of the laryngeal apparatus against the base of the tongue.

Any surgical intervention that interferes with laryngeal elevation or closure will cause dysfunction during stage 2 and will usually result in aspiration. Tracheostomy tethers the larynx in the neck and facilitates aspiration by preventing complete glottic closure. Conservation laryngeal surgery (supraglottic or vertical hemilaryngectomy) also results in aspiration. Patients who have undergone these procedures must relearn the swallowing act. The technique called the *supraglottic swallow* incorporates a cough following every swallow followed by another swallow.[10]

Stage 3

Stage 3 is essentially the esophageal phase; it is effected by the peristaltic movement of the esophageal muscle wall. It should be noted that the upper part of the esophagus is composed of striated muscle of branchial arch origin, whereas the lower esophagus is composed of smooth muscle derived from splanchnic mesoderm.

Impairment of the esophageal phase of swallowing is a rare sequela of head and neck surgery. However, tight pharyngeal closure following total laryngectomy can cause severe debilitating strictures. These may require treatment with completion pharyngectomy and pharyngeal reconstruction.[5]

Some patients experience dysphagia after either total or partial laryngectomy or resection of oral cavity neoplasms. The role of cricopharyngeal myotomy in this setting has not yet been determined. Currently, multicenter clinical trials are investigating the role of cricopharyngeal myotomy in eliminating dysphagia after head and neck cancer surgery.

INNERVATION OF MUSCLES OF PHARYNX AND SOFT PALATE

All of the muscles of the soft palate are supplied by the pharyngeal plexus—with the exception of the TVP, which is supplied by the mandibular branch of the trigeminal nerve. The pharyngeal plexus is usually described as composed of CN IX, X, and XI. CN IX provides only motor innervation to the stylopharyngeus. The vagus and the cranial portion of CN XI carry motor fibers to the superior and middle constrictor muscles as well as to the muscles of the palate through the pharyngeal branch of the vagus. These fibers originate in the nucleus ambiguus, which is a visceral efferent nucleus because the muscles of the pharynx and palate are derived from the branchial arch mesoderm of arches four and six. The inferior constrictor muscle is supplied by the recurrent laryngeal branch of the vagus. The external branch of the pharynx is derived mostly from CN IX, which supplies the nasopharynx and oropharynx. The laryngopharynx and especially the piriform sinuses receive sensory innervation from the internal laryngeal branch of the superior laryngeal nerve.

WALDEYER'S LYMPHATIC RING AND TONSILS

From the area of the eustachian tube to the base of the tongue the pharyngeal mucosa is infiltrated by diffuse lymphatic tissue and organized lymphatic nodules, which in some areas form specific tonsillar masses. When the pharynx is viewed from its posterior aspect, the aggregate of the subepithelial and submucosal lymphatic tissue, including the tubal, pharyngeal, palatine, and lingual tonsils, forms a ring about the pharyngeal wall, which classically has been called *Waldeyer's lymphatic ring*. It purportedly represents the first line of immunologic defense mechanisms.

In 3% to 4% of patients with metastatic carcinoma in the neck, no primary tumor can be found before initiating therapy. These patients are said to have "occult" or "unknown" primary tumors. In nearly 50% of these patients, Waldeyer's ring is found to contain a neoplasm initially thought to be "occult."[1]

Pharyngeal tonsil

As noted earlier, the pharyngeal tonsil lies at the periphery of the pharyngeal bursa in the nasopharynx. Depending on the size and number of lymphatic nodules, the mucosa can be raised into a substantial mass with intervening folds of the surface epithelium. Such folding contrasts with the crypt type of structure seen in the palatine tonsil. The epithelium consists of the columnar type of pseudostratified cells, although occasionally there are areas of stratified squamous epithelium.

Tubal tonsil

The tubal tonsil is formed primarily by an extension of the lymphatic nodules of the pharyngeal tonsil anteriorly in the mucosa of the lateral nasopharyneal wall. The nodules are found particularly in the mucosa of the eustachian tube and Rosenmüller's fossa. These areas of lymphatic tissue, even when they are not particularly elevated, are called the *tubal tonsil* (or Gerlach's tonsil).

Palatine tonsils

The palatine tonsils, unlike the other tonsil tissues, are usually large bulbous masses covered by nonkeratinizing stratified squamous epithelium. Histologic sections reveal deep crypts in the surface with abundant lymph follicles underlying the epithelial surface.

Lingual tonsils

Finally, the lingual tonsils are raised circular papilliform masses on the posterior third of the tongue. Each mass usually has a single opening on the mucosal surface that forms a tubular gland or crypt. Mucous glands are frequently described as opening into the crypt, which is lined by stratified squamous epithelium. In histologic sections the crypt contains a cellular detritus, and bacteria can be observed with appropriate staining techniques.

BLOOD SUPPLY OF TONSILS

The blood supply of the palatine tonsil is derived from many sources. These include (1) the ascending palatine artery and tonsillar artery, branches of the facial artery, (2) a branch from the dorsal lingual artery, (3) the ascending pharyngeal artery, and (4) the descending palatine and its branches, the greater and lesser palatine arteries (Fig. 71-7).

The pharyngeal tonsil (adenoids) receives its blood supply from the ascending palatine artery and the ascending pharyngeal artery, derived from the bifurcation of the common carotid artery. The specific blood supply to other tonsil tissues is not significant surgically, since they are only small regional arteries.

INNERVATION OF TONSILS

Innervation of the palatine tonsil is through the greater and lesser palatine branches of the maxillary division of the trigeminal nerve and lingual branches of the glossopharyngeal nerve. The latter are particularly important, compromising the pathway of referred pain to the ear during tonsillitis.

Patients with severe tonsillitis, peritonsillar abscesses, or oropharyngeal tumors often complain of pain in the ear (referred otalgia). The anatomic basis for this phenomenon is that sensory branches of the glossopharyngeal nerve to the oropharynx have their cell bodies located proximally in the inferior ganglion of CN IX. Also located here are the cell

bodies of the tympanic nerve (Jacobson's nerve), which provides general sensation to the medial surface of the tympanic membrane and the middle ear mucosa. Both the oropharyngeal branches and the tympanic nerve project proximally through the trigeminal (CN V) tract to the ventral posterior medial nucleus of the thalamus. These common central projections account for the simultaneous perceptions of pain in the ear and oropharynx.

APPLIED ANATOMY OF PARAPHARYNGEAL REGION

Many of the anatomic relationships discussed in this chapter are highlighted in Figure 71-8, a cross-sectional view of the pharynx at the level of the tongue. Whether a surgeon places an incision in the mucosa of the oral cavity or oropharynx because of an elective surgical procedure or is exploring a penetrating oral injury caused by assorted objects, such as knitting needles or sharp sticks, the anatomy beyond the mucosal boundary is hazardous territory. Penetration of the posterior wall causes, in addition to obvious hemorrhage, infection and abscess formation in the retropharyngeal space. Because the inferior limit of this space is the diaphragm, infection may spread inferiorly into the thorax, producing a mediastinitis.

Penetrating oral injuries directed posterolaterally traverse the tonsil bed and the superior constrictor muscle and enter the parapharyngeal space. In this region the structures that can be injured include the internal jugular vein, the internal carotid artery, and nerves associated with the carotid sheath at this point (vagus and hypoglossal nerves and sympathetic trunk). If the penetration is slightly more lateral than the previous example, the parotid can be entered, resulting in injury to any of its contents, the posterior facial vein, the external carotid artery, and one of the trunks of the facial nerve. Finally, more direct lateral penetrations may injure the opening of the parotid duct, or after traversing the buccinator muscle, lacerate the duct more proximally in the cheek tissue.

In addition to deficits caused by surgical or other trauma, the otolaryngologist should be aware of other signs and symptoms in the pharynx caused by pathologic conditions in the parapharyngeal regions. For example, trismus may be the result of peritonsillar space infections causing pterygoid myositis or direct infiltration of the pterygoid muscles by tumor extending out of the pterygoid fossa.

Palatal or pharyngeal hypotonia may be caused by vagus or glossopharyngeal CN tumors. A mass in the oropharynx, soft palate, or tonsillar area may represent the medial extension of a parapharyngeal space tumor or an aberrant internal carotid artery. The clinician must use caution in evaluating patients with masses in the pharynx and augment a careful and complete head and neck examination with appropriate imaging studies before obtaining a biopsy specimen.

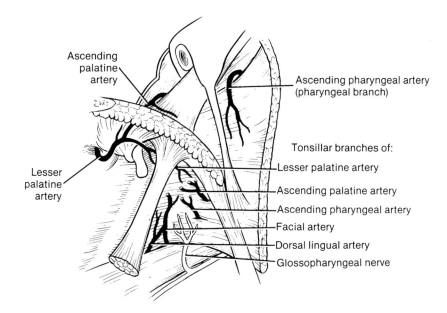

Fig. 71-7. The blood supply of the tonsils.

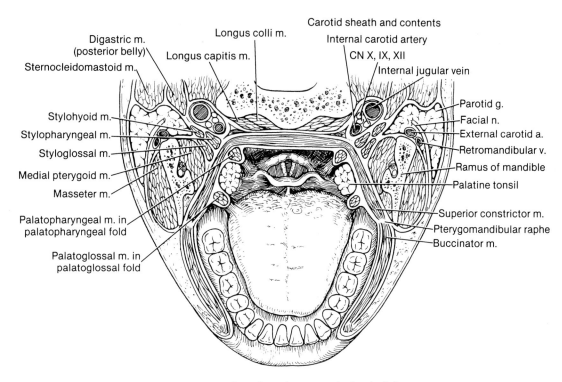

Fig. 71-8. Cross section of oropharynx at the level of the tongue.

REFERENCES

1. Batsakis JG: The pathology of head and neck tumors: the occult primary and metastases to the head and neck, X, *Head Neck Surg* 3:409, 1981.
2. Bosma JF: Deglutition: pharyngeal stage, *Physiol Rev* 37:275, 1957.
3. Calcaterra TC, Ippoliti A: *Neuromuscular disorders of the hypopharynx and upper esophagus.* In English GM, editor: *Otolaryngology,* vol 3, Philadelphia, 1990, JB Lippincott.
4. Casselbrant ML and others: Experimental paralysis of the tensor veli palatini muscle, *Acta Otolaryngol (Stockh)* 106:178, 1988.
5. de Vries EJ and others: Jejunal interposition for repair of stricture or fistula after laryngectomy, *Ann Otol Rhinol Laryngol* 99:496, 1990.
6. Doyle WJ, Cantekin EI, Bluestone CD: Eustachian tube function in cleft palate children, *Ann Otol Rhinol Laryngol* 89(suppl):34, 1980.
7. Doyle WJ, Rood SR: Comparison of the anatomy of the eustachian

tube in the rhesus monkey *(Macaca mulatta)* and man: implication for physiologic modeling, *Ann Otol* 89:49, 1980.

8. Fink BR, Demarest RJ: *Laryngeal biomechanics*, Cambridge, Mass, 1978, Harvard University Press.

9. Komisar A: The functional result of mandibular reconstruction, *Laryngoscope* 100:364, 1990.

10. Logemann JA: *Evaluation and treatment of swallowing disorders,* San Diego, 1983, College-Hill Press.

11. Mendelsohn MS, McConnel FMS: Function in the pharyngoesophageal segment, *Laryngoscope* 97:483, 1987.

12. Misurya VK: Tensor tympani: a "tuner" of tensor palati muscle, *Arch Otolaryngol* 82:410, 1976.

13. Myers EN and others: Effect of certain head and neck tumors and their management on the ventilatory function of the eustachian tube, *Ann Otol Rhinol Laryngol* 93(suppl):3, 1984.

14. Procter B: Anatomy of the eustachian tube, *Arch Otolaryngol* 97:2, 1973.

15. Ramsey GH and others: Cinefluorographic analysis of the mechanism of swallowing, *Radiology* 64:498, 1955.

16. Ross M: Functional anatomy of the tensor palati: its relevance in cleft palate surgery, *Arch Otolaryngol* 93:1, 1971.

17. Saunders JBdeCM, Davis C, Miller ER: Mechanism of deglutition (second stage) as revealed by cine-radiography, *Ann Otol Rhinol Laryngol* 60:897, 1951.

18. Seif S, Dellon AL: Anatomic relationships between the human levator and tensor veli palatini and the eustachian tube, *Cleft Palate J* 15:329, 1978.

19. Warwick R, Williams PL: *Gray's anatomy,* ed 36, Philadelphia, 1984, WB Saunders.

Chapter 72

Physiology

Joseph B. Travers

The oral cavity is a complex organ comprising muscle, glands, teeth, and specialized sensory receptors. For most animals, the orosensory and oromotor apparatus is critical for successful defense, reproduction, exploration, and vocalization.[36] In humans, vocalization has evolved into complex speech production, but other human behaviors depend less on the mouth and tongue than on the eye and hand. In all animals, however, the mouth is essential for the ingestion of nutrients. The incorporation of nutrients by mastication and drinking involves a high degree of coordination within and between different oral motor systems. Chewing requires the reciprocal activation of antagonist trigeminal muscles to open and close the jaws and the tongue to position food between the teeth. A diverse array of highly specialized sensory systems guide these complex oromotor responses. Mechanoreceptors on the tongue, palate, and periodontal ligament all contribute to a three-dimensional (stereognostic) perception of the oral cavity.[13] The sense of taste serves both in food selection and protection from ingesting potentially toxic substances.

Recent reviews provide comprehensive coverage of specific aspects of oral function, including mastication,[53,72,73,75,106] swallowing,[56,82] dental mechanoreception,[18] and the sense of taste.[23,41,81,127] In addition, several recent papers have reviewed oral pain[112] and taste dysfunction.[108,109,119]

This chapter provides a concise overview of orosensory and oromotor function. A brief synopsis of orosensory function describes the innervation and sensitivity of the oral cavity and a summary of central pathways. A section on sensorimotor function includes a discussion of masticatory, lingual, and autonomic reflexes followed by a discussion of mastication and the oral phase of deglutition. The sense of taste is treated separately.

SENSORY FUNCTION

Oral sensitivity

Somatosensory innervation of the oral cavity is provided by the maxillary and mandibular branches of the trigeminal nerve and by the glossopharyngeal nerve. The mandibular nerve branches to innervate the oral mucosa of the cheek, anterior two thirds of the tongue, mandibular dentition, periodontal ligament, gingiva, and anterior mandibular vestibule. Branches of the maxillary nerve innervate the hard and soft palate, the oral mucosa of the maxillary vestibule, and the maxillary dentition, gingiva, and periodontal ligament. Somatosensory innervation of the back of the tongue and oropharynx is provided by the glossopharyngeal nerve. Although the entire oral cavity is densely innervated with sensory fibers, considerable evidence indicates that the innervation is not uniform. Specialized oral tissues, including the lips, teeth, periodontal ligament, tongue, and palate, each display specific patterns of sensitivity. In some instances these sensitivities are associated with specific oral functions.

Overall, the anterior oral cavity displays greater tactile sensitivity than posterior oral structure.[56] The tip of the tongue is particularly sensitive, with a discriminative capability equivalent to that of the digits. Using a two-point discrimination test, Ringel[100] determined that two-point discrimination was greatest for the tongue tip (1.75 mm), followed by the fingertip (2.09 mm), lip (2.42 mm), soft palate (2.88 mm), alveolar ridge (3.02 mm), and thenar region (5.6 mm). The midlines of the palate and tongue were more sensitive than lateral regions. A similar pattern of sensitivity to mechanical stimulation applied to the teeth has also been reported.[76] Adults with complete dentition could detect a 1 g von Frey hair applied to the anterior (midline) teeth but required nearly 10 g to detect stimulation of the first molar. The tearing and piercing functions of anterior teeth require greater sensory control than does the crushing or grinding associated with molar function.

The high degree of sensitivity from structures anterior in the mouth correlates with the physiologic properties of the afferent fibers innervating these structures. Neural responses from afferent fibers innervating the human perioral region had small oval receptive fields (median = 8 sq mm) and low-threshold, slowly adapting responses.[59,60] Two additional cells with receptive fields restricted to a single tooth were directionally sensitive. Maximal response rates and the lowest threshold responses were obtained by forces directed distally and labially. Similar response properties to dental stimulation have been obtained from experimental animals. A study of mechanoreceptors in the lower cat canine revealed that forces applied in the distolingual direction were generally the most effective and that 81% of the responses were slowly adapting.[69] Numerous studies have determined that low-threshold mechanical stimulation directed at the teeth stimulates receptors in the supporting periodontal ligament.[40,68] The preponderance of experimental data indicates that sensations resulting from stimulation of the C- and A-delta fibers innervating the tooth pulp are nociceptive. Sessle,[112] however, points out that small-diameter fibers found elsewhere in the body may mediate touch or temperature sensations.

Studies in experimental animals suggest that specific regions of the perioral and intraoral receptor surface sequentially contribute to oromotor function associated with ingestion. Denervation studies in rats, for example, indicate that cutting trigeminal nerve branches that innervate the perioral region decreases the appetitive response to food.[136] Animals can still chew and swallow if food is placed in their mouths, but they do not actively ingest food. Other trigeminally innervated regions, those of the palate, for example, are low-threshold sites for eliciting the rhythmic oral movements of chewing and drinking.[131] Neither the front of the mouth nor the palate, however, is a particularly sensitive region for eliciting swallowing, the last stage of the ingestive consummatory response. Rather, the posterior aspect of the tongue, fauces, and epiglottis, innervated by the glossopharyngeal and vagus nerves, are low-threshold sites for eliciting a swallow.

A variety of chronic pain syndromes are associated with trigeminal nerve complications of the perioral region associated with maxillofacial surgery, but feeding disorders appear secondary to the loss of masticatory proprioception.[39,47] Nevertheless, experimental animal studies provide insight into the anatomic and physiologic response of the trigeminal nerve to injury.

Trigeminal response to injury

Several studies by Robinson[101,102] have examined the recovery of function and reinnervation of the teeth following injury to the inferior alveolar nerves in the cat. Reinnervation of the teeth was assessed by monitoring the return of a jaw-opening reflex to pulpal stimulation and by recording antidromic responses from the tooth pulp in response to more proximal nerve stimulation.

Evidence for reinnervation and collateral sprouting was clearly evident. Compared with intact animals, the ipsilateral mental nerve and the contralateral inferior alveolar, mental, and lingual nerves all innervated teeth on the side of the severed inferior alveolar nerve. A progressive decrease in both the threshold and latency of the jaw-opening reflex over a 12-week period suggested progressive remyelination of the reinnervating fibers.

A more recent study by Loescher and Robinson[69] showed how the receptive field characteristics of single periodontal mechanoreceptors recovered following crush or section of the cat inferior alveolar nerve. Twelve weeks after nerve damage, periodontal ligament mechanoreceptors responded to stimulation directed at the tooth but were generally less sensitive; that is, they had similar receptive fields and lower response rates. The response properties of recovering afferent fibers also depended on whether the nerve was crushed or severed. Nerve section resulted in greater response thresholds and decreased conduction velocities as compared with animals sustaining the nerve crush.

There is also evidence for changes in the central trigeminal pathway in response to peripheral nerve damage. Damage to the trigeminal nerve in which peripheral reinnervation is blocked can result in transganglionic degeneration of first-order afferent fibers.[2,133] Moreover, following tooth pulp deafferentiation in the cat, neurons in the subnucleus oralis had significantly larger receptive fields and responded atypically to stimulation of more than one division of the trigeminal nerve.[55] These central changes may be associated with the pathophysiology of chronic pain after damage to trigeminal nerves.[47]

Central projections of trigeminal system

Afferent fibers of the trigeminal nerve enter the brainstem in the pons, bifurcate, and terminate in either the principal sensory nucleus in the pons or descend to terminate in the spinal trigeminal complex in the medulla. The bifurcation of the trigeminal nerve at the level of the pons reflects a tendency toward a segregation of function.[64] In general, low-threshold mechanoreceptors predominate in the principal trigeminal sensory nucleus, indicative of a tactile discriminative function. In contrast, considerable evidence implicates the subnucleus caudalis in orofacial pain mechanisms, and many neurons in the subnucleus caudalis respond to noxious stimuli applied to the head and neck.[112] These neurons include those specifically activated by noxious stimuli (nociceptive-specific neurons) and wide dynamic range neurons, responsive to both low- and high-intensity stimulation (Fig. 72-1).

Because the receptive fields for many nociceptive neurons in the subnucleus caudalis are large and include re-

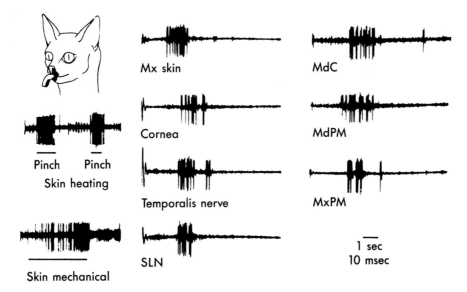

Fig. 72-1. Neuron in subnucleus pars caudalis responds to nociceptive stimulation (pinch or heat) applied to either the tongue or lower lips. This neuron also responds to electrical stimulation of afferent nerves innervating a variety of oral and facial structures, including maxillary skin *(Mx skin)*, cornea, temporalis nerve, and superior laryngeal nerve *(SLN)*. This cell also responds to electrical stimulation of different tooth pulps, including mandibular canine *(MdC)*, second premolar *(MdPM)*, and maxillary second premolar *(MxPM)*. (From Sessle BJ and others: *Pain* 27:219, 1986.)

sponses to nociceptive stimuli applied to the masticatory muscles, tooth pulp, and temporomandibular joint, a role for these neurons in referred pain has been suggested.[113] Anatomic studies confirm that afferent fibers innervating the oral cavity, tooth pulp, oropharynx, temporomandibular joint, masticatory muscles, and superficial skin all converge in the subnucleus caudalis.[10,25,115,133] Other parts of the sensory trigeminal complex, however, also are involved in trigeminal pain. Nociceptive responses have been obtained from extensive areas of the sensory trigeminal complex, and destruction of the subnucleus caudalis does not prevent all trigeminal pain function.[42] Lesions in the subnucleus caudalis, for example, did not interfere with the jaw-opening reflex to pulpal stimulation.[4]

Somatosensory information reaches the ventrobasal complex of the thalamus from all major subdivisions of the trigeminal sensory complex.[112] Many cells in the ventrobasal complex respond to low-intensity stimulation, indicative of a tactile discriminatory function; however, other neurons require high-intensity stimulation. The small receptive fields of both these types of neurons suggest a role in localization. Other nuclei, including the posterior thalamic nuclei and the nucleus submedius, respond preferentially to high-intensity stimulation and may be involved in affective components of pain.[35,112]

MOTOR FUNCTION

Much of what we know about orosensory and motor function has come from the study of oral reflexes and ingestive function in experimental animals. Although a great deal is

known of the synaptic basis for oral reflexes, the role of oral reflexes in complex, integrated oral behavior including either feeding or vocalization remains obscure.[40,106] Oral stimuli not only affect the masticatory, lingual, palatal, and facial muscles, but also elicit autonomic responses involved in chemical digestion. These responses, collectively referred to as the *cephalic phase response*,[99] include salivation, the release of digestive enzymes (amylase), and the pancreatic release of insulin.[44,48,91]

Oral (masticatory muscle) reflexes

A jaw-closing reflex, initiated by stretching muscle spindle afferents in jaw-closing muscles, monosynaptically excites ipsilateral jaw-closing motoneurons.[74] Unlike spinal stretch reflexes, however, there is no corresponding inhibition of antagonist (jaw-opener) motoneurons. The cell bodies for the muscle spindle afferent fibers are located centrally in the mesencephalic trigeminal nucleus. In humans the masseteric reflex is differentially modulated by stimulation of different sites in the oral cavity. Stimulation of the palate decreased masseteric force, but stimulation of the tongue increased it.[118]

The jaw-opening reflex is mediated by a different set of pathways.[74] Although the jaw-opening reflex can be elicited by nonpainful stimuli, because it can be reliably evoked by noxious stimuli, it has been used widely in the study of pain mechanisms.[77] There are few, if any, muscle spindles in the jaw-opening muscles.[40] Thus, during jaw closure when considerable force can be generated to crush objects between the teeth, the corresponding lengthening of the jaw-opener muscles does not provide that afferent signal for a reciprocal reflex. Stimulation of mechanoreceptors located in the periodontal ligament, tongue, and other soft tissues of the mouth, however, initiates reflex jaw opening. The cell bodies for these mechanoreceptors are located in the mesencephalic trigeminal nucleus and in the trigeminal ganglion. The central processes of primary afferent fibers terminate in the supratrigeminal area and in the principal trigeminal sensory nucleus, which in turn inhibit jaw-closer motoneurons and excite jaw openers. Thus, the soft tissues of the mouth are protected against potentially damaging objects through dysynaptic reflex pathways.

Lingual reflexes

Lingual reflexes can be elicited by stimulation of virtually any of the afferent nerves innervating the oral cavity. Depending on the site of stimulation, either a protrusive or a retractive movement of the tongue is produced. An overview by Lowe[71] on the functional significance of lingual reflexes emphasizes a protective role, either for the tongue itself during mastication or for the airway during swallowing.

Compounding the complexity of interpreting lingual reflexes are observations that reflex excitation of the tongue rarely influences a single lingual muscle, and contraction of a single lingual muscle can move the tongue in more than one plane.[70] For example, although a primarily retrusive movement of the tongue is produced by electrical stimulation of the lingual nerve, both protruder and retractor hypoglossal motoneurons are excited.[70]

Electrical stimulation of the glossopharyngeal nerve that innervates mechanoreceptors on the posterior aspect of the tongue and oropharynx also elicits tongue movement. Similar to the lingual nerve, stimulation of the glossopharyngeal nerve excites both protruder and retractor motoneurons, and the movement of the tongue is primarily retrusive. The simultaneous activation of glossopharyngeal nerve afferent fibers by electrical stimulation, however, may mask a more complex reflex organization. Lowe[71] has suggested that stimulation of lingual receptors innervated by the glossopharyngeal nerve elicits a primarily retrusive movement of the tongue, in contrast to lingual protrusion produced by stimulating pharyngeal regions innervated by the glossopharyngeal nerve. Thus, both lingual and glossopharyngeal nerve fibers innervating different regions of the tongue may reflexly protect the tongue during the occlusal phase of mastication with a retrusive movement.

In contrast, electrical stimulation of the superior laryngeal nerve that innervates laryngeal mechanoreceptors produces a protrusive action of the tongue, and protruder motoneurons show depolarizing potentials during this reflex. Mechanoreceptors in the oropharynx and larynx innervated by the superior laryngeal and glossopharyngeal nerves thus preserve airway patency during a swallow with a protrusive tongue movement.

Complex oral reflexes

Oromotor reflexes often involve several motor systems. Electrical stimulation of either the masseteric or anterior digastric nerves, for example, suppressed genioglossus activity, suggesting that proprioceptive or nociceptive signals from the trigeminal musculature inhibited lingual protrusion.[107] In contrast, passively depressing the mandible (in cats) excited the genioglossus muscle, suggesting that lingual protrusion may be reflexly facilitated during jaw opening when the tongue is not subject to occlusal force.[49] Similarly, stimulation of the hypoglossal nerve, which contains some afferent fibers, inhibited the masseteric (jaw-closing) reflex.[92] Thus, there appears to be a tendency for an oral reflex organization that facilitates certain oromotor combinations, that is, jaw opening with tongue protrusion and jaw closing with tongue retraction.

Autonomic reflexes

Studies in both humans and experimental animals indicate that gustatory and mechanical stimuli are effective in eliciting the flow of saliva during mastication.[3] Stimulation of receptors in the periodontal ligament may be one source for reflex salivation. In both rabbits and humans, there is a high correlation between parotid flow and mandibular movement, especially on the working, ipsilateral side (Fig. 72-2). In humans, selective anesthetization of the nerves innervating the periodontal ligament significantly reduced the amount of saliva elicited from crushing a ''Grape Nut'' stimulus.[3]

Both location and stimulus modality influence the release of saliva.[126] Stimulating the anterior part of the tongue is most effective for evoking salivation from the sublingual

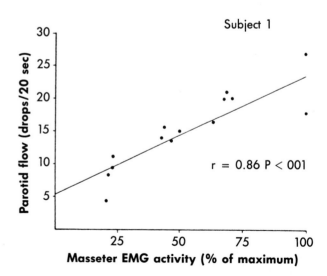

Fig. 72-2. The linear relationship between the amount of masseter electromyography while chewing a piece of Grape Nut cereal and the amount of parotid flow in a single human subject. (From Anderson DJ, Hector J: *Dent Res* 66:518, 1987.)

and submandibular glands, but posterior tongue stimulation is more effective for producing parotid gland flow. Aversive gustatory stimuli such as (sour) acids or (bitter) quinine hydrochloride are more effective for eliciting saliva than is stimulation with weak salt or sucrose solutions. Nevertheless, in experimental animals, sweet stimuli were the most effective stimuli for the release of the enzyme amylase from the parotid gland.[44]

Gustatory receptors also trigger the release of insulin in response to glucose stimulation.[46,48] Oropharyngeal receptors innervated by the superior laryngeal nerve may influence other metabolic or digestive functions.[116] There is increased diuresis in response to drinking a saline solution as compared with the intragastric infusion of the same volume of fluid.[42]

Ingestion

The orosensory apparatus of the mouth and perioral region is an integral part of the regulation of food and fluid intake. In general, the sensory receptors in the mouth are specialized for the consummatory phase of ingestion and play an important role in the sensory evaluation of food and in the sensory control of mastication and deglutition.

Food consumption through the oral cavity can be characterized as a series of stages or phases (Fig. 72-3). Different stages of ingestion have been defined by placing small metal markers in the jaws, hyoid, and tongue of experimental animals. These markers can be detected with high-speed cinefluorographic techniques, allowing the movements of the internal oral apparatus to be monitored during the entire ingestive sequence of the awake preparation.[53] The division of feeding into five dynamic stages by Hiiemae and Crompton[53] is indicated on the second tier of Figure 72-3.

The first stage of putting food into the mouth (ingestion) is followed by intraoral transport and the positioning of food between the molars (second stage) for mastication (third stage). Intraoral transport to the back of the tongue (fourth stage) initiates deglutition (fifth stage). The duration of each stage of feeding is species-specific and variable, depending on what is being ingested.[53] Fluid consumption does not require mechanical breakdown by mastication and thus has only three stages. In humans, drinking uses the same muscles as mastication, but the coupling among the facial, trigeminal, and lingual muscles is different.[73] The orbicularis oris muscle contracts to form a tight seal during human drinking (sucking) but relaxes during mastication.

Mastication

The movements of mastication can be further subdivided. Kinematic measurements during mastication indicate that rhythmic masticatory movements of solid food typically involve several distinct components.[52,75] Beginning the masticatory cycle with an open mandible, the jaw closes rapidly and then more slowly. The transition from fast closure to slow closure occurs when the teeth make contact with solid food and is thought to involve sensory feedback from the periodontal ligament.[73] More detailed analysis of the opening phase of mastication indicates additional complexity. Following the slow-closure phase, when the teeth make maximal intercuspation, the masticatory cycle continues with a slow-opening phase followed by a fast-opening phase. A recent review of mastication suggests a transition phase between slow and fast opening.[73] Pauses during rhythmic mastication are frequent during this transition phase. When mastication commences, it starts with the rapid opening phase, followed by fast and slow closure and ends with a slow opening.

Electromyography. Although mastication involves coordinated activity of the jaws, hyoid apparatus, and tongue,[53] the majority of electromyographic studies of mastication have focused on the jaw musculature. Jaw opening during mastication is associated with activity in the anterior digastric muscles and the inferior head of the lateral pterygoid muscle.[73,75] The closing phase of mastication begins with contraction of the masseter muscle, followed by the temporalis, medial pterygoid, and superior head of the pterygoid, which are recruited during the power stroke (slow closure). Food is typically chewed unilaterally. Although the trigeminal musculature is bilaterally activated during mastication, the ipsilateral (working) side is active earlier.[75]

Food consistency is one factor affecting the masticatory rhythm.[1] In a study of the effects of hardness on chewing, Plesh and others[98] observed that most subjects chewed hard gum at a slightly slower rate than soft gum. The decreased frequency of chewing was associated with significantly longer opening and occlusal phases of chewing rather than with the closing phase, despite the significantly greater electromyographic (EMG) activity in the masseter muscle.

Age is another factor that affects the masticatory rhythm.[62] Older subjects chewed crisp bread at the same frequency as younger subjects (approximately 1.4 Hz), but

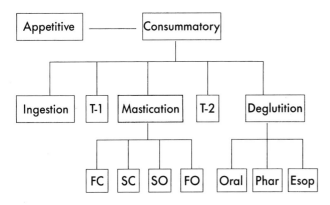

Fig. 72-3. The schematic representation of different stages and substages of ingestive sequence. *T-1* and *T-2*—first and second intraoral transfer; *FC*—fast close; *SC*—slow close; *SO*—slow open; *FO*—fast open.

the structure of the rhythm was different. The older subjects opened and closed their mouths at a slower velocity but achieved the same overall chewing rate by not opening their mouths as far. Movement irregularities during chewing were also observed during the jaw-opening and jaw-closing phases of mastication in patients diagnosed with temporomandibular pain.[122] Unlike the smooth, uninterrupted alteration between opening and closing seen in healthy individuals, patients with temporomandibular pain frequently started reopening their mouths during the closing phase of mastication or reclosed during the opening phase.

Central control. Experimental studies indicate that the masticatory rhythm is centrally programmed; that is, a peripheral stimulus is not necessary to initiate the masticatory rhythm nor is feedback from the active muscles necessary to sustain the response.[73] Fictive mastication evoked by central stimulation in a paralyzed experimental preparation indicates that neither the afferent limb of the jaw-opening reflex nor that of the jaw-closing reflex is necessary to generate the masticatory rhythm. Thus the alternating activation of a jaw-opening reflex followed by a jaw-closing reflex does not explain the origins of the masticatory rhythm.

Nevertheless, both the jaw-opening and jaw-closing reflexes are functionally entwined in rhythmic oral behavior, and the excitability of these reflexes varies as a function of jaw position during rhythmic opening and closing.[74,106] In general, the jaw-opening reflex is attenuated during rhythmic masticatory movements as compared with a stationary mandible. In particular, low-threshold mechanical stimuli are less effective than high-threshold stimuli in producing a jaw-opening reflex when applied during rhythmic masticatory movements (Fig. 72-4). Thus, during the occlusal phase of mastication, a protective jaw-opening reflex can be initiated in the presence of unexpected mechanical forces directed against the teeth or soft tissues, but innocuous mechanical stimulation associated with chewing will not interrupt the masticatory rhythm. Recent studies implicate secondary sensory neurons in the sensory trigeminal complex in jaw-opening reflex modulation.[96] Low-threshold mechanoreceptors in the rostral sensory trigeminal complex had depressed excitability during cortically evoked mastication. High-threshold neuron excitability, in contrast, was clearly phase modulated, with the greatest excitability during the occlusal phase of mastication. The significance of this reflex modulation is still the subject of debate. Are the oral reflexes inhibited to allow voluntary or rhythmic behavior via a central pattern generator, or does reflex modulation reflect the involvement of reflex circuits in the generation of the motor behavior itself?

Transection studies have localized the central pattern generator for mastication to the pontomedullary reticular formation,[27,95] and anatomic and neurophysiologic studies indicate that the medial reticular formation at the pontomedullary junction receives projections from the masticatory cortex.[72]

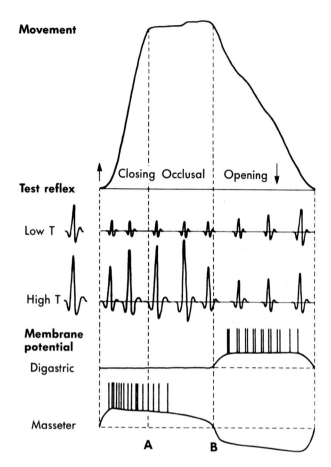

Fig. 72-4. Reflex-evoked jaw opening is modulated during masticatory cycle. During jaw closing, low-threshold afferent stimulation produces smaller motor responses in anterior digastric than when the jaw is at rest. High-threshold afferent stimulation produces high-amplitude anterior digastric responses during occlusion. (From Lund JP, Olsson KA: *Trends Neurosci* 6:461, 1983.)

The basic neural circuitry necessary for the rhythmic alternating contraction of jaw-opening and jaw-closing muscles does not require sensory input. Nevertheless, intraoral sensory receptors are critical for regulating bite force during mastication.

Sensory control. Efficient eating requires that food be reduced in size for swallowing. This requires determining both the hardness and size of the food and correctly positioning food between the occlusal surfaces of teeth. Psychophysical studies in humans indicate that receptors in both the periodontal ligament and temporomandibular joint contribute to the interdental discrimination required during eating.[40] The loss of periodontal ligament receptors associated with complete dentures results in impaired interdental discrimination, as does anesthetization of the dentition in individuals with natural teeth. Receptors in the temporomandibular joint also contribute to size discrimination in the mouth. When the temporomandibular joint is anesthetized, interdental discrimination decreases.

Recent studies have reexamined the morphology, distribution, and innervation of receptors within the periodontal ligament.[19,20] As many as six varieties of receptor morphology were described, ranging from complex Ruffini-like branched endings to free nerve endings. The cell bodies for periodontal ligament receptors were located peripherally in the trigeminal ganglion and centrally in the mesencephalic trigeminal nucleus.[58] Mesencephalic trigeminal innervation of the periodontal ligament was primarily in the apical region near the root and consisted of mostly small myelinated Ruffini-like endings.[21] Trigeminal ganglion innervation extended from the apical region to the more superficial region and included small unmyelinated nerve endings.

The differential innervation of the periodontal ligament by the trigeminal ganglion and mesencephalic trigeminal nucleus has functional significance. Mesencephalic receptors are primarily medium and rapidly adapting receptor types, many with directional sensitivity. The central termination of these mesencephalic force detectors includes inhibitory connections to trigeminal jaw closer motoneurons via the supratrigeminal area.[65] Thus, these receptors serve a protective role in preventing potentially damaging tooth contact during mastication. In contrast, trigeminal ganglion receptors include slowly-adapting mechanoreceptors (position detectors) and high-threshold C fibers (nociceptors) in addition to rapidly adapting mechanoreceptors. Moreover, periodontal receptors from the trigeminal ganglion terminate centrally in the sensory trigeminal complex, the source for the ascending (lemniscal) sensory pathway to the thalamus and cortex. Thus, tooth displacement and dental pain information from the periodontal ligament originates from the sensory trigeminal complex via the trigeminal ganglion pathway.

Although mechanoreceptors in the periodontal ligament are not encapsulated, their response characteristics may be influenced by the elastic properties of the ligament.[20] When the attachment of the ligament is compromised, for example, during periodontitis that loosens the connective attachments of the ligament, a corresponding loss in interdental force discrimination is observed.[130] Periodontal receptors also contribute to the regulation of bite force. Individuals with dentures could not bite as hard as normal dentulous subjects and could not perceive variations in their own bite force.[135] Similar results were obtained by anesthetizing the inferior alveolar nerve.[134] In contrast, anesthetizing the temporomandibular joint does not affect bite force discrimination but does impair jaw-positioning performance. Thus, sensing jaw position and controlling bite force during mastication may be regulated by different populations of oral receptors.

Oral phase of deglutition

After mastication and the intraoral transport of food to the back of the tongue, deglutition is initiated. The oral phase of deglutition consists of an upward movement of the tongue against the soft palate to force the bolus in the direction of the pharynx.[82] The precise nature of the stimulus that triggers the pharyngeal stage of deglutition is unknown. Both the volume and the rate of bolus accumulation interact to trigger swallows in experimental animals.[132] When the rate of licking (intraoral transport) increased in response to increased stimulus delivery, the volume per swallow also increased. Moreover, the physical nature of the bolus can influence the sequence and recruitment of individual muscles involved in the buccal phase of swallowing. In monkeys, the masseter muscle was recruited with the suprahyoid muscles (the anterior digastric, geniohyoid, and mylohyoid) during swallows of solid food in contrast to fluid swallows.[20] Similarly, there is individual variation in the activation sequence of the suprahyoid muscles and genioglossus muscle during voluntary swallows in humans.[54] In summary, the oral phase of swallowing is characterized by the overall movement of a bolus from the dorsal surface of the posterior tongue to the pharynx. The precise motor sequence of individual muscles during the oral phase of deglutition can vary, depending both on the individual and the sensory characteristics of the bolus. Contact of the bolus with sensory receptors in the oropharynx triggers peristaltic contractions of the pharyngeal musculature.

Like mastication, swallowing can be evoked from electrical stimulation of central structures in the absence of peripheral (muscular) feedback and is thus thought to be controlled by a central pattern generator.[82] The location of the central pattern generator for swallowing involves the caudal region of the nucleus of the solitary tract and the medullary reticular formation adjacent to the nucleus ambiguus. Voluntary swallowing is mediated by cortical pathways that reach these medullary regions through descending pathways.

SPECIALIZED SENSORY SYSTEMS: TASTE

Oral sensitivity to chemical stimuli

The oral cavity is sensitive to a wide range of chemical stimuli. Stimulation of the oral cavity with high concentrations of salts, acids, alkaloids, and other compounds elicits sensations ranging from stinging and burning to warm, cool, and painful. This sensitivity of the oral cavity, mediated by nonspecialized free nerve endings and shared by all mucosal membranes, is referred to as the *common chemical sense* and should not be confused with taste. Free nerve endings respond to many traditional gustatory stimuli but typically display a much lower sensitivity. Electrophysiologic recordings from the lingual nerve, for example, indicate that single fibers require concentrations of sodium chloride $1000\times$ higher than those necessary to elicit a response from a gustatory fiber in the chorda tympani nerve.[117] Much lower concentrations of other types of chemical stimuli, for example, menthol (10^{-4}), however, are adequate to elicit a response in trigeminal nerve fibers. The types of chemical stimuli that elicit low-threshold responses in trigeminal fibers suggest that one function of the common chemical sense is to protect the oral cavity.[117] Responses to common chemical stimuli, such as salivating and coughing, diffuse and remove offending stimuli from the mouth. The common chemical sense is not purely protective, however. Spices such as horseradish, ginger, and red pepper are effective stimuli for trigeminal afferent fibers and contribute to the flavor of food.

In contrast to the common chemical sense, taste sensations are evoked by relatively low concentrations of chemical stimuli when applied to the specialized gustatory receptor cells. Most investigators agree that there are a discrete number of taste sensations; the most common and easily recognizable are sweet, salty, sour, and bitter. The Japanese frequently include a fifth taste, ''umami'' (heavenly), associated with the taste of monosodium glutamate.[63] The sensations of flavor while eating are more diverse than those of pure taste and result from the interaction of taste with the smell and texture of food. The confusion between taste and flavor is well documented in taste and smell clinics.[7,119] Self reports of chemosensory dysfunction are highly unreliable; on testing, many individuals reporting loss of taste are frequently found to have impaired olfactory function with no loss in taste sensitivity.

In addition to a sensory-quality dimension with four distinct tastes, taste stimuli can be categorized on a hedonic dimension with stimuli divided into those that are preferred and those that are disliked. The hedonic attribute of taste is concentration dependent and spans the different submodalities of sweet, sour, salty, and bitter. Low and medium concentrations of salt are preferred, but salt becomes aversive at high concentrations. Although there is a strong genetic component to the hedonic values associated with gustatory stimuli, taste preferences are clearly modifiable by experience.[34] Human neonates find bitter solutions strongly aversive, but adults learn to enjoy coffee, alcohol, and other bitter-tasting substances. The hedonic attributes of taste are also subject to metabolic state.

Gustatory structures

Approximately 7900 gustatory receptors in the human mouth are grouped into distinct subpopulations, defined by their intraoral location, gross morphology, and innervation.[128] Gustatory subpopulations differ in sensitivity to chemical stimuli; however, the overall morphology of the taste bud structure within each subpopulation is very similar.[66] Each taste bud contains 50 to 150 neuroepithelial cells arranged in spindle-like clusters. Some of the cells within the taste bud extend microvilli into a nonkeratinized ''pore'' region on the apical surface of the bud. Taste bud cells without microvilli are designated supporting (or basal) cells and may represent a developing receptor cell. Receptor cells die and are replaced over a 10- to 14-day period;[11] however, the lineage of replacement receptor cells within the taste bud remains controversial. Because taste cells undergo continuous differentiation, disruption of cell division by radiation or other agents can disrupt the sense of taste.

The chorda tympani branch of the facial nerve innervates two to five taste buds on each of approximately 400 fungiform papillae on the anterior aspect of the tongue.[84] Fungiform papillae density is greatest at the tip of the tongue and decreases along the dorsal and dorsolateral edges of the tongue. No fungiform papillae are found along the midline. Taste buds on the posterior aspect of the tongue are innervated by the glossopharyngeal nerve and located either in tightly packed clusters distributed along the walls of the trenches surrounding seven to ten circumvallate papillae or in the inner folds of the foliate papillae located along the lateral edges of the posterior part of the tongue. The 2400 taste buds in the circumvallate papillae and 1300 taste buds in the foliate papillae constitute the largest percentage in the human oral cavity. A third large subpopulation of gustatory receptors located in the pharynx and larynx numbers approximately 2400 in humans. These taste buds are not associated with distinct papillae; however, the bud morphology is similar to that found on the tongue. Taste buds of the pharynx are innervated by the glossopharyngeal nerve, and those in the larynx are innervated by the superior laryngeal nerve branch of the vagus. A smaller subpopulation of taste buds (approximately 400 in humans) is found on the soft palate. These taste receptors, also not associated with distinct papillae, are probably innervated by the greater superficial petrosal nerve branch of the facial nerve. In rodent species, small populations of taste buds are also found on the buccal wall and sublingual organ, but these have yet to be characterized in humans.

The specific pattern of innervation of taste buds by a peripheral nerve has been characterized for the fungiform papillae on the front of the tongue. Single fibers of the chorda tympani nerve synapse on multiple receptor cells within a single taste bud and on receptor cells in adjacent taste buds.[83] Likewise, each receptor cell is innervated by more than one fiber of the chorda tympani nerve. Each fiber of the chorda tympani thus receives input from multiple receptor cells, and each bud is innervated by more than one fiber. This pattern of convergence of multiple receptor cells from adjacent taste buds onto a single afferent fiber provides an anatomic substrate for spatial interactions between adjacent taste buds. Successively lower perceptual thresholds in humans may be reached by stimulating multiple adjacent papillae with gustatory stimuli.[86]

Gustatory physiology

A common observation in neurophysiologic studies of the gustatory system is that individual neural elements are usually sensitive to a variety of chemical stimuli. Receptor cells, afferent nerve fibers, and central neurons are often responsive to diverse chemical stimuli that elicit qualitatively different sensations in humans. The central issue in gustatory coding has been to determine how broadly responsive neurons code for such distinct sensations as sweet, salty, sour, and bitter. Recent work has focused on organizing gustatory neurons at different levels of the sensory pathway into neuron types.[127] Although many neurons are multiply sensitive to different-tasting stimuli, these sensitivities are not random. Neurons are not specifically tuned to a single stimulus but typically respond best to one of the stimuli representing the four basic taste qualities. The representation (coding) of quality is thought to be mediated by these classes of neurons.

Sensory transduction

Gustatory receptor cells respond with graded depolarizing (occasionally hyperpolarizing) potentials in response to chemical stimuli. The size of the receptor potential predicts the magnitude of spike discharge in the afferent nerve and may represent the generator potential necessary for the release of a neurotransmitter at the receptor cell/afferent nerve synapse. The neurotransmitter or neurotransmitters released have not been identified.

Several different types of transduction mechanisms have been proposed for the gustatory system.[124,125] Proposed receptor mechanisms include the binding of a stimulus molecule to a receptor macromolecule in the cell membrane that alters membrane permeability and allows ionic flow. Other transduction mechanisms involve the direct movement of stimulus ions across specific membrane channels. Because different receptor mechanisms are associated with different chemical stimuli and individual receptor cells are broadly sensitive, it appears that different receptor mechanisms may coexist for the same cell.

One of the transduction mechanisms for sodium salts (e.g., sodium chloride) involves the direct movement of sodium cations across the cell membrane, which results in depolarization.[37] The passive sodium channel blocker amiloride blocks the depolarization of receptor cells from stimulation with sodium chloride but leaves responses to other chemical stimuli (e.g., sucrose, potassium chloride) largely intact. Further, amiloride selectively blocks responses of afferent fibers optimally responsive to sodium chloride.[51] Psychophysical studies in both humans and rats indicate that the application of amiloride to the tongue is associated with a decrement in perception of Na^+ and Li^+ salts but not K^+ salt.[111] The electrophysiologic and psychophysical response to other salts, for example, potassium chloride, is not blocked by amiloride, nor is the sodium chloride response completely abolished, suggesting multiple receptor mechanisms for salt.

Although monovalent salts do not bind to cell membranes at physiologic concentrations, the binding of a ligand to a receptor on the cell membrane is probably the initial step in the transduction of compounds such as sugars and amino acids, many of which taste either sweet or bitter to humans. The specific binding of L-alanine and L-arginine to a fraction containing catfish taste epithelia suggests distinct amino acid receptors.[125] The binding of amino acids to a membrane receptor either depolarizes the receptor cell directly by opening specific ion channels or alters membrane conductance through second-messenger systems. Although the hydrogen ion concentration of a stimulus correlates with sourness, specific receptor mechanisms are as yet unknown. Recent intracellular studies in mud puppy taste cells, however, indicate that sour stimuli decrease the resting conductance of the membrane to K^+, thereby depolarizing the cell.[67]

Peripheral sensitivity

The broad sensitivity to chemical stimuli observed in single receptor cells of experimental animals is evident following stimulation of single human papillae. Initial observations that single fungiform papillae were sensitive to a single taste quality resulted from stimulus concentrations that were too low.[9] In taste, as in other sensory systems, there is a trade-off between the area stimulated and the threshold concentration. The lingual threshold for a given gustatory stimulus requires progressively higher concentrations for progressively smaller areas. When single papillae are stimulated with sufficiently high concentrations, the majority of fungiform papillae mediate multiple taste sensations. Sixty-six percent of the fungiform papillae tested elicited recognition of at least three of the four standard taste qualities.[9]

Gustatory receptors sample food or fluid as it is ingested, masticated, and transported to the back of the mouth for swallowing. Receptor densities appear greatest at critical junctures of the ingestive sequence outlined in Figure 72-3. Gustatory receptors at the tip of the tongue are contacted immediately as food enters the mouth and are optimally situated to determine whether to continue or abort the ingestive sequence. A second population on the back and sides of the tongue and on the opposing palate is probably stimulated during mastication when food is crushed between the molars. Because subpopulations of gustatory receptors vary in their overall sensitivity to chemical stimuli, subpopulations of gustatory receptors may differentially contribute to oral function.

The chorda tympani nerve in many animal species is highly sensitive to a variety of salts (e.g., sodium chloride). This sensitivity is consistent with human psychophysical studies that show a low threshold to sodium chloride on the anterior aspect of the tongue.[30] Studies in rats indicate that many individual chorda tympani fibers are sensitive to both sodium chloride and hydrochloric acid (which tastes sour to humans) but that only a subset of peripheral nerve fibers are responsive exclusively to sodium salts.[51] When the sodium channel blocker amiloride was applied to the surface of the tongue, only the sodium-specific fibers lost their responsiveness to sodium chloride. Those chorda tympani fibers sensitive to both salts and hydrochloric acid maintained their sensitivity to sodium chloride stimuli in the presence of amiloride, implying that the sodium-specific neurons are particularly important for coding the salty quality of sodium chloride. Moreover, the recognition of sodium chloride decreases following chorda tympani nerve section in rats, further indicating a specialized role for this nerve in sodium recognition.[120]

The high sensitivity of the anterior aspect of the tongue to sweet stimuli in humans is more variable in experimental animals. The chorda tympani of rats, in particular, is not very sensitive to sweet-tasting stimuli; however, a sweet sensitivity is found in the anterior oral cavity in the nasoincisor ducts on the hard palate that lie in apposition to the anterior tongue.[124] The nasoincisor ducts are innervated by the greater superficial petrosal nerve, a branch of the facial nerve. Regardless of the precise location of the "sweet" receptors, many animals have a sensitivity to sugars and other sweet-tasting compounds in the anterior oral cavity. Gustatory receptors in the posterior oral cavity are highly sensitive to aversive stimuli and can initiate powerful rejection responses to unpalatable chemical stimuli. Sectioning the glossopharyngeal nerves in rats attenuates the rejection response to quinine monohydrochloride to a greater degree than sectioning the chorda tympani nerves.[126]

A specific oral function is particularly apparent for the superior laryngeal nerve. Chemoresponsive fibers in the superior laryngeal branch of the vagus nerve differ greatly from facial and glossopharyngeal nerve sensitivities.[126] In general, superior laryngeal nerve fibers are insensitive to sodium chloride and sucrose but respond well to stimulation with potassium chloride, ammonium chloride, and many acid stimuli.[15,38] Moreover, many superior laryngeal nerve fibers are responsive to mechanical and water stimulation.[123] The location of superior laryngeal nerve–innervated taste buds in the larynx and on the epiglottis indicates a protective-reflex role for these receptors, rather than contributing to gustatory quality perception. The superior laryngeal nerve is a particularly low-threshold nerve for eliciting swallows that could protect the airway.[82]

Human psychophysical studies show clear regional variation in the recognition threshold to different gustatory stimuli.[30] The front of the tongue had the lowest threshold for both salty and sweet stimuli; sour stimuli had the lowest threshold when applied to the foliate papillae. Although the front of the tongue also had the lowest threshold for bitter stimuli, such as quinine monohydrochloride, circumvallate papillae stimulation produced a steeper intensity function than obtained by stimulating the front of the tongue. The psychophysical scaling results for quinine monohydrochloride are consistent with the often reported observation that bitter sensations are more intense in the back of the mouth. With the exception of the high sensitivity to sour stimuli on the sides of the tongue, the gradient for threshold to chemical stimuli on the tongue follows the gradient for thresholds to mechanical stimuli, with the anterior region the most sensitive.

Despite these regional variations in threshold and concentration response functions, sensations of sweet, sour, salty, and bitter can be elicited from loci widely distributed within the oral cavity. Moreover, loss of a single gustatory nerve may not be apparent to the individual and can often be ascertained only by specific psychophysical procedures.[5] In general, the high degree of specialization among the different gustatory nerves of experimental animals is not as obvious in humans. Destruction of the chorda tympani from middle ear surgery destroys taste sensitivity from the front of the tongue,[17,57] but there have been no reports of a disruption of salt intake. It is interesting to note, however, that humans with laryngectomies reported thirst less often and were less able to localize thirst compared with a control group, suggestive of a role for the superior laryngeal nerve in mediating thirst.[88] The regional intraoral variation of taste sensitivity of humans may represent only a vestigal form of reflex organization, superseded by a wider distribution of gustatory sensitivities within the oral cavity and by an increase in the voluntary neural control of ingestion.

In general, there is a great deal of individual variation in the absolute thresholds to gustatory stimuli. Several studies have demonstrated as much as a 100-fold variation in detection threshold for both sucrose and sodium chloride over a wide range of ages.[8] Recent studies indicate that some of the variation in perception of gustatory intensity may relate to individual differences in the number of taste buds.[86,87] When the tongues of (live) human subjects were stained with 0.5% methylene blue, taste pores could be counted videomicroscopically and subsequently correlated with individual suprathreshold intensity ratings. Subjects with more taste buds gave significantly higher intensity ratings to standard concentrations of both salt and sucrose solutions applied to the tongue. It is unclear, however, whether the correlation between taste bud number and intensity ratings explains the human loss of gustatory sensitivity with age.[85] The loss of taste sensitivity with age is well established for both detection and recognition thresholds,[90,110] but initial studies showing fewer taste buds with age have not been substantiated in recent human or animal studies.[16,85]

Central gustatory pathways and function

Afferent gustatory fibers in the facial, glossopharyngeal, and vagus nerves synapse in the nucleus of the solitary tract of the medulla with a rostral to caudal organization (Fig. 72-5). An ascending gustatory pathway reaches the cortex via a thalamic projection or an additional synapse in the parabranchial nuclei of the pons, depending on the species.[41] A second gustatory pathway projects to the ventral forebrain, including the hypothalamus, amygdala, and other limbic structures. The thalamocortical pathway may be specialized for perceptual/discriminative gustatory functions; the limbic projections may be more involved in the hedonic/motivational attributes of taste.[97] Local brainstem gustatory pathways, however, have the capacity to mediate basic gustatory discriminative functions. Decerebrate animals and annencephalic human infants discriminate palatable from unpalatable gustatory stimuli.[97]

Gustatory pathways are in close anatomic proximity with

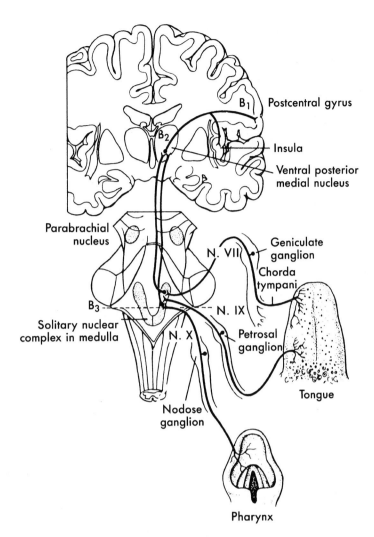

Fig. 72-5. Taste information from different subpopulations of taste buds distributed in oral cavity synapse rostral to caudal in the nucleus of solitary tract in medulla. Ascending projections to the thalamus and the cortex are primarily ipsilateral. (From Castellucci VF. In Kandel ER, Schwartz JH, editors: *Principles of neural science,* ed 2, New York, 1985, Elsevier.)

central pathways controlling autonomic nervous system function. This proximity provides a substrate for interactions between gustatory and autonomic afferent information.[94] Changes in the firing pattern of gustatory-responsive neurons in the nucleus of the solitary tract in response to distension of the gut is indicative of interaction between the autonomic nervous system and the gustatory system.[45] Similarly, hypertonic saline infused into the hepatic portal vein of the rat influences taste responses in the parabrachial nucleus.[104] Both phenomena suggest that visceral signals generated during feeding may influence orosensory perception. Human studies have documented the postingestion effects of feeding on gustatory preference. The preference of specific tastes, such as glucose, for example, diminishes as a function of the amount consumed.[22]

Chronic metabolic conditions also influence the hedonic perceptions of taste stimuli. Obese and slightly overweight individuals rate glucose solutions as more pleasant than do normal-weight individuals, although the perceived intensity of the glucose solutions does not vary between the two groups.[103] Hypoglycemic individuals prefer higher concentrations of sucrose as compared with individuals with high blood glucose,[78] and studies of diabetic patients report elevated psychophysical thresholds to glucose.[114] Loss of gustatory sensitivity in diabetics may result from a systemic lack of glucose receptors and from general neuropathy. Even short-term increases in blood glucose, however, appear to differentially affect neural responses in the nucleus of the solitary tract in response to sugar solutions presented to the tongue of experimental animals.[43]

Systemic electrolyte levels also affect the gustatory system. Sodium chloride thresholds are lower both for individuals on low-sodium diets and in hypertensive patients.[108,109] Physiologically, decreases in the chorda tympani nerve response to sodium chloride flowing over the tongue have been observed in sodium-deprived experimental animals.[33] The convergence between gustatory afferent fibers and visceral interoceptors on central neurons is one explanation for systemic metabolic and electrolyte influences on the gustatory system.[94]

Gustatory-salivary reflexes are another example of an interaction between the gustatory and autonomic nervous systems.[121] Direct gustatory influences over salivation are mediated by short axon pathways between second-order gustatory neurons in the lateral division of the nucleus of the solitary tract and preganglionic parasympathetic salivatory neurons located in more medial portions of the solitary nucleus and the adjacent reticular formation.[94] In addition, the oral cavity provides a peripheral site for interactions between the autonomic and gustatory systems and for general metabolic influences on the gustatory system via the vasculature.

Interaction between saliva and taste

The presence of saliva in the mouth continually stimulates gustatory receptors with low levels of salt ions. Correspondingly, recognition thresholds for sodium chloride are somewhat raised when the tongue is adapted with a solution containing salivary levels of sodium (3.4 millimeter as compared with recognition thresholds using distilled water rinses (0.054 millimeter).[79] By implication, the presence of other salivary constituents as a result of either disease or medication may affect gustatory sensitivity.[28] Salivary concentrations of pirmenol in patients being treated for ventricular arrhythmias, for example, may produce the bitter taste reported by these patients.[61] Increased salivary levels of glucose in diabetics provide one mechanism for the increased detection thresholds for glucose in this patient population.[114]

Saliva may also exert a trophic influence on gustatory receptors. Patients suffering long-term salivary loss as a result of Sjögren's syndrome had increased detection and recognition threshold to many gustatory stimuli.[50] Biopsies of the circumvallate papillae from a subset of these patients indicated a profound loss of taste buds. The effects of desalivation on both taste bud morphology and gustatory sensitivity have also been explored in experimental animals.[24,98] Surgically removing the salivary glands was associated with increased keratosis of the lingual epithelium and shrinking of the circumvallate papillae. Correlated with these morphologic changes was the increased consumption of nonpreferred gustatory stimuli, indicative of a loss of gustatory sensitivity. Electron microscopic observation of the circumvallate papillae showed the infiltration of bacteria, suggesting that the loss of antibacterial agents in saliva permitted degenerative microbial action. Lack of salivation by acute pharmacologic manipulations in experimental human studies, however, had relatively little effect on gustatory sensitivity.[29]

The loss of taste acuity in humans after radiotherapy to the head and neck could result directly from the destruction of taste buds and indirectly from reduced salivary flow.[31,84] Direct irradiation of gustatory structures in experimental animals produced a loss of taste buds.[32] Radiotherapy can also influence the gustatory system through the formation of conditioned taste aversions.[6,12] Clinical observations of hedonic changes in taste may result, in part, from the pairing of a conditioned stimulus (food) with an unconditioned stimulus, the gastrointestinal distress resulting from either chemotherapy or abdominal radiation.[12] An extensive experimental animal literature indicates that such pairings can have a profound impact on gustatory preferences.[26] Experimental animal studies indicate that the formation of a conditioned taste aversion is a central phenomenon that requires an intact forebrain.

Vascular taste

Although the taste pores and microvilli are oriented toward the oral cavity, chemical stimuli gain access to gustatory transduction mechanisms (and ultimately perception) via the vasculature.[14] The extent to which vascular taste mechanisms contribute to the rather extensive number of drugs that have unpleasant gustatory side effects remains to be determined.[105]

REFERENCES

1. Ahlgren J: *Masticatory movements in man*. In Anderson DJ, Matthews B, editors: *Mastication*, Bristol, England, 1976, John Wright & Sons.
2. Aldskogius H and others: The reaction of primary sensory neurons to peripheral nerve injury with particular emphasis on transganglionic changes, *Brain Res Rev* 10:27, 1985.
3. Anderson DJ, Hector MP: Periodontal mechanoreceptors and parotid secretions in animals and man, *J Dent Res* 66:518, 1987.
4. Azerad J and others: Physiological properties of neurons in different parts of the cat trigeminal sensory complex, *Brain Res* 246:7, 1982.
5. Bartoshuk LM: Clinical evaluation of the sense of taste, *Ear Nose Throat J* 68:331, 1989.
6. Bartoshuk LM: Chemosensory alteration and cancer therapies, *NCI Monogr* 9:179, 1990.
7. Bartoshuk LM and others: Clinical evaluation of taste, *Am J Otolaryngol* 4:257, 1983.
8. Bartoshuk LM and others: Taste and aging, *J Gerontol* 41:51, 1986.
9. Bealer SL, Smith DV: Multiple sensitivity to chemical stimuli in single human taste papillae, *Physiol Behav* 14:795, 1975.
10. Beckstead RM, Norgren R: An autoradiographic examination of the central distribution of the trigeminal, facial, glossopharyngeal and vagal nerves in the monkey, *J Comp Neurol* 184:455, 1979.
11. Beidler LM, Smallman RL: Renewal of cells within taste buds, *J Cell Biol* 27:263, 1965.
12. Bernstein IL, Webster MM: Learned taste aversions in humans, *Physiol Behav* 25:363, 1980.
13. Bosma JF, editor: *Second symposium on oral sensation and perception*, Springfield, Ill, 1970, Charles C Thomas.
14. Bradley RM: Electrophysiological investigation of intravascular taste using perfused rat tongue, *Am J Physiol* 224:300, 1973.
15. Bradley RM and others: Superior laryngeal nerve response patterns to chemical stimulation of sheep epiglottis, *Brain Res* 276:81, 1983.
16. Bradley RM and others: Age does not affect numbers of taste buds and papillae in adult rhesus monkeys, *Anat Rec* 212:246, 1985.
17. Bull TR: Taste and the chorda tympani, *J Laryngol Otol* 79:479, 1965.
18. Byers MR: Dental sensory receptors, *Int Rev Neurobiol* 25:39, 1984.
19. Byers MR: Sensory innervation of periodontal ligament of rat molars

consists of unencapsulated ruffini-like mechanoreceptors and free nerve endings, *J Comp Neurol* 231:500, 1985.

20. Byers MR, Dong WK: Comparison of trigeminal receptor location and structure in the periodontal ligament of different types of teeth from the rat, cat, and monkey, *J Comp Neurol* 279:117, 1989.

21. Byers MR and others: Mesencephalic trigeminal sensory neurons of cat: axon pathways and structure of mechanoreceptive endings in periodontal ligament, *J Comp Neurol* 250:181, 1986.

22. Cabanac M: Physiological role of pleasure, *Science* 173:1103, 1971.

23. Cagan RH, editor: *Neural mechanisms in taste*, Boca Raton, Fla, 1989, CRC Press.

24. Cano J, Rodriguez-Echandia EL: Degenerating taste buds in sialectomized rats, *Acta Anat* 106:487, 1980.

25. Capra NF: Localization and central projections of primary afferent neurons that innervate the temporomandibular joint in cats, *Somatosens Res* 4:201, 1987.

26. Chambers KC: A neural model for conditioned taste aversions, *Ann Rev Neurosci* 13:373, 1990.

27. Chandler SH, Tal M: The effect of brain stem transections on the neuronal networks responsible for rhythmical jaw muscle activity in the guinea pig, *J Neurosci* 6:1831, 1986.

28. Christensen CM: *Role of saliva in human taste perception*. In Meiselman HL, Rivlin RS, editors: *Clinical measurement of taste and smell*, New York, 1986, MacMillan Publishing.

29. Christensen CM and others: Effects of pharmacologic reductions in salivary flow on taste thresholds in man, *Arch Oral Biol* 29:17, 1984.

30. Collings VB: Human taste responses as a function of locus of stimulation on the tongue and soft palate, *Percep Psychophys* 16:169, 1974.

31. Conger AD: Loss and recovery of taste acuity in patients irradiated to the oral cavity, *Radiat Res* 53:338, 1973.

32. Conger AD, Wells MA: Radiation and aging effect on taste structure and function, *Radiat Res* 37:31, 1969.

33. Contreras RJ, Frank M: Sodium deprivation alters neural responses to gustatory stimuli, *J Gen Physiol* 73:569, 1979.

34. Cowart BJ, Beauchamp GK: *Factors affecting acceptance of salt by human infants and children*. In Kare MR, Brand JG, editors: *Interaction of the chemical senses with nutrition*, Orlando, Fla, 1986, Academic Press.

35. Craig AD Jr, Burton H: Spinal and medullary lamina I projection to nucleus submedius in medial thalamus: a possible pain center, *J Neurophysiol* 45:443, 1981.

36. Darian-Smith I: *The trigeminal system*. In Iggo A, editor: *Handbook of physiology, vol II. Somatosensory system*, New York, 1973, Springer-Verlag.

37. DeSimone JA and others: The active ion transport properties of canine lingual epithelia in vitro: implications for gustatory transduction, *J Gen Physiol* 83:633, 1984.

38. Dickman JD, Smith DV: Response properties of fibers in the hamster superior laryngeal nerve, *Brain Res* 450:25, 1988.

39. Donoff RB, Colin W: Neurologic complications of oral and maxillofacial surgery, *Oral Maxillofac Surg Clin North Am* 2:453, 1990.

40. Dubner R and others: *The neural basis of oral and facial function*, New York, 1978, Plenum Press.

41. Finger TE: *Gustatory nuclei and pathways in the central nervous system*. In Finger TE, Silver WL, editors: *Neurobiology of taste and smell*, New York, 1987, John Wiley & Sons.

42. Gebruers EM and others: Signals from the oropharynx may contribute to the diuresis which occurs in man to drinking isotonic fluids, *J Physiol* 363:21, 1985.

43. Giza BK, Scott TR: Blood glucose selectively affects taste-evoked activity in rat nucleus tractus solitarius, *Physiol Behav* 31:643, 1983.

44. Gjorstrup P: Taste and chewing as stimuli for the secretion of amylase from the parotid gland of the rabbit, *Acta Physiol Scand* 110:295, 1980.

45. Glenn JF, Erickson RP: Gastric modulation of gustatory afferent activity, *Physiol Behav* 16:561, 1976.

46. Goldfine ID and others: The effect of glucola, diet cola and water ingestion on blood glucose and plasma insulin (33870), *Proc Soc Exp Biol Med* 131:329, 1969.

47. Gregg JM: Studies of traumatic neuralgia in the maxillofacial region: symptom complexes and response to microsurgery, *J Oral Maxillofac Surg* 48:135, 1990.

48. Grill HJ and others: Oral glucose is the prime elicitor of preabsorptive insulin secretion, *Am J Physiol* 246:88, 1984.

49. Hellstrand E: Reflex control of cat extrinsic and intrinsic tongue muscles exerted by intraoral receptors, *Acta Physiol Scand* 115:245, 1982.

50. Henkin RI and others: Abnormalities of taste and smell in Sjögren's syndrome, *Ann Intern Med* 76:375, 1972.

51. Hettinger TP, Frank ME: Specificity of amiloride inhibition of hamster taste responses, *Brain Res* 513:24, 1990.

52. Hiiemae KM: *Masticatory movements in primitive mammals*. In Anderson DJ, Matthews B, editors: *Mastication*, Bristol, England, 1976, John Wright & Sons.

53. Hiiemae KM, Crompton AW: *Mastication, food transport, and swallowing*. In Hildebrand M and others, editors: *Functional vertebrate morphology*, Cambridge, Mass, 1985, Belknap Press.

54. Hrycyshyn AW, Basmajian JV: Electromyography of the oral stage of swallowing in man, *Am J Anat* 133:333, 1972.

55. Hu JW and others: Tooth pulp deafferentation is associated with functional alterations in the properties of neurons in the trigeminal spinal tract nucleus, *J Neurophysiol* 56:1650, 1986.

56. Jean A: *Brainstem control of swallowing: localization and organization of the central pattern generator for swallowing*. In Taylor A, editor: *Neurophysiology of the jaws and teeth*, New York, 1990, MacMillan Publishing.

57. Jeppson P-H, Hallen O: The taste after operation for otosclerosis, *Pract Otolrhinollaryngol* 33:215, 1971.

58. Jerge CR: Organization and function of the trigeminal mesencephalic nucleus, *J Neurophysiol* 26:379, 1963.

59. Johansson RS, Olsson KA: Microelectrode recordings from human oral mechanoreceptors, *Brain Res* 118:307, 1976.

60. Johansson RS and others: Mechanoreceptor activity from the human face and oral mucosa. *Exp Brain Res* 72:204, 1988.

61. Johnson BF and others: Salivary concentrations of pirmenol as a possible cause of unpleasant taste, *Br J Clin Pharmacol* 22:613, 1986.

62. Karlsson S, Carlsson GE: Characteristics of mandibular masticatory movement in young and elderly dentate subjects, *J Dent Res* 69:473, 1990.

63. Kawamura Y, Kare MR, editors: *Umami: a basic taste,* New York, 1987, Marcel-Dekker.

64. Kelly JP: *The trigeminal system*. In Kandel ER, Schwartz JH, editors: *Principles of neural science*, ed 2, New York, 1985, Elsevier Science Publishing.

65. Kidokoro Y and others: Possible interneurons responsible for reflex inhibition of motoneurons of jaw-closing muscles from the inferior dental nerve, *J Neurophysiol* 31:709, 1968.

66. Kinnamon JC: *Organization and innervation of taste buds*. In Finger TE, Silver WL, editors: *Neurobiology of taste and smell*, New York, 1987, John Wiley & Sons.

67. Kinnamon SC, Roper SD: Evidence for a role of voltage-sensitive apical K^+ channels in sour and salt taste transduction, *Chem Sense* 13:115, 1988.

68. Linden RWA: Touch thresholds of vital and nonvital human teeth, *Exp Neurol* 48:387, 1975.

69. Loescher AR, Robinson PP: Properties of reinnervated periodontal mechanoreceptors after inferior alveolar nerve injuries in cats, *J Neurophysiol* 62:979, 1989.

70. Lowe AA: The neural regulation of tongue movements, *Prog Neurobiol* 15:295, 1981.

71. Lowe AA: Tongue movements: brainstem mechanisms and clinical postulates, *Brain Behav Evol* 25:128, 1984.

72. Lund JP: Mastication and its control by the brain stem, *CRC Crit Rev Oral Biol Med* 2:33, 1991.

73. Lund JP, Enomoto S: *The generation of mastication by the mammalian central nervous system.* In Cohen A and others, editors: *Neural control of rhythmic movements in vertebrates,* New York, 1988, John Wiley & Sons.

74. Lund JP, Olsson KA: The importance of reflexes and their control during jaw movement, *Trends Neurosci* 6:458, 1983.

75. Luschei ES, Goldberg LJ: *Neural mechanisms of mandibular control: mastication and voluntary biting.* In American Physiological Society: *Handbook of physiology II,* part 2, Baltimore, 1981, Williams & Wilkins.

76. Manly RS and others: Oral sensory threshold of persons with natural and artificial dentitions, *J Dent Res* 31:305, 1952.

77. Mason P and others: Is the jaw-opening reflex a valid model of pain? *Brain Res Rev* 10:137, 1985.

78. Mayer-Gross W, Walker JW: Taste and selection of food in hypoglycaemia, *Br J Exp Pathol* 65:297, 1946.

79. McBurney DH, Pfaffmann C: Gustatory adaptation to saliva and sodium chloride, *J Exp Psychol* 65:523, 1963.

80. McNamara JA Jr, Moyers RE: Electromyography of the oral phase of deglutition in the rhesus monkey *(Macaca mulatta),* Arch Oral Biol 18:995, 1973.

81. Meiselman HL, Rivlin RS, editors: *Clinical measurement of taste and smell,* New York, 1986, MacMillan Publishing.

82. Miller AJ: Deglutition, *Physiol Rev* 62:129, 1982.

83. Miller IJ Jr: Peripheral interactions among single papilla inputs to gustatory nerve fibers, *J Gen Physiol* 57:1, 1971.

84. Miller IJ Jr: Variation in human fungiform taste bud densities among regions and subjects, *Anat Rec* 216:474, 1986.

85. Miller IJ Jr: Variation in human taste bud density as a function of age. In: Nutrition and the chemical senses in aging: recent advances and current research needs, *Ann NY Acad Sci* 561:307, 1989.

86. Miller IJ Jr, Reedy FE Jr: Quantification of fungiform papillae and taste pores in living human subjects, *Chem Senses* 15:281, 1990.

87. Miller IJ Jr, Reedy FE Jr: Variations in human taste bud density and taste intensity perception, *Physiol Behav* 47:1213, 1990.

88. Miyaoka Y and others: Sensation of thirst in normal and laryngectomized man, *Percept Mot Skills* 64:239, 1987.

89. Mossman KL: Gustatory tissue injury in man: radiation dose response relationships and mechanisms of taste loss, *Br J Cancer* 53(suppl VII):9, 1986.

90. Murphy C: *Taste and smell in the elderly.* In Meiselman HL, Rivlin RS, editors: *Clinical measurement of taste and smell,* New York, 1986, MacMillan Publishing.

91. Naim M and others: Effects of oral stimulation on the cephalic phase of pancreatic exocrine secretion in dogs, *Physiol Behav* 20:563, 1978.

92. Nakamura Y and others: Effects of hypoglossal afferent stimulation on masseteric motoneurons in cats, *Exp Neurol* 61:1, 1978.

93. Nanda R, Catalanotto FA: Long-term effects of surgical desalivation upon taste acuity, fluid intake, and taste buds in the rat, *J Dent Res* 60:69, 1981.

94. Norgren R: Taste and the autonomic nervous system, *Chem Senses* 10:143, 1985.

95. Nozaki S and others: Role of corticobulbar projection neurons in cortically induced rhythmical masticatory jaw-opening movement in the guinea pig, *J Neurophysiol* 55:826, 1986.

96. Olsson KA and others: Modulation of transmission in rostral trigeminal sensory nuclei during chewing, *J Neurophysiol* 55:56, 1986.

97. Pfaffmann C and others: Neural mechanisms and behavioral aspects of taste, *Ann Rev Psychol* 30:283, 1979.

98. Plesh O and others: Effect of gum hardness on chewing pattern, *Exp Neurol* 92:502, 1986.

99. Powley TL: The ventromedial hypothalamic syndrome, satiety, and a cephalic phase hypothesis, *Psychol Rev* 24:39, 1977.

100. Ringel RL: *Oral region two-point discrimination in normal and myo-pathic subjects.* In Bosma JF, editor: *Symposium on oral sensation and perception,* Springfield, Ill, 1967, Charles C Thomas.

101. Robinson PP: Reinnervation of teeth, mucous membrane and skin following section of the inferior alveolar nerve in the cat, *Brain Res* 220:241, 1981.

102. Robinson PP: Reinnervation of teeth after segmental osteotomy in the cat: the effect of segment repositioning and bone grafting, *Int J Oral Maxillofac Surg* 15:152, 1986.

103. Rodin J and others: Relationship between obesity, weight loss, and taste responsiveness, *Physiol Behav* 17:591, 1976.

104. Rogers RC and others: Electrophysiological and neuroanatomic studies of hepatic portal osmo- and sodium receptive afferent projections within the brain, *J Auton Nerv Syst* 1:183, 1979.

105. Rollin H: Drug-related gustatory disorders, *Ann Otolaryngol* 87:37, 1978.

106. Rossignol S and others: *The role of sensory inputs in regulating patterns of rhythmical movements in higher vertebrates: a comparison between locomotion, respiration, and mastication.* In Cohen A and others, editors: *Neural control of rhythmic movements in vertebrates,* New York, 1988, John Wiley & Sons.

107. Sauerland EK, Mizuno N: A protective mechanism for the tongue: supression of genioglossal activity induced by stimulation of trigeminal proprioceptive afferents, *Experientia* 26:1226, 1970.

108. Schiffman SS: Taste and smell in disease (part 1), *N Engl J Med* 308: 1275, 1983.

109. Schiffman SS: Taste and smell in disease (part 2), *N Engl J Med* 308: 1337, 1983.

110. Schiffman SS: *Age-related changes in taste and smell and their possible causes.* In Meiselman HL, Rivlin RS, editors: *Clinical measurement of taste and smell,* New York, 1986, MacMillan Publishing.

111. Schiffman SS and others: Amiloride reduces the taste intensity of Na^+ and Li^+ salts and sweeteners, *Proc Natl Acad Sci U S A* 80:6136, 1983.

112. Sessle BJ: The neurobiology of facial and dental pain: present knowledge, future directions, *J Dent Res* 66:962, 1987.

113. Sessle BJ and others: Convergence of cutaneous, tooth pulp, visceral, neck and muscle afferents onto nociceptive and non-nociceptive neurons in trigeminal subnucleus caudalis (medullary dorsal horn) and its implications for referred pain, *Pain* 27:219, 1986.

114. Settle RG: *Diabetes mellitus and the chemical senses.* In Meiselman HL, Rivlin RS, editors: *Clinical measurement of taste and smell,* New York, 1986, MacMillan Publishing.

115. Shigenaga Y and others: Oral and facial representation within the medullary and upper cervical dorsal horns in the cat, *J Comp Neurol* 243:388, 1986.

116. Shingai T and others: Diuresis mediated by the superior laryngeal nerve in rat, *Physiol Behav* 44:431, 1988.

117. Silver WL: *The common chemical sense.* In Finger TE, Silver WL, editors: *Neurobiology of taste and smell,* New York, 1987, John Wiley & Sons.

118. Smith A and others: Reflex responses of the human jaw-closing system depend on the locus of intraoral mechanical stimulation, *Exp Neurol* 90:489, 1985.

119. Smith DV: *Taste and smell dysfunction.* In Paparella MM and others, editors: *Otolaryngology,* ed 3, Philadelphia, 1988, WB Saunders.

120. Spector AC and others: Chemospecific deficits in taste detection after selective gustatory deafferentation in rats, *Am J Physiol* 258:820, 1990.

121. Spielman AI: Interaction of saliva and taste, *J Dent Res* 69:838, 1990.

122. Stohler CS, Ash MM: Demonstration of chewing motor disorder by recording peripheral correlates of mastication, *J Oral Rehab* 12:49, 1985.

123. Storey AT, Johnson P: Laryngeal water receptors initiating apnea in the lamb, *Exp Neurol* 47:42, 1975.

124. Teeter JH, Brand JG: *Peripheral mechanisms of gustation: physiology*

and biochemistry. In Finger TE, Silver WL, editors: *Neurobiology of taste and smell*, New York, 1987, John Wiley & Sons.

125. Teeter JH, Cagan RH: *Mechanisms of taste transduction*. In Cagan RH, editor: *Neural mechanisms in taste*, Boca Raton, Fla, 1989, CRC Press.

126. Travers JB and others: The effects of glossopharyngeal and chorda tympani nerve cuts on the ingestion and rejection of rapid stimuli: an electromyographic analysis in the rat, *Behav Brain Res* 25:233, 1987.

127. Travers JB and others: Gustatory neural processing in the hindbrain, *Ann Rev Neurosci* 10:595, 1987.

128. Travers SP, Nicklas K: Taste bud distribution in the rat pharynx and larynx, *Anat Rec* 227:373, 1990.

129. Travers SP and others: Convergence of lingual and palatal gustatory neural activity in the nucleus of the solitary tract, *Brain Res* 365:305, 1986.

130. van Steenberghe D and others: The influence of advanced periodonti-
tis on the psychophysical threshold level of periodontal mechanoreceptors in man, *J Periodont Res* 16:199, 1981.

131. van Willigen JD, Weijs-Boot J: Phasic and rhythmic responses of the oral musculature to mechanical stimulation of the rat palate, *Arch Oral Biol* 29:7, 1984.

132. Weijnen JAWM and others: Interaction between licking and swallowing in the drinking rat, *Brain Behav Evol* 25:117, 1984.

133. Westrum LE and others: Transganglionic degeneration in the spinal trigeminal nucleus following removal of tooth pulps in adult cats, *Brain Res* 101:137, 1976.

134. Williams WN and others: The influence of TMJ and central incisor sensory impairment on bite force discrimination, *J Craniomandib Pract* 2:119, 1984.

135. Williams WN and others: Bite force discrimination by individuals with complete dentures, *J Prosthet Dent* 54:146, 1985.

136. Zeigler HP and others: Trigeminal orosensation and ingestive behavior in the rat, *Prog Psychobiol Physiol Psych* 11:63, 1985.

Chapter 73

Odontogenic Infections

Larry J. Peterson

Odontogenic infections are among the most frequently encountered infections afflicting humans. In the vast majority of patients these infections are minor and resolve either by spontaneous drainage through the gingival tissues of the tooth or by extraction of the offending tooth. Chronic sinus tracts from the apex of the tooth to the surface mucosa or skin are not uncommon in populations who receive minimal or no dental care. A great deal of pain and suffering accompany the establishment of these draining sinus tracts. The removal of the offending tooth usually results in rapid resolution of the infection, even without antibiotic therapy. Unfortunately, these minor tooth-related infections occasionally become serious and life threatening. Aggressive surgical and medical care is necessary to prevent disastrous results. This chapter discusses odontogenic infections: their etiology, progression to severe infection, and management.

MICROBIOLOGY OF ODONTOGENIC INFECTIONS

As with infections elsewhere in the body, odontogenic infections usually arise because of normal endogenous flora. The mouth harbors a large number of different bacteria, both aerobes and anaerobes (Table 73-1). The aerobic or facultative anaerobic bacteria are primarily *Streptococcus* species. Notably absent from the mouth are *staphylococci*; *Staphylococcus* organisms rarely cause odontogenic infections. The obligate anaerobic bacteria make up the bulk of the mouth's flora.[29] The predominant bacteria are the anaerobic *Streptococcus*, *Porphyromonas*, *Prevotella*, and *Fusobacterium* organisms.

In most patients normal mouth bacteria cause odontogenic infections. In 1975 the bacteriology of these infections was reported to be primarily *Streptococcus* and *Staphylococcus* organisms,[15,33] however; recent studies performed with careful microbiology techniques under strict anaerobic conditions have produced a different picture of the flora causing these infections.* Based on the results of these investigations, several important conclusions can be drawn regarding the microbiology of odontogenic infections. First, aerobic bacteria alone are rarely the cause. When they are, *Streptococcus* species are usually the offending bacterium. Second, about one half of the infections are caused by anaerobic bacteria (Table 73-2). Third, in most patients, multiple organisms grow from the infection. The average number of different organisms is about five, but as many as 10 can be found. In these mixed infections there is preponderance of anaerobic bacteria.

Table 73-3 lists the bacteria that cause odontogenic infections. These are the bacteria of the normal flora. The most common organisms are *Streptococcus, Peptostreptococcus, Eubacterium, Porphyromonas, Prevotella*, and *Fusobacterium*. Notably absent are group D *Streptococcus* (enterococci), *Staphylococcus* organisms, and *Bacteroides fragilis*. These are important exceptions because their markedly different antibiotic susceptibility requires a major alteration in the choice of antibiotics.

The anaerobic bacteria seen in odontogenic infections are not usually acknowledged as being pathogenic. A more invasive bacterium, such as *Streptococcus* species, probably must accompany them to establish an infection. Of the anaerobes, *Prevotella intermedia* appears to be the most important bacterium of the anaerobic group. Alone or in combination with *Fusobacterium* or *Peptostreptococcus* organisms, *Prevotella intermedia* is the most commonly isolated anaerobic bacterium.

Entry of bacteria into deep tissues to cause an infection

* Refs. 2, 7, 8, 10, 16, 25, 28.

Table 73-1. Normal mouth flora

Aerobic bacteria	Anaerobic bacteria
Gram-positive cocci	**Gram-positive cocci**
Streptococcus species	*Streptococcus* species
	Peptococcus species
	Peptostreptococcus species
Gram-negative cocci	**Gram-negative cocci**
Neisseria species	*Veillonella* species
Gram-positive bacilli	**Gram-positive bacilli**
Corynebacterium species	*Clostridium* species
	Actinomyces species
	Eubacterium species
	Lactobacillus species
Gram-negative bacilli	**Gram-negative bacilli**
Haemophilus species	*Bacteroides* species
	Fusobacterium species

Table 73-2. Etiology of infection

Type of bacteria	Total infections by percent
Aerobic only	<5
Anaerobic only	60
Aerobic/anaerobic	35

Table 73-3. Microbiology of odontogenic infections*

Aerobic bacteria	Anaerobic bacteria
Gram-positive cocci	
Streptococcus species	*Streptococcus* species (C)
α-hemolytic (VC)	*Peptostreptococcus* species (VC)
β-hemolytic (U)	*Peptococcus* species (VC)
Group D (R)	
Staphylococcus species (R)	
Gram-negative cocci	
Neisseria species (R)	*Veillonella* species (C)
Gram-positive bacilli	
Corynebacterium species (R)	*Eubacterium* species (VC)
	Lactobacillus species (U)
Gram-negative bacilli	
Haemophilus influenzae (R)	*Bacteroides* species (VC)
	B. melaninogenicus (VC)
Eikenella corrodens (R)	*B. fragilis* (R)
	Fusobacterium species (VC)

* *VC*—Very common; *C*—Common; *U*—Unusual; *R*—Rare.

results from invasive aerobic bacteria gaining access through a necrotic dental pulp. The aerobic bacteria serve as the initiator of the infection, preparing the local environment for anaerobic bacterial invasion. The anaerobes become predominant, since the reduction-oxidation potential favors anaerobic growth. The clinical picture evolves like this: *Streptococcus* organisms most commonly cause the early stage cellulitis. As the infection progresses, a mixed streptococcal/anaerobic infection occurs. As the local tissue condition changes to a more hypoxic state, the predominant bacteria become anaerobic species, such as *Prevotella* or *Fusobacterium*.

IMPLICATIONS OF MICROBIOLOGY FOR ANTIBIOTIC THERAPY

The primary treatment of odontogenic infections has been surgical for centuries, and this is anticipated to continue into the future. Extraction of the tooth, drainage of the abscess, and release of pressure are fundamental in the treatment of these infections.

Antibiotics are a necessary adjunctive therapy in many infections to hasten resolution. The choice of antibiotics should be made with a clear idea of the antibiotic susceptibility of the bacteria causing the infection. In an uncomplicated infection, the facts presented in the preceding section provide adequate information for choosing an effective antibiotic without the time delay and expense of taking a specimen for culture or antibiotic sensitivity testing. There are two microbiologic factors that should be kept in mind when choosing an antibiotic. First, the antibiotic must be effective against *Streptococcus* organisms, since this bacterium is most commonly encountered. Second, the drug should be effective against a broad range of anaerobic bacteria. Fortunately, the antibiotic susceptibility of the oral anaerobes is great. The outlines that follow provide a summary of the effectiveness of commonly used antibiotics for odontogenic infections. First, the orally administered drugs are listed:

A. Very effective
　1. Penicillin
　2. Clindamycin
　3. Metronidazole (alone or in combination with penicillin)
　4. Amoxicillin/clavulonic acid
B. Effective
　1. Erythromycin
　2. Cephalexin
　3. Tetracycline
C. Less effective
　1. Sulfa drugs
　2. Quinolones

Next the parenterally administered drugs are listed:

A. Very effective
　1. Penicillin

2. Clindamycin
3. Metronidazole
B. Effective
1. Cefazolin
2. Cefoxitin
C. Not effective
1. Gentamicin
2. Tobramycin
3. Amikacin
4. Cephalosporin (third generation)

The very effective drugs can be used with confidence on an empiric basis to treat odontogenic infections. The effective and less effective drugs are less predictable and should be used only when first-line drugs can not be used or when indicated by specific culture and sensitivity testing. Those listed as not effective are not effective against either *Streptococcus* species or anaerobes; therefore, they are not indicated for the routine odontogenic infection. When indicated by specific culture results, they may prove to be quite valuable, but usually in combination with β-lactam antibiotics.

The antibiotics that may be effective in odontogenic infections but should not be routinely employed are: ampicillin, carbenicillin, ticarcillin, piperacillin, azlocillin, mezlocillin, maxolactam, chloramphenicol, and cephalosporins.

The reasons for not using these antibiotics are excess toxicity (chloramphenicol), excess expense (carbenicillin), and a needlessly extended spectrum (third-generation cephalosporins). These antibiotics may be used in specific, serious, life-threatening infections. In general, however, these antibiotics should be held in reserve.

Two final comments concerning recommendation of these antibiotics should be made. First, although penicillin has been an extremely useful drug for anaerobic infections, resistance to it is beginning to emerge.[10] This is especially true with *Prevotella intermedia*, since about 20% of these bacteria are currently reported as resistant to penicillin. This must be remembered when odontogenic infections do not respond to penicillin. Resistance also is being seen with other antibiotics used to treat head and neck infections. This may be the result of more careful testing, especially for anaerobic bacteria, or it may be the result of actual resistance by the bacteria.* Current resistance by percentage to common antibiotics is seen in Table 73-4. Second, the antibiotic metronizadole has become popular recently in the treatment of odontogenic infections. This drug has absolutely no activity against aerobic bacteria but is effective against anaerobes.[27] Since anaerobes alone or in combination with aerobes cause 95% of odontogenic infections, metronidazole may play a major role in such infections. Although it has no effect on the *streptococci* that are likely to be involved, resolution of odontogenic infections treated with metronidazole is usually seen and occurs rapidly.[35] If the drug is to be used in a serious odontogenic infection, it should be combined with

* Refs. 1, 4, 6, 19, 21, 22, 25, 26, 31, 32.

Table 73-4. Antibiotic resistance by percent

Antibiotic	Oral bacteroides	Fuso-bacterium species	Anaerobic cocci	α-Strepto-cocci
Penicillin	25	6	4	0
Erythromycin	0	85	18	0
Clindamycin	4	0	2	0
Metronidazole	0	0	24	100
Cephalexin	10	0	6	18

penicillin because the *Streptococcus* species has a more important role in those situations.

NATURAL HISTORY OF ODONTOGENIC INFECTION

The usual cause of odontogenic infections is necrosis of the pulp of the tooth, which is followed by bacterial invasion through the pulp chamber and into the deeper tissues. Necrosis of the pulp results from deep caries in the tooth, to which the pulp responds with a typical inflammatory reaction. Vasodilation and edema cause pressure in the tooth and severe pain as the rigid walls of the tooth prevent swelling. If left untreated the pressure leads to strangulation of the blood supply to the tooth through the apex and consequent necrosis. The necrotic pulp provides a perfect setting for bacterial invasion into the bone tissue.

Once the bacteria have invaded the bone, the infection spreads equally in all directions until a cortical plate is encountered. During the time of intraosseous spread, the patient usually experiences sufficient pain to seek treatment. Extraction of the tooth (or removal of the necrotic pulp by an endodontic procedure) resolves the infection.

DIRECTION OF SPREAD OF INFECTION

The direction of the spread of infection from the tooth apex depends on the thickness of the overlying bone and the relationship of the bone's perforation site to the muscle attachments of the jaws.

If no treatment is provided, the infection erodes through the thinnest, closest cortical plate of the bone and into the overlying soft tissue (Fig. 73-1). In Figure 73-1, *A*, the closest cortex is the thin labial bone, so the infection erodes through there. In Figure 73-1, *B*, the root apex is closer to the palatal aspect, so the infection goes to the palatal side. If the root apex is centrally located, the infection erodes through the thinnest bone first. In the maxilla the thinner bone is the labial-buccal side; the palatal cortex is thicker.

Once the bone has been perforated, local muscle attachments determine the specific location of the infection in the soft tissue (Fig. 73-2). The most common tooth abscess erodes through the labial bone, occlusal to the muscle attachment, producing a vestibular abscess (see Fig. 73-2). The

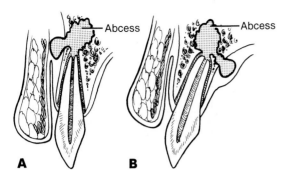

Fig. 73-1. When the infection process is allowed to progress, it erodes through the closest cortical plate. **A,** The tooth apex is near the thin labial bone, so infection erodes onto the labial side. **B,** The apex is near the palatal side and erodes through that side.

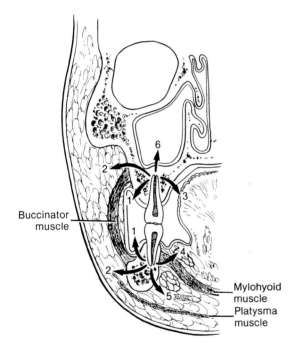

Fig. 73-2. As infection erodes through the bone, it can express itself in variety of places, depending on thickness of overlying bone and the relationship of muscle attachments to the site of perforation. This illustration displays six possible locations: *1,* vestibular abscess; *2,* buccal space; *3,* palatal abscess; *4,* sublingual space; *5,* submandibular space; and *6,* maxillary sinus.

vestibular abscess is seen as a small pouch of pus in the soft tissue overlying the affected tooth (Fig. 73-3). If no treatment is provided, rupture of the abscess occurs and a chronic sinus tract is established (Fig. 73-4).

If the infection perforates the bone above the muscle attachment (see Fig. 73-2, points *2, 4,* and *5*), fascial space involvement occurs. When fascial space involvement occurs, the potential for more severe infection with rapid spread becomes greater.

Table 73-5 lists usual sites for perforation and localization

Table 73-5. Spread of infection from teeth

	Site of bone perforation	Relationship to muscle attachment	Site of laceration
Maxillary			
Incisors	Labial	Below	Vestibule
Canines	Labial	Below	Vestibule
Premolars	Buccal	Below	Vestibule
Molars	Buccal	Below	Vestibule
		Above	Buccal space
Mandibular			
Incisors	Labial	Above	Vestibule
Cuspids	Labial	Above	Vestibule
Premolars	Buccal	Above	Vestibule
First molar	Lingual	Above	Sublingual space
Second molar	Lingual	Above	Sublingual space
Second molar	Lingual	Below	Submandibular space
Third molar	Lingual	Below	Submandibular space

of the infection.[23] These are the usual sites, but variation occurs from patient to patient.

FASCIAL SPACE INVOLVEMENT

Maxillary spaces

Erosion of maxillary tooth infection through the bone usually manifests itself in the labial-buccal surface of the maxilla, most are seen as vestibular abscesses. Some, however, become fascial space infections. The two maxillary spaces that may be involved are the canine space and the buccal space.

The canine space becomes infected almost exclusively as a result of the maxillary canine tooth. The root of the tooth must be long enough so that the apex is superior to the insertion of the levator anguli oris muscle. The canine space is between the anterior surface of the maxilla and the levator labii superioris. When infected, clinically evident swelling lateral to the nose exists, usually obliterating the nasolabial fold (Fig. 73-5).

The buccal space from the maxillary teeth becomes involved when the infection erodes through the bone superior to the attachment of the buccinator muscle. The buccal space lies between the buccinator muscle and the skin and superficial fascia (Fig. 73-6). All three maxillary molars may cause buccal space involvement, but the premolars rarely do. The buccal space swelling is ovoid, below the zygomatic arch, and above the inferior border of the mandible. The buccal space also may be infected from the mandibular molar teeth. This involvement is not common, but it does occur.

In addition to the two maxillary space involvements, maxillary odontogenic infections may ascend to cause orbital cellulitis or cavernous sinus thrombosis. Orbital cellulitis is rarely the result of odontogenic infection but may occur. The clinical picture is similar regardless of the cause. Swelling

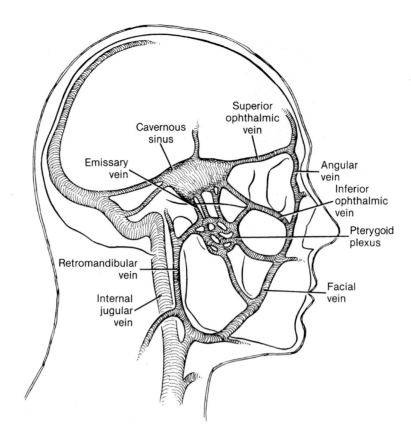

Fig. 73-7. Hematogeneous spread of infection from jaw to cavernous sinus may occur anteriorly through the inferior or superior ophthalmic vein or posteriorly through the emissary veins to the pterygoid plexus.

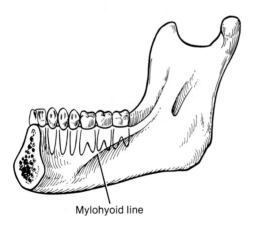

Fig. 73-8. The mylohyoid line is an area of attachment of mylohyoid muscle. Lingual cortical plate perforation by infection from premolars and first molar causes sublingual space infection, whereas perforation from third molar involves submandibular space. The second molar may involve either space.

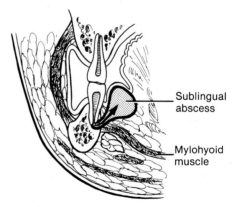

Fig. 73-9. Sublingual space, which exists between oral mucosa and mylohyoid muscle. It is primarily involved by infection from the mandibular premolars and the first molar.

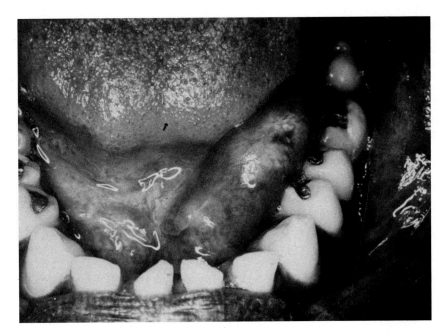

Fig. 73-10. Isolated sublingual space infection, which has produced unilateral swelling of floor of mouth.

(premolars, first molar), the sublingual space is involved. If the apex of the tooth is inferior to the muscle (third molar), the submandibular space is involved. The second molar may involve either or both spaces, since its apex is typically at the mylohyoid line.

The sublingual space is between the oral mucosa and the mylohyoid muscle (Fig. 73-9). Its posterior boundary is open, and it can communicate freely with the submandibular space and the secondary spaces of the mandible. Clinically, when infection of the sublingual space occurs, little extraoral swelling occurs, but much intraoral swelling of the floor of the mouth develops on the affected side (Fig. 73-10). If the infection becomes bilateral, the tongue may become markedly elevated.

The submandibular space lies between the mylohyoid muscle and the skin and superficial fascia (Fig. 73-11). Like the sublingual space, it has an open posterior boundary and can communicate freely with the secondary spaces. When this space becomes infected, the swelling begins at the inferior lateral border of the mandible and extends medially to the digastric area and posteriorly to the hyoid bone (Fig. 73-12).

The three secondary spaces of the mandible are posterior to the tooth-bearing portion of the mandible in the angle-ramus area. They are called *secondary spaces* because they become infected by secondary spread of infection from other anterior spaces. The primary spaces feeding these secondary spaces are the buccal, sublingual, and submandibular spaces.

The masseteric space exists between the lateral aspect of the mandible and the masseter muscle (Fig. 73-13). This space is involved most often by spread from the buccal space or from soft-tissue infection around the third molar. When the masseteric space is involved, the posteroinferior portion

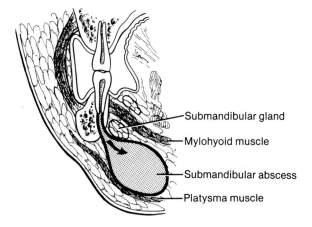

Submandibular gland
Mylohyoid muscle
Submandibular abscess
Platysma muscle

Fig. 73-11. Submandibular space, which lies between the mylohyoid muscle and skin and the superficial fascia. It is infected primarily by the second and third molars.

of the face swells. In addition to the swelling, the patient has mild to moderate trismus caused by inflammation of the masseter muscle.

The pterygomandibular space lies between the medial aspect of the mandible and the medial pterygoid muscle (see Fig. 73-13). This space becomes involved by spread from the sublingual and submandibular spaces and from soft-tissue infection around the third molar. When this space is involved, little or no swelling is evident on either intraoral or extraoral examination. The patient almost always has significant trismus. Thus, trismus without swelling is a valuable diagnostic clue for pterygomandibular space infection.

The temporal space is posterior and superior to the masseteric and pterygomandibular spaces (see Fig. 73-13).

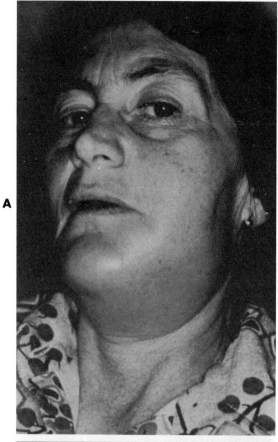

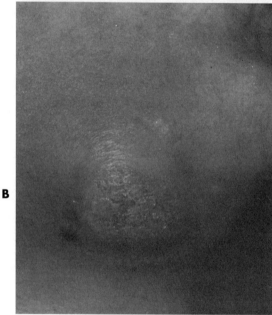

Bounded laterally by the temporalis fascia and medially by the skull, it is divided into two portions by the temporalis muscle. The two sections are known as the *deep* and *superficial temporal pouches*. They are rarely secondarily involved in serious overwhelming infections. Swelling is evident over the temporal area, posterior from the lateral aspect of the lateral orbital rim. Trismus is always a feature of this infection, caused by involvement of the temporalis muscle.

These three secondary spaces of the mandible are collectively known as the *masticator space,* since they are bounded by the muscles of mastication: masseter, medial pterygoid, and temporalis. The three individual spaces communicate freely with one another, so one rarely sees any single space involved alone. Thus, the term *masticator space* does have some clinical usefulness, even if it lacks specific designation.

If all three of the primary mandibular spaces become involved with the infection, the infection is known as *Ludwig's angina*. Ludwig's angina, described in 1936, was a relatively common occurrence until the antibiotic era. It is a rapid, bilaterally spreading, gangrenous cellulitis of the submandibular, sublingual, and submental spaces. It usually spreads posteriorly to the secondary spaces. It produces gross swelling, elevation and displacement of the tongue, and tense, brawny induration of the submandibular region superior to

Fig. 73-12. **A,** Submandibular space infection, which has produced large, indurated swelling of submandibular space. **B,** Submandibular cellulitis may resolve to chronic abscess that alternately drains spontaneously and swells when it closes over.

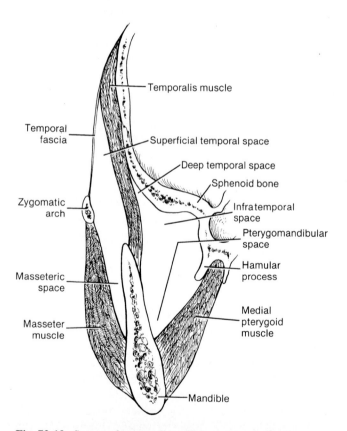

Fig. 73-13. Spaces of ramus of mandible are bounded by the masseter muscle, medial pterygoid muscle, temporal fascia, and skull. Temporal space is divided into two portions, deep and superficial, by the temporalis muscle.

the hyoid bone. There is usually minimal or no fluctuance.[13,30] The patient experiences severe trismus, drooling of saliva, tachypnea, and dyspnea. Impending compromise of the airway produces marked anxiety. The cellulitis can progress with alarming speed, producing an upper airway obstruction that may lead to death. The usual cause of Ludwig's angina is an odontogenic infection, usually from the second or third mandibular molar. The microbes involved are usually *Streptococcus* organisms, oral anaerobes, or both.

Cervical or deep neck spaces

Extension of odontogenic infection beyond the mandibular spaces is an unusual event. When it occurs, spread to the cervical or deep neck spaces from the submandibular, sublingual, or pterygomandibular spaces may have serious, life-threatening sequelae. These sequelae may be the result of locally induced complications, such as upper airway obstruction, or distant problems, such as mediastinitis.

The deep neck spaces can become infected from a variety of sources. Odontogenic infections cause as many as 30% of all deep neck infections.[34] The deep neck spaces have a variety of names and descriptions. Three are relatively consistent through the literature: the lateral pharyngeal space, the retropharyngeal space, and the prevertebral space. The layers of deep cervical fascia form and bind these three spaces.

The lateral pharyngeal space is classically described as having the shape of an inverted pyramid or funnel. The base is the skull base at the sphenoid bone and the apex is at the hyoid bone. It is located between the medial pterygoid muscle laterally and the superior pharyngeal constrictor medially (Fig. 73-14). Anteriorly, the boundary is the pterygomandi-

bular raphe, it communicates with the spaces of the mandible. Posteromedially it extends to and is bounded by the prevertebral fascia and communicates freely with the retropharyngeal space. The styloid process and associated muscles and fascia divide the lateral pharyngeal space into an anterior compartment, which contains muscles, and a posterior compartment, which contains the carotid sheath and cranial nerves (CNs).

When the lateral pharyngeal space is involved in an odontogenic infection, there are several typical findings, foremost of which is severe trismus. This is the result of involvement of the medial pterygoid muscle, but may be caused by involvement of the other muscles of mastication. The severe trismus may interfere with accurate diagnosis and treatment. Lateral neck swelling, especially beyond the angle of the mandible, is usually seen. The lateral pharyngeal wall, if it can be visualized, usually bulges toward the midline. One can differentiate lateral pharyngeal space infection from a primary peritonsillar abscess primarily because the latter rarely has significant trismus. Involvement of the lateral pharyngeal space creates complications for several reasons. First, the odontogenic infection is severe and may be progressing at a rapid rate. Second is the direct effect of the infection on the contents of the space, particularly of the posterior compartment. This includes thrombosis of the internal jugular vein, erosion of the carotid artery or its branches, and interference with CNs IX to XII or the sympathetic chain. Third, the infection may progress from the lateral pharyngeal space to the retropharyngeal space. The retropharyngeal space lies posteromedial to the lateral pharyngeal space. It is bounded anteriorly by the superior pharyngeal muscle and its investing fascia and posteriorly to the alar layer of prever-

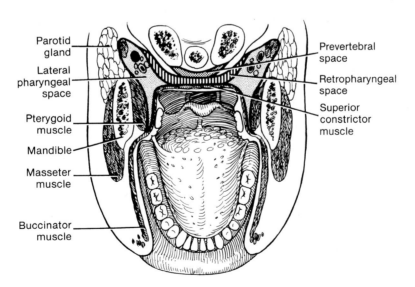

Fig. 73-14. Lateral pharyngeal space, located between medial pterygoid muscle laterally and superior pharyngeal constrictor medially. Retropharyngeal and prevertebral spaces lie between the pharynx and vertebral column. Retropharyngeal space lies between the superior constrictor muscle and alar portion of prevertebral fascia. Prevertebral space lies between the alar and prevertebral layers of prevertebral fascia.

tebral fascia (see Fig. 73-14). The space begins at the skull base at the pharyngeal tubercle and extends inferiorly to the level of C7 to T1, where the two layers of fascia fuse (Fig. 73-15). This level is at the posterosuperior mediastinum. The retropharyngeal space has few contents, except for the retropharyngeal lymph nodes. These nodes are more numerous in the child than in the adult, which may account for the more frequent involvement of this space in children.[3]

When the retropharyngeal space becomes involved secondary to odontogenic infection, the situation is usually grave. Clinical signs and symptoms are those of a severe infection. Trismus is severe in most patients at this stage. Evaluation of the retropharyngeal space is performed successfully by evaluating a lateral radiograph of the neck. Average widths of the prevertebral tissues have been well established.[36] The soft-tissue shadow should be no greater than 7 mm (average, 3.5 mm) at C2 and no greater than 20 mm (average, 14 mm) at C6, i.e., behind the trachea (Fig. 73-16).

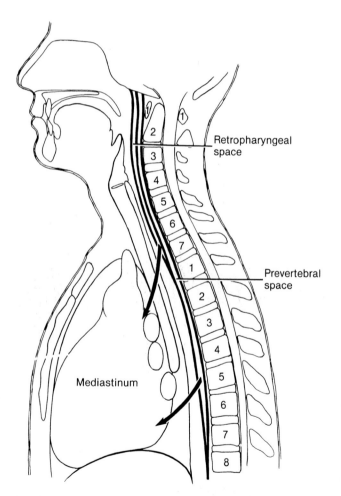

Fig. 73-15. A diagram of fascial spaces. If retropharyngeal space is involved, posterosuperior mediastinum also may become infected secondarily. If prevertebral space is infected, the inferior boundary is the diaphragm, so the entire mediastinum is at risk.

Involvement of the retropharyngeal space also may include the prevertebral space. The prevertebral space is a potential space between the two layers of prevertebral fascia, the alar and prevertebral layers. It extends from the skull base inferiorly to the diaphragm. The space is also known as *danger space No. 4.*[17] When the retropharyngeal space is involved as a result of an odontogenic infection, the patient is seriously ill and in grave danger of death. Three potential complications exist. First, the upper airway is in danger of obstruction because of anterior displacement of the posterior pharyngeal wall into the oropharynx. Narrowing of the upper airway as the retropharyngeal space swells is expected (see Fig. 73-16). Second, when the retropharyngeal spaces are filled with pus, a danger exists of spontaneous rupture of the abscess, resulting in aspiration, pneumonia, and asphyxiation. Rupture also may be caused by attempts at insertion of an endotracheal tube to secure the airway. Third, once the infection has gained access to the retropharyngeal spaces, the posterosuperior mediastinum or the entire posterior mediastinum also may become infected (Fig. 73-17).

MANAGEMENT OF ODONTOGENIC INFECTIONS

The principles of treating odontogenic infections are no different from the principles of treating any other infection. These principles are briefly reviewed in the context of treating odontogenic infections that are serious enough to warrant hospitalization (Fig. 73-18).

Assessment and support of host defenses

Odontogenic infections are usually minor and easily treated. They become serious infections in patients who have some defense compromise, such as diabetes or immunosuppression. Careful review of the patient's defenses should be a routine part of the patient's evaluation.

Patients with moderate or severe odontogenic infections usually have severe pain and dysplasia. This results in a poorly hydrated, exhausted patient. Thus, the infection itself produces a compromised host. Care must be taken to provide proper analgesics, nutrition, and hydration for patients with these infections.

Airway establishment

Fascial space involvement that compromises the airway may be anterior, as in Ludwig's angina, or posterior, as in a retropharyngeal space infection. In either case, rapid severe compromise of the airway may occur. The surgeon should be aware of this and carefully and frequently evaluate airway status to prevent fatal obstruction.

In the uncomplicated odontogenic infection that involves the spaces of the mandible unilaterally, airway problems are rarely seen. If they are seen, nasal endotracheal intubation is the method of choice for airway establishment. Consideration should be given to leaving the endotracheal tube in place for 2 to 3 days to ensure that acute obstruction does not occur in the time shortly after surgical decompression of the infection.

In patients with Ludwig's angina, airway embarrassment is the primary cause of death. Once Ludwig's angina is diagnosed, it is imperative that the patient be monitored frequently and carefully for airway problems. If the decision is made to establish an artificial airway early, intubation by fiberoptic or blind nasal technique can be attempted. These procedures should be performed on awake, unparalyzed patients. The administration of neuromuscular blocking agents may cause airway loss that cannot be regained. Administration of these agents can be safely accomplished only if an experienced anesthesiologist is present. If the decision to establish an artificial airway is delayed, a tracheostomy is the only option. An unhurried approach with a local anesthetic is preferred. If the infection involving a retropharyngeal space abscess has a radiographically enlarged soft-tissue image, an artificial airway should be considered. If the patient has only mild trismus and the anesthesiologist believes that direct laryngoscopy is possible, an endotracheal tube is preferred. However, if the patient has moderate or severe trismus, a planned tracheostomy should be performed. The major concern in this situation is rupturing the abscess while attempting to pass the endotracheal tube into the trachea blindly. If a rupture occurs, aspiration of the pus is possible, with its attendant serious sequelae.

Identification of bacteria

The identification of causative microorganisms in an odontogenic infection is usually not a problem. The usual causes are *Streptococcus* organisms and oral anaerobes. Because the data are so consistent among the various reports and the clinical experience of many surgeons, it is unnecessary to perform cultures for uncomplicated odontogenic infections in uncompromised patients.

However, in compromised patients and in patients with severe fascial space infections, it is wise to get a specimen of pus for culture and antibiotic sensitivity testing. The specimen must be taken in an anaerobic method so that anaerobic culturing can be done. Aspiration with a large-bore needle through intact skin or mucosa is the preferred method.

Choice of antibiotic

The drug of choice for odontogenic infections continues to be parenteral penicillin. Even for serious fascial space infections, including Ludwig's angina,[13,30] penicillin is pre-

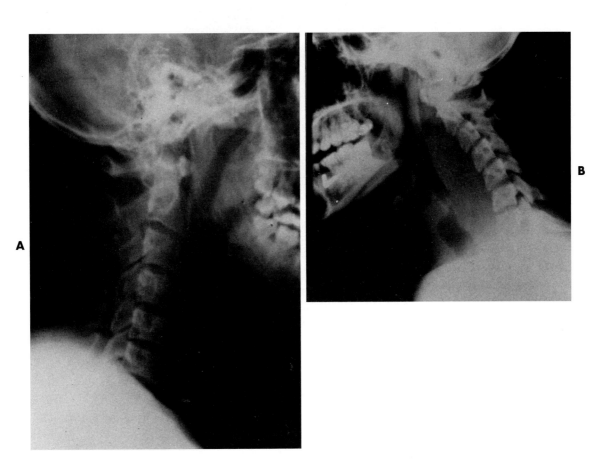

Fig. 73-16. A, Retropharyngeal soft-tissue shadow is narrow (3 to 4 mm) at C2; at C6 retrotracheal soft-tissue shadow is 14 to 15 mm. **B,** Retropharyngeal space is involved, with soft tissue becoming substantially thicker and width of oropharyngeal air shadow decreasing.

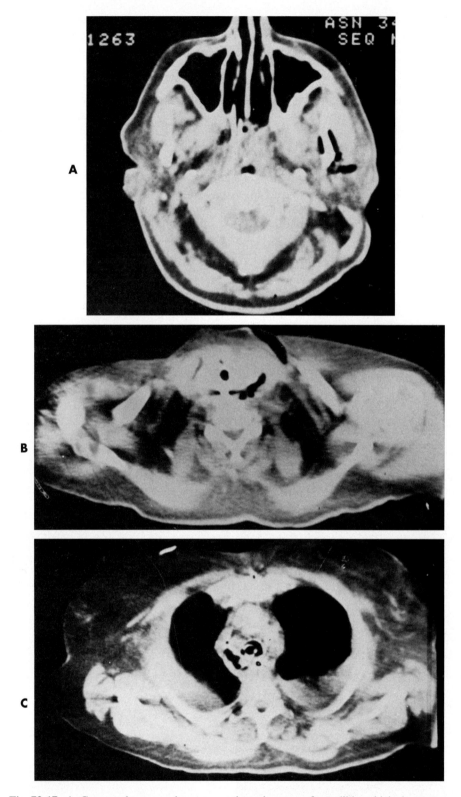

Fig. 73-17. A, Computed tomography scan, cut through ramus of mandible, which shows presence of air space around left ramus of mandible. **B,** Lower section through neck shows progression of gas into retropharyngeal space. **C,** Section through superior thorax shows large abscess formation on posterior wall.

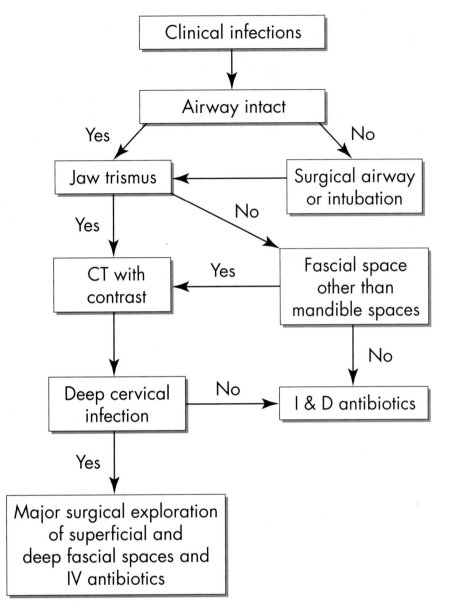

Fig. 73-18. Management of odontogenic infections algorithm.

ferred. Large doses of up to 20 million units daily of intravenous penicillin may be required for serious infections.

In the penicillin-allergic patient, clindamycin is the second drug of choice. It is quite effective against streptococci and anaerobes and has low toxicity. Although clindamycin may cause pseudomembranous colitis, it causes only about one third of the reported cases. Another third of pseudomembranous colitis cases are caused by ampicillin-amoxicillin, and the remaining third are caused by the cephalosporins. The surgeon should be alert to this potential complication and prepared to treat it or to seek consultation if it occurs. Metronidazole alone or in combination with penicillin is also a useful drug. It has minimal toxicity problems and is effec-

tive against anaerobes. Parenteral cephalosporins may be moderately useful. The first-generation cephalosporins have the same effects as penicillin on the microbial population causing odontogenic infections. The second-generation drug cefoxitin is more active against the anaerobic bacteria but loses some of the antistreptococcal activity of the first-generation drugs. The third-generation cephalosporins are generally effective against anaerobes but also have decreased effectiveness against streptococci. Further, they are quite expensive and have no clear additional benefit. Thus, the second- and third-generation drugs are not highly desirable. Ciprofloxacin and metronidazole in combination may be useful in the patient with a severe infection who has had an anaphylactoid reaction to penicillin.

In summary, high doses of parenteral antibiotics with a penicillin-like spectrum are usually effective in treating odontogenic infections. Specific culturing should be done for serious or nonresponsive infections, and the results used accordingly.

Surgical drainage and decompression

Vestibular infections

Odontogenic infections that are confined to the oral vestibule can usually be treated simply. The patient complains of mild to moderate soft-tissue pain and swelling. There may be a mild, but rarely severe, elevation of body temperature. Treatment is primarily surgical, with antibiotic therapy often used adjunctively. Surgical treatment is extraction of the tooth (or removal of the dental pulp of the tooth) and incision and drainage of the vestibular abscess. A small piece of Penrose drain is inserted to maintain drainage for 2 or 3 days. Antibiotic treatment is with penicillin. If the patient is allergic to penicillin, either erythromycin or clindamycin can be used. Antibiotic administration lasts for 7 to 10 days. Such patients can usually be managed as an outpatient. Resolution of the infection is rapid and usually without complications.

Jaw space infections

If the infection spreads to one of the fascial spaces surrounding the maxilla or mandible, treatment must more aggressive. The initial step in therapy is deciding whether hospitalization is necessary. This decision is based on the presence and amount of swelling, the nature of the swelling (soft and doughy, indurated, or fluctuant), and the state of the body's defenses. Infections that appear as chronic abscesses without a major cellulitis component can be surgically drained and the patient observed on an outpatient basis. Similarly, patients with early infections having a soft, doughy swelling can be treated as outpatients with antibiotics and tooth extraction.

However, patients who have moderately increased temperatures with an odontogenic cellulitis that is diffuse and indurated should be treated in the hospital. Support of the host with hydration, antibiotics, and analgesics plays an important role in the overall therapy. Antibiotics should be given parenterally, preferably intravenously.

Surgical treatment should be considered early. If any fluctuance is noted on the physical examination, the patient should be taken to the operating room and drainage procedures should be performed. Aspiration of pus for aerobic and anaerobic cultures is accomplished first. Drainage of the canine and isolated sublingual spaces is usually performed by a transoral approach. The incision is made, an exploration is carried out by blunt dissection to break up all loculations of pus, and the Penrose drains are inserted.

The buccal space can be drained transorally or extraorally, depending on the patient's situation and the preference of the surgeon. Surgery from the mouth side is more difficult, with maintenance of the drainage becoming less predictable. Drainage from the cutaneous side is more likely to leave a scar.

The submental space is drained through a horizontal incision, which parallels the inferior border of the symphysis of the mandible (Fig. 73-19). The area between the anterior belly of the digastric muscles is explored posterior to the hyoid bone.

The buccal, submandibular, masseteric, pterygomandibular, and sublingual spaces can all be drained through a horizontal incision parallel and inferior to the angle of the mandible (see Fig. 73-19). An incision from 0.5 to 5 cm may be used. If the infection is a tense cellulitis that involves several mandibular spaces, a larger incision is indicated. After the incision is made, blunt dissection is used to explore the involved spaces. The most commonly missed space is the pterygomandibular space. In severe submandibular space infections, specific efforts should be made to explore the medial side of the ramus of the mandible in the pterygomandibular space. The inferior portion of the lateral pharyngeal space just medial to the pterygoid muscle also can be explored by this approach. In severe infections, anterior (submental), posterior (submandibular), and superior (superficial temporal) incisions may all be required. Penrose drains are inserted to the extent of the dissection to facilitate drainage. Irrigation/suction catheters may be used in more severe infections.[14] In infections drained by multiple incisions, through-and-through drains should be used. Resolution of these infections depends on several factors: conditions of

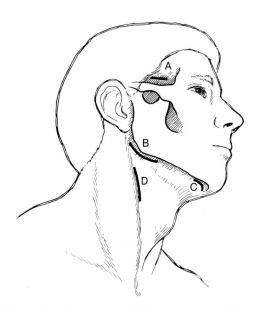

Fig. 73-19. Typical incision and drainage sites for various fascial space infections. *A,* The superficial and deep temporal space. *B,* Submandibular, masseteric, and pterygomandibular spaces. *C,* Submental space. *D,* Lateral pharyngeal and retropharyngeal spaces.

host defenses, seriousness of the original infection, appropriateness of antibiotic therapy, and extensiveness of surgical exploration. Of these, failure to perform adequate surgical drainage is most likely to occur. In severe cellulitis, overlying induration may prevent the clinical diagnosis of an abscess formation. Thus, surgery is critical to successful therapy in those infections characterized by extensive cellulitis.[5,9]

Deep neck spaces

Involvement of the deep cervical spaces as a result of odontogenic infection is an uncommon but life-threatening event. A large proportion of deep neck infections are the result of odontogenic infections.[5] When deep cervical involvement does occur, the fascial spaces of the jaws, particularly of the mandible, are involved initially, usually beginning in the submandibular space and extending through the pterygomandibular space. The major diagnostic goal is to determine whether the lateral pharyngeal and retropharyngeal spaces are involved. The clinical examination, radiography (using anteroposterior [AP] and lateral soft-tissue views of the neck, Figs. 73-16 and 73-20), and computed tomography (CT) (Fig. 73-21) may all be required to make the diagnosis.[11,24] Lateral and AP neck radiographs and CT scans may reveal the presence of gas in the soft tissue as well as soft-tissue swelling. The presence of gas in the tissue usually signifies anaerobic infections and indicates immediate and aggressive surgical therapy.[18]

Initial treatment of a patient with suspected deep neck infection requires immediate hospitalization, host support, maintenance of airway, intravenous antibiotic therapy, and incision and exploration of the involved spaces. Early surgical exploration, even in the absence of palpable fluctuance, is likely to produce more rapid and complete resolution of the infection with minimal mortality. An artificial airway in these patients should usually be established. There should be no hesitation in accomplishing the necessary maneuver, whether it be intubation or tracheostomy. Large doses of parenteral antibiotic therapy should be started immediately. Penicillin with metronidazole is the preferred combination; clindamycin is an adequate alternative. If doubt exists concerning the bacterial cause of the infection, gentamicin or a third-generation cephalosporin may be added.

Medical treatment with antibiotic therapy and host defense support may be employed initially without surgery; however, a rapidly progressing infection of the neck should be explored. If gas emphysema, a foul-smelling discharge, or other signs indicating anaerobic infection exist, the indication for surgical intervention increases. If the infection continues to progress rapidly in spite of aggressive antibiotic therapy, surgical drainage becomes more important. If fluctuance is noted, pus should be drained immedi-

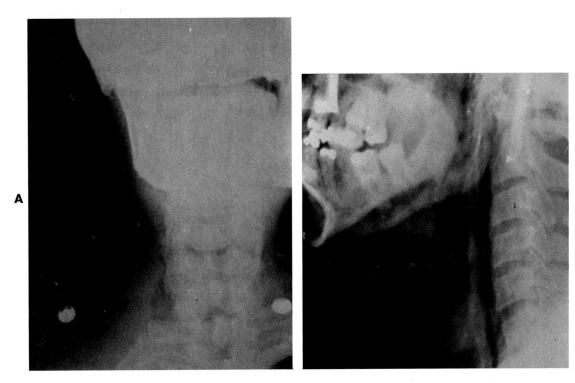

Fig. 73-20. A, Anteroposterior and **B,** lateral neck radiographs showing soft-tissue swelling and emphysema. The gas in tissue usually indicates anaerobic infection.

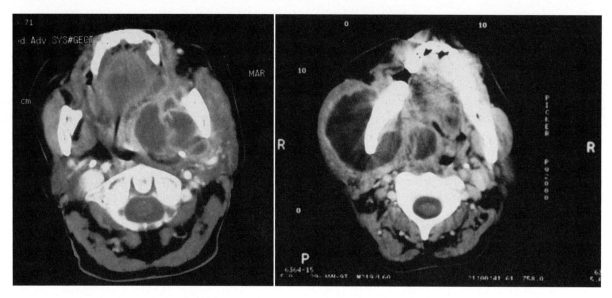

Fig. 73-21. Computed tomography scan taken with intravenous contrast clearly demonstrates the size and location of the abscess formation.

ately.[5,9] Drainage of the lateral pharyngeal space is best accomplished by a combined transoral-extraoral approach. An incision is made lateral to the pterygomandibular raphe, and the space is explored by blunt dissection posterior and inferior to the angle of the mandible with a long Kelly hemostat.

A skin incision is made over the clamp tip along the anterior border of the sternocleidomastoid muscle (see Fig. 73-19). Loculations of pus are disrupted by blunt dissection with the hemostat and by finger pressure. Through-and-through drains are placed.

The retropharyngeal space can be drained through a transoral incision through the posterior pharyngeal mucosa. If this approach is used, a cuffed endotracheal or tracheostomy tube should be in place to prevent any aspiration of pus. Extraoral procedures facilitate dependent drainage. An incision is made along the anterior border of the sternocleidomastoid muscle. The space is explored by blunt dissection between the carotid sheath and pharyngeal constrictor muscle. Deep drains are placed as usual.

When surgical treatment was the only method of therapy (before the antibiotic era), early and aggressive surgery was essential to treat these infections. However, it is important to realize that although aggressive antibiotic therapy may reduce the need for extensive surgical exploration in many patients, antibiotics rarely replace the need for surgery completely.

REFERENCES

1. Aderhold L, Konthe H, Frenkel G: The bacteriology of dentogenous pyogenic infections, *Oral Surg* 52:583, 1981.
2. Baker PF and others: Antibiotic susceptibility of anaerobic bacteria from the human oral cavity, *J Dent Res* 64:1233, 1985.
3. Barratt GE, Koopmann CF, Coulthand SW: Retropharyngeal abscess: a ten-year experience, *Laryngoscope* 94:455, 1984.
4. Bartlett JG, O'Keefe P: The bacteriology of perimandibular space infections, *J Oral Surg* 37:407, 1979.
5. Beck HJ and others: Life-threatening soft-tissue infections of the neck, *Laryngoscope* 94:354, 1984.
6. Chow AW, Roser SM, Brady FA: Orofacial odontogenic infections, *Ann Intern Med* 88:392, 1978.
7. Crook DW and others: Antimicrobial resistance in oral and colonic *Bacteriodes*, *Scand J Infect Dis Suppl* 57:55, 1988.
8. Dornbusch K: Antibiotic susceptibility in oral bacteria, *Swed Dent J* 4:9, 1980.
9. Dzyak WR, Zide MF: Diagnosis and treatment of lateral pharyngeal space infections, *J Oral Maxillofac Surg* 42:243, 1984.
10. Edson RS and others: Recent experience with antimicrobial susceptibility of anaerobic bacteria: increasing resistance to penicillin, *Mayo Clin Proc* 57:737, 1982.
11. Endicott JN, Nelson RJ, Saraceno CA: Diagnosis and management decisions in infections of the deep fascial spaces of the head and neck utilizing computerized tomography, *Laryngoscope* 92:630, 1982.
12. Fielding AF and others: Cavernous sinus thrombosis: report of a case, *J Am Dent Assoc* 106:342, 1983.
13. Finch RG, Snider GE, Sprinkle PM: Ludwig's angina, *JAMA* 243:1171, 1980.
14. Flynn TR, Hoekstra CW, Lawrence FR: The use of drains in oral and maxillofacial surgery: a review and a new approach, *J Oral Maxillofac Surg* 41:508, 1983.
15. Gabrielson ML, Stroh E: Antibiotic efficacy in odontogenic infections, *J Oral Surg* 33:607, 1975.
16. Gilmore WC and others: A prospective double-blind evaluation of penicillin versus clindamycin in the treatment of odontogenic infections, *J Oral Maxillofac Surg* 46:1065, 1988.
17. Grodinsky M, Holyoke EA: The fascia and fascial spaces of the head, neck, and adjacent regions, *Am J Anat* 63:367, 1938.
18. Haug RH, Picard U, Indresano AT: Diagnosis and treatment of retropharyngeal abscess in adults, *Br J Oral Maxillofac Surg* 28:34, 1990.
19. Heimdahl A and others: Clinical appearance of orofacial infections

of odontogenic origin in relation to microbiological findings, *J Clin Microbiol* 22:299, 1985.

20. Karlin RJ, Robinson WA: Septic cavernous sinus thrombosis, *Ann Emerg Med* 13:449, 1984.
21. Konow LV, Nord CE, Nordenram A: Anaerobic bacteria in dentoalveolar infections, *Int J Oral Surg* 10:313, 1981.
22. Labriola JD, Mascaro J, Alpert B: The microbiologic flora of orofacial abscesses, *J Oral Maxillofac Surg* 41:711, 1983.
23. Laskin DM: Anatomic considerations in diagnosis and treatment of odontogenic infections, *J Am Dent Assoc* 69:308, 1964.
24. Lazor JB and others: Comparison of computed tomography and surgical findings in deep neck infections, *Otolaryngol Head Neck Surg* 111:746, 1994.
25. Lewis MAO and others: Prevalence of penicillin resistant bacteria in acute suppurative oral infection, *J Antimicrob Chemother* 35:785, 1995.
26. Lewis MAO, MacFarlane TW, McGowan DA: Quantitative bacteriology of acute dento-alveolar abscesses, *J Med Microbiol* 21:101, 1986.
27. Müller M: Mode of action of metronidazole on anaerobic bacteria and protozoa, *Surgery* 93:165, 1983.
28. Musial CE, Rosenblatt JE: Antimicrobial susceptibilities of anaerobic bacteria isolated at the Mayo Clinic during 1982 through 1987: comparison with results from 1977 through 1981, *Mayo Clin Proc* 64:392, 1989.
29. Newman MG and others: Antibacterial susceptibility of plaque bacteria, *J Dent Res* 58:1722, 1979.
30. Patterson HC, Kelly JH, Strome M: Ludwig's angina: an update, *Laryngoscope* 92:370, 1982.
31. Quayle AA, Russell C, Hearn B: Organisms isolated from severe odontogenic soft tissue infections: their sensitivities to cefotetan and seven other antibiotics, and implications for therapy and prophylaxis, *Br J Oral Maxillofac Surg* 25:34, 1987.
32. Sabiston CB, Grigsby WR: Bacterial study of pyogenic infections of dental origin, *Oral Surg* 44:430, 1976.
33. Sims W: The clinical bacteriology of purulent oral infections, *Br J Oral Surg* 12:1, 1974.
34. Virolainen E and others: Deep neck infections, *Int J Oral Surg* 8:407, 1979.
35. Wallace J: Antibiotics in dentistry, *Curr Med Res Opin* 6:13, 1979.
36. Wholey MH, Bruwer AJ, Baker HL Jr: The lateral roentgenogram of the neck, *Radiology* 71:350, 1958.

Chapter 74

Oral Manifestations of Systemic Disease

Jerry Thomas Guy

Many systemic diseases have manifestations in the yawning abyss that internists call the oral cavity. Most of these manifestations are nonspecific, but they should alert the otolaryngologist to the possibility of concurrent systemic disease or latent systemic disease that may develop subsequently. This chapter discusses most of the oral manifestations of systemic disease encountered in a normal otolaryngology practice.

CONGENITAL AND INHERITED DISEASES

Many congenital malformations are routinely seen in the oral cavity. Bernstein[4] has the best discussion of congenital defects in the oral cavity. A double lip or reduplication of the upper lip's vermilion is sometimes associated with colloid goiters (Ascher's syndrome). The physician may notice that the maxillolabial sulcus is absent or shallow or that frenula exist. This is often associated with chondroectodermal dysplasia, which is a congenital defect in the hair, skin, sweat glands, and cartilage characterized by hyperkeratosis, hypohydrosis, and abnormal shortening of the long bones. Total or partial anodontia frequently coexists.

The teeth may mirror several congenital conditions, including congenital syphilis, which is characterized by notched incisors (Hutchinson's teeth), dome (Moon's) molars, or mulberry molars. The teeth may be stained or mottled if the pregnant mother ingested tetracycline or fluoride during tooth development. The teeth are often brownish green in congenital hemolytic anemia, caused by Rh incompatibility, and in congenital biliary atresia. This reflects staining with bilirubin and its breakdown pigments (Plate 9, *A*).

The bony palate may show (1) a high palatal vault in Turner's syndrome or (2) congenital gonadal dysgenesis, a congenital disease of females characterized by XO chromosome karyotype, infertility, pterygium colli, coarctation of the aorta, a shield chest, and occasionally other developmental defects. A high-arched soft palate is described in the autosomal-dominant Marfan's syndrome, a generalized disorder of connective tissue with skeletal, ocular, and cardiovascular malformations. These patients are characteristically tall and thin with arachnodactyly and joint hypermobility. Subluxated ocular lenses and a proclivity for dissection of the aorta are other important components of this syndrome. Other marfanoid syndromes, including a high-arched palate with crowding of the teeth, have also been described by McKusick[18] and Wyngaarden and Smith.[32] They are listed in Box 74-1.

Homocystinuria is an autosomal recessive disorder of amino acid metabolism that results from a deficiency in cystathionine synthetase and includes osteopenia and premature artherosclerosis, as described by Stanbury and others.[30] A marfanoid habitus is also described in the section on multiple endocrine adenomatosis III.

Ehlers-Danlos syndrome is a group of 11 inherited metabolic disorders of connective tissue that share phenotypic expressions of Marfan's syndrome, extreme laxity of the skin and joints, and easy bruisability. Type VIII Ehlers-Danlos disorder is also characterized by severe periodontal disease.[32]

Mitral valve prolapse was first described to have marfanoid features, but widespread use of two-dimensional Doppler echocardiography has shown that this occurs in many patients without Marfan's disease. Similarly, patients with sickle cell anemia were first characterized by high-arched palates and other phenomena of Marfan's disease, but intensive screening for sickle cell disease has shown this is not usually the case.

Macroglossia with hypertrophic papillae and a cleft or high-arched palate may be noted in mongolism (trisomy 21) or Down syndrome. Also in Down syndrome, the maxilla is hypoplastic; hypodontia or anodontia can occur. These patients are more susceptible to early necrotizing gingivostomatitis and periodontitis. Patients with mongolism have an increased incidence of acute myelogenous leukemia, which may manifest early in the mouth. Atrophy of the fungiform papilla is frequently seen with the Riley-Day syndrome or autosomal recessive familial dysautonomia. This disorder of the autonomic nervous system is characterized by hypertension with postural hypotension and defects in temperature control.

Mucous membranes may show multiple angiomas in a neurocutaneous syndrome called Sturge-Weber syndrome or encephalofacial angiomatosis (listed under the phakomatoses). These patients have port-wine staining of the facial skin and oral mucosa in a unilateral trigeminal distribution. They also have a proclivity for arteriovenous malformations (AVMs) in the brain, with resultant grand mal seizures and mental retardation.

A peculiar syndrome called *phlebectasia of the jejunum*, oral cavity, and scrotum has been described. It is characterized by caviar spots on the tongue, Fordyce's spots on the scrotum, and a propensity for gastrointestinal bleeding caused by the jejunal varicosities.

Rendu-Osler-Weber syndrome or the autosomal dominant hereditary hemorrhagic telangiectasia, is important to recognize. It is characterized by telangiectasia of the tongue, oral cavity, and nasal mucosa, which become apparent at puberty and increase as the patient ages (Plate 9, *B*). It is also associated with multiple telangiectasia of the gastrointestinal tract, which often causes severe blood loss, AVMs of the liver, cirrhosis, and occasionally AVMs of the lung with arterial desaturation, resulting in cyanosis, digital clubbing, and secondary erythrocytosis.

Telangiectasia of the oral cavity may be seen in Fabry's disease (angiokeratoma corporis diffusum universale), an inborn error of glycosphingolipid catabolism characterized by telangiectatic skin lesions; hypohydrosis; corneal opacities; acral pain with paresthesia; renal failure; and cardiovascular, gastrointestinal, and central nervous system disturbances. It is caused by ceramide dihexoside deficiency as described by Stanbury and others.[30]

The physician frequently encounters fibromas of the maxilla, mandible, or tongue. There are five significant systemic syndromes associated with congenital neurofibromas or fibromas of the tongue and jaw: (1) Congenital von Recklinghausen's disease is an autosomal dominant disease associated with multiple neurofibromas of the skin and bone with an increased incidence of sarcomatous degeneration; it also is associated with hypertension caused by bilateral pheochromocytomas or renal artery stenosis, café-au-lait spots on the skin, and oral melanosis. (2) Autosomal dominant multiple endocrine adenomatosis type III is associated with neurofibromas of the tongue and lips, medullary carcinomas of the thyroid, and pheochromocytomas. (3) The peculiar Cowden's disease is dominantly inherited and is characterized by warty papules on the face, arms, and mucous membrane of the mouth. This syndrome has a propensity for the development of carcinomas of the breast, thyroid, endometrium, and cervix. (4) Tuberous sclerosis is another neurocutaneous syndrome characterized by seizures, mental retardation, and sebaceous adenomas. In this syndrome, hypomelanosis, periungal fibromas, and café-au-lait spots also may occur. Intraoral fibromas are frequently observed. (5) The Melkersson-Rosenthal syndrome[27] is a developmental abnormality with unilateral facial paralysis and edema of the periorbital skin, which often progresses to granuloma. The tongue is fissured and has papillary projections, which reveal fibromas at biopsy.

White lesions of the buccal mucosa and tongue are seen in dyskeratosis congenita, which features cutaneous hyperpigmentation, nail dystrophy, and severely hypoplastic bone marrow resembling Fanconi's panmyelopathy. Another interesting syndrome appears in the mouth as self-induced mutilation of the teeth, tongue, and lips. It is associated with choreoathetosis, mental retardation, and striking hyperuricemia (Lesch-Nyhan syndrome) and is caused by a deficiency of hypoxanthine guanine (phosphoribosyltransferase).

Melanosis of the gingiva may occur as a normal variant in the black population but also occurs in hemochromatosis, an autosomal dominant disorder of increased iron absorption from the gastrointestinal tract. See Box 74-2 for various melanoses of the oral cavity.

Hemochromatosis affects middle-aged men and is associated with bronzed skin, arthritis, diabetes, gonadal atrophy, cirrhosis of the liver, congestive heart failure, and sometimes hypopituitarism. Pigmentation of the oral cavity is produced by melanin rather than iron. Albright's disease (the syndrome of precocious puberty, polyostotic fibrous dysplasia, and "coast of Maine" café-au-lait spots) also may show melanosis of the gingiva and migration and mobility of teeth secondary to jaw involvement with the fibrous dysplasia.

lants, such as pokeweed mitogen. AIDS is also characterized by polyclonal hypergammaglobulinemia, often with paraproteins on serum protein electrophoresis. Analysis of the subpopulation of the T-cell lymphocytes in this syndrome invariably discloses a reduced T helper to T-suppressor cell ratio ($T_4:T_8$) that is related to reduction in helper cells and initial proliferation of the suppressor cell population. These patients also manifest high titers of antibodies to Epstein-Barr virus, CMV, toxoplasmosis, and hepatitis. More recently, they have been found to have antibodies to human T-cell leukemia virus type III (HTLV III), in their serum. This is a ribonucleic acid (RNA) retrovirus that infects T_4 lymphocytes and leads to T_4 elimination and nondiscrete immunoproliferation. The p24 antigen can be measured and the viral particle quantitated by the polymerase chain reaction (PCR).

AIDS patients usually pursue one of several courses, although considerable overlap exists. They are very susceptible to many opportunistic infections. Opportunistic infections of the mouth are frequently caused by *Candida* stomatitis involving the tongue and oral mucosa, which is frequently associated with *Candida* esophagitis and not infrequently with systemic candidiasis. When possible, systemic candidiasis should be treated with systemic amphotericin rather than local treatments such as nystatin or fluconazole. Another common oral infection is herpetic gingivostomatitis, which frequently disseminates and should be treated with acyclovir.

Some oral manifestations of HTLV III infection and AIDS are reflections of reduced immune function and are thus oral opportunistic infections. They usually can be diagnosed early and are highly predictive of the development of AIDS. Many of these lesions represent oral manifestations of AIDS.

Candidiasis is the most common oral opportunistic infection and the first to be described. It has several forms; pseudomembranous candidiasis, or thrush, presents as plaques that can be easily removed, leaving an erythematous surface. There is a less common atrophic form of candidiasis seen as patches on the palate, mucosa, or tongue; this form is more difficult to diagnose. The least common form of oral candidiasis in AIDS, *Candida* leukoplakia, presents as hyperkeratosis. These lesions cannot be removed mechanically, but they do regress with treatment. *Candida* leukoplakia can be confused with other forms of leukoplakia.

Candida infection of the mouth can also produce angular cheilitis, producing erythematous fissures of the corner of the mouth. Localized oral candidiasis usually responds to topical antifungal agents.

Other fungal infections in AIDS patients include histoplasmosis, which should be diagnosed by biopsy and often requires systemic therapy; geotrichosis, which can be diagnosed by culture or potassium hydroxide preparation and requires amphotericin therapy, and *Cryptococcus*, which can be cultured or biopsied and requires amphotericin.

Herpes simplex is a very common viral syndrome in AIDS patients. It usually can be diagnosed by clinical appearance or in smears and usually can be readily controlled by oral acyclovir. Herpes zoster is also seen and usually requires intravenous acyclovir.

Hairy leukoplakia is usually grouped with viral infections and is described in all risk groups for AIDS. The differential diagnosis of hairy leukoplakia includes *Candida* leukoplakia; epithelial dysplasia (oral cancer), which is common in these patients; and the white sponge nevus, a plaque form of lichen planus. Biopsy findings are not particularly revealing; they show epithelial hyperplasia and little inflammation. Epstein-Barr virus can be identified in superficial layers of the epithelium using cytochemistry and Southern blot techniques. Hairy leukoplakia is considered to be an Epstein-Barr virus–induced benign epithelial hyperplasia. If this is diagnosed, high-dose oral acyclovir appears to decrease the lesion clinically. Leukoplakia can be sometimes arrested with 13-*cis*-retinoic acid therapy. However, this vitamin A derivative frequently aggravates xerostomia and cheilosis, which usually is unsatisfactory in these patients. When possible, these patients should be counseled to discontinue oral nicotine products.

Unusual forms of gingivitis and periodontitis are frequently seen in patients with AIDS. Periodontal disease in these patients resembles acute necrotizing ulcerative gingivitis. This disease is usually rapidly progressive with loss of periodontal soft tissue and rapid destruction of supporting bone with loss of teeth. The disease may be so fulminating as to resemble noma seen in severely malnourished patients in developing countries. There is no effective treatment for this condition; regimens include thorough débridement and curettage and topical antiseptics, such as povidone-iodine and chlorhexidine mouth rinses. Some authorities recommend short courses of metronidazole in severe cases. CMV is also seen and responds to acyclovir; CMV may be symptomatically synergistic with herpes simplex virus in this condition. *Eikenella corrodens, Wolinella*, and bacterioids agents have been linked in some of these cases, which require consultation with an infectious diseases specialist.

Mycobacterium avium intracellulare (MAI), which can appear in the mouth, is diagnosed by culture and biopsy and requires multiple systemic therapy. This may occasionally be prevented with oral Clarithromycin therapy. Consultation with an infectious diseases specialist or a hematologist skilled in AIDS treatment is recommended.

The course of recurrent opportunistic infections is usually inexorably downward, and death follows from one or more systemic opportunistic infections. The physician should observe strict universal precautions as detailed by the Centers for Disease Control (CDC) when this syndrome is suggested.

Patients with AIDS can develop Kaposi's sarcoma, which was once a very rare disease. Its cell of origin is the endothelial cell. Kaposi's sarcoma is closely linked with AIDS and involves plaque-like lesions of the skin, which on biopsy often are diagnosed as sclerosing hemangiomas until the true nature of the disease is recognized. Kaposi's sarcoma may disseminate viscerally, often to the gastrointestinal tract, bone, lymph nodes, lung, and spleen. Kaposi's sarcoma often first appears as oral hemorrhagic lesions, with eventual development of necrosis and ulceration. This should be considered a forerunner of visceral involvement, and these patients should be referred for endoscopy and colonoscopy to determine the extent of these lesions.

Patients with AIDS can develop aggressive B-cell non-Hodgkin's lymphoma, including Ki-1 large cell non-Hodgkin's lymphoma, with some regularity. They also can develop a strange wasting syndrome characterized by intense polyneuritis, transverse myelitis, or central nervous system abnormalities with dementia. These neurologic abnormalities can be caused by herpes and toxoplasmosis, the retrovirus itself, and progressive multifocal leukoencephalopathy. There are no known specific oral manifestations of the wasting syndrome, although deficiency syndromes are frequent.

HEMATOLOGIC DISEASES

Hematologic diseases with oral manifestations are described here in the order of disturbances of the erythron, myeloid, or megakaryocytic-platelet compartment of the bone marrow.

Plummer-Vinson syndrome,[9] sometimes called *Patterson-Kelly syndrome* or *sideropenic dysphagia*, is a symptom complex caused by iron deficiency. It produces atrophic glossitis caused by the atrophy of the filiform papillae, angular cheilitis, and occasionally hyperkeratotic lesions in the oral mucosa. It also is associated with koilonychia (spoon nails), pagophagia, and esophageal webs that can be premalignant if they are hyperkeratotic.

Megaloblastic anemias, whether caused by a vitamin B_{12} deficiency (commonly coming from pernicious anemia, surgical resection of the ileum, or small intestinal diverticula) or by a folic-acid deficiency (most commonly seen with malnutrition), manifest in the oral cavity as a part of megaloblastic changes in the entire gastrointestinal tract, which are seen morphologically in the bone marrow. Clinically, patients with megaloblastic anemias have painful atrophy of the entire oral mucous membranes and tongue and recurrent aphthous ulcers. "Magenta tongue," which is said to be characteristic, may herald a B_{12} deficiency.

Polycythemia (or erythrocytosis) can be primary (caused by malignant involvement of the bone marrow and a part of the myeloproliferative syndromes) or secondary (caused by hypoxemia of various causes). It often appears with engorged reddish-purple discoloration of the gingiva and tongue. Thalassemia, a congenital disorder of production of the α- or β-globin chain of hemoglobin, is a chronic anemia and may appear in the oral cavity as a mass (caused by extramedullary hematopoiesis) or as a prominent maxilla with severe malocclusion. This is produced by secondary bony overgrowth consequent to chronic bone marrow over-

expansion. Myelofibrosis is categorized as a myeloproliferative disease, either secondary to the spent phase of polycythemia rubra vera or as a primary process. It is a chronic anemia, which after many years may also present with masses in the mandible and maxilla. Biopsy reveals extramedullary hematopoiesis.

The porphyrias are a strange and rare group of disorders that are characterized by defects in the metabolic assembly of the heme portion of the hemoglobin molecule. Congenital erythropoietic porphyria is characterized by erythrodontia secondary to porphyrin deposits in the gums and teeth. Porphyria cutanea tarda, an acquired form of porphyria, is associated with photosensitive vesicles of the skin and oral mucous membranes and frequently is seen in, but not limited to, alcoholics with chronic liver disease.

Thrombocytopenia secondary to collagen vascular disease, disseminated intravascular coagulation, several drugs, or a primary immunologic disorder often appears with oral hemorrhagic bullae in the mucous membrane and petechiae. Occasionally, it is a harbinger of systemic disease.[16]

Agranulocytosis can be produced by several immunologic diseases and drugs (including chemotherapeutic agents); it produces the syndrome of agranulocytic angina. Agranulocytosis also may appear as oral necrotic and ulcerative lesions. A necrotizing gingivitis produced by the fusospirochetal organisms of Vincent's angina may also be seen. Granulocyte colony-stimulating factor has virtually abolished chemotherapy-induced agranulocytic angina.

Hemophilia A is a congenital disorder in the production of factor VIII molecules, which are important in the intrinsic phase of blood coagulation. Factor VIII deficiency is characterized by bleeding from multiple sites that frequently manifests in the mouth, joints, and skin. Hemophilia B, also an X-linked recessive disorder, displays decreased functional factor IX and has similar manifestations.

The most common hereditary coagulation abnormality is von Willebrand's disease (VWD). It is dominantly inherited. VWD is diagnosed by finding a prolonged bleeding time, a low level of factor VIII procoagulant activity, abnormally low levels of factor VIII–von Willebrand protein by immunologic assay, and diminished platelet aggregation in response to ristocetin. The clinical bleeding symptoms of this disorder are notoriously heterogeneous and may range from virtually no symptoms to a disease resembling factor VIII deficiency. If the history suggests VWD and surgery is contemplated, hematologic consultation should be obtained to ascertain the type of VWD. Certain types of VWD respond to desmopressin acetate and obviate the need for blood component therapy. Desmopressin acetate is contraindicated in other types of VWD.

A qualitative defect in granulocytes associated with oral manifestations is chronic granulomatous disease (CGD), an inherited metabolic defect in the oxidative killing of organisms by normal-appearing granulocytes that can phagocytize but not to kill. These patients are afflicted with recurrent bacterial infections with chronic suppurative cervical lymphadenitis; they can present with recurrent aphthous-like ulcers in the mouth, severe acute gingivitis, and peridontitis. Carriers of chronic granulomatous disease can have oral lesions that are clinically and pathologically identical with discoid lupus. Recombinant interferon-γ is strikingly effective in treating this entity.

Chédiak-Higashi syndrome, an inherited disease of the lysosomal membrane of granulocytes, is characterized by large blue lysosomal particles in leukocytes seen on Wright's stain. Partial cutaneous albinism and defects in platelet and coagulation function are other features. Patients also suffer from recurrent bacterial infections and can present with periodontal disease and mouth ulcerations. They also may develop non-Hodgkin's lymphoma if they survive the recurrent infections.

Other enzymatic defects in polymorphonuclear (PMN) leukocytes include hereditary myeloperoxidase deficiency, which disposes patients to recurrent oral and gingival infections with periodontitis, and oral candidiasis. Oral candidiasis has also been described in pyruvate kinase deficiency, which primarily manifests as a severe hemolytic anemia.

The leukocyte adhesion defects denote congenital disorders with normal numbers of PMN leukocytes, but with defects in motility, chemotaxis, and adherence. Gingivitis, oral ulceration, periodontitis, and oral candidiasis are common.

Collagen vascular diseases

Collagen vascular diseases are associated with several oral manifestations; the best review of the subject is by Campbell, Montanaro, and Bardana.[6] Sjögren's syndrome has been a source of controversy and misunderstanding in the literature for years. In reality, it is a tripartite symptom complex consisting of keratoconjunctivitis with xerostomia and arthritis. The triad is diagnostic of Sjögren's (or sicca) syndrome. Sicca syndrome is sometimes associated with lacrimal, parotid, and submandibular gland enlargement caused by benign lymphocytic involvement; it is then referred to as Mikulicz's disease. These patients complain of dry eyes, salivary insufficiency, atrophy, and fissures and ulcers of the tongue, buccal membranes, and lips, particularly at the corners of the mouth. An increased incidence of caries is often seen. Many patients with sicca syndrome have antibodies reactive with nuclear antigens SS-A (Ro) and SS-B (La). They frequently display polyclonal hypergammaglobulinemia on serum-protein electrophoresis. Labial biopsy specimens show an intense infiltration of lymphocytes and destruction of most of the acinar tissue along with islands of epimyoepithelial cells.

If Sjögren's syndrome is not associated with known autoimmune disorder, it is called *primary Sjögren's syndrome*. Few of these patients develop collagen vascular disease during follow-up. If Sjögren's syndrome is associated with other autoimmune diseases—particularly lupus, rheumatoid arthritis, scleroderma, and occasionally dermatomyositis—it

is called *secondary Sjögren's syndrome*. Causes of xerostomia are listed as follows:

1. Acute or chronic renal failure
2. Radiation
3. Chemotherapy
4. Sjögren's syndrome (primary and secondary)
5. Mikulicz's disease
6. Sarcoidosis
7. Lymphoma
8. Anticholinergic drugs
9. Opiate derivatives
10. Graft-versus-host disease

Sjögren's syndrome frequently is symptomatic and associated with caries and periodontal disease. Oral pilocarpine will stimulate the minor salivary glands. Chlorhexidine may improve gingivitis, and fluoride treatment is advised to forestall dental caries.

A recent offering from the Netherlands[17] reports that mucin-containing lozenges (high molecular weight glycoproteins) can reduce the oral symptoms in most patients with Sjögren's syndrome.

Systemic lupus erythematosus (SLE) is an inflammatory condition of small blood vessels that predominantly affects women and is associated with various pronounced autoimmune phenomena, producing a wide spectrum of symptomatology, including skin ulcers and rashes, arthritis, inflammation of serosal surfaces, and involvement of the kidney, heart, lung, and brain. Of patients with SLE, 25% have associated oral lesions, which usually are superficial ulcers with surrounding erythema. Direct and indirect immunofluorescence of these lesions shows granular staining of the basement membrane of the dermal-epidermal junction with immunoglobulins and complement. This is similar to what is seen in the skin lesions. If a patient with lupus develops immunologic thrombocytopenia, the mouth may display petechiae and the characteristic hemorrhagic bullae of immunologic thrombocytopenia. Chronic discoid lupus, which is confined to the skin and mucous membranes and rarely progresses to SLE, can present as ulcerative, vesicular, and white keratotic lesions of the tongue and oral mucosa and as sicca syndrome.

Scleroderma frequently is associated with Sjögren's syndrome. It is idiopathic, characterized by arthritis, calcinosis cutis, esophageal hypomotility, sclerodactyly, and telangiectasia. Fibrosis may involve the entire gastrointestinal tract, leading to malabsorption; it also can produce cardiorespiratory symptoms caused by fibrosis of the lung and heart. One of the most frequent manifestations is Raynaud's phenomenon, particularly of the upper extremities on exposure to cold. Nielsen and others[20] described Raynaud's phenomenon of the tongue, which is associated with peripheral Raynaud's phenomenon and appears as a white tongue associated with dysarthria. Scleroderma victims frequently display a marked inability to open the mouth, (purse-string contractures secondary to fibrosis). Immobility of the tongue, disorders in deglutition, and abnormalities of the periodontal membrane with gingivitis have been described frequently.[1,14]

Polyarteritis nodosa is a disease of middle-aged men associated with inflammatory skin lesions in the medium-sized arteries. It is characterized by chronic skin ulcerations and frequent involvement of the kidney and nerve roots without involvement of the lung; few immunologic markers exist in the blood. Vasculitic ulcerations can be found in the buccal mucosa and soft palate, which on biopsy show a characteristic inflammatory reaction around the adventitia and the media of blood vessels.

Takayasu's syndrome, or pulseless disease, predominates in young females with granulomatous involvement of the aortic arch. It can present as dysphagia, ischemic pain of the mouth during talking and swallowing, and occasionally as fever of unknown origin.

Dermatomyostis-polymyositis is an immunologic disease of muscle usually characterized by the absence of a rash or periungual erythema in adults (but with proximal muscle weakness, elevated creatinine phosphokinase levels, and myopathic electromyelographs) and by interstitial fibrosis of the lung. It also can present as secondary Sjögren's syndrome. The muscle involvement may involve the tongue and upper portion of the esophagus, with difficulties in phonation and deglutition. Stomatitis is not uncommon, and aspiration pneumonia is frequent.

Rheumatoid arthritis usually does not involve the oral cavity except as Sjögren's syndrome, unless the disease evolves into an uncommon subvariant called *rheumatoid vasculitis*. In this situation, mouth ulcers similar to those in polyarteritis nodosa may be seen. Occasionally, arthritis of the temporomandibular joint (TMJ) may interfere with mouth opening. Involvement of the TMJ is most commonly seen in juvenile rheumatoid arthritis (JRA).

DISEASES OF UNCERTAIN CAUSE

Granulomatous diseases

Sarcoidosis, or Mortimer's malady, is a systemic granulomatous disease of unclear cause that predominantly affects black people. It is characterized by the presence of noncaseating granulomas virtually throughout the body, with frequent involvement in the skin, lymph nodes, lung, and liver. It usually pursues a benign, insidious course, but it can have considerable clinical activity and clinically may resemble other granulomatous diseases, such as infectious granuloma, Wegener's granulomatosis, lethal midline granuloma, or even lymphoma. Occasionally, sarcoidosis appears with masses on the tongue, lips, mandible, and maxilla. Biopsy shows characteristic noncaseating granulomas. The diagnosis also can be confused with infectious granulomatous diseases, such as histoplasmosis and blastomycosis.

An identifiable symptom complex syndrome in sarcoidosis is Heerfordt's disease (or uveoparotid fever), which is characterized by the acute onset of uveitis, iritis, parotid enlargement, and fever; it is occasionally associated with Bell's palsy, and frequently Sjögren's syndrome occurs. The course of this disease is decisively benign and usually resolves without specific treatment.

Wegener's granulomatosis is a rare disorder that histologically is characterized by granulomatous inflammation and vasculitis. The destructive granulomatous inflammation most commonly involves the paranasal sinus mucosa, lungs, synovia, skin, and kidneys. This was originally a chronic progressive disease with no treatment, but cytotoxic agents, particularly cyclophosphamide, have greatly improved the prognosis. Recently, the development of serum antineutrophil cytoplasmic antibodies has added to early diagnosis of this syndrome.

Handlers and others[15] reviewed 10 cases of Wegener's granulomatosis manifesting in the oral cavity. The most common early oral lesion is a hyperplastic gingiva, which is red to purple and has many petechiae (Plate 11, *B*). Tooth mobility, loss of teeth, and failure of the wound to heal are common manifestations. The disease may remain localized to the oral cavity for an unusually long time before multiorgan involvement occurs. Oral biopsy tissue may not exhibit the characteristic feature of granulomatous vasculitis seen elsewhere. Diagnostic histologic patterns include pseudoepitheliomatous hyperplasia, epithelial histiocytes, giant cells, and eosinophils. Failure to recognize these diagnostic and clinical features delays diagnosis and treatment of this progressive disease.

Lethal midline granuloma, a very rare disease characterized by destructive granulomas, often leads to mutilation of the upper respiratory tract and face. This disease resembles Wegener's granulomatosis, except it does not involve the lungs, kidneys, or skin. Histologically, lethal midline granulomas display no vasculitis. Cultures for mycobacterium and fungi are negative. Early radiotherapy is the treatment of choice, and satisfactory results require early recognition. Lethal midline granuloma should be carefully separated from lymphomatoid granulomatosis and malignant midline reticulosis because therapy and prognosis differ. Hematologic consultation is strongly suggested.

Dimitrakopoulos, and others[10] described two cases of tuberculosis in the oral cavity in young immunologically-competent women. Both presented with painless ulcers of the gingiva with enlarged regional lymph nodes. The underlying bone was not involved. The diagnosis was made by histologic examination with noncaseating granulomas, negative acid-fast bacilli stain, elevated erythrocyte sedimentation rates, and positive purified protein derivative (PPD) (Mantoux skin test). No evidence of tuberculosis was found elsewhere. Both patients responded to antituberculosis therapy. Both patients were Greek with a history of ingestion of unpasteurized milk, so this probably represents *Mycobacterium bovium*.

Histiocytoses X are a group of congenital, rare, and arcane maladies characterized by relatively uncontrolled proliferation of histiocytes. These disorders have recently been renamed *Langerhans' cell histiocytosis* (LCH). However, the clinical separation—Letterer-Siwe disease (acute disseminated LCH resembling an acute leukemia), eosinophilic granuloma (a chronic lung and bone disease), and Hand-Schüller-Christian disease (the chronic disseminated form characterized by multiple osteolytic cholesterol-laden histiocytes involving the bone of the skull, face, and mouth)—remains intact. Langerhans' cells are dendritic antigens processing and presenting cells and are potent initiators of primary T-cell–dependent immunologic processes. Pringle and others[22] described six cases of periapical inflammatory disease that showed aggregates of Langerhans' cells on biopsy. These authors postulated that these lesions represented incipient eosinophilic granuloma or a more minimally destructive form of LCH. These observations are worth noting and pursuing.

Nongranulomatous inflammatory diseases

Dermatitis herpetiformis is a dermatologic condition associated with malabsorption and characterized by a recurrent eruption of closely cropped vesicles with erythematous haloes, resembling herpes, on the skin of the extremities and buttocks; these vesicles do not form the characteristic dermatome pattern commonly seen in herpes. Occasionally, the oral mucosa is involved, with erythematous macules and papules, purpura, and superficial erosions, which are nonspecific; direct immunofluorescence may demonstrate immunoglobulin A (IgA) in the basement membrane area of the bullous lesions.

Psoriasis is a little-understood dermatologic condition characterized by scaly, silver plaques on an erythematous base that produce bleeding when stripped off. Biopsy of these lesions shows parakeratosis, acanthosis, and intraepithelial microabscesses. Rarely, psoriasis appears in the mouth with white, crusted, hyperkeratotic lesions on the oropharynx; the surrounding buccal mucosa is usually brightly erythematous.

Behçet's syndrome is an idiopathic condition that consists of recurrent oral and genital ulcers, arthritis, and inflammatory disease of the eyes and gastrointestinal tract. The skin, central nervous system, and coronary blood vessels may be involved. Often, Behçet's syndrome appears as recurrent aphthous ulcers, which may also be found in the genital area and skin. Eye lesions consist of iritis, retinal vasculitis, optic neuritis, conjunctivitis, and keratitis. Involvement of the central nervous system with meningitis is a particularly distressing complication. Behçet's syndrome is virtually limited to persons of Middle Eastern descent.

Patients with inflammatory bowel disease—regional enteritis (Crohn's disease) and ulcerative colitis—may present with recurrent aphthous ulcers, which are extraintestinal manifestations. With ulcerative colitis, the aphthous ulcers are frequently associated with other mucous membrane in-

volvement, iritis, arthritis, and erythema nodosum. Regional enteritis is a noncaseating granulomatous disease of the gastrointestinal tract from the mouth through the anus. Occasionally, masses resembling granulomas can be seen in the mouth; biopsy shows noncaseating granulomas. Ramsdell, Shulman, and Lifschitz[23] described, in addition to aphthous ulcers in regional enteritis, oral ulcerations that may be deep and extensive. Additional manifestations include thickened, edematous buccal mucosa, producing a cobblestone appearance similar to that found in the gut, swelling of the lips, and granulomatous cheilitis. Ulcerative colitis also may manifest pyostomatitis, which is a particularly distressing progressive necrotic and inflammatory involvement of the entire oral mucous membranes. Causes of aphthous ulcers are listed as follows:

1. Primary causes
2. B_{12} deficiency
3. Gluten-sensitive enteropathy (celiac disease or nontropical sprue)
4. Chronic granulomatous disease
5. Behçet's syndrome
6. Inflammatory bowel disease

Reiter's syndrome is a recurrent arthritis condition characterized by conjunctivitis, asymmetric oligoarticular lower extremity arthritis, urethritis, circinate balanitis, and keratoderma blennorrhagia, particularly on the soles of the feet. Reiter's syndrome can follow *Yersinia* enterocolitic infections, or it can occur in the absence of this infection. It is closely associated with the human leukocyte antigen B27 phenotype. Painless oral ulcers and gingival lesions with hemorrhagic crusts and exudates can be seen in this syndrome, which may be confused with disseminated gonococcemia or the infectious enterarthropathy most commonly seen with *Salmonella* or *Shigella* infections.

Kawasaki's disease (mucocutaneous lymph node syndrome) is an acute multisystem illness that predominantly affects children but has been described in adults. It is characterized by a triphasic course. The initial phase of acute illness is marked by high fever, conjunctival injection, and oral changes producing a strawberry tongue and desquamative rash (Plate 12, *A*). The second phase begins with a decline in the acute findings and includes heart disease and joint manifestations. The third phase is usually asymptomatic.[29]

IMMUNOLOGIC DISEASES

In idiopathic polychondritis, the cartilage is thought to be the autoimmune target tissue because antibodies against chondroitin sulfate have been found in the blood. It is characterized by progressive destruction of the cartilage of the ears, nose, and upper respiratory tract. Arthritis and aortic insufficiency may occur. The patient may have extensive difficulty with breathing and talking, yet nothing will be seen on examination of the oral cavity.

Although much has been written in the past 15 years about the oral lesions in AIDS, less attention has been paid to congenital (primary) immunodeficiency disorders. Severe combined immunodeficiency (SCID) is a congenital genetic disorder associated with decreased serum immunoglobulins and decreased T-cell function caused by a maturation defect in T and B cells. Patients with severe combined immunodeficiency usually have no detectable tonsillar tissue and a proclivity for oral candidiasis, oral ulcerations, and even necrotizing gingivostomatitis (noma). Fluconazole, acyclovir, and intravenous immunoglobulin ameliorate many symptoms but do not attack the primary disorder; nothing has been found to ameliorate the T-cell dysfunction.

Oral candidiasis and lack of tonsillar tissue are characteristics of adenosine deaminase deficiency and purine nucleoside phosphorylase deficiency, which produce T- and B-cell defects and T-cell defects, respectively, from accumulation of toxic metabolites inherent on the lacking enzymes.

Combined immunodeficiency as a result of major histocompatibility complex (MHC) class II deficiencies can present as severe infection with *Candida* and herpes simplex viruses I and II. Sex-linked recessive (Bruton's) agammaglobulinemia is a congenital defect in the production of all classes of serum immunoglobulins and is associated with atrophy of lymphoid tissue of the mouth, soft palate, tonsils, and lips. The availability of intravenous γ globulin has substantially improved this disorder.

Selective IgA deficiency, which is common, is caused by a failure in terminal differentiation of IgA B cells. It is characterized by tonsillitis and gingival enlargement, oral ulceration, and lichenoid changes in the buccal mucosa. A host of autoimmune (systemic lupus erythematosus) and allergic (atopy and anaphylaxis) disorders are described in this disorder. A hematologist or immunologist should be consulted before attempting any replacement therapy in these patients.

Common variable immunodeficiency is very common and is caused by failure of B-cell differentiation, antibodies to B cells, or defects on CD4 function. Oral manifestations include oral candidiasis (pharyngitis), aphthous ulcerations, and enamel hypoplasia.

Wiskott-Aldrich syndrome is an X-linked recessive inherited disease characterized by eczema, chronic thrombocytopenia with purpura of the skin and oral mucous membranes, low IgM concentrations with later development of cellular immunodeficiency, and a propensity to develop infections. Non-Hodgkin's lymphoma develops later in the course.

Ataxia–telangiectasia (AT) is a rare, inherited abnormality of chromosomal instability or clonal evolution characterized by low serum IgA (sometimes immunoglobulin M [IgM]), decreased T-cell function, and a propensity to develop lymphoid malignancies. Clinically, these patients present with widespread telangiectasia that may involve the palate and oral mucosa, cerebellar ataxia, and a characteristic dull expression with drooling. Severe oral ulcers have been described, and the resultant lymphomas can involve the face and mouth.

DiGeorge syndrome is caused by embryonic maldevelopment of the third and fourth pharyngeal pouches. This results in thymic dysfunction with decreased T-cell function and hypoparathyroidism. A peculiar orofacial syndrome occurs in these patients, with prominent forehead, hypertelorism and low-set ears, a fish-like mouth, and palatal clefts. Severe chronic mucocutaneous candidiasis is a result of the T-cell dysfunction, and enamel hypoplasia is a result of the hypocalcemia.

Chronic mucocutaneous candidiasis is a recurrent disorder occasionally associated with the autoimmune disorders hypoparathyroidism and pernicious anemia. It also probably has an autoimmune basis and is characterized by depressed cellular immunity and recurrent candidiasis in the mouth, esophagus, and skin. Treatment with fluconazole is very effective. The candidiasis rarely disseminates internally.

Some mucositis in bone marrow transplant recipients is mediated by graft-versus-host (GVH) disease or treatment, which often includes methotrexate. Methotrexate stomatitis can be ameliorated in some cases with leucovorin mouthwash. Mucosal graft-versus-host reactions can last for years and are characterized by erythematous atrophy and lichenoid changes in the mucosa. There is no known treatment for this problem. It is often symptomatic and resembles Sjögren's syndrome.

GVH disease is an acute and chronic disorder seen after bone marrow transplantation and blood transfusion presumably with immunocompetent lymphocytes in patients with SCID syndrome or Swiss agammaglobulinemia. Oral manifestations have been well described by Schubert and others[26] and Barrett and Bilous.[2] They very frequently are seen after allogeneic bone marrow transplantations, may occur very early, and are characterized by painful mucosal atrophy, erythema, and licheniform lesions in the buccal and labial mucosa. Biopsy may show the pathologic findings described previously in the sicca syndrome. Other manifestations of GVH disease resemble scleroderma, primary biliary cirrhosis, hepatic veno-occlusive disease, nephrosis, rheumatoid arthritis, systemic lupus erythematosus, and lichen planus with erythematous skin lesions and later atrophy. These changes are not associated with but resemble congenital or acquired immunosuppression; they should be caused by the injection of immunocompetent cells into an immunosuppressed host.

Pemphigus vulgaris and pemphigus vegetans are serious bullous skin disorders that affect the oral cavity in about two thirds of cases.[21] In about one half of cases, the mouth initially is affected with later involvement of the skin. The immunology of this disease has been well described. On biopsy, the lesions show bullae in the suprabasal layer of the epithelium. Direct immunofluorescence displays intracellular deposits of immunoglobulin in the affected area, and indirect immunofluorescence shows autoantibodies in the serum and bullae fluid against the epithelial intracellular substance. Many believe that these antibodies are directly involved in the reaction against epithelial cellular material, with the release of proteolytic enzymes leading to bullae formation. This disease also involves all areas of the gastrointestinal tract, and sepsis is the usual mode of death. Systemic corticosteroids are the treatment of choice in pemphigus but are not particularly effective.

There are two pemphigoid diseases: bullous pemphigoid and benign mucous membrane pemphigoid. In the latter, the lesions are virtually confined to the eye and oral cavity. Oral lesions are seen in about one third of cases with bullous pemphigoid. In these two diseases, a biopsy shows subepithelial bullae, and direct immunofluorescence shows autoantibodies against the basement membranes of the surface epithelia. Anti–basement membrane antibodies are detected in the serum and fluid of the lesions. The lesions in bullous pemphigoid and benign mucous membrane pemphigoid are thought to be caused by an autoimmune reaction against the basement membrane of surface epithelial cells. The treatment of these diseases is much more satisfactory than that of pemphigus, and they usually can be controlled by intermittent systemic corticosteroid therapy. A reaction similar to pemphigoid can be seen when penicillamine is used in the treatment of primary biliary cirrhosis or systemic rheumatoid vasculitis.

Erythema multiforme[3] is a heterogeneous symptom complex characterized by pleomorphic skin lesions that are often symmetric. The most characteristic lesions are concentric lines of erythema interspersed with healthy skin, in the center of which is usually a papule. This is frequently associated with a systemic symptomatology such as fever, malaise, and arthritis; when it involves the mucous membranes, it is frequently called the *Stevens-Johnson syndrome* (Plate 12, *B*).

The cause of this disease is multifactorial. It can be seen after streptococcal illness and infections such as herpes and mycoplasma. Penicillin and sulfa are the most common drugs implicated. Occasionally, patients with a splenectomy develop recurrent erythema multiforme, but it is idiopathic in 50% of the patients.

Oral manifestations of erythema multiforme are frequently estimated at about 50% and consist of bullae, ulcerations, and hemorrhagic crusts, particularly around the lips. Histologically, oral lesions exhibit degenerative changes of the epithelium, with epithelial vacuolation of the basal layer and inflammation mostly with mononuclear cells. Associated with such changes are deposits of immunoglobulin and complement, which have been found in subepithelial vessels. Systemic corticosteroids are indicated for very symptomatic cases.

Lichen planus[21] is a dermatologic condition that affects the mucous membranes of the lips, tongue, and tonsils. Mucous membrane lesions are the sole manifestation in one third of cases, mucous membranes and skin are involved in another third, and involvement of the skin alone occurs in another third. The mucous membrane lesions are asymptomatic papules that range in color from white to blue to gray and whose morphology may be reticular, linear, annular, or even plaque-like (Plate 13, *A*). Occasionally, bullous lesions are seen and seem to indicate mucous membrane pemphigoid. The skin lesions are violaceous papules on the extensor surface of the forearms and neck; they are chronic and heal with some atrophy. The oral lesions tend to be more chronic than the skin lesions. The pathogenesis of this disease is not clear, but it is thought to be an immunologic disease because of reports of fibrin and complement deposition in the basement membrane zone with infiltration of inflammatory cells just below the dermis. Also, this disease can be seen after bone marrow transplantation and in association with systemic lupus erythematosus (SLE). Findings indicate that a combined type IV (delayed) and III (antigen-antibody) hypersensitivity reaction occurs in the lesions in response to locally produced or released epidermal or mucosal antigens.

A study prospectively linked erosive and nonerosive lichen planus with nonsteroidal anti-inflammatory drugs and antihypertensive drug ingestion.[24] For especially chronic and symptomatic oral lichen planus, cyclosporine mouthwash may be beneficial.[11]

Urticaria is an eruption of common skin wheals, or hives. When the edema extends into the deep portions of the dermis and the subcutaneous or submucosal tissues, it is called *angioedema*. Angioedema also may involve the lung, gastrointestinal tract, and cardiovascular system. Angioedema frequently occurs in the mouth, tongue, uvula, and soft palate and may seriously impair breathing. See Box 74-3 for classifications.

Box 74-3. Classification of angioedema

IgE-dependent activation of mast cells

Atopy
Specific antigen sensitivity (foods, drugs)
Physical stimuli (cold)

Complement-mediated activity

Hereditary and acquired C_1 esterase inhibitor deficiency
Serum sickness
Hypersensitivity vasculitis
Reaction to blood products

Agents with direct action on mast cells

Radiation contrast media

Agent altering arachidonic acid pathways of inflammation

Aspirin

TOXIC AND DRUG EFFECTS ON ORAL CAVITY

Diphenylhydantoin, which should be renamed Dreyfuss' remedy, is used in the treatment of epilepsy and various types of neuralgia and is associated on prolonged use with gingival hyperplasia of the maxillary and mandibular areas. This is seen only at sites of tooth formation and probably is related to less-than-adequate oral hygiene (Plate 13, *B*). Staining of the teeth during ingestion of tetracycline and fluoride during tooth development has already been described in the section on congenital lesions. Mercury, bismuth, lead, and arsenic can produce dark gray or black pigment at gingival margins; the latter two metals may also produce changes in the nails and may mimic obscure hematologic, gastrointestinal, or neurologic illness. Iodides and bromides may produce idiosyncratic granulomas in the oral cavity. Various drugs have anticholinergic activity, major ones are listed as follows:

1. Atropine
2. Dicyclomine
3. Propantheline
4. Antiarrhythmics
5. Phenothiazine tranquilizers
6. Tricylic antidepressants
7. Antiparkinsonian drugs

These drugs produce mouth and eye dryness, which can be treated with oral pilocarpine to stimulate the minor salivary glands. The most common allergic reaction to drugs in the oral mucosa is the vesicular bullous reaction, which was discussed in the section on erythema multiforme.

Botulism, a disease produced by ingestion of the toxin *Clostridium botulinum*, makes acetylcholine transmission at the neuromuscular junction difficult. Difficulty with eyesight and dilated, fixed pupils may be the first signs of this disease, followed by dry mouth, inability to swallow, and poor phonation caused by involvement of the bulbar musculature.

The many medical diseases associated with gastroesophageal reflux disease (GERD) now include oral and gingival erosions and inflammation thought to be caused by acid. The reflux can be nocturnal and asymptomatic and usually is controlled with Prilosec, a potent acid cation-pump inhibitor that does not help in cases of achlorhydria of the eldery. A properly interpreted serum gastrin is a good substitute for a gastric acid analysis.

NEUROLOGIC DISORDERS

Parkinson's disease and Shy-Drager syndrome (idiopathic orthostatic hypotension) are thought to be similar if not the same disease. Besides having extrapyramidal symptoms, both are associated with idiopathic atrophy of the autonomic nervous system, which produces hypohydrosis, orthostatic hypotension without compensatory tachycardia, and dry mouth and eyes. The tremor of Parkinson's disease can involve the lips and tongue. Bradykinesia may affect the masticatory muscles. Esophageal motility disturbances may affect deglutition and frequently lead to aspiration pneumonia, a major cause of morbidity.

Myasthenia gravis is an autoimmune disease with antibodies directed against the acetylcholine receptors of the neuromuscular junction. It may present with difficult swallowing and phonation, with resultant muscular atrophy. The availability of serum acetylcholine receptor antibodies has greatly facilitated early diagnosis of this condition. Similarly, amyotrophic lateral sclerosis (Lou Gehrig's disease), a progressive degeneration of the pyramidal tract involving the bulbar motor neurons, may produce difficulty with deglutition, mastication, and phonation. Fasciculations of the tongue with later atrophy are characteristic.

Syringobulbia is a developmental cavitary defect in the cervical spinal cord, often extending into the medulla. It is manifested by weakness of the tongue, palatal paralysis, and unilateral vocal cord involvement. Nuclear magnetic resonance imaging (MRI) has greatly facilitated this diagnosis.

Wallenberg's lateral medullary plate syndrome is produced by thrombosis of the posterior inferior cerebellar artery. Dysphagia and palatal paralysis are seen and are caused by involvement of the glossopharyngeal and vagus nerves. Involvement of the solitary tract produces a loss of taste.

Bell's palsy (unilateral facial nerve paralysis) may be idiopathic or postviral; it may be associated with diabetes mellitus, sarcoidosis, non-Hodgkin's lymphoma, leptomeningeal carcinomatosis, or deep benign parotid tumors such as oncocytoma. It appears as a peripheral facial paralysis with disorders in phonation and mastication and hyperacute hearing. If the chorda tympani nerve is involved, taste on the anterior two thirds of the tongue is lost.

Multiple sclerosis is an idiopathic demyelinating disorder characterized by optic neuritis, nystagmus, ataxia, tremor, peripheral neuropathy, and transverse myelitis. Dysarthria (scanning speech) secondary to cerebellar dysfunction and difficulty with breathing and swallowing are extremely common. Although multiple sclerosis remains a clinical diagnosis, MRI has led to earlier diagnosis, and interferon-β is a promising new therapy.

Myotonic dystrophy is an autosomally dominant disease characterized by distal myotonia (difficulty in muscular relaxation). It frequently is associated with ocular and oropharyngeal muscle involvement, producing facial weakness, dysarthria, and difficulties with phonation and mastication. Cataracts, hypogonadism, baldness, atrophy of the sternocleidomastoid muscles, and cardiac disease are common.

A variant of the Pickwickian syndrome, sometimes called the Alfred Hitchcock syndrome, is idiopathic alveolar hypoventilation. Although originally seen in massively obese[5] patients, this is not always the case. This syndrome is associated with changes on the electroencephalogram, idiopathic alveolar hypoventilation with chronic partial pressure of carbon dioxide (artery) retention, snoring, and a history of sleep apnea and daytime sleepiness. These patients may have headaches, secondary polycythemia, and often digital clubbing and pulmonary hypertension. They frequently exhibit cardiac arrhythmias and syncope. The site of upper airway obstruction is in the oropharynx and the velopharyngeal sphincter. These patients frequently respond to progesterone, tricyclic antidepressants, and aminophylline. An otolaryngologist should always be consulted, and removal of excess adenoids and tonsils and a uvulopalatopharyngoplasty are often helpful. A tracheostomy is sometimes indicated. The diagnosis of sleep apnea–idiopathic hypoventilation syndromes has become so complex that consultation with a neurologist specializing in sleep disorders is recommended before therapeutic or surgical intervention.

DEFICIENCY STATES

Deficiency states in the United States are virtually limited to alcoholics, food faddists, and patients with malabsorption. Malabsorption produces deficiencies of vitamins A, D, E, and K and calcium and folate. The oral manifestations of hypocalcemia are detailed in the section on acquired endocrine-metabolic diseases; folate deficiencies are discussed in the hematology section. Common causes of malabsorption are listed as follows:

I. Maldigestion
  A. Exocrine pancreatic insufficiency
  B. Biliary tract disorders and primary biliary cirrhosis
  C. Bacterial overgrowth with deconjugation of bile salts
    1. Blind loops
    2. Jejunal diverticulae
    3. Scleroderma with intestinal motility disorders
II. Malabsorption
  A. Congenital
    1. Hartnup disease
    2. Abetalipoproteinemia
  B. Gluten-sensitive enteropathy (celiac disease or nontropical sprue)
  C. Whipple's disease
  D. Amyloidosis
  E. Crohn's disease
  F. Tropical sprue
  G. Non-Hodgkin's lymphoma or α-chain disease
  H. Agammaglobulinemia (usually with *Giardia lamblia* infestation)

Vitamin K deficiency leads to deficient assembly of competent procoagulants of the prothrombin complex (factors II, VII, IX, and X), leading to a hemorrhagic diathesis that often presents with oral hemorrhagic bullae. This also may be produced with warfarin anticoagulation.

Besides the oral manifestations produced by the lack of vitamin B_{12} and folate (mentioned in the section on hematology), these two deficiencies may produce recurrent aphthous ulcers. Recurrent aphthous ulcers can also be seen in gluten sensitivity with malabsorption (celiac disease).

Vitamin A deficiency produces nyctalopia (night blindness), dyskeratotic changes of the skin and mucous membranes, angular cheilitis, and defects in the dentin and enamel of developing teeth. A biopsy reveals pseudoepitheliomatous hyperplasia carcinoma *in situ*. These problems revert with administration of vitamin A.

Vitamin B_2 (or riboflavin) deficiency is associated with angular cheilitis and burning pain in the lips, mouth, and tongue. Later changes include atrophy of the mucous membranes of the mouth. Scurvy, or vitamin C deficiency, is associated with perifollicular hemorrhages and petechiae in the mouth caused by vascular integrity compromise, gingival hyperplasia, and stomatitis.

Pellagra, an acquired disorder caused by dietary niacin (nicotinic acid or nicotinamide) deficiency, is associated with hyperkeratotic dermatitis (a bronze rash), diarrhea, and dementia. It also can present with oral mucous membrane atrophy and painful erythematous, edematous angular cheilitis. Deficiencies of vitamins B and C, niacin, and folate frequently occur concomitantly.

Acrodermatitis enteropathica is characterized by psoriaform lesions, especially about the mouth; candidiasis of the oral cavity; and diarrhea. It is caused by a zinc deficiency (often caused by a congenital deficiency in zinc ligand, a prostaglandin necessary for its absorption). Secondary causes include prolonged hyperalimentation without zinc supplementation. Symptoms can be completely reversed with zinc supplementation.

ACKNOWLEDGMENT

My thanks to Jennifer L. Guy for reading this manuscript 10^6 times, and thanks to Sherri Starrett (Munch) for considerable help in the second revision.

REFERENCES

1. Alexandridis C, White SC: Periodontal ligament changes in patients with progressive systemic sclerosis, *Oral Surg Oral Med Oral Pathol* 58:113, 1984.
2. Barrett AP, Bilous AM: Oral pattern of acute and chronic graft-vs-host disease, *Arch Dermatol* 120:1461, 1984.
3. Bean SF, Quezada RK: Recurrent oral erythema multiforme, *JAMA* 249:2810, 1983.
4. Bernstein L: *Congenital malformations of the oral cavity.* In Paparella M, Shumrick D, editors: *Otolaryngology,* Philadelphia, 1972, WB Saunders.
5. Burock B: The hypersomnia-sleep apnea syndrome: its recognition in clinical cardiology, *Am Heart J* 107:543, 1984.
6. Campbell SM, Montanaro A, Bardana EJ: Head and neck manifestations of autoimmune disease, *Am J Otolaryngol* 4:187, 1983.
7. Carl W: Oral complications in cancer patients, *Am Fam Physician* 27:161, 1983.
8. Damm DD and others: Intraoral sebaceous carcinoma, *Oral Surg Oral Med Oral Pathol* 72:709, 1991.
9. DeWeese DD, Saunders WH: *Textbook of otolaryngology,* ed 6, St Louis, 1982, Mosby.
10. Dimitrakopoulos I and others: Primary tuberculosis of the oral cavity, *Oral Surg Oral Med Oral Pathol* 72:712, 1991.
11. Eisen D and others: Cyclosporin wash for oral lichen planus, *Lancet* 335:535, 1990.

12. Eisenbud L and others: Oral presentations in non-Hodgkin's: review of thirty-one cases (data analysis), *Oral Surg* 56:151, 1983.

13. Epstein JB, Voss NJS, Stevenson-Moore P: Maxillofacial manifestations of multiple myeloma, *Oral Surg* 57:267, 1984.

14. Eversole LR, Jacobson PL, Stone CE: Oral and gingival changes in systemic sclerosis (scleroderma), *J Periodontal* 55:175, 1984.

15. Handlers JP and others: Oral features of Wegener's granulomatosis, *Arch Otolaryngol Head Neck Surg* 111:167, 1985.

16. James WD, Guiry CC, Grote WR: Acute idiopathic thrombocytopenic purpura, *Oral Surg* 57:149, 1984.

17. Johannes's-Gravenmade E, Vissink A: Mucin-containing lozenges in the treatment of intraoral problems associated with Sjögren's syndrome, *Oral Surg Oral Med Oral Pathol* 75:466, 1993.

18. McKusick VA: *Heritable disorders of connective tissue,* ed 4, St Louis, 1972, Mosby.

19. Nadimi H: Subclasses of extranodal oral B-cell lymphomas express cIgM, plasmacytoid, and monocytoid differentiation, *Oral Surg Oral Med Oral Pathol* 77:392, 1994.

20. Nielsen HV and others: Paroxysmal dysarthria and Raynaud's phenomenon in the tongue, *Acta Med Scand* 216:431, 1984.

21. Pedersen A, Klausen B: Glucocorticosteroids and oral medicine, *Oral Surg Oral Med* 13:1, 1984.

22. Pringle GA and others: Langerhans' cell histiocytosis in association with periapical granulomas and cysts, *Oral Surg Oral Med Oral Pathol* 74:186, 1992.

23. Ramsdell WM, Shulman RJ, Lifschitz CH: Unusual appearance of Crohn's disease, *Am J Dis Child* 138:500, 1984.

24. Robertson WD, Wray D: Ingestion of medication among patients with oral keratoses including lichen planus, *Oral Surg Oral Med Oral Pathol* 74:183, 1992.

25. Rusthoven JJ, Fine S, Thomas G: Adenocarcinoma of the rectum metastatic to the oral cavity, *Cancer* 54:1110, 1984.

26. Schubert MM and others: Oral manifestations of chronic graft-vs-host disease, *Arch Intern Med* 144:1591, 1984.

27. Shklar G, McCarthy PL: *The oral manifestations of systemic disease,* Woburn, Mass, 1976, Butterworths.

28. Smith RJH, Evans JNG: Head and neck manifestations of histiocytosis X, *Laryngoscope* 94:395, 1984.

29. Soman M, Faulkner S, Snively GG: Kawasaki disease, *J Fam Pract* 16:723, 1983.

30. Stanbury JB and others: *The metabolic basis of inherited disease,* ed 5, New York, 1983, McGraw-Hill.

30a.Toker C: Trabecular carcinoma of the skin, *Arch Dermatol* 105:107, 1972.

31. Vigneswaran N and others: Merkel cell carcinoma of the labial mucosa, *Oral Surg Oral Med Oral Pathol* 74:193, 1992.

32. Wyngaarden JB, Smith LH: *Textbook of medicine,* Philadelphia, 1985, WB Saunders.

SUGGESTED READINGS

Ballenger JJ: *Diseases of the nose, throat, ear, head, and neck,* ed 13, Philadelphia, 1985, Lea & Febiger.

Brown RB, Clinton D: Vesicular and ulcerative infections of the mouth and oropharynx, *Postgrad Med* 67:107, 1980.

Dilley DH, Blozis GG: Common oral lesions and oral manifestations of systemic illnesses and therapies, *Pediatr Clin North Am* 29:585, 1982.

Greenspan JS, Greenspan D, Winkler JR: Oral manifestations of HIV infection and AIDS, *Opportun Infect Patients AIDS* 1, 1991.

Kelly WN and others: *Textbook of rheumatology,* ed 2, Philadelphia, 1985, WB Saunders.

Moschella SL, Hurley HJ: *Dermatology,* ed 2, Philadelphia, 1985, WB Saunders.

Paparella MM, Shumrick DA: *Otolaryngology,* Philadelphia, 1972, WB Saunders.

Porter SR, Scully C: Orofacial manifestations in the primary immunodeficiency disorders, *Oral Surg Oral Med Oral Pathol* 78:4, 1994.

Powell FC, Rogers RS: A practical approach to oral lesions, *Prim Care* 10:495, 1983.

Rodnam GP, Schumaker HR: *Primer on the rheumatic diseases,* ed 8, Atlanta, 1983, Arthritis Foundation.

Chapter 75

Facial Trauma: Soft-Tissue Lacerations and Burns

Kevin A. Shumrick

Facial soft-tissue injuries are common and always have existed.[15] Because the face is in the lead position, it is often the first recipient of any hostilities or unfortunate events. Many possible facial soft-tissue injuries exist, ranging from the uncomplicated pediatric laceration to massive disruptions with deforming sequelae. The physician should keep in mind that facial wounds consist of a physical injury and a strong psychologic component. The psychologic sequelae arise from the important social and self-image role physical appearance plays in our society. Additionally, the trauma of repairing a facial laceration in the emergency room may have a tremendous negative psychologic effect on a pediatric patient, leaving life-long negative feelings regarding hospitals or physicians. Facial wounds that fail to achieve optimal results (with scarring or deformity) may cause self-image and self-confidence problems that may alter the patient's, personality and impact the course of the patient's life. This chapter provides an overview of the management of facial soft-tissue injuries and burns and addresses effective methods for managing the physical damage and minimizing the psychologic trauma.

CLINICAL HISTORY

An accurate clinical history regarding the cause of facial trauma is invaluable for completely and accurately assessing a wound and, most importantly, planning appropriate treatment. Unfortunately, many facial injuries, particularly pediatric injuries, are not witnessed, or the patient has an altered sensorium from the trauma or pharmacologic agents; thus, the traumatic event should be reconstructed retrospectively. Much valuable information may be lost regarding the

wounding agent, degree of contamination, and other associated injuries. Additionally, the clinician treating pediatric facial trauma should keep in mind the possibility that the facial injuries were not accidental but intentionally inflicted; it is the physician's responsibility to investigate any unusual or suspicious injuries to a child.

HISTORY OF TRAUMATIC EVENT

The history should consider the following questions: What was the mechanism of injury? Was the patient mobile, restrained, or stationary? Was the impacting object mobile or stationary? Was the injury the result of blunt trauma, penetrating trauma, or both? Can the degree of energy transfer (high versus low) be estimated? Were there coincident fatalities? Were associated thermal or chemical injuries present?

ASSESSMENT OF SOFT-TISSUE INJURIES

Several types of soft-tissue facial injuries are possible, including contusions and avulsions, but the most common soft-tissue injuries, particularly in children, are lacerations. Lacerations may range from simple, superficial wounds that are easily repaired to injuries that involve deeper structures, including muscles, nerves, and ducts. Major lacerations, improperly treated, can leave dysfunctional and deforming sequelae. The most important factor in treating any injury is proper initial evaluation and assessment so that relevant concerns are identified and a comprehensive treatment plan formulated.

Chart documentation also is an integral part of medical care for follow-up and medicolegal concerns. The follow-

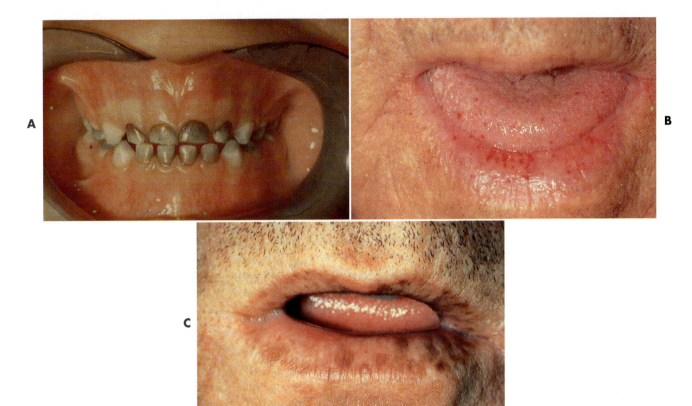

Plate 9. **A,** Staining of teeth as seen in patients with congenital biliary atresia or severe Rh incompatibility. **B,** Large telangiectasia of the tongue as seen in hereditary hemorrhagic telangiectasia (Weber-Rendu-Osler syndrome). **C,** Melanin deposits in the lip, mucous membrane, and skin, as seen in Peutz-Jeghers syndrome. (**A,** From Davis JM, Law DB, Lewis TM: *An atlas of pedodontics,* ed 2, Philadelphia, 1981, WB Saunders. **B** and **C,** Courtesy of AF Morgan, MD, Seattle.)

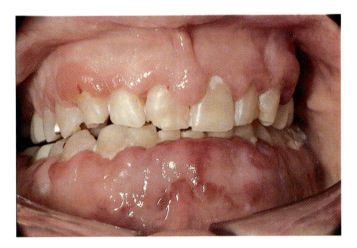

Plate 10. Leukemic infiltrate of the gingiva in an elderly patient with acute myelogenous leukemia. (Courtesy of Carl M Allen, DDS.)

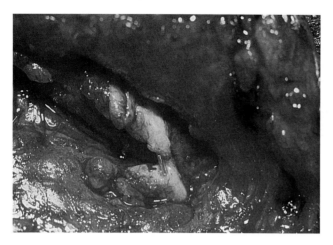

Fig. 75-1. Deep cheek laceration with transection of the parotid duct. A Silastic tube has been passed intraorally connecting the proximal and distal ends of the duct. Note the severed buccal branch of the facial nerve lateral to superior and the duct. Both nerve and duct were repaired with 8-0 monofilament.

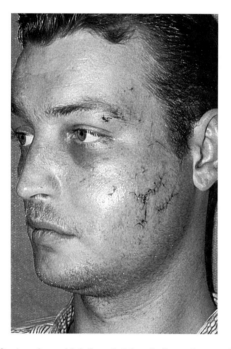

Fig. 75-2. A patient with infected sialocele from a lacerated parotid duct that was not diagnosed at the time of primary repair. Treatment consisted of anticholinergics and pressure dressings. The salivary drainage stopped after 3 to 4 weeks.

itself.[17,18,22] If the fistula persists, a superficial parotidectomy may be required.

Lacrimal apparatus

There should be a high index of suspicion for injury to the lacrimal drainage apparatus with any laceration involving the medial portion of the upper or lower eyelid in the region of the medial canthus laceration (Fig. 75-3 *A* through *C*). The major sequela of a lacrimal canalicular laceration is epiphora, which may not be obvious in the acute setting because of associated pain and edema. If a canalicular laceration or lacrimal duct laceration may be present, the lacrimal punctum and duct should be cannulated with lacrimal probes and the laceration examined to see if they appear in the wound. A laceration should be repaired over Silastic stents under magnification with fine sutures (8-0).

Retained foreign body

The treating physician should consider the possibility of a retained foreign body in penetrating injuries involving glass or wood or resulting from striking the ground (Fig. 75-4 *A* through *C*). The phenomenon of debris tattooing results from particulate matter being imbedded in the dermis and not appropriately removed (Fig. 75-5). Typically, this occurs as a result of abrasions sustained from falling and sliding along the ground or pavement. The epidermis is denuded, and dirt, stones, and other debris implanted in the dermis. The epidermis will then resurface the wound, and the retained material will be visible externally. Once the epidermis has sealed the wound, it is virtually impossible to remove the visible debris short of full-thickness excision of the affected area (late dermabrasion has been disappointing; laser vaporization may eventually prove useful). Therefore, it is important to identify wounds with the potential for debris tattooing because the optimum time to treat this condition is at the time of injury when the epidermis is still open and the foreign material can be removed by scrubbing, irrigation, or dermabrasion. It is extremely difficult to achieve adequate local anesthesia for débridement of large areas of abraded tissue; these cases are probably best performed in the operating room with general anesthesia.

REPAIR OF SOFT-TISSUE INJURIES

After ruling out injuries to associated deep structures, attention may be turned to repair of the superficial soft-tissue injury. As noted, the treating physician should meticulously remove all foreign bodies from the wound. A wound that appears grossly contaminated should be irrigated with copious quantities of saline under mild pressure. With regard to débridement of tissue in acute wounds, it is generally accepted that conservative removal of only obviously devitalized tissue should be performed. The specific method of repair or treatment depends primarily on the wound morphology and etiology and other relevant factors noted during the wound evaluation.

When repairing a straight forward uncomplicated laceration, the aim should be to provide an anatomically accurate, secure repair. This aim is best accomplished with complete anesthesia, fine instruments, excellent lighting, and comfortable working conditions for the surgeon. These conditions often are not met in the usual emergency room setting, and the surgeon has a duty to the patient to assure that the proper

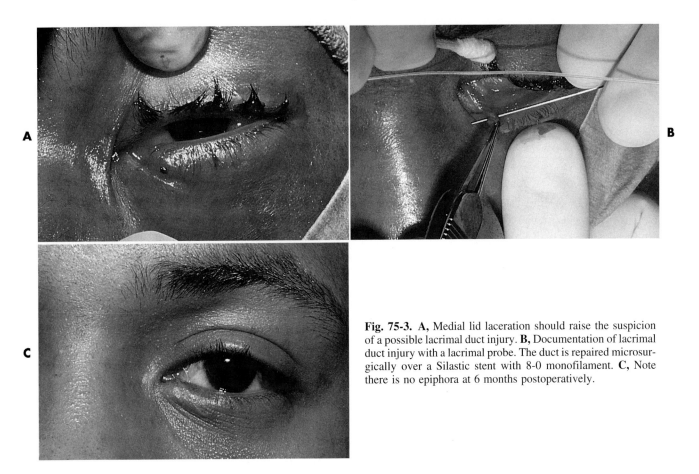

Fig. 75-3. A, Medial lid laceration should raise the suspicion of a possible lacrimal duct injury. **B,** Documentation of lacrimal duct injury with a lacrimal probe. The duct is repaired microsurgically over a Silastic stent with 8-0 monofilament. **C,** Note there is no epiphora at 6 months postoperatively.

conditions and resources are available before beginning a repair. This may mean taking the patient to the operating room and using monitored sedation or general anesthesia, particularly if the patient is uncooperative.

INSTRUMENTS AND SUTURE MATERIAL

Often, the physician repairing a facial wound in the emergency room is faced with the prospect of using rather crude instruments that do not lend themselves to atraumatic soft-tissue handling and optimal soft-tissue repair. Although accurate soft-tissue co-adaption may be of little consequence on the hand or trunk, scars on the face are of significant cosmetic, social, and psychologic importance, and every effort should be made to minimize the visibility of a facial scar. An accurate primary repair is the first step to minimize facial scarring. To achieve an accurate repair, the surgeon requires instruments commensurate with the fine work to be accomplished. The two most important instruments involved in fine suturing are a fine pair of tissue forceps and a fine-needle holder. Unfortunately, these two instruments are most commonly lacking in emergency room suture packs. Typically, the emergency room provides a thick pair of Addison toothed forceps and a long-handled, thick-jawed needle holder. These bulky instruments are inadequate for fine soft-

tissue work, and every effort should be made to upgrade the available instruments, even going so far as to have plastic instruments brought from the operating room. Many facial plastic surgeons own a few key instruments and bring them to the emergency room for facial repairs (Fig. 75-6). Additionally, some authors believe that wound repair under magnification (2.5× loupes) significantly enhances the final result.

The next issue to consider is that of suture material. As with instrumentation, the results achieved are directly related to the caliber of the suture material (the finer the suture, the better the results). Larger-caliber sutures significantly increase the incidence of crosshatching or railroad track appearance of facial scars. Additionally, large-caliber sutures do not provide as accurate skin approximation and the quality of the final scar is compromised.

Rarely is anything larger than a 6-0 suture used on the face, especially in pediatric cases. The only time a 5-0 suture would be used is in the scalp or on nonvisible soft-tissue surface. For skin sutures, a 7-0 monofilament suture is used. Although somewhat fine, 7-0 suture provides excellent soft-tissue approximation and does not require a microscope (although loupe magnification is helpful). Also, external nonabsorbable sutures are used only on patients who will likely

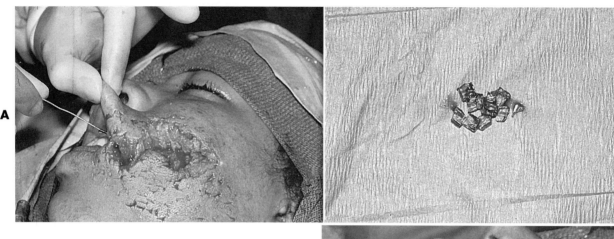

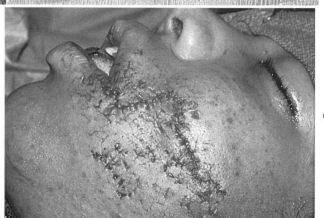

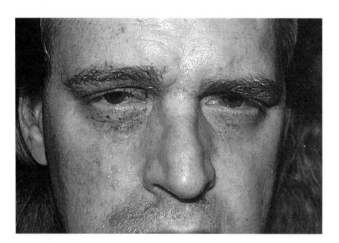

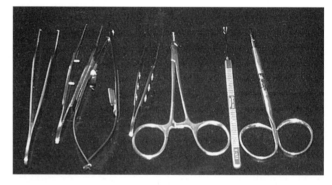

Fig. 75-4. A, Cheek laceration from an automobile windshield. Note the lacrimal probe intraorally being used to check the integrity of the parotid duct. **B,** Glass particles removed from wound. Automobile windshield lacerations are notorious for leaving embedded glass fragments. **C,** The results after foreign body removal and meticulous reapproximation of lacerations.

Fig. 75-5. Right periocular debris tattooing after a blast injury. The epithelium has sealed the wound, trapping the foreign material and making removal difficult. Note that dermabrasion of the thin eyelid skin is extremely dangerous.

Fig. 75-6. A basic set of plastic soft-tissue instruments for emergency repair of facial lacerations.

return for suture removal and be cooperative. Perhaps the only thing more frustrating than performing a suture repair on an uncooperative child is trying to remove sutures from an uncooperative child. Additionally, adults who do not return for suture removal within an appropriate time will often have a worse scar (because of crosshatching or festering of the suture) than if nothing had been done to the wound. Therefore, in children who may be uncooperative during suture removal or in adults whose follow-up is questionable, a 6-0 Absorbing Gut suture is used (Fig. 75-7). This suture is different than the commonly available mild chromic sutures, which often persist longer than needed and have needles that are not ideal. Absorbing Gut suture has a needle conducive for soft-tissue repair, and the suture will usually be gone from the wound in 3 to 5 days.

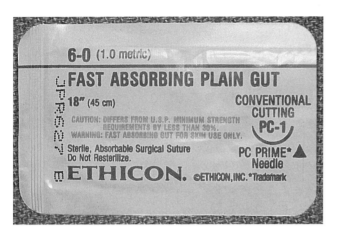

Fig. 75-7. A packet of Absorbing Gut suture, which has a good needle for soft-tissue repair, handles easily, and is gone from the wound in 3 to 5 days. It is often the preferred suture for uncooperative children or noncompliant adults.

Some authors believe that absorbable subcutaneous sutures are used excessively and often inappropriately. Although the commonly available subcutaneous sutures (most of them are a variant of polyglycolic acid) are said to dissolve, they in fact elicit an inflammatory reaction and are broken down. This inflammatory reaction prolongs the proliferative and maturation phases of wound healing and may lead to more prominent scarring. Therefore, the least number of the finest caliber subcutaneous sutures that will adequately approximate the soft tissues should be used. Usually, this entails using 6-0 or 5-0 sutures. Furthermore, muscle or fat does not have the tensile strength to effectively support a suture, and sutures placed in these tissues add little or no tensile strength to the wound and simply act as foreign bodies. The only facial tissues that will reliably support a suture with some tension are dermis and fascia covering muscle.

Dermal sutures that are placed too superficially increase the possibility of extrusion. When subcutaneous sutures extrude, they significantly degrade the quality of the scar, and therefore, subcutaneous sutures should be placed in the deep dermis.

ANESTHESIA FOR FACIAL LACERATIONS

The most important determinant of a positive experience for the patient and physician during the management of a facial laceration is obtaining adequate anesthesia with minimal trauma, especially in pediatric patients. In the past, the most commonly used method of obtaining anesthesia for facial laceration repair was to infiltrate the local anesthetic into the wound through a needle. Anesthetic infiltration had two negative psychologic effects. First, the patient's anticipation of a needle being stuck into an open wound is enough to generate extreme anxiety, which heightens the perception of pain for any stimuli subsequently encountered. Second, infiltration of the local anesthetic, as expected by the patient, is painful because of the hydrostatic and chemical properties of the anesthetic. This combination of heightened expectation followed by painful stimuli makes anesthetic injection the most unpleasant aspect of facial laceration repair. Anesthetic injection may cause a child to become completely uncooperative on any subsequent endeavors, even if adequate anesthesia has been obtained. This hysterical response requires placement of restraints, which further aggravate the child; the following repair is an ordeal for all involved. If the physician can achieve anesthesia of the wound without inflicting additional anxiety or pain, the suture repair is usually fairly simple. To minimize the pain of anesthetizing facial lacerations, TAC (tetracaine [0.5%], adrenaline [1:2000], cocaine [11.8%])[5] anesthesia has been developed and effectively used in the management of facial lacerations.[2,25]

TAC anesthesia is applied topically into a facial wound and usually obviates the need for injected anesthetics. The primary advantage of TAC anesthesia is that the patient never experiences pain. If the physician can avoid creating pain to the patient initially, even small infants can be sutured without requiring restraints such as the papoose board.

A variant of TAC, LAT (lidocaine [4%], adrenaline [1:2000], tetracaine [1%]) uses lidocaine instead of cocaine.[12] Ernst and others[12] reported that LAT seemed to better control pain than TAC and that the cost per dose for LAT was $3 versus $35 for TAC. Because the chance for systemic toxicity with LAT is small and the potential for abuse is low, LAT may become the topical anesthesia of choice.

TECHNIQUE OF TETRACAINE, ADRENALINE, AND COCAINE ANESTHESIA

The application of TAC anesthesia is straightforward. The wound can be briefly cleaned, but no attempt should be made to perform a complete scrubbing because children may interpret this as being potentially painful. It is necessary to remove any clots from the wound so that the solution has a chance to diffuse into the surrounding tissue. The TAC solution comes in 3-ml vials; some have found that the simplest way to apply TAC solution is to place it in a medicine cup, use sterile cotton-tipped applicators to absorb the solution, and then place the applicators directly into the wound (Fig. 75-8). The applicators should then be completely saturated with the TAC solution (Fig. 75-9 A, B). Once the applicator is in the wound, it is generally changed every 4 to 5 minutes to ensure that the concentration of the TAC solution is maximal within the wound. It generally takes 7 to 12 minutes for the TAC solution to become effective. However, the duration to achieve anesthetic effect can vary; perhaps the most reliable sign is the presence of a ring of blanching around the wound margin, which indicates that the solution has moved out into the surrounding tissues and has now become effective (see Fig. 75-9, B). Once this blanching has occurred, the anesthetic has taken effect and repair can begin.

INDICATIONS AND CONTRAINDICATIONS OF TETRACAINE, ADRENALINE, AND COCAINE ANESTHESIA

TAC anesthesia has been used on lacerations involving the entire face and head and neck region. However, TAC is probably contraindicated in several areas. Because TAC contains cocaine, a major concern regarding its use has been about systemic absorption of cocaine sufficient to cause toxic symptoms. The fact that TAC is mixed with a vasoconstrictor lessens the possibility of a systemic dose. However, there have been instances of toxic symptoms, but they occurred when TAC was used around mucosal membranes. The proposed explanation for the increased toxicity of TAC when used on mucous membranes is that, because of the high blood flow in mucosal membranes, enough of the cocaine

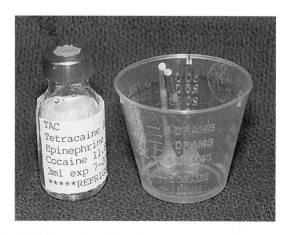

Fig. 75-8. Tetracaine, adrenaline, and cocaine (TAC) in a 3-ml vial. TAC is often applied with cotton-tipped applicators, but dental pledgets can also be used.

is picked up to cause systemic symptoms. Therefore, it is generally recommended that TAC anesthesia not be used on significant mucosal lacerations of the lips or nose. Additionally, because of its vasoconstrictive effect, TAC should be used with care in end-arterial situations, such as the tip of the nose or ear or when pedicled flaps of tissue are encountered.

Also, TAC administration will cause a positive urine or blood test for cocaine.[1] Although this is rarely of concern in children, it may cause significant difficulty for adults undergoing routine drug testing.

MINIMIZING PAIN WITH INJECTABLE ANESTHETICS

TAC anesthesia has been extremely effective, and many pediatric patients have been managed with it as the only anesthesia. However, TAC anesthesia is not advised for lip lacerations extending onto the mucosa, lacerations in which a flap has been raised, or lacerated areas in which the vascularity is in question. Additionally, TAC anesthesia may not be available in all emergency rooms, particularly at smaller community hospitals. In these situations, the physician may need to use the standard injectable anesthetic. Injection of a local anesthetic is painful; however, most of the pain associated with local anesthetic injection is not from the injection procedure, but from the chemical properties of the anesthetic. Specifically, the pH of most commercially available anesthetics is in the range of 4.0. This acidic pH causes most of the stinging encountered with local anesthetic injection. If the anesthetic solution is buffered so that the pH is increased to the physiologic range, the pain of the local injection considerably diminishes. Neutralization of the anesthetic solution may be achieved by mixing sodium bicarbonate with the local anesthetic solution. Generally, 1

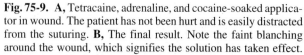

Fig. 75-9. A, Tetracaine, adrenaline, and cocaine-soaked applicator in wound. The patient has not been hurt and is easily distracted from the suturing. **B,** The final result. Note the faint blanching around the wound, which signifies the solution has taken effect.

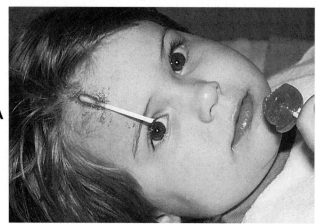

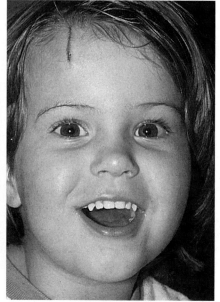

ml of 8.4% sodium bicarbonate is mixed with 9 ml of 1% lidocaine with 1:100,000 epinephrine, which will raise the pH to approximately 7.0. Sodium bicarbonate solution is available in multiple-use bottles or may be obtained from the pharmacy in single-use vials for injection on emergency resuscitation carts (Fig. 75-10). The cost of a sodium bicarbonate vial is approximately $2. If 10 ml of injection is not needed, a proportional solution may be used (e.g., 0.5 ml sodium bicarbonate with 4.5 ml local anesthetic). Using this buffered anesthetic solution with a fine needle (27 or 30 gauge) can significantly diminish, and often eliminate, the pain of local anesthetic injection. If done properly with concealment of the needle, slow injection technique, and some

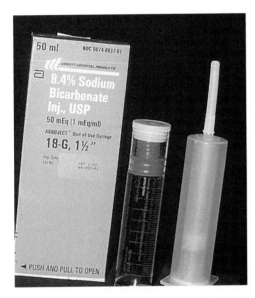

Fig. 75-10. Commonly available vials of 8.4% sodium bicarbonate, which may be used for buffering local anaesthetics. One ml of sodium bicarbonate is mixed with 9 ml of 1% lidocaine with 1:100,000 epinephrine to achieve a pH of approximately 7.0.

form of distraction, the anesthesia can be administered with little or no discomfort to the patient.

However, buffered local anesthetic solution should be used with caution because the duration of effective anesthesia is lessened by neutralizing the solution. However, the treating physician can expect at least 30 to 45 minutes of substantial anesthetic effect, which should be sufficient for most uncomplicated facial lacerations.

VASOCONSTRICTORS IN LOCAL ANESTHETICS

Although the vascular supply of the facial skin is probably the best of the entire body, necessitating the addition of a vasoconstrictor to the lidocaine, vasoconstrictor use may be inappropriate in some situations. In particular, vasoconstrictors should probably be avoided when the pedicle type blood supply is limited (e.g., injury to the tip of the nose or ear, an avulsion type injury in which a pedicled flap of skin has been raised). In these types of injuries, consideration should be given to using a solution with a reduced concentration of epinephrine (e.g., 0.5% lidocaine with 1:200,000 epinephrine), using a plain anesthetic without epinephrine, or performing the repair under regional or general anesthesia.

MANAGEMENT ISSUES WITH COMPLICATED WOUNDS

Soft-tissue contusions

Blunt trauma often presents with an associated stellate laceration resulting from the skin being caught between the striking object externally and the facial skeleton internally. In these situations, the skin is actually ripped rather than cut, giving rise to widespread surrounding tissue disruption. These wounds often do poorly from an aesthetic standpoint, even with the most meticulous repair (Fig. 75-11 *A, B*). The scars are irregular, often widen, and tend to become depressed. Initial treatment should be directed at obtaining as

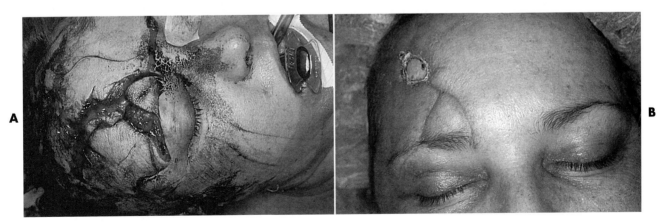

Fig. 75-11. A, Severe facial contusion resulting from a train-auto accident. Soft-tissue disruption extends beyond the borders of the laceration. This wound has a prognosis for an aesthetic outcome. **B,** The result at 6 months. Note the loss of skin centrally and the depressed scar. Also note the pin cushioning of the triangular segment of skin above the brow.

Fig. 75-12. A, Significant soft-tissue contusion with stellate lacerations. **B,** The result at 1 year. No tissue was débrided. Instead, meticulous attention was paid to accurate soft-tissue realignment with fine suture (7-0).

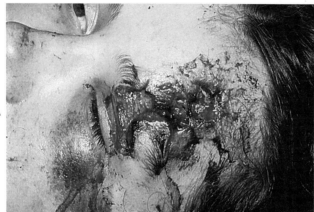

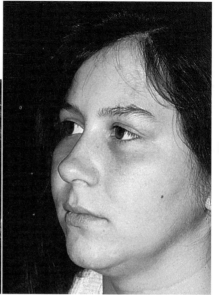

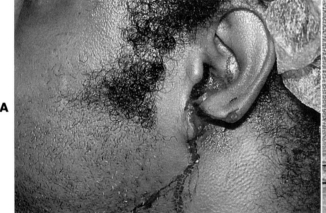

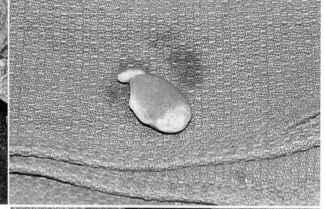

Fig. 75-13. A, Human bite to the ear, with avulsion of the lobule. **B,** Recovered lobule before replantation. **C,** Replanted lobule. The patient was managed with antibiotics and hyperbaric oxygen with complete survival of lobule.

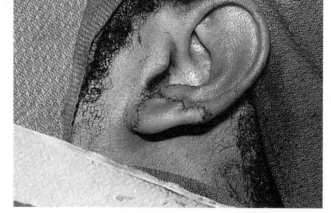

accurate a repair as possible (Fig. 75-12 *A, B*). As a general rule, extensive débridement should not be performed at the time of primary repair because of the difficulty in assessing what tissue will be important for the final outcome. When the wound has fully matured (in at least 6 months or ideally 1 year), a scar revision may be considered.

Soft-tissue avulsions

Actual loss of soft tissue represents one of the most difficult wound management situations. If soft tissue is available, it is not unreasonable to try and reattach it as a full-thickness graft (Fig. 75-13 *A* through *C*). Some authors believe hyperbaric oxygen may facilitate the survival of these grafts. Adjunctive treatment might include some form of anticoagulation or platelet inhibition. If the portion of tissue is large with identifiable blood vessels (e.g., scalp, ear), microvascular reattachment may be considered. If the reattached portion survives long enough to develop venous stasis, surgical leeches have been used with some success to provide temporary venous decompression until the peripheral circulation reestablishes itself.[6] If the avulsed tissue is not available, the surgeon should manage the wound in its absence. If the defect is not too wide, an attempt at primary closure with undermining can be considered (Fig. 75-14 *A* through *C*). However, if excessive tension on the wound distorts anatomic landmarks (e.g., lip, eyebrow), it is probably best to allow the wound to granulate and heal by secondary intention with a revision when the wound is stable (Fig. 75-15 *A* through *D*).

No matter how tempting, split- or full-thickness skin grafting is indicated in few situations (except perhaps massive tissue loss or third-degree burns) (Fig. 75-16 *A, B*). Placement of a skin graft in situations where soft tissue has been avulsed or lost stops secondary healing of the wound (which can be helpful in closing a wound) and almost always provides a poor tissue match. This is particularly true in cases in which full-thickness skin and subcutaneous tissue has been lost. For situations in which there has been loss of skin and subcutaneous tissue, placement of a skin graft, even a full-thickness one, will result in a poor tissue match and leave a noticeable contour defect. It is usually best to allow these wounds to stabilize and plan a local or regional flap repair with facial skin that matches the skin surrounding the wound.

Lacerations involving a margin or border

Special consideration should be given to any laceration that extends through an anatomic margin or border because of the aesthetic and functional importance of these junctional structures. Aesthetically, the eye is attracted to discrepancies

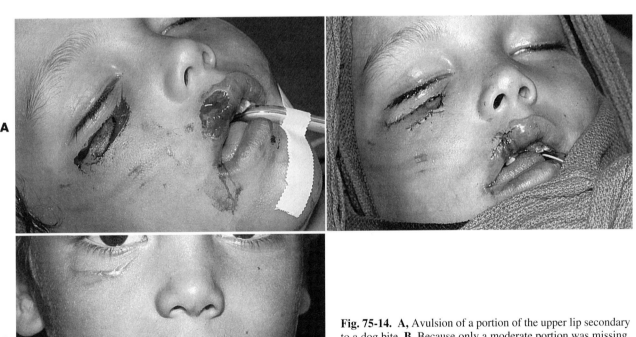

Fig. 75-14. A, Avulsion of a portion of the upper lip secondary to a dog bite. **B,** Because only a moderate portion was missing, soft-tissue undermining and closure was performed. **C,** The results at 1 year showing an acceptable lip scar.

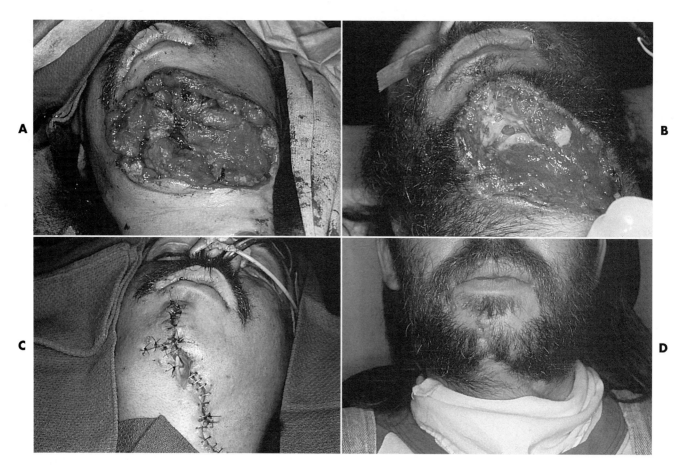

Fig. 75-15. **A,** Massive soft-tissue loss secondary to a shotgun blast. **B,** The wound is stable and beginning to granulate. It is now ready for wide undermining and closure. **C,** The wound is closed without the need for flaps or skin grafts. **D,** An acceptable chin scar 4 months after closure.

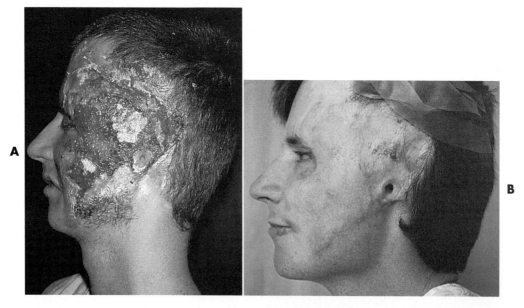

Fig. 75-16. **A,** Massive abrasion injury of the left side of the face with loss of the auricle. **B,** Because the defect was large and relatively superficial, it was skin grafted. No attempt was made to reconstruct the auricle.

in facial lines and contours, and a misaligned margin or border will immediately be noticed. Technically, these structures are somewhat more demanding to repair because they have an internal and external surface, both of which may be involved with the laceration. If an optimal repair is to be performed, all three layers (internal, middle, external) should be completely and accurately realigned. In particular, if the internal surface of the laceration is not repaired, the wound contraction associated with secondary wound healing may cause distortion of the external surface or margin. The sites that merit attention include:

Vermilion border of the lip

The smooth line of transition between the pale, external, cutaneous lip skin and the red mucosa is a critical facial landmark, and any malalignment, even as small as 1 mm, will be quite noticeable (Fig. 75-17). With any lip repair, the vermilion border should be a primary focus of attention, and the continuity of the border should be accurately realigned first to assure that repair of the rest of the lip structures will not distort the vermilion border (Figs. 75-18 A through C and 75-19 A, B). With the vermilion border aligned and stabilized, the rest of the lip layers (inner mucosal, muscular, cutaneous) are repaired in the standard fashion. Generally, the inner mucosa is closed loosely with 4-0 plain gut sutures, the muscular layer with 6-0 polyglycolic acid, and the external skin and mucosa with a fine monofilament (7-0).

Nostril margin

Lacerations involving the margin of the nostril need to be accurately repaired to ensure that unsightly notching does not occur. Additionally, in the medial portion of the nostril and superior columella, the lower lateral cartilages are quite close to the margin and relatively superficial. If a coincident laceration of the lower lateral cartilage is not recognized and

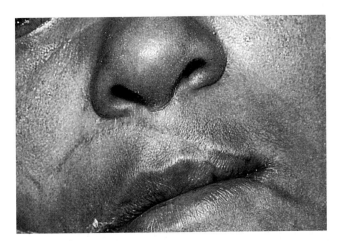

Fig. 75-17. A poorly aligned vermilion border distorts the lip contour.

repaired, the likelihood is high that the nose will shift and twist as the forces of healing put stress on the ipsilateral nose and as the ends of the lower lateral cartilage slip over one another (Fig. 75-20 A, B). If the inner mucosa is not repaired, the contraction resulting from secondary wound healing may cause superior retraction of the nostril margin. Because the nose is aesthetically important and secondary repair of the complications is so difficult, significant lacerations that involve the nostril margin are often best repaired in the operating room. The principal of a three-layer closure is followed with the exception that a laceration of the lower lateral cartilage is identified and repaired with 5-0 or 6-0 clear monofilament nylon to impart some permanent strength to the wound (Fig. 75-21 A through C).

Auricular helical rim

Lacerations of the helical rim traverse two skin surfaces and as cartilage and require a three-layer repair with accurate reapproximation of the auricular cartilage, as in the nose, to avoid notching. The cartilage is repaired by placing 5-0 or 6-0 clear monofilament through the perichondrium and cartilage. The skin is repaired with a 6-0 or 7-0 monofilament (Fig. 75-22 A through C).

Eyelids

While laceration or injury of the globe is a primary concern (and should be ruled out with appropriate ophthalmologic consultation or examination), other structures may be involved with eyelid trauma and should be considered. With upper eyelid lacerations, the surgeon should consider the possibility of injury to the levator palpebrae, which could cause ptosis of the upper lid if not repaired. The lacrimal gland may be involved with lacerations of the lateral portion of the upper lid and may be mistaken for orbital fat. There are reports of the lacrimal gland being excised under the mistaken assumption that orbital fat was being débrided. In the lower eyelid, the possibility of a laceration to the lacrimal system should be considered with any medial lid laceration (Fig. 75-23 A through C). In the upper and lower eyelids, special concern should be given to lacerations that involve the lid margin (see Fig. 75-23). If lacerations involving margins elsewhere on the face are improperly repaired, unsightly notching may occur. Briefly, repair of a lid margin laceration involves a three-layer closure with a fine plain gut suture (6-0 or 7-0) on the conjunctival side (to avoid irritation of the scleral conjunctiva), a fine absorbable suture in the tarsal plate, and a fine monofilament on the external surface.

FACIAL BURNS

General comments

Burns are a separate category of soft-tissue facial injuries. Although the term *burn* implies a thermal injury, other causes are cold or freezing temperatures, electrical current, chemicals, or ionizing radiation. Regardless of the cause,

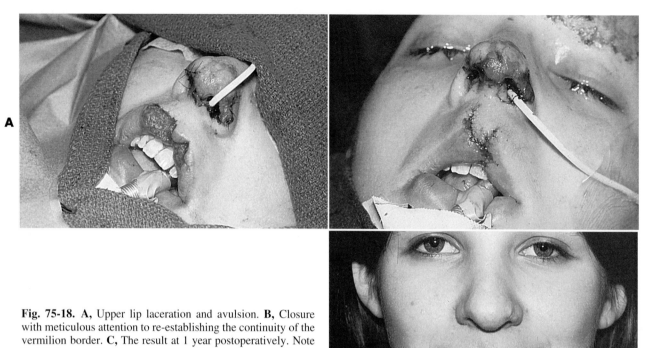

Fig. 75-18. **A,** Upper lip laceration and avulsion. **B,** Closure with meticulous attention to re-establishing the continuity of the vermilion border. **C,** The result at 1 year postoperatively. Note that if the vermilion border is reestablished, the rest of the lip will adjust to regain normal symmetry.

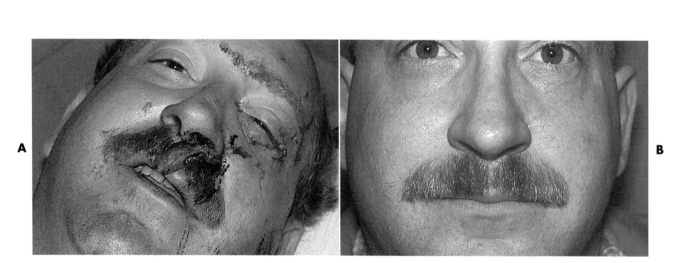

Fig. 75-19. **A,** Upper lip laceration from striking a steering wheel. **B,** The result at 6 months postrepair following the principle of accurate vermilion border realignment and three-layer closure.

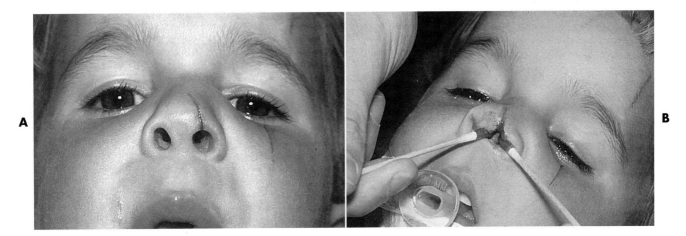

Fig. 75-20. A, Initially benign appearing laceration of left nostril in a 2-year-old patient. **B,** However, further investigation shows a full-thickness injury with a laceration of the lower lateral cartilage. A three-layer closure with reapproximation of the cartilage was performed.

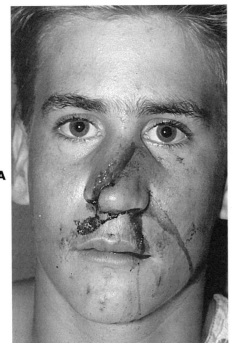

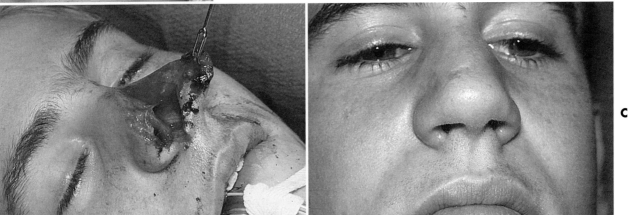

Fig. 75-21. A, Full-thickness nasal injury from a boat propeller. **B,** Because this injury is extensive, it is best repaired in the operating room under general anesthesia. Mucosal and cartilaginous lacerations were accurately realigned. **C,** The result at 1-year postrepair. Note the continuity of the nostril margin and integrity of the nasal skeleton support.

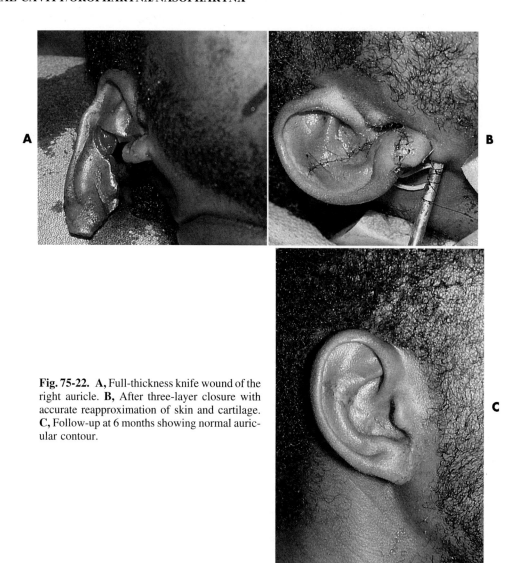

Fig. 75-22. A, Full-thickness knife wound of the right auricle. **B,** After three-layer closure with accurate reapproximation of skin and cartilage. **C,** Follow-up at 6 months showing normal auricular contour.

the common histologic picture of a burn is that of widespread cell death in the affected tissue. Typically, cell death extends from the external skin surface internally for a variable depth. In fact, burns are classified on the basis of the depth of extension of cell death into the soft tissue and are referred to as first-degree, second-degree, or third-degree burns.

First-degree burns are defined as a superficial injury involving just the epidermis. They result in pain and redness but little significant tissue damage, and they heal without scarring.

Second-degree burns extend into the dermis for a variable distance. The identifying features of a second-degree burn are pain (often severe), erythema, and blistering (Fig. 75-24). Second-degree burns will re-epithelialize spontaneously and generally have limited scarring (unless they are deep into the dermis). A deep second-degree burn may be converted to a full-thickness injury by improper wound management or infection.

Third-degree burns extend through (or nearly through)

the full thickness of the dermis and destroy all the adnexal structures, which are the source of epithelial regeneration, blood vessels, and nerve endings. Severe third-degree burns can extend through the dermis into the subcutaneous tissue and can even involve bone. Clinical evaluation of third-degree burns is deceptive as to the severity of this type of injury. By definition, in a third-degree burn, blood vessels and nerves are destroyed so there is no bleeding, inflammation, blistering, or pain in the area of full-thickness injury, although pain may occur in surrounding areas with just partial thickness injury (Fig. 75-25). Pricking a third-degree burn with a needle elicits no bleeding or pain. The initial relatively benign appearance of a third-degree burn belies the serious nature of this injury. Because the full thickness of the dermis has been lost, there is no possibility of regeneration or re-epithelization of this portion of skin (as there is in a second-degree burn). A third-degree burn of the skin results in an eschar, which will eventually slough or require débridement, leaving a full-thickness wound that can only

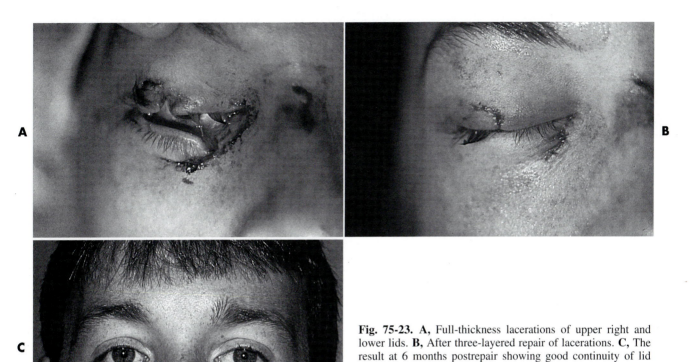

Fig. 75-23. A, Full-thickness lacerations of upper right and lower lids. **B,** After three-layered repair of lacerations. **C,** The result at 6 months postrepair showing good continuity of lid margins.

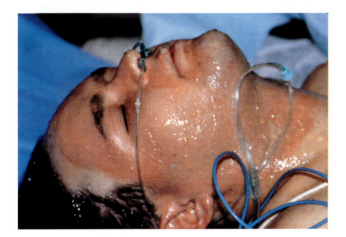

Fig. 75-24. A patient with second-degree burns of most of the face sparing the upper forehead. Note the redness and blistering of the skin, indicating that it is still viable.

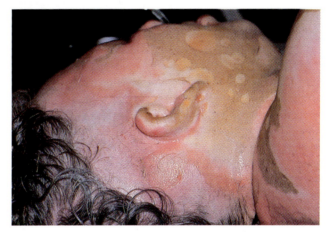

Fig. 75-25. Second- and third-degree burns juxtaposed. Note the gray leather-like appearance of the third-degree burns of the cheek skin compared with the second-degree injury of the postauricular skin.

heal by secondary wound contraction (which invariably causes severe hypertrophic scarring).

Acute treatment

The major concern with the acute treatment of facial burns relates to making sure that systemic life-threatening issues are addressed. Third-degree burns of any size are seri-ous and may be fatal with as little as 20% of the body surface burned. Formerly, the major cause of death in burn patients was ''burn shock'' resulting from massive extravascular fluid shifts. With modern physiologic monitoring and im-proved replacement fluids, mortality from burns has been steadily decreasing over the past several decades.

Respiratory concerns

Types of respiratory burns

Any patient with a significant facial burn should be considered to have a possible coincident burn of the respiratory system. Although most patients with inhalation injuries have extensive burns (> 50% of their body), Cudmore and Vivori[8] pointed out that it is possible to sustain severe damage to the larynx and lungs from the inhalation of hot fumes and gases without there being any significant degree of body-surface injury.[7,19,24]

Three major factors should be kept in mind when considering the cause of inhalation burn injury: (1) hot, dry gas, (2) steam, and (3) smoke. These three by-products of combustion are often found together in a fire, but each produces a distinct injury to the respiratory tract.

Hot, dry gas primarily affects the nasal cavity, nasopharynx, oropharynx, and supraglottis. These structures absorb most of the heat, and little damage is done to the glottis, subglottis, trachea, or lung parenchyma. The protective effect of this rapid dissipation of heat is enhanced by the anatomic barrier of the vocal cords and the reflex closure of the cords to heat stimulus.[21]

Steam, on the other hand, with its superheated water vapor, has 4000 times the heat-bearing capacity of air. The large amount of latent heat released during steam condensation overwhelms the cooling capacity of the upper air passages, and thermal burns may result down to the level of the bronchioles. More commonly, steam burns are confined to the subglottis and trachea, with severe subglottic stenosis a frequent sequela.

Smoke inhalation produces a chemical injury to the respiratory tract that usually affects the entire airway and pulmonary tissue. The effects of smoke inhalation may be confined to the epithelial lining, or they may be systemic, as with carbon monoxide and cyanide. This chemical toxicity causes intense inflammation and edema of the upper airway and larynx. In the trachea, the mucosa sloughs and denudes the cartilages. The cilia are paralyzed, and debris accumulates with plug and cast formation. The alveoli also are damaged, with loss of surfactant and increased capillary permeability. The result is atelectasis and a picture similar to adult respiratory distress syndrome. Finally, the damaged airways are susceptible to infection with the development of bronchopneumonia several days later.

Symptoms of inhalation injury

Burns occurring in confined areas or with steam or other superheated gases should raise concern over the possibility of inhalation injury. Common symptoms of inhalation injury are a sensation of choking, a metallic taste in the mouth, dizziness, wheezing, hoarseness, odynophinia, dysphagia, coughing, and increasing respiratory difficulty. Typically, an inhalation injury has an evolving nature, and careful attention should be paid to the development of new symptoms or a changing physical examination.

Physical signs of inhalation injury

Physical findings suggestive of an inhalation injury include facial burns, particularly around the mouth or nose; singed nasal vibrissae; soot in the nasal cavities or oropharynx; and swelling and hyperemia of the nasal or oropharyngeal mucosa (Fig. 75-26). Laryngeal findings depend on the nature and extent of the injury and may vary with time. With direct thermal injuries to the larynx secondary to dry heat, hyperemia and moderate to marked firm edema of the larynx are present. Bronchoscopy often shows soot-stained sputum and mucus plugs, edema, and necrosis of mucosa. Wheezing, rales, or rhonchi present on admission or developing later also are signs of respiratory tract injury and should prompt further investigation.

Inhalation injury to the respiratory tree is diagnosed almost exclusively by history and physical examination. Hypoxemia, hypercapnia, and increased carboxyhemoglobin levels are laboratory indicators that should prompt further clinical investigations. The most reliable test to detect early inhalation injury to the larynx, subglottis, and trachea is endoscopy, usually with a flexible bronchoscope.

Treatment of inhalation injuries

With regard to the treatment of inhalation injuries to the larynx and subglottis, some basic tenets exist: (1) awareness of the possibility of an inhalation injury in any burn patient,

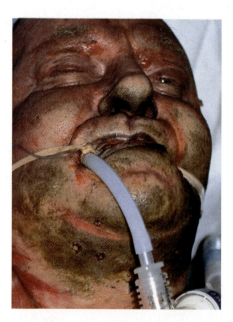

Fig. 75-26. A patient with third-degree burns over most of the face. Note the singed nasal vibrissae and soot around the nostrils, which indicate that this patient inhaled hot gases and smoke. Patients with these findings are at high risk for burns of the respiratory tree.

particularly in patients who were burned in a confined area with facial burns or soot around the nose; (2) the laryngeal injury may not immediately manifest itself and may evolve over 6 to 12 hours with eventual respiratory obstruction; and (3) oxygen through nasal prongs or a face mask, a cool mist, and systemic rehydration are generally agreed on. Corticosteroid use is controversial, but the trend appears to avoid their routine use in inhalation injury.

Finally, what is the best way to manage respiratory obstruction in inhalation injury? This complicated issue depends, to a large extent, on the overall status of the patient. Sataloff and Sataloff[21] detailed general guidelines for dealing with pediatric inhalation burn injuries. Patients with extensive burns and coincident inhalation injury are best managed with intubation. Patients with generalized lower respiratory tract inhalation injury that does not affect the larynx are best managed with intubation. Patients with severe upper airway obstruction and laryngeal burns are best managed with tracheotomy to avoid the additional trauma of an endotracheal tube. Patients with severe facial burns sparing the neck, with or without inhalation injury, are often best managed with tracheotomy. Tracheotomies are best avoided in patients with significant coincident neck burns because of the adverse wound healing of burns in the presence of a tracheotomy and the potential for pulmonary sepsis from the infected burn eschar. Obviously, these guidelines are general, and treatment should be tailored to the patient's situation and needs.

Definitive treatment

A generally accepted treatment principle for facial burns is that the sooner burns of the face and neck are sealed by spontaneous re-epithelization or skin graft, the better will be the ultimate cosmetic and functional outcome. Complete closure of the wound should be accomplished by the third or fourth week after the injury. If a burn spontaneously heals within 10 to 14 days, there will usually be little scarring and the skin quality will be good. However, if healing has not taken place by 2 weeks, the chances of unsatisfactory hypertrophic scarring increase dramatically. Therefore, at approximately 10 days, the wound is assessed with regard to its ability to heal spontaneously. If it is determined that healing will be significantly delayed, the burn eschar is tangentially excised until viable tissue is reached and the wound is skin grafted. While awaiting eschar excision and grafting, a major source of potential morbidity lies with colonization and superinfection of the eschar. In the past, a major cause of burn sepsis was the heavily infected eschar having direct access to the bloodstream through the adjacent viable tissues. Topical antimicrobial agents have significantly reduced the dangers of eschar superinfection and the most commonly used preparation is silver sulfadiazine applied twice daily.

When planning skin grafts to the face, it is important to consider the unit theory of facial reconstruction by Gonza-

lez-Ullola[13,14] and replace entire facial units (i.e., perioral region, cheek, forehead, nose) rather than just portions of a unit. Failure to follow the unit concept of facial reconstruction will result in a patchwork appearance with diminished aesthetic results. As a general rule, the thicker the skin graft, the closer the results will be healthy to skin color and texture, but full-thickness skin grafts create more donor site morbidity; therefore, split-thickness grafts of 0.015 to 0.035 inches are the most common alternative.

Postgrafting care is directed at avoiding scar contracture through vigorous physical therapy, splints, and pressure garments. A major source of long-term facial burn morbidity is hypertrophic scarring with scar contracture and distortion of anatomic structures such as the neck, lip, eyelid, and nostril margin. Pressure garments and anatomically contoured acrylic splints are beneficial for keeping hypertrophic scars soft and thin and for lessening scar contracture. However, no technique will completely rehabilitate a severely burned face, and long-term management with various techniques (skin grafts, contracture releases, local flaps, possibly free microvascular flaps, cosmetic camouflage) at an experienced institution is required for maximum patient benefit.[20]

Special considerations

Eyelids

With thermal injuries to the periorbital region, direct injury to the eye is rare, but there may be severe long-term ocular sequelae. The major concern in patients with eyelid burns is maintenance of adequate corneal covering. Corneal exposure typically does not occur until the initial periorbital swelling subsides and scar contracture begins to occur with ectropion formation. Treatment consists of early eschar removal and skin grafting (thick split-thickness grafts for the upper lids and full-thickness for the lower lids) with meticulous attention to corneal lubrication using ointment and appropriate ophthalmologic consultation. Tarsorrhaphy, once routinely recommended, is now reserved for difficult cases with a high chance of corneal ulceration.[7]

Ears

Because of their exposed position and thin skin, ears are often severely injured in any major facial burn. Of all burns of the face, 90% involve the ears.[11,16] Conservatism is the best course of therapy in acute care of the burned ear. Previously, a major source of morbidity in burned ears was progressive chondritis caused by infection of the exposed cartilage, which led to the admonition of early radical débridement and closure of all ear burns regardless of size. With the addition of topical antimicrobials, the complication of progressive chondritis has virtually disappeared. The presently recommended treatment is liberal use of silver sulfadiazine, continuous conservative débridement, and grafting when a suitable recipient bed is available.

Reconstruction of the ear depends on the type of deformity, but classically the ear periphery is most affected and the concha the least. With moderate injuries involving the helical rim, conchal transposition has proven useful.[9] More severe injuries may require rib grafts with temporoparietal fascial flaps or a prosthesis.[3,23]

Oral commissure burns

A characteristic pediatric burn is of the oral commissure from an electric current. These injuries occur most commonly in children 2 to 3 years of age. Typically, oral commissure burns result from the child biting an electric cord, causing an arc of electric energy at the oral commissure where the cord was in contact with the lip. Because this injury results from the electric current passing through the tissue rather than from heat applied to the skin surface, the initial injury may seem limited, but progressive necrosis becomes evident over the next 36 to 48 hours. Because of the difficulty in distinguishing viable from nonviable tissue, early débridement and primary closure is generally not recommended. Instead, it is advocated that the wound be treated conservatively with topical antibiotics and progressive gentle débridement. Earlier literature attached considerable importance to the possible complication of delayed hemorrhage from the labial artery when the eschar separates, but several large recent series have had a 0% incidence of this complication.[4,10] Treatment of the resultant oral commissure deformity is somewhat controversial. For some time, oral splints were routinely advocated, but Donelan[10] and Canady[4] question the benefit of splints and believe they may do some harm. Presently, the consensus appears to be to treat the wounds conservatively until the scar matures and softens and then perform the definitive repair with one of various commissureplasties.

REFERENCES

1. Altieri M, Bogema S, Schwartz RH: TAC topical anesthesia produces positive urine tests for cocaine, *Ann Emerg Med* 19:577, 1990.
2. Anderson AB and others: Local anesthesia in pediatric patients: topical TAC versus lidocaine, *Ann Emerg Med* 19:519, 1990.
3. Brent B: Auricular repair with autogenous rib cartilage grafts: two decades of experience with 600 cases, *Plast Reconstr Surg* 90:355, 1992.
4. Canady JW, Thompson SA, Bardach J: Oral commissure burns in children, *Plast Reconstr Surg* 97:738, 1995.
5. Cannon RC, Chouteau S, Hutchinson K: Brief communications: topically applied tetracaine, adrenalin, and cocaine in the repair of traumatic wounds of the head and neck, *Otolaryngol Head Neck Surg* 100:78, 1989.
6. Chalain T, Jones G: Replantation of the avulsed pinna: 100 percent survival with a single arterial anastomosis and substitution of leeches for a venous anastomosis, *Plast Reconstr Surg* 95:1275, 1995.
7. Constable JD: *Thermal injuries of the head and neck.* In Stark RB, editor: *Plastic surgery of the head and neck,* ed 1, vol 1, New York, 1987, Churchill Livingstone.
8. Cudmore RE, Vivore E: Inhalation injury to the respiratory tract of children, *Prog Pediatr Surg* 14:173, 1981.
9. Donelan MB: Conchal transposition flap for postburn ear deformities, *Plast Reconstr Surg* 83:641, 1989.
10. Donelan MB: Reconstruction of electrical burns of the oral commissure with a ventral tongue flap, *Plast Reconstr Surg* 95:1155, 1990.
11. Dowling JA, Foley FD: Chondritis in the burned ear, *Plast Reconstr Surg* 42:115, 1968.
12. Ernst AA and others: LAT (lidocaine-adrenaline-tetracaine) versus TAC (tetracaine-adrenaline-cocaine) for topical anesthesia in face and scalp lacerations, *Am J Emerg Med* 13:151, 1995.
13. Gonzalez-Ulloa M: A quantum method for the appreciation of the morphology of the face, *Plast Reconstr Surg* 34:241, 1964.
14. Gonzalez-Ulloa M and others: Preliminary study of the total restoration of the facial skin, *Plast Reconstr Surg* 13:151, 1954.
15. Gore R: The dawn of humans: neandertals, *National Geographic* 189: 2, 1996.
16. Hammond JS, Ward CG: Burns of the head and neck, *Otolaryngol Clin North Am* 16:679, 1983.
17. Levine CL, Berger JR, Lazow SK: Parotid salivary fistula secondary to external pin fixation: case report, *J Craniomaxillofac Trauma* 2:20, 1996.
18. Parekh D and others: Posttraumatic parotid fistulae and sialoceles. A prospective study of conservative management in 51 cases, *Ann Surg* 209:105, 1989.
19. Phillips AW, Cope O: Burn therapy: III. Beware the facial burn, *Ann Surg* 156:759, 1962.
20. Rose EH: Aesthetic restoration of the severely disfigured face in burn victims: a comprehensive strategy, *Plast Reconstr Surg* 96:1573, 1995.
21. Sataloff DM, Sataloff RT: Tracheotomy and inhalation injury, *Head Neck Surg* 6:1024, 1984.
22. Tachmes L and others: Parotid gland and facial nerve trauma: a retrospective review, *J Trauma* 30:1395, 1990.
23. Tjellstrom A: Osseointegrated implants for replacement of absent or defective ears, *Clin Plast Surg* 17:355, 1990.
24. Trunkey DD: Inhalation injury *Surg Clin North Am* 58:1133, 1978.
25. White WB, Iserson KV, Criss E: Topical anesthesia for laceration repair: tetracaine versus TAC (tetracaine, adrenaline, and cocaine), *Am J Emerg Med* 4:319, 1986.

Chapter 76

Benign Tumors and Tumor-Like Lesions

Isaäc van der Waal
Gordon B. Snow

Benign tumors occur more frequently in the oral cavity than in the oropharynx and nasopharynx. A distinction, however, between neoplasms in the oral cavity and those in the other sites would be rather artificial.

Tumors arising from adjacent nerves or tumors of the deep lobe of the parotid gland may indent the lateral wall of the oropharynx and appear as symptomless swellings. However, this chapter discusses reactive, cystic, and developmental lesions.

CYSTS

This chapter only discusses cysts arising in the soft tissues.

Epidermoid and dermoid cysts

An epidermoid cyst is lined by stratified squamous epithelium without the adnexal structures in the fibrous wall that a dermoid cyst has. Sometimes, the term *dermoid cyst* is used clinically, using histologic subdivisions such as dermoid type, epidermoid type, and teratoid type.

An epidermoid cyst may result from traumatic implantation of epithelial cells into surface epithelium, whereas in a dermoid cyst, entrapment of epithelium during the embryologic phase seems to be the most likely explanation.

Epidermoid and dermoid cysts may occur in the floor of the mouth, the lips, and the cheek mucosa. A few cases of lingual involvement have been reported. The clinical aspect is not characteristic and consists of cystic swelling (Fig. 76-1). When adnexal structures (such as sebaceous glands) exist, a dermoid cyst can be diagnosed.

In most instances, epidermoid and dermoid cysts can be enucleated. Only in very large cysts should marsupialization be considered. Recurrence is rare.[17]

Nasolabial cyst

The nasolabial cyst is a developmental cyst probably derived from epithelial remnants of the nasolacrimal duct. It usually appears as an asymptomatic, extremely slow-growing swelling of the soft tissues in the nasal vestibule, the nasolabial fold, or the mucobuccal fold of the upper jaw. Only in large cysts may radiography show some erosion of the underlying bone. The cyst may be confused clinically with other lesions, especially those of an odontogenic nature, so a careful dental examination should be carried out.

Various types of epithelial cells—often ciliated cells and goblet cells—may form the lining of the cyst lumen.

In almost all cases, the cyst can be removed through an intraoral approach. A small perforation of the nasal mucosa can be left alone.

EOSINOPHILIC GRANULOMA OF MUCOSA

Eosinophilic granuloma of the oral mucosa (also called *traumatic granuloma*) is a benign idiopathic lesion. It has no relation to eosinophilic granuloma of bone. Perhaps a giant cell arteritis (e.g., of the lingual nerve) is the underlying disorder in some cases, which should be diagnosed by histologic examination, which is further supported by an elevated erythrocyte sedimentation rate.

Eosinophilic granuloma may occur at any age and does not show a preference for either sex. The tongue is a site of

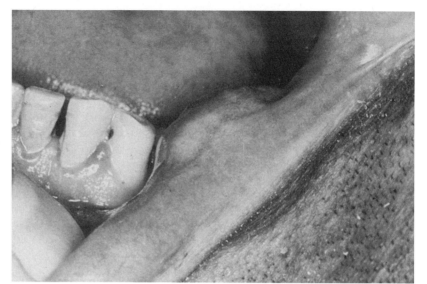

Fig. 76-1. An epidermoid cyst on the labial mucosa of the lower lip.

predilection.[12] Most eosinophilic granulomas that have been reported were ulcerative, not indurated, and rather well circumscribed. The lesion may be confused clinically with squamous cell carcinoma.

Histopathologic examination shows varying numbers of eosinophilic granulocytes, neutrophils, plasma cells, and histiocytes. No true granuloma formation exists. Eosinophilic granulomas heal spontaneously in a matter of weeks; therefore, surgical intervention is not indicated.

FIBROMA

Almost all fibromas in the oral cavity are not true neoplasms but fibrous overgrowths caused by chronic irritation. Many authors prefer the term *fibroepithelial polyp* or *fibrous hyperplasia* for this type of lesion. They rarely occur before the fourth decade and show no preference for either sex.

A fibroma has a smooth overlying mucosa and is often pedunculated. The size may vary from a few millimeters to some centimeters. The consistency may vary from soft and myxomatous to firm and elastic. A fibroma is asymptomatic and can be located at all sites of the oral and oropharyngeal mucosa (Fig. 76-2).

The microscopic picture may show a collagenous stroma and a varying number of inflammatory cells. The fibroblasts may have a giant cell appearance, justifying in some cases the term *giant cell fibroma*, which does not have any clinical implication.[10] A fibroma is not demarcated or encapsulated. Vascularity may be scarce or abundant. In the latter case, it may be difficult to differentiate the lesion from a hemangioma with secondary inflammatory signs or from a pyogenic granuloma. In some cases, myxoid changes and osseous and chondroid metaplasia can be observed.

Treatment consists of conservative excision, during which any possible irritating factor should be removed. Recurrences are exceptional.

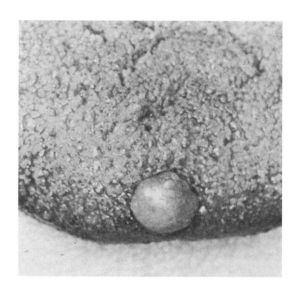

Fig. 76-2. A fibroma at the tip of the tongue.

GRANULAR CELL TUMOR

A granular cell tumor, formerly called *granular cell myoblastoma*, is a benign lesion of the soft tissues whose origin and nature are not fully understood. For a long time, the lesion was considered a benign neoplasm related to muscles, but a neurogenic origin seems to be more likely. Moreover, evidence is increasing that the lesion is not a true neoplasm but a benign proliferation of peripheral neurogenic elements of the Schwann cell[11] or a degenerative alteration of this cell. It has no preference for race, sex, or age. The tumor may occur in children and may be present at birth.

The granular cell tumor occurs everywhere in the body, especially in the oral cavity. Most oral cases are located in the tongue. In rare instances, multiple tumors have been

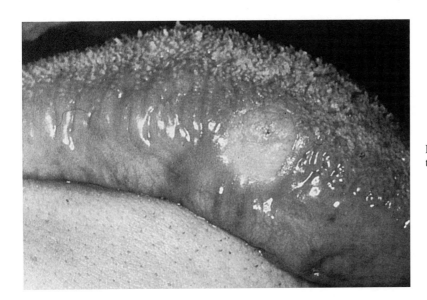

Fig. 76-3. A granular cell tumor on the border of the tongue.

reported, in the oral cavity or elsewhere. In congenital cases, the tumor is located on the alveolar ridge and is called *epulis of the newborn.*[8]

The granular cell tumor usually appears as a firm, submucosal nodule. Its size varies, from a few millimeters to a few centimeters. The color of the overlying mucosa may be unchanged but also may be somewhat yellow or pink. Ulceration of the epithelium is rare (Fig. 76-3).

Histologic examination shows a somewhat circumscribed but not encapsulated mass of large cells with a coarse, granular, slightly eosinophilic cytoplasm. No signs of cellular or nuclear polymorphism or any mitotic activity exist. In about 50% of cases, the overlying epithelium shows pseudoepitheliomatous hyperplasia, which may be mistaken for differentiated squamous cell carcinoma.

Treatment of a granular cell tumor consists of conservative surgical removal. Recurrences are rare, even when the excision has not been radical. Radiotherapy of a granular cell tumor has not been shown to be successful.

HEMANGIOMAS AND ALLIED LESIONS

A hemangioma is a benign lesion of blood vessels or vascular elements. Most oral and oropharyngeal hemagiomas are of a developmental nature and are located in the soft tissues. In rare instances, a hemangioma is located intraosseously.

Hemangiomas often are present at birth or shortly thereafter. They tend to occur in the tongue and the floor of the mouth (Fig. 76-4). A hemangioma of the tongue may affect a part of the tongue or the entire tongue, producing macroglossia. The color of a hemangioma may vary from bluish to purple or fiery red. The texture of the mucosa may be unchanged, showing only increased vascularity on the surface; other cases, however, have a pebbly appearance. Pain is not a prominent feature, except in cases of traumatization or secondary inflammation. Bleeding spontaneously or from mechanical irritation can be serious. Angiography may be an aid in diagnosing a hemangioma that has a pulsatile component. In most cases, the diagnosis of hemangioma is clinical. Magnetic resonance imaging (MRI) can be helpful in the evaluation of the extent of the lesion.[21]

A nonpulsatile hemangioma may histologically consist of numerous irregular, blood-filled spaces lined by endothelial cells and surrounded by connective tissue. When many proliferating endothelial cells line small capillaries, the lesion is referred to as a *capillary hemangioma.* In the case of large dilated blood sinuses, the term *cavernous hemangioma* is applied. A third histologic variant is the cellular (juvenile) hemangioma. In the case of ulceration (and thereby the presence of inflammatory cells), distinguishing a hemangioma from a pyogenic granuloma may be impossible.

Most hemangiomas do not require treatment and regress spontaneously during childhood. When hemangiomas undergo regression, extensive sclerosis can occur, sometimes followed by calcification. Such concretions are called *phleboliths.*

Therapeutic management of a large, persisting, or even growing hemangioma is difficult. A conservative approach seems justified (i.e., managing only the areas that produce bleeding). In large, diffuse lesions, cryosurgery or carbon dioxide laser therapy may be helpful. Injection of sclerosing agents has been advocated has not been shown to be effective. Selective percutaneous embolization before surgery has emerged as a valuable adjunct to surgery in the management of such lesions. Radiotherapy should be avoided because of possible late adverse sequelae.

Hemangiopericytoma

A hemangiopericytoma is a complex neoplasm that should be regarded as malignant, not in terms of 5-year survival but over the lifetime of the host. A distinction is made between an adult and an infantile hemangiopericytoma.[2] Oc-

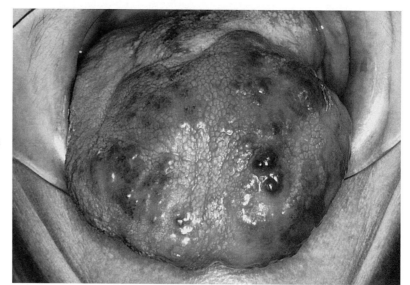

Fig. 76-4. A large, diffuse hemangioma of the tongue.

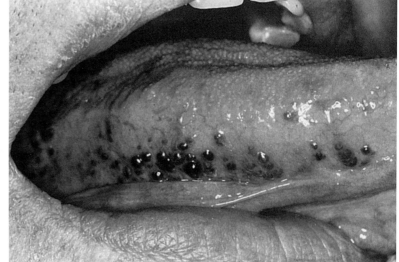

Fig. 76-5. Phlebectasias (varicosities) at the border of the tongue.

currence in the oral cavity and the oropharynx is extremely rare. The clinical appearance is a firm, usually well-circumscribed swelling of the mucosa.

Phlebectasias

In patients older than 40 to 50 years, single or multiple, bluish, hemangioma-like changes may occur in the oral and lingual mucosa as the result of vein widening (Fig. 76-5). These phlebectasias also are referred to as *varicosities*. No treatment is required.

Caliber-persistent labial artery

A unilateral swelling of the lower lip may be caused by a visible or palpable pulsatile swelling, also referred to as *caliber-persistent labial artery*. Treatment consists of ligation of the artery.[9]

Angina bullosa haemorrhagica

Angina bullosa haemorrhagica is a benign phenomenon characterized by the sudden appearance of a blood blister on the oral mucosa in the absence of an identifiable cause or systemic disorder; local trauma has been suggested to be the most likely contributory factor (Fig. 76-6). Angina bullosa haemorrhagica affects mainly middle-aged and elderly patients. There is no strong predilection for men or women. No treatment is required.[6]

KERATOACANTHOMA

A keratoacanthoma, also called *molluscum sebaceum*, is a benign cutaneous lesion that is believed to arise from hair follicles. Its cause is unknown. Men are affected twice as often as women.

A keratoacanthoma is usually solitary, rapidly growing,

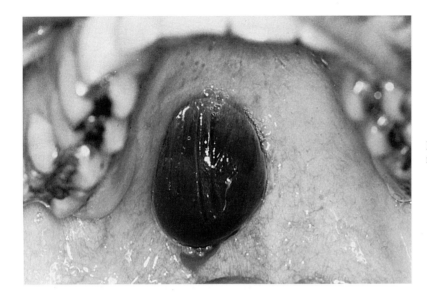

Fig. 76-6. A blood blister (angina bullosa haemorrhagica) on the palate.

well-circumscribed, slightly elevated, and rarely measures more than 1 cm. Centrally, a crateriform excavation can be seen with slighty indurated borders. Clinically, the lesion may mimic squamous cell carcinoma. Occurrence on the lower lip is not uncommon; intraoral and oropharyngeal locations are exceptional.[19]

Histologic examination of a keratoacanthoma shows hyperplastic epithelium with carcinoma-like features. No distinct features histologically substantiate the diagnosis. Spontaneous regression occurs within a few months.

LEIOMYOMA

A leiomyoma is a benign neoplasm composed of smooth muscle cells. The source of a smooth muscle tumor is believed to be the walls of blood vessels or undifferentiated mesenchymal cells. Occurrence of a leiomyoma in the oral cavity is rare.[1] Most reported leiomyomas of the oral cavity and oropharynx are small, circumscribed, and asymptomatic swellings covered with an apparently intact mucosa. They are single or multiple.

A leiomyoma is composed of whorls of smooth muscle cells. Leiomyoma can be difficult to diagnose on just light microscopic examination. The tumor should be differentiated from fibromatosis, schwannoma, and leiomyosarcoma. Treatment consists of surgical removal.

LINGUAL OSTEOCHONDROMA

An osteoma of the soft tissues is a benign lesion that consists of bone. A chondroma is similar. In some cases, an intermingling of the two lesions occurs, leading to the term *osteochondroma*. The osteochondroma represents a choristoma rather than a neoplasm.

It has no predilection for race, but is frequent in women aged 20 to 40 years. About 70 cases have been reported in the literature.[3]

Although osteochondroma may occur everywhere in the oral cavity, the tongue the most common site. Clinically, the

lesion appears as a pedunculated swelling of about 1 cm, usually in the posterior part of the dorsum of the tongue near the foramen cecum. Dysphagia may be the only symptom. Clinically, the differential diagnosis includes a lingual thyroid and a salivary gland tumor.

The histology shows a well-circumscribed lesion of mature lamellar bone or cartilage or a mixture of these tissues. Haversian canals may exist in the bone. Blood-forming elements are rarely present. Treatment consists of surgical removal.

LINGUAL THYROID

Lingual thyroid is a condition in which thyroid tissue is found in the foramen cecum area of the tongue. Approximately 400 cases have been reported in the literature.[7]

Ectopic thyroid tissue becomes clinically manifest almost exclusively in women and is perhaps the result of hormonal influences. The age of onset ranges from birth to the sixth decade, with a peak in the second decade. No racial or geographic predilection exists.

The lesion appears as a nodule or mass in the foramen cecum area, reaching a size of a few centimeters. The overlying mucosa may show an increased vascularity. The patient may experience dysphagia, dysphonia, and a feeling of fullness or pain. In some cases, the lingual thyroid tissue is the only functioning thyroid tissue. Therefore, a thyroid scan is mandatory.

The histopathologic findings of lingual thyroid are similar to those of cervical thyroid tissue. The chance of malignant degeneration in a lingual thyroid is rather small. A few cases have been reported.

Treatment of lingual thyroid is not always necessary and largely depends on the complaints. Most patients are in an euthyroid state, with normal thyroxine (T_4), triiodothyronine (T_3), and free thyroxine factor (T_7) determinations. The serum thyroid-stimulating hormone concentration may be increased. Some patients have hypothyroidism. Hyperfunction is exceptional. When the mass is causing functional impairment, suppressive doses of thyroid hormones may be sufficient; when it is not, total excision should be considered. This usually can be done through an intraoral approach, which may require midline splitting of the tongue.

LIPOMA

A lipoma is a benign neoplasm composed of fat cells. Its cause is unknown. Trauma and metaplasia of perivascular connective tissue have been suggested to have a role. Oral and oropharyngeal lipomas are rather rare. There is no predilection for either sex. An oral lipoma rarely occurs before the second decade.

A lipoma appears as a sessile, soft, and asymptomatic swelling (Fig. 76-7). When it is located superficially, a yellowish texture can be seen. In rare instances, bilateral or multiple occurrence has been reported.

Histologic examination of a lipoma shows a well-delineated mass of lobules of fat cells with interpersed fibrous septa. In rare instances, a benign ''infiltrative'' lipoma occurs and should not be confused with a liposarcoma. The distinction between a benign lipoma and a low-grade liposarcoma may be difficult in some cases. When fibrous tissue is a substantial part of a lipoma, the term *fibrolipoma* can be applied. When vascularity is a prominent feature, the term *angiolipoma* is used. Spindle cell lipoma is another histologic variant. Surgical removal is the treatment of choice. Recurrences have not been reported.

LYMPHANGIOMA

A lymphangioma is a benign lesion characterized by proliferation of lymphatic vessels. It is a hamartoma rather than a neoplasm. In some cases, distinguishing between a lymphangioma and hemangioma is difficult, in which case the term *angiomatosis* may be used.

Occurrence in the oral cavity and oropharynx is rather rare; the tongue is a usual site (Fig. 76-8). The size may vary from pinhead to massive dimensions. The typical lymphangioma is characterized by irregular nodularity of the mucosa, with gray and pink grape-like projections.

Histologically, endothelium-lined spaces are found in the connective tissue. In some cases, the spaces contain elements of blood, making the distinction between lymphangioma and hemangioma difficult or even impossible. No true encapsulation occurs, and often the proliferation of lymphatic vessels spreads diffusely into the surrounding soft tissues.

During infectious episodes, the combined use of corticosteroids and antibiotics may be required. Small lesions can be excised. With extensive, symptomatic lymphangiomas, surgical removal of the bulk of the lesion may be the only possible treatment. Complete surgical removal is difficult to obtain because of the multiple finger-like projections extending into the adjacent tissues. Corticosteroids and antibiotics should be administered during and after surgery. Recurrences are common.

LYMPHOID PATCHES

Lymphoid patches are localized, solitary or multiple lymph follicles occurring in the oropharynx, including the base of the tongue, where they are called *lingual tonsils*. Lymphoid patches are to be regarded as physiologic rather than pathologic and can be seen in most persons.

Lymphoid patches are often found in the posterior pharyngeal wall, appearing as single or multiple slightly elevated projections of the mucosa. Their size may vary from a few millimeters up to 1 cm. The color is usually yellowish or grayish. During a cold, the lymphoid patches may cause slight irritation but are otherwise asymptomatic.

Enlargement of the lingual tonsils may occur after tonsillectomy, probably because of a compensatory mechanism. In rare instances, lingual tonsillitis and abscess formation may occur.

Occasionally, single or multiple lymphoid patches are en-

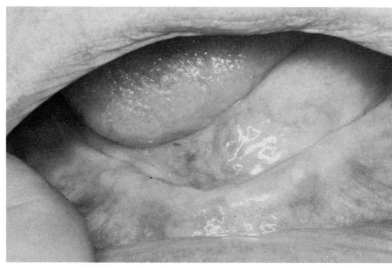

Fig. 76-7. A lipoma of the floor of the mouth, appearing as circumscribed swelling.

countered in the oral cavity, especially in the floor of the mouth (Fig. 76-9). These are sometimes called *oral tonsils*.[4] The diagnosis usually is based on clinical judgment. Only in doubtful cases is a biopsy indicated. A few cases have been described of benign lymphoid hyperplasia of the hard palate, which may simulate malignant non-Hodgkin's lymphoma.[13] Treatment is usually not required.

MESENCHYMOMA

A mesenchymoma is composed of two or more mesenchymal tissues and fibrous tissue that is actually always present in mesenchymal growths. Smooth or striated muscular tissue and fat, chondroid, or osseous tissues may be found. Whether a mesenchymoma is a true neoplasm or a hamartoma is not always clear.

Very few oral and oropharyngeal mesenchymomas have been reported. The ages of the reported patients range from 2.5 months to 23 years.

A mesenchymoma is usually a single, well-circumscribed lesion appearing as a submucosal nodule. Of reported cases, a few were located in the base of the tongue. Treatment consists of simple excision.

NEUROGENIC TUMORS

Although the distinction between a schwannoma (neurilemoma) and a neurofibroma may be debatable, most authors believe that these are separate entities.

Schwannoma

A schwannoma (neurilemoma) is a benign neurogenic neoplasm composed of Schwann's cells. The tumor may occur at all ages and does not show a preference for men or women.

A schwannoma is a slowly growing, rather circumscribed, submucosally located tumor that may be painful. No characteristic clinical features appear. It may occur at

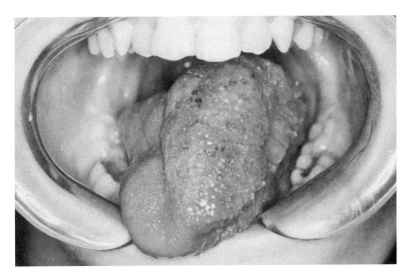

Fig. 76-8. Lymphangioma of the left side of the tongue.

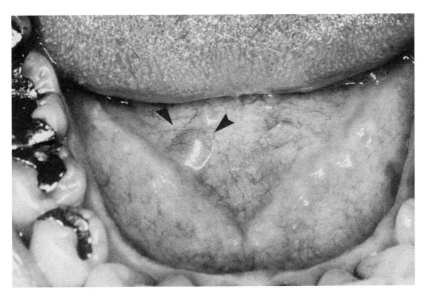

Fig. 76-9. An oral tonsil on the right side of the floor of the mouth (*arrows*).

any site in the oral cavity and rarely involves the oro-pharynx.[20]

Histologically, the encapsulated tumor is composed of two cell types: Antoni type A and Antoni type B cells. The A cells have elongated nuclei and are often arranged in a palisade pattern, including hyalinized material between them (Verocay bodies). Treatment consists of conservative surgical removal. Recurrences are rare.

Neurofibroma

A neurofibroma similar to a schwannoma, is derived from sheath cells. Is is usually not painful and rarely occurs as a single lesion. Most often neurofibromas are part of Reckling-hausen's disease (Fig. 76-10). The tongue is often involved, sometimes resulting in unilateral macroglossia. Also, the possibility of hereditary neuropoly–endocrine syndrome (consisting of mucosal neuromas, pheochromocytoma of the adrenal glands, and medullary thyroid carcinoma) should be taken into account. In general, the mucosal neuromas are already present at childhood, being the first manifestation of the syndrome.

In contrast to the schwannoma, a neurofibroma is not encapsulated. Proliferating Schwann's cells are haphazardly arranged, not showing the palisade arrangement of schwannomas.

With a single neurofibroma, management consists of surgical removal. With multiple or massive involvement, surgical removal may be impossible and is indicated only when malignant changes are suspected. With Recklinghausen's disease, there is a 5% to 15% risk of malignant degeneration.

Traumatic neuroma

A traumatic neuroma is a reactive hyperplasia caused by injury of a nerve. Traumatic neuromas may occur anywhere in the oral cavity. Occurrence in the oropharynx is exceptional. The lesion usually manifests as a small submucosal nodule that may be painful at palpation. No characteristic clinical features appear.

Histologically, masses of irregularly arranged nerve fibers and Schwann's cells are spread diffusely throughout the tissue, mimicking, to some extent, a neurofibroma.[5] Treatment consists of conservative surgical removal, if possible, followed by coagulation of the adherent nerve. Recurrence is rare.

PAPILLOMA AND ALLIED LESIONS

Papilloma

A papilloma is a benign epithelial neoplasm composed of finger-like projections of squamous epithelium. Some authors use the term *squamous papilloma*. The cause is unknown, although a human papillomavirus is most likely.

The prevalence of oral papillomas is less than 0.1%. Oral and oropharyngeal papillomas may occur as single or multiple, sessile, warty lesions, seldom measuring more than a few millimeters. When they involve the oropharynx, the soft palate and the uvula are the usual sites. The clinical differential diagnosis of a papilloma includes verruca vulgaris, fibroepithelial polyp, focal epithelial hyperplasia, and condyloma acuminatum.

The histology of a papilloma shows finger-like projections of squamous epithelium above the level of the surrounding mucosa. In most cases, a mild hyperorthokeratosis occurs. Epithelial dysplasia is not a feature of papilloma. Carcinomatous changes in a papilloma are exceptional, if ever proven. Treatment consists of surgical excision. Recurrences are rare.

Condyloma acuminatum

Condyloma acuminatum is a papillomatous growth that occurs most frequently on anogenital skin and mucosa and is caused by a papillomavirus of the papovavirus group. Con-

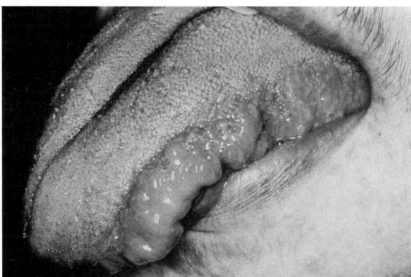

Fig. 76-10. Neurofibroma of the border of the tongue in a patient with neurofibromatosis.

dyloma is a common venereal disease. One probable reason for the few reports on oral condylomas is that they have been diagnosed as papillomas, verrucae, or fibroepithelial polyps.

They start as multiple, small, whitish-pink nodules that often proliferate and coalesce to form soft, sessile, or pedunculated papillary growths. They may occur anywhere in the oral mucosa and in the upper aerodigestive tract.[15] The lesions show a hyperplastic epithelium arranged in a papillomatous pattern but without keratinization. There is often spongiosis of the epithelium, which has a benign appearance. Treatment consists of surgical removal. Recurrences are rare.

Focal epithelial hyperplasia

Focal epithelial hyperplasia, also called *Heck's disease*, is a benign disorder of the oral mucosa. The condition is characterized by multiple, more or less papillomatous lesions, possibly caused by a virus of the papovavirus group. When first reported in 1965, focal epithelial hyperplasia was thought to be an extremely rare entity, occurring exclusively in children of American Indian origin. It has been shown, however, that focal epithelial hyperplasia occurs worldwide and is not limited to young adults.[16]

The lesions measure several millimeters and have a papillomatous or fibroma-like appearance and consistency (Fig. 76-11). They are asymptomatic and may occur everywhere in the oral mucosa. A biopsy is usually not required to confirm the diagnosis.

The histologic picture of focal epithelial hyperplasia is more or less pathognomonic. It comprises hyperplastic epithelium without keratosis and broadening and clubbing of the rete ridges. No dysplasia occurs. In the upper spinous layer of the epithelium, mitosoid cells may be observed. The lamina propria occasionally shows signs of inflammation. No specific treatment is required.

Verruciform xanthoma

Verruciform xanthoma is a benign lesion of the oral mucosa, histologically characterized by the presence of numerous foam cells in the connective tissue papillae. The cause is unknown. Some speculate that epithelial cells implanted by trauma or inflammation become necrotic and that the cell membrane lipids are ingested by macrophages that form the characteristic foam cells. More than 100 cases have been reported. No sex predilection exists. The patient is usually older than the second decade.[18]

A verruciform xanthoma clinically manifests as an asymptomatic, slowly growing, somewhat raised, papilloma-like lesion with a normal or somewhat reddish or yellowish color. Crateriform surfaces also have been reported. The lesion may occur anywhere in the oral cavity.

Histologically, the lesion is characterized by a papillomatous surface with elongated rete processes. The more or less pathognomonic feature is the presence of foam cells in the lamina propria. Treatment consists of conservative surgical removal. Recurrence is highly unlikely.

EXTRAMEDULLARY PLASMACYTOMA

Plasmacytoma, also called *plasma cell myeloma* or *multiple myeloma*, is primarily a neoplasm of bone. Extramedullary location without bony involvement may occur in the nasopharynx, nasal cavity, and paranasal sinuses and rarely in the oral cavity and oropharynx. Whether such soft-tissue plasmacytomas are related to the intrabony lesions is debatable.

The oral and oropharyngeal lesions have been described as reddish, pedunculated, or diffuse, without ulceration or any characteristic features. The disease usually involves a single lesion. In a few patients, regional metastases may develop.

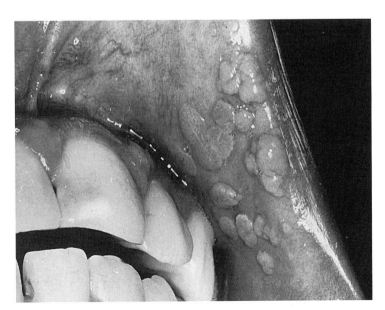

Fig. 76-11. Focal epithelial hyperplasia involving the upper lip.

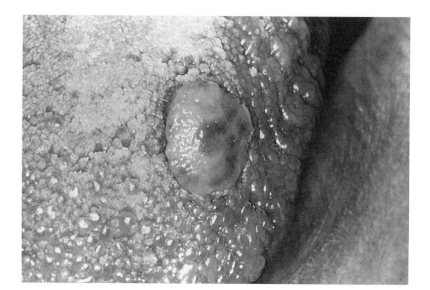

Fig. 76-12. Pyogenic granuloma on the tongue.

The histologic picture shows a homogeneous picture of densely packed plasma cells and is indistinguishable from the bony lesion in multiple myeloma.

For localized extramedullary plasmacytomas, surgery seems to be the management of choice. Radiotherapy also may be considered. In general, the prognosis is good unless the lesion is the initial sign of multiple myeloma.

PYOGENIC GRANULOMA

A pyogenic granuloma is a benign, elevated, and capillary-rich lesion occurring on the skin and mucous membranes. The pyogenic granuloma is thought to be the result of an overreaction to minor trauma rather than to infection. Hormonal changes may be another cause. It has no predilection for either sex or any age group.

An oral pyogenic granuloma most frequently involves the gingiva. The lower lip and the dorsal surface of the tongue also are common sites. The lesion is usually pedunculated or sessile, and the surface is often ulcerated (Fig. 76-12). The lesion's diameter may vary from 0.5 to 2 cm or more.

Histologically, a pyogenic granuloma does not consist of true granulomas. Many vascular spaces can exist together with numerous inflammatory cells, sometimes raising the question of whether the granuloma is a vascular lesion with secondary signs of inflammation or an inflammatory condition. Mitotic activity may be abundant and should not be mistaken as a sign of malignancy. Surgery is the management of choice. With the exception of the gingival lesions, recurrence of a pyogenic granuloma is rare.

RHABDOMYOMA

A rhabdomyoma is a benign neoplasm of striated muscles. It is exceedingly uncommon. The male:female ratio is more than 2:1. The mean age of patients with a rhabdomyoma is about 40 years.

Although extracardiac rhabdomyomas show a preference for the head and neck, occurrence in the oral cavity and oropharynx is rare. The floor of the mouth is the most common site.[14] Multifocal appearance is exceptional. The clinical presentation is a submucosal swelling without any specific signs or symptoms.

A rhabdomyoma is a well-circumscribed tumor. Based on histopathologic characteristics and gross morphology, two types are recognized: fetal and adult. The adult type is composed of large, round or polygonal cells with a slight granular cytoplasm. The cytoplasm may contain lipoid material. Cross striations may be found in a few cells. The fetal type almost exclusively occurs in the first few years of life. Histologically, this type is characterized by immature skeletal muscle in varying stages of development and by undifferentiated mesenchymal cells. Differentiating a rhabdomyoma from a rhabdomyosarcoma may be difficult. Treatment of a rhabdomyoma consists of surgical removal.

PALATINE TORUS AND MANDIBULAR TORUS

The palatine torus and mandibular torus are exostoses rather than neoplasms of the palatal and the mandibular bone, respectively; both are common. The palatal protuberance is located in the midline of the hard palate, having a unilobular or multilobular shape (Fig. 76-13). The consistency is bony hard. There are no symptoms. Clinically, a palatine torus may be confused with a firm, indurated neoplasm and vice versa. However, the bony consistency is more or less diagnostic. In rare instances, additional radiographic examination is needed for diagnostic support. The mandibular torus is less common than the palatal exostosis. Usually, this torus is seen bilaterally at the lingual aspect of the bicuspid region.

The histologic picture of a torus shows healthy vital bone without any further characteristics. Surgery is indicated in cases of the construction of dental appliances.

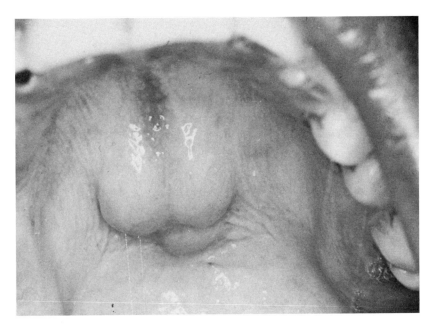

Fig. 76-13. The multilobular palatine torus.

REFERENCES

1. Baden E and others: Leiomyoma of the oral cavity: a light microscopic and immunohistochemical study with review of the literature from 1884 to 1992, *Eur J Cancer* 30B:1, 1994.
2. Baker DL and others: Intraoral infantile hemangiopericytoma: literature review and addition of a case, *Oral Surg Oral Med Oral Pathol* 73: 596, 1992.
3. Blum MR and others: Soft tissue chondroma of the cheek, *J Oral Pathol Med* 22:334, 1993.
4. Buchner A, Hansen LS: Lympho-epithelial cysts of the oral cavity: a clinicopathologic study of 38 cases, *Oral Surg* 50:441, 1980.
5. Chauvin PJ and others: Palisaded encapsulated neuroma of oral mucosa, *Oral Surg Oral Med Oral Pathol* 73:71, 1992.
6. Deblauwe BM, van der Waal I: Blood blisters of the oral mucosa (angina bullosa haemorrhagica), *J Am Acad Dermatol* 31:341, 1994.
7. Douglas PS, Baker AW: Lingual thyroid, *Br J Oral Maxillofac Surg* 32:123, 1994.
8. Kaiserling E and others: Congenital epulis and granular cell tumor: a histologic and immunohistochemical study, *Oral Surg Oral Med Oral Pathol* 80:687, 1995.
9. Lovas JGL, Goodday RHB: Clinical diagnosis of caliber-persistent labial artery of the lower lip, *Oral Surg Oral Med Oral Pathol* 76:480, 1993.
10. Magnusson BC, Rasmussen LG: The giant cell fibroma: a review of 103 cases with immunohistochemical findings, *Arch Odont Scand* 53: 293, 1995.
11. Mazur MT and others: Granular cell tumor: immunohistochemical analysis of 21 benign tumors and one malignant tumor, *Arch Pathol Lab Med* 114:692, 1990.
12. Movassaghi K and others: Ulcerative eosinophilic granuloma: a report of five new cases, *Br J Oral Maxillofac Surg* 34:115, 1996.
13. Napier SS, Newlands C: Benign lymphoid hyperplasia of the palate: report of two cases and immunohistochemical profile, *J Oral Pathol Med* 19:221, 1990.
14. Napier SS and others: Sublingual adult rhabdomyoma: report of a case, *Int J Oral Maxillofac Surg* 20:201, 1991.
15. Nash M and others: Condylomatous lesions of the upper aerodigestive tract, *Laryngoscope* 97:1410, 1987.
16. Pilgard G: Focal epithelial hyperplasia: report of nine cases from Sweden and review of the literature, *Oral Surg Oral Med Oral Pathol* 57: 540, 1984.
17. Shear M: *Cysts of the oral regions*, ed 3, Oxford, 1992, Wright.
18. Toida M, Koizumi H: Verruciform xanthoma involving the lip: a case report, *J Oral Maxillofac Surg* 51:432, 1993.
19. de Visscher JGAM and others: Giant keratoacanthoma of the lower lip: report of a case of spontaneous regression, *Oral Surg Oral Med Oral Pathol* 81:193, 1996.
20. Williams HK and others: Neurilemmoma of the head and neck, *Br J Oral Maxillofac Surg* 31:32, 1993.
21. Yonetsu K and others: Magnetic resonance imaging of oral and maxillofacial angiomas, *Oral Surg Oral Med Oral Pathol* 76:783, 1993.

Chapter 77

Malignant Neoplasms of the Oral Cavity

Pramod K. Sharma
David E. Schuller
Shan R. Baker

Approximately 20,000 new cases of cancer of the oral cavity are diagnosed each year, with 4000 deaths annually.[1] The relatively small number of deaths is offset by the severe functional and cosmetic disabilities that many of these patients endure in coping with their disease, which is primarily preventable. Unfortunately, when first seen, most patients have an advanced tumor—partly because of self-neglect and partly because of the primary physician's lack of training in the early detection of oral cancer. The oral cavity is one of the most accessible areas for inspection and palpation. A sore or lump that persists, especially if it is nontender, or evidence of nerve dysfunction should alert the physician to the probable existence of a malignant neoplasm rather than an inflammatory process. The dental profession is conscious of oral cancer and often discovers intraoral malignancies even before the patient suspects their presence.

ANATOMY

The oral cavity is divided into a number of distinct sites that allow formulation of treatment modalities and prognosis in a more defined fashion (Fig. 77-1). Classification also enables more accurate statistical collection and evaluation. The oral cavity extends from the cutaneous vermilion junction of the lips to the junction of the hard and soft palate above and to the line of the circumvallate papillae below. It is divided into the lips, buccal mucosa, upper and lower alveolar ridges, retromolar trigone, floor of the mouth, hard palate, and anterior two thirds of the tongue. This chapter considers each of these sites separately.

Lymphatics of the oral cavity

Several important groups of lymph nodes act as first-echelon nodes in the oral cavity (Fig. 77-2). Two or three submental nodes lie on the mylohyoid muscle in the submental triangle. This triangle is bounded by the anterior bellies of the digastric muscles and the hyoid bone. Six or more submandibular nodes lie on the anterior surface of the submandibular gland or between the gland and the lower jaw adjacent to the facial artery. The nodes on the surface of the gland are preglandular nodes; those adjacent to the facial artery are facial nodes. They extend upward along the course of the facial artery and are subdivided into prevascular and retrovascular nodes, depending on their relationship to the facial artery. With the exception of one or two at the lower border of the jaw, the facial nodes are small and inconstant.

Another important first-echelon nodal group that receives afferent vessels from the oral cavity is the upper deep jugular nodes located along the upper internal jugular vein, between the levels of the digastric and omohyoid muscles. The uppermost node is the jugulodigastric or tonsillar node; the lowest is the jugulo-omohyoid node. The jugulocarotid node, the principal node of the tongue, is located between these nodes just below the level of the greater horn of the hyoid bone at the level of the bifurcation of the common carotid artery. Additional but less common nodal groups receiving primary lymphatics from the oral cavity include the lateral retropharyngeal lymph nodes and nodes adjacent to the inferior portion of the parotid gland (periparotid nodes).

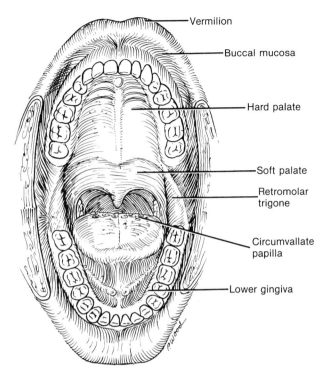

Fig. 77-1. The oral cavity includes the lips, floor of the mouth, anterior two thirds of the tongue, buccal mucosa, hard palate, upper and lower alveolar ridge, and retromolar trigone.

In general, regional metastatic squamous cell carcinoma (SCC) of the oral cavity demonstrates an orderly progression from neck nodes located in the upper regions of the neck toward nodes in the lower region. Malignancies of the lips and anterior floor of the mouth as well as adjacent gingiva and buccal mucosa tend to metastasize to submandibular lymph nodes first. Tumors situated more posteriorly in the oral cavity usually metastasize initially to the upper deep jugular lymph nodes. As multiple cervical nodes become involved with metastatic disease, spread to the middle and lower deep jugular nodes occurs. It is unusual for a single metastatic node from an oral cavity cancer to metastasize to the lower or posterior cervical nodes initially. However, there are lymphatic channels that directly connect oral cavity sites with lower jugular nodes, which provide an anatomic basis for lower jugular lymphadenopathy independent of other lymphadenopathy.

Lips

The lips begin at the junction of the vermilion border with the skin and form the anterior boundary of the oral vestibule. The lip includes only the vermilion surface, or that portion of the lip that comes into contact with the opposing lip.

Lip musculature is derived from the second branchial arch, which migrates to the facial processes. The orbicular

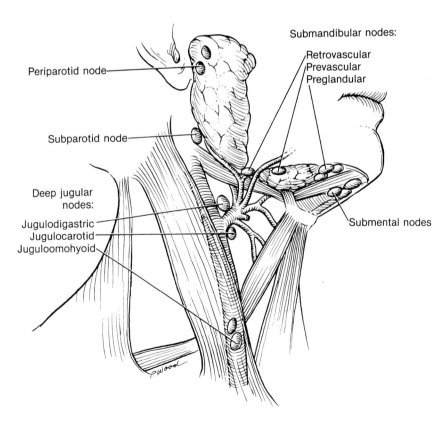

Fig. 77-2. First-echelon lymph node groups of the oral cavity.

mouth muscle is the sphincter lying within the lip and encircling the oral aperture. This muscle extends upward almost to the columella of the nose and downward to the mental crease. The muscle fibers decussate in the midline and occasionally form a raphe in the lower lip (Fig. 77-3).

The infraorbital branch of the maxillary nerve (V2) supplies sensation to a major portion of the skin and mucous membrane of the upper lip. The buccal branch of the mandibular nerve (V3) supplies the oral commissure area. Portions of this nerve pierce the buccinator muscle to supply the mucous membrane of the commissure. The mental branch of the mandibular nerve emerges through the mental foramen to supply the skin and mucous membrane of the lower lip and provides an important pathway for spread of lip cancer into the interior of the mandible.

The seventh cranial (facial) nerve (CN VII) is the motor supply to the muscles of the lip. The buccal branch of the facial nerve is superficial to the masseter muscle but runs in the same direction as the buccal branch of CN V to supply the upper-lip musculature.

The major blood supply of the lips is from branches of the facial artery including the inferior and superior labial arteries. These vessels, along with those of the opposite side, encircle the mouth between the orbicular mouth muscle and the submucosa of the lip. The anterior facial vein runs posterior to the facial artery and gives off branches corresponding to the artery, providing venous return from the lip.

The lymphatic drainage of the lips has been well described.[77,96] The upper and lower lips have a cutaneous and a mucosal system of lymphatics, both arising from a fine capillary network beneath the vermilion border. The medial portion of the lower lip drains to submental lymph nodes, whereas the lateral portion drains into submandibular lymph nodes (Fig. 77-4). Numerous anastomoses from the lymphatic vessels of the two lip halves are present near the midline and account for bilateral metastases from tumors that are close to or cross the midline. Collecting lymphatic trunks have been shown to enter the mental foramen in 22% of lip cancer cases.[119] The upper-lip lymphatics drain to preauricular, infraparotid, submandibular, and submental lymph nodes. In contrast to the lower lip, only a few of the upper-lip cutaneous lymph trunks drain to contralateral nodes. No crossing of the midline has been documented for the mucosal lymphatics of the upper lip. Lymphatic channels from nodes located in the submental, submandibular, and periparotid areas drain into the lymph nodes of the upper and occasionally the middle deep jugular lymphatic chain.

Buccal mucosa

The buccal mucosa includes the entire membrane lining of the interior surface of the cheek and lips, from the opposing lip's line of contact to the pterygomandibular raphe posteriorly and to the line of attachment of the alveolar ridge mucosa above and below. The buccal mucosa forms the lateral wall of the oral vestibule. The buccinator muscle is the lateral muscular wall of the oral cavity and, along with the orbicular mouth muscle, helps to determine oral competence. It extends from the superior constrictor of the pharynx and blends with orbicular muscle fibers in the upper and lower lips. Tumors of the buccal mucosa may extend laterally through the buccinator muscle to involve the buccal fat pad posteriorly or subcutaneous tissues and skin of the cheek.

The buccal branch of CN VII is the motor supply to the buccinator muscle. It runs in the same direction as the buccal branch of CN V (V3), which provides sensory innervation to the cheek. The infraorbital (V2) and mental (V3) nerves

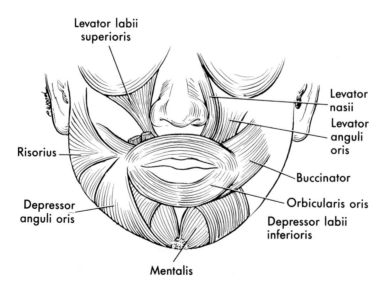

Fig. 77-3. Musculature of the lips.

provide additional sensory innervation to the anterior buccal mucosa.

The vascular supply of the buccal mucosa is derived from branches of the facial artery and the transverse facial artery and their respective companion veins. Lymphatics of the buccal mucosa arise from a submucosal capillary network and drain to lymph nodes located in the submental and submandibular triangles.

Upper and lower alveolar ridges

The alveolar ridges include the alveolar processes of the mandible and maxilla and their mucosal covering that, in the case of the lower alveolar ridge, extends from the line of attachment of mucosa in the buccal gutter to the line of free mucosa in the floor of the mouth. Posteriorly, the lower alveolar ridge's mucosa extends to the ascending ramus of the mandible. The upper alveolar ridge's mucosa extends from the line of attachment of mucosa in the upper buccal gutter to the junction of the hard palate. Its posterior margin is the upper end of the pterygopalatine arch. Malignancies of the upper gingiva readily invade underlying bone and may extend upward into the floor of the nasal cavity or into the maxillary antrum. Lateral spread will result in involvement of the upper buccal sulcus and buccal mucosa. Medial extension will involve the hard palate.

The maxillary nerve (V2) provides innervation to the teeth of the upper jaw through the posterosuperior and anterosuperior alveolar nerves. Different sensory branches of the maxillary nerve innervate the lingual and labial gingiva of the upper alveolus. The greater palatine nerve supplies the lingual side of the alveolus behind the premaxilla. The naso-

palatine nerve supplies the lingual gingiva of the premaxilla; two different branches of the maxillary nerve innervate the labial surface of the upper alveolar gingiva. The posterosuperior alveolar nerve, which descends on the infratemporal surface of the maxilla, supplies the gingiva posterior to the premaxilla. Branches of the infraorbital nerve supply the labial gingiva.

The mandibular nerve (V3) innervates the teeth and gingiva of the lower jaw. The teeth are also innervated by the inferior alveolar nerve, which enters the mandibular foramen and runs the length of the mandible in the mandibular canal to exit the mental foramen. Malignancies arising on the alveolus may infiltrate bone and reach the mandibular canal, where the tumor may follow the mandible along the nerve toward the skull base or through the mental foramen and into the skin of the lower lip and chin. In edentulous persons the alveolar bone is absorbed, and the mandibular canal may be only a few millimeters from the mandible's upper margin, providing for early access of the tumor into the mandible's medullary portion.

Branches of the lingual nerve supply the entire lingual gingiva of the lower alveolus. The buccal nerve (V3) supplies the labial surface behind the canine tooth; the mental nerve supplies the surface in front of the canines.

The posterosuperior alveolar artery and vein provide the blood supply to the upper alveolus. The greater palatine artery and vein also contribute to the lingual aspect. The inferior alveolar artery and vein primarily supply the lower alveolus.

Lymphatics of the buccal aspect of the upper and lower alveolar ridges drain to submental and submandibular lymph

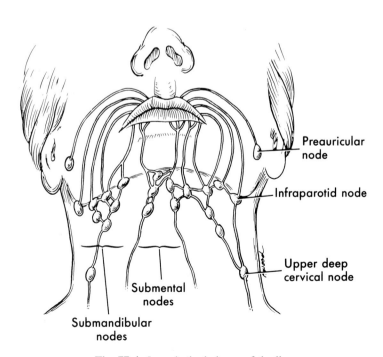

Fig. 77-4. Lymphatic drainage of the lips.

nodes. Lymphatics from the lingual aspect of the upper and lower gingiva pass chiefly to upper deep jugular and lateral retropharyngeal lymph nodes. Some channels may drain to lymph nodes adjacent to the tail of the parotid gland (subparotid). Lymphatics from the lingual surface of the lower alveolus also may end in submandibular nodes.

Retromolar trigone

The retromolar trigone is the attached gingiva overlying the ascending ramus of the mandible. The distal surface of the last lower molar forms the base of this triangular area, and its apex terminates at the maxillary tuberosity. The upward extension of the oblique line of the mandible to the coronoid process forms the triangle's lateral side, and a line connecting the distal lingual cusp of the last molar and the coronoid process forms the medial side. The triangle's base is continuous laterally with the gingivobuccal sulcus and medially with the gingivolingual sulcus. The triangle's lateral side is continuous with the buccal mucosa, and the medial side blends into the anterior tonsillar pillars.

The mucosa adheres closely to the underlying bone in the region of the retromolar trigone, and malignant tumors arising in this area may readily infiltrate the mandible. The inferior alveolar nerve enters the mandibular foramen at a point just posterior to the midpoint of the trigone's medial side and may be affected by neoplasm early in the course of disease.

Nerve twigs from the ninth cranial (glossopharyngeal) nerve and branches of the lesser palatine nerve (V2) provide sensory innervation to the retromolar triangle. The contribution of CN IX accounts for the referred ear pain that may be observed in patients with cancer arising in this region.

The tonsillar and ascending palatine branches of the facial artery supply blood to the retromolar trigone. The dorsal lingual, ascending pharyngeal, and lesser palatine arteries also may contribute to this region's vascularity. Venous drainage is through the tonsillar bed to the pharyngeal plexus of veins and to the common facial vein.

The lymphatic drainage of the retromolar trigone is similar to that of the tonsillar fossa, passing to the upper deep jugular chain of lymph nodes. Some lymph channels may also end in subparotid and lateral retropharyngeal lymph nodes.

Hard palate

The hard palate is a semilunar area consisting of mucous membranes covering the horizontal laminae of the palatine bones (Fig. 77-5). The upper alveolar ridge partly surrounds the hard palate, which extends from the inner surface of the superior alveolar ridge to the posterior edge of the palatine bone. Each palatine bone is somewhat L-shaped. The palate's horizontal lamina meets the other side's lamina in the midline, forming the secondary palate, and the perpendicular lamina runs upward, forming the posterolateral wall of the nasal passage. The fusion of the palatine processes of the two maxillae, known as the primary palate, forms the bony palate in front of the palatine bone's horizontal laminae. The primary palate is part of the premaxilla, or the bone that bears the incisor teeth. Its union with the posterior portion of the hard palate is marked in the midline by the incisive fossa.

Two or more foramina are located posterolaterally on either side near the junction of the hard and soft palate. The larger is the greater palatine foramen, and behind this are one or two lesser palatine foramina. These foramina represent the lower end of the pterygopalatine canal, through which nerves and vessels are conducted from the pterygopalatine fossa to supply the hard and soft palate. The foramina provide access for tumor spread into the pterygopalatine fossa and regions of the skull base. Likewise, the incisive fossa and canal provide a pathway for tumor extension into the nasal cavity.

Similar to the alveolar ridge, the periosteum of the hard palate adheres more intimately to the mucosa than to the bone; thus, the two are referred to as *mucoperiosteum*. The mucoperiosteum acts as a temporary barrier to the deep spread of tumor; however, cancers of the hard palate frequently extend into the underlying bone as the disease progresses. Contiguous spread of tumor may involve the upper gingiva laterally and the soft palate posteriorly.

The hard palate receives its vascular supply from the greater palatine artery and vein, which are terminal branches of the sphenopalatine vessels. They gain access to the palate through the greater palatine foramen. The greater palatine nerve supplies the secondary palate and exits the foramen. The nasopalatine nerve, a branch of the maxillary nerve (V2) that descends through the incisive canal from the nasal passage, innervates the primary palate.

Lymphatics of the hard palate are sparse compared with other sites in the oral cavity. Drainage is similar to that of the lingual surface of the upper alveolus. Most of the lymphatics drain into upper deep jugular (subdigastric) or lateral retropharyngeal nodes. Lymph channels draining the primary palate may terminate in the prevascular and retrovascular group of submandibular nodes.

Floor of the mouth

The floor of the mouth is a crescent-shaped region of mucosa overlying the mylohyoid and hyoglossus muscles, extending from the inner aspect of the lower alveolar ridge to the underside of the anterior two thirds of the tongue. Posteriorly, the floor of the mouth is continuous with the base of the anterior tonsillar pillar, and anteriorly the frenulum of the tongue divides it into two sides. On either side of the frenulum is the sublingual caruncle, marking the orifices of the submandibular duct. Posterolaterally from the orifices is a rounded ridge called the sublingual fold, which overlies the upper border of the sublingual salivary glands.

The paired mylohyoid muscles constitute a muscular diaphragm and provide the structural support of the anterior floor of the mouth. They arise from the mylohyoid lines of

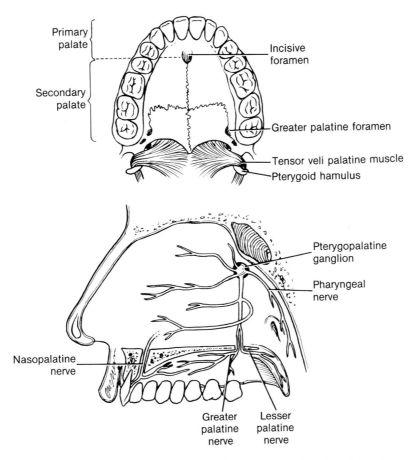

Fig. 77-5. Primary and secondary hard palates. Incisive fossa marks the union of the primary palate, which is innervated by the nasopalatine nerve, and secondary palate, which is innervated by the greater palatine nerve.

the mandible and insert into the hyoid bone. Their borders unite in the midline as a median raphe that extends from the symphysis of the mandible to the hyoid bone (Fig. 77-6). The hyoglossus muscle partly supports the extreme posterior floor of the mouth; it is a flat, quadrilateral muscle extending upward into the tongue from the body and greater horn of the hyoid, partly above and partly behind the mylohyoid muscle. An important point of surgical anatomy is that the lingual nerve, submandibular duct, sublingual gland, and twelfth cranial (hypoglossal) nerve lie lateral to the hyoglossus muscle, whereas the lingual artery runs deep (medial) to it.

Medially, the space between the mylohyoid muscle and the mucosa of the floor of the mouth contains the three extrinsic muscles of the tongue: the hyoglossus, genioglossus, and the styloglossus (see Fig. 77-6). Laterally, this space contains the sublingual gland, the submandibular gland duct, the lingual nerve, and branches of the lingual artery.

The lingual artery and vein supply the floor of the mouth. The artery arises from the external carotid and enters the oral cavity deep to the hyoglossus muscle (Fig. 77-7). After giving rise to the dorsal lingual artery, which supplies the

base of the tongue, the lingual artery terminates in the sublingual and deep lingual arteries, which supply the floor of the mouth. A branch of the mandibular nerve (V3) supplies the mylohyoid muscle. Branches of the lingual nerve provide sensory innervation to the floor of the mouth.

The lymph vessels of the floor of the mouth spring from an extensive submucosal plexus that forms two discrete systems: a superficial mucosa and a deep collecting.[96] The superficial system has crossing afferent lymphatic vessels in the anterior floor of the mouth, where no definite midline exists. These channels drain into the ipsilateral and contralateral preglandular lymph nodes. The deep collecting system drains into the ipsilateral preglandular nodes. Only the most anterior collecting vessels of the deep system cross the midline. Lymph channels from the posterior portion of the floor of the mouth drain directly into the jugulodigastric and jugulocarotid nodes.

Malignant tumors of the floor of the mouth usually occur anteriorly near the midline and spread to such contiguous structures as the root of the tongue and the mandible. Tumors near the orifice of the submandibular duct frequently track along the duct. Tumors may also extend far along the lingual

In contrast to leukoplakia, other white patches involving the oral mucosa are not considered premalignant. These lesions include white spongy nevus, leukoedema, candidiasis, systemic lupus erythematosus, and psoriasis. Leukoedema is filmy white, transparent, nonpalpable, and not raised above the level of the surrounding mucosa. Candidiasis is more frequently observed in infants or immunologically suppressed individuals. It consists of heaps of white aggregates that appear to be stuck to the underlying mucosa.

Erythroplakia is a nonwhite, premalignant lesion of the oral cavity. It has a much greater potential for malignancy than leukoplakia, and many are already carcinoma *in situ*. It appears as a slightly raised, red granular area that bleeds easily when scraped with an instrument. It typically occurs on the retromolar trigone, anterior tonsillar pillars, and soft palate. Additional nonwhite lesions of the oral mucosa include inflammatory papillary hyperplasia of the palate, inflammatory fibrous hyperplasia, pyogenic granuloma, papillomas, and pigmented nevi. Other conditions in the oral cavity that occasionally produce a reddened appearance are Kaposi's sarcoma, leukemia, hemangiosarcomas, mycosis fungoides, and polycythemia vera.

Gross pathology

Three gross morphologic growth patterns of SCC occur in the oral cavity: exophytic, ulcerative, and infiltrative. Malignancies often display more than one of these manifestations. The exophytic form is least common, except on the lip. It tends to grow more superficially and metastasize later than the other types. This form begins as an area of thickened epithelium, which heaps up and can protrude 1 cm or more above the surrounding mucosa (Fig. 77-10). Ulceration occurs early in its development. Exophytic carcinomas gradually become deeply infiltrative in more advanced cases. On the lip this form of tumor may reach a size of 6 or 7 cm, with little local destruction of tissue.

The ulcerative type is the most common form of SCC in the oral cavity. It begins as a round or oval ulcer with a gray, shaggy base that bleeds readily (Fig. 77-11). Ulcerative types manifest a greater tendency for rapid infiltration and usually have a higher histologic grade than the exophytic type. The ulcer eventually may heap up and become exophytic or remain lower than surrounding mucosa.

Infiltrative malignancies are common in the tongue and initially appear as a firm mass or plaque covered by mucosa. This type of tumor extends deeply into underlying tissues, with minimal elevation above the surrounding mucosa. As the neoplasm progresses, ulceration and exophytic manifestations may be observed.

A fourth morphologic type of oral cancer is verrucous carcinoma, which is a clearly defined but uncommon variant of SCC. It typically occurs in elderly patients who have poor oral hygiene or ill-fitting dentures and most commonly affects the buccal mucosa of men and women with a history of tobacco chewing or snuff dipping (Table 77-1).[57] The tumor has a warty, bulky, elevated, and fungating appear-

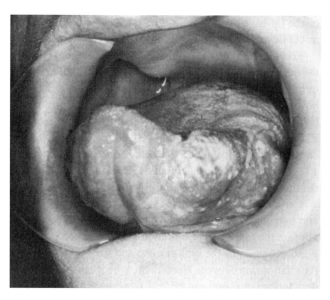

Fig. 77-10. Exophytic squamous cell carcinoma of the tongue.

ance. It may grow considerably through lateral spread and occasionally may be multifocal; it does not invade deeply into underlying tissue. Verrucous carcinomas have an indolent biologic behavior and do not metastasize. The characteristic histologic pattern is an undulating, densely keratinized outer layer covering large papillary fronds and a sharply circumscribed, deep margin composed of rows of bulbous, well-oriented rete ridges. The advancing margin appears to push through rather than invade and infiltrate deep tissue. Tumors must be sectioned serially so that the entire specimen is examined for a more invasive SCC (Fig. 77-12).

Histopathology

In 1920 Broders established a microscopic grading of carcinoma of the lip. He later made a slight revision, and for the most part this system is used today in assessing SCC, not only of the lip but also elsewhere in the oral cavity.[15] Broders classified tumors into one of four groups depending on cellular differentiation, as based on the percentage of total cellular elements (Table 77-2; Fig. 77-13).[50] The presence of minimal pleomorphism and few mitoses indicates a well-differentiated grade I neoplasm. Poorly differentiated neoplasms show extreme pleomorphism, minimal or no keratinization, and frequent mitoses and are classified as grade IV. Most oral cavity cancers are grade I or II.

Regional metastases

Regional metastases portend a worse prognosis for patients with oral cancer. The 5-year survival rate in patients with cervical metastasis is approximately 50% lower than that in patients without clinical evidence of metastases. The prognosis is further worsened in patients with multiple cervical metastases. In addition to the correlation of clinical metastases with decreased survival, histopathologic evaluation

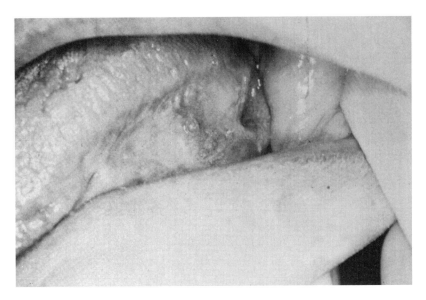

Fig. 77-11. Ulcerative squamous cell carcinoma of the tongue.

Table 77-1. Verrucous carcinoma of oral cavity: location of 77 tumors

Location	Patients, n(%)
Buccal mucosa	50 (65)
Gingiva	21 (27)
Tongue	3 (4)
Retromolar region	1 (1)
Hard palate	2 (3)
TOTAL	77 (100)

Modified from Kraus FT, Perez-Mesa C: *Cancer* 19:26, 1966.

Table 77-2. Broders' classification of squamous cell carcinoma

Cellular differentiation expressed in percentage of total cellular elements	Grade of malignancy	Histopathologic terminology
Near 75-100	I	Well differentiated
50-75	II	Moderately well differentiated
25-50	III	Moderately differentiated
0-25	IV	Poorly differentiated

of the metastatic lymph nodes is also significant. Patients found to have extracapsular spread of carcinoma in cervical lymph nodes have been shown to have a statistically lower rate of survival.[50,82] Despite the extracapsular spread being directly related to the size of cervical nodes, it is apparent that spread is more common in small (N1) cervical nodes than previously appreciated. Extracapsular spread may indicate depressed immunologic surveillance and failure to contain tumor spread. Several studies indicate that the survival rate of patients with cervical metastases in which the tumor is limited to the node ranges from 50% to 70% for 5 years. If extracapsular spread of neoplasm occurs, however, the number of patients who survive for 5 years is reduced to 25% to 30%.[51,82,103]

Regional metastases are present on initial evaluation in approximately 30% of patients with oral cavity cancer, excluding cancers of the lip and hard palate. The incidence of regional metastases is related to the size of the primary tumor, with larger tumors manifesting a higher incidence. Contralateral or bilateral metastases may develop when the primary tumor is near or crosses the midline. Approximately 25% of patients who show no evidence of regional metastases when first evaluated will eventually develop nodal disease despite control of their original primary tumor.

Clinically apparent cervical lymph node metastases occur in 10% to 15% of patients with SCC of the lip[5] and 15% to 25% of patients with cancer of the hard palate.[23] Subsequent development of regional metastases following control of lip cancer ranges from 5% to 15%. The lower incidence of metastases from hard palate tumors is related to the rather sparse lymphatic supply to this region. The lower metastatic rate of lip cancer occurs because most lip cancers are small and well differentiated when first evaluated.

Distant metastases

Until advanced stages, metastatic disease from carcinoma of the oral cavity tends to remain above the level of the clavicle. General dissemination of the tumor eventually occurs in 15% to 20% of patients dying of oral cavity cancer. In such instances regional cervical metastases have been

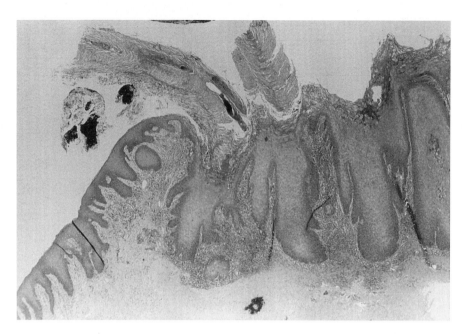

Fig. 77-12. Verrucous carcinoma of the oral cavity. The outer, undulating, densely keratinized layer covering large papillary fronds and a sharply circumscribed deep margin composed of rows of bulbous, well-oriented rete ridges are characteristic.

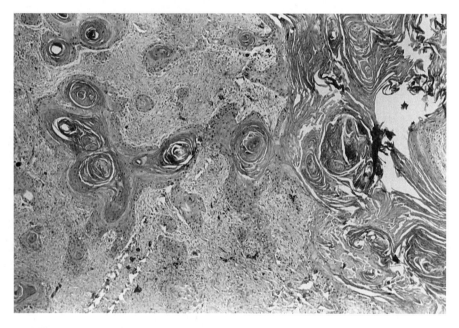

Fig. 77-13. Squamous cell carcinoma of the oral cavity. Keratin pearls can be seen throughout the specimen.

present for prolonged periods. Disseminated neoplasm affects bone and lungs most frequently.

Multiple primary neoplasms

The occurrence of multiple primary neoplasms in patients with head and neck cancer is believed to be as high as 30%. These tumors are described as simultaneous if diagnosed with the primary tumor, synchronous if diagnosed within 6 months, or metachronous if diagnosed more than 6 months after diagnosis of the primary tumor. The frequency of second primary tumors in patients with oral cancer is approximately 18%.[10,38] The second primary tumor occurs in the upper aerodigestive tract in 50% to 75% of cases and is related to the effects of alcohol and tobacco on the mucosa.

It appears that the patients at greatest risk of developing a second primary tumor are those who smoke and drink heavily for many years.[98,124] The risk of developing additional malignancies in patients who discontinue smoking after control of their first malignancy is one sixth the risk for those who continue to smoke.[76] However, this risk does not appear to decrease until 5 years after ceasing the habit, suggesting that carcinogenic factors are long-term influences. The greatest risk of developing a second primary tumor occurs within the first 3 years after therapy for the first cancer.[65,84]

DIAGNOSIS

The most common symptom of cancer of the oral cavity is a persistent sore in the mouth. The diagnosis is frequently delayed, however, probably because pain associated with ulceration occurs rather late in the course of disease. Dentists usually see patients first because of loosening of the teeth or pain around the teeth or in the jaw. Occasionally, dysphagia may be seen, particularly if the tumor is located in the posterior oral cavity or is extending into the oropharynx. A neck mass is seen in one third of patients. Weight loss eventually occurs as the disease progresses, interfering with deglutition.

Physical examination is the key to diagnosing and evaluating oral cavity cancer. Thorough inspection and bimanual palpation assist the physician in assessing the extent of the tumor, particularly in the tongue musculature and the floor of the mouth. Pharyngoscopy and laryngoscopy should be performed to evaluate the tumor's extension into regions of the oropharynx. An adequate biopsy of the lesion allowing assessment of histopathology and invasiveness is mandatory prior to any therapeutic intervention.

Radiologic evaluation is an important adjunct in assessing oral cavity carcinoma that encroaches on the mandible or involves the hard palate. Computed tomography (CT) can be helpful in assessing soft tissue and bony extension of the tumor, particularly when it occurs on the hard palate and concern exists about the tumor extending into the maxillary sinus or the floor of the nose. The pterygopalatine fossa is an important pathway for spread of neoplastic disease originating in the posterior hard palate (Fig. 77-14). The soft-tissue structures and bony landmarks of this region are well demonstrated by CT.

CT is also helpful in assessing extension into the tongue base by tumors arising in the tongue or posterior floor of the mouth. The anatomy of the tongue and floor of the mouth is readily discernible by CT because of low-density fascial planes that outline the extrinsic musculature, lingual arteries, and hypoglossal nerves (Fig. 77-15). The physician must note, however, that normal variation in the structures of the oral pharynx and floor of mouth and particularly the lingual and faucial tonsils may be potential sources of asymmetry and may lead to misinterpretation of the CT scan.[79]

Evaluation of the neck for possible cervical lymph node

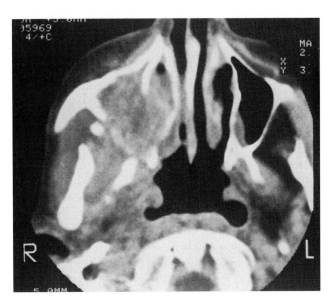

Fig. 77-14. Computed tomography of a patient with cancer of hard palate. Tumor extension into the pterygopalatine fossa is noted, with erosion of the medial and lateral pterygoid plates and posterior aspect of maxillary sinus.

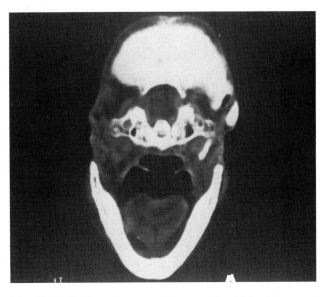

Fig. 77-15. Horizontal computed tomography (CT) of a normal tongue. The anatomy of the tongue and floor of the mouth is readily discernible by CT analysis.

metastases is essential. Physical examination of the neck remains the most common method of staging neck disease. However, palpation has been reported to have a sensitivity of only about 75%. Sensitivity is increased with the use of imaging studies. CT and magnetic resonance imaging have an approximately equal sensitivity (85% to 95%) for diagnosis of nodal metastases.[34a,45] Ultrasound evaluation can identify lymph nodes not palpable by clinical examinations.[12] The criteria used to define a pathologic node will vary the sensitivity and specificity of this technique. Criteria allowing the sensitivity of about 90% can result in specificity as low as 30%.[45] Fine-needle aspiration cytology can be combined with ultrasound to increase specificity to 90%.[144] A recently introduced imaging modality, positron emission tomography (PET), has also been evaluated for identification of cervical nodal metastases. In PET, the radionuclide glucose analog fluorodeoxyglucose is used to identify rapidly dividing cells such as tumor cells. Comparison between PET and standard techniques revealed that PET had an accuracy of 82%, CT 84%, and physical examination 71%.[70] Therefore, PET currently provides no additional information compared with conventional imaging techniques and remains more expensive. With improvements in imaging resolution and the use of agents with greater tumor specificity, PET may become a more important imaging modality in the future.

Differential diagnosis

A number of benign and malignant lesions occasionally may be confused with SCC of the oral cavity. Melanoma of the oral cavity is rare. Melanin-producing melanomas must be differentiated from benign melanosis of mucous membranes. Melanomas demonstrate less tendency for necrotic ulceration than do SCCs. Sarcomas and lymphomas arising anew in soft tissues of the oral cavity are rare and appear as painless, smooth, mucosa-covered masses. Malignant minor salivary gland tumors have a similar appearance and most often occur on the hard palate or floor of the mouth.

Pyogenic granulomas, tuberculous ulcers, and primary or secondary chancres are benign diseases but may be confused occasionally with cancer. Pyogenic granuloma has a bluish-red tint and occurs on the gingiva or tongue protruding above the epithelium similar to a cupola (Fig. 77-16). It bleeds copiously when manipulated and has a softer consistency than cancer.

Extragenital chancres or tuberculous ulcers, which may appear on the lips and the tip of the tongue, can present diagnostic difficulties. The history of a rapidly developing, ulcerated, firm lesion with evidence of spirochetes on dark-field examination should establish the diagnosis of syphilis. Acute tuberculous ulcers can occur on the buccal mucosa and tongue and are associated with an active pulmonary focus. Tuberculous ulcers tend to be less shaggy, more painful, and have less debris in the depth of the ulcer than chancres.

Benign papillomas and keratoacanthomas are typically confused with lip cancer because they are exophytic and occur on the vermilion border or adjacent skin. Papillomas are more exophytic for their size than are carcinomas and tend to be pedunculated. Because the base of the papilloma is situated chiefly in the epithelium of the lip, minimal induration of the lip occurs.

Keratoacanthoma (molluscum sebaceum) can occur on the cutaneous aspect of the lip and can resemble an SCC (Fig. 77-17). These lesions are usually circular with a central crater and may grow rapidly. They have a tendency to regress spontaneously, but malignancy should be suspected until growth has ceased and signs of involution appear. Histologically, they are well circumscribed and have a central keratinizing core.

Two benign lesions of the hard palate may be misinterpreted as malignant: follicular lymphoid hyperplasia and necrotizing sialometaplasia. Follicular lymphoid hyperplasia appears as a slowly growing, nonpainful mass of the hard palate that represents a reactive lymphoid proliferation. Histologically, it closely resembles follicular lymphoma, and both diseases display similar clinical findings. It is impera-

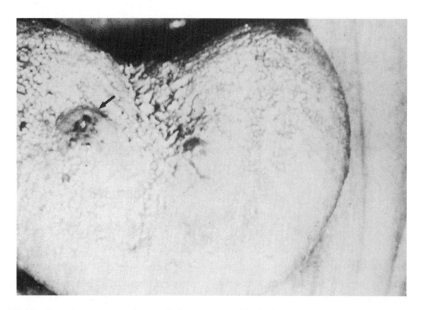

Fig. 77-16. Granuloma pyogenicum of the tongue. This lesion (*arrow*) bleeds copiously when manipulated and has a softer consistency than cancer.

tive that the pathologist be familiar with the features that separate these two entities. In equivocal cases, immunoperoxidase staining helps determine whether the lesion is monoclonal (neoplastic) or polyclonal (reactive).[122]

Similar to follicular lymphoid hyperplasia of the hard palate, necrotizing sialometaplasia is a reactive lesion involving the hard palate and is most frequently is observed in smokers. The lesion may also occur in the floor of the mouth or the buccal mucosa and appears as an ulcerative lesion that is sometimes confused clinically and histologically with SCC. A biopsy differentiates it from SCC and shows inflammation and metaplasia of minor salivary gland tissue with no evidence of malignancy. Necrotizing sialometaplasia is a self-limiting disease that regresses over several weeks.

Granular cell tumor may be seen anywhere in the oral cavity but most frequently occurs in the tongue. This benign tumor consists of pleomorphic cells with granular cytoplasm and has the gross appearance of a firm, nontender, pedunculated or sessile mass.[7] Its most significant feature is the presence of extensive hyperplasia of the overlying surface epithelium in 50% to 65% of cases. This hyperplasia can be misdiagnosed as SCC, particularly if the biopsy is shallow (Fig. 77-18).

CLINICAL STAGING

Grading and staging of neoplasms provide the physician with information regarding the prognosis of cancer. Grading designates the relative differentiation of cells that compose the tumor and has not been found to be highly correlated with prognosis in patients with head and neck cancer. Staging refers to the extent of tumor spread and has been standardized into the tumor, nodes, metastases (TNM) system

by the International Union Against Cancer. The American Joint Committee on Cancer Staging and End Results Reporting (AJCC) was organized in 1959 under the auspices of several professional organizations. Since 1982, cooperation between the two groups has led to a uniform staging system. All references to TNM and staging in this chapter are to the AJCC system (1997).

The purpose of staging cancer of the head and neck is to determine management planning and provide common terminology in reporting end results and in comparing treatment methods. The various TNM categories are grouped into stages that reflect both the extent and prognosis of the tumor. The categories are based almost entirely on the anatomic extent of the tumor determined by inspection, physical examination, imaging studies, and other diagnostic methods. In contrast to staging of cancers in other sites, head and neck cancers are staged before treatment begins and surgical pathologic information is not considered. Regardless of subsequent findings, the original clinical classification cannot be altered if the staging system is to have any clinical significance. Although surgical and pathologic classifications are possible, they are less important in the overall management of cancer.

For the oral cavity the system provides for staging only SCCs. No staging system is perfect because clinical examination requires human judgment with the potential for inherent imperfections. In addition, the present staging system considers only anatomic factors. Other factors such as tumor biology and the immunologic and nutritional status of the host may play an important role in prognosis. These parameters may become important components of future staging systems. Table 77-3 presents the ''T'' classification of oral cavity cancer, which indicates extent of the primary tumor

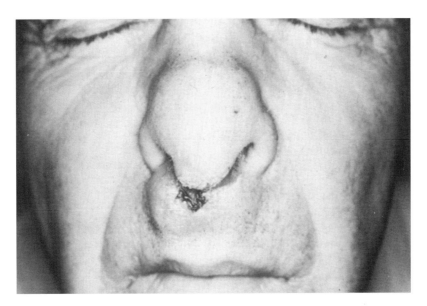

Fig. 77-17. Keratoacanthoma of the upper lip. These lesions often resemble squamous cell carcinoma and may demonstrate rapid growth.

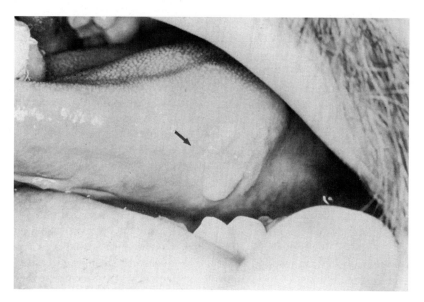

Fig. 77-18. Epithelial hyperplasia (*arrow*) overlying a granular cell tumor of the tongue.

Table 77-3. Primary tumor classification of oral cavity cancer

TNM classification	Description
Primary tumor (T)	
Tx	No available information on primary tumor
T0	No evidence of primary tumor
Tis	Carcinoma *in situ*
T1	Greatest diameter of primary tumor 2 cm or less
T2	Greatest diameter of primary tumor more than 2 cm but not more than 4 cm
T3	Greatest diameter of primary tumor more than 4 cm
T4	Massive tumor more than 4 cm in diameter with deep invasion involving antrum, pterygoid muscles, base of tongue, and skin of neck

Data from Fleming ID, editor: *AJCC cancer staging manual,* ed 5, Philadelphia, 1997, Lippincott-Raven.

Table 77-4. Metastatic tumor classification of oral cavity cancer

TNM classification	Description
Nodal involvement (N)	
NX	Regional lymph nodes cannot be assessed
N_0	No regional lymph node metastases
N_1	Metastases in a single ipsilateral lymph node, 3 cm or less in greatest dimension
N_2	Metastases in a single ipsilateral lymph node, more than 3 cm but not more than 6 cm in greatest dimension; or none more than 6 cm in greatest dimension; or in bilateral or contralateral lymph nodes, none more than 6 cm in greatest dimension
N_{2a}	Metastases in single ipsilateral lymph node, more than 3 cm but not more than 6 cm in greatest dimension
N_{2b}	Metastases in multiple ipsilateral lymph nodes, none more than 6 cm in greatest dimension
N_{2c}	Metastases in bilateral or contralateral lymph nodes, none more than 6 cm in greatest dimension
N_3	Metastases in a lymph node more than 6 cm in greatest dimension

Data from Fleming ID, editor: *AJCC cancer staging manual,* ed 5, Philadelphia, 1997, Lippincott-Raven.

as determined by its size. T_1 tumors are 2 cm or less in greatest diameter, T_2 are between 2 and 4 cm, T_3 are larger than 4 cm, and T_4 represent massive tumors larger than 4 cm in diameter with deep invasion involving structures outside the oral cavity.

Clinical classification of cervical lymph nodes is the same for oral cavity cancer as for carcinoma of all other head and neck areas (Table 77-4). The clinical evaluation is based on the actual size of the nodal mass as measured, recognizing that most nodes larger than 3 cm in diameter are not single but confluent nodes or represent direct tumor extension into soft tissues of the neck. Clinically positive nodes are classified as N_1, N_2, or N_3. Midline nodes are considered ipsilateral. Metastases to lymph nodes peripheral to the head

and neck, such as the axilla or mediastinum, are considered distant metastases. The status of distant metastatic disease is denoted by the "M" classification (Table 77-4). Distant metastases are uncommon among patients who first have oral cavity cancers.

The clinical stage grouping for oral cavity cancer is depicted in Table 77-5. Stages I and II represent tumors con-

Table 77-5. Clinical stage groupings of oral cavity cancer

Stage	Description		
Stage 0	Tis	N0	M0
Stage I	T1	N0	M0
Stage II	T2	N0	M0
Stage III	T3	N0	M0
	T1	N1	M0
	T2	N1	M0
	T3	N1	M0
Stage IVA	T4	N0	M0
	T4	N1	M0
	Any T	N2	M0
Stage IVB	Any T	N3	M0
Stage IVC	Any T	Any N	M1

Data from Fleming ID, editor: *AJCC cancer staging manual,* ed 5, Philadelphia, 1997, Lippincott-Raven.

fined to the primary site. Stage III denotes large primary tumors or represents a single ipsilateral cervical metastases 3 cm or less in diameter. Stage IV disease represents massive primary tumor or more extensive regional or distant metastases.

MANAGEMENT

A number of therapeutic modalities are currently available for the management of oral cavity cancer. The most important of these include surgical excision, radiotherapy, chemotherapy, or a combination of these modalities. The treatment employed depends on the tumor's extent and location, the patient's physical and social status, and the physician's experience and skill. Generally, either surgery or irradiation is successful in controlling small tumors confined to the site of origin (stage I). The main advantage of radiotherapy is the avoidance of surgery, anesthesia, and their associated risks. Radiotherapy is particularly advantageous for ill-defined neoplasms located posteriorly that make surgical exposure and resection more difficult. The major disadvantage of radiotherapy is the often permanent xerostomia and dysgeusia. Full-mouth tooth extractions may be required before instituting therapy to avoid the risk of progressive deterioration of the teeth (Fig. 77-19) and the development of osteoradionecrosis. Xerostomia may prevent some patients from wearing dentures following radiotherapy. Radiotherapy can also have a significant social and economic impact as a result of the daily treatments required for an extended period.

Small, anteriorly located cancers of the oral cavity may be surgically resected even with the patient under local anesthesia. This procedure is often easier on the patient and requires less time than radiotherapy. The surgical defect may be closed primarily, skin grafted, or allowed to heal by secondary management without significant functional impairment. The advantages of surgery include the avoidance of xerostomia and the rapid rehabilitation of the patient. The major disadvantage is the functional disability, which is di-

rectly related to the extent of resection of the mandible or tongue.

Radiotherapy

There are four general principles governing the use of radiotherapy in the management of oral cancer[118]: (1) most SCCs are radioresponsive, although high doses of radiation are required for local control; (2) well-oxygenated neoplasms are more radioresponsive than hypoxic ones; (3) bone or deep muscle invasion decreases radiocurability; and (4) large cervical metastases are better managed by neck dissection, with or without adjunctive radiotherapy.

Radiotherapy is indicated when survival is equal to and morbidity is less than surgery alone or combined therapy. Radiotherapy can be given as external-beam management, interstitial therapy (brachytherapy), or a combination of the two. The total dose of radiotherapy for oral carcinomas is usually in the range of 65 to 75 Gy. The dose may be modified according to the tolerance level of the patient. The goal is to maximize local control but minimize complications such as osteoradionecrosis.

Conventional fractionation external-beam radiotherapy is usually administered at a dose of 1.8 to 2.0 Gy per fraction five times per week. The fractionation schedule may have a significant impact on locoregional control. Fraction size is known to be the major factor in determining late effects or complications. Altered fractionation is used to improve locoregional control while decreasing the risks of late complications. Hyperfractionation involves smaller than conventional dose fractions given twice a day to a greater total dose. A prospective, randomized comparison of conventional fractionation versus hyperfractionation showed a significant improvement in locoregional control in the hyperfractionation group.[42] In contrast, another randomized trial showed no difference in locoregional control but did show an increased rate of complications associated with hyperfractionation.[66] Results from the Radiation Therapy Oncology Group (RTOG) randomized study of standard fractionation compared with three different methods of hyperfractionation (RTOG 9003) are pending. Presently, it is unclear whether hyperfractionation enhances locoregional control, and there are indications that it may even increase the incidence of late complications.

The dose of external-beam radiotherapy used for head and neck carcinoma is often limited by the exposure and tolerance of surrounding normal tissues. Computer based three-dimensional conformal treatment planning can be used to limit the dose given to surrounding normal tissue while increasing the dose to the tumor. Theoretically, this should allow increased tumor control with decreased complications. Further studies are needed to determine whether a clear benefit exists compared with traditional two-dimensional treatment planning.

Interstitial irradiation (brachytherapy) is frequently used in combination with external radiotherapy to treat cancers

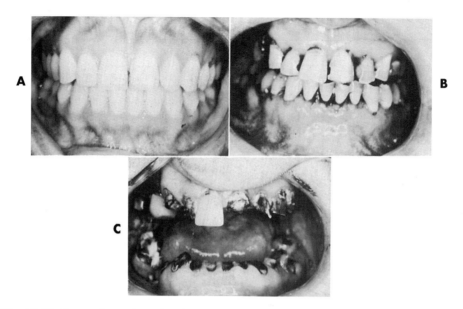

Fig. 77-19. Progressive carious deterioration of the teeth after full-course radiotherapy for the treatment of oral cancer. **A,** Before radiotherapy. **B,** Twelve months after radiotherapy. **C,** Twenty-four months after treatment. The single remaining tooth is a cap. (Courtesy of John G Knapp, DDS, MS, Livonia, Mich.)

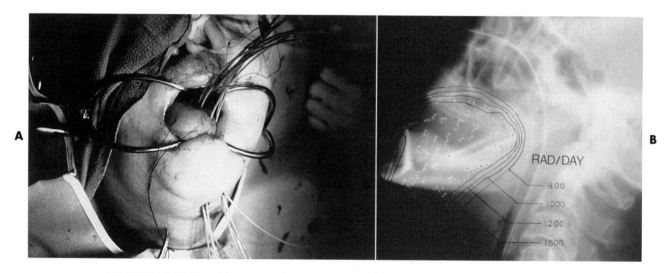

Fig. 77-20. A, Patient with squamous cell carcinoma of the tongue treated with brachytherapy using hollow tubes that are later loaded with a radiation source. **B,** Simulation film with isodose distribution. (Courtesy of Subir Nag, MD, Columbus, Ohio.)

of the tongue and floor of the mouth (Fig. 77-20). Much larger doses are given to the tumor than to the surrounding region with use of temporary implants of iridium-192 via hollow catheters and afterloading techniques.

Prophylactic neck irradiation

Management of the clinically negative neck in patients with primary SCC of the oral cavity remains an active debate. Occult metastases consist of microfoci tumors in cervical nodes that are not clinically detectable. The incidence of occult metastases varies with site and size of the primary tumor in the oral cavity and ranges from 15% to 60%.[62,120] Prophylactic neck irradiation can be used for the treatment of occult metastases. Reports indicate that radiotherapy of the clinically negative neck to a level of 50 to 55 Gy will control occult disease and prevent later occurrence of cervical metastases.[30,73] Provided the primary cancer remains controlled, development of cervical nodal disease occurs in less than 5% of oral cavity cancer patients undergoing prophylactic neck irradiation.[3,72,91] This statistic is in contrast to an expected 25% failure rate in patients initially having N0 classified necks and receiving no neck treatment.

Prophylactic irradiation of the neck relieves the patient of the functional and cosmetic deformity of neck dissection. Neck fibrosis is not a serious problem when 50 Gy are administered over 5 weeks; however, xerostomia may occur as a result of encompassing submandibular and parotid glands in the irradiated fields. Although prophylactic neck irradiation appears to be at least as effective as elective neck dissection in the management of occult neck disease, prospective randomized studies are needed for conclusive evidence in support of one modality or the other.

Surgery

Local surgical excision may be used for malignancies of the oral cavity measuring 2 cm or less. Most small oral cavity cancers can be exposed and resected perorally. Tumors extending toward or into the oropharynx may require a mandibulotomy for adequate exposure. Improved local control may be obtained by the use of Mohs' histographic surgical resection of the primary lesion.[26] In the previously untreated lesion, this technique may allow identification and resection of contiguous tumor extensions that are missed by gross surgical margins and standard frozen-section analysis. Prospective, randomized trials are needed to determine the efficacy of this technique.

Surgical resection is often recommended for patients with oral carcinoma who use excessive tobacco and alcohol and who admit that they will not reduce or stop this consumption after treatment. Persistent severe mucositis and edema of the mucous membranes are observed when such patients are treated with radiotherapy. These patients are at high risk for developing additional primary tumors of the upper aerodigestive tract. If the initial tumor is small, surgery alone would reserve radiotherapy for use in a combined regimen to manage subsequent primary neoplasms that might warrant management of greater magnitude.

Carcinomas of the oral cavity with invasion of the mandible are less radiocurable than are neoplasms confined to soft tissue. Thus when a neoplasm directly invades the mandible, surgery is the preferred treatment. Conventional radiography, including dental panorex views, is helpful in determining invasion of bone, although normal radiographic findings do not preclude bone involvement. As many as 30% of patients who have oral cavity cancer encroaching on the mandible and normal radiographic findings have microscopic invasion of bone. Bone scanning with technetium-99m–phosphate is sensitive enough to be positive in bone involved with tumor before these lesions can be detected by conventional radiographic examination. However, specificity to differentiate between tumor, infection, trauma, and inflammation is lacking.

The high incidence of microscopic invasion of the periosteum and cortical layer of the mandible even with normal radiographic findings has warranted guidelines for surgical management of the mandible. Tumors that encroach on the mandible and do not provide a margin of 1.5 cm of normal tissue between tumor and bone usually require resection of at least a portion of the mandible (Fig. 77-21). Depending on the location of the neoplasm, a marginal resection of the upper portion of the mandible or resection of the inner or outer cortical plate of the jaw may provide an adequate margin around the tumor while still preserving mandibular continuity. Direct invasion of the mandible demonstrable by radiography requires a full-thickness segmental resection of the mandible. Samples of the inferior alveolar nerve from the remaining mandibular segment along with samples of cancellous bone should be submitted for frozen-section analysis to check for tumor tracking in the medullary portion of the mandible. These specimens can be evaluated by standard frozen-section analysis for carcinoma. This method has been shown to have an excellent correlation to permanent section analysis of the decalcified mandibular specimen.[32]

Preservation of the bony architecture of the jaw is particularly important in the region of the anterior arch to preserve facial contour and deglutitional function through continued support of the lip, tongue, and floor of the mouth. The arch is preserved when possible by marginal resection. Complete preservation of the mandible is possible using pull-through resections when it is not necessary to include a portion of the mandible to conform to *en bloc* procedures (Fig. 77-22). Combining the peroral and transcervical approaches obviates the need to perform a mandibular osteotomy for surgical access when performing an *en bloc* resection of oral cavity cancer.

In other instances, mandibular osteotomy is performed to allow improved exposure and access to oral cavity lesions. The advantages include wide surgical exposure enabling complete *en bloc* resection of the lesion and reconstruction of the defect while maintaining sensation to the lower lip. Disadvantages include a lip-splitting incision, the need to fixate the mandibular osteotomy site, and the possible loss of teeth. Although a variety of lip-splitting incisions have been advocated, the midline and circummental incisions are the most common. The midline incision creates the least amount of alteration of sensation because of its ability to avoid damage to the mental nerve and its branches (Fig. 77-23). Good cosmetic results can be obtained with either incision with good surgical technique (Fig. 77-24). The mandibular osteotomy can be performed in the midline or paramedian position. Location of the tumor and gaps in dentition guide the location of the osteotomy. Care must be taken to avoid injuring tooth roots when cutting the mandible. A variety of osteotomies including a stair step, chevron style, or vertical have been championed in the past. However, with the use of modern plating systems and surgical saws, this is no longer a major issue.

Resection of the anterior arch of the mandible results in disability that is directly related to the amount of bone re-

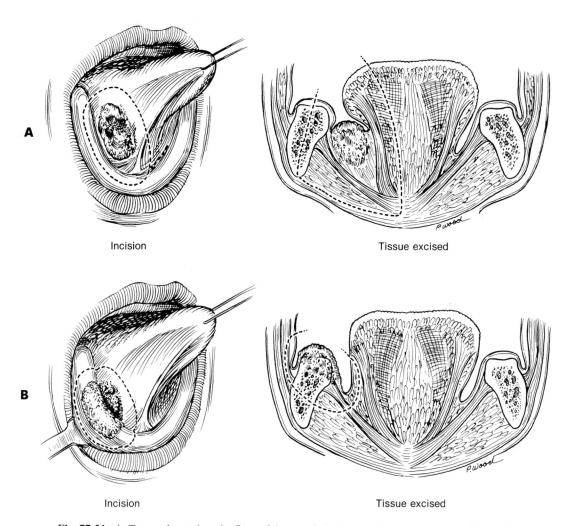

Fig. 77-21. **A,** Tumors located on the floor of the mouth that encroach on mandible usually require resection of at least the inner cortical plate of the mandible to ensure adequate surgical margins. **B,** Tumor extension onto the gingiva without evidence of bone erosion on radiographic examination may be resected with the upper margin of the mandible while still preserving continuity of jaw.

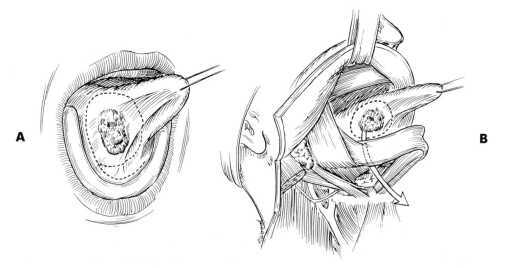

Fig. 77-22. Complete preservation of the mandible is possible using pull-through resections when it is not necessary to include a portion of mandible to conform to *en bloc* procedures. **A,** Tumor in the tongue and floor of the mouth. **B,** Pull-through resection.

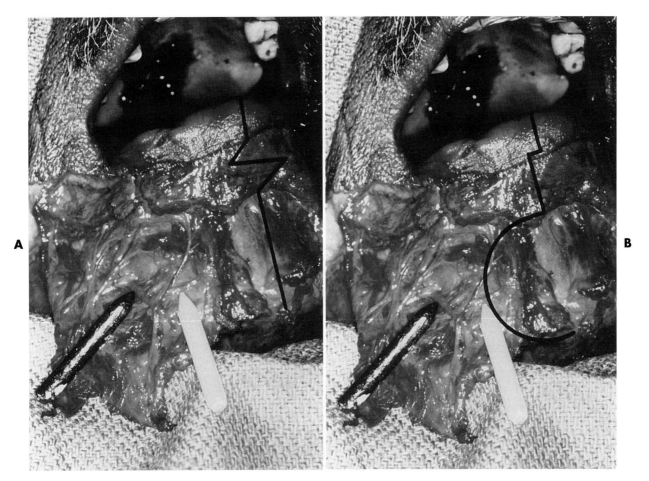

Fig. 77-23. A, Midline incision avoids the mental nerve (V3) and its branches as shown in this dissection. **B,** Circummental incision avoids V3 but will sever the medial branches. (Courtesy of Michael Sullivan, MD, Columbus, Ohio.)

moved (Fig. 77-25). In most instances, primary reconstruction of the mandible is necessary to restore function and cosmesis. In contrast, lateral resection of the mandible produces only moderate disability, and reconstruction for restoration of function is easily performed. A reconstruction bar can be used to span the bony defect maintaining proper alignment of the mandibular fragments. This allows accurate occlusion to be maintained.

Largely because of the potential for bony involvement, cancers of the hard palate are generally managed by surgery. Removal of portions of the maxilla and upper alveolus may be necessary to encompass the neoplasm. Small tumors can be resected perorally. Subtotal maxillectomy may require an extended sublabial incision that allows mobilization of the upper lip and cheek on both sides to expose the entire maxilla (Fig. 77-26). Full-thickness resection of the hard palate results in a fenestration of the nasal passage or maxillary sinus. Oral prostheses are very effective in obturating the hard palate and can be attached to removable partial or full upper dentures (Fig. 77-27).

Surgery is indicated in patients who have completed a full course of radiotherapy and demonstrate persistent tumor or suffer recurrence at the primary site or in the neck. Incomplete healing of the primary site immediately following full-course radiotherapy should be observed closely, allowing 8 to 12 weeks to elapse before biopsy. If tumor is persistent, *en bloc* resection is indicated, including the entire area of the original tumor. If clinically positive lymphadenopathy was present before irradiation, neck dissection is also performed. If radiotherapy controls the primary tumor but the patient continues to have palpable lymphadenopathy, neck dissection without resection of the primary site is indicated.

Neck dissection

The clinical distribution of cervical lymph node metastases from SCC of the upper aerodigestive tract was described by Lindberg.[60] Oral cavity lesions were found most commonly to have subdigastric (upper jugular), submaxillary triangle, and midjugular lymph node involvement. Low jugular and posterior triangle lymph node metastases were

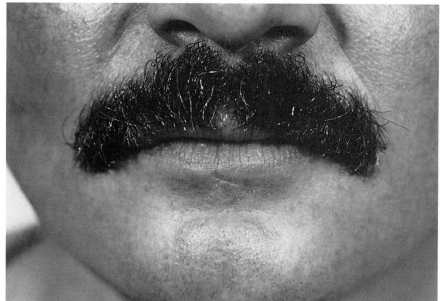

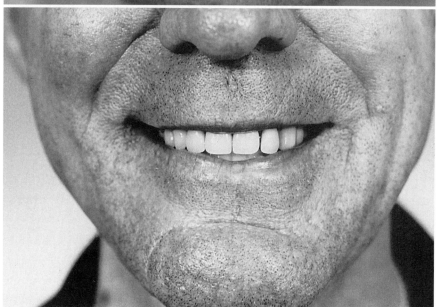

Fig. 77-24. Midline and circummental incisions have good cosmetic results when good surgical technique is used. (Courtesy of Michael Sullivan, MD, Columbus, Ohio.)

rarely found. This predictable pattern of cervical metastases in previously untreated patients allows for modifications of the classic radical neck dissection.

Patients with clinically negative necks but extensive primary lesions (T2, T3, or T4) have a high probability of neck metastases. Selective *en bloc* removal of the lymph nodes most likely to harbor metastases is performed by a supraomohyoid neck dissection (zone I, II and III). Patients with no evidence of metastases can be spared radiotherapy. Patients found to have metastases have improved regional control of disease with the addition of radiotherapy.[71] A recent report described patients with oral cavity cancers who developed cervical node metastases at zone IV without evidence of metastases at zone I, II, or III.[17] These ''skip metas-

tases'' were found in 15.8% of the patients. The authors recommended an extended supraomohyoid neck dissection (zones I through IV) as the most effective staging neck dissection. In the clinical N0 neck, an extended supraomohyoid neck dissection provides the same information as a radical neck dissection in directing postoperative radiotherapy with lower morbidity and equivalent disease control.

Patients with clinically detectable neck disease (N1, N2, or N3) require a comprehensive neck dissection for optimal disease control. A modified neck dissection sparing the spinal accessory nerve can be performed if the neck disease is not in the proximity of the nerve. However, with oral cavity lesions, cervical lymph node metastases are often located in the upper jugular region, preventing the preservation

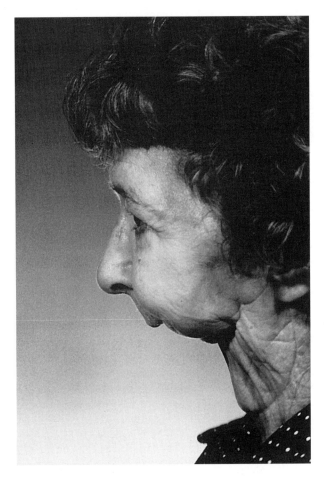

Fig. 77-25. "Gump" deformity created by mandibular resection. Reconstruction is necessary to maintain oral function.

of the spinal accessory nerve. Patients with clinically detectable neck disease should undergo postoperative radiotherapy to optimize regional disease control.

Lesions located in the midline may cause bilateral metastases. It is therefore important to address both sides of the neck. If both are clinically N0, bilateral extended supraomohyoid neck dissections can be performed as staging procedures. Bilateral comprehensive neck dissections should be performed if bilateral disease is noted.

Combined therapy

Most physicians have advocated the combination of radiotherapy and surgery in treating advanced stage III and IV disease of the oral cavity in hopes of reducing local recurrence and improving survival rates. Preoperative radiotherapy has been shown to reduce neck recurrence.[109] Improved results also have been noted when using preoperative radiotherapy in the management of supraglottic laryngeal and pharyngeal carcinoma.[9,39] Postoperative radiotherapy has also been shown to be effective in increasing locoregional control in advanced (stage III or IV) SCC of the head and neck.[116]

Preoperative irradiation usually consists of 45 to 50 Gy delivered at 2.0 Gy per day. Surgery is initiated after a 4-week interval following radiotherapy. Resection encompasses a 1.5-cm margin of normal tissue around the entire area of the neoplasm, as determined before the administration of radiotherapy. Theoretic advantages of preoperative irradiation in combined therapy include the following: (1) tumor cells may have better oxygenation before surgery and thus be more sensitive to irradiation; (2) malignant cells at the periphery of the neoplasm are destroyed; (3) tumor seeding at the time of resection may be decreased; and (4) there

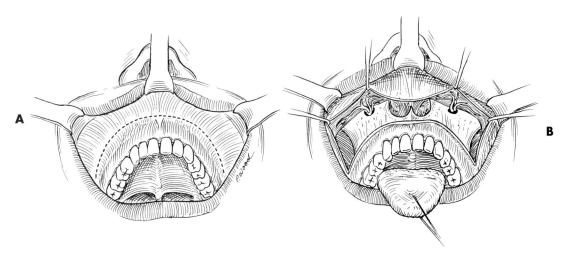

Fig. 77-26. A, Extended sublabial incision allows mobilization of the upper lip and cheek on both sides for excellent exposure of the entire hard palate. **B,** Elevation of tissue, exposing the maxilla.

may be fewer and less viable cells intravascularly and within lymphatics at the time of surgery, which could lower the frequency of distant metastases.

The disadvantages of preoperative radiotherapy center around wound healing problems, which increase as preoperative doses exceed 40 Gy. An increased incidence of tissue necrosis, wound infection, and fistula formation occurs when surgery is performed in a radiated region. Because of fibrosis, inflammation, and decreased blood supply, reconstruction usually is more difficult. An additional disadvantage of preoperative radiotherapy is that changes in the size of the neoplasm as well as general inflammatory responses elicited by the radiotherapy may obscure tumor margins.

Postoperative radiotherapy is begun 3 to 4 weeks following surgery. Theoretic advantages of postoperative irradiation include (1) safer administration of a higher total dose of irradiation; (2) destruction of subclinical residual tumor, which may remain following surgery; (3) fewer wound infections; (4) distinct tumor margins, facilitating more accurate and complete surgical removal; and (5) the ability to direct radiation to specific areas observed intraoperatively where tumor-free surgical margins are questionable.

The major disadvantage of postoperative radiation is that theoretically surgery may interrupt the blood supply of the remaining tumor cells and lessen their sensitivity to radiotherapy. Wound breakdown or other operative complications may delay the onset or prevent the delivery of radiotherapy.

The RTOG undertook a prospective randomized trial (RTOG 73-03) that compared planned preoperative versus planned postoperative radiotherapy for locally advanced SCC of the oral cavity and oropharynx.[56] Analysis of the data revealed a significant advantage in locoregional dis-

ease control for postoperative radiotherapy as compared with preoperative radiotherapy. There was also a trend in improving overall survival. Conventional treatment of advanced carcinoma of the head and neck in the United States currently involves surgical resection with postoperative radiotherapy.

Special precautions are taken for patients with oral cavity cancer who undergo combined therapy. Dental evaluation, including instruction in oral care, should be done before radiation. When the mouth or pharynx is exposed in combination with neck dissection, dermal grafting of the carotid artery is indicated.

Early complications of combined therapy include mucositis and poor nutritional maintenance. In the case of preoperative radiotherapy, wound infection, fistula, flap necrosis, and carotid rupture may occur. Late complications are usually chronic and the result of radiotherapy. These include xerostomia, rampant dental caries, and osteoradionecrosis.

Chemotherapy

Chemotherapy for head and neck carcinoma can be given in a variety of settings. Chemotherapy can be given alone as a curative treatment, although this has not been shown to be effective and is not recommended. Chemotherapy can be used for palliation for unresectable disease or distant metastases although the toxicities can have a significant impact on quality-of-life. Combined therapy with the use of surgery, radiotherapy, and chemotherapy for advanced lesions is an area of active investigation. A variety of agents have been used, including cisplatin, 5-fluorouracil, methotrexate, bleomycin, paclitaxel, and topotecan.

Chemotherapy given before other methods of treatment is called *neoadjuvant* or *induction chemotherapy*. The South-

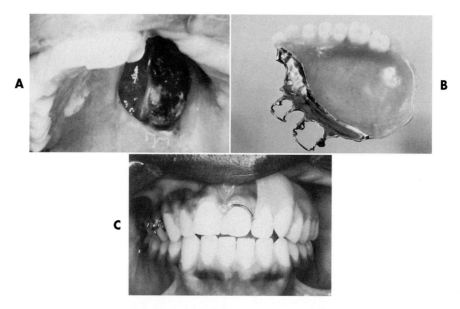

Fig. 77-27. A, Palatal defect following resection of cancer of the hard palate. **B,** Oral prosthesis used to obturate a palatal defect. **C,** Prosthesis in place.

west Oncology Group conducted a prospective randomized trial of 158 patients with advanced SCC of the head and neck.[98a] The conventional treatment group received surgery and postoperative radiotherapy. The experimental arm received induction chemotherapy consisting of cisplatin, vincristine, methotrexate, and bleomycin followed by surgical resection and postoperative radiotherapy. The final analysis demonstrated no benefit in survival with the use of induction chemotherapy. Other randomized studies evaluating induction chemotherapy have also failed to show any survival benefit.[43]

Adjuvant chemotherapy involves the use of chemotherapy in conjunction with other treatments. The Head and Neck Cancer Intergroup compared conventional surgery and postoperative radiotherapy with surgery and three cycles of cisplatin and 5-fluorouracil followed by radiotherapy.[58] This adjuvant chemotherapy trial failed to show any difference in survival between the groups. However, this study did reveal a decreased incidence of distant metastases in the experimental group.

Chemotherapy agents can also be given concurrently with radiotherapy. This may result in a radiosensitizing effect and improved locoregional control. Trials have shown improvement in local control with a trend toward improved survival, but with significantly increased toxicity.[41]

CANCER OF THE LIP

The incidence of carcinoma of the lip in the United States is 1.8 in 100,000.[113] The disease occurs most frequently on the lower lip of elderly men. Cancer most frequently originates in the exposed vermilion border just outside the line of contact with the upper lip. Tumors on the upper lip, which frequently arise near the midline, account for 2% to 8% of all lip cancers.[53,119] Tumors arising from the commissure represent less than 1% of reported cases.[61,121] More than one third of patients with carcinoma of the lip have outdoor occupations[4]; prolonged exposure to sunlight has been implicated as a major etiologic factor. The lip is susceptible to actinic changes because it lacks a pigmented layer for protection. Blacks have pigment in the lips, which may explain the rare occurrence of carcinoma of the lip in this population.

Most neoplasms of the lip are SCC. The remainder of the malignant epithelial neoplasms originate from the minor salivary gland, predominantly adenoid cystic carcinoma, adenocarcinoma, or mucoepidermoid carcinoma.

The two most common morphologic types of SCC of the lip are exophytic and ulcerative. The exophytic type is slightly more common than the ulcerative, grows superficially, and tends to metastasize late. The superficial portion of the tumor eventually becomes necrotic, and frank ulceration usually occurs when the lesion has reached 1 cm. The ulcerative type begins like the exophytic type, as an epithelial thickening; however, ulceration occurs earlier (Fig. 77-28). The tumor manifests a relatively greater tendency for rapid infiltration and invasion and is usually of a higher histologic grade than the exophytic type.

Diagnosis

Carcinoma of the lip tends to have a protracted course. In early stages it usually demonstrates rather indolent behavior, and frequently the only symptom is a blister or induration arising in an area of leukoplakia. A history of recurrent lip crusting that bleeds readily on removal is characteristic of this lesion. Such crusting may exist for many years before evidence of infiltration develops.

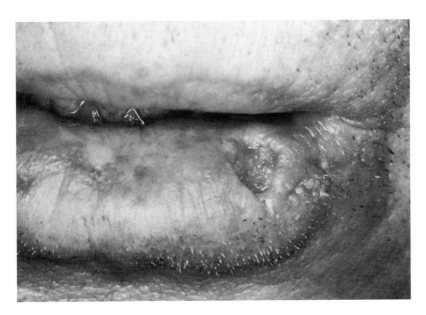

Fig. 77-28. Ulcerative squamous cell carcinoma of the lower lip.

As carcinoma of the lip progresses, involvement of the mandible may occur. The patient must be closely examined for hypesthesia in the distribution of the mental nerve. Even in the absence of cortical bone destruction, tumor may grow along the mental nerve into the medullary portion of the mandible. Perineural invasion or direct extension from mandibular involvement may spread the neoplasm to the mental nerve.

Carcinomas of the upper lip and commissure grow more rapidly, ulcerate sooner, and metastasize earlier than lower lip cancer. Lesions larger than 2 cm or involving the upper lip or extending to the lateral commissure thus have a poorer prognosis. Mandibular involvement with the tumor also results in a poor prognosis and a higher incidence of regional metastases.

Cervical metastases occur in less than 10% of patients with SCC of the lower lip.[53,63] Approximately 20% of patients with cancer of the commissure have cervical metastases on initial evaluation.[63] Subsequent development of cervical metastases following treatment of carcinoma of the lip ranges from 5% to 15%.[53] Most metastases appear within 2 years following treatment of the primary tumor. The likelihood of their occurrence increases with increased duration and size of the primary tumor and with repeated local recurrences.

As a rule, metastases occur later in the course of disease with lip cancer than with malignancies found in other sites within the oral cavity; further dissemination also tends to occur later. When tumors occur in the midportion of the lower lip, the submental nodes are usually involved first; whereas when tumors arise on the lateral portion of the lip, the submandibular triangle nodes are involved most frequently. Metastatic spread from upper-lip carcinomas tends to occur first to the preauricular and periparotid lymph nodes. Spread then occurs to the submandibular nodes and upper deep jugular nodes more rapidly than is seen with lower-lip tumors. Contralateral or bilateral metastases may develop when the primary lesion is near or crosses the midline of the lip.

Management

Small carcinomas of the lip may be managed successfully by either surgery or radiation; the results are cosmetically acceptable with both methods. Radiation treatment consists of brachytherapy or external beam radiotherapy. Regardless of the form of radiotherapy used, care must be taken to protect uninvolved tissues by the use of a cutout lead shield. The shield limits the beam to the desired region of the tumor and confines the side effects of radiomucositis and radiodermatitis to a minimal area of the lip.

Small tumors of the lip may be treated surgically by making a V-shaped excision and performing primary closure. A full-thickness, wedge-shaped excision of a tumor with at least a 0.5-cm normal tissue margin beyond the recognized limits of the tumor can be performed with the patient under local anesthesia. Larger lesions can be excised by making a W-shaped excision and closing primarily. Surgery offers the advantage of eradication of disease, pathologic survey of margins, and reconstruction of the defect in a single procedure and avoids radiation-induced complications. Advanced tumors should be managed by a combination of surgery and radiotherapy.

Cervical metastases should be managed surgically, which offers a 5-year control rate of 50%. If neck dissection confirms the presence of histologically positive nodes, postoperative radiotherapy should be considered. Elective neck dissection for occult metastatic disease is not indicated because the percentage of patients who subsequently develop cervical metastases following treatment of the primary tumor is less than 10%.[25,37,61]

Results

The extent of disease governs the prognosis for cure in carcinoma of the lip. Tumors less than 2 cm in diameter that involve the lower lip have an excellent prognosis. Cure rates for T1 and T2 lesions without evidence of cervical node metastases generally are greater than 90% when surgery or radiotherapy is performed (Table 77-6).[5] If the population with lip cancer is considered as a total group, the 5-year disease-specific survival rate is approximately 80% in a combined series of 10,230 patients.

The incidence of recurrent disease increases and the cure rate drops significantly in large cancers of the lip (Fig. 77-29).[5] This is partly a result of the magnitude of the primary tumor and the higher incidence of metastases. Control of cervical metastases is more difficult. The overall curability of patients with cancer of the lip and regional metastases approaches 50%.[25,53,64,74] The poorest results are obtained when radiographic evidence of mandibular involvement by the primary tumor exists and when cervical node metastases are fixed to the deep structures of the neck. A statistical review of 3166 patients with confirmed SCC demonstrated that when regional nodes were not involved on the patient's admission, the primary tumor was controlled in 93% of patients. Of the patients with lymph node involvement on admission, the primary tumor was controlled in 75%; however, control of cervical metastases was achieved only in 59% of patients.[63]

Table 77-6. Relationship between treatment and survival for T_{1s}, T_1, and T_2 squamous cell carcinoma of lip

	Patients (n)	Determinate survival (%)	
		3 years	5 years
Surgery	143	96.7	95.3
Radiation	108	95.8	95.2

Adapted from Baker SR, Krause CJ: *Laryngoscope* 90:19, 1980; and American Joint Committee on Cancer, 1980.

CANCER OF THE ORAL TONGUE

The oral tongue is the mobile portion of the tongue anterior to the circumvallate papillae. It is the second most common site, after the lip, of oral cavity malignancies. Three fourths of all tongue cancers occur in the oral tongue. SCC comprises 97% of all malignant tumors. The disease predominates in men and has a peak incidence in the sixth and seventh decades of life. Cancer of the tongue has been correlated with poor oral hygiene, alcohol and tobacco use, and syphilitic glossitis. It is also associated with cirrhosis and Plummer-Vinson syndrome.[113a]

Infiltrative and exophytic are the two most common morphologic types of cancer involving the oral tongue. Exophytic types have less tendency to infiltrate deeply. Early in the disease they appear as an area of focal thickening or clinical leukoplakia or as a painless superficial ulceration. The infiltrative type may show minimal or no surface ulceration until late in its development. SCC of the oral tongue tends to be better differentiated than cancers of the tongue base and is usually grade I or II (moderately well differentiated).

Carcinoma of the oral tongue most commonly arises from the lateral border of the middle third of the tongue; approximately 45% of all tongue cancers occur here (Fig. 77-30). In contrast, 20% of cancers occur in the anterior third and only 4% on the dorsum of the tongue.[34]

Cervical metastases occur more frequently from cancer of the tongue than from any other site within the oral cavity. Forty percent of patients have nodal metastases on admission.[128] In contrast to tumors of the tongue base, bilateral or contralateral metastases are uncommon, but they may be present when the tumor involves the midline of the tongue.

Metastases usually occur first in the upper deep jugular (subdigastric) lymph nodes and then spread downward along the jugular chain. Tumors arising from the anterior third of the tongue tend to metastasize slightly less frequently than those arising from the middle third.[7] Unlike in the lip, the size of the primary lesion in tongue cancer is not necessarily correlated with the presence or likelihood of cervical metastases.

Diagnosis

The intrinsic musculature of the tongue provides a minimal barrier to tumor growth (Fig. 77-31), and thus malignancies may grow to considerable size before causing symptoms. In the early stages, carcinoma of the tongue often is asymptomatic. Pain usually is not an early symptom and does not occur until branches of the lingual nerve become directly involved with neoplasm. Pain may either occur in the tongue or be referred to the ipsilateral ear. Referred ear pain is caused by the common origin from the trigeminal nerve (V3) of the lingual nerve, which supplies sensation to the oral tongue, and the auriculotemporal nerve, which supplies sensation to the external auditory canal and tympanic membrane.

Overall, approximately 30% of patients initially have symptoms of pain.[34] In 10% of cases growth is rapid with minimal discomfort, so initial symptoms are a lump or mass in the mouth. Approximately 5% of patients complain of dysphagia, and 6% note an enlarged cervical lymph node. The presence of bleeding, slurred speech, and dysphagia suggest far-advanced disease.

Most cancers of the tongue are at least 2 cm in diameter when first seen. Neoplasms arising from the ventral aspect

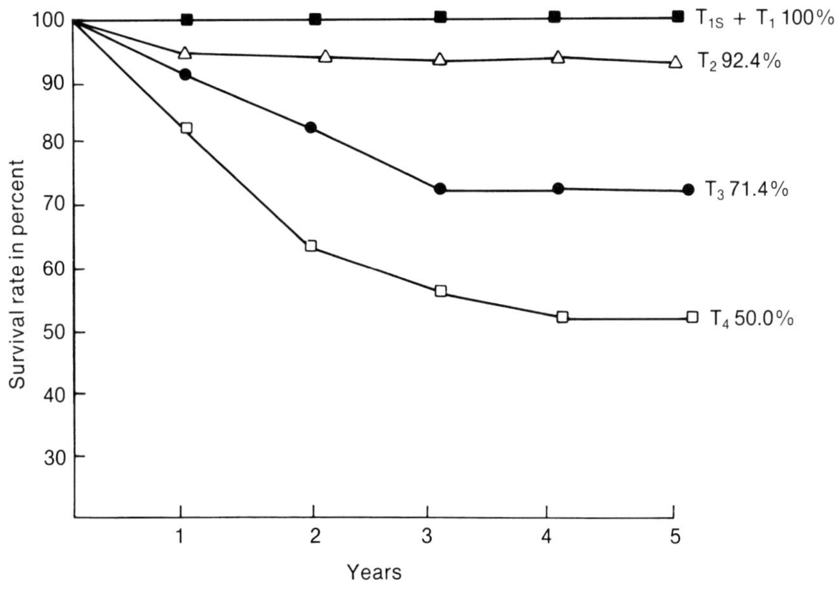

Fig. 77-29. Determinant survival curves for T1 to T4 squamous cell carcinoma of lips. (From Baker SR, Krause CJ: *Laryngoscope* 90:19, 1980.)

Table 77-8. Local control at 2 years in patients with squamous cell carcinoma of the oral tongue

T Stage	Radiotherapy alone	Surgery alone or combined with radiotherapy	P Value
T1	79%	76%	.76
T2	72%	76%	.86
T3	45%	82%	.03
T4	0%	67%	.08

Adapted from Fein DA and others: *Head Neck* 16:360, 1994.

managed by brachytherapy and external beam radiotherapy. Surgery was the most common method used to manage neck nodes.

A comparison of curative radiotherapy versus surgical resection (with or without radiotherapy) was recently reported.[31] The rates of local control were equivalent in patients with T1 and T2 lesions. However, patients with T3 or T4 lesions had a lower rate of local control when treated by radiotherapy alone (Table 77-8). The authors concluded that surgical resection was the best option for T1 and T2 lesions and combined therapy was indicated for advanced lesions or those early lesions with unfavorable pathologic findings.

Trends in survival rates of patients with cancer of the oral tongue were reported in a clinical study from Memorial Sloan-Kettering Cancer Center.[80] The authors reported determinate 5-year survival rates of 82% and 49% for stages I and II and stages III and IV, respectively, for 297 patients treated between 1978 and 1987. This was compared with determinate 5-year survival rates of 75% for stages I and II and 37% for stages III and IV for patients treated between 1969 and 1978. The authors attributed the improvement in survival to more aggressive management of the neck for early-stage tumors (stage II) and the addition of postoperative radiotherapy for advanced-stage tumors (stage III and IV).

Only 10% to 15% of patients who develop local recurrence at the primary site following management of oral tongue cancer are amenable to surgical resection. Even when feasible, salvage surgery for recurrence of the primary tumor is usually not successful, controlling disease in only 30% of cases.[33,42] This is related partly to confusing residual tumor with scar, resulting in delayed diagnosis of recurrent disease.

CANCER OF THE FLOOR OF THE MOUTH

Cancers of the floor of the mouth predominate in men in the fifth and sixth decades of life. The male to female ratio of occurrence is between 3:1 to 4:1.[80,86] Two thirds of patients are moderate to heavy smokers, and approximately 50% are heavy alcohol consumers. Many have poor nutritional habits.

Multifocal carcinomas are more common in patients with cancer of the floor of the mouth than in those with cancer of other oral cavity sites. A 20% incidence of second primary tumors occurs, with the majority in the head and neck area.[80]

Most cancers of the floor of mouth are SCCs. The majority are grade I or II (well or moderately well differentiated) tumors. The most common morphologic type is a superficial exophytic tumor. As the tumor enlarges, ulceration occurs. The loose connective tissues in the submental and submandibular spaces facilitate tumor extension. Advanced cancers frequently appear with direct extension into the soft tissues and skin of the submandibular triangle (Fig. 77-33). Fixation of tumor to bone shows mandibular involvement with the neoplasm. Spread along the periosteum is common once the infiltrative growth has reached the mandible. Restricted mobility marks invasion into the root of the tongue. The tumor may descend into the tissue plane between the tongue and the mouth floor as far as the hyoid bone.

Metastases to cervical lymph nodes from cancer of the mouth are observed in approximately 50% of patients when first evaluated. The submandibular lymph nodes are involved most frequently, followed by the upper deep jugular nodes.[80] Submental nodes are rarely involved with metastases. Tumors classified as T2N0 have a 40% occult metastatic rate, and 70% of T3N0 tumors have occult metastases. Table 77-9 shows the distribution according to stage from a series of 273 patients with cancer of the mouth floor.[2,40,86] Primary lesions located in the midline may metastasize to both necks. Half of the patients have advanced stage III and IV disease.

DIAGNOSIS

Carcinoma of the mouth floor is located most frequently in the anterior portion of the floor and usually extends to the root of the tongue and into the mandible (Fig. 77-34). Posterior extension along the gutter of the mouth is less common. Palpation demonstrates the depth of infiltration. Similar to tongue carcinoma, cancers of the mouth floor usually do not cause pain until they become deeply infiltrative enough to involve periosteum or branches of the lingual nerve. The most common symptom encountered on initial evaluation, however, is a painful mass in the mouth. Patients occasionally complain of ill-fitting dentures. A lump in the neck and impairment of speech are late symptoms.

Cancers located near the midline may spread along the duct of the submandibular gland or obstruct the duct. When obstruction occurs, the gland swells and becomes indurated and may be difficult to discern from metastases or direct tumor extension. Fine-needle aspiration and cytologic examination may be helpful in determining whether the submandibular mass represents a metastatic node or an enlarged submandibular gland.

Radiographic evaluation of the mandible is unreliable in detecting early bone involvement by cancer. This involvement is best assessed clinically by thorough palpation of the tumor. Immobility related to the lingual cortex of the mandible suggests at least involvement of the periosteum. Tumor invasion of the gingiva is automatically restricted

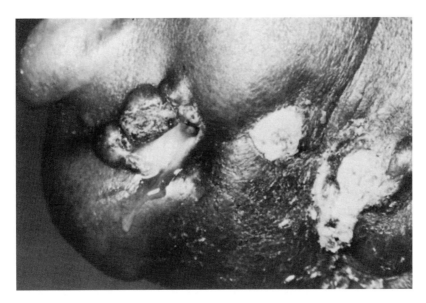

Fig. 77-33. Advanced squamous cell carcinoma of the floor of the mouth resulting in direct extension of tumor through the soft tissues and the skin of submandibular triangle.

Table 77-9. Squamous cell carcinoma of the mouth floor by stage: 273 patients

Stage	Patients (n (%)
I	68 (25)
II	64 (23)
III	85 (31)
IV	56 (21)

in mobility because the gingiva adheres to the underlying alveolar bone. In these situations the physician must rely on radiographic findings and histologic assessment at the time of surgery. When floor-of-the-mouth cancers involve the mucosa of the mandible, bone involvement by the neoplasm is common, occurring in approximately 7% of T1, 55% of T2, and 63% of T3 tumors. Among T2 cancers demonstrating bone erosion on radiography, approximately 70% show only destruction of the compact layer with a superficial bone defect, whereas 75% of T3 tumors having bony erosion show extensive basin-like defects or complete rarefaction of the mandible.[85] Whenever bone erosion is noted before treatment, the prognosis is poorer and a T4 designation is given.

Management

Early-stage (I and II) SCCs of the mouth floor involving mucosa alone may be managed effectively by either surgery or irradiation with equal results. Peroral, wide local resection of stage I tumors usually is more convenient than radiother-

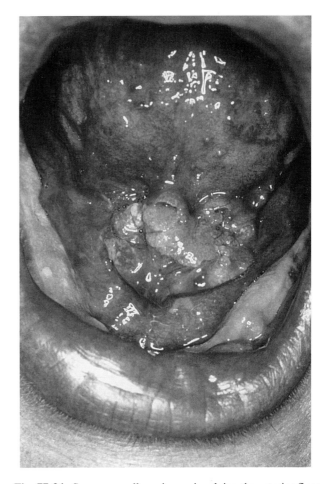

Fig. 77-34. Squamous cell carcinoma involving the anterior floor of the mouth.

apy. Defects are closed primarily or with the help of skin grafts. Radiotherapy can be administered as external-beam therapy alone, brachytherapy alone, or a combination of the two.

Stage I and II cancers of the floor of the mouth that are attached to or invade the mandible should be managed surgically because bone involvement by the tumor compromises radiotherapy. Tumors that appear to involve periosteum or superficially invade the mandible usually can be excised along with a partial-thickness resection of the mandible. Depending on the site of tumor attachment, either the superior half or the lingual cortical plate of the bone is removed (see Fig. 77-21). If evidence of bone destruction exists, a full-thickness segmental resection of the mandible should be performed (Fig. 77-35). Frozen-section control of the inferior alveolar nerve and cancellous bone at the resected mandibular margins should be obtained.

Stage II malignancies of the mouth floor managed by surgery usually require resection via a lip-splitting incision and mandibulotomy or a transcervical approach. An *en bloc* resection should remove the contents of the entire submandibular triangle, anterior belly of the digastric muscles, portions of the mylohyoid and hyoglossus muscles, and the floor-of-the-mouth tumor together. The high occult metastatic rate (40%) of stage II floor-of-the-mouth cancers warrants elective neck dissection or prophylactic neck irradiation. Combined surgery and radiotherapy is the preferred treatment of stage III and IV cancer of the floor of the mouth.

Advanced tumors frequently require segmental resection of the anterior arch of the mandible and neck dissection. Functional disability associated with loss of the anterior arch is significant and is directly related to the amount of bone removed. The optimal method of reconstruction for this type of defect involves the use of composite free flaps. Successful reconstruction of arch defects with fibular and iliac free flaps is now performed routinely. Subtotal mandibular defects require fibular free-flap reconstruction due to the length of bone necessary. Innervated soft tissue and skin can also be harvested with these flaps for sensated oral reconstruction.

Neck dissection is indicated when clinical evidence of regional metastases exists. Tumors of the anterior floor of the mouth near the midline with unilateral metastases also require management of the contralateral neck by either elective neck dissection or radiotherapy. Simultaneous bilateral radical neck dissections carry a high morbidity.[94] When possible, dissection should be staged at an interval of 4 to 6 weeks.

Results

Survival rates comparing radiotherapy versus surgical therapy are difficult to document as a result of the heterogeneous treatments found in most retrospective studies. However, some studies with almost exclusive use of radiation or surgery for early stage (I and II) lesions have been published. One such study with predominately surgical therapy reveals 5-year disease-free survival rates of 95% for stage I and 86%

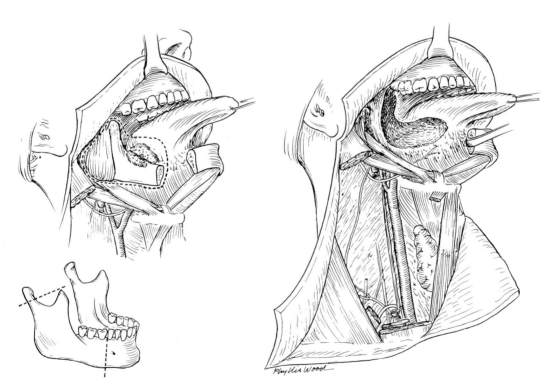

Fig. 77-35. Full-thickness segmental resection of the jaw is indicated when cancer has invaded the depths of the mandible.

for stage II lesions of the floor of the mouth.[44] Another study that evaluated patients treated with radiotherapy documented 5-year disease-free survival rates of 88% for T1 and 47% for T2 lesions.[89] This study did not report survival by clinical stage. Stage III and stage IV disease have a worse prognosis despite aggressive combination therapy. The 5-year disease-free survival rates have been reported to be 66% for stage III and 32% for stage IV tumors.[100]

Overall, approximately 65% to 75% of all patients with floor-of-the-mouth cancers are cured.[44,100] Ipsilateral node involvement markedly reduces survival rates to 25%. Other factors that appear to lessen survival are involvement of the tongue and mandible with neoplasms. Tumor extension out of the oral cavity posteriorly or anteriorly is a serious prognostic factor (Table 77-10).[86] Approximately 90% of recurrences occur within 2 years following treatment.

Table 77-10. Five-year survival in patients with squamous cell carcinoma of the mouth floor, according to tumor extent

Tumor extent	Patients (n)	5-year survival (%)
Localized	33	82
Across midline	24	59
Tongue and mandible	30	52
Bone destruction	9	50
Posterior out of oral cavity	6	17
Anterior out of oral cavity	4	0

Adapted from Panje WR, Smith B, McCabe BF: *Otolaryngol Head Neck Surg* 88:714, 1980.

CANCER OF THE ALVEOLAR RIDGE

Squamous cell carcinoma of the gingivae (gum, alveolar ridge) is an uncommon oral cavity malignancy when compared with cancer arising from the lip, tongue, or floor of the mouth. It represents approximately 10% of all oral cancers. More women than men are affected by gingival SCC as compared with other oral SCCs that affect men more frequently. Studies have revealed male to female ratios of gingival SCC ranging from 1.4:1 to 1:1.4.[6,105] Patients are seen most often in the sixth decade of life. Approximately 65% of patients use tobacco products, and 15% consume alcoholic beverages daily.[105]

Seventy percent of gingival carcinomas occur on the lower gum. Most tumors are seen in the molar area of the posterior third of the dental arch (Fig. 77-36). Most gingival cancers develop in edentulous areas. Because the gingival mucosa adheres directly to the periosteum of the mandible, tumors arising from this region are likely to invade the underlying bone. From 35% to 50% of patients will have neoplastic destruction of the mandible that is demonstrable radiographically or histologically.[18,112] Similarly, because the gingiva represents a small region of the oral cavity, 90% of cancers extend beyond the gum to involve adjacent structures.

Carcinoma of the gingiva is commonly associated with leukoplakic changes and may arise from areas of leukoplakia or severe periodontal disease. Most malignancies are well-differentiated grade I neoplasms. The typical morphologic type is an exophytic papillary (Fig. 77-37) or ulcerating tumor with a tendency toward peripheral spread rather than deep extension into the soft tissues. Some tumors may appear as a nodular or disk-like lesion.

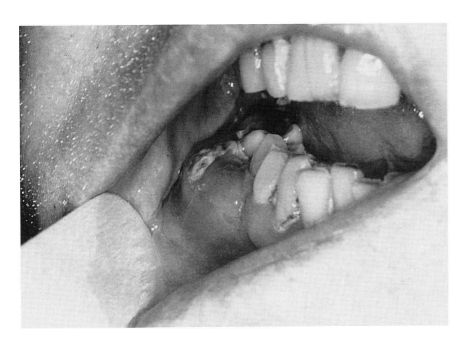

Fig. 77-36. Squamous cell carcinoma involving the posterior mandibular gingiva.

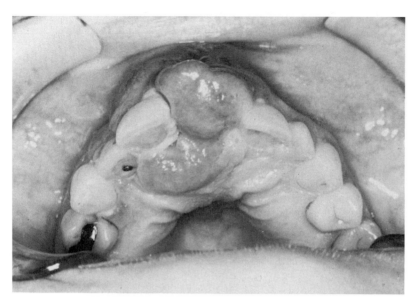

Fig. 77-37. Squamous cell carcinoma of the upper gingiva with an exophytic papillary morphology.

Cancers of both the upper and the lower gingivae metastasize first to the submandibular lymph nodes. Upper gingival cancers may spread initially to the upper deep jugular lymph nodes. Clinical evidence of neck metastases on presentation was noted in 32% of patients with lower gingival lesions and in 14% of patients with upper gingival lesions.[105]

Diagnosis

The clinical diagnosis of alveolar ridge cancer may be more difficult than diagnosis of tumors elsewhere in the oral cavity because of confusion with benign inflammatory or reactive gum lesions. Occasionally, maxillary sinus cancers may appear as upper gingival lesions (Fig. 77-38). In certain circumstances, discerning whether the tumor is of gingival or antral origin may be impossible. Radiographic evaluation with CT is helpful not only in this regard, but it also provides precise information concerning the extent of bone involvement.

Cancers arising from the alveolar mucosa in regions bearing teeth appear to occur at the free gingival margin adjacent to the tooth surface. In such instances the first clinical sign may be loosening of the tooth. In edentulous patients the first symptom is usually an inability to obtain proper denture fitting or difficulty with mastication. Pain is an early symptom of gingival cancer because of neoplastic involvement of the periosteum as the tumor progresses. Late symptoms include bleeding and a complaint of a mass in the mouth.

Radiographs of the mandible are required to assess lower gingival malignancies. Smooth, erosive pressure defects of the alveolar bone or upper cortical surface of the mandible should be distinguished from the moth-eaten type of bone destruction that tumor infiltration of bone causes. The latter finding suggests tumor extension toward the medullary portion of the mandible and usually necessitates segmental resection. Normal radiographic findings must be interpreted with caution. One third of patients without radiographic evidence of bone erosion will have histologic evidence of tumor involving bone.[112]

Management

Management of gingival cancer is governed by the extent of tumor, the degree of bone involvement, and the status of cervical lymph nodes. Most physicians prefer surgery for stage I and II disease. Small, localized (stage I) tumors of the lower alveolus may be excised perorally in conjunction with a marginal resection of the mandible. Neoplasms requiring segmental resection of the mandible are best approached externally. Upper alveolar cancers may also be removed perorally. An alveolectomy or partial maxillectomy may be accomplished in most cases without the need for facial incisions. In 60% of surgically treated patients with gingival cancers, less than a full segment of bone is necessary for adequate tumor resection with little cosmetic or functional impairment.[18] Radiotherapy is contraindicated due to the decreased response rate when there is bony involvement and due to the risk of osteoradionecrosis.

Combined surgery and radiotherapy have been advocated for the management of stage III and IV cancers of the gingivae. Neck dissection is indicated in all patients with clinically positive nodes. If nodes are found to contain tumors, postoperative radiotherapy is warranted. Elective neck dissection is probably unwarranted in the initial management of stage II gingival cancer because of the low incidence of occult metastases. Patients with T3N0 and T4N0 neoplasms, however, should be considered for elective neck dissection or prophylactic neck irradiation.

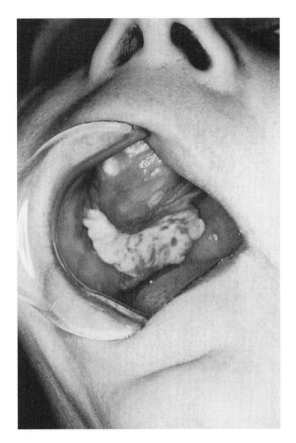

Fig. 77-38. Maxillary sinus cancer appearing as an upper gingival tumor.

Results

Overall 5-year survival rates for all patients with carcinoma of the gingivae range from 50% to 65%. No significant difference in survival exists between malignancies of the upper and lower jaw. Five-year determine survival has been reported to be 77% for stage I, 70% for stage II, 42% for stage III, and 24% for stage IV disease.[105] Patients with a history of dental extractions or histopathologic evidence of bony invasion or positive surgical margins have a significantly worse prognosis. Surgical results appear clearly superior to those cases managed by radiotherapy alone, probably because of the frequent early bone involvement by these neoplasms.

CANCER OF THE BUCCAL MUCOSA

Buccal carcinoma is an uncommon form of oral cavity cancer, representing 5% of all oral cancers diagnosed in the United States. In patients with more advanced disease, buccal cancer generally occurs in the seventh decade of life.[83] It occurs more often in men, at a 3:1 to 4:1 ratio over women. Buccal carcinoma is more common in the southeastern United States compared with the rest of the country. Snuff dipping by rural southern women is a common habit and is believed to be responsible for the higher incidence in this region. In support of tobacco chewing as the main etiologic factor, women in the southeastern United States have almost the same incidence of buccal cancer as men. Another etiologic factor may be local irritants from poor oral hygiene. Jagged carious teeth causing chronic irritation may explain why many buccal carcinomas occur in the area of the cheek mucosa marked by the occlusal plane.[68] Most recent studies, however, implicate tobacco and alcohol consumption as the major causative factors for buccal cancer.

Buccal carcinomas often arise with leukoplakia and frequently occur in the central posterior portion of the cheek (Fig. 77-39). In tobacco chewers, tumors may be located more frequently in the lower sulcus of the buccal mucosa where the quid is retained. Most tumors are well-differentiated grade I or II SCCs. Three distinctive morphologic types are recognized: exophytic, ulceroinfiltrative, and verrucous.[7] The exophytic type is more common, appearing as a heap of soft, white outgrowth, often in an area of leukoplakia. Exophytic tumors are papillary, have a benign appearance, and usually do not ulcerate until they have reached 3 to 4 cm. Ulceroinfiltrative carcinomas penetrate into the deep, soft tissues of the cheek early and appear as deep, excavating ulcers surrounded by diffuse induration. They are more destructive than the exophytic type and may ulcerate through the skin of the cheek or invade adjacent bone or masticatory muscles.

Although it is the least common morphologic type of buccal cancer, verrucous carcinoma occurs more frequently in the cheek mucosa than at other sites within the oral cavity. It is a low-grade SCC that rarely metastasizes. It has an indolent growth pattern, often arising in regions of leukoplakia, and therefore may be misdiagnosed as a benign hyperplasia. The clinical appearance of verrucous carcinoma is described earlier in this chapter. Briefly, it appears as a piled-up growth or papillary mass with considerable keratinization that usually gives it a whitish appearance. Verrucous carcinoma grows by progressive enlargement as a single mass and penetrates the soft tissue to invade underlying bone and muscle and may extend to the skin of the cheek.

Approximately 65% of patients with cancer of the buccal mucosa have extensive disease beyond the cheek mucosa.[68,83] From 40% to 50% of patients have stage I and II disease.[11,24] Clinically, regional lymph nodes are involved, with metastases in about 50% of cases.[11,88] The occult metastatic rate approaches 10% overall and is near 20% for stage II disease.[11] Metastases to the submandibular lymph nodes occur first. Tumors located posteriorly in the cheek, however, may spread initially to upper deep jugular lymph nodes.

Diagnosis

Cancer of the buccal mucosa clinically tends to be insidious. Until ulceration occurs, pain may not be a symptom. Many tumors arise in regions of leukoplakia that presumably are less sensitive to pain as a result of hyperkeratosis. By the time pain or bleeding occurs, the tumor may be so advanced as to involve the entire cheek from the superior to the inferior gingival buccal sulcus. Extension beyond the buccal mucosa occurs most commonly on the upper or lower alveolus, particularly in edentulous patients (Table 77-11).[11] Additional regions of extension include the floor of the mouth, the retromolar trigone, and the hard palate.

Symptoms of buccal cancer include a complaint of a painful ulcer or roughening of the cheek mucosa. If the tumor arises posteriorly, infiltration of the masseter or pterygoid musculature may cause trismus and swelling of the posterior face. Tumors occurring anteriorly may appear as a white mass near the oral commissure or inner aspect of the lip. Late symptoms include swelling of the cheek with induration, a through-and-through defect of the cheek, a foul-smelling, bleeding intraoral mass, or a mass in the submandibular triangle.

The frequent concomitants of leukoplakia and buccal cancer may necessitate multiple biopsies to assess the possibility of multiple cancers in the buccal region. Excisional biopsies with removal of large areas of leukoplakia may be necessary if cancer is suspected. Patients with a tumor extending on the mandible or hard palate should have appropriate radiographs to look for bone involvement by neoplasm. Trismus is an ominous sign and may require CT to assess the possibility of tumor extension into the pterygoid fossa or infratemporal fossa.

Management

Management of stage I and II cancer of the buccal mucosa may be by surgery or radiotherapy. Surgical excision and reconstruction can be performed more conveniently than radiotherapy. Trismus of varying severity may follow the administration of full tumorcidal doses of irradiation to fields that encompass the masseter and pterygoid musculature. Brachytherapy may be an effective method of treating larger buccal cancers that have not invaded the alveolus or pterygoid fossa.

Surgery is the management of choice for stage II tumors that have encroached on the bone of the upper or lower jaw or have extended posteriorly into the masseter muscle. Smaller stage II tumors are excised perorally, and closure is primarily by split-thickness skin graft or local oral mucosal flaps. Stage II tumors may require a cheek flap for proper exposure to allow for a marginal mandibulectomy, segmental mandibulectomy, or partial maxillectomy, depending on the extent of the malignancy. Elective neck therapy for stage I buccal carcinoma is not warranted because of the relatively low incidence of occult metastases.[11] Stage II, III, and IV disease with N0 necks should undergo ipsilateral elective neck therapy.

Combined therapy consisting of surgical resection and postoperative radiotherapy is preferred for stage III and IV

Table 77-11. Squamous cell carcinoma of buccal mucosa: extent of primary tumor

Tumor extent	T_1	T_2	$T_{3,4}$	Total	%
Confined to cheek mucosa	15	22	3	40	43
Gingivae	2	20	7	29	31
Retromolar region	0	7	7	14	15
Skin	1	1	3	5	5
Lip or commissure	0	4	0	4	4
Multiple structures	0	0	1	1	1

Adapted from Bloom ND, Spiro RH: *Am J Surg* 140:556, 1980.

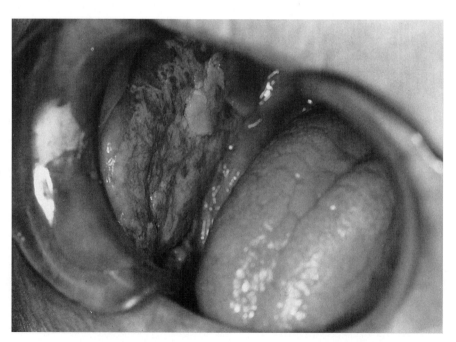

Fig. 77-39. Squamous cell carcinoma involving the buccal mucosa.

lesions. Primary reconstruction can be performed using skin grafts, local flaps, myocutaneous flaps, or free flaps depending on the nature of the defect.

Neck dissection is indicated in patients with clinically positive cervical nodes. An *en bloc* resection along with neck dissection is performed and may necessitate partial mandibulectomy or partial maxillectomy for advanced tumors. Total parotidectomy may be indicated for tumors extending posterolaterally toward the masseter muscle. Postoperative radiotherapy should be considered if lymph nodes are confirmed to contain metastases.

Results

As with other cancers of the oral cavity, results of management depend on the extent of the primary tumor and the presence or absence of nodal metastases. Overall survival in patients with carcinoma of the buccal mucosa has improved from 28%,[68] when most tumors were treated primarily with radiotherapy, to 50%, when surgery replaced irradiation as the preferred treatment for most tumors.[83] Nodal status is the most important prognostic factor.[11] Only 25% to 30% of patients developing cervical metastases are cured.[11,83]

Surgery is effective when the tumor is confined to the cheek mucosa. The approximate 5-year determinate survival rates for stage I and II disease are 75% and 65%, respectively. In contrast, 5-year determinate survival is near 30% for stage III and 20% for stage IV tumors.[11] Local recurrences affect 40% of patients.[24,83] Retreatment for cure, when feasible, yields a 25% cure rate.

CANCER OF THE HARD PALATE

The hard palate is the site of various malignant neoplasms, although the incidence of primary malignancies is low. Malignant salivary gland tumors of the hard palate occur about as frequently as SCC. Salivary gland malignancies are discussed elsewhere in this chapter. Statements concerning palatal cancer in this section refer to SCC of the hard palate occurring in the western hemisphere.

Squamous cell carcinoma of the hard palate is rare, comprising only 0.5% of oral cancers in the United States.[81] Although uncommon in Western cultures, it is prevalent in India, representing approximately 40% of all oral cancers.[92] This difference undoubtedly is related to the habit of reverse smoking, in which the lighted end of a cigarette is held within the mouth.

In the United States, SCC of the hard palate is a disease of elderly men, usually appearing in the seventh decade of life. Tobacco use and alcohol consumption are associated with epidermoid carcinoma of the palate as with other sites in the head and neck.[28]

Most carcinomas of the hard palate are well-differentiated to moderately well-differentiated grade I and II SCCs. A granular superficial ulceration is the predominant morphologic type seen on the hard palate. Despite proximity to bone, periosteum of the palate acts as a barrier to early tumor involvement. Initial growth tends to be superficial, and tumors usually grow to considerable size before bony destruction is observed (Fig. 77-40). A less common morphologic type of hard palate cancer is an exophytic, heaped-up tumor. Approximately half of all patients with cancer of the hard palate have neoplasm extending beyond the palate into adjacent regions of the oral cavity.

Approximately 10% to 25% of patients with hard palate carcinoma show clinical evidence of cervical metastases.[23,93] Metastases from cancers located in the primary palate occur first to the prevascular and retrovascular group of submandibular lymph nodes. From the secondary palate, metastases occur initially to the upper deep jugular (subdi-

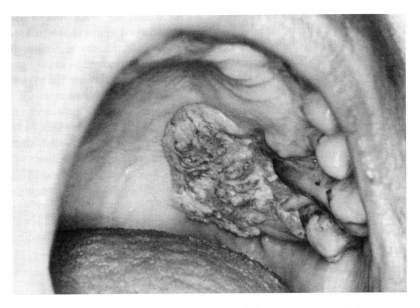

Fig. 77-40. Squamous cell carcinoma of the posterior hard palate.

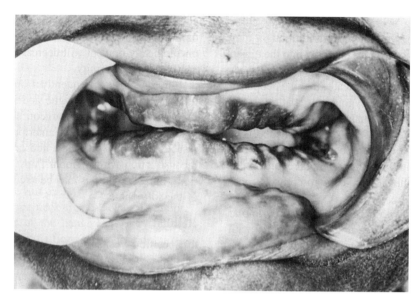

Fig. 77-41. Pigmentation of the gingivae is a common phenomenon in blacks.

often remain asymptomatic until ulceration and bleeding occur. Melanoma of the oral cavity characteristically occurs in men between 50 and 70 years of age. Mucosal melanoma must be differentiated from other benign pigmented lesions of the oral cavity. The most common oral pigmentation includes iatrogenic amalgam tattooing, which may result from the filling of a tooth. Physiologic pigmentation in the oral cavity is also seen in different racial groups (Fig. 77-41). It is imperative that pigmented lesions of the oral cavity undergo excisional (preferred) or incisional biopsy for possible melanoma.

The management of melanoma of the oral cavity is wide surgical excision. Neck dissection is indicated in patients with clinical findings of cervical metastases. Elective neck dissection remains controversial for the neck without clinically evident disease. Survival rates are extremely poor, with only 5% to 15% of patients surviving 5 years.[22,99] Most patients die within 1 to 2 years after onset of disease, with local recurrence and often concurrent regional and distant metastases.

Kaposi's sarcoma

Kaposi's sarcoma was classically found in elder Jewish or Mediterranean men with an indolent course involving the lower extremities. With the emergence of autoimmunodeficiency syndrome (AIDS) in 1981, widespread Kaposi's sarcoma metastases with multiple organ involvement have been commonly seen. Kaposi's sarcoma is the most common malignancy associated with AIDS and often involves the oral cavity.

The lesions appear as multiple red-purple nodules or plaques involving the skin or mucosa. Histologically, interwoven bands of spindle cells with atypical vascular clefts are seen in a background of collagen fibers (Fig. 77-42).

Lesions often involve the perioral skin, hard palate, gingiva, or tongue. Oral lesions range from asymptomatic plaques to ulcerated nodules. These lesions may cause difficulty with eating and speaking and may bleed. Asymptomatic lesions may be followed up clinically. Local therapy of symptomatic lesions includes surgical excision, laser ablation, cryotherapy, intralesional injection of chemotherapy agents, or radiotherapy. Systemic chemotherapy can be used in patients with widespread Kaposi's sarcoma with multiple organ involvement.[107]

Minor salivary gland malignancies

Minor salivary gland malignancies are an uncommon form of oral cavity cancer. Approximately 70% of all minor salivary gland tumors of the oral cavity are malignant (Table 77-12), and most commonly occur on the hard palate.[107]

Irradiation of the head and neck may result in both benign and malignant salivary gland tumors. A fivefold increase is expected in the incidence of salivary gland neoplasms in survivors of the Hiroshima and Nagasaki nuclear disasters.[8] Most malignant minor salivary gland tumors, however, are of unknown etiology.

The most common clinical setting of minor salivary gland cancer is a slowly enlarging, painless, mucosa-covered mass. In the oral cavity most tumors occur in the posterior aspect of the hard palate near the greater palatine foramen. Midline tumors are rare. Pain is inconsistent, and ulceration is uncommon. Except for those of the hard palate, tumors are usually mobile. Pain or hypesthesia may occur when perineural or bone invasion is present. Tumors occurring on the palate may appear as only a small neoplasm; however, CT may show extensive invasion into the paranasal sinuses or pterygopalatine fossa (Fig. 77-43). Only 14% of patients with

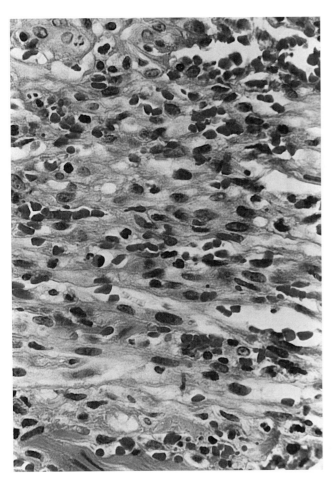

Fig. 77-42. Kaposi's sarcoma with interwoven bands of cells with cleft-like vascular spaces in a background of reticular and collagen fibers.

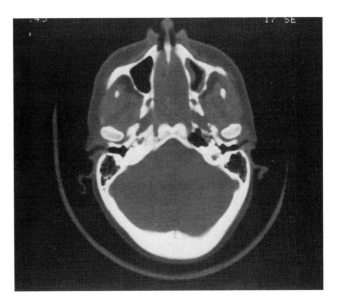

Fig. 77-43. Computed tomography of the paranasal sinuses of a patient with adenoid cystic carcinoma of the hard palate. Note extensive tumor extension into the ethmoid sinuses.

Table 77-12. Minor salivary gland malignancies

Site	Incidence (%)	Malignant (%)
Palate	49	66
Tongue	18	97
Cheek	13	81
Gingiva	6	100
Floor of the mouth	6	100
Lip	5	69
Retromolar trigone	3	100

Adapted from Spiro RH and others: *Am J Surg* 162:330, 1991.

minor salivary gland cancer have initial evidence of cervical metastases.[108]

Adenoid cystic carcinoma is the most common minor salivary gland malignancy, comprising 30% of all such cancers. The tumor exhibits slow growth and recurs locally, sometimes after many years. Adenoid cystic carcinoma is prone to follow the routes of cranial nerves in the vicinity of the neoplasm (Fig. 77-44), and thus local recurrence is almost inevitable. Distant metastases are common, occurring to the lung, brain, and bone in more than 50% of patients by the time of death.

Mucoepidermoid carcinoma also represents approximately 30% of minor salivary gland malignant tumors. It occurs more frequently in women, with a peak age in the fifth decade of life. From 50% to 65% are histologically considered low-grade tumors, which have an excellent prognosis with a low probability of recurrence and a low propensity for cervical metastases. High-grade tumors have aggressive local growth patterns and frequently recur at the primary site. Metastases are more common but tend to be confined to cervical nodes.

Adenocarcinoma represents approximately 20% of all minor salivary gland cancers. They are firm, locally aggressive malignancies occurring more often in patients over 60 years of age. Low-grade tumors have a good prognosis in contrast to high-grade adenocarcinoma, which has a poor prognosis.

Wide-field surgical excision is indicated for malignancies of minor salivary gland origin. Surgical procedures are similar to those employed for SCC of the oral mucosa. Therapeutic neck dissections are performed for histologically confirmed cervical metastases. Elective neck dissection is not warranted because only 9% of patients later develop cervical metastases.

Radiotherapy to the primary tumor site is indicated when the tumor is unresectable or when gross or microscopic surgical margins are involved with neoplasm. Many surgeons also favor postoperative radiotherapy for high-grade malignancies and for adenoid cystic carcinoma because of their

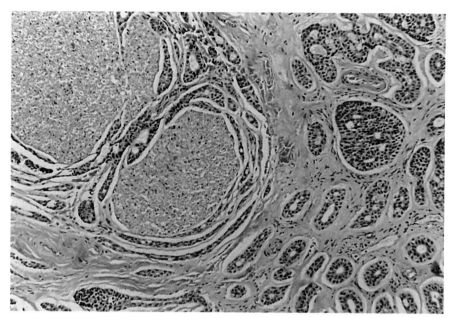

Fig. 77-44. Adenoid cystic carcinoma has a predilection for perineural spread. The cribriform pattern of adenoid cystic carcinoma is clearly seen here along with infiltration of a nerve.

proclivity for local recurrence. No controlled study has demonstrated the superiority of treating such malignancies with combined therapy.

Five-year survival in patients with oral cavity cancer of minor salivary gland origin is 40%.[8] Because nearly 15% of malignant tumors recur more than 5 years after diagnosis, long-term follow-up is essential. Taking all minor salivary gland malignancies of the head and neck into consideration, 5, 10, 15, and 20 year survival rates are 75%, 62%, 57%, and 51%, respectively.[13]

The AJCC does not provide for the staging of minor salivary gland malignancies. Survival is related to histology, tumor size, and the presence of regional or distant metastases. Poor survival is associated with adenoid cystic carcinoma, high-grade mucoepidermoid carcinomas, and high-grade adenocarcinomas. Cervical metastases are observed less frequently in minor salivary gland malignancies than in SCC. When metastases do occur, however, they are more likely to be associated with a fatal outcome. Management failure is usually at the primary site initially, and later nodal and distant metastases occur.[35]

REFERENCES

1. American Cancer Society: *Cancer facts and figures,* Atlanta, 1996, American Cancer Society.
2. Appelbaum EL, Callins WP, Bytell DE: Carcinoma of the floor of the mouth: surgical therapy vs. combined therapy vs. radiation therapy, *Arch Otolaryngol Head Neck Surg* 106:419, 1980.
3. Bagshaw MA, Thompson RW: Elective irradiation of the neck in patients with primary carcinoma of the head and neck, *JAMA* 217:456, 1971.
4. Baker SR: Risk factors in multiple carcinomas of the lip, *Otolaryngol Head Neck Surg* 88:248, 1980.
5. Baker SR, Krause CJ: Carcinoma of the lip, *Laryngoscope* 90:19, 1980.
6. Barasch A and others: Squamous cell carcinoma of the gingiva, *Oral Surg Oral Med Oral Pathol* 80:183, 1995.
7. Batsakis JG: *Tumors of the head and neck: clinical and pathological considerations,* Baltimore, 1974, Williams & Wilkins.
8. Belsky JL and others: Salivary gland tumors in atomic bomb survivors, Hiroshima-Nagasaki 1957-1970, *JAMA* 219:864, 1972.
9. Biller HF and others: Planned preoperative irradiation for carcinoma of the larynx and laryngopharynx treated by total and partial laryngectomy, *Laryngoscope* 79:1387, 1969.
10. Black RJ, Gluckman JL, Shumrick DA: Multiple primary tumors of the upper aerodigestive tract, *Clin Otolaryngol* 8:277, 1983.
11. Bloom ND, Spiro RH: Carcinoma of the cheek mucosa: a retrospective analysis, *Am J Surg* 140:556, 1980.
12. Boatenburg de Jong RJ and others: Metastatic neck disease: palpation vs ultrasound examination, *Arch Otolaryngol Head Neck Surg* 115:689, 1989.
13. Buchbinder A, Friedman-Kien AE: Clinical aspects of Kaposi's sarcoma, *Curr Opin Oncol* 4:867, 1992.
14. Burkell CC: Cancer of the lip, *Can Med Assoc J* 62:28, 1950.
15. Broders AC: Squamous cell epithelioma of the lip: a study of five hundred and thirty-seven cases, *JAMA* 74:656, 1920.
16. Brusenina ND, Rudakova AT: Immunoglobulin levels in serum and saliva of patients with precancerous diseases of the mouth mucosa, *Stomatologia (Mosk)* 61:30, 1982.
17. Byers RM and others: Frequency and therapeutic implications of "skip metastases" in the neck from squamous carcinomas of the oral tongue, *Head Neck Surg* 19:14, 1997.
18. Byers RM and others: Results of treatment of squamous carcinoma of the lower gum, *Cancer* 47:236, 1981.
19. Byers RM and others: Treatment of squamous carcinoma of the retromolar trigone, *Am J Clin Oncol* 7:647, 1984.
20. Reference deleted in pages.
21. Chase M: Health journal, *Wall Street Journal,* B1, October 28, 1996.
22. Chaudhry AP, Hampel A, Gorlin RJ: Primary malignant melanoma of oral cavity: review of 105 cases, *Cancer* 11:923, 1958.
23. Chung CK and others: Radiotherapy in the management of primary malignancies of the hard palate, *Laryngoscope* 90:576, 1980.
24. Conley J, Sadoyama JA: Squamous cell cancer of the buccal mucosa, *Arch Otolaryngol Head Neck Surg* 94:330, 1973.
25. Cross JE, Guralnick E, Daland EM: Carcinoma of the lip: a review of 563 case records of carcinoma of the lip at the Pondville Hospital, *SGO* 87:153, 1948.

26. Davidson TM and others: Mohs' for head and neck mucosal cancer: report on 111 patients, *Laryngoscope* 98:1078, 1988.

27. Ebenius B: Cancer of the lip, *Acta Radiol Suppl* 48:1, 1943.

28. Evans JF, Shah JP: Epidermoid carcinoma of the palate, *Am J Surg* 142:451, 1981.

29. Fein DA and others: Carcinoma of the oral tongue: a comparison of results and complications of treatment with radiotherapy and/or surgery, *Head Neck Surg* 16:358, 1994.

29a. Fleming ID, editor: *AJCC cancer staging manual,* ed 5, Philadelphia, 1997, Lippincott-Raven.

30. Fletcher GH: Elective irradiation for subclinical disease in cancers of the head and neck, *Cancer* 29:1450, 1972.

31. Fletcher GH, Jesse RH: The contribution of supervoltage roentgentherapy to the integration of radiation and surgery in head and neck squamous cell carcinoma, *Cancer* 15:566, 1962.

32. Forrest LA and others: Rapid analysis of mandibular margins, *Laryngoscope* 105:475, 1995.

33. Franceschi D and others: Improved survival in the treatment of squamous carcinoma of the oral tongue, *Am J Surg* 166:360, 1993.

34. Frazell EL, Lucas JC: Cancer of the tongue: report of the management of 1,554 patients, *Cancer* 15:1085, 1962.

34a. Frichman M, Mafee MF, Pacella BL: Rationale for elective neck dissection in 1990, *Laryngoscope* 100:54, 1990.

35. Fuk K and others: Cancer of the major and minor salivary glands: analysis of treatment results and sites and causes of failure, *Cancer* 40:2882, 1977.

36. Fukano H and others: Depth of invasion as a predictive factor for cervical lymph node metastases in tongue carcinoma, *Head Neck Surg* 19:205, 1997.

37. Gladstone WS, Kerr HD: Epidermoid carcinoma of the lower lip: results of radiation therapy of the local lesions, *Am J Roentgenol* 79:101, 1958.

38. Gluckman JL, Crissman JD, Donegan JO: Multicentric squamous cell carcinoma of the upper aerodigestive tract, *Head Neck Surg* 3:90, 1980.

39. Goldman JL, Friedman WH: High dose preoperative irradiation in cancer of the larynx, *Otolaryngol Clin North Am* 2:473, 1969.

40. Guillamondegui OM, Oliver B, Hayden R: Cancer of the anterior floor of mouth: selective choice of treatment and analysis of failures, *Am J Surg* 140:560, 1980.

41. Gupta NK, Pointon RC, Wilkinson P: A randomized clinical trial to contrast radiotherapy with radiotherapy and methotrexate given synchronously in head and neck cancer, *Clin Radiol* 28:575, 1987.

42. Hariot JC and others: Hyperfractionation versus conventional fractionation in oropharyngeal carcinoma: final analysis of a randomized trial of the EORTC cooperative group of radiotherapy, *Radiother Oncol* 25:23, 1992.

43. Head and neck contracts program: adjuvant chemotherapy for advanced head and neck squamous carcinoma. Final report, *Cancer* 60:301, 1987.

44. Hicks WL and others: Squamous cell carcinoma of the floor of mouth: a 20 year review, *Head Neck Surg* 19:400, 1997.

45. Hillsamer PJ, Schuller DE, McGhee RB: Improving diagnostic accuracy of cervical metastases with computed tomography and magnetic resonance imaging, *Arch Otolaryngol Head Neck Surg* 116:1297, 1990.

46. Hirsch JM, Johansson SL: Effect of long term application of snuff on the oral mucosa: an experimental study in the rat, *J Oral Pathol* 12:187, 1983.

47. Hirsch JM, Thilander H: Snuff induced lesions of the oral mucosa: an experimental model in the rat, *J Oral Pathol* 10:342, 1982.

48. Incze J and others: Premalignant changes in normal appearing epithelium in patients with squamous cell carcinoma of the upper aerodigestive tract, *Am J Surg* 144:401, 1982.

49. Jenson AB and others: Papillomavirus etiology of proliferative squamous epithelial lesions of the skin, oral tracheolaryngeal and anogenital mucosa: papilloma viruses, Cold Spring Harbor, NY, Sept 14-18, 1982, Cold Spring Harbor Laboratory (abstract).

50. Johnson JT and others: Cervical lymph node metastases: incidence and implications of extracapsular carcinoma, *Arch Otolaryngol Head Neck Surg* 111:534, 1985.

51. Johnson JT and others: The extra-capsular spread of tumors in cervical node metastases, *Arch Otolaryngol Head Neck Surg* 107:725, 1981.

52. Jones K and others: Prognostic factors in the recurrence of stage I and II squamous cell carcinoma of the oral cavity, *Arch Otolaryngol Head Neck Surg* 118:483, 1992.

53. Jørgensen K, Elbrond O, Andersen AP: Carcinoma of the lip: a series of 869 cases, *Acta Radiol* 12:177, 1973.

54. Kennett S: Recognizing premalignant conditions in the mouth, *Consultant* 20:32, 1980.

55. Kissin B and others: Head and neck cancer in alcoholics, the relationship of drinking, smoking and dietary patterns, *JAMA* 224:1174, 1973.

56. Kramer S and others: Combined radiation therapy and surgery in the management of advanced head and neck cancer: final report of study 73-03 of the Radiation Therapy Oncology Group, *Head Neck Surg* 10:19, 1987.

57. Kraus FT, Perez-Mesa C: Verrucous carcinoma: clinical and pathologic study of 105 cases involving oral cavity, larynx and genitalia, *Cancer* 19:26, 1966.

58. Laramore GE and others: Adjuvant chemotherapy for resectable squamous cell carcinoma of the head and neck: report on intergroup study, *Int J Radiat Oncol Biol Phys* 23:705, 1992.

59. Leonard JR and others: Combined radiation and surgical therapy: tongue, tonsil and floor of mouth, *Ann Otol Rhinol Laryngol* 77:514, 1968.

60. Lindberg R: Distribution of cervical lymph node metastases from squamous cell carcinomas of the upper respiratory and digestive tracts, *Cancer* 29:1446, 1972.

61. Longenecker CG, Ryan RF: Cancer of the lip in a large charity hospital, *South Med J* 58:1459, 1965.

62. Lyall D, Schetlin CF: Cancer of the tongue, *Ann Surg* 135:489, 1952.

63. MacKay EN, Sellers AH: A statistical review of carcinoma of the lip, *Can Med Assoc J* 90:670, 1964.

64. Mahoney LJ: Resection of cervical lymph nodes in cancer of the lip: results in 123 patients, *Can J Surg* 12:40, 1969.

65. Marchetta FC, Sako K, Camp F: Multiple malignancies in patients with head and neck cancer, *Am J Surg* 110:537, 1965.

66. Marcial VA and others: Hyperfractionated photon radiation therapy in the treatment of advanced squamous cell carcinoma of the oral cavity, pharynx, larynx, and sinuses using radiation therapy as the only planned modality: (preliminary report) by the Radiation Therapy Oncology Group (RTOG), *Int J Radiat Oncol Biol Phys* 13:41, 1987.

67. Martin HE, MacComb WS, Blady JV: Cancer of the lip, *Ann Surg* 114:226, 1941.

68. Martin HE, Pflueger OH: Cancer of the cheek (buccal mucosa), *Arch Surg* 30:731, 1935.

69. Mascres C, Franchebois P: The ultrastructure of the buccal mucosa in the non-smoking cirrhotic patient, *Ann Anat Pathol (Paris)* 24:285, 1979.

70. McGuirt WF and others: A comparative diagnostic study of the head and neck nodal metastases using positron emission tomography, *Laryngoscope* 105:373, 1995.

71. Medina JE, Byers RM: Supraomohyoid neck dissection: rationale, indications, and surgical technique, *Head Neck Surg* 11:111, 1989.

72. Million RR: Elective neck irradiation for TxNo squamous carcinomas of the oral tongue and floor of mouth, *Cancer* 34:149, 1974.

73. Million RR, Fletcher GH, Jesse RH: Evaluation of elective irradiation of the neck for squamous cell carcinoma of the nasopharynx, tonsillar fossa and base of tongue, *Radiology* 80:973, 1963.

74. Modlin J: Neck dissections in cancer of the lower lip: five-year results in 179 patients, *Surgery* 28:404, 1950.

75. Molnar L, Ronay P, Tapolcsanyi L: Carcinoma of the lip: analysis of the material of 25 years, *Oncology* 29:101, 1974.

76. Moore C: Cigarette smoking and cancer of the mouth, pharynx and larynx, *JAMA* 218:553, 1971.

77. Most A: *Die topographic des Lymphgefassaparates des koopfes and des hales in iher Bedeutung jue die Chirurgie*, Berlin, 1906, Verlag Von August Hirschwald.

78. Morency R, Laliberte H, Delamarre R: Focal epithelial hyperplasia of the oral mucosa, *J Otolaryngol* 11:29, 1982.

79. Muraki AS and others: CT of the oropharynx, tongue base, and floor of mouth: normal anatomy and range of variations, and applications in staging carcinoma, *Radiology* 148:725, 1983.

80. Nakissa N and others: Carcinoma of the floor of the mouth, *Cancer* 42:2914, 1978.

81. New GB, Hallberg OE: The end results of treatment of malignant tumors of the palate, *SGO* 73:520, 1941.

82. Noone RB and others: Lymph node metastases in oral carcinoma (a correlation of histopathology with survival), *Plast Reconstr Surg* 53:158, 1974.

83. O'Brien PH, Catlin D: Cancer of the cheek (mucosa), *Cancer* 18:1392, 1965.

84. Odette J, Szymanowski R, Nichols R: Multiple head and neck malignancies, *Trans Am Acad Ophthalmol Otolaryngol* 84:805, 1976.

85. Otten JE, Duker J: Bone involvement in x-rays in carcinomas of the oral mucosa, *Dtsch Zahnarztl Z* 2:741, 1981.

86. Panje WR, Smith BS, McCabe BF: Epidermoid carcinoma of the floor of the mouth: surgical therapy vs. combined therapy vs. radiation therapy, *Otolaryngol Head Neck Surg* 88:714, 1980.

87. Parken DM, Laara E, Muir CS: Estimates of the worldwide frequency of sixteen major cancers in 1980, *Int J Cancer* 41:184, 1988.

88. Paymaster JC: Cancer of the buccal mucosa, *Cancer* 9:431, 1956.

89. Pernot M and others: Epidermoid carcinomas of the floor of mouth treated by exclusive irradiation: statistical study of a series of 207 cases, *Radiother Oncol* 25:177, 1995.

90. Petzoldt D, Dennin R: The isolation of virus-like particles from Heck's focal epithelial hyperplasia, *Hautarzt* 31:35, 1980.

91. Rabuzzi DD, Chung CT, Sagerman RH: Prophylactic neck irradiation, *Arch Otolaryngol Head Neck Surg* 106:454, 1980.

92. Ramulu C, Reddy CRRM: Carcinoma of the hard palate and its relationship to reverse smoking, *Int Surg* 57:636, 1972.

93. Ratzer ER, Schweitzer RJ, Frazell EL: Epidermoid carcinoma of the palate, *Am J Surg* 119:294, 1970.

94. Razack MS, Baffi R, Sako K: Bilateral radical neck dissection, *Cancer* 47:197, 1981.

95. Rodriguez-Perez I, Banoczy J: Oral leukoplakia: a histological study, *Acta Morphol Hung* 30:289, 1982.

96. Rouviere H: *Anatomy of the human lymphatic system*, Ann Arbor, Mich, 1938, Edwards Brothers (translated by MJ Tobias).

97. Schmidt W, Popham RE: The role of drinking and smoking in mortality from cancer and other causes in male alcoholics, *Cancer* 47:1031, 1981.

98. Schottenfeld D, Gantt R, Wyner EL: The role of alcohol and tobacco in multiple primary cancers of the upper digestive system, larynx and lung: a prospective study, *Prev Med* 3:277, 1974.

98a. Schuller DE and others: Preoperative chemotherapy in advanced resectable head and neck cancer: final report of the Southwest Oncology Group, *Laryngoscope* 98:1205, 1988.

99. Shah JP, Huvos AG, Strong EW: Mucosal melanomas of the head and neck, *Am J Surg* 134:531, 1977.

100. Shaha AR and others: Squamous cell carcinoma of the floor of mouth, *Am J Surg* 148:455, 1984.

101. Shumrick DA, Quenelle DJ: Malignant disease of the tonsillar region, retromolar trigone, and buccal mucosa, *Otolaryngol Clin North Am* 12:115, 1979.

102. Silverman S, Griffith M: Smoking characteristics of patients with oral carcinoma and the risk for second oral primary carcinoma, *J Am Dent Assoc* 85:637, 1972.

103. Snow GB and others: Prognostic factors of neck nodule metastases, *Clin Otolaryngol* 7:185, 1982.

104. Snow GW, von der Waal I: Mucosal melanomas of the head and neck, *Otolaryngol Clin North Am* 19:537, 1986.

105. Soo KC and others: Squamous carcinoma of the gums, *Am J Surg* 156:281, 1988.

106. Spiro RH and others: Predictive value of tumor thickness in squamous cell carcinoma confined to the tongue and floor of the mouth, *Am J Surg* 152:345, 1986.

107. Spiro RH and others: The importance of clinical staging of minor salivary gland carcinomas, *Am J Surg* 162:330, 1991.

108. Spiro RH and others: Tumors of the minor salivary origin: a clinico-pathologic study of 492 cases, *Cancer* 31:117, 1973.

109. Strong EW: Preoperative radiation and radical neck dissection, *Surg Clin North Am* 49:271, 1969.

110. Strong MS, Ditroia JF, Vaughan CW: Carcinoma of the palatine arch: a review of 73 patients, *Trans Am Acad Ophthalmol Otolaryngol* 75:957, 1971.

111. *Surgeon General's Report*, 1982.

112. Swearingen AG, McGrew JP, Palumbo VD: Roentgenograph pathologic correlation of carcinoma involving the mandible, *Am J Roentgenol Radium Ther Nucl Med* 96:15, 1966.

113. Szpak CA, Stone MJ, Frenkel SK: Some observations concerning the demographic and geographic incidence of carcinoma of the lip and buccal cavity, *Cancer* 40:343, 1977.

113a. Trieger N and others: Cirrhosis and other predisposing factors in carcinoma of the tongue, *Cancer* 11:357, 1958.

114. van den Brekel MWM and others: Modern imaging techniques and ultrasound-guided aspiration cytology for the assessment of neck node metastases: a prospective comparative study, *Eur Arch Otorhinolaryngol* 250:11, 1993.

115. Vas Kovskaia GP, Abramova EI: Cancer development from lichen planus on the oral and labial mucosa, *Stomatologiia (Mosk)* 60:46, 1981.

116. Vikram B and others: Elective postoperative radiation therapy in stages III and IV epidermoid carcinoma of the head and neck, *Am J Surg* 140:580, 1980.

117. Waldron CA, Shafer WG: Leukoplakia revisited, a clinicopathologic study of 3256 oral leukoplakias, *Cancer* 36:1386, 1975.

118. Wang CC: Radiation therapy in the management of oral malignant disease, *Otolaryngol Clin North Am* 12:73, 1979.

119. Ward GE, Hendrick JW: Results of treatment of carcinoma of the lip, *Surgery* 27:321, 1950.

120. Ward GE and others: Cancer of the oral cavity and pharynx and results of treatment by means of the composite operation in continuity with radical neck dissection, *Ann Surg* 150:202, 1959.

121. Wilson JSP, Kemble JVH: Cancer of the lip at risk, *Br J Oral Surg* 9:186, 1972.

122. Wright JM, Dunsworth AR: Follicular lymphoid hyperplasia of the hard palate: a benign lymphoproliferative process, *Oral Surg* 55:162, 1983.

123. Wynder EL, Klein UE: The possible role of riboflavin deficiency in epithelial neoplasia, *Cancer* 18:167, 1965.

124. Wynder EL, Mushinski M, Spival J: Tobacco and alcohol consumption in relationship to the development of multiple cancers, *Cancer* 40:1872, 1977.

125. Wynder EL and others: Environmental factors in cancer of the upper alimentary tract, a Swedish study with special reference to Plummer-Vinson (Patterson-Kelly) syndrome, *Cancer* 10:470, 1957.

126. Wynder EL, Stellman SD: Comparative epidemiology of tobacco related cancers, *Cancer Res* 37:4608, 1977.

127. Yves D, Ghossein NA: Experience of the Curie Institute in treatment of cancer of the mobile tongue. I. Treatment policies and results, *Cancer* 47:496, 1981.

128. Yves D, Ghossein NA: Experience of the Curie Institute in treatment of cancer of the mobile tongue. II. Management of neck nodes, *Cancer* 47:503, 1981.

Chapter 78

Malignant Neoplasms of the Oropharynx

Eric M. Genden
Stanley E. Thawley
Michael J. O'Leary

Proper evaluation and treatment of tumors of the oropharynx require knowledge of (1) the anatomy, staging, etiology, histopathology, and clinical behavior of the cancer; (2) the various options for treatment; and (3) the proper management of immediate and long-term complications. Generally, a team approach including an otolaryngologist, radiation therapist, medical oncologist, prosthodontist, speech therapist, and nursing specialist, offers the most comprehensive treatment.

ANATOMY

The oropharynx includes four different sites: (1) the base of the tongue, (2) the soft palate, (3) the tonsillar area (fossa and pillars), and (4) the posterior pharyngeal wall. The oropharynx extends from the plane of the hard palate superiorly to the plane of the hyoid bone inferiorly and is continuous with the oral cavity (Figs. 78-1 and 78-2). The faucial arch includes both surfaces of the entire soft palate and the uvula, the anterior border of the base of the anterior tonsillar pillar, and the line of the circumvallate papilla. The base of the tongue extends from the line of the circumvallate papilla to the junction with the base of the epiglottis (the vallecula) and includes the pharyngoepiglottic and glossoepiglottic folds.

The lateral wall of the oropharynx is made up largely of the tonsil and tonsillar fossae. The posterior tonsillar pillar, the narrow lateral wall, and the posterior wall comprise the pharyngeal wall. The tonsillar fossa, which harbors the palatine tonsil, is an area bounded anteriorly by the anterior tonsillar pillar (palatoglossus muscle) and posteriorly by the posterior tonsillar pillar (palatopharyngeal muscle). The soft palate includes the uvula and is continuous laterally with the tonsillar pillars. Lateral to the tonsil region are the pharyngeal constrictor muscles, the mandible, and the lateral pharyngeal space. The internal carotid artery is just lateral and posterior to the tonsillar fossa (Fig. 78-3).

The posterior pharyngeal wall of the oropharynx begins at the inferior limit of the nasopharynx around the soft palate and extends inferiorly to the epiglottis. This wall is composed of mucosa, submucosa, pharyngobasilar fascia, underlying superior constrictor muscle, and buccopharyngeal fascia. Loose areolar tissue occupies the space between the buccopharyngeal fascia and the prevertebral fascia. The buccopharyngeal fascia acts as a natural barrier to prevent posterior extension of carcinoma. A tumor often will invade the muscle but not penetrate this fascia, thereby allowing a clear margin of resection. In larger and more aggressive tumors, however, the buccopharyngeal fascia may be penetrated; if this occurs, the prevertebral fascia is involved with the tumor fixating to the vertebra. This tumor usually cannot be resected.

The mucosa at the base of the tongue is irregular, and the lingual tonsil lies on the base's surface. Generally, these tonsillar masses are more concentrated toward the lateral areas. Palpation may confuse this irregular area with disease. A midline mucosal fold, the glossal epiglottic fold, divides the vallecula and connects the base of the tongue to the epiglottis (see Fig. 78-3). Deep to the tonsillar fossa lie the superior constrictor muscle and upper fibers of the middle

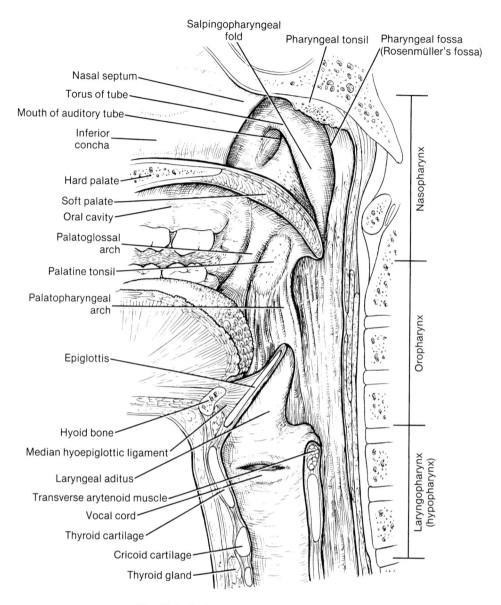

Fig. 78-1. Surface anatomy of the oropharynx.

constrictor muscle. Other muscles that affect this area are the palatoglossus, palatopharyngeal, salpingopharyngeal, and stylopharyngeal. The major blood supply to the tonsil is the tonsillar branch of the facial artery. The ascending pharyngeal and dorsal lingual arteries and the palatine branches of the internal maxillary and facial arteries also are involved. The peritonsillar veins pierce the inferior constrictor muscle and drain into the common facial vein and pharyngeal plexus (see Fig. 78-2).

The posterior wall of the oropharynx is related to the second and third cervical vertebrae. Tumors of the oropharynx may extend to the parapharyngeal space, which extends from the base of the skull to the hyoid bone (Fig. 78-4). It is bounded anteriorly by the pterygomandibular raphe and posteriorly by the prevertebral fascia. The lateral boundary

is the internal pterygoid muscle, mandible, and deep surface of the parotid. The medial boundary is the tonsillar area and superior constrictor muscle. Tumor invading this space may involve the carotid artery and the internal jugular vein and cranial nerves (CN) IX, X, XI, and XII. Once the nerves are involved, the tumor may spread peripherally or extend closely along the nerves to the base of skull area. Involvement of the pterygoid muscles will produce trismus. The most common lymph node initially involved with a lesion of the oropharynx is the jugulodigastric. Lesions of the base of the tongue and lateral oropharyngeal walls also may drain to the retropharyngeal and parapharyngeal nodes. These nodes drain into the jugulodigastric and posterior cervical group. The base of the tongue and midline palate areas may drain bilaterally.

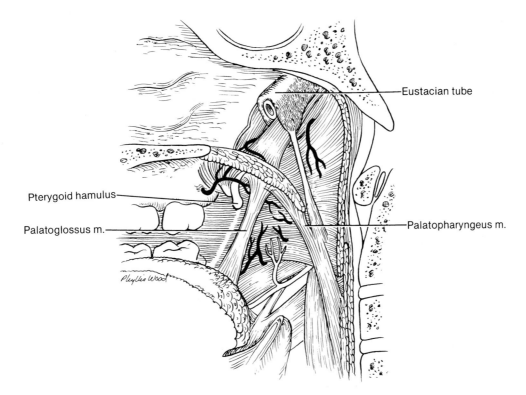

Fig. 78-2. Deep anatomy of the oropharynx muscles, nerves, and blood vessels.

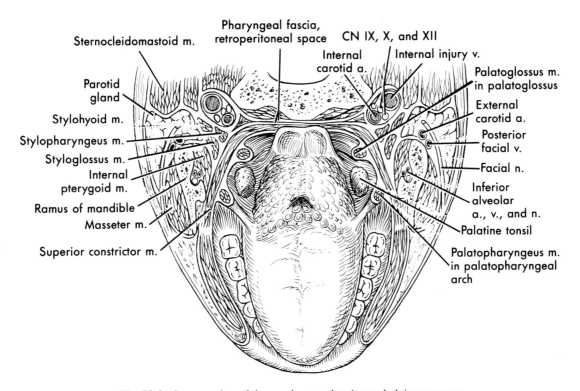

Fig. 78-3. Cross section of the oropharynx showing underlying anatomy.

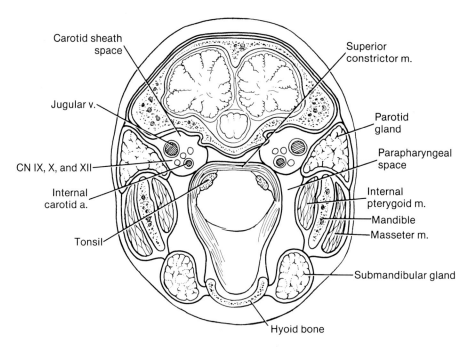

Fig. 78-4. Oropharyngeal anatomy showing parapharyngeal space.

HISTOPATHOLOGY

As in the oral cavity, precancerous lesions may occur in the oropharynx, but to a lesser extent. These lesions include leukoplakia secondary to hyperkeratosis with or without atypical changes, erythroplasia, lichen planus, and nicotine mucositis. In the oropharynx, the palate is most likely to be involved with any of these changes.

Any white plaque may be described by the term *leukoplakia*, which is clinically descriptive and has no pathologic meaning unless qualified by a biopsy. Leukoplakia may reveal hyperkeratosis, with or without atypical cellular changes, or early invasive carcinoma. Most cases of benign leukoplakia are secondary to smoking. Erythroplasia is a flat or slightly elevated, circumscribed injected plaque that is likely to be associated with underlying carcinoma or leukoplakia with very atypical changes. *Lichen planus* is usually a delicate, white, lacy lesion on the buccal mucosa; however, it may occur on the soft palate. *Nicotine mucositis* may produce changes on the palate that range from leukoplakia, hyperkeratotic areas to injected flap plaques or small, raised lesions. At times, many palatal mucosal changes may involve different appearances, and distinguishing changes that are clinically significant is difficult. Nicotine mucositis is often seen in patients who are heavy smokers and drinkers and often reveals extensive mucosal changes in the oral cavity and oropharynx.

Squamous cell carcinoma

More than 90% of malignant tumors in the oropharyngeal region are squamous cell carcinoma. Grossly, these tumors may be exophytic and bulky or ulcerative and deeply infiltra-

tive. Histologically, squamous cell carcinoma may be classified as nonkeratinizing, keratinizing, verrucous, spindle cell, and adenoid squamous carcinoma.

Nonkeratinizing and keratinizing carcinoma

Nonkeratinizing carcinomas may be well or poorly differentiated. Classically, they spread submucosally and have a "pushing" margin. They are derived from a respiratory tract mucosa, which originates endodermally. Keratinizing squamous cell carcinomas are considered to derive more often from ectodermally derived tissue. Generally, these lesions tend to be ulcerative and fungating, have less of a tendency for submucosal spread, and have infiltrating margins. The keratinization characteristics of a squamous cell carcinoma do not affect the rate of lymph node metastases or survival of the patient. In general, the degrees of differentiation and keratinization of the primary tumor are less relevant than the primary tumor's location, size, stage, and extent of deep invasion.

Verrucous carcinoma

Verrucous carcinoma occurs rarely in the oropharynx and more often in the oral cavity. It is a histologic variant of a well-differentiated squamous cell carcinoma. Histology reveals well-differentiated, keratinized epithelium in long, papillomatous folds. Growth is usually slow, producing few symptoms. Regional lymph nodes may be confusingly enlarged because of the inflammatory response and may masquerade as metastatic tumor. The lesion may erode underlying structures, including bone, but does not show widespread surface involvement. Cellular atypism and mitosis are rare,

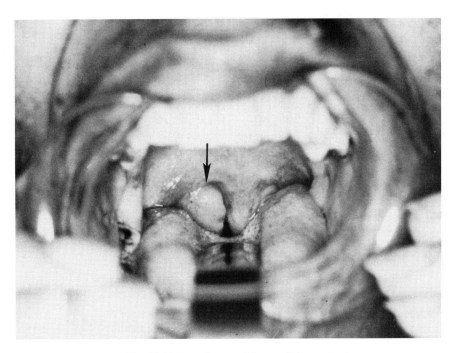

Fig. 78-5. Lymphoma of the tonsil (*arrow*).

and therefore multiple biopsies usually are required for definitive diagnosis. A deep biopsy showing invasion of the deeper structures is helpful; having the pathologist look at the lesion clinically is especially beneficial to correlate the histopathology with the clinical pathology. Recommended treatment is wide surgical excision. Radiotherapy is not recommended because transformation to a more anaplastic aggressive form has been reported.

Spindle cell carcinoma

The histopathology of spindle cell carcinoma reveals a spindle-shaped mesenchymal cell resembling anaplastic sarcoma, with various mixtures of squamous cells. The epidermoid component may be overlooked unless many sections are reviewed. Electron microscopy reveals that these are variants of squamous cell carcinoma and are not primary connective tissue tumors. These tumors spread to regional lymph nodes; generally, treatment is the same as that for squamous cell carcinoma.

Adenoid squamous cell carcinoma

The adenoid squamous cell carcinoma is a rare variant of squamous cell carcinoma and occasionally occurs in the base of tongue. These lesions should be distinguished from adenoid cystic tumors, which originate in the minor salivary glands in this area. They are treated the same as routine squamous cell carcinoma.

Lymphocytic lesion

The large amount of lymphoid tissue in the oropharyngeal area is sometimes involved in malignant transformation. The most common lymphocytic lesion is *lymphoma*, which oc-

Table 78-1. Malignant neoplasms affecting the tonsil (Armed Forces Institute of Pathology Registry)

Neoplasm	Cases (%)
Squamous cell carcinoma	72
Lymphoma (non-Hodgkin's)	14
Lymphoma (Hodgkin's)	2
Others	12

From Crawford BE and others: *Otolaryngol Clin North Am* 12:29, 1979.

curs especially in both palatine tonsils (Fig. 78-5) and may occur in the base of the tongue. Lymphoma may be unifocal or may involve many areas. The lesions are likely to be large and bulky, with a relatively brief history of symptoms. These tumors usually do not appear as ulcerating lesions. Typically, the tonsil is grossly enlarged. In many cases, the entire tonsil is involved with homogeneous disease, and no evidence of healthy tonsil is present. Lymphoma of the tonsil and the base of the tongue may be the first symptom of systemic lymphoma, which may be widespread throughout the body. In other cases, the disease may be diagnosed early, and only the palatine tonsil or base of the tongue may be involved or the disease may be limited to the primary oropharyngeal area and cervical sites (Table 78-1).

Salivary gland carcinoma

Because minor salivary glands are scattered throughout the soft palate and base of the tongue, occasionally adenoid cystic carcinomas and other salivary gland carcinomas may involve the oropharyngeal area. They behave as their counterparts in other head and neck areas, with local growth, perineural invasion, and metastasis to the lung. Other rare malignant tumors also may occur in the oropharyngeal area.

ETIOLOGY

The most significant etiologic factor associated with squamous cell carcinoma of the oropharynx is use of tobacco, although the correlation is less than with squamous cell carcinoma of the oral cavity. The oropharynx has fewer dependent drainage areas compared with the oral cavity, which has several mucous reservoirs that pool and concentrate to dissolve carcinogens, promoting prolonged contact with mucosa.

Tobacco may vary in its carcinogenic activities, depending on use. For example, "reserve" smoking, which is practiced in certain countries, consists of placing the lighted end of the cigarette or cigar inside the mouth. Smoking inexpensive cigarettes with high concentrations of toxins and chewing tobacco combined with slate, lime, or betel nut leaves also seem to increase tobacco's carcinogenic potential.

Most tumors of the oropharynx occur in patients who are heavy drinkers and smokers, and separating the effects of each agent is impossible. Alcohol irritates the mucosa directly and indirectly by promoting malnutrition and sclerosis. These side effects may stimulate activity of carcinogens in this area indirectly and may change mucosal reactivity to various carcinogenic stimulants. Patients who are heavy drinkers and smokers typically have extensive mu-

cositis of the entire oropharyngeal and laryngeal area, manifested by injection of the mucosa. Other areas may be raised and injected and may present a confusing picture to the physician trying to distinguish simple irritative mucositis from a tumor (Fig. 78-6).

In some patients, papillomavirus and cancers of the tonsil appear to be related. Deoxyribonucleic acid (DNA) changes associated with papillomavirus have been shown in some patients with tonsillar carcinoma.[12]

Cases of oropharyngeal cancer are increasing, and the age of patients is decreasing. Previously, it was diagnosed most often in 60- to 70-year-old patients; however, cases appearing in the fourth and fifth decades of life are now common. The incidence is higher in males, and the male to female ratio is approximately 4:1. The incidence of oropharyngeal cancer is low compared with the incidence of overall cancers in the body. Of the almost 1 million new cancers diagnosed each year in the United States, approximately 7000 to 9000 are in the oropharynx.

STAGING

Staging of oropharyngeal cancer is based on the American Joint Committee on Cancer system (Box 78-1).[1] In this system, clinical staging is defined before therapy, and the initial classification does not change after response to subsequent treatment.

Staging tumors in the oropharynx may be difficult. The measurements usually are performed on the lesion's surface; however, this may not give an accurate definition of the tumor's size. A base of the tongue lesion may be greater

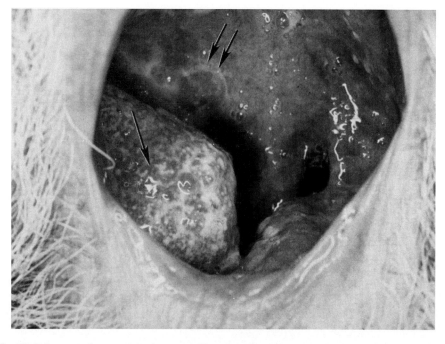

Fig. 78-6. Large oral cancer (*single arrow*). Note the adjacent extensive mucositis of the soft-palate area (*double arrow*).

Box 78-1. TNM Classification for oropharyngeal cancer staging

Primary tumor (T)

T_x Tumor cannot be assessed
T_0 No evidence of primary tumor
T_{is} Carcinoma *in situ*
T_1 Tumor 2 cm or less in diameter
T_2 Tumor larger than 2 cm but not larger than 4 cm in diameter
T_3 Tumor larger than 4 cm in diameter
T_4 Tumor larger than 4 cm in diameter with deep invasion into antrum, pterygoid muscles, root of tongue, or skin of neck

Nodal involvement (N)

N_x Nodes cannot be assessed
N_0 No clinically positive node
N_1 Single clinically positive ipsilateral node less than 3 cm in diameter
N_2 Single clinically positive ipsilateral node but not larger than 6 cm in diameter
  N_{2a} Single clinically positive ipsilateral node, 3 to 6 cm in diameter
  N_{2b} Multiple clinically positive ipsilateral nodes, none larger than 6 cm in diameter
N_3 Massive ipsilateral node(s), bilateral node(s), or contralateral node(s)
  N_{3a} Clinically positive ipsilateral nodes, none larger than 6 cm in diameter
  N_{3b} Bilateral clinically positive nodes (each side of neck should be staged separately; i.e., N_{3b}; right, N_{2a}; left, N_1)
  N_{3c} Contralateral clinically positive node(s) only

Distant metastasis (M)

M_x Not assessed
M_0 No (known) distant metastasis
M_1 Distant metastasis present
  Specify sites according to the following notations:

  Pulmonary — Pul   Bone marrow — Mar
  Osseous — Oss   Pleura — Ple
  Hepatic — Hep   Skin — Ski
  Brain — Bra   Eye — Eye
  Lymph nodes — Lym   Other — Oth

Staging

  Stage I $T_1N_0M_0$
  Stage II $T_2N_0M_0$
  Stage III $T_3N_0M_0T_1$-T_3, N_1, M_0
  Stage IV T_4, N_0 or N_1, M_0
               Any T, N_2 or N_3, M_0
               Any T, any N, M_1
  Residual tumor (R)
    R_0 No residual tumor
    R_1 Microscopic residual tumor
    R_2 Macroscopic residual tumor

than 2 cm. The same applies to tonsillar lesions, especially if the lesion originates in the epithelium in the depths of one of the crypts. The surface lesion may be deceptive, and if palpation is not performed, the extent may be misjudged. Distinguishing between T_3 and T_4 lesions may be difficult; at times, distinguishing between a lymph node and a direct extension of the primary tumor into the neck's soft tissues is impossible. Bimanual palpation to evaluate these lesions is mandatory. Computed tomography (CT) may help determine the depth and extent of tumor. Most tumors of the palate are easily visible, and staging is more accurate in these cases. Judging the location of the tumor's primary origin sometimes is difficult. Lesions of the tonsillar area frequently extend to and involve the retromolar trigone and palate and the inferior lateral pharyngeal wall. Base of the tongue lesions may involve the vallecula and epiglottis, and distinguishing between a supraglottic primary lesion and a base of the tongue primary lesion may be impossible. Thus, the physician should be careful in interpreting the data regarding tumors in this area.

MECHANISM OF CANCER BEHAVIOR AND CLINICAL PRESENTATION

As elsewhere in the body, oropharyngeal tumors spread along tissue planes of least resistance and along neurovascular structures in the head and neck. They extend to lymphatics and lymph nodes, erode into the blood vessels, and metastasize systemically to distant areas of the body. Microvascular invasion has a significant impact on survival. It is correlated with local and neck recurrences and distant metastasis.[16] Most squamous cell carcinomas of the oropharynx originate on the surface and generally spread along the mucosal surface (Fig. 78-7).

As the lesion enlarges, deeper structures may be involved, and base of the tongue tumors classically have a more vertical, deep growth pattern. When tumors involve the pharyngeal wall, submucosal spread is common, but the prevertebral fascia usually is not involved until an advanced stage. Generally, tumors spread along preformed pathways, such as fascial planes. This method of growth is more common than deep muscle invasion, at least initially. Perineural invasion by tumor may occur at any time but classically occurs early and frequently in adenoid cystic carcinoma. The functions of the involved nerve may be compromised. Generally, bone and cartilage are considered to be barriers to tumor spread and usually are not involved until an advanced stage. Periosteum and perichondrium are also natural tumor barriers because of their density and their lack of many capillaries. Once tumors in the oropharynx invade deeply, the parapharyngeal space may be involved, which allows tumors to spread up and down the neck from the base of the skull to the lower neck and even into the upper mediastinum (see Fig. 78-4).

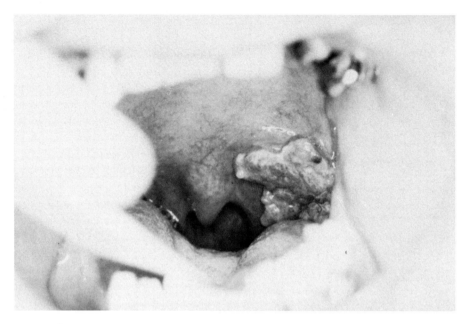

Fig. 78-7. Carcinoma of the soft palate and tonsillar area with spread along the surface.

Lymphatic metastasis

Lymphatic metastasis typically occurs in oropharyngeal carcinoma and most often is related to the depth of tumor invasion, the size of the tumor, and the amount of lymphatic channels supplying the primary site. Although the occurrence of cervical metastasis is reasonably predictable, some unpredictability is present with any primary site (Table 78-2), such as variability in terms of filtering and trapping of the lymph nodes, which may be modified by inflammation and fibrosis from past disease or radiation. Generally, cancers of the oropharynx metastasize superiorly to interiorly, from the high cervical lymph nodes downward to the midcervical and lower cervical lymph nodes; however, this is not true in all cases. ''Skipped'' metastases may bypass the upper cervical nodes and may appear first as a lower cervical node. The lower cervical node may be clinically involved on the gross examination, and the physician might assume that intervening lymph channels also may be skipped. For treatment, however, the physician should assume that the intervening lymph channels and lymph nodes are probably involved microscopically and should be treated. The physician cannot safely assume that no microscopic involvement of the cervical lymph nodes has occurred if no palpable first-echelon nodes exist.

Primary lymph node drainage from the oropharynx is to the upper deep jugular chain (Fig. 78-8). The superior parapharyngeal nodes lie medial to the posterior belly of the digastric muscle deep to the sternocleidomastoid and to the tail of the parotid gland. The jugular chain of lymph nodes extends from the upper neck downward to the clavicle area; these nodes lie very close to the internal jugular vein. A chain of lymph nodes also is distributed along CN XI in the

Table 78-2. Incidence of cervical lymph node metastases based on clinical examination of 1155 patients

Area	Primary tumor (T)	Incidence (%)		
		N_0	N_1	N_{2-3}
Tonsillar fossa	T_1	29	41	29
	T_2	32	14	53
	T_3	30	18	52
	T_4	10	13	76
Base of the tongue	T_1	30	15	55
	T_2	29	14	56
	T_3	25	23	51
	T_4	15	8	76
Soft palate	T_1	92	0	8
	T_2	63	12	24
	T_3	35	26	39
	T_4	33	11	56

Adapted from Lindberg R: *Cancer* 37:1901, 1976.

posterior neck triangle. These nodes tend to be somewhat superficial; as CN XI enters the anterior neck triangle very superiorly, however, the nerve and its associated lymph nodes are deep and closely associated with the internal jugular vein at the base of the skull.[82] The posterior triangle contains fewer lymph nodes than the anterior triangle, but these posterior nodes may be involved with oropharyngeal tumors more often than with tumors of the oral cavity. Although present staging schemes account for lymph node size, recent evidence suggests that the level of nodal involvement may serve as a prognostic indicator. Jones and others[43] examined 3419 patients with head and neck squamous cell

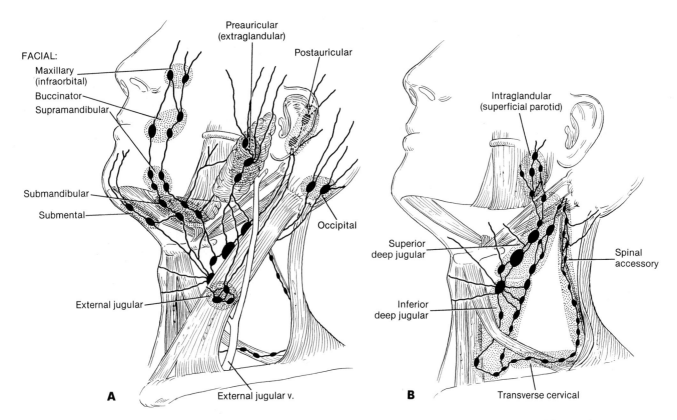

Fig. 78-8. Lymph node chains of neck that may be involved with cervical metastatic spread from oropharyngeal tumors. **A,** Superficial cervical and facial lymph nodes. **B,** Deep cervical and intraparotid lymph nodes.

carcinoma, of whom 947 had neck nodes metastases. A relationship between 5-year survival and the level of nodal disease was found; survival fell with decreasing nodal level. The 5-year survival was 37% for nodal disease at the upper jugular 32% for deep cervical nodes, and 25% for lower deep cervical nodes. Supraclavicular and posterior triangle nodal metastasis had the worse prognosis.

Bilateral metastasis

Bilateral metastasis from tumors of the oropharynx may occur, especially from the soft palate and base of the tongue area. Bilateral neck metastases occur more often from midline primary lesions and from tumors with bilateral lymphatic drainage. Contralateral lymph node metastases may occur from crossed primary afferent lymphatic vessels or after the primary ipsilateral nodes are involved and secondary collateral lymphatic flow develops. This is especially true in patients who have had neck surgery or been treated with irradiation. These modalities typically change the lymph flow, and collateral circulation increases. Tumor involvement of the upper cervical nodes also may change lymph flow.[26] Unusual lymphatic involvement may represent a peculiar pattern of metastases from the obvious primary tumor; however, the physician should remember that "unusual" lymph node metastases may represent metastatic

Table 78-3. Incidence of distant metastasis in head and neck squamous cell carcinoma in 5019 patients*

Primary site	Incidence of distant metastasis (%)
Faucial arch	6.7
Hypopharynx	23.6
Nasopharynx	28.1
Oral cavity	7.5
Oropharynx	15.3
Paranasal sinuses and nasal cavity	9.1
Supraglottic larynx	15.0
Vocal cord	3.1

Adapted from Merino OR, Lindberg RD, Fletcher GH: *Cancer* 40:145, 1977.
* At least 2-year follow-up. Excludes 41 patients in whom distant metastasis was found only at autopsy.

spread from a second primary tumor that may not have been obvious initially. As with regional metastases, distant metastases occur with increasing frequency with larger tumors (Tables 78-3 and 78-4).[8]

The initial cervical lymph node involvement and the development of distant metastases are correlates. The most common site of distant metastases are lungs, liver, and bones.[109]

Base of the tongue

Primary squamous cell carcinomas of the base of the tongue are relatively rare. The ratio of lesions in the anterior two thirds of the tongue to lesions in the base of the tongue is approximately 4:1. Base of the tongue carcinomas are notorious for deep infiltration into the muscular tissues. Symptoms frequently do not appear until these lesions are at an advanced stage. They may produce a sore throat or a sensation of a mass in the throat. The soreness may increase with swallowing, coughing, or any movement of the tongue. Referred otalgia may be the first symptom. Otalgia without obvious ear pathologic findings demands thorough examination of the entire oropharyngeal, hypopharyngeal, and laryngeal areas. The referred otalgia is mediated through CN IX or X, with both nerves peripherally distributed in the oropharyngeal and the ear areas (Fig. 78-9).

As the disease advances, the pterygoid muscles may be invaded, producing trismus. Base of the tongue tumors may extend anteriorly to involve the oral cavity portion of the tongue. They may also extend superiorly and laterally to involve the tonsil (Fig. 78-10). Inferior growth results in extension into the lateral pharyngeal wall with involvement of the epiglottis and preepiglottic space.

Base of the tongue tumors typically appear at a more advanced stage than tumors of the anterior two thirds of the tongue. Thus, they have been considered very invasive, wildly metastatic, and anaplastic. The concept that base of the tongue tumors are more aggressive may be a misconception and may only indicate that these tumors are found at a later stage because of the lack of symptoms. Asymptomatic early lesions are rarely diagnosed because the base of the tongue is not visualized by direct examination and requires a mirror to be inspected adequately. Internal bleeding and necrosis may produce rapid enlargement and pain. Some patients may have the sensation of a mass in the throat and may palpate it themselves. Many of these tumors may not be diagnosed until palpation of the base of the tongue area is performed, and in many cases the physician is surprised at the size of the lesion when first encountered. Extensive deep invasion may exist with only a very small surface lesion (Fig. 78-11). As the tumor enlarges, lymph node metastases

Table 78-4. Risk of distant metastasis according to stage

Stage	Risk (%)	T stage	Risk (%)	N stage	Risk (%)
I	2.0	T_1	5.2	N_0	4.9
II	5.7	T_2	9.6	N_1	11.8
III	8.5	T_3	12.7	N_2	21.8
IV	19.5	T_4	19.5	N_3	27.1

Adapted from Merino OR, Lindberg RD, Fletcher GH: *Cancer* 40:145, 1977.

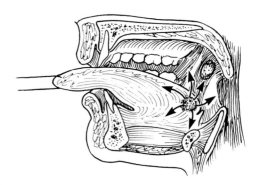

Fig. 78-10. Pathways of tumor spread in the base of the tongue. These lesions may extend inferiorly toward the larynx, deep into tongue muscles, anteriorly toward mobile portions of the tongue, or laterally toward the tonsillar and pharyngeal areas.

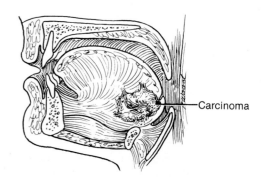

Fig. 78-11. Base of the tongue carcinoma with extensive involvement of deep muscles from a very small surface lesion.

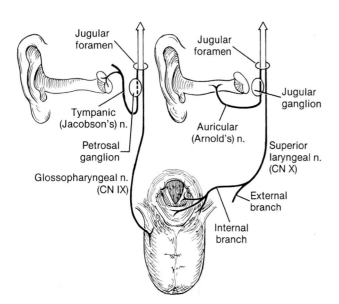

Fig. 78-9. Pathways for referred pain from the oropharynx to the ear.

are common. The base of tongue is rich in lymphatics, and the tumor's propensity for early invasion of the muscle predisposes it to early lymphatic involvement. The muscular contractions on the involved tumor may help propel the malignant cells at an earlier rate into the lymphatic system. The primary node is the subdigastric (jugulodigastric) node (Fig. 78-12), with the metastatic path extending inferiorly to the midjugular and lower jugular nodes. The submaxillary and posterior cervical nodes also may be involved. Lymph node metastases at the initial appearance of this disease are extremely common, and the first symptom is often an enlarged high cervical node. Approximately 60% to 75% of patients with cancer of the base of the tongue have a clinically positive cervical node at the initial visit, and 20% to 30% have bilateral nodes (Fig. 78-13). Incidence of occult nodes in clinically negative necks is approximately 20%, but because of the effectiveness of treatment with surgery and/or radio-

therapy, the actual risk for occult disease probably is closer to 50% or 60%.[9,56,70] Furthermore, a common site of occult disease lies between the site of the primary lesion and the easily accessible lymph nodes, namely nodal levels II, IV, and V.[50] Treating nodes in this area adequately should be emphasized.

Anterior tonsillar pillar and the tonsil

The anterior tonsillar pillar and the tonsil are the most common locations for tumors within the oropharynx. Rarely, a primary tumor is limited to the posterior pillar. Frequently, lesions on the anterior tonsillar pillar may appear as areas of leukoplakia or may be raised and infected. Asymptomatic lesions may not be noticed until observed in the mirror by the patient, or they may be diagnosed by a routine oral examination.

As the lesions enlarge, the central portion may ulcerate and the borders may rise. They may spread to the retromolar trigone and extend laterally to the buccal mucosa (Fig. 78-14). Once they involve the buccal mucosa, occult spread to the buccal fat pad may occur, appearing as a subtle fullness in the cheek (Fig. 78-15). Some anterior tonsillar pillar lesions extend superiorly and medially to involve the soft palate and may even extend to the hard palate. As the lesions extend medially, they involve the tongue, which worsens prognosis. The anterior tonsillar pillar is reasonably close to the medial aspect of the mandible, and lesions adhering to the mandible and eventually invading the periosteum and bone are not unusual. Inferior alveolar nerve involvement in these tumors may occur at an earlier stage in elderly patients because in edentulous mandibles the inferior alveolar nerve is more superficial and therefore is more prone to involvement from overlying mucosal cancers (Figs. 78-16 and 78-17). Tumors of the anterior tonsillar pillar eventually may spread posteriorly to involve the tonsil tissue. As these lesions erode deeply, the pterygoid muscles may be involved, producing trismus and pain (see Fig. 78-15).

Lesions arising primarily in the tonsillar fossa are less likely to appear as leukoplakia and frequently are exophytic

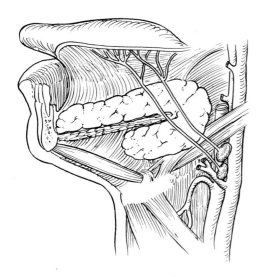

Fig. 78-12. Lymphatics of the base of the tongue, with the jugulodigastric node involved first.

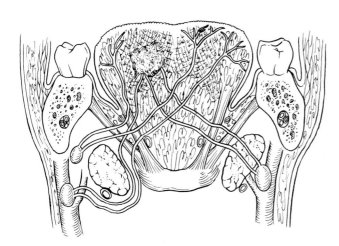

Fig. 78-13. Bilateral base of the tongue lymphatic drainage.

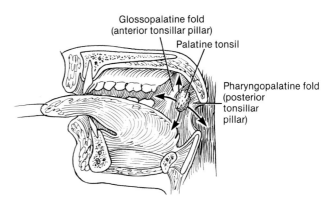

Fig. 78-14. Pathways of spread from the tonsil and tonsillar pillar lesions.

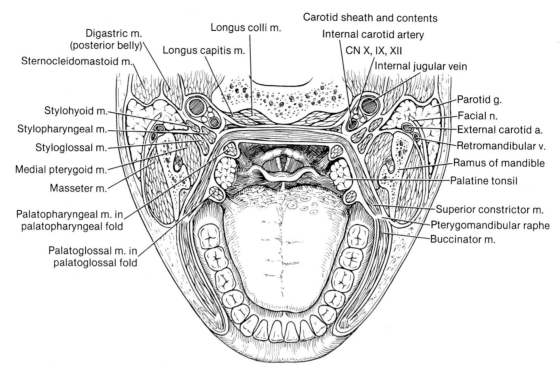

Fig. 78-15. Deep invasion from tonsillar lesions showing possible routes of extension to the buccal fat pad, pterygoid muscle (producing trismus), and parotid and cranial nerves.

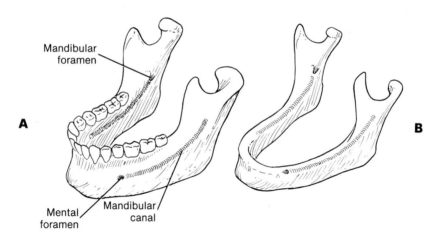

Fig. 78-16. A, A healthy mandible with alveoli protected by thick bone. **B,** Absorption of the mandible in elderly patients places the alveolar nerve closer to the intraoral cavity, increasing the possibility of its involvement with spread from oropharyngeal tumors.

or ulcerative (Fig. 78-18). These lesions usually extend posteriorly to the posterior pillar, interiorly to the lateral oropharyngeal wall, and inferiorly and medially to involve portions of the base of the tongue. As these lesions enlarge, they extend laterally and penetrate the parapharyngeal space and may extend superiorly toward the base of the skull with neurologic involvement. Once these lesions extend inferiorly to involve the lateral pharyngeal wall, they may extend down to the piriform fossa. Lesions that arise primarily in the pos-

terior tonsillar pillar may spread inferiorly along the palatal pharyngeal muscle, extending into the pharyngeal constrictor muscle, the pharyngeal epiglottic fold, and the posterior aspect of the thyroid cartilage. Because these lesions are more posterior, the spinal accessory lymph nodes and the posterior triangle lymph nodes are more likely to be involved.

Lesions of the tonsillar and pillar areas drain to the upper cervical nodes. Cancers involving the anterior tonsillar pillar

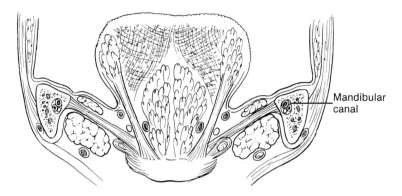

Fig. 78-17. Cross section of the mandible in an elderly person showing absorption of the alveolar bone and proximity of the alveolar nerve to the alveolus.

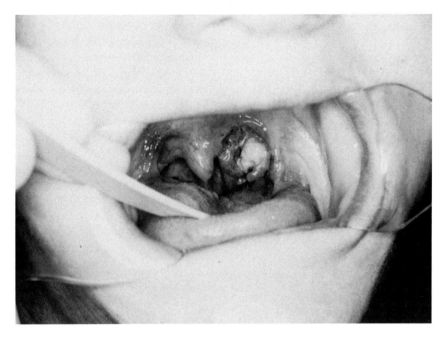

Fig. 78-18. Ulcerated tonsillar cancer.

have less risk of forming clinically positive lymph nodes compared with lesions limited to the tonsillar fossa. The anterior tonsillar pillar drains into the upper internal jugular vein lymph nodes and the submaxillary gland lymph nodes (Fig. 78-19). The risk of involvement of the spinal accessory and posterior triangle lymph nodes is low. Contralateral spread infrequently occurs in early lesions, but the risk of occult metastases in clinically negative necks is significant.[6,67]

Tonsillar fossa lesions have a higher risk of lymph node involvement compared with lesions of the anterior tonsillar pillar. The lymph node distribution for the tonsil includes the upper cervical, spinal accessory, and posterior triangle nodes (see Fig. 78-19). Contralateral neck metastases also may occur, and the risk of this involvement increases as more structures are involved (e.g., soft palate, base of the tongue). The risk also increases with enlarging ipsilateral neck nodes, which may produce obstruction and retrograde lymphatic flow. Although primary lesions of the posterior tonsillar pillar are rare, their lymph node metastatic direction also would be more posterior, with involvement of the high cervical, spinal accessory, and upper posterior triangle nodes (see Fig. 78-19).

Unlike base of the tongue lesions, tonsillar and anterior tonsillar tumors may be easily visualized, and dentists and physicians frequently diagnose them on routine oral examinations (Fig. 78-20). The patient may notice a sore throat and may see the lesion while looking in the mirror. As the tumors enlarge, they produce increasing pain; dentures may not fit, which may be an initial symptom. With their spread to other structures, these lesions may produce trismus, bleeding, fixation of the tongue, and referred otalgia. Primary lesions of the tonsillar fossa usually are large before symptoms manifest (see Fig. 78-18). This area seems to be less sensitive than the anterior tonsillar pillar. Lesions that occur primarily at the inferior pole may be difficult to visualize by direct examination, and visualization using mirrors may be necessary. Again, bimanual palpation is mandatory to determine the extent of these lesions. The tonsillar tissue

may harbor a hidden primary tumor that originates deep in one of the tonsillar crypts. In evaluation of an unknown primary tumor with known metastatic squamous cell carcinoma in a high cervical node, tonsillectomy probably should be by routine biopsy as opposed to by simple biopsy if no other lesion is obvious. A primary tumor deep in the tonsillar crypts may be missed by routine biopsy.

Soft palate

Soft-palate carcinomas occur almost exclusively on the anterior surface of the palate. They rarely involve the posterior surface until advanced stages. Lesions appear with leukoplakia, or they may be raised or flattened injected lesions (Fig. 78-21). At times, heavy smokers may have many areas of leukoplakia and injection; thus, distinguishing the significant lesions can be difficult. Even if a biopsy reveals squamous cell carcinoma, accurately delineating the borders of the lesion may be difficult (see Fig. 78-21).

Occasionally, several small primary tumors occur in the same patient, with large areas of intervening healthy mucosa. Most lesions are diagnosed at a reasonably early stage, when limited to the anterior soft palate. As the lesions enlarge, they spread to the tonsillar pillars and extend into the tongue area (Fig. 78-22). They also may extend laterally and then superiorly into the nasopharynx. Larger lesions may appear with large, ulcerative defects of the soft palate. The constrictor muscles of the pharynx and pterygoid muscles may be involved at a later stage, with resultant pain and trismus.

As the tumor enlarges, it may involve the palatine nerves, with resulting pain and extension of tumor along the nerve toward the cranial area (Fig. 78-23). These lesions produce a

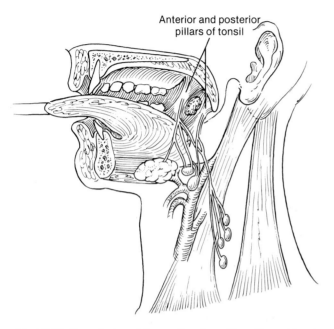

Fig. 78-19. Lymphatics of the tonsil and tonsillar pillars with primary drainage routes to upper cervical nodes.

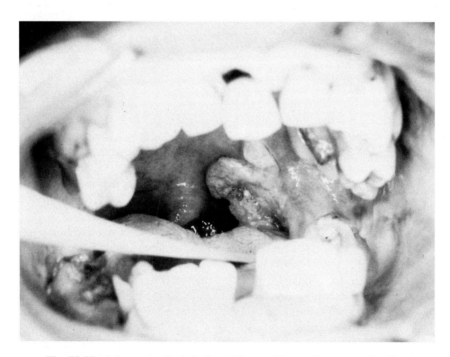

Fig. 78-20. A large, exophytic lesion of the tonsil extending onto soft palate.

sore throat, and bleeding may occur. Changes in swallowing, speech, and voice may be initial symptoms. Most of these tumors are easily visualized by the patient and physician.

Soft palate lesions metastasize to the digastric nodes and then into the upper cervical nodes (Fig. 78-24). The spinal accessory and posterior triangle nodes are involved less often. As the tumor extends laterally into the tonsillar areas and base of the tongue, the metastatic rate increases, along with the rate of spinal accessory and posterior triangle node involvement. Tumors close to the midline have a significant

bilateral metastatic rate, and soft palate lesions in general have a higher contralateral metastatic rate than tonsillar and anterior pillar lesions. Of patients, 40% to 50% have clinically positive lymph nodes at the initial examination, and approximately 15% have bilateral nodes.

DIAGNOSTIC EVALUATION

Thorough examination is mandatory in patients who have symptoms related to the oropharynx (e.g., sore throat, bleeding, voice changes, dysphagia). This includes direct exami-

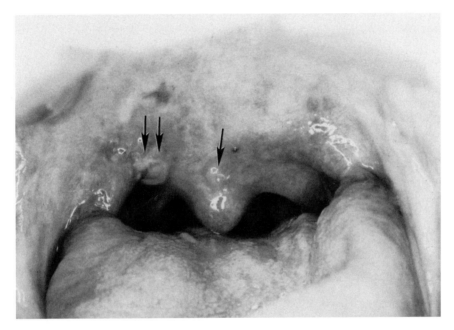

Fig. 78-21. A small carcinoma of lateral soft palate at the junction of the tonsillar area. Note the indistinct borders *(double arrow)* and leukoplakia secondary to hyperkeratosis with atypical changes *(single arrow)*.

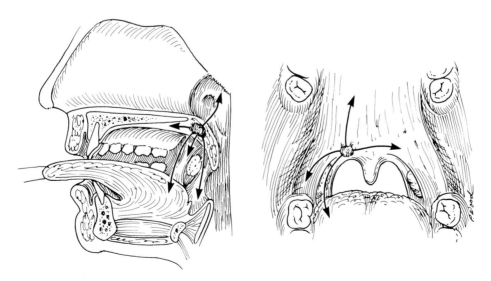

Fig. 78-22. Routes of spread from soft-palate carcinomas.

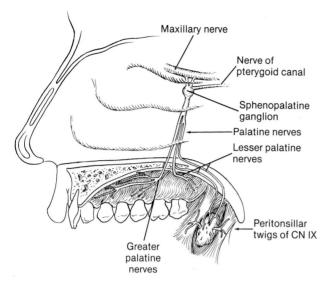

Fig. 78-23. Nerves supplying the soft palate that may be involved with spread of tumor.

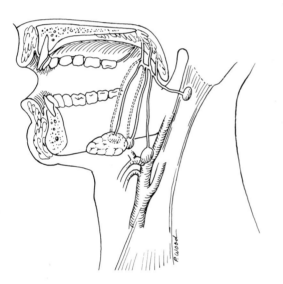

Fig. 78-24. Lymphatics of the soft palate.

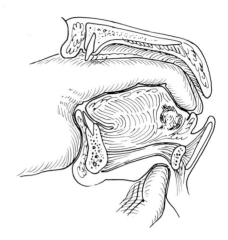

Fig. 78-25. Bimanual palpation of the oropharynx.

nation and indirect examination using laryngeal and nasopharyngeal mirrors. Bimanual palpation of the oropharynx is necessary (Fig. 78-25). The primary lesions should be accurately delineated, and a drawing or sketch should be made for the patient's permanent medical record. Panendoscopy, including nasopharyngoscopy, laryngoscopy, esophagoscopy, and bronchoscopy, should be performed routinely, even when the primary lesion is obvious and easily delineated. Panendoscopy also is needed to search for other primary tumors. The incidence of second primary tumors occurring with primary tumors of the oropharynx is significant.[63]

With the patient under general anesthesia, the physician carefully palpates the neck for lymph nodes (Fig. 78-26). At times, cervical lymph nodes may become palpable during general anesthesia with muscle relaxation. The physician also should determine whether the lymph nodes are fixed. The lesions should be biopsied with sharp instruments to avoid crushing artifact, and necrotic central areas of the tumor generally should be avoided. Multiple biopsies in questionable areas help define the exact limits of the tumor. Specifically, in lesions of the base of the tongue, several deep biopsies may be necessary because the surface lesion may be small. Excisional biopsy may be appropriate if the physician suspects the lesion is benign (Fig. 78-27). Tatooing tumor margins with India ink is helpful, especially in patients who received some type of therapy before surgical intervention. If a lymphoma is suspected, then larger biopsies usually should be performed to help the pathologist make a more accurate diagnosis; in many cases, the macroscopic pattern of the tumor helps diagnose lymphoma. Careful palpation of the primary tumor should yield information concerning whether the primary lesion is fixed to an underlying structure, such as the mandible or pterygoid muscles. It is also helpful to patients with deep lobe parotid tumors in the oropharynx (Fig. 78-28).

Barium swallow examinations may help to delineate the inferior extent of the lesion. Mandibular radiography and bone scanning frequently reveal useful information concerning possible tumor involvement of the mandible.

CT may determine the extent of the lesion, especially around the base of the skull (Fig. 78-29). Because of its close anatomic proximity to the oropharynx, the carotid artery may also require evaluation to rule out tumor involvement. Advances in magnetic resonance imaging (MRI) and magnetic resonance angiography offer promise regarding the noninvasive evaluation of the vascular system.[78] Presently, definitive diagnosis of carotid involvement requires angiography. Neurophysiologic evaluation for possible carotid resection involves balloon test occlusion of the internal carotid, followed by xenon CT blood flow mapping[42] or single photon emission CT brain scanning.[86] Results from these experimental techniques help predict the propensity for neurologic se-

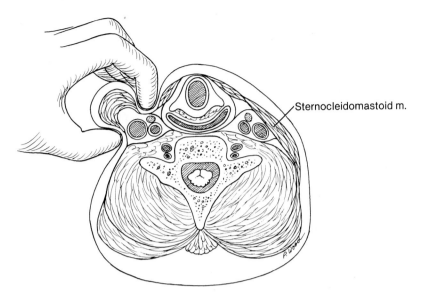

Fig. 78-26. Palpation of the lymph node. The sternocleidomastoid muscle is grasped between the thumb and index finger, allowing structures beneath the muscle to be palpated.

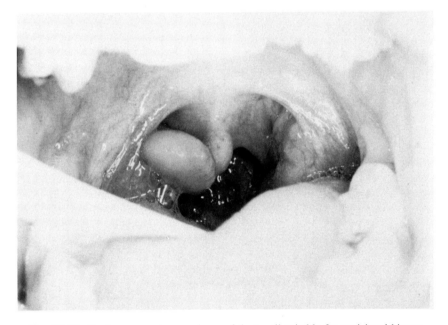

Fig. 78-27. Benign pyogenic granuloma of the tonsil suitable for excisional biopsy.

quelae if the internal carotid artery requires ligation intentionally or after iatrogenic injury.

MRI may help determine overall extent of the tumor and impingement or invasion of contiguous structures. It may help distinguish tumor persistence from delayed fibrosis.[76]

MANAGEMENT PHILOSOPHY

The literature frequently separates tumors of the oropharynx into several smaller groups, such as those of the soft palate, tonsil, anterior tonsillar pillar, and base of the tongue.

In fact, these lesions are derived from a common mucosal covering that blends to form one area. These cancers frequently extend from one area to the next without restrictions. Although the literature on the results of treatment discusses the sites of origin with a degree of certainty, the site of origin may be uncertain when the tumor involves adjacent areas. For example, when a tumor involves the superior laryngeal area and the base of tongue and vallecula, determining the exact site of origin is often impossible, even at the initial diagnosis. This distinction is impossible to make by a physi-

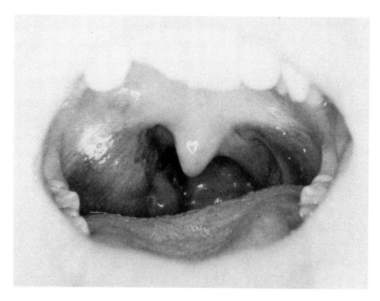

Fig. 78-28. A deep lobe tumor of the parotid gland appearing as an oropharyngeal mass.

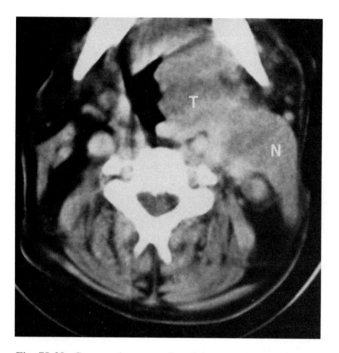

Fig. 78-29. Computed tomography of the oropharynx showing a large carcinoma of the base of the tongue and tonsillar area (*T*) extending into the lateral neck area (*N*).

cian reviewing charts retrospectively; the treatment results may be skewed, depending on the reviewer's assignment of the tumor to a specific site.

The biggest problem with oropharyngeal cancers is late diagnosis. Often, these tumors do not produce symptoms until a late stage and appear with a cervical metastasis at the initial examination. In the past, oropharyngeal cancers were considered more aggressive and anaplastic than tumors

of the anterior oral cavity. Some authors believed that the only difference between oropharyngeal and anterior oral cavity cancers is the more advanced stage of disease of oropharyngeal lesions at first appearance. The concepts of treatment of tumors in this area have changed over time. Initially, these tumors were approached with surgery to the primary and metastatic site. Later, the emphasis shifted to radiation as the primary treatment modality and, over the past several years, to combined therapy with radiation and surgery. Changing and improving techniques in radiotherapy and in surgical resection and reconstruction have improved the cure rates and have allowed patients to maintain more physiologic functions of the oropharyngeal area.

The role of chemotherapy in the treatment of these lesions continues to evolve.[81] Chemotherapy aimed at increasing locoregional control rates in advanced lesions has been used with good response in some patients without additional morbidity after surgical resection or postoperative radiotherapy.[38] The use of preoperative cisplatin and 5-fluorouracil has been efficacious in select patients,[59] and continued work in this area is promising. No difference is apparent between the induction and sequential groups.[39] A pathology specimen that reveals microvascular invasion indicates a worse prognosis, and adjuvant chemotherapy is recommended.[16]

In the literature, data on the treatment of these tumors are difficult to interpret because of different methods of reporting. For example, some radiotherapists use the term *locally controlled*, whereas others use *locally cured*. Kaplan, Million, and Cassisi[45] reported that T_1 and T_2 tumors did well with radiation alone, but the failure rate with T_3 and T_4 tumors was significant. They also acknowledged that early growths could be treated by surgery. Tong and others,[95] in a series of 104 patients treated by radiation alone, reported that 100% of the T_1 lesions and 74% of the T_2 lesions were

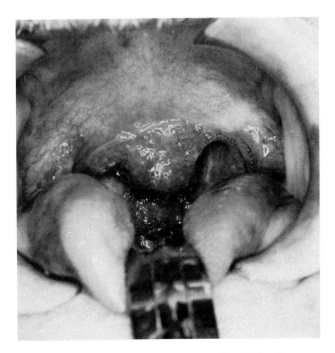

Fig. 78-32. Uvula carcinoma extending bilaterally.

elderly patients whose entire soft palate mucosa is injected and shows changes related to nicotine stomatitis; several biopsies may be necessary to determine the exact extent of the primary lesion. This reason explains why radiation generally is the primary treatment. It treats the primary lesion and local area, including epithelium that may have malignant changes not obvious to the physician. Radiation also treats the local lymphatics, which is important if the incidence of bilateral neck disease is to decrease.

Surgical resections of early lesions usually are recommended only for small carcinomas of the uvula. Larger resections of the palate for more advanced lesions without radiotherapy increase the chances for locoregional metastases. The functional disability from soft palate resection is significant; therefore, surgery is uncommonly recommended as the only therapy for soft palate lesions. If surgery is performed initially, postoperative radiation usually is planned as combined therapy. The irradiation technique generally involves parallel opposed external beam portals to include the primary lesion and the upper neck nodes bilaterally because even small T_1 soft palate lesions may have occult bilateral cervical metastases. If the lesion is small and discrete, a radioactive seed implant may be used initially, followed by external beam therapy. The implant may permit a reduced external beam dose, may decrease radiation side effects, and may improve local control because of a higher biologic dose.

Carcinomas involving the soft palate generally produce cervical metastases in at least one third of cases. Generally, the cure rates with radiation alone for T_1 lesions with N_0 necks are 80% to 90% and for T_2 lesions with N_0 necks,

70% to 80%; for T_3 and T_4 lesions, the cure rates drop dramatically to 20% to 30%. Because of the low survival rates for advanced T_3 and T_4 lesions, these tumors generally are managed by combined therapy of surgical resection followed by postoperative radiation.[79] Leemans and others[53] reviewed 52 patients with squamous cell carcinoma of the soft palate and the anterior tonsillar pillar treated by surgery, radiotherapy, and a combination of the two. Compared with tumor stages I and II, stages III and IV decreased survival by half. Leemans and others concluded that surgery followed by radiation is the most effective form of treatment for lesions in this area. Recurrent disease after primary radiotherapy should be treated with surgery if the lesion is resectable. If the lesion is not amenable to surgical resection, cryotherapy and laser treatment may give temporary local control; chemotherapy is frequently useful.

Base of the tongue

Carcinoma of the base of the tongue generally is considered to be more formidable than carcinoma of the palate or tonsil. These lesions frequently are large at the initial diagnosis (Fig. 78-33). Many patients have obvious neck metastases and bilateral neck metastases at the initial evaluation. Most series include few patients who are T_1; most usually are T_3 or T_4. The overall cure rate for most series, regardless of therapeutic modality, is usually about 30%.

Treatment regimens vary according to different institutions. Some centers initially use radiation as a primary modality and reserve surgery for irradiation failures.[93] However, surgery after irradiation failure only improves the cure rate by about 10%; thus, initial surgery followed by postoperative radiation frequently is recommended in an attempt to improve the prognosis. Although surgical resections of the base of the tongue involve significant functional morbidity, surgical reconstruction has improved significantly over the past years, and patients tolerate surgical resections better. Because of the improved use of myocutaneous flaps, postoperative radiation is more likely to be tolerated without complications at this site. Surgical resection is seldom used as a single modality because of the aggressive nature of this tumor, the advanced stage of disease, and the frequent cervical metastases.

Irradiation of cancer of the base of the tongue is delivered by parallel opposed external beam portals to the primary site, which also includes the bilateral regional lymph nodes (Fig. 78-34). The areas treated include the base of the tongue, portions of the oral tongue, the vallecula, pharyngeal walls, suprahyoid epiglottis, and the superior portion of the preepiglottic space. The cervical nodes, including the spinal accessory nodes bilaterally, are treated up to the base of the skull. Care should be taken to ensure an adequate portal for the anterior portion of the base of the tongue because many of these tumors extend deeply and anteriorly into this area. Because base of the tongue tumors have a significantly high rate of bilateral metastasis, both sides of the neck routinely

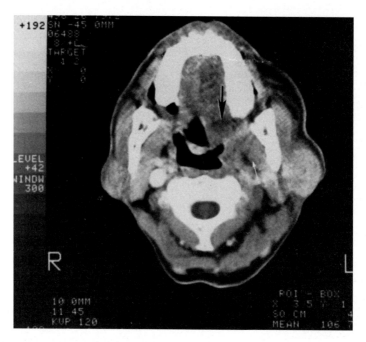

Fig. 78-33. Large carcinoma of the left tonsil (*white arrow*) extending to the left palate (*black arrow*).

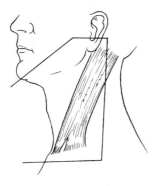

Fig. 78-34. Radiotherapy portals for base of the tongue carcinoma.

are treated. The amount of radiation may be boosted by the submental route. This is more effective for central rather than lateral lesions. Interstitial implants may be used if the lesion is in the anterolateral base of the tongue. Planned preoperative radiotherapy usually is not recommended except for large, fixed neck nodes. If radiation is used as a primary therapeutic modality, surgery may be recommended if significant improvement does not occur with 5000 rad. Attempting to improve the prognosis, the physician usually uses planned initial surgical resection with reconstruction, followed by irradiation after about 3 weeks. Recurrent disease usually is treated by surgical resection if this was not performed initially; however, the survival rates are low except for very small lesions. Regardless of the modality chosen, the 5-year cure rates are low (20% to 50%) because most lesions are treated at advanced stages.[41,79]

SURGICAL THERAPY

The principles of surgical resection and reconstruction for the oropharynx are generally the same whether the tumors involve the tonsillar area, the soft palate, the base of the tongue, or various combinations of these areas. Surgical management mandates a careful initial examination. During endoscopy, which is usually performed with the patient under general anesthesia, the surgeon takes care to map the extent of the primary lesion by visualization and by manual palpation. Other areas of the upper respiratory and gastrointestinal tract are examined during endoscopy to rule out tumor extension and to search for other primary lesions in this area. CT and nuclear MRI scans may help determine the extent of the primary lesions, especially when the surgeon is looking for pterygoid and base of the skull extension (Fig. 78-35).[79] Biopsies should be performed at the time of endoscopy. Necrotic centers of tumors should be avoided, and biopsies generally are taken at the periphery to include the tumor and healthy tissue. Questionable areas of tumor are biopsied, and the tumor area may be tattooed with ink, especially if patients are going to be treated initially with radiation.

Limited intraoral excision of oropharyngeal tumors generally is condemned except in unusual circumstances. If surgical resection is considered, the surgeon should plan resection of the primary lesions along with the appropriate lymphatic drainage areas. Most often this involves resection of the primary site and some type of neck dissection. In planning the resection and reconstruction, the surgeon should consider the extent of primary lesion and the locoregi-

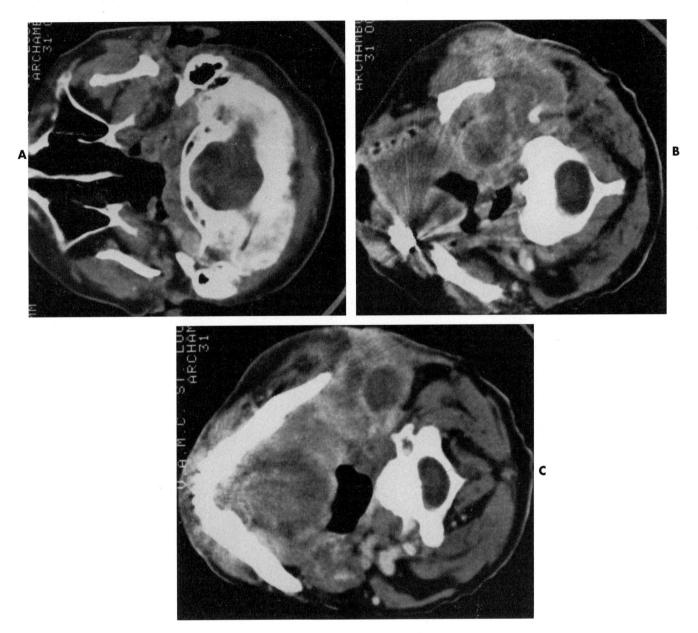

Fig. 78-35. A, A tonsillar lesion extending to the pterygoid area. **B,** The same lesion extending farther inferiorly, with a large mass in the left tonsil area. **C,** The same lesion at a more inferior site showing extension of the tumor into the pharynx and direct extension into the lateral neck tissues.

onal metastases. The surgeon also should consider any past and possible future treatment, assess the functional deformity, and plan for reconstruction of functional defects and for cosmesis. Most local excisions in the soft palate and tonsillar area can be closed primarily by split-thickness skin or dermal graft. Usually, palatal reconstruction for small defects is unnecessary because a prosthesis can remedy any functional defect.

The approach to resection of larger primary tumors of the oropharynx involves consideration of the mandible. Previously, with most surgical resections of oropharyngeal tu-

mors, a portion of the mandible was removed. Resection of a section of this bone dates back to the development of the classic commando operation (Fig. 78-36).[79] Removing a portion of the mandible along with the primary lesion was considered necessary, and neck dissection was considered necessary to ensure the *en bloc* resection. Surgical techniques have changed over the years, however; surgeons now try to preserve the mandible when it is considered safe in terms of tumor resection. Marchetta, Sako, and Murphy[61] showed that malignant cells were not found in the periosteal lymphatics unless the gross tumor lesions were in direct contact with the mandibular mucoperiosteum. Partial marginal mandibular resections may be performed for lesions close to but not directly involving the lingual surface of the mandible. These resections ensure an adequate margin yet preserve the continuity of the mandible (Fig. 78-37).

Multiple techniques are available to determine bone involvement, including nuclear scanning, plain radiographs, and CT; however, none seems more accurate for assessing bone involvement than direct intraoperative inspection. If the periosteum strips cleanly from the bone, then invasion of the bone is unlikely. In the past, a portion of the mandible was removed with the tumor to facilitate closure (Fig. 78-38). If the mandible is left intact, the closure is more difficult because less collapse of the surrounding tissue occurs and some reconstruction in this area usually is necessary. The use of flaps, especially the myocutaneous type, has greatly improved reconstruction and allows more patients to retain intact mandibles.

Approaches for combined primary tumor and neck resection

Planning the approach for combined primary tumor and neck resection should include whether the mandible will be spared, such as in the lateral or transhyoid pharyngotomy, or whether the mandible will be transected. If the mandible will be transected, it may be split in the anterior midline or laterally. The mandible may not be completely transected but only partially, allowing maintenance of the arch support of the mandible. The approach to the lesion and neck disease should consider approach, resection, and closure. Multiple options exist in each case, and decision-making should consider many variables.

The neck incisions for combined primary tumor and neck resections should allow for good blood supply to the neck skin flaps and good access to the area of resection (Fig. 78-39, *A*). Generally, the neck incision includes an upper horizontal limb, which usually starts in the area of the mas-

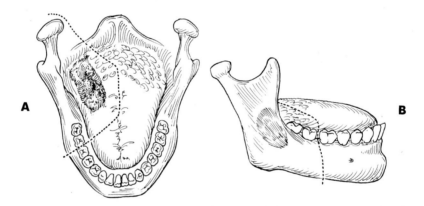

Fig. 78-36. A, Composite resection of the tonsillar and base of the tongue area, including the primary lesion and mandible. **B,** Composite resection, including primary lesion, mandible, and neck dissection, to include appropriate lymphatic drainage field. Note that neck dissection is based superiorly at the inferior border of the mandible.

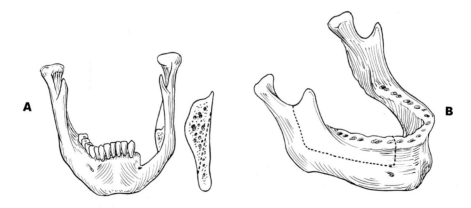

Fig. 78-37. A, Partial mandibulectomy, including the inner table of the mandible. The body of the mandible is intact. **B,** More extensive partial mandibulectomy, maintaining continuity of the mandible.

toid tip, extends inferiorly, and parallels the lower border of the mandible. This incision is made approximately 2 to 3 cm inferior to the mandible to avoid the marginal mandibular nerve. The anterior limb of the horizontal incision may curve superiorly to extend up through the submental, chin, and lower lip areas, or it may continue for a few centimeters to the opposite side of the neck, allowing the surgeon to perform a visor flap for the chin and lower lip (Fig. 78-39, *B*). A lower limb is dropped from the posterior portion of the horizontal incision, extending inferiorly down the neck posteriorly and allowing access to the contents of the anterior and posterior neck triangles. The junction of the vertical and horizontal limbs of this incision should be planned so that it is not over the carotid area; thus, if the tip of the flap becomes necrotic at the junctional area, the carotid artery will not be exposed. The junctional angles should be at 90° to maintain maximal blood supply to the tip of each flap. The upper limb of the incision allows access to the oropharyngeal area through (1) a lip-splitting incision,[61] allowing a lip and cheek flap to be elevated (Fig. 78-40), or (2) by allowing creation of a visor flap (Fig. 78-41), thus preserving the continuity of the chin and lip area.

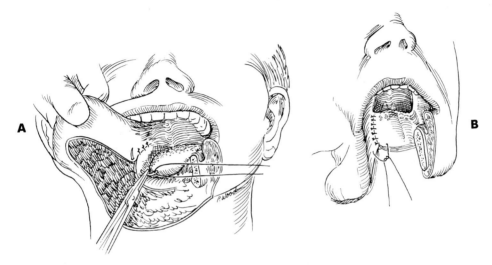

Fig. 78-38. A, In composite resections involving the mandible, closure is usually easier if the mandible is removed, thus allowing the lateral buccal flap to be sutured to the lateral border of the resected area. **B,** Closure of defect. Resection of the mandible allows the lateral buccal area to be closed more easily to the tongue area.

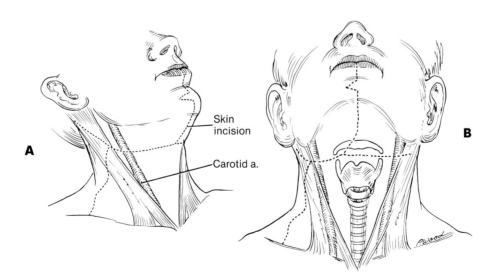

Fig. 78-39. A, Incision for composite resection of the oropharyngeal area. Incision allows good access to the neck and adequate exposure of the oropharynx and mandible. **B,** Medial superior extent of the incision may be extended superiorly, splitting lip, or extended to the contralateral side to create a visor flap.

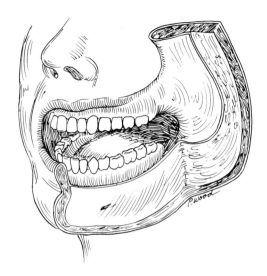

Fig. 78-40. Lip-splitting incision with extension to create a buccal cheek flap. This allows access to the mandible and oropharyngeal site.

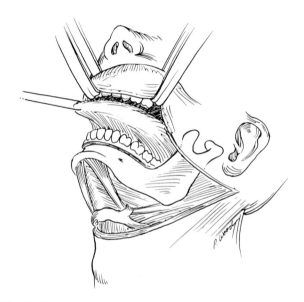

Fig. 78-41. Visor flap. This allows good access to the mouth and oropharyngeal area.

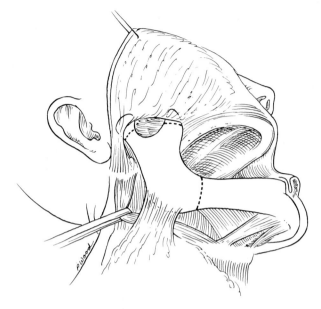

Fig. 78-42. After the flap is elevated, mandibular cuts are made across the body of the mandible anteriorly and at the coronoid and condyloid processes superiorly. With this exposure, partial mandibulectomy also may be performed. Neck dissection is based at the angle of the mandible.

If the surgeon wishes to gain access to the oropharyngeal area without splitting the lower lip, the upper horizontal limb of the cervical incision may be extended across the midline approximately 2 cm. An intraoral incision is made along the anterior buccal gingival sulcus, extending from the contralateral mental foramen area anteriorly and then posteriorly on the ipsilateral side. The soft tissue between the upper cervical incision and the buccal gingival incision is joined to create a visor lip and cheek flap, which may be elevated superiorly, allowing access to the oropharyngeal area. The major limitation of this approach is failure to extend the flap far enough to the contralateral side (see Fig. 78-39, *B*). If a neck dissec-

tion is done in continuity with a primary resection, the base of the neck dissection is generally anchored at the area of the angle of the mandible at the inferior medial surface (Figs. 78-36, *B*, and 78-42). This most closely approximates the area of lymphatic drainage from the areas of the oropharynx.

By splitting the lip or using a visor flap, the surgeon carries the incision along the ipsilateral gingival buccal sulcus posteriorly, and a lateral lip and cheek flap is created and elevated (see Fig. 78-40). This permits access to the lateral border of the mandible posteriorly, and the surgeon may perform an osteotomy in this area for access to the oropharynx (Fig. 78-43) with preservation of the mandible. If the mandible is to be included in the resection, it is transected anterior to the tumor, and superior mandible cuts are performed, generally in the area of the condyloid and coronoid processes (see Fig. 78-42). An alternate osteotomy may be performed anteriorly by swinging the ipsilateral mandible laterally and extending a medial incision along the ipsilateral glossal gingival sulcus back to the anterior portion of the planned resection (Fig. 78-44). This allows the mandible to be rotated laterally and the contralateral tongue to be pulled to the opposite side, thus permitting access to the primary site of resection. The anterior osteotomy is joined together during closure (Fig. 78-45).

If a marginal mandibulectomy is to be performed, the bony cuts are made before starting the soft-tissue intraoral incisions around the tumor (Fig. 78-46). As the resection continues, the anterior resection of the tumor is begun and extended posteriorly and inferiorly so that visualization is

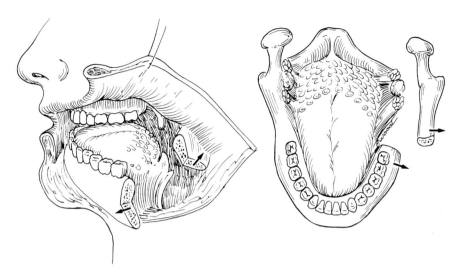

Fig. 78-43. Mandibulotomy allows good access to oropharyngeal area. Mandibular segments are rotated, allowing adequate access to the base of the tongue, tonsil, and palate. Mandibular segments are wired together at the end of the procedure. *Arrows* indicate direction of tissue retraction.

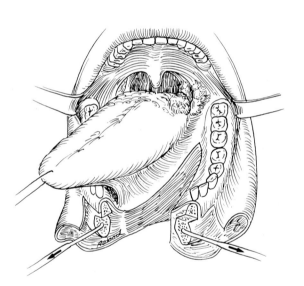

Fig. 78-44. Anterior mandibulotomy may be used to expose the oropharynx. Incision along the medial aspect of the mandible is made to obtain posterior exposure. *Arrows* indicate direction of tissue retraction.

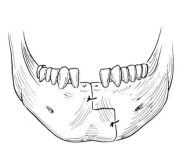

Fig. 78-45. Reapproximation of anterior mandibulotomy with wires. Making bony cuts in steps creates more stable approximation.

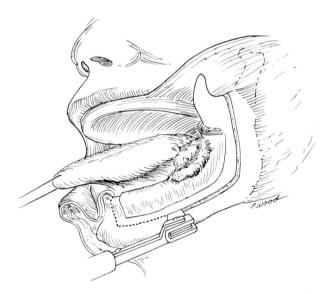

Fig. 78-46. Elevation of the buccal cheek flap and partial mandibulectomy to encompass the primary lesion.

always adequate. Typically, a portion of the tongue is resected to obtain a surgical margin. This anterior tongue incision is extended to the medial aspect of the resection and then extended posteriorly (Fig. 78-47). At the same time, the lateral resection is extended posteriorly and superiorly to include adequate portions of the mandible, if it is to be part of the resection. As primary tumor resection continues, traction is placed on this area to pull it anteriorly and laterally out of the oropharyngeal site. If the tumor is primarily limited to the tonsillar and soft palate areas, the portion of the tongue resected may be small and the posterior limits of the resection are easily reached (Fig. 78-48). Usually the tissue is still attached around the pterygoid muscles lying directly over the internal carotid artery (Fig. 78-49). If the tumor does not involve the pterygoids, they are cut off of the mandible, usually superiorly to inferiorly. The primary tumor is then dissected from the internal carotid artery, generally inferiorly to superiorly.

Palate removal

Depending on the extent of the tumor, various portions of the palate may require removal. If the tumor extends onto the hard palate, chisels are used to make appropriate hard palate cuts, and this area is removed along with the resection (Fig. 78-50). In patients with trismus whose tumor involves the pterygoids, the pterygoids are removed and the pterygoid plates are transected with a chisel to ensure their removal

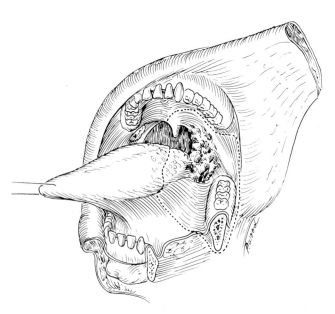

Fig. 78-47. The mandible is rotated laterally, and the tongue is pulled to the contralateral side, allowing adequate access to the oropharynx. Resection should proceed anteriorly to posteriorly, permitting easy visibility of primary resection.

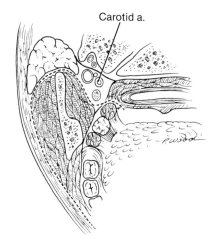

Fig. 78-49. Cross section of the tonsillar area showing primary resection. Surgeon should take care not to injure the carotid artery because deep cuts are made for primary resection.

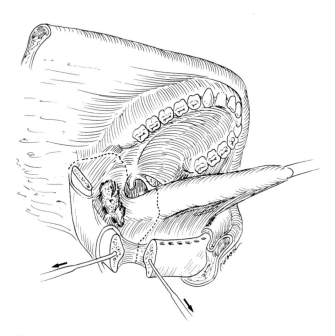

Fig. 78-48. If the medial incision extends more posteriorly and superiorly, the base of the primary area close to the carotid artery generally remains. *Arrows* indicate direction of tissue retraction.

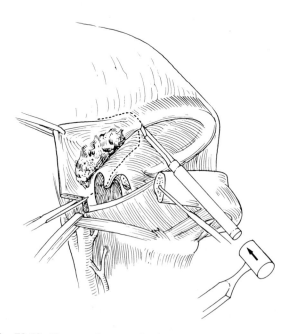

Fig. 78-50. If an oropharyngeal primary tumor extends onto soft palate or hard palate, appropriate cuts should be made and incision extended up to encompass this area for composite resection. *Arrow* indicates direction of hammer.

(Fig. 78-51). If the tumor involves the base of the tongue, a greater portion of the tongue will have to be removed; extreme care is necessary to obtain an adequate margin around the tumor's deep extent by palpating the base of the tongue to determine the areas to be resected. The surgeon should also be careful to ensure preservation of the contralateral lingual artery.

Median translingual pharyngotomy

An alternate approach to the primary tumor involves a median translingual pharyngotomy (Fig. 78-52). The midline of the tongue is incised, bisecting the tongue into bilateral equal segments and extending back to the area of the tumor in the base of the tongue (Fig. 78-53). This approach

is generally only useful for small, limited midline base of the tongue lesions.

Transhyoid pharyngotomy

Transhyoid pharyngotomy is another approach to base of the tongue lesions (Figs. 78-54 through 78-56). This technique has the advantages of maintaining mandibular and occlusal integrity, avoiding cosmetic deformity, and preventing scarring in the anterior oral cavity for maximal mobility of the tongue remnant.[4,68] The danger of this approach is that the vallecula is entered blindly, and the surgeon should be sure that the tumor is not transected during the approach. The hyoid bone may be transected or, often, removed. The vallecula is entered, and the resection is performed from the

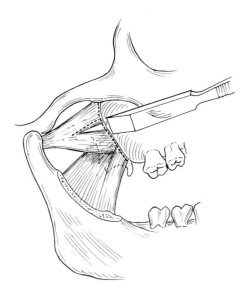

Fig. 78-51. If trismus is present and the tumor involves pterygoid muscles, pterygoid plates may have to be removed by transecting them at the base of the skull to ensure adequate margin around the tumor.

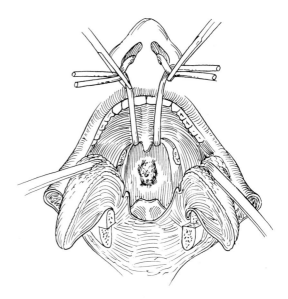

Fig. 78-53. Median translingual pharyngotomy allows good access for limited lesions of the midline of the base of the tongue or of the posterior pharyngeal wall. If limits of this procedure are extended, the hypoglossal nerve (cranial nerve XII) and the lingual artery are at risk for injury. For most tumors of the oropharynx, this approach is not indicated.

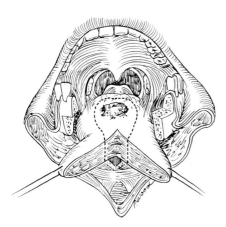

Fig. 78-52. For midline base of the tongue lesions, the anterior midline glossotomy approach may be indicated.

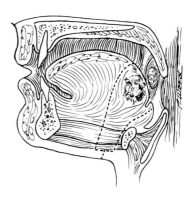

Fig. 78-54. The transhyoid or suprahyoid approach allows access to the base of the tongue from the neck area.

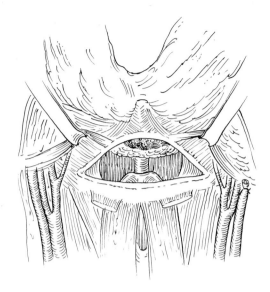

Fig. 78-55. Base of the tongue may be approached by dissecting just superiorly to hyoid bone, or bone may be removed and included in resection.

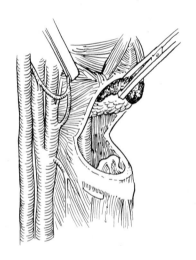

Fig. 78-56. Lateral view following the removal of a small base of the tongue tumor through anterior approach. The surgeon should be careful using this approach to avoid transection of the tumor when entering the primary site.

neck area. Care should be taken to avoid injury to the lingual artery and hypoglossal nerve (CN XII). The defect is closed primarily. This procedure has only limited applicability.

Lateral pharyngotomy

Lateral pharyngotomy may be useful for small lesions of the posterior and lateral pharyngeal wall. The pharynx is entered laterally by retracting the thyroid ala, entering the superior portion of the piriform fossa, and extending superiorly. The superior laryngeal nerve should be spared. This approach is limited superiorly by the mandible. Surgeons should be cautious in using this approach because most lesions require more exposure for adequate resection.

Associated laryngectomy procedures

Supraglottic laryngectomy

Base of the tongue tumors may extend inferiorly and laterally to involve the vallecula, epiglottis, and other portions of the supraglottic larynx. If tumors are small and inferior in the base of the tongue, approaching these tumors through a supraglottic laryngectomy may be appropriate. This basically involves a supraglottic resection with extension into the base of the tongue.

The surgeon should consider the postoperative function in relation to the amount of the base of the tongue resected. With a supraglottic laryngectomy and loss of the epiglottis and false vocal cords, the base of the tongue is critical to allow adequate swallowing and prevent aspiration. Factors involved in this decision include the age and respiratory status of the patient, the extent of the tumor, and the amount of tongue to be resected. Generally, no more than one half of the base of the tongue should be removed in a supraglottic laryngectomy (Fig. 78-57). The surgeon should ascertain that the remaining hypoglossal nerve (CN XII) and lingual artery are intact. An associated cricopharyngeal myotomy should be performed. Reconstruction with a flap (see Fig. 78-57) is useful if much of the base of the tongue is resected with a supraglottic laryngectomy. If a flap is not used, a tight, tenuous closure with resultant fistula is common.[75]

Total laryngectomy

If a large portion of the base of the tongue requires excision, or if both hypoglossal nerves are sacrificed, usually patients will aspirate with an associated supraglottic laryngectomy. In these patients, a concomitant total laryngectomy should be performed. In poor-risk patients, an associated total laryngectomy may be required, even if a supraglottic laryngectomy is technically feasible. This is especially true in patients with excessive alcohol intake and poor pulmonary functions.[83] Some patients may have excessively bulky tumors of the tongue that may involve the base of the tongue to such an extent that a total glossectomy is necessary (Fig. 78-58). Patients requiring a total glossectomy are at high risk to aspirate, and concomitant total laryngectomy is usually performed (Fig. 78-59).[85] Some patients, however, can learn to swallow effectively without aspiration. With the use of more bulky myocutaneous flaps and microvascular reconstruction, more patients with total glossectomies may be able to retain their larynx.[10,23] Functional results after total or near-total glossectomy with laryngeal preservation may be improved with ancillary procedures of laryngeal suspension, palatal augmentation, and videofluoroscopy to improve swallowing.[103]

Near-total laryngectomy

Near-total laryngectomy may be used in some base of the tongue tumors that extend inferiorly. This preserves portions of the larynx and laryngeal speech and allows for ade-

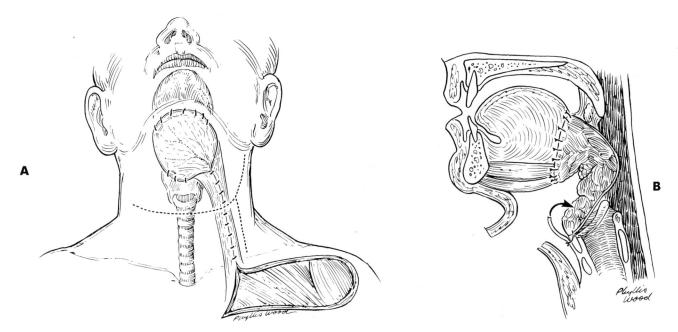

Fig. 78-57. Extended supraglottic laryngectomy approach for tumor at the base of the tongue. **A,** Use of a deltopectoral skin flap for reconstruction of an extended supraglottic laryngectomy defect. **B,** Reconstruction of the base of the tongue and supraglottic area allows anterior shelf to deflect bolus during deglutition.

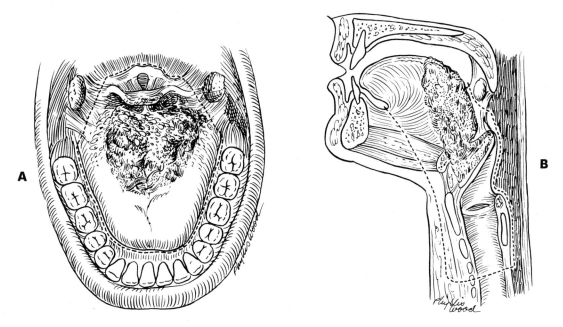

Fig. 78-58. A, Extensive tumor at the base of the tongue that requires total glossectomy and **B,** total laryngectomy.

quate tumor resection.[19] This technique demands careful patient selection, precise surgical technique, and intense postoperative rehabilitation.

Closure

A small defect produced by the resection can frequently be closed primarily, especially if a portion of the mandible has been removed, allowing the tissues to collapse and mak-

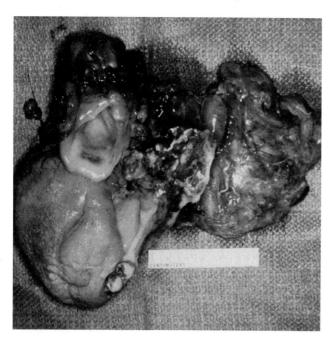

Fig. 78-59. Large tumor at the base of the tongue managed with total glossectomy and laryngectomy.

ing primary closure possible (see Fig. 78-38). If the resected area is more extensive or if osteotomies have been performed and the mandible may be reapproximated, primary closure is more difficult and some type of reconstruction is necessary. Primary closure usually includes suturing the lateral pharyngeal wall to the base of the tongue; the more anterior portions of the tongue are sutured to the lateral posterior buccal area at the previous site of the resected tonsil (Fig. 78-60). This produces some tethering of the tongue and thus limited tongue mobility; however, many patients function very well with good speech and adequate swallowing. If one third of the width of the tongue or more has been resected, primary closure may significantly limit speech, tongue mobility, and swallowing. The surgeon seldom can resect a significant portion of the base of the tongue and perform a primary closure without risking complications. If the closure heals, the patient usually will be oropharyngeally crippled, with an inadequate ability to swallow. Tight primary closure in the base of the tongue typically results in postoperative dehiscence with a resultant fistula; thus, some type of flap reconstruction usually is necessary for base of the tongue tumors.

Carotid artery protection

If neck dissection is part of surgery and the sternocleidomastoid muscle is removed, proper protection of the carotid artery is necessary. Measures may involve a dermal graft (Fig. 78-61), a local scalene muscle flap, or the muscle pedicle of a myocutaneous flap (see Fig. 78-72) or microvascular flap. Before wound closure, hemostasis should be meticulous to avoid postoperative bleeding and hematoma.

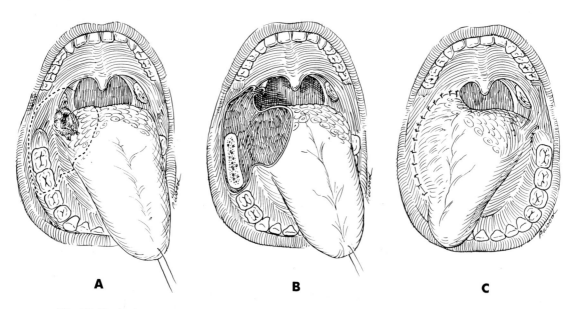

A **B** **C**

Fig. 78-60. A, Area of resection for the primary tonsil and the base of the tongue tumor. **B,** The defect after resection. **C,** Primary closure of the defect by suturing the lateral edge of the resected tongue to the buccal border. If this is excessive, the tongue may have limited mobility because it attaches directly to the buccal flap.

Reconstruction

Free skin or dermal graft

If the primary site is to be reconstructed, several choices are available. Free skin grafts[25] or dermal grafts[13] are useful in closing defects of the tonsil and lateroposterior tongue areas (see Fig. 78-61). These grafts are sutured in place and generally held with a sutured bolster. Usually, the skin graft reconstruction should be generous to allow for shrinkage.[83] Generally, a pouch is produced laterally to improve tongue mobility and create a lateral gutter to improve control of oral secretions (Fig. 78-62). Intermaxillary fixation assists in graft immobilization, improving the success of the graft. Partial loss of the graft is not unusual; however, enough of the graft is usually retained to be beneficial, and frequently the area of lost graft will granulate, with stimulation of epithelial regrowth and healing by secondary intention.[51]

Tongue flaps

Tongue flaps are another alternative to reconstruction and are frequently used in reconstruction of the tonsillar area.[21,84] The most common approach involves dividing the tongue longitudinally in the midline and rotating it 180° to close the defect in the tonsillar lateral palate area (Fig. 78-63). Occasionally, less tongue has to be used as a flap, and more than one half may be retained for functional use. The advantages of the tongue flap are its ease of accessibility, its excellent blood supply, and its lack of cosmetic defect. Despite these advantages, the resultant speech defects and deglutition problems limit the usefulness of the tongue flap in oropharyngeal reconstruction.

Regional flaps

Regional flaps allow a larger volume of healthy tissue for reconstruction. These flaps may be skin, muscular, or myocutaneous.

Regional skin flaps. Some skin flap choices include postauricular flap, forehead flap, deltopectoral flap, and nape of neck flap. The postauricular flap was recently reintroduced as another candidate for reconstruction of moderately sized oropharyngeal defects (Fig. 78-64). Available as either a pedicled or microvascular free transfer, the pedicled flap is particularly well suited for defects of the oropharynx. Based on the postauricular branch off the external carotid artery, the venous drainage via the postauricular vein is more often the limiting aspect. Variation in the outflow of this superficial system prevents elevation of a healthy pedicle in up to 15% of cases. The skin paddle offers a unique, pliable surface comparable with the lining of the oral cavity. Inclusion of the greater auricular nerve offers the potential for neurosensory restoration, although a resultant functional benefit has yet to be shown. Donor site morbidity is minimal, as expected in the postauricular area.[47,55]

The forehead flap is based on the superficial temporal artery (Fig. 78-65); it may be brought directly through a cheek incision to repair more anterior defects or brought

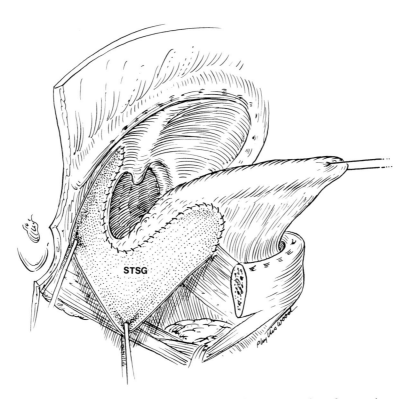

Fig. 78-61. Placement of a skin or dermal graft for reconstruction of resected area.

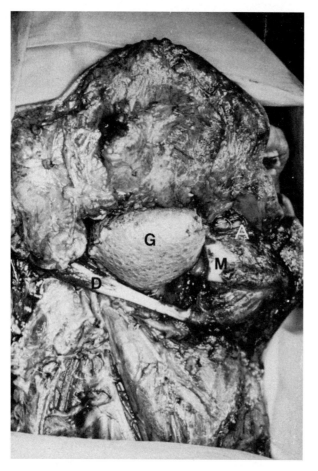

Fig. 78-62. Inferior view of reconstructed area using dermal graft *(G)*. Note digastric muscle *(D)* and anterior transected edge of mandible *(M)*. Note also arch bars *(A)* used for intermaxillary fixation.

under the zygomatic arch for reconstruction of more posterior defects (Fig. 78-66). Usually, this flap provides more than adequate tissue for repair of even large defects in the tonsillar or base of the tongue area. In 2 to 3 weeks, the unused portion of the flap is returned to the forehead, or it may be severed, allowing the forehead defect to granulate to elevate this area. A split-thickness skin graft is placed on the donor site. The forehead flap is excellent for reconstruction of the oropharyngeal area. Its disadvantages are the resultant forehead cosmetic deformity and the requirement of two stages. It cannot be considered a high-priority flap because of the cosmetic disfigurement.

The deltopectoral flap also may be used to repair oropharyngeal defects. This flap is most often based medially (Fig. 78-67). Its blood supply is more tenuous than the forehead flap, and delaying the flap with an initial extra stage may be necessary. This flap, if created properly by extending to or including portions of the shoulder, usually is long enough to reach the tonsillar and base of the tongue area. The flap procedure involves two stages: suturing the flap in the defect and creating a controlled pharyngostome. After 2 to 3 weeks, the pharyngostome is closed and the flap is severed.

Nape of neck flaps are also useful for repair of the oropharyngeal defect; however, these almost always require a delaying procedure to ensure adequate blood supply (Fig. 78-68). The amount of tissue available for use is limited, and this flap is not commonly used.

Regional muscular flaps. Several regional muscular flaps are available for closure of moderately large oropharyngeal defects. The masseter flap with its overlying fascia can be swung over the mandible after release of its inferior mandibular attachments. Defects should be limited to the palatoglossal fold, tonsillar fossa, tonsillolingual sulcus, or

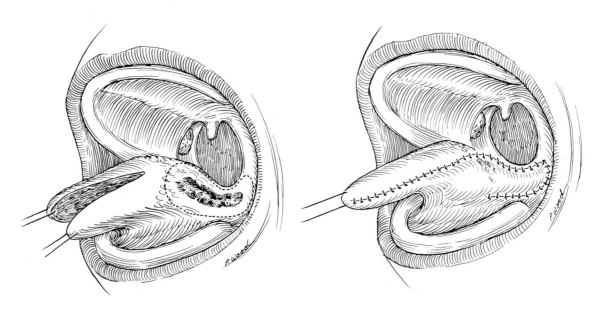

Fig. 78-63. A tongue flap used for reconstruction of the lateral oropharynx.

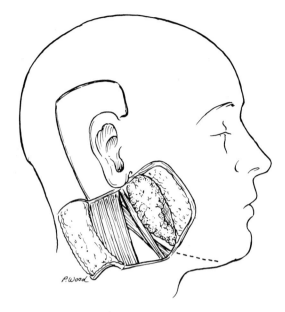

Fig. 78-64. Postauricular flap. (Courtesy of Dr. Richard Hayden.)

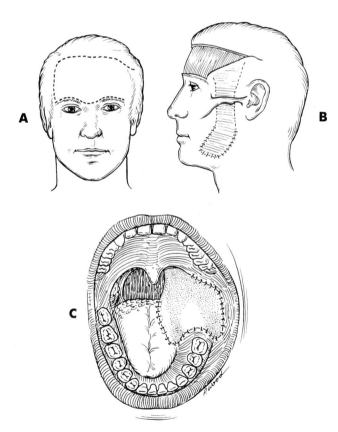

Fig. 78-65. A, Forehead flap based on the superficial temporal artery and portions of the occipital artery. **B,** Rotation of the forehead flap medial to the zygomatic arch for reconstruction of the oropharynx. The flap is pulled inferiorly to fill the resected area. **C,** Completion of forehead flap reconstruction.

lateral tongue base. In these select cases, morbidity is minimal, as is the cosmetic defect.[94] The temporalis muscle can also be rotated into the oral cavity in a similar fashion, again including the overlying fascia for an eventual double-layer closure. Transection of the coronoid process facilitates access to the oral cavity. Care should be taken not to compromise the maxillary artery, which is critical to sustain the flap via the paired deep temporal branches. Epithelialization of the fascia occurs within 2 weeks, and functional impairment is minimal. Cosmetically, the depression over the zygoma is well hidden by the overlying hair-bearing tissue and may be obliterated using an implant if desired. Injury to the temporal branches of the facial nerve as they cross the zygoma is avoided through gentle retraction in this area.[36,48]

The levator scapulae muscle flap was formerly used to protect the carotid artery after neck dissection. It may also be used in oropharyngeal reconstruction to provide soft tissue for bulk and to buttress suture lines.[32,69]

Regional myocutaneous flaps. The development of myocutaneous flaps has made reconstruction of the oropharynx and base of the tongue somewhat more predictable.[2,80] Use of these flaps has generally replaced use of skin flaps. The myocutaneous flaps have the advantages of supplying a large amount of healthy tissue with an excellent blood supply and of usually allowing one-stage reconstruction. For larger oropharyngeal composite defects, the pectoralis major flap is most often used (Fig. 78-69); however, the trapezius flap also provides adequate tissue for oropharyngeal reconstruction (Fig. 78-70).[101] Although the trapezius flap is successful, loss of a portion of this muscle creates more functional disability than loss of the pectoralis flap; therefore, the trapezius flap is not used as often. The sternocleidomastoid flap is not used frequently because concomitant neck surgery interferes with its development (Fig. 78-71). In addition, reliable survival of the cutaneous portion occurs in less than 50% of cases.

The pedicle of the myocutaneous flap is beneficial because it provides bulkiness in the neck (Fig. 78-72) and serves a cosmetic and a protective function for the underlying structures. In some patients, the flaps may be too bulky because of excessive adipose tissue; however, the flaps usually thin with time, and this problem is seldom permanent. If bulkiness is a problem, the skin may be removed from the flap, the fat resected, and the skin grafted to the underlying muscle. This produces a thinner piece of tissue and has proved to be a reliable technique.[88]

Innervated latissimus dorsi and pectoralis major flaps[99] retain their bulk and provide excellent closure of tongue base defects, often avoiding the need for concomitant laryngectomy. For moderately sized tumors with mandibular sparing, large myocutaneous flaps (e.g., pectoralis and trapezius flaps) may actually be too bulky. As discussed, several smaller regional flaps may be applied to such cases.

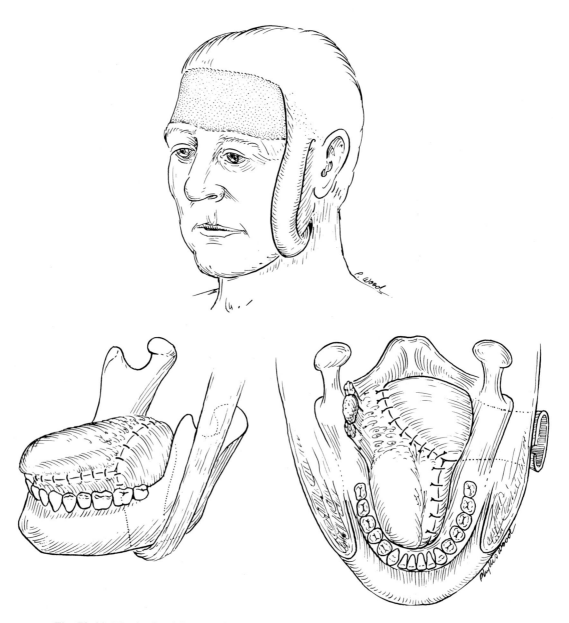

Fig. 78-66. The forehead flap may be rotated inferiorly to the mandible for reconstruction at the base of the tongue.

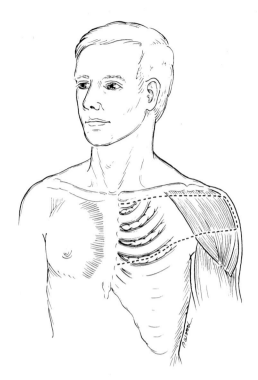

Fig. 78-67. The deltopectoral flap is supplied by perforating branches of internal mammary arteries. This is usually based on second, third, and fourth intercostal spaces. Extension over shoulder usually allows adequate tissue for reconstruction of oropharynx.

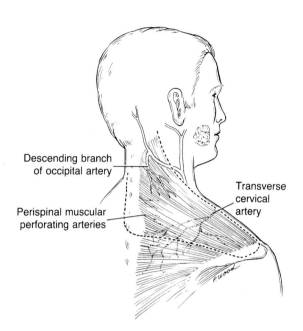

Fig. 78-68. Nape of the neck flap, which may be extended laterally to include portions of the shoulder. This flap is useful for reconstruction of oropharynx but usually requires a delaying procedure.

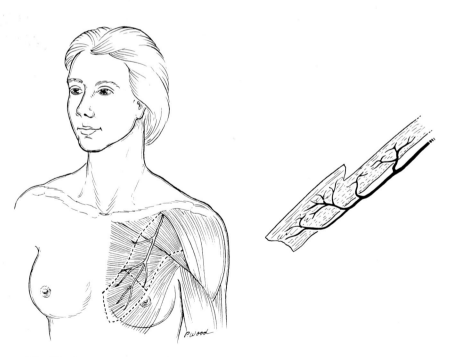

Fig. 78-69. An example of pectoralis myocutaneous flap showing its blood supply.

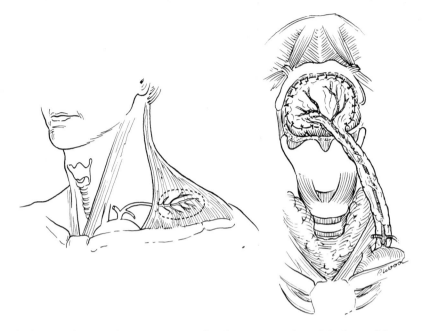

Fig. 78-70. Use of a trapezius myocutaneous flap for reconstruction of the base of the tongue.

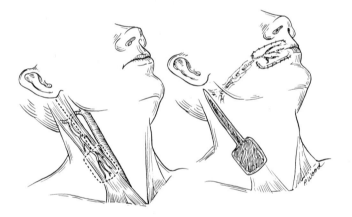

Fig. 78-71. A superiorly based sternocleidomastoid myocutaneous flap.

Microvascular free flaps

The use of free flaps with microvascular anastomosis is a viable technique and may be indicated in certain circumstances. The advantage of this technique is the large amount of tissue available and the flexibility of usage in difficult oropharyngeal reconstruction. In some cases, the flap can incorporate bone, allowing free flap reconstruction of the mandible and the surgical defect. The disadvantages of the technique are that it requires extra time, which lengthens an already long surgical procedure, and requires a two-team approach with personnel well trained in microvascular techniques. The recipient defect site should have an appropriate artery and vein available, which can be problematic after prior neck dissection and radiotherapy. Various options

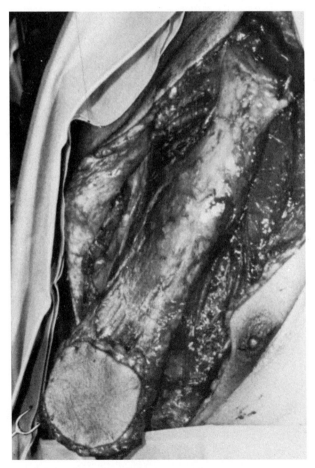

Fig. 78-72. A bulky pectoral flap pedicle, which provides carotid protection and improves cosmesis.

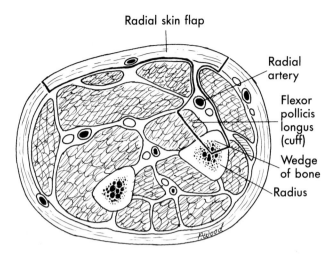

Fig. 78-73. Radial forearm flap.

exist, and the choice of graft varies with each patient and the experience of the surgeon.

The radial forearm fasciocutaneous free flap offers thin, pliable skin with a capacity for neurosensory restoration (Fig. 78-73). Inclusion of the medial and lateral antebrachial cutaneous nerves provides vascularized nerve grafts for repair to the glossopharyngeal nerve or branches of the cervical plexus. Morbidity consists of a skin graft to the volar surface of the forearm; this graft can be removed after adjacent skin expansion. Harvesting from the extremity facilitates a two-team approach, reducing operative time and morbidity.[92,100]

For complicated oropharyngeal lesions, such as radiation treatment failures in the tonsillar fossa, the greater omentum free flap offers several unique features. It may include a portion of the greater curve of the stomach with its attached omentum (Fig. 78-74). The flap is relatively easy to harvest; offers large-bore, long pedicle vessels; is available in various sizes; and has a tenacious adhesiveness and resilience, even in anoxic tissue beds. It provides moist, non–hair-bearing, soft, pliable tissue that is easily tailored to fit complex soft-tissue defects. The omentum provides carotid artery protection, soft-tissue augmentation, good lymph node drainage, and a smooth surface that does not collect food particles.[72,73]

Finally, when a large oropharyngeal malignancy necessitates composite resection, including segmental mandibulectomy, an osteocutaneous free flap may be indicated. At present, the fibula free flap offers the advantage of a neurosensory skin paddle potential and minimal donor site morbidity. As a truly ''accessory'' bone, all but a 10-cm distal segment of the fibula may be transferred without significant functional or cosmetic donor site morbidity. In cases requiring excision of the dentulous mandible, osseointegrated implants may be placed at the primary reconstruction; integration proceeds despite ongoing postoperative radiotherapy.

Other flaps include the rectus abdominis based on the

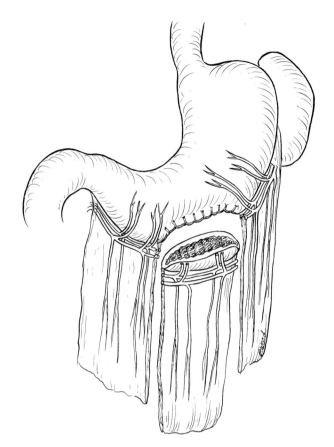

Fig. 78-74. Gastric omental flap.

deep inferior epigastric vessels[98] and the latissimus dorsi scapular flap based on the subscapular vessels. This flap includes the scapular and parascapular skin flaps, the serratus and latissimus dorsi muscle flaps, and the lateral scapular bone flap (Fig. 78-75). A segment of vascularized rib can be included with the serratus. The advantage of this combined flap is the independent vascular pedicles of its components, which allow freedom in orientation of the various portions of this flap. It has a disadvantage of being difficult to harvest simultaneously with the primary resection.[3,34]

Composite free flaps offer the advantage of providing skin, soft-tissue bulk, and bone for mandibular reconstruction. There are many donor sites, including iliac crest, scapula, metatarsus, rib, radius, fibula, ulna, and humerus. No donor site provides ideal replacement for missing oral cavity soft tissue. Perhaps the best overall reconstruction is attained with an iliac crest–internal oblique osteomyocutaneous flap, which provides excellent bone and two soft-tissue flaps for mucosal and cutaneous defects. The best approach may require the combination of two free flaps: a vascularized bone flap and a sensate soft-tissue flap.[97]

Mandible reconstruction

Mandible reconstruction has always been challenging. In some cases, resection of the posterior mandible with primary closure without bone reconstruction may result in minimal

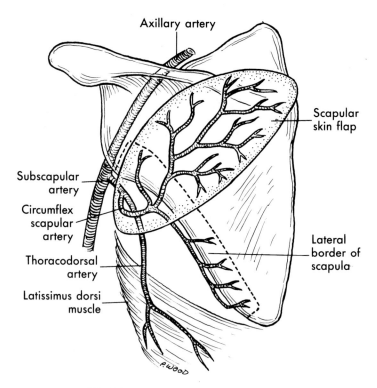

Fig. 78-75. Scapular latissimus dorsi flap.

disability. In other cases, there is significant cosmetic deformity and functional mastication, speech, and swallowing disabilities. Implanting metal mandibular prostheses in preoperatively radiated tissue commonly led to infection requiring removal of the implant. Use of postoperative radiation contributes to a higher success rate with metal implants.

Bone may be incorporated in a myocutaneous or free microvascular flap. The success and versatility of the microvascular techniques have led to increased use of bone grafts, including rib, fibula, radius, metatarsus, ulna, scapula, and iliac crest. Currently, the iliac crest and fibula seem to be the best overall grafts (Fig. 78-76). An important factor in selection is availability of bone with enough mass and height for placement of dental implants.[22,97] Dental implants may be placed into the grafted bone at the initial reconstruction with later fitting of a dental prosthesis (Fig. 78-77). The rate of loss of peri-implant bone in vascularized bone grafts is unknown, but osteointegration of the implants appears to be good. A technique that may have future use is mandibular reconstruction using human recombinant bone-inducing factor that stimulates bone formation.[96]

Rehabilitation

Rehabilitation of patients undergoing surgical resections of the oropharynx involves a team approach. The motivation of the patient is extremely important. Many patients are elderly and in poor general health with marginal nutritional status. The addition of radiotherapy and large surgical resec-

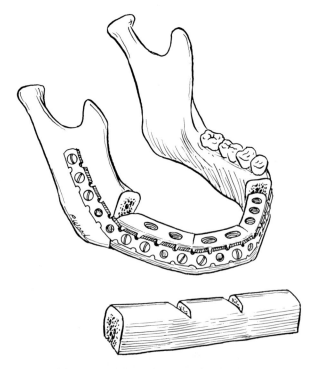

Fig. 78-76. Mandible reconstruction with dental implants. (Courtesy of Dr. Richard Hayden.)

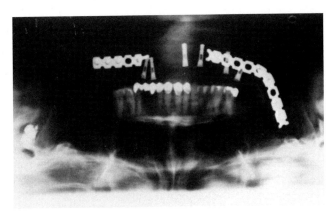

Fig. 78-77. Dental implants in grafted mandible reconstruction. (Courtesy of Dr. Allan Sclaroff.)

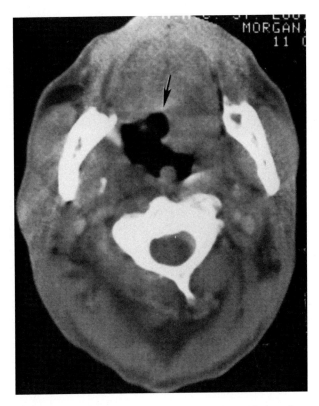

Fig. 78-78. Computed tomography showing postradiation ulceration *(arrow)* of the base of the tongue.

tions with reconstruction alters swallowing and speech and possibly appearance. These factors place patients under great physical and emotional strain. The team approach, with the physician in charge, is extremely useful for encouragement of the patient during the months of required therapy and rehabilitation. Nursing staff, speech therapists, physical therapists, social workers, and prosthodontists all play an active role to accomplish consistent, satisfactory rehabilitation. Rehabilitation is enhanced by the prevention of complications. Cosmetic appearance, speech, deglutition, and mastication depend on proper preoperative planning by the surgeon (in terms of resection and reconstruction) and by the prosthodontist and radiotherapist.

COMPLICATIONS

Irradiation

Patients receiving therapy typically develop mucositis in the oropharyngeal area. This is manifested by injection and irritation of the involved mucosa. Mucositis generally changes the quality and quantity of mucus produced, and the long-term results usually involve some dryness in the involved area and thickening of mucus. Typically, this problem is not difficult and is managed with topical care of the involved area. Taste also may be affected, with temporary loss of taste and with some foods tasting the same. Again, usually this resolves over time, but some patients have permanent taste changes.

Dysphagia from the resultant mucositis may occur during radiotherapy. It also may develop after radiotherapy as the area heals with scarring and fibrosis and may be severe enough to interfere with swallowing. Dysphagia may produce weight loss, and weight should be monitored carefully, especially with preoperative radiotherapy. Weight loss with resulting negative nitrogen balance may adversely affect the healing potential during and after the operation. Fibrosis of the treated primary tumor area and of the neck also may produce a stiffness in the soft tissues, which may be uncomfortable for patients and may make follow-up more difficult

because neck stiffness may mask an underlying tumor for a significant time. The stiffness in the soft tissue may limit the mobility of the neck, and intensive physical therapy should be ongoing. Scarring and fibrosis of the palate may produce poor function with resultant nasopharyngeal regurgitation. Occasionally, perforations of the palate develop, especially if the tumor involves full thickness of the palate.

Ulcerations may occur in the palate, tonsil, and base of the tongue (Fig. 78-78) after radiotherapy. These ulcerations may be painful and associated with hemorrhage. Diagnosis is difficult because they could harbor persistent or recurrent tumor. In patients with total laryngectomies, postoperative radiation may induce a tracheitis in the stoma area, which usually responds to topical humidification and local medical therapy. Rarely, CN XII palsies may result from radiotherapy to oropharyngeal tumors.

The potential for tissue necrosis always exists when radiotherapy is used. This consideration is important when skin flaps are being designed. The relationship of the vascular supply to the flap should be carefully planned to minimize future breakdown of a flap. Dermal grafts over the carotid artery should be used if the risk of skin necrosis is significant (Fig. 78-79). Mandibular radionecrosis may occur with external beam radiotherapy but is much more common if therapy involves supplemental interstitial implants. This may represent a therapeutic dilemma and often appears as a draining necrotic area on the medial aspect of the mandible intra-orally (Fig. 78-80). Continued exposure to saliva and food often prevents healing; therapy involves local topical care. Occasionally, local intraoral flaps may be used to cover the radionecrotic area and stimulate healing. Hyperbaric oxygen therapy may be useful; however, many patients require some type of partial mandibular resection of the necrotic area.

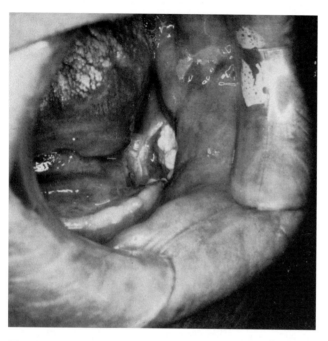

Fig. 78-79. Radionecrosis of the mandible after radiation implants.

Dental and alveolar disease should be resolved before the initiation of radiotherapy. Failure to do this will result in a high rate of dental complications.

Medical-surgical complications

Many patients who have oropharyngeal tumors are elderly and have general medical problems that should be properly managed by an appropriate specialist. A history of a previous myocardial infarct, possible arrhythmias, cardiac failure, hypertension, or emphysema should alert the surgeon to potential management problems. A careful preoperative treatment medical evaluation is usually a routine part of planning management for these patients. The nutrition status of patients may be borderline.[89,90] Hypokalemia, unless recognized and treated, may predispose these patients to poor healing. During the course of radiation, patients may have decreased appetites; supplemental feedings are necessary. Patients with large tumors, dysphagia, and weight loss may require supplemental nasogastric tube feedings or gastrostomy feedings.

Anesthesia management may be difficult for several reasons. During induction of anesthesia, a potential for airway obstruction exists in some patients with bulky tumors. With relaxation, inability to ventilate the patient properly may result in obstruction. Early recognition of this eventuality allows for a controlled, stepwise establishment of airway control. Patients with oropharyngeal tumors may have decreased ability to open the mouth, and intubation via the oral route may be difficult; nasal endotracheal intubation should be considered. Manipulation of the base of the tongue area with a laryngoscope may result in bleeding and difficult intu-

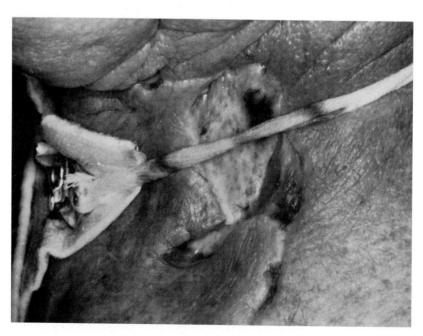

Fig. 78-80. Dermal graft covering the carotid artery for protection. (From Conley J: *Complications of head and neck surgery*, Philadelphia, 1979, WB Saunders.)

bation. Preoperative anesthetic consultation is necessary to prevent catastrophes during the induction of anesthesia. Performing a tracheostomy with the patient under local anesthesia may be preferable.

The key to treating surgical complications is in their prevention. Careful planning at each step of the therapeutic process will decrease complications dramatically. Tumors should be mapped carefully so their exact extent is well known before therapy. Surgical resection of the tumor should be planned carefully, and the reconstruction should be part of the initial plan.

Cosmesis

The skin incisions should be designed to allow easy access to the primary area and the neck. They should be planned so that local or regional skin flaps can be used. Although adequate resection of the tumor is the most important consideration, postoperative cosmetic appearance is included in planning. Attempts are made to hide scars in natural skin lines. Loss of bulk is restored with soft-tissue flaps, and mandible contour is replaced with implants or bone. Routine skin incisions and skin flaps may have to be modified, depending on the patient's irradiation or surgical history.

Oropharyngeal dysfunction

An important part of surgical planning involves the prevention of oropharyngeal dysfunction. The oropharyngeal inlet and lumen should be prepared to avoid stricture, otherwise, dysphagia, poor swallowing, and drooling will result in a patient who is oropharyngeally crippled.[17,22] With any treatment of the oropharynx, the mouth function should be considered to prevent problems with speech and mastication.

Mastication

Resection of part of the mandible without replacement commonly results in drift of the remaining mandible with poor dental occlusion and interference with mastication. Oral prostheses may prevent or decrease horizontal deviation. The best treatment is prevention of the mandibular drift by flap reconstruction or replacement with a plate or bone graft. Mastication is further enhanced by dental implants on the grafted bone.

Deglutition

Swallowing is most dependent on base of the tongue function and prevention of aspiration. If the resected defect is tightly closed, a stricture may result, producing dysphagia. Closure of the defect should be planned so that no tightness results. If excessive tension exists in the closure, wound breakdown, necrosis, and fistula will predictably occur. Proper flap design ensures adequate tissue for reconstruction and maintains proper flap circulation. A planned pharyngotomy as an alternative to a tenuous closure is a valid consideration; in most cases, it relieves the pressure on the suture line

and may make the difference between success and failure in healing. Tethering of this area and loss of bulk and function may allow the bolus of food to descend quickly into the hypopharynx, resulting in aspiration. If a significant amount of the base of the tongue is resected, it should be replaced with some type of flap reconstruction. A certain amount of bulk in this area is necessary for prevention of aspiration and for successful swallowing. Anesthesia of the flap is a detriment to swallowing but may be overcome with swallowing therapy.

Aspiration may occur postoperatively if planning and reconstruction are improper. The loss of a substantial portion of the base of the tongue combined with loss of the supraglottis puts the patient at high risk for aspiration. In some cases, a cricopharyngeal myotomy may help prevent aspiration by facilitating swallowing. If aspiration is severe enough, resulting in chronic pulmonary complications, total laryngectomy may be necessary. Most patients require nasogastric tube feedings for at least 2 weeks postoperatively or until healing is complete and deglutition achieved. Swallowing may be aggravated by leakage of liquid into the nose from resection of the palate. This is usually easily corrected with a prosthesis.

Speech

The amount of tongue resected and the resultant tongue mobility are the most important factors in the quality of postoperative speech. If possible, the tongue should be able to touch the incisors and the hard palate. Although the tongue may be satisfactorily used to close a defect, resultant tethering should be avoided. A common error is to suture the tongue too high or too laterally on the remnant soft palate. Mobility may be improved by tongue release with skin grafting or prevented by proper use of flap reconstruction. Velopharyngeal incompetence results from resection of the soft palate and produces a more nasal speech. The soft-palate defect may be surgically reconstructed but is usually corrected by a prosthesis. The long-term surgical complications primarily relate to dealing with oropharyngeally crippled patients. As stated, this problem should be dealt with at the initial planning and treatment to minimize its effects. The success rate of rehabilitation and the prevention of complications are enhanced if these patients are managed by a team approach.

Tumor recurrence

The recurrence of tumors (Fig. 78-81) after treatment is the most difficult therapeutic complication. Most patients have had extensive resections and radiation; therefore, therapy options are limited. Preventive planning and execution at the initial treatment will diminish recurrence. If the initial evaluation is inaccurate and the resection and reconstruction are planned improperly, local recurrence of tumor will occur at a predictably higher rate.

The options include resection (Fig. 78-82), external beam

30. Givene CD, Johns ME, Cantrell RW: Carcinoma of the tonsil, *Arch Otolaryngol Head Neck Surg* 107:730, 1981.

31. Goepfert H, Jesse RH, Ballantyne AJ: Posterolateral neck bisection, *Arch Otolaryngol Head Neck Surg* 106:618, 1980.

32. Goodman AL, Donald PJ: Use of the levator scapulae muscle flap in head and neck reconstruction, *Arch Otolaryngol Head Neck Surg* 116:1440, 1990.

33. Haagensen CE and others: *The lymphatics in cancer*, Philadelphia, 1972, WB Saunders.

34. Haughey BH, Fredrickson JM: The latissimus dorsi donor site, *Arch Otolaryngol Head Neck Surg* 117:1129, 1991.

35. Ho CM and others: Occult lymph node metastasis in small oral tongue cancers, *Head Neck* 14:359, 1992.

36. Huttenbrink KB: Temporalis muscle flap: an alternative in oropharyngeal reconstruction, *Laryngoscope* 96:1034, 1986.

37. Jackson RM, Rice DH: Blood transfusions and recurrence in head and neck cancer, *Ann Otol Rhinol Laryngol* 98:171, 1989.

38. Jacobs JR, Pajak TF: Induction chemotherapy in advanced head and neck cancer, *Arch Otolaryngol Head Neck Surg* 113:193, 1987.

39. Jacobs JR, Ru KD: 5-Year results of cisplatin and fluorouracil infusion in head and neck cancer, *Arch Otolaryngol Head Neck Surg* 117:288, 1991.

40. Jesse RH, Ballantyne AJ, Larson DL: Radical or modified neck dissection: therapeutic dilemma, *Am J Surg* 136:516, 1978.

41. Jesse RH, Lindberg RD: The efficacy of combining radiation therapy with a surgical procedure in patients with cervical metastasis from squamous cancer of the oropharynx and hypopharynx, *Cancer* 35:1163, 1975.

42. Johnson DW, Stringer WA, Marks MP: Stable xenon CT cerebral blood flow imaging: rationale for and role in clinical decision making, *Am J Neuroradiol* 12:201, 1991.

43. Jones AS and others: The level of cervical lymph node metastasis: their prognostic relevance and relationship with head and neck squamous cell carcinoma primary sites, *Clin Otolaryngol* 19:63, 1994.

44. Jones KR, Weissler MC: Blood transfusion and other risk factors for recurrence of cancer of the head and neck, *Arch Otolaryngol Head Neck Surg* 116:304, 1990.

45. Kaplan R, Million RR, Cassisi NJ: Carcinoma of the tonsil: results of radical irradiation with surgery reserved for radiation failure, *Laryngoscope* 87:600, 1977.

46. Khafif RA, Rafle S: Effectiveness of radiotherapy with radical neck dissection in cancers of the head and neck, *Arch Otolaryngol Head Neck Surg* 117:196, 1991.

47. Kohle PS, Leonard AG: The posterior auricular flap: anatomical studies, *Br J Plast Surg* 40:562, 1987.

48. Koranda FC, McMahon MF: The temporalis muscle flap for intraoral reconstruction: technical modifications, *Otolaryngol Head Neck Surg* 98:315, 1987.

49. Krause CJ: Carcinoma of the oral cavity a comparison of therapeutic modalities, *Arch Otolaryngol Head Neck Surg* 97:354, 1973.

50. Kurita H and others: Pitfalls in the treatment of delayed lymph node metastases after control of small tongue carcinomas, *Int J Oral Maxillofac Surg* 24:356, 1995.

51. LaFerriere KA and others: A functional approach to composite resection and reconstruction for cancer of the oral cavity and oropharynx, *Arch Otolaryngol Head Neck Surg* 106:103, 1980.

52. Lee WR and others: Carcinoma of the tonsillar region: a multivariate analysis of 243 patients treated with radical radiotherapy, *Head Neck* 15:283, 1993.

53. Leemans CR and others: Carcinoma of the soft palate and inferior tonsillar pillar, *Laryngoscope* 104:1477, 1994.

54. Lele PP: *Local hyperthermia for advanced squamous carcinoma of the head and neck*. In Wolf G, editor: *Head and neck oncology*, Boston, 1984, Martinus Nighoff.

55. Leonard EG: The posterior auricular flap: intra-oral reconstruction, *Br J Plast Surg* 40:570, 1987.

56. Lindberg RD: Distribution of cervical lymph node metastases from squamous cell carcinoma of the upper respiratory and digestive tract, *Cancer* 29:1446, 1972.

57. Lindberg RD, Jesse RH, Fletchr GH: *Radiotherapy before or after surgery?* In *Neoplasia of head and neck*, Chicago, 1974, Mosby.

58. Lingemann RE and others: Neck dissection: radical or conservative, *Ann Otolaryngol* 80:737, 1977.

59. Lore JM and others: Improved survival with preoperative chemotherapy followed by resection uncomprimised by tumor response for advanced squamous cell carcinoma of the head and neck, *Am J Surg* 170:506, 1995.

60. Mantravadi RVP, Liebner EJ, Ginde JV: An analysis of factors in the successful management of cancer of tonsillar region, *Cancer* 41:1054, 1978.

61. Marchetta FC, Sako K, Murphy JB: The periosteum of the mandible and intraoral carcinoma, *Am J Surg* 122:711, 1971.

62. Martin J: Neck dissection, *Cancer* 4:441, 1951.

63. McGuirt WF: Panendoscopy as a screening examination for simultaneous primary tumors in head and neck cancer: a prospective sequential study and review of the literature, *Laryngoscope* 92:569, 1982.

64. Mendenhall WM, Million RR, Cassisi NJ: Elective neck irradiation in squamous cell carcinoma of the head and neck, *Head Neck Surg* 3:25, 1980.

65. Million RR, Cassisi NJ: *Oropharynx*. In Million RR, Cassisi NJ, editors: *Management of head and neck cancer*, Philadelphia, 1984, JB Lippincott.

66. Million RR, Fletcher GH, Jesse RH: Evaluation of elective irradiation of the neck for squamous cell carcinoma of the nasopharynx, tonsillar fossa, and base of tongue, *Radiology* 80:973, 1963.

67. Million RR: Elective neck irradiation for TX N0 squamous carcinoma of the oral tongue and floor of the mouth, *Cancer* 34:149, 1974.

68. Moore DM, Calcaterra T: Cancer of the tongue base treated by a transpharyngeal approach, *Ann Otol Rhinol Laryngol* 99:300, 1990.

69. Netterville JL, Wood DE: The lower trapezius flap, *Arch Otolaryngol Head Neck Surg* 117:73, 1991.

70. Northrop M and others: Evolution of neck disease in patients with primary squamous cell carcinomas of the oral tongue, floor of mouth and palatine arch and clinically positive neck neither fixed nor bilateral, *Cancer* 29:23, 1972.

71. Pacheco-Ojeda L, Marandas P: Salvage surgery by composite resection for epidermoid carcinoma of the tonsillar region, *Arch Otolaryngol Head Neck Surg* 118:181, 1992.

72. Panje WR, Little AG: Immediate free gastro-omental flap reconstruction of the mouth and throat, *Ann Otol Rhinol Laryngol* 96:1187, 1988.

73. Panje WR, Piitcock JK: Free omental flap reconstruction of complicated head and neck wounds, *Otolaryngol Head Neck Surg* 100:588, 1989.

74. Parsons JT, Million RR, Cassisi NJ: Carcinoma of the base of the tongue: results of radical irradiation with surgery reserved for irradiation failure, *Laryngoscope* 92:689, 1982.

75. Pearson BW, Donald PJ: *Larynx*. In Donald PJ, editor: *Head and neck cancer*, Philadelphia, 1984, WB Saunders.

76. Piiolet H, Steckel RT: Magnetic resonance imaging to distinguish tumor persistence from delayed fibrosis in carcinoma of the tongue and floor of the mouth, *Ann Otol Rhinol Laryngol* 99:753, 1990.

77. Rollo J, Rozenbaum CV, Thawley SE: Squamous carcinoma of the base of the tongue: a clinical pathologic study of 81 cases, *Cancer* 47:333, 1981.

78. Ross JS, Masaryk TJ, Modic MT: Magnetic resonance angiography of the extracranial carotid arteries and intracranial vessels: a review, *Neurology* 39:1369, 1989.

79. Schaefer SO, Muerkel M: Computed tomographic assessment of squamous cell carcinoma of oral and pharyngeal cavities, *Arch Otolaryngol Head Neck Surg* 108:688, 1982.

80. Schuller DE, Platz DE, Krause DJ: Spinal accessory lymph nodes: a prospective study of metastatic involvement, *Laryngoscope* 88:439, 1978.

81. Schuller DE: Do otolaryngologist-head and neck surgeons and/or chemotherapy have a role in the treatment of head and neck cancer? *Arch Otolaryngol Head Neck Surg* 117:498, 1991.

82. Schuller DE: *Myocutaneous flaps in reconstructive surgery of the head and neck.* In Wolf G, editor: *Head and neck oncology*, Boston, 1984, Martinus Nighoff.

83. Sessions DG, Dedo DD, Ogura JH: Tongue flap reconstruction following resection for cancer of the oral cavity, *Arch Otolaryngol Head Neck Surg* 101:166, 1975.

84. Sessions DG: Surgical resection and reconstruction for cancer of the base of the tongue, *Otolaryngol Clin North Am* 16:309, 1983.

85. Sessions DG and others: Total glossectomy for advanced carcinoma of the base of the tongue, *Laryngoscope* 83:39, 1973.

86. Sharp PF, Smith FW, Gemmell HG: Technetium-99m Hm-PAQ steroisomers as potential agents for imaging regional cerebral blood flow: human volunteer studies, *J Nucl Med* 27:171, 1986.

87. Shrewsbury D and others: Carcinoma of the tonsillar region: a comparison of radiation therapy with combined preoperative radiation and surgery, *Otolaryngol Head Neck Surg* 89:979, 1981.

88. Smith PG, Collins SL: Repair of head and neck defects with thin and double-lined pectoralis flaps, *Arch Otolaryngol Head Neck Surg* 110:468, 1984.

89. Sobol SM and others: Nutritional concepts in the management of the head and neck cancer patient: II. Management concepts, *Laryngoscope* 89:962, 1979.

90. Sobol SM and others: Nutritional concepts in the management of the head and neck cancer patient: I. Basic concepts, *Laryngoscope* 89:794, 1979.

91. Spiro JD, Spiro RH: Carcinoma of the tonsillar fossa, *Arch Otolaryngol Head Neck Surg* 115:1186, 1989.

92. Takato T, Kiyonori H: Oral and pharyngeal reconstruction using the free forearm flap, *Arch Otolaryngol Head Neck Surg* 113:873, 1987.

93. Thawley SE and others: Preoperative irradiation and surgery for carcinoma of the base of tongue, *Ann Otol Rhinol Laryngol* 92:485, 1983.

94. Tiwari RM, Snow GB: Role of masseter crossover flap in oropharyngeal reconstruction, *J Laryngol Otol* 103:298, 1989.

95. Tong D and others: Carcinoma of the tonsillar region: results of external irradiation, *Cancer* 49:2009, 1982.

96. Toriumi DM, Kotler HS: Mandibular reconstruction with a recombinant bone-inducing factor, *Arch Otolaryngol Head Neck Surg* 117:1101, 1991.

97. Urken ML, Weinberg H: Oromandibular reconstruction using microvascular composite free flaps, *Arch Otolaryngol Head Neck Surg* 117:757, 1991.

98. Urken ML, Naidu RK: The lower trapezius island musculocutaneous flap revisited, *Arch Otolaryngol Head Neck Surg* 117:502, 1991.

99. Urken ML, Weinberg H: The neurofasciocutaneous radial forearm flap in head and neck reconstruction: a preliminary report, *Laryngoscope* 100:161, 1990.

100. Urken ML, Turk JB: The rectus abdominis free flap in head and neck reconstruction, *Arch Otolaryngol Head Neck Surg* 117:857, 1991.

101. Urken ML: Composite free flaps in oromandibular reconstruction, *Arch Otolaryngol Head Neck Surg* 117:724, 1991.

102. Wang CC, Montgomery W, Efird J: Local control of oropharyngeal carcinoma by irradiation alone, *Laryngoscope* 105:529, 1995.

103. Weber RS, Ohlms L: Functional results after total or near total glossectomy with laryngeal preservation, *Arch Otolaryngol Head Neck Surg* 117:512, 1991.

104. Weissler MC, Weigel MT: Treatment of the clinically negative neck in advanced cancer of the head and neck, *Arch Otolaryngol Head Neck Surg* 115:691, 1989.

105. Weller SA and others: Carcinoma of the oropharynx: results of megavoltage radiation therapy in 305 patients, *Am J Roentgenol* 126:236, 1976.

106. Wetmore SJ, Swen JW: *Clinical management of regional metastases.* In Wolf G, editor: *Head and neck oncology*, Boston, 1984, Martinus Nighoff.

107. Wolf GT, Schmaltz S: Alteration in T-lymphocyte subpopulations in patients with head and neck cancer, *Arch Otolaryngol Head Neck Surg* 113:1200, 1987.

108. Wong CS, Ang KK, Fletcher GH: Definitive radiotherapy for squamous cell carcinoma of the tonsillar fossa, *Int J Radiat Oncol Biol Phys* 16:657, 1989.

109. Zbaren MP, Lehmann W: Frequency and sites of distant metastases in head and neck squamous cell carcinoma, *Arch Otolaryngol Head Neck Surg* 113:762, 1987.

Chapter 79

Benign and Malignant Tumors of the Nasopharynx

H. Bryan Neel, III
Willard E. Fee, Jr.

BENIGN TUMORS

The nasopharynx or "epipharynx" is the cephalic end of the tubular aerodigestive tract. Various epithelia—keratinized and nonkeratinized squamous, pseudostratified, ciliated, and columnar—comprise its internal surface, along with glandular and lymphoid tissues. Deeper tissues are composed of connective tissue, including fascia and muscle. Diverse benign tumors that arise from epithelia and lymphoid, glandular, and connective tissue are occasionally encountered.

Benign tumors of the nasopharynx are rare. Fibromyxomatous polyps, pedunculated fibromas, papillomas, and teratomas are occasionally seen, as are extracranial tumor-like entities that may present in the nasopharynx—craniopharyngiomas, extracranial meningiomas, encephaloceles, hemangiomas, and chordomas (not always benign). Antral-choanal polyps should be added to this list because they often present as nasopharyngeal "tumors." In contrast, other benign tumor-like neoplasms (e.g., adenoids, Tornwaldt's cysts of the pharyngeal bursa, choanal polyps, mucosal cysts) are common.

No recent incidence or prevalence data list epithelial tumors; however, Fu and Perzin[19] reviewed the records from a 35-year period for a clinicopathologic study of nonepithelial tumors of the nose, paranasal sinuses, and nasopharynx. The histologic classification and distribution are shown in Table 79-1. The number and distribution of tumors in the nasopharynx alone were not noted, except for vascular tumors; as expected, angiofibromas were the most common benign tumors, and all occurred in the nasopharynx.

Angiofibroma

Angiofibroma is a benign tumor that affects young males. The triad of nasal obstruction, a nasopharyngeal mass, and recurrent epistaxis usually indicates the presence of the tumor, which is morphologically benign but aggressive and destructive.[52] Although angiofibromas are the most common benign tumors of the nasopharynx, they account for less than 0.05% of head and neck tumors.[38,63] The low frequency of occurrence has made it difficult to accumulate a sufficiently large series for an in-depth prospective or retrospective study. The term *angiofibroma* is most appropriate because the tumor is not often limited to the nasopharynx and usually has extensions (e.g., into the nose, paranasal sinuses, pterygomaxillary fossa, and other adjacent regions).[9,52,59] The term *juvenile angiofibroma* is inaccurate because the neoplasm also occurs in older patients.

Angiofibromas may grow considerably, causing significant structural and functional damage. They often erode bone and push into and through regional structures. Many grow insidiously to a substantial size, sometimes into the cranium, before symptoms occur; the symptoms are often attributed to more common problems before an accurate diagnosis is established.* Surgical therapy is recommended by most authors, and the tumors are a challenge for even the most experienced otolaryngologists.

Important issues relate to the choice of diagnostic procedures, adjunctive measures, and surgical approach and the role of radiotherapy.[9,34,52]

---

* Refs. 5, 7, 9, 32, 34, 52, 55, 62.

Table 79-1. Benign nonepithelial tumors of the nasal cavity, paranasal sinuses, and nasopharynx in 156 cases

Type of tumor	Cases (n)
Vascular	81
Capillary hemangioma	30
Cavernous hemangioma	5
Venous hemangioma	3
Benign hemangioendothelioma	3
Angiomatosis	1
Glomus tumor	1
Angiofibroma	38
Osseous and fibroosseous	52
Osteoma	31
Fibrous dysplasia	9
Ossifying fibroma	7
Osteoblastoma	1
Giant cell tumor	4
Chondroma	7
Myxoma	7
Fibroma	5
Leiomyoma	2
Lipoma	1
Rhabdomyoma	1

(From Fu YS, Perzin KH: Non-epithelial tumors of the nasal cavity, paranasal sinuses, and nasopharynx: a clinicopathologic study. I. General features and vascular tumors, *Cancer* 33:1275, 1974. By permission of the American Cancer Society.)

Gross and histologic morphology

Angiofibromas are pale blue, smooth, and often lobulated. The overlying mucosa is rarely ulcerated unless the patient has had previous biopsy or therapy.[52] Often, dry blood and mucus may be on the surface of the tumor.

Light microscopy reveals angiofibroma to be composed of spindle or stellate fibrocytes in various connective tissue stroma. The two striking microscopic features, a fibrostroma and a rich vascular network, may vary in pattern.[5,52] Vascular channels may be small and of capillary size or very large and of a venous size; the channels are lined with endothelial cells that lie directly against stromal cells. There is no intervening smooth muscle between these two cell types, and this feature undoubtedly contributes to the capacity for massive bleeding that occurs with biopsy or removal (Fig. 79-1). Batsakis[5] noted that the classic histologic appearance of the tumor is generally found in the interior portions; some investigators believe that surface biopsy specimens of the tumor mass may be misleading.

Clinical findings and point of origin

In a study of 150 white male patients aged 7 to 29 years at diagnosis (median age, 15 years), angiofibromas were not

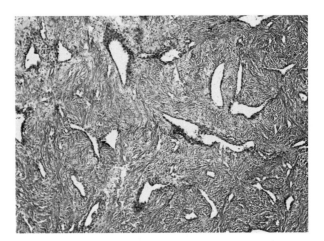

Fig. 79-1. Typical juvenile angiofibroma. (Hematoxylin-eosin, ×30.) (From Neel HB III and others: Juvenile angiofibroma: review of 120 cases, *Am J Surg* 126:547, 1973. By permission of Reed Publishing USA.)

Table 79-2. Symptoms and signs of angiofibroma in 150 patients, according to year of study

Symptom or sign	1945–1971 Patients (n = 120)		1972–1983 Patients (n = 30)	
	(*n*)	(%)	(*n*)	(%)
Epistaxis	84	70	26	87
Nasal obstruction	110	92	24	80
Nasal drainage	25	21	1	3
Facial deformity	23	19	4	13
Deafness, otitis	15	13	1	3
Bulging palate	12	10	1	3
Proptosis	10	8	4	13
Other*	24	20	6	20

(From Bremer JW and others: Angiofibroma: treatment trends in 150 patients during 40 years, *Laryngoscope* 96:1321, 1986. By permission of the Triological Foundation.)
* Other symptoms and signs, in one patient each, included breathing through the mouth, noisy sleeping, orbital pain, allergy, sinusitis, and female habitus.

more "aggressive" nor more likely to show intracranial spread in younger patients.

Nasal obstruction and epistaxis occurred in more than 80% of patients (Table 79-2). The typical patient was young and had occasional epistaxis and nasal obstruction. There may have been some bulging of the face or eye, and examination showed a pale blue, smooth mass in the nasopharynx and often in the posterior aspect of the nose. In most patients, the tumor was located on the side of the nasopharynx. This observation confirms the surgical observation that the specific point of origin is at the posterolateral wall of the roof of the nose where the sphenoid process of the palatine bone meets the horizontal ala of the vomer and the root of the

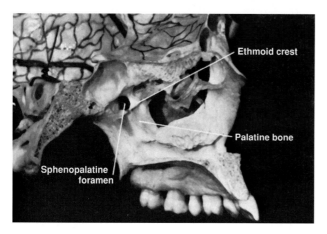

Fig. 79-2. Left nasal cavity showing the point of origin, which lies near the superior margin of the sphenopalatine foramen at the attachment of the posterior end of the middle turbinate. (From Neel HB III and others: Juvenile angiofibroma: review of 120 cases, *Am J Surg* 126:547, 1973. By permission of Reed Publishing USA.)

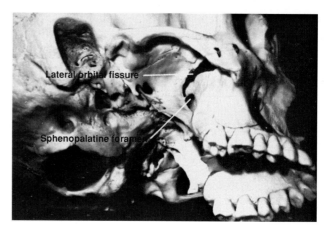

Fig. 79-3. Right side of the skull showing infratemporal, temporal, and pterygomaxillary fossae and their relationship to the sphenopalatine foramen, pterygomaxillary fissure, and posterior wall of maxillary antrum. (From Neel HB III and others: Juvenile angiofibroma: review of 120 cases, *Am J Surg* 126:547, 1973. By permission of Reed Publishing USA.)

pterygoid process of the sphenoid bone (Fig. 79-2). This junction forms a superior margin of the sphenopalatine foramen, and the ethmoid crest or attachment of the posterior end of the middle turbinate lies on or above the foramen.

Understanding the point of origin of the tumor helps explain the pathways of extension of the tumor. From the point of origin, the tumor may extend into the nose, the nasopharynx, the paranasal sinuses, the temporal fossa,[9,52] the infratemporal fossa, and the cranium (Fig. 79-3).

Diagnostic evaluation

Diagnosis is based on a thorough history, physical examination, and radiographic studies. Patients with diagnoses such as sinusitis, rhinitis, or antral choanal polyps may be observed. During the past 40 years, the duration of symptoms before management has decreased from a mean of 20 months to a mean of 6 months.[9] This decrease probably reflects a greater awareness of this rare tumor and improved diagnostic methods.

The trend in the application of radiography for diagnosis has changed from plain sinus radiographs to tomography, to a combination of tomography and computed tomography (CT) of the head, and to CT of the head alone, with and without contrast medium. The classic radiographic findings for angiofibroma are combinations of the following: (1) nasopharyngeal mass, (2) anterior bowing of the posterior wall of the antrum, (3) erosion of the sphenoid bone, (4) erosion of the hard palate, (5) erosion of the medial wall of the maxillary sinus, and (6) displacement of the nasal septum. Anterior bowing of the posterior wall of the maxillary sinus has been considered pathognomonic of angiofibroma, but other lesions such as fibromyxomatous polyps may rarely cause similar radiologic findings.[29,52,60] As noted, CT of the head with contrast medium has supplanted hypocycloidal

tomography for the diagnosis of angiofibroma. Magnetic resonance imaging (MRI) is indicated in some patients, particularly those who may have intracranial extension and those whose soft-tissue planes require clearer delineation.

Angiography has been unnecessary in most patients.[9,34] It has been used for patients in whom intracranial extension has been suspected or when the diagnosis remains in question, usually for patients in whom previous management has failed. The technique and technology of angiography have improved a great deal in recent years; however, risks are associated with angiography, especially when embolization is used.[52,55,64,65]

CT has improved the capacity to define the extent of the tumor clearly and safely. CT defines precisely the extent of the tumor, bony destruction, sinus involvement, and other extensions. CT of the head is now an integral part of the preoperative diagnostic evaluation.

Finally, at the time of planned surgical resection, a biopsy of the tumor is performed (with the patient under general anesthesia) to establish a definitive diagnosis; however, the need for biopsy has been challenged.[59]

Clinical staging systems

Sessions and others[58] proposed a staging system based on tumor location and extension. They proposed that CT should be used for the standardized reporting and staging of patients with angiofibroma after a clinical investigation in which angiofibroma is suspected. A description of the stages is provided in Table 79-3.

From the surgeon's viewpoint, stages IIC and III are the most difficult to manage. Indeed, 75% of recurrences occur in stage III patients (see Table 79-3).

Chandler and others[11] described a four-stage system.

Table 79-3. Staging* of angiofibroma and incidence of recurrence in 30 patients

Stage	Patients (*n*)	Recurrence
IA Tumor limited to posterior nares or nasopharyngeal vault	1	0
IB Extension into one or more paranasal sinuses	2	0
IIA Minimal lateral extension through sphenopalatine foramen into medial PMF	10	0
IIB Full occupation of PMF, displacing posterior wall of antrum forward; superior extension eroding orbital bones	6	1
IIC Extension through PMF into cheek and temporal fossa	3	0
III Intracranial extension	_8_	_4_
Total	30	5

(From Bremer JW and others: Angiofibroma: treatment trends in 150 patients during 40 years, *Laryngoscope* 96:1321, 1986. By permission of the Triological Foundation.)
PMF—Pterygomaxillary fossa.
* Based on radiographic and surgical findings.

Management

Various surgical approaches have been described recently: the facial degloving procedure and the extensive intracranial and extracranial approaches.[11,32,62] The approach may depend on the surgeon's experience with the technique. However, the lateral rhinotomy approach and its variations is the most direct route to the body of the tumor and is versatile so the surgeon can reach all extensions of the tumor.[9,34,52] Other surgical approaches provide limited, inadequate exposure, as noted in a detailed review of the various approaches.[52]

Given the point of origin of the tumor (described above), it is clear that the lateral rhinotomy incision provides an excellent approach to the tumor. The incision can be extended down the center of the upper lip when lateral exposure is required beyond the infraorbital foramen (Fig. 79-4); this method provides better superior and lateral exposure than does the facial degloving approach. The skin incision begins or ends within or just beneath the medial aspect of the brow and curves downward to within 5 mm of the inner canthus. The portion of the incision near the depression of the inner canthus should be curved so that a web of scar does not form. It then curves forward and downward on the side of the nose *midway* between the nasal dorsum and the nasal facial angle. It is carried down through the periosteum. The incision is carried down the side of the nose to the base of the ala, where it may terminate if the rhinotomy is limited. Because most angiofibromas extend beyond the nose and the nasopharynx, the incision is continued around the base of the nose to the base of the columella, where it turns and

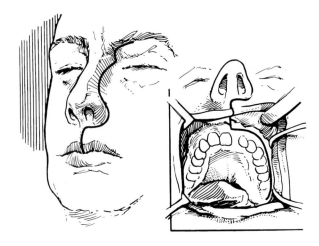

Fig. 79-4. Lateral rhinotomy incision with alternative extensions. (From Neel HB III and others: Juvenile angiofibroma: review of 120 cases, *Am J Surg* 126:547, 1973. By permission of Reed Publishing USA.)

runs down the center of the upper lip. The incision on the mucosal surface of the upper lip has a **Z** incorporated into it. The incision reaches the depth of the alveolobuccal sulcus and continues in the sulcus to the maxillary tuberosity.

Once the incision is completed, the underlying bone should be adequately removed to get good exposure, and this should be completed before the tumor is touched. The nasal bone is removed to the midline and to its junction with the frontal bone. The frontal process of the maxilla and the facial surface of the maxilla are removed. A small margin of bone around the infraorbital nerve at the level of the foramen is preserved. By this time, the antrum is opened and the posterior wall is inspected. If the antrum is bulging forward excessively, more exposure is needed. The infratemporal surface of the maxilla should be removed along with the eggshell of bone on the posterior wall of the antrum. The terminal branches of the internal maxillary artery usually can be identified and are ligated, clipped, or electrocoagulated. The internal maxillary artery is invariably the main source of blood supply to the tumor.

As Neel and others[52] noted in a detailed description of the surgical procedure, the tumor can be extracted from the pterygomaxillary fossa, infratemporal fossa, temporal fossa, sinuses, and middle fossa by pushing the tumor medially with packing. The middle fossa can also be approached through the incision (Fig. 79-5). Most angiofibromas are not intracranial; rather, they are pericranial, having destroyed the bony floor of the middle cranial fossa. The tumor can be carefully removed from the middle cranial fossa, dura, and the cavernous sinus.[34] Ideally, all of the lobulations of the tumor should be extracted and should be seen to communicate with each other and with the body of the tumor.[7-9,23,52] All intervening bone that interferes with the removal of the tumor should be removed. Most large angiofibromas extend

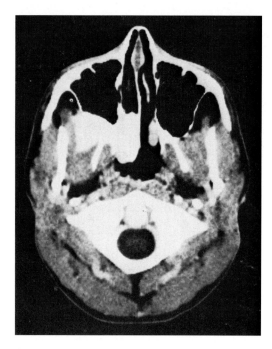

Fig. 79-5. Computed tomography with contrast shows angiofibroma in the right pterygopalatine fossa and in the posterior nasal cavity. Note that the posterior wall of the maxillary sinus has been pushed forward by tumor (a typical Holman-Miller sign). The tumor was separated and removed from the middle fossa dura by way of a lateral rhinotomy.

beneath the adenoid pad on the side of the lesion. Once the tumor is firmly grasped with a strong forceps, it is necessary to work with an elevator or index finger around the base of the tumor to aid in avulsion.

On removal of the tumor, a search is made for any residual fingers, lobules, or pseudopods remaining in the body of the sphenoid bone. The cavity is packed; the packing is removed in 5 to 7 days with the patient under general anesthesia. Tracheotomy tubes and feeding tubes are unnecessary. Postoperatively, patients have healed well and cosmesis has been satisfactory, even in patients in whom the incision is used for reoperation.

Intracranial extension and residual tumor

Intracranial extension has been reported in approximately 20% to 25% of cases.[9,32,34,36,62] Intracranial extension is a result of anatomic proximity and not of a more aggressive tumor. In general, the surgeon can carry out adequate extracranial resection by way of the lateral rhinotomy and its extensions and manage any residual tumor expectantly. Recurrence is managed only when symptoms justify the added risk.[9,34]

The tumor has two major routes into the cranial cavity[52]: by way of the middle fossa anterior to the foramen lacerum and lateral to the cavernous sinus and carotid artery, or through the sella medial to the carotid artery and lateral to the pituitary gland. The latter form of intracranial extension

is difficult and hazardous to remove; it occurs in a few patients. Often, these tumors are intimately associated with the branches of the internal carotid artery and the cavernous sinus within the cranium and are difficult to manage surgically. These few patients with central tumor extension into the cranium probably should be managed with a combination of surgery and radiation or with external radiation only, whereas tumors may be safely removed from the middle fossa and may be considered pericranial.

At operation, the posterior wall of the maxillary sinus is carefully removed, and the tumor often can be found in the pterygomaxillary fossa. The tumor may destroy the root of the pterygoid process of the sphenoid bone posteriorly. Large tumors extend into the infratemporal fossa through the pterygomaxillary fissure, where they expand and induce the classic facial fullness and bulging of the cheek. More enlargement leads to extension into the lower part of the temporal fossa, which results in swelling above the zygoma. When this occurs, the tumor usually extends into the infraorbital fissure; the inferior orbital fissure opens into the upper anterior part of the pterygomaxillary fossa and is an entrance into the lower end of the superior orbital fissure, which meets the inferior (lateral) orbital fissure in the posterosuperior wall of the pterygomaxillary fossa. At this point, the tumor may destroy the greater wing of the sphenoid bone, forming the characteristic widening along the lower lateral margin of the superior orbital fissure and producing proptosis. If the tumor enlarges in the infratemporal and pterygomaxillary fossae, it can destroy the bone that forms the base of the pterygoid process where the body and the great wing of the sphenoid bone meet; the tumor then rests against the dura of the middle fossa, anterior to the foramen lacerum but lateral to the cavernous sinus.

The mean volume of blood replacement in one series was 1400 ml (range, 0–4000 ml).[9] Hypotensive anesthesia did not reduce the volume of blood transfusion.

Some authors have relied on intraarterial embolization to decrease the vascularity of the tumors.[55,59] Embolization has been used for the management of angiofibromas on a limited basis, usually in patients who have epistaxis at some time after surgical resection and in whom no gross tumor is obvious at the time of reexploration but a tumor blush is noted at angiography. Waldman and others[63] used preoperative embolization routinely. Biller[7] limited the use of embolization to large tumors that had an arterial blood supply from the internal and external carotid arteries or to tumors with intracranial extension that were thought to be resectable.

McCombe and others[40] found that the strongest predictor of recurrence was preoperative embolization. There was no greater predominance of large tumors in the embolized subgroup. They postulated that embolization shrinks the tumor but makes identification of tumor extensions more difficult so that the incidence of residual tumor is greater. They added that MRI has made angiography ''redundant'' as a diagnostic and therapeutic method and has eliminated the morbidity of angiography and exposure to radiation.

An outstanding exception to primary surgical management is a series of patients in whom external radiation was advocated as the primary method of management in most instances.[10,12–14,18] Radiation as primary management is of much concern, especially in young patients, because thyroid carcinomas and radiation-induced sarcomas of bone and soft tissue are small but definite risks after radiation.[13,63,67] Also, lifelong follow-up may be necessary. Radiation induces more profound local changes, such as atrophic rhinitis and occasionally osteomyelitis or soft-tissue necrosis. Radiotherapy may affect growth centers in the face, particularly in male adolescents, in whom growth is rapid.[11,53] Goepfert and others[20] suggested that chemotherapy may be of some value in selected patients.

Outcome

Of the 30 patients studied from 1972 to 1983, 29 had lateral rhinotomies and one had a small tumor removed by the transpalatal route.[9] The overall recurrence rate in this series was 17%; 5% (1 of 22) of patients with extracranial tumors had recurrences, and 50% of patients (4 of 8) with intracranial involvement had recurrences (Tables 79-3 and 79-4). The surgeon believed that the tumor was completely removed in 28 cases. Two patients had preoperative angiography, one of whom had preoperative embolization. Both patients had evidence of intracranial extension (stage III disease), and the embolization was by way of the internal maxillary artery and was performed 1 day before operation.

Five patients had recurrent tumor and two had nasal lacrimal duct obstruction requiring a secondary procedure. Of the five patients with recurrent tumor, two had operation followed by embolization because of evidence of recurrent tumor and bleeding, one had embolization for recurrent tumor on angiography, one had postoperative external radiation (3000 cGy) for recurrent tumor 3 years after operation, and one had recurrent tumor removed elsewhere 1 year after the initial operation. The two patients with nasolacrimal duct obstruction had dacrylocystorhinostomies.

All 30 patients had long-term follow-up: 28 were alive without disease and two were alive with known residual disease but no symptoms. None of the patients have died of their disease. The natural history of this tumor, based on close follow-up after resection, indicates that small residual tumors can regress. Several patients in this series and in a previous series with known residual tumor have not required management and have not had significant symptoms or signs of recurrence.[9,52] There is no clear relationship between the age of the patient and the outcome. Hemorrhage, nasal obstruction, and orbital encroachment are sometimes present with a primary tumor; however, many cases of residual tumor are asymptomatic. The surgeon should attempt to remove the entire tumor, but incomplete resection is not life-threatening and can be managed expectantly. When symp-

Table 79-4. Outcome after lateral rhinotomy for angiofibroma in 86 patients according to year of study

Status	1945–1971 Patients (n = 56)		1972–1983 Patients (n = 29)	
	(*n*)	(%)	(*n*)	(%)
Alive				
Without disease	45	80	27	93
With disease	5	9	2	7
Dead	5	9	0	0
Lost to follow-up	1	2	0	0
Total	56	100	29	100

(From Bremer JW and others: Angiofibroma: treatment trends in 150 patients during 40 years, *Laryngoscope* 96:1321, 1986. By permission of the Triological Foundation.)

toms develop, appropriate secondary management of residual tumor can be successful.

In a review of management trends and outcome in 150 cases, it was concluded that surgery is the best primary form of management for most patients, including many with intracranial extension.[9] The lateral rhinotomy and its variations, in one procedure, allow exposure of all the projections of the tumor. It has not been show that intracranial extension justifies a craniotomy. The use of adjunctive procedures—hypotensive anesthesia and preoperative embolization—has increased although there is no evidence that they reduce bleeding or improve the capability to remove the tumor in its entirety. Hormones, cryotherapy, or external carotid artery ligation does not seem to be of value in the control of the tumor or hemorrhage at operation. In any surgical series the trend was toward more complete removal at the time of operation and fewer recurrences postoperatively. Mortality declined from 9% in the previous surgical series[52] to 0% in the most recent series.[9]

MALIGNANT TUMORS

Patients with malignant tumors of the nasopharynx have a bewildering array of signs and symptoms. Sometimes the nasopharynx is difficult to examine, even by experienced physicians. Scanlon and others[57] described the consequences:

Always a challenging problem, both from the diagnostic and therapeutic standpoint, malignant lesions of the nasopharynx are perhaps the most commonly misdiagnosed, most poorly understood, and most pessimistically regarded of all tumors of the upper part of the respiratory tract.

In addition to the clinical challenge, there are other matters of interest on which worldwide attention has been focused: the wealth of biologic, biochemical, and immunologic evidence that supports both an association between the Epstein-Barr virus (EB virus) and certain forms of nasopharyngeal carcinoma and the fact that genetic environmental, and viral factors seem to play a part in the genesis of certain histologic types of nasopharyngeal carcinoma.*

Nasopharyngeal carcinoma

Until recently, there has been little agreement in the literature about correct and acceptable pathologic classification of tumors of the nasopharynx. In one tumor registry, malignant tumors of the nasopharynx have been subdivided by light microscopy into three main groups: squamous cell carcinomas (keratinizing, nonkeratinizing, and undifferentiated); lymphomas; and a miscellaneous group consisting of adenocarcinomas, plasma cell myelomas, cylindromas, rhabdomyosarcomas, melanomas, fibrosarcomas, carcinosarcomas, and unclassified spindling malignant neoplasms (Table 79-5). The nonglandular, nonlymphomatous epithelial malignancies, collectively called *nasopharyngeal carcinomas*, are the most common tumors of the nasopharynx.

Various epithelia—including keratinized and nonkeratinized squamous, pseudostratified, ciliated, and columnar—are found in the nasopharynx along with lymphoid tissue and glandular tissue. Therefore, various benign and malignant tumors can arise from the minor salivary glands, lymphoid tissue, and connective tissue in the nasopharyngeal region. These are excluded from the epithelial tumors by definition, but the epithelial tumors show different degrees of differentiation and morphology.

Epidemiology

Nasopharyngeal carcinoma is a relatively rare tumor in most parts of the world; in North America it comprises about 0.25% of all cancers. However, it accounts for approximately 18% of all malignant cancers among the Chinese. The incidence is even higher among southern Chinese of Guangdong province, the northern provinces, and Taiwan. Hsu and others[31] estimated from surgical specimens in Taiwan that nasopharyngeal carcinoma is the most common cancer in males and the third most common cancer in females.

For populations in which Chinese genes have been introduced, the incidence of nasopharyngeal carcinoma rises. The marker for genetic susceptibility to nasopharyngeal carcinoma among Chinese has been suggested to be at the human leukocyte antigen (HLA)-A2 histocompatibility locus. Even after migration, the Chinese have a higher frequency of nasopharyngeal carcinoma than other populations. Emigration from high-incidence to low-incidence areas (e.g., United States, Canada) reduces the incidence of nasopharyngeal carcinoma in the first generation, but it is still greater than that in whites. Dickson,[15] in a unique, racially balanced series of 209 nasopharyngeal carcinoma cases, found that the incidence of nasopharyngeal carcinoma among Chinese born in China was 118 times the rate in whites and that in Chinese

* Refs. 1, 16, 23–26, 37, 39, 43, 44, 46, 48–50, 53.

Table 79-5. Malignant tumors of nasopharynx from the Mayo Clinic Tissue Registry, 1972 to 1981

Tumor type		No.	%
Squamous cell carcinoma*		120	71
Lymphoma		31	18
Miscellaneous		18	11
Adenocarcinoma	6		
Plasma cell myeloma	3		
Cylindroma	2		
Rhabdomyosarcoma	2		
Melanoma	2		
Fibrosarcoma	1		
Carcinosarcoma	1		
Unclassified spindling	1		
malignant neoplasm		___	___
Total		169	100

* Combined World Health Organization types 1, 2, and 3.

born in North America it was seven times the rate in whites. The biologic behavior of the disease appeared to be the same in Chinese and non-Chinese persons. Other factors implicated as causes of this disease include Epstein-Barr virus (EBV), polycyclic hydrocarbons, nitrosamines from dry salted fish, chronic nasal sinus infection, and poor hygiene.

Histopathology

Using light microscopy, pathologists can consistently divide nasopharyngeal carcinoma into three types based on the predominant histologic type in the primary lesion. These types are the basis of a broad classification by the World Health Organization (WHO) that is fairly well accepted by pathologists: squamous cell carcinoma (WHO type 1, Fig. 79-6); nonkeratinizing carcinomas, that is, transitional cell carcinomas (WHO type 2, Fig. 79-7); and undifferentiated carcinomas, that is, lymphoepitheliomas and anaplastic carcinomas (WHO type 3, Fig. 79-8).[6,61,66] Electron microscopy shows ultrastructural characteristics (desmosomes, tonofibrils) of squamous (epidermoid) carcinomas in the entire spectrum of these tumors, which at one extreme are well-differentiated keratinizing types and at the other extreme are undifferentiated anaplastic variants.

WHO type 1 carcinomas show distinct intercellular bridges and abundant keratin production. Various degrees of these differentiating features can be observed. The tumor is similar microscopically to other squamous carcinomas of the upper aerodigestive tract and does not appear to be unique to the nasopharynx. About 25% of tumors in North American patients fall into this category.[43] WHO type 2 and type 3 tumors have a greater degree of tumor pleomorphism than the keratinizing type of tumors. Several microscopic patterns may exist: spindle cell, transitional cell, lymphoepithelioma, clear cell, anaplastic, and others; combinations of these patterns are fairly common. These combinations, in conjunction with the ultrastructural features common to all

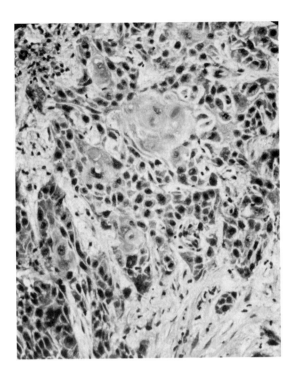

Fig. 79-6. Nasopharyngeal carcinoma World Health Organization type 1 squamous cell. (Hematoxylin-eosin; ×175.) (From Pearson GR and others: *Cancer* 51:260, 1983. By permission of the American Cancer Society.)

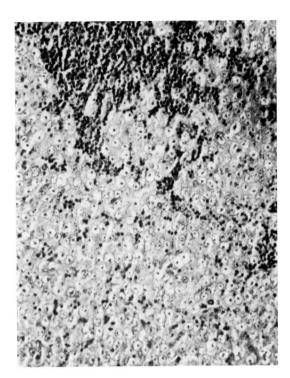

Fig. 79-8. Nasopharyngeal carcinoma World Health Organization type 3 undifferentiated. (Hematoxylin-eosin; ×175.) (From Pearson GR and others: *Cancer* 51:260, 1983. By permission of the American Cancer Society.)

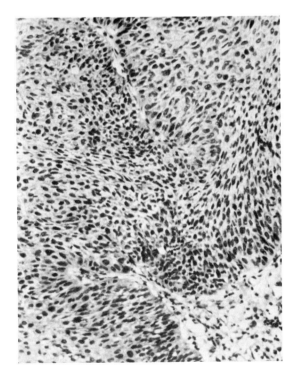

Fig. 79-7. Nasopharyngeal carcinoma World Health Organization type 2 nonkeratinizing, transitional cell. (Hematoxylin-eosin; ×175.) (From Pearson GR and others: *Cancer* 51:260, 1983. By permission of the American Cancer Society.)

WHO type 2 and type 3 tumors, are the reason why these tumors are considered variants of nonkeratinizing nasopharyngeal carcinoma rather than distinct tumor entities. Indeed, a substantial body of clinical and serologic evidence supports the theory that carcinomas of the nasopharynx can be classified as two distinct diseases: squamous cell carcinomas (WHO type 1) and a combined group of nonkeratinizing undifferentiated carcinomas (WHO types 2 and 3).[43,44,46,48,53]

Other classifications have been complicated and impractical and have failed to acknowledge the heterogeneity within the nonkeratinizing and undifferentiated groups. Nevertheless, both groups appear to be unique to the nasopharynx or, at most, to the lymphoepithelial tissue of Waldeyer's tonsillar ring. The criteria for these categories have been reviewed in detail.[61,66]

Clinical findings

Complaints of nasopharyngeal carcinoma patients are related to the location of the primary tumor and the degree of spread. Generally, subtle symptoms and signs are confusing to primary care physicians, otorhinolaryngologists, neurologists, ophthalmologists, and other specialists until the disease has reached advanced stages. Late diagnosis accounts for the poor outcome in many cases.

Hearing loss and a lump in the neck are the most common reasons for seeking medical attention.[15,46,54,57] A tumor in

three-fold higher in WHO types 2 and 3 sera, respectively, than in WHO type 1 sera.

In cases of occult and early nasopharyngeal carcinoma—stage I, in groups staged by one of three systems—anti–early antigen titers were positive in 100%, and positive IgA anti–viral capsid antigen titers ranged from 90% to 94% (Table 79-8). In all cases, the nasopharyngeal tumor was small and limited to a small area in the nasopharynx. The early antigen and viral capsid antigen tests can complement diagnosis and are especially useful in directing attention to the nasopharynx in patients with occult nasopharyngeal carcinoma.[45] They might be considered for screening programs in high-incidence areas of the world.

Antibody-dependent cellular cytotoxicity (ADCC) titers obtained at diagnosis often predict the clinical course of WHO types 2 and 3 nasopharyngeal carcinoma.[46] Figure 79-10 shows freedom from progression (clinically detectable metastatic disease) in a high-titer group and a low-titer group. The association between low titers and known progression was strongly significant at 3 years; with longer follow-up, the association with death was strongly significant.[48] This association, however, was found only in cases of WHO types 2 and 3 and not in well-differentiated WHO type 1. At diagnosis, ADCC titers appear to identify patients who could be candidates for systemic therapy from the outset.

Most patients with the poorly differentiated types of nasopoharyngeal carcinoma have IgA antibodies to EBV antigens in their sera. Mathew and others[39] found that IgA antibodies purified from the sera of patients with nasopharyngeal carcinoma blocked the ADCC reaction, which is mediated by IgG anti-EBV antibodies directed against membrane antigens. Furthermore, an inverse relationship exists between specific IgA and ADCC antibody titers. Perhaps blocking of the IgG antibody-mediated cytotoxic reaction by IgG antibodies or by IgA antigen-antibody complexes is the reason that ADCC titers are low in cases of nasopharyngeal carcinoma. This also presumes that the ADCC reaction occurs

in vivo—a supposition that may or may not be true but does not detract from the specificity of the test.

In Chinese populations, nasopharyngeal carcinoma has been associated with certain HLA alleles: A2, Bw46, and B17. The associations with A2 and Bw46 appear to be additive. Bw46 is an extremely uncommon antigen among whites. In a study of HLA and nasopharyngeal carcinoma in whites, no significant associations were found.[41] This finding may mean that no HLA allelic association with nasopharyngeal carcinoma exists in whites, or that HLA associations are weak and were not detected.

Clinical staging systems

Traditional systems. Although no international agreement exists on the best staging system, several are well known: the American Joint Committee for Cancer Staging (AJCC),[3] the Union Internationale Contre le Cancer (UICC),[22] and the Ho system.[27,28,51]

The AJCC system is used most commonly in the United States by institutions concerned with cancer and the reporting of results. Major criticisms of this system relate to the description of the extent of the primary tumor and of the regional lymph nodes.

Determination of the extent of nasopharyngeal carcinoma can be difficult, even for expert examiners and even when the nasopharynx is well visualized with mirrors or endoscopic instruments because submucosal extension beneath a normal appearing surface mucosa is common. Furthermore, the definition of posterosuperior and lateral walls is a problem. The posterior part of Rosenmüller's fossa is in part the meeting point of the lateral and posterior walls. Tumors often arise in this site, and attempts to designate their extent as Tis (*in situ*), T_1, or T_2—as is done in the AJCC and UICC sys-

Table 79-8. Incidence of positive anti–Epstein-Barr virus titers in cases (World Health Organization types 2 and 3) of stage I nasopharyngeal carcinoma (by various staging systems)

System	Patients (n)	Early antigen, % positive	Viral capsid antigen (IgA), % positive
AJCC	10	100	90
UICC	11	100	91
Ho	17	100	94

(From Neel HB III and others: Application of Epstein-Barr virus serology to the diagnosis and staging of North American patients with nasopharyngeal carcinoma, *Otolaryngol Head Neck Surg* 91:255, 1983. By permission of the American Academy of Otolaryngology—Head and Neck Surgery.) EA—Early antigen; VCA—Viral capsid antigen; AJCC—American Joint Committee on Cancer; UICC—Union Internationale Contre le Cancer.

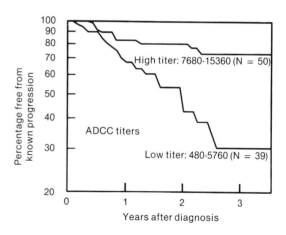

Fig. 79-10. Freedom from progression of nasopharyngeal carcinoma in groups whose antibody-dependent cellular cytotoxicity titers at diagnosis were high and low. At 3 years, the difference in incidence of progression was significant ($P < 0.001$). N—Number of patients. (From Neel HB III and others: *Otolaryngol Head Neck Surg* 91:255, 1983. By permission of the American Academy of Otolaryngology-Head and Neck Surgery.)

tems—are likely to be ambiguous. Indeed, no appreciable difference in survival exists in these subgroups.[48,50] The Ho system recognizes this. Of further concern is the fact that T_4 refers to tumor invasion of the skull, cranial-nerve involvement, or both. Also, stage IV embraces patients with T_4, N_2, M_1 disease; no patient with M_1 disease survives 5 years, whereas some patients with T_4 and N_2 disease do survive. Therefore, patients with M_1 disease should be staged separately (as recommended by Ho).

Another point of controversy in the AJCC system is cervical node classification as it relates to level, involvement of one or both sides of the neck, nodal mobility, and size of the metastatic deposit or deposits. The AJCC and UICC classifications were designed primarily as guides for surgical management and not for radiotherapy. Both systems place more emphasis on whether the nodal involvement is unilateral or bilateral and on whether the nodes are mobile than on the level of the nodal involvement. These issues need clarification; it is hoped that within the next few years an internationally accepted classification system can be devised and adopted.

It appears that nodes low in the neck indicate a poor prognosis.[15,27,48,51,57] In the study by Scanlon and others,[57] if the involved upper cervical nodes were mobile, their unilaterality or bilaterality did not seem to affect survival. But involvement of lower jugular nodes was more unfavorable regardless of whether it was unilateral or bilateral. These data reflect well on Ho's system, in which involvement of nodes low in the neck is designated stage III and involvement of supraclavicular nodes is stage IV. Ho's system[27,28] appears to give the best correlation of stages with survival.

Changes in technology and serologic testing may help refine all the staging systems. Originally, radiologic study of the skull base used only plain radiography. Tomography was then added; currently, MRI of the head is the primary imaging study. The thoroughness of the radiologic investigation sometimes has a bearing on the clinical staging of a case. It also appears that serologic testing may be useful in the staging of nasopharyngeal carcinoma.

A new view of staging. Traditional cancer staging systems (e.g., TNM) mainly describe and classify the extent of disease and are not based on other characteristics or variables that could have an important bearing on management. A combination of variables, including some of the traditional characteristics of extent of disease, provides a more accurate prediction of prognosis using Cox regression methods.[48,50] These variables form the basis of a new staging system in terms of a prognosis score called *score to death* (Table 79-9). A simplified working formulation for staging by score is shown in Table 79-10.[48] A second system that includes antibody-dependent cellular cytotoxicity titer (i.e., score to death, including the titer) was developed because a high titer correlated strongly with a good prognosis, although a commercial assay is not available.

The two new systems are better predictors of outcome than are the traditional staging systems.

Management

Management of nasopharyngeal carcinoma consists primarily of supervoltage irradiation. The primary tumor and the primary echelon of lymph nodes are included in large

Table 79-9. Components of prognosis score* in nasopharyngeal carcinoma

Risk factor	Score If yes†	If no
Score to death		
Seven or more symptoms	+ 1.14	0
Nodes positive in lower neck or supraclavicular region‡	+ 1.10	0
WHO type 1 tumor	+ 1.04	0
Extensive tumor in nasopharynx	+ 0.53	0
Symptoms for <2 mo	− 0.63	0
Score to death, including ADCC		
ADCC titer ≤1:960	+ 1.36	0
Seven or more symptoms	+ 1.28	0
Nodes positive in lower neck or supraclavicular region	+ 1.19	0
WHO type 1 tumor	+ 1.14	0
Extensive tumor in nasopharynx	+ 0.56	0
ADCC titer ≥1:15,360	− 0.86	0
Symptoms for <2 mo	− 1.05	0

(From Neel HB III, Taylor WF: New staging system for nasopharyngeal carcinoma: long-term outcome, *Arch Otolaryngol Head Neck Surg* 115: 1293, 1989. By permission of Mayo Foundation.)
WHO—World Health Organization; ADCC—Antibody-dependent cellular cytotoxicity.
* Prognosis score is equal to sum of scores.
† Regression weights. Negative value reflects better survival (lower score).
‡ Nodes below skin crease extending laterally and backward from the laryngeal eminence and including the supraclavicular fossa (Ho's line).

Table 79-10. Working formulation for staging* by score

Characteristics	Score If yes	If no
Seven or more symptoms	+ 1	0
Nodes in lower neck or supraclavicular region	+ 1	0
WHO type 1	+ 1	0
Extensive tumor in nasopharynx	+ 0.5	0
Symptoms for <2 months	− 0.5	0

(From Neel HB III, Taylor WF: New staging system for nasopharyngeal carcinoma: long-term outcome, *Arch Otolaryngol Head Neck Surg* 115: 1293, 1989. By permission of Mayo Foundation.)
WHO—World Health Organization.
* Stage A: total score, <0; stage B: total score, ≤0.99; stage C: total score, 1–1.99; stage D: total score, ≥ 2.

lateral opposed portals. Encompassing this volume with fields that average 10 × 13 cm can induce local control in all cases of T_1 and T_2 disease.[30] Small primary tumors may be sterilized with 6500 cGy at rates of 175 to 200 cGy/day, but large tumors or tumors involving cranial nerves of the base of the skull require doses of 7000 cGy or more, usually with smaller fields or electron beam supplements. As the radiation dose is increased, the incidence of complications increases significantly.

Prophylactic irradiation of the lower cervical and supraclavicular lymph nodes to 5000 cGy by direct anterior fields with similar fractionation has prevented the extension of tumor to lymph nodes in those regions.

Radical neck dissection is seldom necessary. This surgical procedure is reserved for the occasional case in which radiotherapy has controlled the primary tumor but has failed to control cervical metastasis. Operation of the skull base for recurrent or residual nasopharyngeal carcinoma after radiation failure at the primary site may be of value in a few carefully selected patients.[17]

Cervical node biopsies may reduce survival.[15] This underscores the desirability of a thorough otorhinolaryngologic examination. Diagnosing nasopharyngeal carcinoma by examination of tissue from the nasopharynx and by serologic testing rather than by biopsy of the neck is safer and certainly advisable.

Intracavitary radioactive implants may supplement external irradiation to the nasopharynx as part of primary management, or they may be reserved for management of recurrent or residual tumors. Occasionally, cryotherapy is applied in the nasopharynx as management for recurrence. Although the use of chemotherapy is limited, it is sometimes helpful for palliation after radiotherapy fails. Even after a recurrent or residual tumor becomes apparent, life may continue for years, and patients may suffer intractable pain. In the future, irradiation and immunotherapy in combination may yield better results.

The remarkable immunologic associations of nasopharyngeal carcinoma encourage the belief that with better understanding of immunologic mechanisms, immunotherapy will become a management option for this disease in the near future.[42] Optimism regarding this development is based in part on the premise that ADCC occurs *in vivo*; if in fact it does, then a high-titered serum containing IgG antibodies directed against EBV membrane antigens may have a good effect on patients with circulating IgA blocking antibody. This therapeutic approach should be considered with plasmapheresis to remove a specific IgA-blocking antibody.

New therapeutic approaches are usually studied in patients with large recurrences, but in general, immunotherapy and perhaps chemotherapy most likely benefit patients with minimal, clinically nonapparent, residual disease.

Prevention

One of the most controversial issues in EBV-associated diseases is related to the development and use of vaccine.[1]

Already the major EBV-specific membrane glycoprotein from infected cells has been purified and shown to induce neutralizing and cytotoxic antibodies. Someday it may be possible to study the efficacy of a vaccine in high-incidence areas of the world.

Outcome

By life-table analysis, survival of 182 contemporary patients with and without recurrence after conventional radiotherapy was 60% at 3 years and 50% at 5 years after diagnosis.[48] Of patients with WHO type 1 tumors, 37% survived 3 years and 10% 5 years; of those with WHO types 2 and 3 tumors, 65% survived 3 years and 52% 5 years.[48,46] Thus a definite trend existed toward more deaths being caused by nasopharyngeal carcinoma in the WHO type 1 group than in the others. The unique WHO type 2 and 3 morphologic forms of nasopharyngeal carcinoma appear to be chronic diseases because the risk of death does not level off with time (beyond 5 years) as it does with most other cancers.

Dickson[15] found very similar results in study of Chinese and white patients. In most studies, overall 5-year survival is 30% to 48%; among the survivors, attrition in the next 5 years is about 10%.[31,57] Most of the recurrences after 5 years are in cases of WHO types 2 and 3 disease. The outcome depends on the histopathology of the tumor and on the type and technique of radiotherapy, the stage of the tumor, and the age of the patient. Patients at the extremes of age have poorer survival.[4,31,44,57]

Many of the differences in survival in the various staging systems are not significant, but every system shows a clear trend to poorer survival with higher stage of disease. As expected, comparison of the AJCC and UICC systems showed no difference in survival between the small stage I and stage II group.[48,50]

ACKNOWLEDGMENTS

Nasopharyngeal carcinoma is of tremendous interest internationally to otolaryngologists, immunologists, virologists, radiation oncologists, epidemiologists, and persons in other disciplines. The reference list by no means reflects all of the important work done by the many prominent investigators throughout the world.

REFERENCES

1. Ablashi DV and others: Fourth international symposium on nasopharyngeal carcinoma: application of field and laboratory studies to the control of NPC, *Cancer Res* 43:2375, 1983.
2. Ackerman LV, del Regato JA: *Cancer: diagnosis, treatment, and prognosis*, ed 4, St Louis, 1970, Mosby.
3. American Joint Committee for Cancer Staging and End-Results Reporting: *Manual for staging of cancer*, Chicago, 1977, American Joint Committee.
4. Applebaum EL, Mantravadi P, Haas R: Lymphoepithelioma of the nasopharynx, *Laryngoscope* 92:510, 1982.
5. Batsakis JG: *Tumors of the head and neck: clinical and pathological considerations*, ed 2, Baltimore, 1979, Williams & Wilkins.
6. Batsakis JG, Solomon AR, Rice DH: The pathology of head and neck

tumors: carcinoma of the nasopharynx, part II, *Head Neck Surg* 3:511, 1981.

7. Biller HF: Juvenile nasopharyngeal angiofibroma, *Ann Otol Rhinol Laryngol* 87:630, 1978.

8. Boles R, Dedo H: Nasopharyngeal angiofibroma, *Laryngoscope* 86: 364, 1976.

9. Bremer JW and others: Angiofibroma: treatment trends in 150 patients during 40 years, *Laryngoscope* 96:1321, 1986.

10. Briant TDR, Fitzpatrick PJ, Berman J: Nasopharyngeal angiofibroma: a twenty-year study, *Laryngoscope* 88:1247, 1978.

11. Chandler JR and others: Nasopharyngeal angiofibromas: staging and management, *Ann Otol Rhinol Laryngol* 93:322, 1984.

12. Cummings BJ: Juvenile nasopharyngeal angiofibroma: control rates and treatment costs, *Head Neck Surg* 3:169, 1980 (editorial).

13. Cummings BJ: Relative risk factors in the treatment of juvenile nasopharyngeal angiofibroma, *Head Neck Surg* 3:21, 1980.

14. Cummings BJ: The treatment of juvenile nasopharyngeal angiofibroma: the case for radiation therapy, *J Laryngol Otol Suppl* 8:101, 1983.

15. Dickson RI: Nasopharyngeal carcinoma: an evaluation of 209 patients, *Laryngoscope* 91:333, 1981.

16. Epstein MA, Achong BG: Recent progress in Epstein-Barr virus research, *Annu Rev Microbiol* 31:421, 1977.

17. Fee WE Jr, Gilmer PA, Goffinet DR: Surgical management of recurrent nasopharyngeal carcinoma after radiation failure at the primary site, *Laryngoscope* 98:1220, 1988.

18. Fitzpatrick PJ, Briant TDR, Berman JM: The nasopharyngeal angiofibroma, *Arch Otolaryngol Head Neck Surg* 106:234, 1980.

19. Fu Y-S, Perzin KH: Nonepithelial tumors of the nasal cavity, paranasal sinuses, and nasopharynx: a clinicopathologic study. I: General features and vascular tumors, *Cancer* 33:1275, 1974.

20. Goepfert H and others: Chemotherapy of locally aggressive head and neck tumors in the pediatric age group: desmoid fibromatosis and nasopharyngeal angiofibroma, *Am J Surg* 144:437, 1982.

21. Hara HJ: Cancer of the nasopharynx: review of the literature report of 72 cases, *Laryngoscope* 79:1315, 1969.

22. Harmer MH: *TNM classification of malignant tumours*, ed 3, Geneva, 1978, Union Internationale Contre le Cancer.

23. Henle G, Henle W: Epstein-Barr virus specific IgA serum antibodies as an outstanding feature of nasopharyngeal carcinoma, *Int J Cancer* 17:1, 1976.

24. Henle W, Henle G: The immunological approach to study of possibly virus-induced human malignancies using the Epstein-Barr virus as example, *Prog Exp Tumor Res* 21:19, 1978.

25. Henle W and others: Antibodies to Epstein-Barr virus in nasopharyngeal carcinoma, other head and neck neoplasms, and control groups, *J Natl Cancer Inst* 44:225, 1970.

26. Henle W and others: Nasopharyngeal carcinoma: significance of changes in Epstein-Barr virus-related antibody patterns following therapy, *Int J Cancer* 20:663, 1977.

27. Ho JH: Stage classification of nasopharyngeal carcinoma: a review, *IARC Sci Publ* 20:99, 1978.

28. Ho JH (moderator): Clinical staging, *IARC Sci Publ* 20:594, 1978. ·

29. Holman CB, Miller WE: Juvenile nasopharyngeal fibroma: roentgenologic characteristics, *Am J Roentgenol* 94:292, 1965.

30. Hoppe RT, Goffinet DR, Bagshaw MA: Carcinoma of the nasopharynx: eighteen years' experience with megavoltage radiation therapy, *Cancer* 37:2605, 1976.

31. Hsu M-M and others: The survival of patients with nasopharyngeal carcinoma, *Otolaryngol Head Neck Surg* 90:289, 1982.

32. Jafek BW and others: Juvenile nasopharyngeal angiofibroma: management of intracranial extension, *Head Neck Surg* 2:119, 1979.

33. Jafek BW and others: Surgical treatment of juvenile nasopharyngeal angiofibroma, *Laryngoscope* 83:707, 1973.

34. Jones GC and others: Juvenile angiofibromas: behavior and treatment

35. Klein G: *The Epstein-Barr virus.* In Kaplan AS, editor: *The herpesviruses*, New York, 1973, Academic Press.

36. Krekorian EA, Kato RH: Surgical management of nasopharyngeal angiofibroma with intracranial extension, *Laryngoscope* 87:154, 1977.

37. Lanier AP and others: Association of Epstein-Barr virus with nasopharyngeal carcinoma in Alaskan native patients: serum antibodies and tissue EBNA and DNA, *Int J Cancer* 28:301, 1981.

38. Lee DA, Sessions DG: Juvenile nasopharyngeal angiofibroma, *Surg Rounds* 3:38, 1980.

39. Mathew GD and others: Immunoglobulin A antibody to Epstein-Barr viral antigens and prognosis in nasopharyngeal carcinoma, *Otolaryngol Head Neck Surg* 88:52, 1980.

40. McCombe A, Lund VJ, Howard DJ: Recurrence in juvenile angiofibroma, *Rhinology* 28:97, 1990.

41. Moore SB and others: HLA and nasopharyngeal carcinoma in North American caucasoids, *Tissue Antigens* 22:72, 1983.

42. Neel HB III, Huang AT: *Session Vc: treatment of NPC.* In Grundmann E, Krueger GRF, Ablashi DV, editors: *Cancer campaign, vol 5, Nasopharyngeal carcinoma*, Stuttgart, 1981, Fischer Verlag.

43. Neel HB III, Pearson GR, Taylor WF: Antibodies to Epstein-Barr virus in patients with nasopharyngeal carcinoma and in comparison groups, *Ann Otol Rhinol Laryngol* 93:477, 1984.

44. Neel HB III and others: Anti-EBV serologic tests for nasopharyngeal carcinoma, *Laryngoscope* 90:1981, 1980.

45. Neel HB III and others: Immunologic detection of occult primary cancer of the head and neck, *Otolaryngol Head Neck Surg* 89:230, 1981.

46. Neel HB III and others: Application of Epstein-Barr virus serology to the diagnosis and staging of North American patients with nasopharyngeal carcinoma, *Otolaryngol Head Neck Surg* 91:255, 1983.

47. Neel HB III, Taylor WF: *Clinical presentation and diagnosis of nasopharyngeal carcinoma: current status.* In Prasad U and others, editors: *Nasopharyngeal carcinoma: current concepts*, Kuala Lumpur, 1983, University of Malaya Press.

48. Neel HB III, Taylor WF: New staging system for nasopharyngeal carcinoma: long-term outcome, *Arch Otolaryngol Head Neck Surg* 115: 1293, 1989.

49. Neel HB III, Taylor WF: Epstein-Barr virus-related antibody: changes in titers after therapy for nasopharyngeal carcinoma, *Arch Otolaryngol Head Neck Surg* 116:1287, 1990.

50. Neel HB III, Taylor WF, Pearson GR: Prognostic determinants and a new view of staging for patients with nasopharyngeal carcinoma, *Ann Otol Rhinol Laryngol* 94:529, 1985.

51. Neel HB III and others: *Clinical staging of patients with nasopharyngeal carcinoma.* In Grundmann E, Krueger GRF, Ablashi DV, editors: *Cancer campaign, vol 5, Nasopharyngeal carcinoma*, Stuttgart, 1981, Fischer Verlag.

52. Neel HB III and others: Juvenile angiofibroma: review of 120 cases, *Am J Surg* 126:547, 1973.

53. Pearson GR and others: Application of Epstein-Barr virus (EBV) serology to the diagnosis of North American nasopharyngeal carcinoma, *Cancer* 51:260, 1983.

54. Prasad U: Fossa of Rosenmüller and nasopharyngeal carcinoma, *Med J Malaysia* 33:222, 1979.

55. Roberson GH and others: Presurgical internal maxillary artery embolization in juvenile angiofibroma, *Laryngoscope* 82:1524, 1972.

56. Scanlon PW, Devine KD, Woolner LB: Malignant lesions of the nasopharynx, *Ann Otol Rhinol Laryngol* 67:1005, 1958.

57. Scanlon PW and others: Cancer of the nasopharynx: 142 patients treated in the 11-year period 1950–1960, *Am J Roentgenol* 99:313, 1967.

58. Sessions RB and others: Radiographic staging of juvenile angiofibroma, *Head Neck Surg* 3:279, 1981.

59. Sessions RB, Humphreys DH: *Angiofibroma.* In Gates GA, editor: *Current therapy in otolaryngology head and neck surgery 1984–1985*, St Louis, 1984, Mosby.

60. Shaffer K and others: Pitfalls in the radiographic diagnosis of angiofibroma, *Radiology* 127:425, 1978.

61. Shanmugaratnam K: *Histological typing of upper respiratory tract tumours (International Histological Classification of Tumours, No. 19)*, Geneva, 1978, World Health Organization.

62. Standefer J and others: Combined intracranial and extracranial excision of nasopharyngeal angiofibroma, *Laryngoscope* 93:772, 1983.

63. Waldman SR and others: Surgical experience with nasopharyngeal angiofibroma, Arch Otolaryngol Head Neck Surg 107:677, 1981.

64. Ward PH: The evolving management of juvenile nasopharyngeal angiofibroma, *J Laryngol Otol Suppl* 8:103, 1983.

65. Ward PH and others: Juvenile angiofibroma: a more rational therapeutic approach based upon clinical and experimental evidence, *Laryngoscope* 84:2181, 1974.

66. Weiland LH: The histopathological spectrum of nasopharyngeal carcinoma, *IARC Sci Publ* 20:41, 1978.

67. Witt TR, Shah JP, Sternberg SS: Juvenile nasopharyngeal angiofibroma: a 30-year clinical review, *Am J Surg* 146:521, 1983.

Chapter 80

Oral Mucosal Lesions

Carl M. Allen
George Gordon Blozis

This chapter discusses nonneoplastic lesions that involve the oral mucous membranes. Only the more common lesions seen in the oral cavity are considered; there is no attempt to be comprehensive. More complete and detailed information about these and the less common lesions can be found elsewhere.[10,37,39,53]

The principal emphasis of this chapter is on the clinical features of the lesions and their management, when appropriate. Of the several different formats that can be used to classify lesions, the authors consider the clinical appearance to be the most useful. Thus, lesions are grouped into the three classic clinical presentations that have been described: color change, raised, and depressed. Lesions that show a color change and are raised are discussed under the raised category. Vesiculobullous lesions that initially appear as raised lesions but usually are seen as ulcerations also are discussed in the raised category. Lesions occurring on the gingiva are identified as a specific group; because many of the entities are unique to this area, they are recognized largely by their clinical appearance and their location. The authors believe this format is the most practical when trying to identify clinical disease.

LESIONS SHOWING A COLOR CHANGE

Predominantly white mucosal lesions

The term *leukoplakia* has been used in many contexts in the past, ranging from a general description of any white mucosal lesion to a histologic diagnosis implying premalignant change. As defined by the World Health Organization, leukoplakia should be used as a clinical diagnosis to indicate a white lesion that cannot be removed by gentle scraping and that cannot be diagnosed clinically or histopathologically as

any other lesion. Therefore, several oral mucosal lesions may appear as white patches but should not be diagnosed clinically as leukoplakia.

Leukoedema

Leukoedema is a benign condition that most likely represents a variation of healthy mucosal appearance, although smoking may accentuate its features. Almost 90% of blacks and 45% of whites exhibit the filmy, opalescent quality of the buccal mucosa that characterizes leukoedema. Fine folds occasionally are observed in the affected mucosa and superficially may resemble other conditions, such as lichen planus (Fig. 80-1). Leukoedema is asymptomatic and has no malignant potential. Histologically, the epithelial cells appear edematous and swollen, with no evidence of epithelial atypia. Stretching or everting the buccal mucosa causes the white, filmy character to disappear. Because this condition is completely benign, no treatment is necessary.

White sponge nevus

Initially described by Cannon[9] in 1935, white sponge nevus is a benign mucosal disorder inherited as an autosomal dominant trait. Usually the lesions appear in childhood and are seen as thick, white, typically corrugated folds involving primarily the buccal mucosa, although other areas of the oral mucosa and the vaginal and rectal mucosa may be affected.[26] The characteristic histologic appearance is not pathognomonic. A ragged surface parakeratin layer is seen with a remarkable increase in the epithelial thickness. The cells of the spinous layer exhibit marked intracellular edema and small, pyknotic nuclei. Exfoliative cytology reveals keratinized squamous epithelial cells that exhibit an eosinophilic, perinuclear condensation of the cytoplasm. The diagnosis is

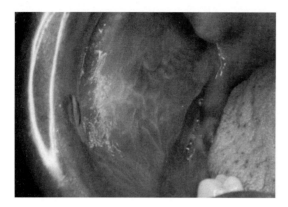

Fig. 80-1. Leukoedema. Buccal mucosa of this patient shows characteristic filmy appearance of leukoedema. Fine folds that may develop when mucosa is relaxed could suggest a diagnosis of lichen planus; however, they disappear when mucosa is stretched.

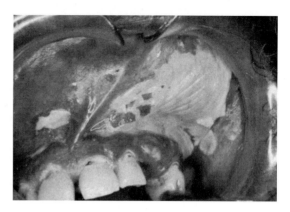

Fig. 80-2. An aspirin burn. Extensive distribution of epithelial damage is evidence of caustic effect of aspirin on oral mucosa.

made on the basis of history, clinical distribution of lesions, and cytologic or histologic findings. Because there is no malignant potential, no treatment is necessary.

Keratosis follicularis

Oral lesions may be seen in patients affected by keratosis follicularis (Darier's disease), although the skin manifestations of this autosomal dominant genodermatosis are more striking. These patients typically exhibit numerous erythematous, crusted papules distributed primarily over the skin of the face and trunk. Intraorally, ragged white papules are seen on the gingivae, the alveolar mucosa, and the dorsal tongue.[31] Histologic evaluation shows the characteristic suprabasilar epithelial clefting, acantholysis, corps ronds, and grains. Diagnosis usually can be made on the basis of the skin lesions, although exfoliative cytology or biopsy will support the clinical impression. The oral lesions typically are asymptomatic and therefore do not require treatment.

Chemical injury

Application of caustic substances to the oral mucosa may produce varying degrees of epithelial necrosis, which clinically appears as a white, sloughing membrane. Perhaps the most commonly seen injury of this type results from the inappropriate use of aspirin as a topical anesthetic for toothache pain (Fig. 80-2). The clinical appearance of such lesions may be dramatic, although obtaining a good history should confirm the clinical impression.

Nicotine stomatitis

Nicotine stomatitis frequently is seen among patients who smoke, particularly those who smoke pipes. Although the name implies that nicotine is responsible for the lesion, a more likely etiologic factor is the heat, which produces tissue injury. These patients primarily are middle-aged men with a long history of smoking. The lesion is seen clinically as a diffuse, whitened palatal mucosa, which serves as a back-

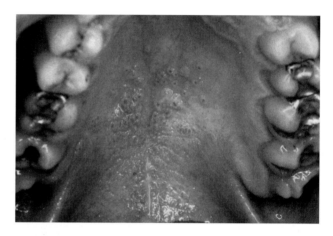

Fig. 80-3. Nicotine stomatitis. The 1- to 2-mm papules represent inflamed orifices of minor salivary glands.

ground for a variable number of 1- to 2-mm papules with erythematous centers (Fig. 80-3). These papular structures represent the inflamed orifices of the palatal minor salivary glands. Usually these changes are restricted to the hard palate and anterior soft palate, and occasionally keratinization may extend to involve the entire soft palate and buccal mucosa. Although the appearance of this condition is so typical that a clinical diagnosis usually is sufficient, at times, one of the papules will enlarge to such an extent that a biopsy may be needed to rule out a salivary gland lesion. Nicotine stomatitis is considered a benign mucosal reaction, but these patients should be encouraged to reduce their tobacco use.

Candidiasis

Infection of the oral mucosa by the yeast *Candida albicans* is common and frequently is overlooked because of the range of clinical appearances. The classic description of candidiasis mentions white, curd-like flecks of material that can be wiped off, leaving a raw, bleeding surface. This definition is limited because it describes only the pseudomem-

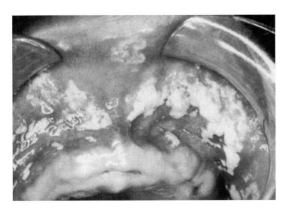

Fig. 80-4. Acute pseudomembranous candidiasis. This is typical appearance of *thrush*. White flecks of candidal organisms and desquamated epithelial cells can be removed relatively easily, leaving erythematous mucosal base.

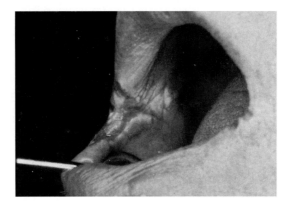

Fig. 80-5. Chronic hyperplastic candidiasis. Unlike acute pseudomembranous form, "candidal leukoplakia" cannot be removed by scraping. At times, there may be associated erythematous mucosa. Anterior buccal mucosa is a common site for this lesion.

branous form of the disease, also termed *thrush*. In addition, the description is not accurate because a "bleeding" surface rarely is encountered, although the mucosa may appear erythematous (Fig. 80-4). The patients affected usually are very young or very old—age groups whose immune systems are not functioning optimally. Patients infected with the human immunodeficiency virus (HIV) often exhibit pseudomembranous oral candidiasis because of their immunologic deficits. Patients who recently have taken corticosteroids or broad-spectrum antibiotics also are affected. Immune suppression and elimination of competing bacteria are believed to cause the overgrowth of the yeast.

Diagnosis can be made by examining a potassium hydroxide preparation of the lesion's scrapings. The characteristic ovoid yeasts mixed with the hyphal forms of this dimorphic organism are seen. A routine cytologic smear may be stained using the periodic acid–Schiff method. These studies can be confirmed by culturing the organism on a mycologic medium, such as Sabouraud's, Pagano-Levin, or BiGGY agar, although a culture alone should not be used for diagnosing candidiasis because patients who are simply carriers of the yeast may have a positive culture.

Treatment of oral candidiasis consists of 7 to 14 days of topical antifungal agent therapy, such as with nystatin or clotrimazole, or systemic drug therapy, such as with ketoconazole or fluconazole. Signs and symptoms typically abate in 1 to 3 days, and recurrence is not uncommon.

A less frequently encountered form of oral candidiasis that appears as a white lesion is *chronic hyperplastic candidiasis.*[11] Because these lesions manifest as a white patch that will not rub off, they have been termed *candidal leukoplakia.*[4] The anterior buccal mucosa, just posterior to the angle of the mouth, is a typically affected site (Fig. 80-5). Unless such a lesion is mentioned in the clinical impression, the pathologist may overlook the candidal hyphae in the parakeratin layer and simply diagnose the lesion as hyperkeratosis and chronic inflammation. Some degree of atypia may be

seen microscopically within the lesion's epithelium, and some investigators have suggested that chronic hyperplastic candidiasis may represent a premalignant lesion.[18] Although a large percentage of these lesions are removed completely with biopsy, those treated with antifungal agents frequently do not regress fully and need to be excised.

Lichen planus

Erasmus Wilson initially described lichen planus as a dermatologic condition in 1869. Since then, little information has been added to the understanding of its etiology. The skin lesions appear as pruritic, violaceous papules distributed over the forearms and medial thigh. Oral lesions may be seen with or without skin lesions. Patients affected by oral lichen planus are typically middle-aged adults, and most series have reported a female predilection.[40] Several clinical forms of the disease have been described, although the reticular and erosive types are seen most frequently.

Reticular lichen planus generally exhibits such a characteristic clinical pattern that biopsy is seldom necessary to establish the diagnosis. The lesions typically are seen on the buccal mucosa, often bilaterally, and consist of an interlacing network of white, slightly raised striae (Fig. 80-6). Gingival involvement also may be observed, although the floor of the mouth and palatal mucosa usually are not affected. Lichen planus may occur on the dorsum of the tongue, but these lesions usually do not exhibit the characteristic linear pattern. Instead, a flattened, well-delineated area of mucosal involvement is seen, characterized by a patchy, streaked pattern of atrophic, erythematous, and keratotic areas (Plate 14, *A*). *Erosive* lichen planus typically is painful, unlike the reticular form. The most commonly affected areas include the buccal mucosa, the gingivae, and the lateral tongue. Clinically, these lesions exhibit an erythematous or ulcerated central area surrounded by a keratotic periphery (Plates 14 and 15). Close inspection shows the peripheral keratosis forming fine, delicate striae radiating away from the center of the lesion. Occasionally, these lesions may mimic those of lupus erythematosus. If biopsy is necessary to differentiate between the two, the specimen should be taken from the periphery of the lesion to obtain diagnostic tissue. The ulcerated center will not provide the necessary histologic information. The clinician also should be aware that 25% to 30% of lichen planus lesions will have a superimposed candidal infection.

Microscopically, oral lichen planus exhibits varying degrees of hyperorthokeratosis or hyperparakeratosis, irregular acanthosis and atrophy, degeneration of the basal cell layer, and a band-like infiltrate of predominantly T lymphocytes. Immunofluorescence shows a coarsely granular deposition of fibrinogen at the basement membrane zone.[14]

The reticular form of the condition requires no treatment because the lesions are asymptomatic. Erosive lichen planus is best managed by corticosteroid therapy. With smaller, focal ulcerations, topical application of fluocinonide or betamethasone dipropionate gel may be used to control symptoms. More diffuse lesions may require a corticosteroid syrup, such as betamethasone, which can be applied topically or can be swallowed to provide systemic effect. Once the lesions are controlled, the dosage can be tapered, although the condition rarely is eliminated.

Chronic cutaneous lupus erythematosus

Approximately 25% of patients with chronic cutaneous lupus erythematosus (CCLE), a dermatologic condition, exhibit oral manifestations; oral lesions rarely are observed without skin lesions. The etiology of CCLE and its relationship to systemic lupus erythematosus remain unclear. The oral lesions clinically and histologically resemble erosive lichen planus. Clinically, the presence of skin lesions should assist in the diagnosis. Histologically, a perivascular lymphocytic infiltrate in the deeper submucosal tissue should suggest CCLE.

Leukoplakia

As stated previously, the term *leukoplakia* should represent a clinical diagnosis only and should apply to white lesions that cannot be scraped off or recognized as any other disease process. Leukoplakic lesions tend to occur in an older age group, and men are affected more than women.[50] Approximately 80% of these lesions microscopically show a benign histology consisting of either hyperorthokeratosis, hyperparakeratosis, acanthosis, or a combination of these. The remaining 20% represent premalignant epithelial dysplasia, carcinoma *in situ*, or frank invasive squamous cell carcinoma. Obviously, biopsies of these lesions should be done to establish a diagnosis. Biopsy particularly is indicated for a leukoplakic lesion that has no apparent cause, such as a source of irritation, or for a lesion that does not resolve once the irritating factor is removed. Lesions that are found on the lower lip, the lateral tongue, and the floor of the mouth also should be viewed with much more suspicion.

Chapter 77 discusses the premalignant aspects of leukoplakia in more detail.

Hairy leukoplakia

In 1984, Deborah Greenspan and others described an oral lesion that appeared to be strongly associated with patients who were infected with HIV. Because the lesion often exhibited a shaggy white surface and could not be wiped off, it was termed *hairy leukoplakia*. Initially, hairy leukoplakia was thought to be caused by a chronic candidal infection because the organism frequently colonized the lesion; however, research indicates that hairy leukoplakia is caused by infection of the epithelium by Epstein-Barr virus.[21] In the majority of patients, hairy leukoplakia occurs on the lateral/ventral tongue of those with HIV (Fig. 80-7). Infrequently, other immunosuppressed patients may develop the condition, and rarely, an otherwise healthy person can be affected. The lesions may be unilateral or bilateral and un-

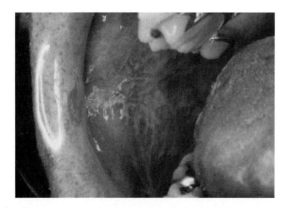

Fig. 80-6. Lichen planus. Reticular form of condition is commonly found on buccal mucosa and is characterized by interlacing pattern of white striae.

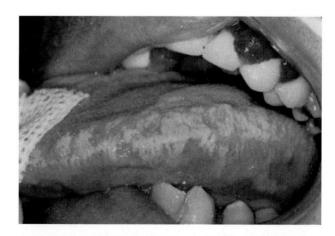

Fig. 80-7. Hairy leukoplakia. Whereas the more developed lesions may show ragged surface keratin, earlier lesions typically are more plaque-like.

commonly extend onto the dorsal surface of the tongue, the buccal mucosa, or the soft palate. Incipient lesions often do not exhibit the ragged, hair-like projections of more fully developed hairy leukoplakia. The microscopic features of hairy leukoplakia are characteristic, but not pathognomonic. Ideally, demonstration of Epstein-Barr virus by deoxyribonucleic acid (DNA) hybridization studies would confirm the diagnosis.

Unlike classic leukoplakia, hairy leukoplakia shows no known tendency for malignant transformation. It is important because its appearance correlates well with the rapid development of acquired immunodeficiency syndrome (AIDS) in HIV-infected patients. A majority of these patients will proceed to the end-stage of their disease within a 3-year period after the onset of hairy leukoplakia. Treatment of hairy leukoplakia generally is not necessary, although it will regress with anti-herpesvirus therapy.

Predominantly red mucosal lesions

As with the white oral mucosal lesions, the etiologic agents associated with red lesions are numerous, representing a broad spectrum of disease. Most of these lesions are inflammatory and frequently nonspecific, although these should be distinguished from specific microbial infections and preneoplastic conditions.

Benign migratory glossitis

Benign migratory glossitis (geographic tongue) is relatively common, affecting approximately 1% of the population. The etiology is unknown, although histologically, the lesion resembles psoriasis of the skin. No particular age, race, or sex predilection is observed. Clinically, the lesions are asymptomatic or, much less frequently, associated with a mild burning sensation from hot or spicy foods. A spectrum of clinical appearances exists because the lesions tend to appear and then regress, only to appear in another site and repeat the pattern. At their peak, the lesions consist of an erythematous central area of atrophic mucosa. The tongue papillae commonly are lost in this area, resulting in a flat but nonulcerated mucosal surface. The erythematous area usually is surrounded by a serpiginous keratotic border, although this can vary in degree (Fig. 80-8). Frequently, the tongues of these patients also show evidence of fissuring, an asymptomatic developmental condition seen on the dorsum. An infrequent finding is the appearance of similar lesions on other oral mucosal surfaces.

Benign migratory glossitis may occur on mucosal sites other than the tongue, such as the buccal and labial mucosa. These lesions have been reported under a variety of names, including *erythema migrans, stomatitis areata migrans,* and *ectopic geographic tongue.* Because these lesions are benign and usually asymptomatic, no treatment is recommended. In the occasional patient whose lesions are symptomatic, topical corticosteroid therapy sometimes is beneficial.

Vascular proliferations

The hemangioma is a fairly common lesion composed of a benign aggregation or proliferation of blood vessels. Whether these lesions represent true neoplasms or simply hamartomatous structures is open to debate. Frequently, hemangiomas are present at birth, although at times they may appear later. The clinical size of the lesion and the histologic size of the vascular components may vary considerably. Usually these lesions blanch when pressure is applied, a phenomenon most easily observed by diascopy.

Treatment of hemangiomas varies according to their size and site and the patient's age. Many congenital lesions regress dramatically during childhood. Smaller lesions can be removed surgically. In patients with larger, cosmetically deforming lesions, treatment is more difficult, although sclerosing agents, cryotherapy, and laser therapy have been used with varying degrees of success.

Encephalotrigeminal angiomatosis, or *Sturge-Weber syndrome,* is a developmental disorder characterized by hemangiomas affecting the leptomeninges or the skin and mucosal surfaces innervated by the trigeminal nerve. The condition does not seem to be inherited but occurs sporadically, probably because the cephalic vascular plexus fails to regress during the ninth week of gestation.

Hereditary hemorrhagic telangiectasia is inherited as an autosomal dominant trait and is characterized by the appearance of multiple, 1- to 2-mm vascular dilations. These surface lesions are traumatized easily and can be a source of bothersome hemorrhage. Although such blood loss occasionally has resulted in death, this is uncommon. Epistaxis frequently is the patient's initial complaint. Conditions to be considered in the differential diagnosis include Ehlers-Danlos syndrome and calcinosis, Raynaud's phenomenon, esophageal dysmotility, sclerodactyly, telangiectasia (CREST) syndrome. Treatment has included cryosurgery, skin grafting, and corticosteroid therapy.

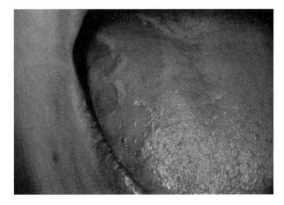

Fig. 80-8. Benign migratory glossitis. Note areas of uniform erythema and loss of papillae, which are surrounded by slightly raised, white borders.

Candidiasis

Although candidiasis is regarded more frequently as a white lesion, it also may manifest as an erythematous one. This generally is associated with broad-spectrum antibiotic therapy, such as with tetracycline. The patient frequently reports a burning sensation on the tongue, and clinically, the tongue may show a diffuse redness over the entire dorsum. A culture and exfoliative cytology should establish the diagnosis.

Another commonly observed red lesion associated with *C. albicans* is *denture stomatitis*. This condition involves only the denture-bearing mucosa of a patient who wears a complete or partial upper denture. In contrast to what the name implies, most patients are completely asymptomatic. Certain authors also have suggested the term *chronic atrophic candidiasis*. Even though *C. albicans* may be cultured from either the denture or the mucosa, this is not a consistent finding. Marked improvement of the mucosa may occur if the patient removes the denture while sleeping. Otherwise, oral nystatin rinses and weak sodium hypochlorite solution soaks for the denture usually restore the mucosa's normal appearance.

Median rhomboid glossitis

Median rhomboid glossitis (central papillary atrophy) appears as an asymptomatic, well-defined erythematous area involving the midline posterior dorsum of the tongue (Fig. 80-9). Loss of the lingual papillae is a prominent feature in the area of the lesion, which has prompted some investigators to suggest the term *central papillary atrophy*.[16] The lesion's surface usually is smooth but may appear somewhat uneven or mammillated. The etiology of median rhomboid glossitis is controversial. For many years, median rhomboid glossitis was thought to be a developmental lesion resulting from a failure of the lateral processes of the tongue to cover the midline tuberculum impar during embryologic formation. Median rhomboid glossitis, however, is seen almost exclusively in adults, which would not be expected if the lesion was truly developmental.

Perhaps the most widely accepted etiologic hypothesis is that median rhomboid glossitis results from a chronic candidal infection.[13] *C. albicans* often can be cultured from these lesions and identified in cytologic smears; also, antifungal therapy may result in regression of the lesion with regeneration of the lingual papillae. Such findings unfortunately are not consistent, and further study is necessary to better define the pathogenesis of median rhomboid glossitis.

The management of median rhomboid glossitis consists of establishing the presence of *C. albicans* and treating the patient accordingly. If the lesion shows a tendency to recur after antifungal therapy, then immunologic evaluation may be indicated because such lesions are common in HIV-infected patients. The dorsal tongue mucosa is a rare location for malignancy, and the patient can be reassured that the lesion has no precancerous potential.

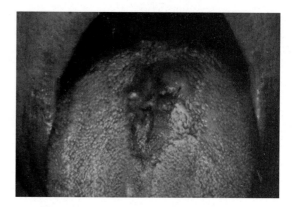

Fig. 80-9. Median rhomboid glossitis (central papillary atrophy). This asymptomatic, erythematous lesion of the midline posterior dorsum of the tongue is often caused by chronic candidal infection.

Histoplasmosis

Although uncommon, oral lesions of histoplasmosis should be included in the differential diagnosis of erythematous lesions. Infection by the fungal organism *Histoplasma capsulatum* is confined primarily to the lower respiratory tract. In areas wherein the disease is endemic, such as the Ohio and Mississippi River valleys, as many as 80% to 100% of the population show evidence of past infection, usually identified as calcified perihilar lymph nodes on chest radiographs. Oral lesions usually occur in debilitated patients with disseminated disease. The lesion may appear as an ill-defined erythematous patch with an irregular, granulomatous surface, or it may exhibit ulceration, simulating malignancy (Fig. 80-10).[34] Biopsy and a culture are necessary to establish a diagnosis. Treatment for disseminated disease previously was limited to administration of amphotericin B, although good results have been reported with ketoconazole[48] particularly in those patients with minimal immune dysfunction, and itraconazole appears to be even more effective.

Allergy

Allergy symptoms may be more widespread than generally realized. Patients with allergic reactions usually are adults with a history of a burning or stinging sensation of the oral mucosa. Sometimes the signs are localized, but diffuse involvement of the mucosa may occur. Often, the symptoms wax and wane with no readily apparent pattern. The lesions are characterized by an erythematous color and may have a velvety texture. A white, keratotic surface may be superimposed on the erythematous base, clinically suggesting candidiasis (Fig. 80-11). Careful history taking usually reveals that the patient routinely uses a particular brand of chewing gum, mouthwash, breath mint, or other flavored material. Frequently, the flavoring agent at fault is cinnamon.[5] Withdrawal of the offending agent results in complete resolution within 3 to 4 days. Other materials, particularly drugs, may elicit an allergic response from the oral mucosa. Such lesions

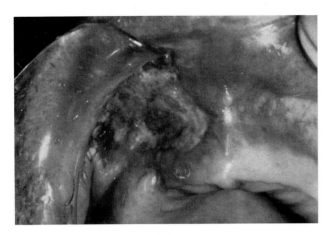

Fig. 80-10. Histoplasmosis. This large ulceration with an irregular surface suggested malignancy to the clinician, although histologic examination of biopsy material established the diagnosis of histoplasmosis. Ketoconazole therapy produced complete resolution in 2 months.

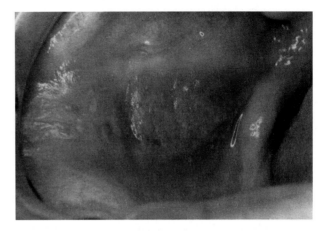

Fig. 80-11. Reaction from cinnamon-flavored chewing gum. This lesion appears to be clinically similar to candidiasis, although no organisms were found on cytology or culture. It was later found that patients could induce lesions by chewing a particular brand of chewing gum.

may appear as a lichenoid mucositis, superficial ulcerations, or a vesiculobullous process.

Anemia

Erythematous oral lesions have been described in association with various anemias. The most commonly involved site is the dorsal tongue mucosa, which clinically appears atrophic and reddened. Such lesions should not be confused with benign migratory glossitis, which also appears as atrophic dorsal tongue lesions. Benign migratory glossitis typically is sharply demarcated and often exhibits a slightly raised white border. Pernicious anemia (vitamin B_{12} deficiency) classically has been associated with elderly patients of northern European origin, although recent reports suggest that the disorder also may be common in black women.[20] In these patients, the lesions may not be restricted to the tongue mucosa; they also may be found on the buccal and labial mucosa. As with a candidal infection or allergy, the patient may complain of a burning sensation. Blood studies should confirm the diagnosis, and the lesions usually clear after appropriate therapy for the anemia.

Systemic lupus erythematosus

Systemic lupus erythematosus (SLE) affects multiple organ systems through damage induced by circulating immune complexes. Kidney involvement usually is seen and represents the most serious aspect of the disease. Skin lesions also are common, typically described as a butterfly-shaped rash distributed over the malar eminences and the bridge of the nose. SLE has a distinct female predilection and generally appears in the third and fourth decades of life. Oral lesions are seen occasionally in those with SLE and consist of erythematous and hyperemic lesions of the buccal mucosa or palate that may appear macular or somewhat granuloma-

tous. Infrequently, the oral lesions may represent the initial signs of the disease. Histologic findings are characteristic but not diagnostic, and the oral lesions usually resolve with systemic therapy.

Erythroplakia

The term *erythroplakia* literally means "red patch" and is used to denote erythematous lesions of the oral mucosa that cannot be diagnosed as any other lesion. Although the term should be used as a clinical diagnosis, microscopically these lesions likely represent premalignant or malignant disease. Shafer and Waldron[41] found that 90% of these lesions exhibited severe epithelial dysplasia, carcinoma *in situ,* or invasive squamous cell carcinoma. Thus, even though erythroplakia is seen much less than leukoplakia, its presence is much more ominous. Once inflammatory processes have been ruled out, biopsy of the erythroplakic lesion is mandatory.

Burning tongue

Burning tongue (glossopyrosis, burning mouth syndrome) is a source of frustration to patients and clinicians. The different terms used to identify the problem, such as *painful tongue (glossodynia), oral dysesthesia,* and *orolingual paresthesia,* reflect the uncertain nature of the problem. Most patients are women and often are postmenopausal,[22] some have denture trauma, oral candidiasis, anemia, diabetes mellitus, psychogenic problems, and folic acid or vitamin B_{12} deficiencies.[29] After appropriate management of these problems, the patient's symptoms often resolve. Patients usually complain of a burning sensation similar to that caused by drinking extremely hot liquids such as coffee. Occasionally, it may be described as a soreness, pain, or stinging sensation that often is constant and may vary in intensity. Some patients indicate that the sensation is not present in the morning but becomes apparent during the course of the day and increases in severity at the end of the day. The problem often is limited to the tongue but may involve the lips, anterior palate, gingiva, or buccal mucosa. Clinical examination typically shows no evidence of mucosal abnormality.

Treatment of these patients should focus on identifying local factors, systemic disease, or psychogenic causes. When these have been eliminated, patients should be reassured that no apparent evidence of major disease exists; then they should be treated with supportive measures. Cancer phobia has been associated with burning sensations, and reassurance is extremely important for these patients.

Mucosal lesions characterized by yellow, brown, blue, or black pigmentation

Hairy tongue

The "coated" tongue is a common condition that has a characteristic white color caused by an accumulation of keratin associated with the filiform papillae. Occasionally, for poorly understood reasons, the keratin is either produced more quickly or desquamated less rapidly, resulting in a marked elongation of the filiform papillae. These elongated keratinaceous papillae resemble hair and frequently assume various colors, ranging from yellow to black because of colonization with chromogenic bacteria. The condition is harmless, although the patient may complain of a gagging sensation. Treatment consists of having the patient use a tongue scraper to help remove the accumulated keratin.

Melanotic lesions

Melanin pigmentation of the lips and oral mucosa is a relatively common finding. In those of darker races, such pigmentation is considered normal, although its distribution may vary from person to person. The usual sites for normal oral pigmentation include the attached gingival mucosa, the buccal mucosa, and the palate. Occasionally, the fungiform papillae of the tongue also are pigmented. Focal areas of melanin deposition may be seen as brown macular pigmentation that can involve any oral mucosal site but particularly the vermilion zone of the lips, the gingiva, palate, and buccal mucosa. When on the lips, such lesions may represent ephelides (freckles) or lentigines. Ephelides darken with sun exposure, whereas lentigines do not. Such focal pigmentation also may represent posttraumatic melanosis, although often a specific history of trauma cannot be elicited. Some investigators[52] have termed these lesions *melanotic macules* because they do not fit well into any other category: the lack of change with sun exposure rules out ephelis; the lack of melanocytic aggregation at the tips of the rete ridges rules out lentigo; and the absence of a history of trauma rules out posttraumatic melanosis (Fig. 80-12). These lesions should be removed and evaluated histologically to rule out the pos-

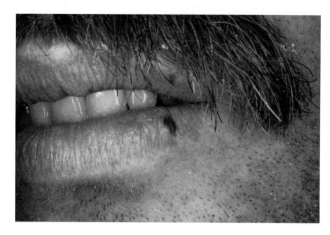

Fig. 80-12. Melanotic macule. Such lesions should be excised and examined microscopically if the patient gives history of recent enlargement or increase in pigmentation.

sibility of melanoma, particularly if the patient has noticed an increase in the size of the lesion or density of its pigmentation.[28]

With more diffuse areas of pigmentation, other conditions should be considered in the differential diagnosis. If the pigmentation has developed recently, a careful history should be taken. Certain drugs may induce melanin pigmentation. Addison's disease (chronic adrenocortical insufficiency) also may show disorders of pigmentation as a prominent feature. A history of weakness, salt craving, diarrhea, and vomiting suggests this diagnosis. The "bronzing" of the skin often is described as the classic sign of Addison's disease, although the oral pigmentation involving the buccal mucosa, lips, tongue, and gingiva frequently is the initial manifestation of this disorder.

If diffuse melanin pigmentation of the oral mucosa has been present since early childhood, particularly if accompanied by freckling of the perioral, perinasal, and periorbital skin, then Peutz-Jeghers' syndrome should be considered as a diagnostic possibility. Patients with this syndrome frequently have a history of gastrointestinal problems caused by multiple intestinal polyps. Although these polyps are considered benign with only sporadic reports of malignant transformation, the problem of intestinal intussusception with its attendant complications may have to be resolved. Other family members should be investigated because this syndrome is inherited as an autosomal dominant trait with a high degree of penetrance.

Exogenous pigmentation

The most common form of exogenous pigmentation of the oral mucosa results from the implantation of silver amalgam during dental restorative procedures. The resulting amalgam "tattoo" may exhibit a range of color (brown, blue, black), depending on the amount of material embedded, the depth, and the duration of implantation (Fig. 80-

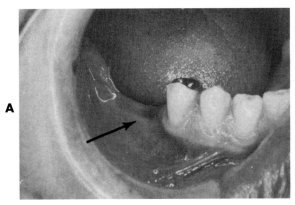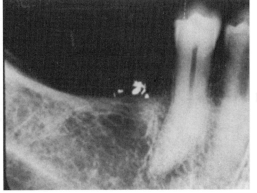

Fig. 80-13. Amalgam tattoo. **A,** Clinically, color may range from faint blue to black *(arrow)*. **B,** Dental radiograph usually shows embedded metallic fragments as radiopaque flecks.

13, *A*). These lesions are invariably asymptomatic, although occasionally a patient may notice the pigmentation and, fearing cancer, anxiously seek professional evaluation. Generally, the area of discoloration is no more than 5 mm in diameter, and the usual location is the gingiva, although buccal mucosa, palate, tongue, and floor of the mouth are potential sites.[8] A dental radiograph of the lesion area (Fig. 80-13, *B*) may show fine, radiopaque remnants of the filling material, and histologic examination reveals granular foreign material, usually with minimal reaction between the host and foreign body. Silver amalgam often can be detected positively in microscopic sections because of the characteristic staining of the connective tissue reticulin fibers by the silver salts.

If the lesion can be verified by radiography, then no treatment is required because the material is inert. If positive identification cannot be made, excisional biopsy is indicated. Lesions to be considered in the differential diagnosis include other forms of exogenous pigment such as graphite, focal melanosis, the various melanocytic nevi, and malignant melanoma.

Varix

The varix seen on the oral mucosa is essentially the same lesion that affects the subcutaneous tissues of the lower leg, so-called varicose veins. Varices typically develop in middle-aged or elderly persons and occur on the lower lip, labial mucosa, buccal mucosa, and ventral tongue. Because the lesions are basically dilated venous structures, they are deep blue or purplish blue. Varices usually are elevated slightly and may appear multilobular. Palpation typically reveals a soft consistency, although some degree of firm nodularity may exist because of thrombus formation within the vascular lumen. Thrombus formation, probably caused by stasis, is relatively common and has little or no adverse influence. Varices usually are characteristic enough to be diagnosed clinically. Excisional biopsy may be performed if the lesion is traumatized periodically or if the patient is concerned.

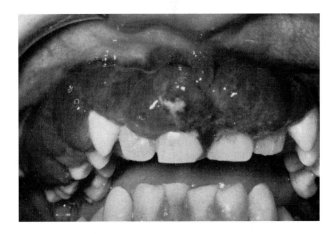

Fig. 80-14. Acquired immunodeficiency virus-related Kaposi's sarcoma. These gingival lesions exemplify the tumor stage of Kaposi's sarcoma and certainly pose an esthetic problem for this patient.

Such a procedure generally is not associated with major bleeding because the intravascular pressure is low.

Kaposi's sarcoma

The development of Kaposi's sarcoma in an HIV-infected patient is one manifestation that heralds the onset of AIDS. Although the incidence of AIDS-related Kaposi's sarcoma seems to be decreasing (now affecting approximately 15% of patients with AIDS), 50% of those patients with Kaposi's sarcoma will have oral lesions. Not infrequently, the oral lesions are the initial manifestation of AIDS-related Kaposi's sarcoma.[17] The palate and gingivae are the most common sites of oral involvement of AIDS-related Kaposi's sarcoma. Clinically, the lesions will present initially as red or purple macules or plaques that enlarge to form tumor masses (Fig. 80-14). The lesions usually are asymptomatic, although they may ulcerate or become so bulky as to interfere with speech or swallowing. Esthetics also may be a consideration in some patients. Diagnosis is established by means of histologic examination of biopsy material. The purple color seen clinically can be correlated with numerous extravasated erythrocytes that have leaked from incompetent vascular spaces formed by the neoplastic endothelial cell proliferation. Treatment of AIDS-related Kaposi's sarcoma can include surgical excision, radiotherapy, or intralesional vinblastine injections.[15]

LESIONS WITH A RAISED SURFACE

Papilloma

Papillomas of the oral cavity are relatively common and easily recognized. Human papillomavirus antigen and DNA have been identified in a large percentage of patients with these lesions, suggesting an etiologic role for the virus. Papillomas tend to occur more frequently in the third, fourth, and fifth decades of life but may be found at any age without an obvious sex predilection. The lesion may be comprised of soft fronds or appear warty and cauliflower-like. Most are less than 1 cm in size, pedunculated, and either pink or white, depending on the extent to which they are keratinized. Papillomas appear most often on the soft and hard palates, uvula, tongue, and lips.[1]

Lesions that may have a similar appearance are verruca vulgaris, condyloma acuminatum, verruciform xanthoma, and early verrucous carcinoma. Although the papilloma's appearance usually is sufficiently characteristic to make a diagnosis, a biopsy should be taken to confirm it. An excisional biopsy provides a diagnostic and a therapeutic service. Recurrences, presumably because of inadequate excision, have been reported infrequently.

Verruca vulgaris

Occasionally, warts appear on the oral mucous membranes; these are identical to skin warts caused by the human papillomavirus. Oral verrucae tend to occur most often in children and young adults. Cutaneous lesions of verruca vulgaris frequently are present and serve as a source of autoinoculation. The lips, labial mucosa, and tongue are affected.

A differential diagnosis should include papilloma, condyloma acuminatum, verruciform xanthoma, and verrucous carcinoma. In typical patients, the last two usually can be discounted because of the lesion's location or the patient's age. A biopsy is necessary at times to make a diagnosis. Histologically, elongated rete ridges that are pointed inward and contain large, vacuolated cells with basophilic nuclei help distinguish this papillary lesion from others. Reports indicate that 50% of cutaneous lesions disappear spontaneously within 2 years. Simple excision or cryosurgery is the usual treatment.

Condyloma acuminatum

Condyloma acuminatum, a venereal wart, once was seen infrequently in the oral cavity and was considered a problem primarily of the anogenital region. In some locales, this human papillomavirus-induced lesion now is perceived as a relatively common lesion of the oral mucosa because of changing sexual practices. Often, a history of oral–genital sex can be elicited from the patient. Lesions usually are found on the labial and buccal mucosae, tongue, gingiva, and palate. They begin as small, pink, papillary lesions and progress to white, cauliflower-like growths measuring 0.5 to 1 cm. Often patients have multiple lesions.[45] The occurrence of condyloma acuminatum in HIV-infected patients also is recognized. Depending on its stage of evolution, condyloma acuminatum may resemble an enlarged papilla of the tongue or a small papilloma. Later stages appear similar to papillomas, verruciform xanthomas, and verrucous carcinoma (Fig. 80-15). A biopsy is necessary to establish a definitive diagnosis. Simple local excision and cryosurgery have been the most effective forms of therapy. Recurrent disease is not uncommon.

Verruciform xanthoma

Although the nature and cause of verruciform xanthoma is unknown, speculation suggests that it represents a reactive lesion. Verruciform xanthoma tends to occur mainly in middle-aged persons, with a slight predilection for women. The lesions range in size from a few millimeters to 1 or 2 cm and appear granular or wart-like. The color may be normal, red, yellow, or white. They may occur anywhere in the oral cavity but most often are found on the gingiva or alveolar mucosa.[36] Lesions of verruciform xanthoma are similar in appearance to papillomas, verruca vulgaris, and squamous cell carcinoma. A biopsy is necessary to make the diagnosis. The principal histologic features include a papillary, parakeratotic surface epithelium that exhibits uniform elongation of the rete ridges. Large, foamy xanthoma cells fill the connective tissue papillae between the rete ridges. Reports show serum lipid levels of these patients to be normal. Therapy consists of simple excision of the lesion, and recurrence is rare.

Papillary hyperplasia

Papillary hyperplasia occurs primarily in patients who wear maxillary dentures. No specific factor has been identified as producing this lesion, but it tends to be found in patients who wear their dentures continuously or have ill-fitting ones. Occasionally, papillary hyperplasia affects patients who are not wearing any dental appliance, and usually they have a candidal infection. The lesions typically are confined to the hard palate. They appear as multiple, small, red, edematous papules with a cobblestone appearance. The lesion may involve only a small focal area, multiple areas, or the entire hard palate (see Plate 14, *C*).

Because of its characteristic appearance and its association with dental appliances, papillary hyperplasia usually is not confused with other lesions. Occasionally, a granulomatous infection or carcinoma *in situ* may have a similar appearance. The histologic changes may be striking, showing

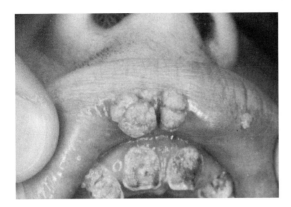

Fig. 80-15. Condyloma acuminatum. This cauliflower-like lesion appeared on upper labial mucosa in a young man who practiced oral–genital sex. Note early lesion on the left side.

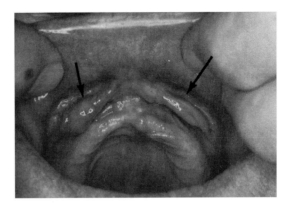

Fig. 80-16. Epulis fissuratum. There are two linear folds of tissue *(arrows)* on facial aspect of alveolar process, which are caused by ill-fitting denture.

a marked pseudocarcinomatous hyperplasia with abundant keratin pearl formation. Perhaps because of this histologic pattern, it once was thought to represent a precancerous lesion, although no good evidence exists to support this concept.

Treatment involves resolving the previously identified factors. The patient who wears a denture continuously should remove it a few hours each day, preferably while sleeping, and soak it in a denture cleaner. Ill-fitting dentures should be relined or remade. Complete resolution of the connective tissue hyperplasia usually does not occur; when extensive, it should be considered for surgical removal.

Epulis fissuratum

Epulis fissuratum is an *inflammatory fibrous hyperplasia* caused by ill-fitting dentures. The denture flange produces a low-grade chronic irritation of the mucosa in the fornix, which results in a proliferation of soft tissue. This inflammatory hyperplasia is a relatively slow process. The lesions most often occur in the facial region of the anterior jaws but can be found in any area. They usually have linear fissures and may be bosselated or ulcerated (Fig. 80-16). The inflammatory response is variable; some swellings are fibrotic, whereas others appear edematous and red. Occasionally, the swellings can be large and can be mistaken for tumors. The lesions should be excised, and new dentures should be fabricated for the patient.

Irritation fibroma

Irritation fibroma (traumatic fibroma) is one of the most common soft-tissue lesions in the oral cavity and represents a reactive fibrous hyperplasia. It usually occurs in the third, fourth, and fifth decades of life and can affect any area, usually the buccal mucosa, and less frequently the tongue, gingiva, and palate. The lesion usually appears as a sessile nodule with a smooth surface (Fig. 80-17). It may be pale pink or slightly keratotic, with a soft to rather firm consis-

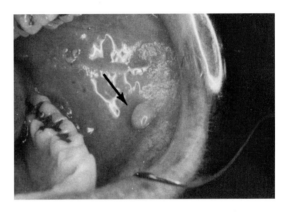

Fig. 80-17. Irritation fibroma. Smooth-surfaced small nodule *(arrow)* on left buccal mucosa.

tency. The fibroma grows slowly and may range in size from a few millimeters to 1 or 2 cm.

Any mesenchymal or glandular tumor may look similar and should be considered in a differential diagnosis. Microscopically, the lesion consists of relatively acellular collagenous connective tissue that may contain foci of chronic inflammatory cells. The irritation fibroma should be excised because it will not regress and usually continues to enlarge.

Pyogenic granuloma

Pyogenic granuloma is a reactive lesion, an overgrowth of granulation tissue that can occur at any age but is found more often in those in the second through fifth decades of life, with a slight predilection for women.[7] The lesion is a red or reddish purple mass with a smooth or slightly nodular surface. This mass is soft, usually is ulcerated, and tends to bleed with minimal provocation. The lesion may be found anywhere in the oral cavity, but many occur on the gingival tissue. The facial regions of the anterior jaws are affected frequently; other sites include the tongue, buccal mucosa, and lips. These lesions may grow rapidly, a feature that mimics malignancy. The size may range from a few millimeters to several centimeters. During pregnancy a clinically and histologically identical lesion may be found on the gingiva and is referred to as a *pregnancy tumor*. An endocrine imbalance may predispose the patient to this lesion. Other gingival swellings similar to pyogenic granuloma include peripheral ossifying fibroma and peripheral giant cell granuloma. In other sites, the pyogenic granuloma may appear similar to Kaposi's sarcoma. Histologically, the pyogenic granuloma has numerous dilated, blood-filled, endothelium-lined vascular spaces and shows marked proliferation of fibroblasts and budding endothelial cells. An infiltrate of acute and chronic inflammatory cells of variable intensity also is seen.

The pyogenic granuloma should be removed surgically. At times, the lesions, especially gingival ones, recur because of inadequate excision or persistence of an inciting factor, such as dental calculus.

Mucocele

The mucocele, or *mucous retention phenomenon*, is thought to occur because of traumatic injury to a minor salivary gland duct that allows saliva to escape into the surrounding connective tissue. However, all lesions cannot be explained by trauma, and other factors seem to play a pathogenic role. Mucoceles may occur at any age but more frequently appear in the first three decades of life. They may be seen in any area where salivary gland tissue is found but occur most often on the mucosa of the lower lip, although they rarely appear on the upper lip. The second most common site is the floor of the mouth; the lesion here is called a *ranula*. A variant called the "plunging ranula" may produce a neck mass.[32]

The mucocele appears as a soft, compressible swelling that may have a bluish color (Fig. 80-18). It ranges from a few millimeters to 1 or 2 cm; when small and superficial, it resembles a vesicle. The swelling occurs rather rapidly and persists for weeks to months, depending on its location. Superficial lesions tend to rupture, drain, and then recur.

Deeper lesions usually persist, and their consistency may cause them to be mistaken for a lipoma. On occasion, patients are seen after the swelling ruptures, discharging a thick, mucoid material, and only a tag of tissue remains. Because of the mucocele's compressible nature and bluish cast, it may be suspected as representing a vascular lesion or a mucoepidermoid carcinoma, which also may be mistaken for a mucocele. The histology shows a cavity filled with an eosinophilic coagulum and lined by connective tissue that consists of granulation tissue. A mucocele occasionally ruptures and does not recur, although it usually is recurrent or persistent and should be excised. Marsupialization generally has proved unsatisfactory.

Retention cyst

Retention cysts involving the minor salivary glands are found infrequently in the labial or buccal mucosa. They typically are detected on palpation of the mucosa and are noted as small nontender, firm nodules. Often, an erythematous, slightly dilated duct orifice can be seen on the mucosa overlying the nodule. Slight pressure on the nodule usually expresses a cloudy, mucoid saliva from the orifice.

Small sialoliths may be associated with these retention cysts or may occur as separate entities. They also appear as small, firm, asymptomatic nodules. These may be demonstrated readily on a dental radiograph with a soft-tissue exposure. Excisional biopsy should be performed because minor salivary gland tumors have similar clinical features. Recurrence would be unlikely.

Palatal and mandibular tori

Bony tori are found on the palate and mandible with some frequency. Although not conclusive, the evidence suggesting that these are hereditary conditions is strong.[19] Palatal tori appear in approximately 20% of the population, more frequently in women. Typically, they are midline swellings that range from a small nodule to diffuse enlargements that involve almost the entire palate. A torus may be smooth, lobu-

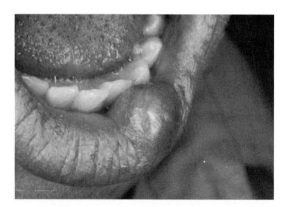

Fig. 80-18. Mucocele. Typical smooth-surfaced swelling showing less bluish tinge than usual.

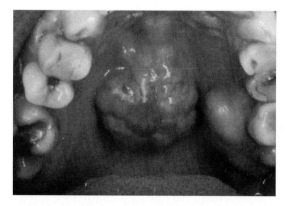

Fig. 80-19. Palatal torus. This is slightly larger and more nodular than usual. Also note exostosis on left palatal surface.

lated, sessile, or pedunculated (Fig. 80-19). Surprisingly, patients often are unaware of its presence. A palatal torus may appear similar to the swelling produced by a minor salivary gland tumor, although the bony hardness and consistent midline location of the torus help confirm its diagnosis.

Mandibular tori occur less frequently but are still rather common. They may or may not be associated with a palatal torus. The tori usually appear as smooth swellings on the lingual surface of the mandible in the bicuspid region. As with the palatal torus, they also can vary in size and shape. Infrequently, only a unilateral exostosis may exist. Because of their unique and consistent location, mandibular tori should not pose a diagnostic problem.

Occasionally, bony exostoses occur elsewhere on the alveolar process of the jaws and produce a nodular excrescence of bone. These develop bilaterally and usually involve the facial alveolus in the molar region. The tori and exostoses are asymptomatic unless the overlying mucosa is traumatized and becomes ulcerated. Healing may take longer than usual because of the location. Removal of tori or exostoses usually is not necessary unless they interfere with dental prosthetic appliances.

Pemphigus vulgaris

Current evidence suggests that pemphigus vulgaris is an autoimmune disease characterized by serum antibodies directed against desmoglein 3, a transmembrane glycoprotein component of the desmosomes of the epidermis and mucosa. Of the various types of pemphigus, *pemphigus vulgaris* is the only form seen with any frequency in the oral cavity. It is likely that nearly all affected patients have oral lesions as the initial manifestation of the disease, and these may precede the cutaneous lesions by as much as 2 years. In most patients, the oral lesions have a slow and mild onset; often several months pass before multiple sites are involved. The average age of patients is 55 years, with those in the fifth, sixth, and seventh decades affected most often. A slight female predilection exists. The characteristic bulla usually is

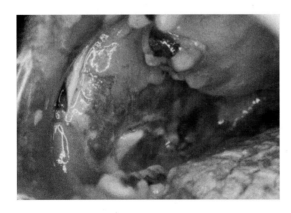

Fig. 80-20. Pemphigus vulgaris. Note diffuse superficial erosion with shaggy remnants of covering mucosa.

present only a short time. The lesion then appears as a rather superficial, ragged, eroded area. The surrounding mucosa is friable and can be dislodged with minimal pressure or trauma (Fig. 80-20). Lesions most often involve the palate, buccal mucosa, and tongue.[30] At times, the disease waxes and wanes in severity, creating the impression that it may be resolving. Diseases to be considered in a differential diagnosis are cicatricial pemphigoid, bullous lichen planus, erythema multiforme, and drug reactions. Histologically, the diagnostic features are suprabasilar acantholysis, with acantholytic cells present in the bulla that develops. Direct and indirect immunofluorescence, which primarily show immunoglobulin G (IgG) directed against the intercellular spaces of the epithelium, should be used to verify the diagnosis.

Pemphigus vulgaris usually can be controlled with systemic corticosteroids. Unfortunately, high doses often are necessary, and patients develop complications of corticosteroid therapy. To reduce the likelihood of this problem, gold, methotrexate, cyclophosphamide, and azathioprine may be used with the corticosteroid so that therapeutic corticosteroid levels can be reduced.

Cicatricial pemphigoid

Because deposits of IgG and C3 complement are found in the basement membrane zone of cicatricial pemphigoid (benign mucous membrane pemphigoid [BMMP], ocular pemphigoid), it has been speculated that this also is an autoimmune disease. Pemphigoid is seen in an older age group of patients; the average age of patients is 66 years, and women are affected more frequently. Lesions occur most often in the oral cavity, with the conjunctiva being the second most likely site. Skin lesions are seen less frequently. The initial oral lesion is a blister of variable size that may be clear or hemorrhagic, with a surrounding erythematous mucosa.

After the blister ruptures, the mucosa may persist as a shaggy membrane covering the blister site, or it may be lost, leaving an erythematous, eroded area (Plate 15, *A*). The buccal mucosa, gingiva, and palate are involved most often.[30] The gingival lesions may be present with other mucous membrane involvement or may be the only manifestation of the disease. Gingival involvement appears as a diffuse, edematous redness. The gingival mucosa is extremely friable and hemorrhagic. Areas of necrosis and sloughing also may be seen (Plate 15, *B*).

Oral lesions may be relatively asymptomatic, even though they appear painful. The disease may improve slightly but seldom goes into remission; usually it becomes more severe with time. A differential diagnosis should include pemphigus vulgaris, bullous pemphigoid, bullous lichen planus, and erythema multiforme. Histologically, subepithelial clefting is seen. Direct immunofluorescence is necessary to make a diagnosis and shows linear deposits of IgG and C3 in the basement membrane zone.

Topical corticosteroids have been used with some success in treatment of milder cases of cicatricial pemphigoid. Systemic corticosteroids combined with other immunosuppressive drugs usually are necessary to control the disease, particularly if ocular involvement is present. Dapsone also has been used with some success.[3]

Primary herpetic gingivostomatitis

The herpes simplex virus is responsible for an initial or primary infection of the oral cavity, herpetic gingivostomatitis. Either type 1 or type 2 virus may cause such a ''primary'' infection, although type 1 is much more frequently responsible for oral disease, whereas type 2 is seen in the genital region. Primary herpetic gingivostomatitis once was considered mainly a pediatric disease, occurring most often in patients aged between 2 and 6 years. Presumably, because of improved hygiene and living standards, fewer adults have antibodies to the herpes simplex virus and thus may have primary infections caused by the herpes virus. Approximately 10% of the population has a clinical history of primary herpetic gingivostomatitis.[27]

The disease course is variable, ranging from a patient who has a few, mildly painful ulcers to one who is ill and complains of fever, malaise, sore throat, headache, and cervical lymphadenopathy. Vesicles appear 1 to 2 days after onset of symptoms and persist for another 1 to 2 days; they may affect any area of the oral cavity. The gingiva usually becomes red and edematous.

Patients often are not seen during the vesicular stage. When examined, they have numerous 1- to 3-mm ulcers with a tan–yellow base and erythematous halo. Some ulcers coalesce to produce larger lesions. At this stage, the oral lesions of herpes essentially are identical to those seen in patients with aphthous ulcers (Fig. 80-21). This similarity has resulted in the misdiagnosis of recurrent aphthous ulcers as recurrent herpes.

Diseases that may have oral lesions similar to primary herpes are herpangina, varicella, herpes zoster, and hand-

foot-and-mouth disease. Often other clinical features, such as cutaneous lesions, help distinguish one from the other. Several recurrent diseases also have oral lesions similar to those of primary herpes and should be included in a differential diagnosis because a patient with an initial episode of one of these diseases could not provide a history of recurrent episodes. Additional diseases that should be included are minor aphthous ulcers, herpetiform ulcers, Behçet's syndrome, cyclic neutropenia, and erythema multiforme. A diagnosis of herpes can be verified by exfoliative cytology, a culture for the virus, or immunofluorescence for the herpes antigen. The clinical course of primary herpetic gingivostomatitis usually lasts from 1 to 2 weeks. Supportive care may be necessary for patients with severe infections. *Recurrent intraoral herpes* appears to be an infrequent problem. The lesions are characteristic and usually can be distinguished from others. They occur as a cluster of 10 to 20 small vesicles, which rupture within a few hours. The only evidence of disease often is a cluster of small, superficial ulcerations (Fig. 80-22). The lesions restriction to keratinizing tissue (the attached gingiva and hard palate) has diagnostic importance because recurrent aphthous ulcerations (''canker sores'') would not occur at these sites. Patients may have some mild discomfort, but the lesions often are relatively asymptomatic. The lesions may persist for 3 to 10 days.[51]

Hand-foot-and-mouth disease

Hand-foot-and-mouth disease usually is caused by a group A coxsackievirus and primarily affects children. It is characterized by a vesicular eruption that appears in specific sites on the skin of the hands, feet, and occasionally the buttocks. Oral lesions are found in 90% of the patients and may be the only evidence of disease in 15%.[2] The intraoral vesicles most often are found on the palate, tongue, and buccal mucosa. The degree of involvement may vary from a few isolated lesions to a marked stomatitis. Clinical symp-

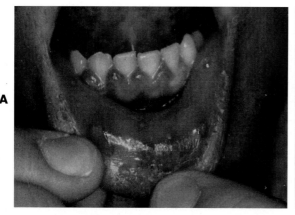
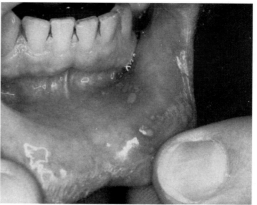

Fig. 80-21. Primary herpetic gingivostomatitis. **A,** Lesions of primary herpes with associated gingival swelling; other areas of oral mucosa were involved. **B,** Lesions of recurrent aphthous ulcers that are clinically similar to those of primary herpes, found in same location. Lesions were localized to this area.

toms may include fever, malaise, coryza, diarrhea, abdominal pain, conjunctival infection, and headache; cervical lymphadenopathy is an uncommon finding. When the disease is confined to the oral cavity, it cannot be distinguished from primary herpetic gingivostomatitis. To confirm a diagnosis, it is necessary to culture for the virus or examine the serum for antibody titers during the acute phase of the disease.

Herpangina

Herpangina has characteristic oropharyngeal lesions but is not a specific disease because several different coxsackieviruses and enteric cytopathogenic human orphan (ECHO) viruses have been associated with it. It primarily affects children and typically occurs during the summer and early autumn. The condition usually is mild, but patients may complain of sudden fever, anorexia, neck pain, and headache. Multiple, small, gray–white papules and vesicles with an erythematous base appear and usually are confined to the soft palate, uvula, and tonsillar pillars. The vesicles rupture within 2 or 3 days, leaving ulcers that may enlarge. The cervical nodes may be enlarged and tender. Oral lesions seldom persist for more than 1 week. The diagnosis is made primarily on a clinical basis.[12]

Erythema multiforme

The specific cause of erythema multiforme is unknown, but several precipitating factors have been identified, including recurrent herpes simplex infections, *Mycoplasma pneumoniae* infections, and drugs such as sulfonamides. The disease has been separated into two forms: the classic disease, initially described by Hebra, is the *minor* form; the more severe disease, reported by Stevens and Johnson[44] and characterized by marked mucosal involvement, is the *major* form. The oral mucosa is more likely to be involved in the major than the minor form.

Erythema multiforme is a disease of younger persons; most patients are aged between 10 and 30 years.[24] It is much more common in male patients. The oral lesions have been described as progressing through five stages: macular, bullous, sloughing, pseudomembranous, and healing.[54] Although new lesions may develop during the course of the disease, the macular and bullous stages seldom are observed. The sloughing stage is marked by the collapsed covering mucosa, which is white and friable; it usually can be removed, leaving a red, raw surface. A fibrinous exudate appears on this surface, producing the pseudomembranous stage. The erosive areas vary in size and may range from several millimeters to diffuse involvement of a mucosal surface. Any area of the oral cavity may be affected, but the most common sites are the lips, buccal mucosa, and tongue. The gingivae usually are spared, whereas the lips frequently have a hemorrhagic crust, a distinctive feature of the disease.[43]

Oral lesions occur in the absence of skin involvement in 25% or more of these patients. This makes establishing a diagnosis difficult because no specific test exists for erythema multiforme. The diagnosis should be made from the history and clinical features. Other diseases with similar oral lesions include pemphigus vulgaris, bullous pemphigoid, cicatricial pemphigoid, and bullous lichen planus.

Erythema multiforme is a self-limiting disease, with the mild form lasting 2 or 3 weeks and the more severe form lasting up to 6 weeks. Therapy usually is not necessary for the mild form. In patients with more severe forms, corticosteroids have been used to provide symptomatic relief.

LESIONS WITH A DEPRESSED SURFACE

Most lesions with depression of their surface morphology are clinically ulcerations. Color changes usually are associated with such lesions because of the yellowish white fibrinous exudate, which fills the epithelial defect, and because of the peripheral erythema, which is characteristic of the accompanying inflammation. Other conditions may exhibit ulceration as a result of a vesiculobullous process and are considered elsewhere.

Traumatic ulcer

Ulcers resulting from trauma are common and not restricted to any particular age, sex, or racial group. These may be caused by injury from biting, from coarse foods, or from an external object. The patient often can remember the initial injury. Clinically, these lesions frequently exhibit an irregularly shaped, slightly elevated or rolled, erythematous border. The central portion of the lesion usually is depressed and may appear either granular and erythematous, because of granulation tissue, or yellowish white, because of a fibrinous pseudomembrane. Sometimes pain is present, although tenderness is more characteristic. These lesions usually heal spontaneously within 1 or 2 weeks, although they may persist for as long as several months, particularly if the patient continually irritates the lesion or if other problems exist, such as xerostomia or immunosuppression.

Administration of a protective agent, such as carboxy-

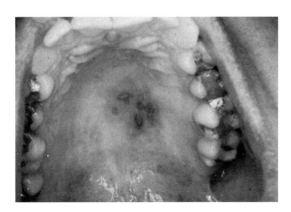

Fig. 80-22. Recurrent intraoral herpes. A cluster of small superficial ulcerations that show more inflammatory response than usual.

methylcellulose paste or hydroxypropylcellulose gel, or an antibiotic, such as tetracycline syrup, may aid healing. Corticosteroids probably should not be used to treat these lesions because many steroidal properties can inhibit healing. Excisional biopsy of the lesion may be necessary if the lesion has been present for 2 weeks or longer. Microscopic evaluation helps rule out other lesions in the differential diagnosis, such as squamous cell carcinoma, syphilis, histoplasmosis, or tuberculosis. Primary closure of the biopsy wound usually results in healing of the lesion site.

Primary syphilis

Although the majority of primary syphilitic lesions, also known as *chancres*, are seen in the genital region, perioral and oropharyngeal lesions are being identified with increasing frequency. Approximately 3 weeks after exposure to the causative organism, *Treponema pallidum*, an ulcerated papule develops at the site of the spirochete's initial penetration. Such lesions typically are painless and are associated with significant regional lymphadenopathy. Diagnosis at this stage may be difficult because results of serology frequently are negative. If dark-field microscopy is used as a diagnostic aid, care should be taken to avoid contaminating the material with saliva because *Treponema microdentium* is a common inhabitant of the oral microflora that may be mistaken for *T. pallidum.* Examination of biopsy material reveals an ulceration with an intense plasmacytic infiltrate. A special silver stain, such as the Warthin-Starry, should be used to identify the organism in tissue sections.

Perlèche

The term *perlèche* has been used since the mid-nineteenth century to describe fissured lesions at the corners of the mouth. Also called *angular cheilitis,* this condition is seen with some frequency, particularly in elderly patients whose dentures do not provide the appropriate support for the facial contours. As a result, creases in the facial skin develop at the commissures. These creases remain continually moist with saliva, creating an environment that is favorable to infection by yeasts, primarily *C. albicans,* and other microorganisms such as *Staphylococcus aureus.*[38] Frequently, the condition clears after treatment with an antifungal cream such as nystatin, although if the skin crease is allowed to persist, the condition will return. Lesions of perlèche also should suggest the presence of other candidal lesions of the oral mucosa. Recurrence may be expected if the oral reservoir of *C. albicans* is not treated.

Recurrent aphthous ulcers

Recurrent aphthous ulcers, known as ''canker sores'' in lay terminology, are a common problem that usually affects a younger population, but no age group is immune. The etiology of recurrent aphthous ulcers is unknown, although cell-mediated hypersensitivity to oral mucosa has been suggested as a probable cause. Alternatively, aphthous ulcers may represent several entities with a similar clinical appearance. One study has shown that the tendency to develop these lesions may be inherited.[33] Other suggested etiologic or contributing factors include microbial agents (L form of streptococcus), hormonal changes, nutritional deficiencies (vitamin B_{12}, folic acid, iron), hypersensitivity states (gluten-sensitive enteropathy), and stress.[49]

Clinically, aphthous ulcers may appear as solitary lesions, or several may develop simultaneously. The frequency of episodes and the size of the lesions may vary considerably from patient to patient, and three categories have been described based on the clinical presentation. *Minor aphthae* are by far the most commonly seen form, appearing as 2- to 10-mm ulcerations that exhibit a yellowish white central fibrinous pseudomembrane and an erythematous periphery. The central area frequently is depressed, and the rim of the ulcer usually is smooth (Fig. 80-23). The ulcer typically is painful, and although mild cervical lymphadenopathy may be found, these patients rarely have a fever. Healing occurs over 10 to 14 days. Sometimes the patient can attribute the development of aphthous ulcers to such factors as stress, minor trauma, or menses.

In contrast to minor aphthae, the *major aphthous ulcer* typically is much larger, at times attaining a size of 2 or 3 cm (Fig. 80-24). These patients often are afflicted constantly with these lesions; when one resolves, another begins. Scarring may be seen after healing, and this probably relates to the size rather than any intrinsic property of the lesion.

Herpetiform ulcerations, as the name suggests, may mimic a primary herpes simplex infection. These lesions appear as numerous 1- to 2-mm ulcerations, which may be clustered in one area of the mucosa or distributed more widely (Plate 15, *C*). Unlike primary herpes, the lesions typically recur periodically. Viral cultures are consistently negative, and cytologic or histologic examination shows no evidence of viral cytopathic effect.

Differentiation of aphthous ulcerations from herpetic and other viral infections is important but may be difficult at

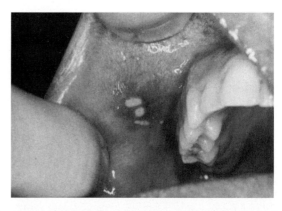

Fig. 80-23. Aphthous ulcer. Typical lesions with cream-colored center and erythematous halo. ''Canker sore'' may be differentiated from herpetic infection in part by its location. Notice that this lesion is situated on mucosa that is not tightly bound to periosteum.

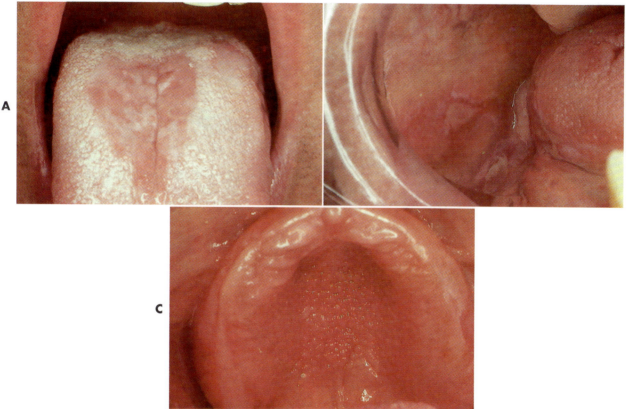

Plate 14. **A,** Lichen planus. Lesions of lichen planus that involve dorsal tongue mucosa frequently do not exhibit typical lack-like pattern. Patchy keratotic and erythematous change is seen instead, which replaces normal papillary mucosa. **B,** Lichen planus. Lesions of erosive lichen planus should be examined carefully to discern characteristic keratotic periphery surrounding central atrophic and ulcerated portion of lesion. **C,** Papillary hyperplasia. This patient has multiple small papules in midportion of the palate because of ill-fitting denture.

apical periodontitis because of marked pulp disease or severe periodontal involvement. It usually is found on the facial gingiva or alveolar mucosa near the involved tooth. A papule or small nodule that may be umbilicated is the typical lesion (Fig. 80-25). The inflammatory response can vary, resulting in little or marked redness of the fistula and surrounding tissue. A purulent discharge may be expressed from the lesion. A small abscess, referred to as a "gum boil" or parulis, occasionally develops on the alveolar process. This ruptures and persists as a fistula. To resolve these lesions, the offending tooth should be treated with either surgical extraction or endodontic or periodontal management, depending on the situation.

Gingival enlargement

The gingival tissues may show marked and diffuse enlargement because of a variety of conditions, some of which reflect systemic disease. Poor oral hygiene and local factors often contribute to the problem. Because of endocrine changes during puberty and pregnancy, gingival enlargement may occur. A more regional enlargement of the gingiva also may be seen in patients with diabetes mellitus and regional enteritis (Crohn's disease). A diffuse and boggy swelling affects patients with myelomonocytic leukemia.

A marked and extensive proliferation of the gingival tissues may be seen in patients who are taking phenytoin or who have fibromatosis gingivae. This proliferation may be so extensive that the crowns of the teeth are covered. Two other drugs that also have been shown to produce gingival hyperplasia are cyclosporin A and the calcium channel-blocking agents such as nifedipine.[47] Fibromatosis gingivae, also known as *hereditary gingival fibromatosis*, may have an autosomal dominant mode of inheritance, although several different forms of this condition are recognized.

A pebbly enlargement of the gingiva that may have an associated fine papillomatosis of the oral mucosa is seen in patients with *multiple hamartoma syndrome* (Cowden's syndrome; Fig. 80-26). Multiple facial trichilemmomas usually are present. These patients may have fibrocystic disease of the breast, thyroid goiters or adenomas, multiple polyposis of the gastrointestinal tract, and ovarian cysts. In women, there is an increased prevalence of malignant disease in the breasts and thyroid gland.[46]

The patient's oral hygiene habits and local factors such as calculus and irregular restorations influence many of these gingival enlargements. Good oral care often stabilizes the condition or results in some improvement. If the gingival proliferation is marked, surgical excision (gingivectomy) is necessary to restore the tissues to normal.

Acute necrotizing ulcerative gingivitis

Acute necrotizing ulcerative gingivitis (Vincent's angina, trenchmouth) has been attributed to a fusiform bacillus and a spirochete, *Borrelia vincentii*. Stress often has been implicated as a modifying factor.[25] Young adults and teenagers are affected most often, and an increased frequency of this condition is seen in HIV-infected patients. The classic feature of the disease is ulceration of the interdental papillae,

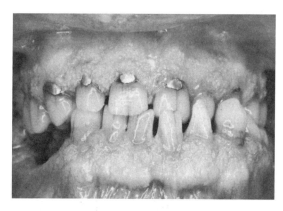

Fig. 80-26. Cowden's disease. Diffuse enlargement of gingiva with finely papillary surface.

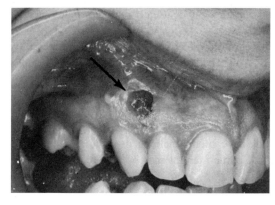

Fig. 80-25. Fistula. Slightly red, umbilicated swelling *(arrow)* drains apical area of lateral incisor, which was nonvital.

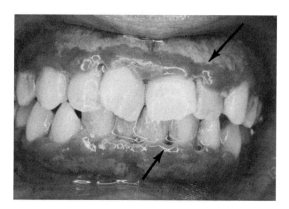

Fig. 80-27. Acute necrotizing ulcerative gingivitis. Diffuse swelling and erythema of gingiva with multiple areas of ulceration in interdental papilla areas *(arrows)*.

which has been described as having a "punched out" appearance. The problem may be limited to a few areas or may be generalized. When the disease is more extensive, the free gingival margins also become ulcerated and covered by a necrotic membrane (Fig. 80-27). The adjacent gingiva often is edematous and erythematous. Patients frequently complain of severe pain. The problem can spread to the adjacent soft tissues, producing areas of erythema and ulceration. When the condition is mild, débridement and cleaning of the affected dentition usually is sufficient to resolve the disease. In patients with more severe cases, rinses and systemic broad-spectrum antibiotics are necessary.

REFERENCES

1. Abbey LM, Page DS, Sawyer DR: The clinical and histopathologic features of a series of 464 oral squamous cell papillomas, *Oral Surg* 49:419, 1980.
2. Adler JL and others: Epidemiologic investigation of hand, foot, and mouth disease, *Am J Dis Child* 120:309, 1970.
3. Ahmed AR, Kurgis BS, Rogers RS: Cicatricial pemphigoid, *J Am Acad Dermatol* 24:987, 1991.
4. Allen CM: Diagnosing and managing oral candidiasis, *J Am Dent Assoc* 123:77, 1992.
5. Allen CM, Blozis GG: Oral mucosal reactions to cinnamon-flavored chewing gum, *J Am Dent Assoc* 116:664, 1988.
6. Allen CM and others: Wegener's granulomatosis: report of three cases with oral lesions, *J Oral Maxillofac Surg* 49:294, 1991.
7. Angelopoulos AP: Pyogenic granuloma of the oral cavity: statistical analysis of its clinical features, *J Oral Surg* 29:840, 1971.
8. Buchner A, Hansen LS: Amalgam pigmentation (amalgam tattoo) of the oral mucosa, *Oral Surg* 49:139, 1980.
9. Cannon AB: White nevus of the mucosa (naevus spongiosus albus mucosae), *Arch Dermatol Syph* 31:365, 1935.
10. Cawson RA, Binnie WH, Eveson JW: *Color atlas of oral disease.* In *Clinical and pathologic correlations,* ed 2, London, 1994, Wolfe Publishing.
11. Cawson RA, Lehner T: Chronic hyperplastic candidiasis-candidal leukoplakia, *Br J Dermatol* 80:9, 1968.
12. Cherry JD, Jahn CL: Herpangina: the etiologic spectrum, *Pediatrics* 26:632, 1965.
13. Cooke BED: Median rhomboid glossitis: candidiasis and not a developmental anomaly, *Br J Dermatol* 93:399, 1975.
14. Daniels TE, Quadra-White C: Direct immunofluorescence in oral mucosal disease: a diagnostic analysis of 130 cases, *Oral Surg* 51:38, 1981.
15. Epstein JB and others: Oral Kaposi's sarcoma in acquired immunodeficiency syndrome: review of management and report of the efficacy of intralesional vinblastine, *Cancer* 64:2424, 1989.
16. Farman AG and others: Central papillary atrophy of the tongue, *Oral Surg* 43:48, 1977.
17. Ficarra G and others: Kaposi's sarcoma of the oral cavity: a study of 134 patients with a review of the pathogenesis, epidemiology, clinical aspects, and treatment, *Oral Surg* 66:543, 1988.
18. Field EA, Field JK, Martin MV: Does *Candida* have a role in oral epithelial neoplasia? *J Med Vet Mycol* 27:277, 1989.
19. Gould AW: An investigation of the inheritance of torus palatinus and torus mandibularis, *J Dent Res* 43:159, 1964.
20. Greenberg MS: Clinical and histologic changes of the oral mucosa in pernicious anemia, *Oral Surg* 52:38, 1981.
21. Greenspan JS, Greenspan D: Oral hairy leukoplakia: diagnosis and management, *Oral Surg Oral Med Oral Pathol* 67:396, 1989.
22. Grushka M, Sessle BJ: Burning mouth syndrome, *Dent Clin North Am* 37:33, 1993.
23. Helm TN and others: Clinical features of Behcet's disease: a report of four cases, *Oral Surg Oral Med Oral Pathol* 72:30, 1991.
24. Hurwitz S: Erythema multiforme: a review of its characteristics, diagnostic criteria, and management, *Pediatr Rev* 11:217, 1990.
25. Johnson BD, Engel D: Acute necrotizing ulcerative gingivitis: a review of diagnosis, etiology and treatment, *J Periodontol* 57:141, 1986.
26. Jorgenson RJ, Levin LS: White sponge nevus, *Arch Dermatol* 117:73, 1981.
27. Juretic M: Natural history of herpetic infection, *Helv Paediatr Acta* 21:356, 1966.
28. Kaugars GE and others: Oral melanotic macules: a review of 353 cases, *Oral Surg Oral Med Oral Pathol* 76:59, 1993.
29. Lamey PJ, Lewis MAO: Oral medicine in practice: burning mouth syndrome, *Br Dent J* 167:197, 1989.
30. Laskaris G, Sklavounou A, Stratigos J: Bullous pemphigoid, cicatricial pemphigoid, and pemphigus vulgaris, *Oral Surg* 54:656, 1982.
31. Macleod RI, Munro CS: The incidence and distribution of oral lesions in patients with Darier's disease, *Br Dent J* 171:133, 1991.
32. McClatchey KD and others: Plunging ranula, *Oral Surg* 57:408, 1984.
33. Miller MF and others: The inheritance of recurrent aphthous stomatitis, *Oral Surg* 49:409, 1980.
34. Miller RL and others: Localized oral histoplasmosis, *Oral Surg* 53:367, 1982.
35. Neuwelt CM, Borenstein DG, Jacobs RP: Reiter's syndrome: a male and female disease, *J Rheumatol* 9:268, 1982.
36. Neville BW: The verruciform xanthoma: a review and report of eight new cases, *Am J Dermatopathol* 8:247, 1986.
37. Neville BW and others: *Oral and maxillofacial pathology,* Philadelphia, 1995, WB Saunders.
38. Ohman SC and others: Angular cheilitis: a clinical and microbial study, *J Oral Pathol* 15:213, 1986.
39. Regezi JA, Sciubba JJ: *Oral pathology: clinical-pathologic correlations,* ed 2, Philadelphia, 1993, WB Saunders.
40. Scully C, El-Kom M: Lichen planus: review and update on pathogenesis, *J Oral Pathol* 14:431, 1985.
41. Shafer WG, Waldron CA: Erythroplakia of the oral cavity, *Cancer* 36:1021, 1975.
42. Sklavounou A, Laskaris G: Frequency of desquamative gingivitis in skin diseases, *Oral Surg* 56:141, 1983.
43. Stampien TM, Schwartz RA: Erythema multiforme, *Am Fam Physician* 46:1171, 1992.
44. Stevens AM, Johnson FC: A new eruptive fever associated with stomatitis and ophthalmia, *Am J Dis Child* 24:526, 1922.
45. Swan RH and others: Condyloma acuminatum involving the oral mucosa, *Oral Surg* 51:503, 1981.
46. Takenoshita Y and others: Oral and facial lesions in Cowden's disease: report of two cases and a review of the literature, *J Oral Maxillofac Surg* 51:682, 1993.
47. Thomason JM, Seymour RA, Rice N: The prevalence and severity of cyclosporin and nifedipine-induced gingival overgrowth, *J Clin Periodontol* 20:37, 1993.
48. Toth BB, Frame RR: Oral histoplasmosis: diagnostic complication and treatment, *Oral Surg* 55:597, 1983.
49. Vincent SD, Lilly GE: Clinical, historic, and therapeutic features of aphthous stomatitis, *Oral Surg Oral Med Oral Pathol* 74:79, 1992.
50. Waldron CA, Shafer WG: Leukoplakia revisited, *Cancer* 36:1386, 1975.
51. Weathers DR, Griffin JW: Intraoral ulcerations of recurrent herpes simplex and recurrent aphthae: two distinct clinical entities, *J Am Dent Assoc* 81:81, 1970.
52. Weathers DR and others: The labial melanotic macule, *Oral Surg* 44:219, 1977.
53. Wood NK, Goaz PW: *Differential diagnosis of oral lesions,* ed 4, St Louis, 1990, Mosby.
54. Wooten JW and others: Development of oral lesions in erythema multiforme exudativum, *Oral Surg* 24:808, 1967.

Chapter 81

Sleep-Disordered Breathing

Jay F. Piccirillo
Stanley E. Thawley

Manifestations of sleep-disordered breathing (SDB) have been present in our society for many years. Snoring, apnea, restless sleep, and daytime drowsiness have been well recognized by the lay public, but until recently the understanding, evaluation, and treatment of these symptoms have largely eluded physicians. During the past 10 to 15 years, epidemiologic information concerning SDB has increased tremendously.[9,17,79,153] The prevalence of obstructive sleep apnea in adults has been estimated to be around 4% for men and 2% for women.

SDB is a broad term that encompasses obstructive sleep apnea, obstructive sleep hypopnea, snoring, and upper airway resistance syndrome. Symptoms of SDB include snoring, restless, sleep disruption, choking during sleep, esophageal reflux, nocturia, and heavy sweating.[40] Physical findings may include obesity, tonsillar hypertrophy, elongated uvula, redundant pharyngeal folds, thickened tongue, and retro- or micrognathia.[6,69] Associated medical conditions may include cardiac and pulmonary hypertension, cardiac arrythmias, chronic obstructive pulmonary disease, and anoxic seizures. With the availability of more information, it has become obvious that SDB apnea has great importance to a range of cardiopulmonary and other medical problems.[51,53,85,131] The lay public is becoming more educated concerning the importance of snoring, restless sleep, and daytime drowsiness and consequently, otolaryngologists are increasingly being asked to evaluate SDB symptoms.

SLEEP PHYSIOLOGY

Polygraphic recordings during sleep, consisting of an electroencephalograph (EEG), electrooculograph (EOG), and chin electromyograph (EMG), have shown sleep to be a complex state.[2,93] During various stages of sleep, the EEG may show patterns of activity compatible with cortical sedation and intervals compatible with cortical activation. The cortical sedation phase of sleep is termed *nonrapid eye movement* sleep (NREM, pronounced non-REM). NREM sleep is divided into four stages that roughly correspond to a depth of sleep continuum. NREM can be thought of as a relatively inactive, yet actively regulating, brain in a moveable body. The cortical activation phase of sleep is termed *rapid eye movement* sleep (REM). In contrast to NREM sleep, REM sleep presents an episodic burst of REM, muscle atonia, and twitching. The mental activity of REM sleep is associated with dreaming. REM sleep can be thought of as highly activated brain in a paralyzed body.[22]

During REM sleep associated with intercostal muscle inhibition, thoracic respiration may decrease, leading to a degree of mechanical instability that, during certain clinical circumstances, may produce decreased lung volume and greater susceptibility to hypoxemia. Decreased muscular activity during REM sleep has been shown in some of the upper respiratory tract muscles, creating an increased susceptibility to airway occlusion during sleep.[68,141] Decrease in the activity of the genioglossus and medial pterygoid muscles may allow for major jaw retrusion during sleep, making the airway considerably more susceptible to occlusion through a prolapse of the tongue.[112]

Apnea is defined as the cessation of airflow at the nostrils and mouth for at least 10 seconds. The *apnea index* (AI) is defined as the number of apneas per hour. Systematic investigations of healthy volunteers with no evidence of obesity, maxillofacial deformities, or other medical problems established that the upper range of "normality" was defined by an AI of 5.[43] Although an AI greater than 5 is defined as the upper limit of normal, clinically symptomatic patients

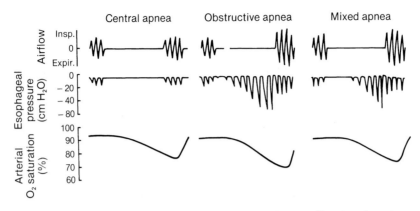

Fig. 81-1. Representation of apneas: patterns of airflow, respiratory effort (esophageal pressure), and arterial oxygen saturation in central, obstructive, and mixed apneas. Central apnea is diagnosed by absence of airflow and lack of respiratory effort. Obstructive apnea is characterized by absence of airflow and presence of continued respiratory effort. Mixed apnea is present when there is absence of airflow associated with lack of respiratory effort initially, followed by respiratory effort usually at end of apneic episode. Note corresponding drop in arterial oxygen saturation with all types of apnea. (From Thawley SE: In Cummings CW and others, editors: *Otolaryngology—head and neck surgery: update I*, St Louis, 1989, Mosby.)

usually have an AI greater than 20. In general, periods of apnea last 20 to 30 seconds, seldom exceed 100 seconds, and are longer during REM sleep than during NREM sleep.[42]

Three general types of apnea have been described. *Obstructive apnea* (OSA) is a cessation of airflow in the presence of continued inspiratory effort. *Central apnea* is the absence of airflow and inspiratory effort. *Mixed apnea* is a combination of both components, beginning as central apnea followed by the onset of inspiratory effort without airflow (Fig. 81-1).[14] OSA is the most common type of SDB condition.[44]

Normal airway patency is maintained as a result of the dilating action of the respiratory muscles of the upper airway. Airway occlusion may ensue if this dilating force is overcome by a sufficient negative intrathoracic pressure; thus the normal function of the upper airway depends on the normal phasic inspiratory activity of the several muscles in this area.[123] Measurements of ventilation during normal sleep show various changes and responsiveness to the carbon dioxide and oxygen drives. During NREM sleep, there is a depressed carbon dioxide responsiveness, and the hypoxic drive also appears to be decreased during NREM sleep and REM sleep in humans. In addition, the threshold for arousal from REM sleep to the hypoxic stimulus appears to be substantially increased.

PATHOPHYSIOLOGY OF SLEEP-DISORDERED BREATHING

The correct evaluation of SDB requires careful monitoring of airflow at the nose and mouth and monitoring of thoracic breathing movements. These measurements also are combined with standard monitoring of the electrocardiograph (ECG) and ear oximetry. Basic data from an over-

night sleep study include the type and frequency of apneic episodes, the relationship of these apneic episodes to cardiac arrhythmias and oxygen desaturation, and the incidence of the apneic episodes during REM and NREM sleep.

Snoring and OSA result from the narrowing or complete occlusion of the oropharynx related to the effects of sleep. Snoring may originate at different anatomic levels and may be intermittent or continuous and mild or loud. Snoring may occur as soon as the patient falls asleep and progresses with the deepening of NREM sleep. It reaches a peak during stage 4 NREM and may decrease during REM sleep. Pulmonary arterial pressure increases during snoring, sometimes even above the upper limits of normal. Systemic arterial pressure increases instead of decreasing, as usually is the case during sleep. The increase in systemic arterial pressure is thought to be a result of the mechanical effects of the increased negative endothoracic pressure during snoring.[74]

Upper airway resistance syndrome[41] manifests by repetitive transient arousals, increase in snoring just before an arousal, and an increase in inspiratory time and a decrease in expiratory time. No major change in oxygen administration in arterial blood (Sao_2) is seen, and the respiratory distress index (RDI) remains low (usually <5). Because of the repetitive arousals, major sleep fragmentation can occur, and excessive daytime sleepiness can result. The diagnosis can be confirmed with the use of nasal continuous positive airway pressure as a therapeutic test.

Three variables are important in the development of the collapse and obstruction of the upper airway in those with SDB: the decreased activity of the muscle dilators of the pharyngeal airway, the relative vacuum generated in the upper airway during inspiration, and the surgical anatomy of the upper airway.[96] In patients who have obstructive apnea, the site of the predominant airway obstruction has been localized to the supralaryngeal portion of the airway. This has been shown by simultaneous recording of the pressure in the esophagus and in the supraglottic airway and by fluoroscopic and direct fiberoptic observation.[15,106,134]

The occlusion typically begins in the oropharynx with the tongue contacting the soft palate and posterior pharyngeal wall (Fig. 81-2), followed by progressive collapse of the lower pharyngeal airway. In addition to obstruction in the anteroposterior direction, progressive collapse of the lateral oropharyngeal walls also has been shown. Periods of OSA usually are terminated by brief arousals that increase pharyngeal muscular activity sufficiently to maintain airway patency.[116,138,140]

Disorders producing anatomic narrowing of the upper airway and thereby necessitating the generation of more negative inspiratory pressures to maintain ventilation have been found to be associated with the development of OSA. Major structural narrowing of either the oral or hypopharyngeal airway, or both, has been confirmed by computed tomography (CT) in many patients with OSA.[19,73] These findings often correlate with the clinical finding of large tonsils, excessive tissue in the soft palate, a large uvula, and a large base on tongue area (Fig. 81-3). In many patients, excessive tissue in the pharynx with multiple folds of pharyngeal mucosa also is clinically noted. The OSA event is characterized by collapse of the pharyngeal airway at the level of the oropharynx and hypopharynx. There has been some question as to whether this collapse is passive or active. The patency of the pharyngeal airway is under partial control of the central nervous system, and involuntary adjustments in muscle tone are responsible for maintaining an adequate airway. The pharyngeal muscles should increase their tone to resist the tendency of the walls of the pharynx to collapse in the inspiratory airstream. Factors that may contribute to the collapse of the pharyngeal airway include atmospheric pressure, weight of cervical tissue, compliance of the airway walls, and inspiratory negative pressure within the airway (Fig. 81-4).

Compliance of the walls of the pharyngeal airway is variable, depending on local factors and, most important, on the tone of the musculature of the pharynx. Negative pressure within the lumen of the airway essentially is controlled by the resistance to airflow and the opening pressure within the alveoli. Any lesion increasing resistance to airflow, whether in the upper or lower airway, would necessarily increase the amount of effort required to maintain airflow. This in turn increases negative intraluminal pressures and the tendency of the airway to collapse. The small size of the oropharynx in patients with sleep apnea has been shown by CT scans (Fig. 81-5).[47] Correlations of direct fiberoptic videoscopic evaluation and polysomnographic sleep recordings have shown that during OSA events, the glottis remains widely patent at all times. Collapse of the airway seems to be passive and primarily related to the high intraluminal negative pressures associated with hypotonic pharyngeal walls and disproportionate anatomy in the oropharynx, the hypopharynx, or both. The disproportionate anatomy consists of any combination of a large base of tongue, large soft palate, shallow palatal arch, narrow mandibular arch, or retrognathic mandible. The collapse of the pharyngeal airway appears to be a passive event because it can be stopped when the predisposing condition or disproportionate anatomy is bypassed by tracheotomy.

During apneic events, corresponding arterial carbon dioxide pressure ($Paco_2$) increases, and corresponding arterial oxygen pressure (Pao_2) decreases (Fig. 81-6). Apneic episodes of 60 seconds generally will decrease the Pao_2 concentration by as much as 35 to 50 mm Hg. Because lung volume

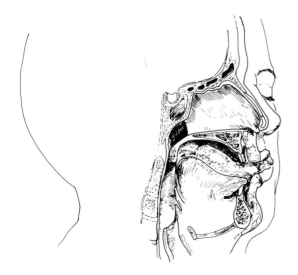

Fig. 81-2. Narrow oropharyngeal airway secondary to tongue approaching excessive tissues of soft palate. (From Thawley SE: Surgical treatment of obstructive sleep apnea, *Med Clin North Am* 69: 1337, 1985.)

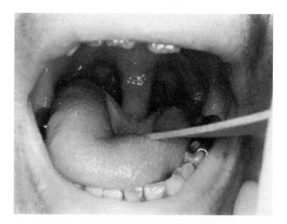

Fig. 81-3. Large uvula in obstructive sleep apnea. (From Thawley SE: In Cummings CW and others, editors: *Otolaryngology—head and neck surgery: update I*, St Louis, 1989, Mosby.)

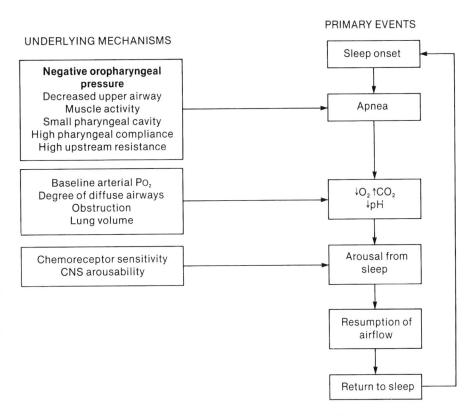

Fig. 81-4. Primary sequence of events in patients with obstructive sleep apnea and pathogenetic mechanisms that contribute to these events. (From Bradley D, Phillipson E: Pathogenesis and pathophysiology of the obstructive sleep apnea syndrome, *Med Clin North Am* 69:1170, 1985.)

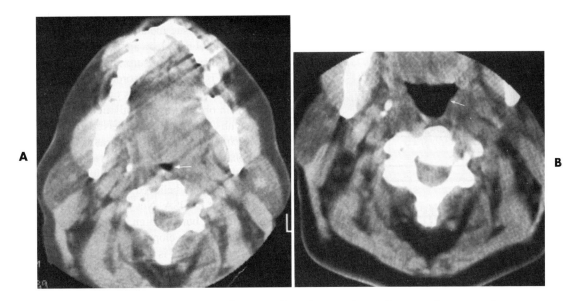

Fig. 81-5. A, Computed tomography scan of oropharyngeal area demonstrating narrow lumen *(arrow).* **B,** Same patient after enlargement of oropharyngeal area by uvulopalatoplasty. Note enlargement of oropharyngeal airway. (From Thawley SE, Shepard JW. Understanding of the sleep apnea syndrome: causes and treatment, *VA Practitioner* 2:60, 1985.)

nal hypoxemia also is an important contributing factor. Daytime hypersomnolence clearly impairs cognitive function and motor task performance. It is not unusual that patients or spouses describe intellectual deterioration, increasing inattentiveness, and difficulty in concentrating. Many experience personality change and morning headaches. Although present in many patients, hypersomnolence is not present in all patients with an ostensible major degree of OSA.[76] Symptoms rarely volunteered, but frequently elicited from a careful history, are intermittent nocturnal enuresis[146] and impotence. Patients with this affliction commonly fall asleep while talking with someone or when sitting for a few minutes (Fig. 81-7). In addition, falling asleep while driving a vehicle is not uncommon, and interference with social and professional life frequently occurs. The Epworth Sleepiness scale is a valid, patient-based measure of daytime sleepiness.[58] The scale describes eight situations wherein a person might fall asleep (i.e., sitting and reading, watching television). The patient rates how likely he or she is to doze off or fall asleep in each of the eight situations (0—would never doze; 3—high chance of dozing). The score range is from 0 to 24, with scores above 16 indicating major sleepiness.

Everyone who snores does not necessarily have OSA, although virtually all patients with OSA have major snoring problems. Finally, the history may indicate nasal, facial, or pharyngeal trauma that may, in retrospect, have triggered the later onset of snoring or OSA. This trauma may have produced nasal septal deviation with complete or partial obstruction of the nasal cavity. Lesions in the pharynx may produce dysphagia or a "lump in the throat" sensation. Patients should be questioned specifically regarding appearances or changes in neck masses, especially in the thyroid area. A history of recent weight gain and symptoms related to myotomic dystrophy should be specifically sought.

Physical findings

Approximately 70% of patients with OSA are 15% heavier than their ideal body weights, and many have short, thick necks (Fig. 81-8) with excessive cervical tissue.[43] Systemic hypertension has been reported in 30% to 50% of patients.[139] Clinically evident pulmonary hypertension seldom is present unless the patients have either concomitant chronic lung disease or alveolar hypoventilation.[16] Cardiomegaly with right and left ventricular failure occurs in patients with severe OSA, but obesity, hypertension, or underlying heart disease frequently coexists as a predisposing cause. In addition, detection of polycythemia usually, but not always, implies daytime and nocturnal hypoxemia.

The examination should include the mouth, nasal, pharyngeal, laryngeal, and neck areas. The pharynx and larynx should be examined indirectly with a laryngeal mirror, and direct fiberoptic examination through the nose should be performed in the sitting and reclining positions. The physician may note obstruction caused by a deviated nasal septum. Occasionally, there may be a mass in the nasopharynx such

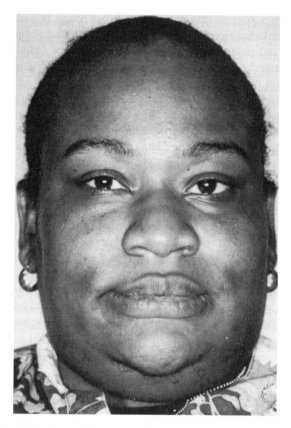

Fig. 81-8. A typical patient with obstructive sleep apneas with short, thick neck. (Modified from Thawley SE: Surgical treatment of obstructive sleep apnea, *Med Clin North Am* 69:1337, 1985.)

as a cyst, tumor, or antral choanal polyp.[105] Obstructions in the hypopharynx include cysts of the base of the tongue, vallecula, and epiglottis (Fig. 81-9). Tumors in the hypopharynx also may be noted. In most patients with typical classic OSA, a specific obstructive lesion is not noted. Frequently, these patients have an excessive amount of tissue in the oropharynx, characterized by a low-hanging redundant palate (Fig. 81-10), large tonsils, and excessive pharyngeal mucosal folds. Examination of the oropharynx frequently reveals enlargement of the uvula, prominant oropharyngeal folds, and a small oropharyngeal orifice. Commonly, the base of the tongue is large in these patients, and frequently the tongue simply appears too large for the mouth.

A minority of patients with major OSA are thin and have no apparent anatomic abnormalities on physical examination, and their oropharyngeal inlet appears widely patent.

Several authors have attempted to combine patient history and physical examination findings to predict the presence of polysomnographic-documented OSA.[34a,54a,142a] The most consistent characteristics suggestive of OSA include loud snoring, witnessed apnea, excessive daytime sleepiness, obesity, male gender, age greater than 45 years, and large neck circumference. Although the combination of patient history and physical examination findings can predict fairly well the

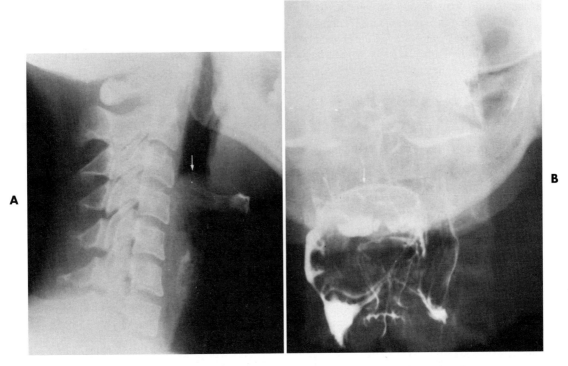

Fig. 81-9. A, Large cyst of epiglottis and valleculla that was producing obstructive sleep apnea *(arrow)*. **B,** Contrast laryngogram demonstrating same vallecular cyst *(arrow)*. (From Thawley SE: Surgical treatment of obstructive sleep apnea, *Med Clin North Am* 69:1337, 1985.)

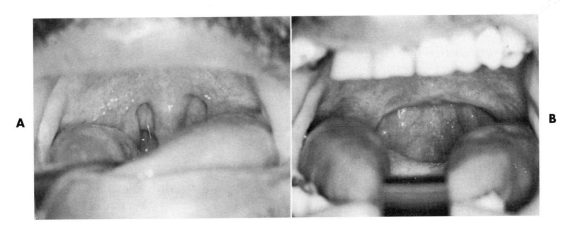

Fig. 81-10. A, Narrowing of oropharyngeal airway secondary to excessive folds of soft palate *(arrow)*. **B,** Same patient after uvulopalatoplasty. Note enlargement of airway. (From Thawley SE: Surgical treatment of obstructive sleep apnea, *Med Clin North Am* 69:1337, 1985.)

presence of major sleep apnea, many researchers recommend formal sleep studies for all patients suspected of a SDB problem. These authors cite the problem of relatively low sensitivity of screening and thus the potential to miss the diagnosis of sleep apnea.

Polysomnograph

A laboratory-based polysomnograph (PSG) is the gold standard for the diagnosis of sleep apnea and defines its severity.[38,107] This study is performed overnight in a sleep laboratory, and the patient's sleep is monitored. The minimum diagnostic evaluation of the sleep study should include determination of the stages of sleep, identification of the types of apneic events, continuous monitoring of arterial oxygen saturation, and documentation of cardiac arrhythmias in relationship to the apneic events and oxygen desaturation (see Fig. 81-4).[81] Additional parameters, such as monitoring of esophageal pH for evaluation of gastroesophageal reflux disease, may be used in certain clinical situations. PSG is helpful in allowing physicians to decide on a correct course of management. It also is helpful for patients to educate them regarding the magnitude and potential seriousness of the problem. Some patients simply do not understand the potential seriousness of the problem until it can be shown to them on a sleep study that they are intermittently apneic and that their oxygen saturation is decreasing during these episodes. The presence and severity of OSA should be determined before initiating surgical therapy.[5]

In some sleep centers, the night's study is divided between a diagnostic portion and a continuous positive airway pressure (CPAP) titration therapeutic trial for patients with moderate or severe OSA.[109] The first few hours of the study are dedicated to establishing a baseline measure of the degree of SDB. Once the diagnosis of OSA has been made, the remaining portion of the night is spent titrating the CPAP to correct OSA.

The role of home, or unmonitored, sleep studies (portable PSG) remains controversial.[3,34] It seems likely that when home monitoring is performed by a validated agency with experienced sleep technicians and professionals, accurate results can be obtained. In patients with one or more risk factors for OSA (e.g., body mass index over 30, habitual snoring, and witnessed apnea) home study is particularly accurate for the diagnosis of OSA. The drawback of home monitoring is that sleep stage architecture is not available (in most cases, information describing whether the patient is asleep or not is missing). In addition, for the patient with moderate-to-severe sleep apnea for whom CPAP therapy is indicated, a subsequent laboratory-based study will be required. The use of nocturnal O_2 monitoring alone is only sufficient to serve as a crude screening tool for SDB.

Multiple sleep latency test

The multiple sleep latency test (MSLT) provides an objective assessment of the tendency to sleep. It correlates well with the subjective feelings of excessive daytime sleepiness. It basically measures the amount of time required for a patient to fall asleep. The mean sleep onset latency in normal persons is 10 to 15 minutes. Patients with OSA, who have excessive daytime sleepiness, commonly have a much reduced sleep onset time.[81]

Other diagnostic studies

Inspiratory and expiratory flow volume loops determine if a sawtooth pattern is present or if the ratio of expiratory-to-inspiratory flow, at 50% of vital capacity, exceeds one in the absence of obstructive airway disease.[111] Videoendoscopic examination during obstructive sleep periods may provide objective dynamic evidence of mechanical structural narrowing of the upper airway.[106] Arterial blood gas analysis yields important information concerning the adequacy of alveolar ventilation, severity of hypoxemia, and acid–base status during wakefulness. A blood count is useful to determine the presence of polycythemia. Other blood studies evaluate thyroid function. Patients identified in the sleep study as

having predominantly central sleep apnea should be carefully examined for lesions involving the brainstem. CT evaluation of the upper airway has been used in patients with predominantly OSA to determine the level and severity of the anatomic narrowing (see Fig. 81-6). Recently, cine CT scans with multiple-level rapid-sequence scans have been used to determine the site of airway obstruction.[28] This may represent an improved method to study with pathophysiology of the upper airway in this syndrome. Three-dimensional CT reconstructions of the upper airway, tongue, and soft palate volume may provide information concerning the areas most likely obstructed.[72] Fluoroscopy also may be helpful to confirm the area of obstruction.[145] Cephalometry may be useful to determine the anatomic relationships of the soft palate, pharynx, tongue, hyoid, and mandible and may be used to help decide which surgical procedure may be indicated and successful.[108] Rhinomanometry may measure the amount of nasal resistance, and acoustic rhinometry may determine the size and location of the different stenoses in the nasal cavity that contribute to the increased nasal resistance.[70]

Differential diagnosis

The differential diagnosis of SDB in adults usually is not difficult when the classic history and typical physical findings are present. Because of the daytime hypersomnolence, this condition may be confused with narcolepsy.

Narcolepsy is a sleep disorder characterized by episodes of sudden onset of sleep of short duration. These episodes may occur at any time, usually last about 15 minutes, and occur 1 to several hours apart. The onset of this disease usually takes place between the ages of 10 to 20 years. Both sexes are equally affected. Narcolepsy may be associated with episodes of cataplexy, a sudden loss of tone in the major striated muscles that occurs at the onset of sleep, and hypnogogic hallucinations (auditory, visual, or tactile hallucinations that occur at the onset of sleep) also are seen in those with narcolepsy. Nocturnal sleep problems frequently coexist. The diagnosis is confirmed by the presence of REM-onset sleep during a daytime sleep study.[8]

Patients with heart disease, congestive heart failure, chronic obstructive lung disease, and pulmonary fibrosis may have some of the same symptoms as those with OSA obstructive sleep apnea, but these conditions usually can be diagnosed with a good history and physical examination combined with pulmonary function and cardiac function tests. These conditions may coexist in patients with OSA and contribute to the symptoms and physical findings. Obesity may produce alveolar hypoventilation, hypercapnia, hypoxemia, right-sided heart failure, and daytime hypersomnolence (pickwickian syndrome).[142] The excessive tissue in the oropharynx may predispose to collapse or the oropharynx during sleep so that OSA may be a factor.

Medical management

Medications that decrease the amount of time a patient is in REM sleep are considered helpful because sleep apnea is worse during REM sleep with its associated muscle relaxation. *Progesterone*, a recognized respiratory stimulant, increases alveolar ventilation and Pao_2 concentration; its reported effects on apnea frequency are variable, and in the absence of hypoventilation, progesterone probably has no major therapeutic effect.[75,82] Decreased libido, impotence, and alopecia are major side effects that frequently limit its long-term usefulness. The carbonic anhydrase inhibitor *acetazolamide*, which stimulates ventilation by increasing the hydrogen ion concentration of arterial blood, has been reported to decrease apnea frequency, apnea-associated arousals, and the severity of oxygen desaturation in patients with central sleep apnea.[135,150] The effects of acetazolamide in patients with OSA have not yet been reported. *Theophylline*, which increases hypoxic, but not hypercapnic, ventilatory drive in healthy adults, has been successfully used to treat apnea in premature infants, but a thorough study of its effects in adults with sleep apnea has not been reported.

Protriptyline, a nonsedating tricyclic antidepressant, produces variable but generally beneficial clinical results in patients with mild-to-moderate OSA.[24] Protriptyline decreases the percentage of time spent in REM sleep, thereby reducing the severity of nocturnal hypoxemia by decreasing the frequency of the more severe REM-related apneas.[18,129] Side effects of protriptyline that frequently limit its use include dry mouth, urinary retention, constipation, and impotence.

Although *oxygen therapy* has a well-established role in the treatment of hypoxemic patients with chronic lung disease, its role in the treatment of those with sleep apnea is more controversial.[78] It has been reported that the administration of oxygen has the adverse effect of prolonging apnea duration, thereby increasing the severity of hypercapnia and acidosis during NREM and REM sleep.[77] Patients with an intact ventilatory drive may show severe CO_2 retention when nocturnal oxygen therapy removes the major stimulus maintaining ventilation.

The risk of hypercapnic acidosis mandates that all patients receiving nocturnal oxygen therapy be carefully monitored, although oxygen limited to a flow rate of 2 l/min usually improves nocturnal oxygen saturation with little risk of inducing serious hypercapnia, acidosis, or arrhythmias in the majority of patients. The treatment of such coexisting disorders as hypothyroidism, hypertension, congestive heart failure, and chronic lung disease cannot be neglected.

Because respiratory efforts continue during OSA, various methods have been recommended to maintain upper airway patency during sleep. *Nasopharyngeal intubation* at night has been successful in a few patients[1] but is inacceptable in terms of comfort to a majority of patients. A *tongue-retaining device* that uses suction to hold the tongue in a protruded position has been somewhat successful, but discomfort also limits its practical widespread use.[23]

A dental appliance is intended to eliminate the obstruction at the base of the tongue by advancing the mandible forward while the patient is sleeping.[72] There are more than 10 different dental appliances. Each of the devices has primary action in one or more of three critical areas: moving the mandible anteriorly, changing the position of the soft palate, or changing the position of the tongue. In two studies, the sleep splint was effective at reducing snoring and produced a major improvement in AI and the longest duration of apnea, oxygen saturation, and symptoms.[55,114] Dental appliances should not be used in patients with arthritis, crepitus, or temporomandibular joint symptoms.

Continuous positive airway pressure

Nasally applied CPAP is a highly effective form of treatment and is considered to be the major form of nonsurgical treatment for most types of SDB.[5] It is delivered while the patient is asleep with a mask over the nasal area. This mask is connected through a tube to a device that produces a CPAP in the range of 5 to 15 cm of water. This pressure acts as a pneumatic splint and passively opens the airway to prevent the obstructive episodes (Fig. 81-11). In many patients, this technique is effective in eliminating obstructive apneic episodes, improving arterial oxygen saturation, and producing a decrease in daytime hypersomnolence.* Its use over the past few years has increased. It may be used as the sole therapeutic measure or may be combined with surgery and weight loss. In many patients, it is effective in relieving the sluggish feelings and thereby allows the patient to become more effective in a weight reduction and exercise program. It also may be used to allow the patient to sleep safely and to improve the cardiopulmonary status so that surgery can be safely performed at a later date. Patients who have had surgery for sleep apnea with poor results may find CPAP effective. Its disadvantage is that patients have to sleep with a mechanical device. Consequently, patient compliance is a problem. Some patients simply do not tolerate the mask discomfort or the nasal dryness and congestion. Causes for discontinuation of CPAP therapy include insomnia, noise from the machine, poor mask fit, otitis media, and nasal mucosal irritation. The reported compliance rate of continued usage at home over many months varies from 53% to 83%.[67a] CPAP commonly is used as initial therapy in patients with no clinically apparent causes for obstruction because of the predictability of success and lower costs and complication rates when compared with surgical therapy.[7]

SURGICAL MANAGEMENT

Surgery is indicated for patients who have an underlying specific surgically correctable abnormality that is causing SDB or for whom other noninvasive treatments have been unsuccessful or rejected by the patient.[5]

---

* Refs. 57, 95, 110, 130, 132, 143.

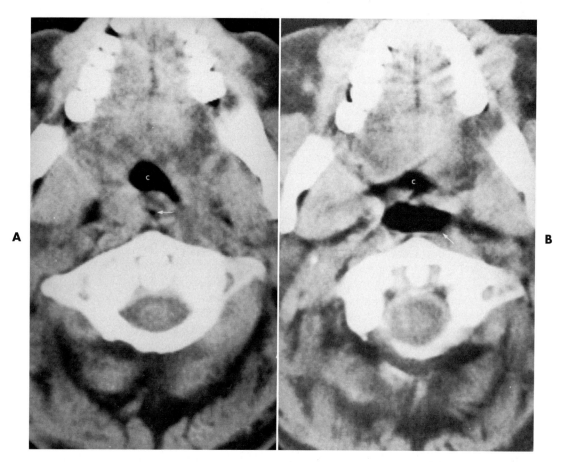

Fig. 81-11. A, Computed tomography (CT) of oropharynx in patient with obstructive sleep apnea. Note almost complete obstruction of airway *(arrow). c,* Oral cavity. **B,** CT at same level with continous positive airway pressure. Note dilation of airway *(arrow).* (From Thawley SE: In Cummings CW and others, editors: *Otolaryngology—head and neck surgery: update I,* St Louis, 1989, Mosby.)

General anesthesia

General anesthetic management in these patients frequently is difficult. The combination of obesity and low oxygen saturation creates an increased risk of problems. These obese, short, thick-necked patients may be difficult to intubate, and in a reclining state, the oropharyngeal tissues may collapse posteriorly, creating difficulty in ventilating these patients adequately by mask alone. Along with excessive tissues in the hypopharynx, the large mass of the tongue in these patients combined with the inflexibility of the thick neck may produce a difficult if not impossible situation for intubation. Supplemental inhaled oxygen may be used during light anesthesia before intubation. The use of oxygen may depress the ventilatory stimulus in these patients, who may have a chronically low oxygen saturation. The routine use of paralytic agents before intubation may lead to further collapse of the airway and an inability to ventilate by mask or to intubate.

Intubations of these patients commonly are difficult, and the experienced anesthesiologist should be prepared to use an alternative technique of intubation, such as nasal intubation while the patient is awake or intubation using a fiberoptic laryngoscope within the endotracheal tube.

Preoperative sedation is not given so that the respiratory drive is not further depressed. Unless an adequate airway is ensured, paralytic agents usually are not used. In some patients, a long nasal hypopharyngeal tube may be inserted into the nose and down into the hypopharyngeal area just above the epiglottis to facilitate maintenance of an airway during intubation. During these intubations, the surgeon and the operating room staff should be prepared for an emergency tracheotomy if intubation cannot be achieved and if mask ventilation is inadequate.

Patients should only be extubated when fully awake. If the patient has had some type of oropharyngeal procedure, the endotracheal tube may be left in place longer than usual postoperatively to ensure an adequate airway. The tube may be removed in the recovery room or even left in place until the next morning, depending on the alertness of the patient and the patency of the oropharyngeal airway. Patients with severe preoperative OSA may be treated with CPAP immediately after extubation and postoperatively to assist with airway patency and oxygen saturation. This treatment has been shown to be effective in maintaining oxygen saturation at levels of 90% when using CPAP on room air.[92]

Intravenous steroids may be used during surgery and postoperatively to decrease the edema in the operative area. Postoperatively, the respiratory drive may remain depressed because of the high Po_2 and low Pco_2 after anesthesia. The surgeon should be alert to the possibility of early postoperative extubation, leading to obstruction and difficulty in ventilating with a mask, similar to what occurs during induction. Use of intraoperative narcotics should be avoided when possible. Sleep medication postoperatively is routinely withheld, and narcotics and hypnotics should be used cautiously postoperatively for fear of further respiratory depression. Patients with arrhythmias or low minimum oxygen saturation on their preoperative sleep study should be monitored for arrhythmias postoperatively.

Factors that predispose to postoperative airway problems and arrhythmias are lower minimum oxygen saturation and higher AI on the preoperative sleep study and the amount of intraoperative narcotic administration. Patients with intubation complications tend to weigh more, whereas patients with extubation complications receive more narcotic analgesia intraoperatively.[31]

Surgical treatment

Because there may be three different regions of anatomic obstruction (i.e., nose, palate, and base of tongue), surgical interventions may take place at different anatomic levels. Powell, Guilleminault, and Riley[90] divided the various surgical procedures into two groups based on their complexity. The most straightforward or conservative procedures, referred to as phase 1 surgeries, should be attempted first. Phase 1 surgeries included nasal reconstruction, uvulopalatopharyngoplasty, and inferior mandibular sagittal osteotomy with geniohyoid advancement. Phase 2 surgeries are more complex and should be used only after phase 1 surgeries have failed. Phase 2 surgeries include bimaxillary advancement, subapical mandibular osteotomy, and base of tongue surgery.

Unfortunately, the published reports of the efficacy of surgical treatment for SDB have important methodologic weaknesses and limitations. These weaknesses were identified during a literature review of 175 articles on the efficacy of surgical treatment for OSA.[122] The weaknesses and limitations included (1) study designs that did not incorporate randomization of treatment or use of contemporaneous control patients, (2) failure to obtain thorough and long-term follow-up, (3) lack of uniformity in reporting results of PSG, and (4) lack of valid measures of sleep-related health status and quality-of-life. These methodologic weaknesses and limitations make it difficult to truly define the benefits and risks of the various surgical procedures to be discussed.[113]

Phase 1 procedures

Nasal reconstruction

Nasal obstruction may be a contributing factor to OSA. Experience teaches that even a simple cold with nasal obstruction leads to restless sleep. Although nasal obstruction may be a contributing cause, in most patients with major OSA, the nasal obstruction is not the major factor.[10] The nasal obstruction may be a result of deviation of the nasal septum, narrowing of the angle between the septum and lateral nasal cartilages, nasal polyps, or hypertrophy of the turbinate tissues caused by infection or allergies. If the patient and surgeon believe that the nasal obstruction may be a contributing factor, appropriate measures such as nasal septal reconstruction or nasal polypectomy or measures to reduce the size of the turbinates should be performed. Generally, it is unusual (unless the nasal obstruction is severe) that correction of a nasal septal deformity leads to an objective improvement of the quality of sleep in patients with major OSA. These procedures frequently will relieve the symptomatic nasal obstruction, but objective evidence of improvement on a sleep study usually is not seen.[115]

In some patients, nasal surgery and oropharyngeal surgery are performed at the same time. Because nasal packing itself can produce apnea even in healthy persons and can aggravate it in patients with apnea, a less risky approach in some patients is to separate nasal and oropharyngeal operations into two stages, allowing recovery from one before the other is undertaken.[32]

Pediatric tonsillectomy and adenoidectomy

It is not unusual that parents of children with enlarged tonsils and adenoids describe loud, sonorous respirations with retractions and restless sleep patterns. Many of these patients also have recurrent episodes of tonsillitis. In most patients, removal of the tonsils and adenoids will result in symptomatic improvement in nighttime respirations.[67] A few morbidly obese children with severe OSA may require the more standard type of uvulopalatopharyngoplasty. It is well known that adenotonsillar hypertrophy with upper airway obstruction may lead to cor pulmonale if not properly treated.

Pharyngeal surgery

Laser-assisted uvulopalatopharyngoplasty (LAUP) was first described by Kamami as a procedure for those who snore and who have sleep apnea in 1993. LAUP is performed with the CO_2 laser during local anesthesia in the outpatient setting. A specially designed handpiece is used to protect the posterior pharyngeal wall. LAUP incises the soft palate and excises the inferior rim of the soft palate and uvula. The procedure does not remove or alter tonsils or lateral pharyngeal wall tissues. Multiple sessions may be required. Indications for the procedure include snoring and mild sleep apnea.[3,21,60,61] Surgical candidates for LAUP should undergo preoperative clinical examinations that include an objective measure of respirations during sleep. For those patients who undergo LAUP, postoperative objective examination also should be obtained. At present, limited objective data exist regarding outcomes for patients undergoing LAUP for snoring or OSA. Postoperative swelling can result in airway complications for patients who have marginal airways preoperatively. Because of the potential for airway compromise, patients should be cautioned about using sedatives, hypnotics, and narcotics postoperatively. Because adequate controlled studies regarding LAUP were not found in peer-reviewed journals, the Standards of Practice Committee of the American Sleep Disorders Association recommended that patients be advised that the risks, benefits, and complications of the procedure have not been established.[3,4]

Uvulopalatopharyngoplasty is designed to enlarge the retropalatal airway through the excision of the tonsils, if present, to trim and reorient the posterior and anterior tonsillar pillars, and to excise the uvula and posterior portion of the palate.[119] It was first described by Ikematsu[56] for correction of snoring. It has been popularized by Fujita and others,[37] Gislason and others,[39] Katsantonis, Miyazake, and Walsh,[64] Katsantonis and Walsh,[65] and Simmons, Guilleminault, and Silvestri.[126] Uvulopalatopharyngoplasty should be considered if the patient cannot tolerate CPAP or if the symptoms are refractory to CPAP. The decision regarding surgical therapy is made by a team of medical specialists and otolaryngologist. When life-threatening cardiac arrhythmias are identified in association with OSA, a tracheostomy should be performed, at which time uvulopalatopharyngoplasty also may be considered. If a uvulopalatopharyngoplasty is concomitantly performed, the effectiveness of this surgical procedure can be evaluated after 6 to 8 weeks (when healing is complete) by repeating the sleep study with the tracheostoma occluded.

Such patients have to be monitored closely during the postoperative healing phase to ensure that postoperative swelling of the oropharynx does not lead to upper airway obstruction. For some patients with severe narrowing of the upper airway, intubation management during anesthesia can be a serious problem. In such patients, a tracheotomy may be necessary at the beginning of the uvulopalatopharyngoplasty procedure to maintain a safe airway during the early postoperative healing phase. After the patient has healed satisfactorily, the tracheotomy tube may be removed. Enlargement of the oropharyngeal airway has been shown after the uvulopalatopharyngoplasty by comparing preoperative and postoperative CT scans.[120] This has confirmed the major enlargement of the oropharyngeal airway and is correlated with improvement of oxygen saturation and reduction of the number of apneic episodes per hour.

During the uvulopalatopharyngoplasty, the tonsils, if present, are excised, and excessive tissue along the posterior

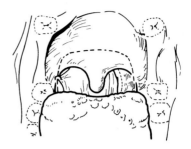

Fig. 81-12. Technique of uvulopalatopharyngoplasty. Dotted line on right indicates partial resection of posterior tonsillar pillar. On left, mucosa of posterior pharyngeal wall has been stretched to remove excessive mucosal folds, and posterior tonsillar pillar has been partially attached to anterior tonsillar pillar, thus producing enlargement of horizontal plane. *Dotted line* on palate indicates area of palate and uvula to be excised. (From Thawley SE: Surgical treatment of obstructive sleep apnea, *Med Clin North Am* 69:1337, 1985.)

tonsillar pillar is removed (Fig. 81-12). Posterior tonsillar pillars are sutured anteriorly to the anterior tonsillar pillar, which removes any excessive tissue and enlarges the oropharyngeal opening in the horizontal plane. The uvula also is excised, and a portion of the inferior edge of the soft palate frequently is removed. This area then is closed on itself, and the anterior wall of the nasopharynx, which is a posterior wall of the soft palate, is rotated anteriorly to enlarge the nasopharyngeal outlet into the pharynx. The resection of the uvula and portions of the palate enlarge the oropharynx in a vertical and a horizontal fashion, which results in a dramatic increase in the size of the oropharyngeal inlet (Figs. 81-6, 81-10, 81-13, and 81-14).

Fujita and others[36] have reported in detail the postoperative results of this surgery. Before surgery, their patients had the sleep disturbance characteristics of OSA. The percentage of stage 1 sleep was increased, and that of stage 2 sleep was decreased. After surgery, the percentage of stage 1 sleep was decreased, and the percentage of stage 2 sleep was significantly increased. Preoperative and postoperative objective measurements of excessive daytime sleepiness were performed. (Short latencies indicate pathologic sleepiness. A healthy adult falls asleep with the MSLT in 10 to 12 minutes, and a sleep-deprived healthy subject falls asleep in 6 to 7 minutes.) Preoperatively, the MSLT latency period was 3.9 minutes compared with 6.6 minutes postoperatively.

Although major post-uvulopalatopharyngoplasty improvements were found in the total group of patients, there was great variability in the degree to which patients responded. Patients were divided into responders and nonresponders, depending on the AI (number of apneic episodes/hour). The AI was selected as a key parameter because it is the measurement used to make the diagnosis of sleep apnea syndrome. Patients showing a minimum of a 50% decrease in AI were placed in the responder group, and all others were placed in the nonresponder group. Half of the total

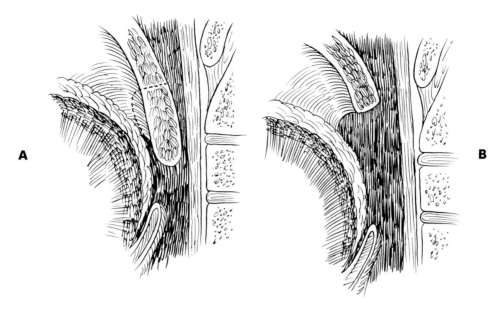

Fig. 81-13. A, Oropharynx with excessive soft palate and large base of tongue producing narrowness of airway. *Dotted line* indicates incision for palatoplasty. **B,** Postoperative view of the same area. Note enlargement produced in oropharyngeal airway. (Modified from Thawley SE: Surgical treatment of obstructive sleep apnea, *Med Clin North Am* 69:1337, 1985.)

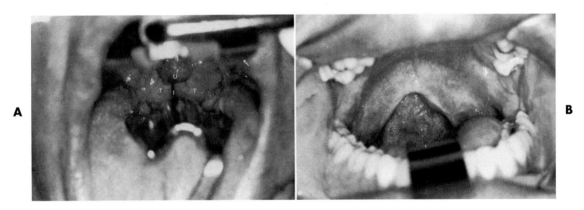

Fig. 81-14. A, Preoperative oropharynx with excessively enlarged tonsils *(T). U,* Uvula; *I,* airway. **B,** Postoperative view with enlarged oropharynx. (From Thawley SE: In Cummings CW and others, editors: *Otolaryngoly—head and neck surgery: update 1,* St Louis, 1989, Mosby.)

number of operative patients were considered to be responders. The decrease in AI for responders to surgery ranged from 9.5% to 58.3%, with an 84% decrease in AI. In nonresponders, the mean duration of the apneic episodes remaining after surgery was significantly shorter than before surgery. The number of times oxygen saturation was below 85% decreased significantly in responders but not as dramatically for nonresponders. There was no major change in any sleep parameter for nonresponders. In contrast, the sleep of responders improved markedly after surgery. The percentage of stage 2 sleep increased significantly to a normal level, and the percentage of stage 1 sleep decreased significantly.

Daytime sleepiness, as measured by the MSLT, increased significantly from 3.4 to 9.6 minutes in responders.

Generally, the variables that distinguish the responder from the nonresponder group were body weight and the oropharynx as the major site of airway compromise. All patients whose body weight was greater than 125% of the ideal body weight did not respond to uvulopalatopharyngoplasty. The majority of patients at each level of body weight less than 125% of ideal body weight responded to the uvulopalatopharyngoplasty. The majority of patients whose major site of airway compromise was the oropharynx responded to the surgery. The oropharyngeal obstruction included a large uvula, wide tonsillar pillars and mucosal folds, redundant posterior pharyngeal mucosa, and a low-arched soft palate. In contrast, the majority of the patients who had oropharyngeal and hypopharyngeal abnormalities did not respond to surgery. Hypopharyngeal obstructions included a large base of tongue, omega-shaped epiglottis, and redundant aryepiglottic folds. It was shown in this study that uvulopalatopharyngoplasty decreased excessive daytime sleepiness, improved the quality of nocturnal sleep and respiration during sleep, decreased nocturnal hypoxemia, and decreased the number of apneic episodes per hour.

It is to be noted that in the nonresponder group, even though the AI was not dramatically decreased, nocturnal oxygenation showed major improvement in some patients, and a decrease in excessive daytime sleepiness frequently was noted. It has been my experience and the experience of other surgeons that patients undergoing uvulopalatopharyngoplasty report improvement in their symptoms whether they fall into the responder or nonresponder group as defined by the 50% decrease in AI. Postoperative questioning reveals that most patients are pleased with the surgical results and would undergo the surgery again if given the option. Simmons, Guilleminault, and Miles[125] reported similar results in 155 patients by showing that uvulopalatopharyngoplasty is about 50% effective in curing or considerably decreasing sleep apnea.

Simmons, Guilleminault, and Miles[125] reported that snoring was eliminated or decreased in 93% of all their patients and in 95% of patients without serious OSA. It is important to note that in their series, two thirds of the patients with complaints of snoring and with none of the classic symptoms of sleep apnea actually did have OSA as shown by the polysomnograph. Katsantonis and Friedman[63] reported that 86% of patients indicated that their snoring was either completely eliminated or markedly decreased. Pelausa and Tarshis[87] reported elimination or improvement of snoring in 76% of their patients. It has been the author's experience that virtually all patients who have major snoring report dramatic improvement in their symptoms after the uvulopalatopharyngoplasty. The main complaint of patients who undergo uvulopalatopharyngoplasty for snoring is postoperative pain, which usually persists for about 10 days but may linger for weeks.

The decrease in snoring and daytime sleepiness after uvulopalatopharyngoplasty is most predictable. Less predictable is the ability to decrease the number of apneic events per hour and to improve the oxygen saturation.[154] In a study by Wetmore and others,[149] using a number of factors, 30% of postoperative uvulopalatopharyngoplasty patients were judged markedly improved, 33% showed some improvement, and 37% were believed to have experienced no major improvement. Another study has shown that patients with more than 70 apneic events per hour experienced the most improvement.[20] In a study that rated success by decreasing the number of apneic episodes with oxygen saturation below 85%, 66% were good responders.[63] It generally is agreed that when reporting results of treatment that the apnea–hypopnea index and some measure of oxygen deprivation should be used. A 50% improvement in the AI, commonly used as a bench mark for improvement, is not necessarily reflective of oxygen desaturation.[127] Sleep architecture and respiratory indices are improved in the majority of patients after uvulopalatopharyngoplasty, particularly in the lateral sleep position.[63]

CT confirmed the velopharynx to be the site of maximal preoperative narrowing in the majority of patients with OSA. Maximal narrowing was observed at 10 and 20 mm below the level of the hard palate in 87% of patients. Uvulopalatopharyngoplasty produced maximal increases in cross-sectional area at these two levels in patients with successful results.[121]

Sher, Schechtman, and Piccirillo[122] performed a meta-analysis of 37 previously published studies regarding uvulopalatopharyngoplasty. They included papers providing mean preoperative and postoperative PSG data on at least nine patients. Of the 37 papers, 17 contained raw PSG data for 345 patients. When success was defined as a 50% decrease in AI, the overall response rate was 65.8% (129/196). Nonresponders had a higher baseline AI (51.7 ± 32.5) than responders (43.1 ± 27.9), although this difference did not reach statistical significance ($P = 0.055$). Nonresponders had a lower baseline body weight (271 ± 53.4 lb) than did responders (240 ± 69.4) ($P = 0.094$). When defined as a 50% decrease in respiratory distress index (RDI), the response rate was 52.8% (114/216). With this definition of success, baseline RDI was significantly higher in nonresponders (60.5 ± 25.0) than in responders (52.1 ± 30.8) ($P = 0.028$). When response was defined as a 50% decrease in AI or RDI, with consequent achievement of an AI of less than 10 or an RDI of less than 20, the response rate was 40.7% (137/337). Nonresponders had a higher baseline AI (56.6 ± 30.5) than did responders (31.2 ± 23.3) ($P = 0.0001$) and a higher baseline RDI (65.7 ± 26.7) than did responders (43.1 ± 26.3) ($P = 0.0001$) (Table 81-1).

Classification of the site of collapse was established in 9 of the 17 papers (168 patients) that had raw PSG data. The number of patients in each category of collapse was as follows: 111 patients with retropalatal collapse (type I) and 57 patients with retrolingual collapse alone (type II) or retrolingual and retropalatal collapse. The percentage change after uvulopalatopharyngoplasty in AI (−22.8 ± 29%) and RDI (−6.5 ± 47%) in patients with type II or III collapse was significantly smaller than the decreases in AI (−74.6 ± 27%) ($P < 0.0001$) and in RDI (−32.7 ± 61%) ($P = 0.002$) in patients with type I collapse (Table 81-2). For all definitions of success, response rates were far higher in patients with type I collapse than in patients with type II or type III collapse (Table 81-3). The percentage of patients who attained a 50% decrease in RDI and a postoperative RDI of less than 20 (or a 50% decrease in AI and a postopera-

Table 81-1. Results of analysis of group 3 papers: baseline characteristics of responders and nonresponders

Baseline characteristic	Response defined by 50% drop in apnea index (AI)			Response defined by 50% drop in respiratory disturbance index (RDI)			Response defined by a 50% drop in either AI with final AI less than 10 or RDI with final RDI less than 20		
	Responders (n = 129)	Non-responders (n = 67)	P value	Responders (n = 114)	Non-responders (n = 102)	P value	Responders (n = 137)	Non-responders (n = 200)	P value
Age (years)	48.7 ± 12.5 (n = 72)	50.1 ± 11.2 (n = 47)	0.568	45.9 ± 12.1 (n = 49)	46.6 ± 11.8 (n = 49)	0.768	47.2 ± 12.8 (n = 68)	49.1 ± 11.4 (n = 129)	0.302
Apnea index	43.1 ± 27.9 (n = 129)	51.7 ± 32.5 (n = 67)	0.055	34.2 ± 24.4 (n = 53)	35.3 ± 27.8 (n = 27)	0.518	31.2 ± 23.3 (n = 92)	56.6 ± 30.5 (n = 109)	0.0001
Respiratory disturbance index	54.5 ± 28.9 (n = 59)	61.8 ± 33.4 (n = 19)	0.358	52.1 ± 30.8 (n = 114)	60.5 ± 25.0 (n = 102)	0.028	43.1 ± 26.3 (n = 100)	65.7 ± 26.7 (n = 119)	0.0001
Minimum O_2 saturation	63.9 ± 18.0 (n = 68)	63.4 ± 9.1 (n = 21)	0.896	66.0 ± 19.1 (n = 71)	63.0 ± 18.0 (n = 56)	0.369	66.9 ± 19.0 (n = 76)	60.0 ± 18.2 (n = 66)	0.030
% Rapid eye movement	6.7 ± 5.3 (n = 8)	7.7 ± 5.2 (n = 4)	0.762	17.0 ± 6.7 (n = 21)	15.7 ± 7.5 (n = 9)	0.645	14.8 ± 8.0 (n = 24)	12.6 ± 7.2 (n = 18)	0.346
Weight (lb)	240 ± 69.4 (n = 78)	217 ± 53.4 (n = 31)	0.094	231 ± 52.8 (n = 46)	225 ± 55.3 (n = 39)	0.612	233.0 ± 67.0 (n = 67)	229.0 ± 60.0 (n = 88)	0.761
Body mass index (kg/m²)	31.7 ± 6.7 (n = 39)	29.8 ± 6.2 (n = 16)	0.317	31.0 ± 4.1 (n = 33)	33.3 ± 6.9 (n = 20)	0.184	31.4 ± 5.7 (n = 48)	32.7 ± 6.9 (n = 40)	0.316

Table 81-2. Baseline and percentage-change data based on location of pharyngeal narrowing or collapse, expressed as mean ± standard deviation

Variable	Type I (n = 111)	Type II or III (n = 57)	Unknown location (n = 177)	P value[a]
Apnea index (AI)				
Baseline	38.9 ± 26 (n = 80)	59.9 ± 29 (n = 21)	46.4 ± 32 (n = 102)	0.004
Percentage change[b]	−74.6 ± 27 (n = 77)	−22.8 ± 29 (n = 20)	−53.6 ± 47 (n = 94)	<0.0001
Respiratory disturbance index (RDI)				
Baseline	56.6 ± 29 (n = 72)	64.5 ± 24 (n = 39)	47.8 ± 30 (n = 103)	0.096
Percentage change[b]	−32.7 ± 61 (n = 68)	−6.5 ± 47 (n = 37)	−32.1 ± 58 (n = 96)	0.002
Minimum O_2 saturation				
Baseline	63.0 ± 15.8 (n = 55)	61.9 ± 20 (n = 20)	66.9 ± 20 (n = 68)	0.935
Percentage change	24.7 ± 45 (n = 55)	12.7 ± 45 (n = 12)	32.3 ± 79 (n = 67)	0.049

Some papers reported AI and RDI as responses; consequently, the two subgroups add up to more than the sum of the two groups individually.

[a] Compares patients having type I narrowing or collapse with patients having type II or III narrowing or collapse and does not compare unknown location. Chi-square tests are used for response-rate comparisons, Wilcoxon's two-tailed rank-sum test for percentage-change comparisons and Student's t tests for baseline comparisons.

[b] Sample sizes for percentage changes in AI and RDI are less than sample sizes in corresponding response-rate data because of the deletion of outliers in computing means.

tive AI of < 10, if that index was given) was much higher for patients with type I collapse than for patients with type II or type III collapse (52.3 versus 5.3%) ($P < 0.0001$). Further, the mean baseline AI for those patients with type I collapse who achieved this degree of improvement was significantly lower than for patients with type I collapse who did not respond to the procedure (30.4 ± 18.6 versus 56.2 ± 25.9, respectively) ($P < 0.0001$).

The obvious dilemma to overcome is to predict those patients who are going to be significant responders to uvulopalatopharyngoplasty and those who will not respond adequately.[11] This is a difficult decision and one not easily an-

swered. Despite careful preselection of patients for upper airway narrowing and collapse in the oropharynx, uvulopalatopharyngoplasty does not always produce successful results. The reasons for failure in these patients are unclear, but they could include a poor technical result, persistent collapse at the same level, or shift in the site of collapse to another region. If the majority of the obstruction is occurring in the retropalatal area, it can be reasonably predicted that the results of uvulopalatopharyngoplasty will be good (52.3% success rate). However, if the major portion of the obstruction is occurring in the retrolingual area, the results of uvulopalatopharyngoplasty are likely to not be good (5.3% success

Table 81-3. Response rates correlated to definition of response based on location of pharyngeal narrowing or collapse

	Response rates (%)			
Variable used to measure response	Type I (n = 111)	Type II or III (n = 57)	Unknown location (n = 177)	P value*
50% Decrease in apnea index (AI)	65/78 (83.3)	4/21 (19.0)	60/97 (61.9)	<0.0001
50% Decrease in respiratory distress index (RDI)	47/70 (67.1)	9/38 (23.7)	56/97 (57.7)	<0.0001
50% Decrease in either AI or RDI	83/109 (76.1)	12/57 (21.1)	100/171 (58.5)	<0.0001
50% Decrease in RDI and a postoperative RDI less than 20 or a 50% decrease in AI and a postoperative AI less than 10	57/109 (52.3)	3/57 (5.3)	77/171 (45.0)	<0.0001

Some papers reported AI and RDI as responses; consequently, the two subgroups add up to more than the sum of the two groups individually.

* Compares patients having type I narrowing or collapse with patients having type II or III narrowing or collapse and does not compare unknown location. Chi-square tests are used for response-rate comparisons, Wilcoxon's two-tailed rank-sum test for percentage-change comparisons and Student's *t* tests for baseline comparisons.

rate). Fluoroscopic studies of the oropharynx and hypopharynx during sleep have shown that obstructions may occur predominantly in the oropharynx or hypopharynx or in a combination of multiple areas.[124] To isolate a specific area of obstruction is, at times, impossible. In a large percentage of patients, there probably are multiple areas of obstruction, and it may be shown in the future that a diagnostically important point is to distinguish the area that initiates the collapse. Once the initial site of collapse develops, all area of the oropharynx and hypopharynx may be prone to obstruction.

When the palate is modified in a uvulopalatopharyngoplasty, there is a possibility of complications related to changes in palatal function. The possible complications include velopharyngeal insufficiency (VPI) for more than 1 month, postoperative bleeding, nasopharyngeal stenosis, voice change, successfully managed perioperative upper-airway obstruction, vague foreign-body sensation, and death resulting from airway obstruction. Fortunately, the incidence of these complications appears to be low.[31,32,50,122] If the modification resection is excessive, palatal incompetence will result in nasal air leakage during speech and nasal regurgitation during swallowing.[66,137] Initially, during the early postoperative healing period, palatal incompetence will occur for several days to 2 weeks, but permanent major palatal incompetence is unusual unless an excessive resection is performed (Fig. 81-15).

Excessive resection particularly of the midline should be avoided. Palatal closure depends on the central mounding action of the musculus uvulae and on the lifting action of the levator palati muscles, which course from the eustachian tube downward (posteriorly) and medially to interdigitate in the midline. A midline defect, surgical or congenital, disrupts the function. Ideally, the uvula should be shortened to a level slightly below the trailing edge of the rest of the shortened soft palate.[32]

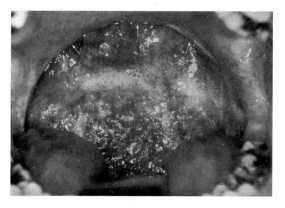

Fig. 81-15. Excessive palatal excision *(arrows)* that resulted in nasal air leakage and regurgitation of liquid and food into nasal area. (From Thawley SE: Surgical treatment of obstructive sleep apnea, *Med Clin North Am* 69:1337, 1985.)

An unusual complication may be the occurrence of nasopharyngeal–palatal stenosis (Fig. 81-16). This complication should be avoided because it is difficult to correct. This is more likely to occur with excessive resection of the posterior tonsillar pillars, the excessive use of cautery, and the undermining of the mucosa of the posterior pharyngeal wall.[66] Other factors may be wound dehiscence, infection, necrosis, scarring and nasopharyngeal packing, and the concomitant performance of an adenoidectomy.[137]

The uvulopalatopharyngoplasty is designed to avoid nasopharyngeal stenosis. The incision lines should face forward, and away from the nasopharynx. Excision should involve the anterior pillar (palatoglossal arch) and not the posterior pillar. When the redundant posterior pillar is advanced laterally, forward, and upward (for suturing), the soft palate will be pulled forward along with it, and the nasopharyngeal space will be expanded. If the posterior pillar were

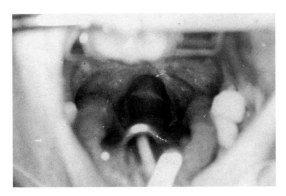

Fig. 81-16. Postoperative nasopharyngeal stenosis *(arrow)*, an unusual complication of palatoplasty. (From Thawley SE: Surgical treatment of obstructive sleep apnea, *Med Clin North Am* 69:1337, 1985.)

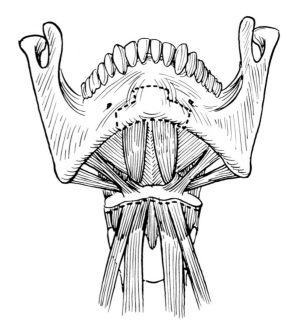

Fig. 81-17. Anteroinferior sagittal mandibular osteotomy. Note also transection and release of infrahyoid muscles. This allows hyoid to move forward, enlarging hypopharyngeal airway. (Redrawn from Thawley SE: Surgical treatment of obstructive sleep apnea, *Med Clin North Am* 69:1337, 1985; Courtesy of RW Riley, Stanford, Calif.)

to be excised, then the anterior pillar and the soft palate would be pulled backward (either by suturing or scarring), and the nasopharyngeal space would become narrowed or stenotic. Injury to the posterior pharyngeal membranes, either by undermining or cautery, is best avoided altogether. Passavant's ridge should be left uninjured. If adenoidectomy is necessary, great care should be taken to avoid any injury to the posterior (nasal) surface of the soft palate.[32]

Patients may complain of mild dryness in the throat and a sensation of persistent mucus in the oropharynx, which may be caused by decreased flow of nasal secretions over the scarred inferior edge of the soft palate.

Inferior sagittal mandibular osteotomy and genioglossal advancement with hyoid myotomy and suspension

In genioglossal advancement with hyoid myotomy (GAHM) the genioid tubercle of the mandible is advanced by means of a limited mandibular osteotomy[100] Riley and Powell[101,102] described a mandibular technique in which an anterioinferior sagittal osteotomy is performed to include the geniotubercle on the inner cortex. This is the site of attachment for the genioglossus muscle. This procedure involves forward advancement of the anteroinferior portion of the mandible, maintenance of the general continuity of the mandible, and repositioning of the genioglossus-attached segment of the mandible more anteriorly (Fig. 81-17). This theoretically should pull the tongue forward and improve the hypopharyngeal airway. Concomitantly with this procedure, the infrahyoid muscles are transected, allowing the hyoid bone to be pulled more anteriorly and superiorly. This bone is held in position by attaching it with pieces of fascia to the remaining intact mandible. Although the number of patients on which this procedure has been performed is small, postoperatively the patients have had fewer symptoms of OSA. The long-term results of inferior sagittal osteotomy are as yet unknown. This procedure has the advantage of

obviating the need for intermaxillary fixation, and it does not affect dental occlusion.

Newer modifications involve stabilization of the hyoid bone anteriorly and inferiorly by attachment to the thyroid cartilage.[97] Fifty-five patients were reported by Riley and Powell,[100] and 67% (37/55) were in the responder group. The response rate for those patients who had previously undergone failed uvulopalatopharyngoplasty was 85.7% (6/7). Factors that appeared to differentiate nonresponders from responders were degree of obesity and mandibular-skeletal deficiency; nonresponders were more obese and more severely mandibular-deficient. Another study[59] reported a response rate of 77.8% in nine patients who underwent inferior sagittal mandibular osteotomy and genioglossal advancement without hyoid myotomy and suspension.

Phase 2 surgery

Midline glossectomy

Midline glossectomy involves laser resection of the midline of the base of the tongue. This has been performed primarily on patients who have failed uvulopalatopharyngoplasty and who were considered to have major hypopharyngeal collapse on physical examination and Mueller's maneuver.[122] In two separate articles, one group of investigators evaluated the effects of tongue operations.

The first study[35] described 12 patients who underwent the laser midline glossectomy (LMG) procedure. All patients had major retrolingual narrowing or collapse on physical examination and dynamic cephalometric radiographs. With response defined as a reduction in RDI of at least 50%, the response rate was 41.7% (5/12). For the responder group, the RDI decreased from 60.6 to 14.5. Nonresponders were significantly more obese than responders (body mass index = 37.9 ± 6.3 kg/m² versus 30.6 ± 4.6 kg/m², respectively) ($P < 0.05$).

The second study[152] described patients with a modification of LMG called *lingualplasty*. Lingualplasty resulted in a higher proportion of responders than did LMG. For the entire group, the mean RDI decreased from 58.6 ± 36.6 to 16.3 ± 17.2. Response was defined as a postoperative RDI of less than 20 per hour and at least a 50% reduction from preoperative RDI. Seventy-seven percent of patients (17/22) were responders; the mean RDI in the responder group decreased from 58.8 ± 39.5 to 8.8 ± 6.2 postoperatively. Age, body mass index, and cephalometric variables did not differentiate responders from nonresponders. The possible complications include bleeding and swallowing and speech problems. Although this technique, or other modifications, may have applicability in the future, more results need to be reported before this technique is widely recommended.

Mandibular advancement techniques

It has long been recognized that conditions associated with a receding mandible predispose to the development of sleep apnea. This may occur in pediatric patients who have the Pierre Robin syndrome, and it occurs in older patients who have a somewhat small, retrognathic mandible. This retrognathia may be congenital or acquired through trauma or iatrogenic means. It has been reported after partial mandibular resection for tumors.[84] Most of these patients have nonobtuse mentocervical angle (neck-to-chin angle), a chin deficiency, and usually a class II dental malocclusion. The tongue posture is more posterior because the genioglossus muscles are not attached as far anterior as in patients with normal occlusion and mandibular position. The tongue position in the oropharynx, which is determined partially by the function of the genioglossus muscle and is related to the position of the mandible, may be an important consideration in patients who have obstruction in the base of the tongue–hypopharyngeal area.[151] This problem has been addressed by advancing the mandible anteriorly.[27] Patients who are candidates for this procedure may or may not have obvious mandibular retrognathism on clinical examination. Cephalometric radiographic studies should be performed on all patients who are considered potential candidates for this approach.[19,104] Cephalometric radiographic analysis should confirm the retrognathic position of the mandible and should show a narrowing of the hypopharyngeal airway.[139]

Bimaxillary advancement

This procedure consists of bilateral bony cuts in the area posterior to the last molar (Fig. 81-18). This is done bilaterally, and the entire anterior segment of the mandible is ad-

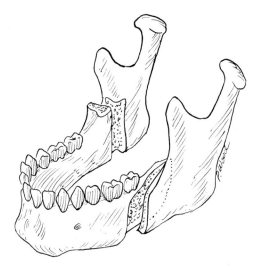

Fig. 81-18. Mandibular advancement with mandible being displaced forward. (Redrawn from Thawley SE: Surgical treatment of obstructive sleep apnea, *Med Clin North Am* 69:1337, 1985.)

vanced anteriorly. Preoperatively, an acrylic splint is made to recreate the predicted normal occlusion, and the anterior advanced portion of the mandible is wired into position and held in intermaxillary fixation by wiring the mandible to the splint and then attaching all of this to the maxilla. Healing takes place over a period of 6 weeks, and intermaxillary fixation is required during that time. When healing is complete, the wires and splint are removed, the mandible is positioned more anteriorly, which in turn pulls the genioglossus muscle and the tongue more anteriorly, thus enlarging the hypopharyngeal airway.[91] Problems with this are the need of intermaxillary fixation and the resultant change in dental occlusion.

Maxillomandibular osteotomy and advancement

A Le Fort I maxillary osteotomy advancing the maxilla forward is combined with mandibular advancement and hyoid suspension.[101] The initial results of this surgery were reported in 25 patients who were selected because of morbid obesity, severe mandibular deficiency, and failure of other surgical procedures. All patients showed good results.[103] Subsequent reports from these same group of investigators[98,99] established a two-stage surgical treatment protocol. The overall response rate for 91 patients who underwent maxillomandibular osteotomy after unsuccessful uvulopalatopharyngoplasty (n = 84) or who had primary skeletal deformities (n = 7) was 97.8% (89/91) at a mean follow-up time of 9 months. The mean preoperative RDI decreased from 68.3 ± 23 to 8.4 ± 5.9.

Waite and others[144] reported their treatment of 23 patients. They devised a protocol in which maxillomandibular osteotomy was the primary surgical approach for those patients with abnormal anatomy (as determined by cephalometric measurements) and performed other adjunctive procedures only if they believe further treatment was indicated. Adjunctive procedures included sliding geniotomy (n = 15), partial glossectomy (n = 8), and uvulopalatopharyngoplasty (n = 7). Seventy-eight percent of patients (18/23) had adjunctive procedures, and 52.2% (12/23) had two adjunctive procedures. The response rate for the group that had maxillomandibular osteotomy with no adjunctive procedure was 20% (1/5). The response rate for the group having maxillomandibular osteotomy and at least one adjunctive procedure was 77.8% (14/18). The response rate for the patients who had maxillomandibular osteotomy and uvulopalatopharyngoplasty as their only adjunctive procedure, or as one of at least two adjunctive procedures, was 100% (7/7). There was no statistical difference between the responders and nonresponders in terms of cephalometric measures, weight loss, apnea severity, or degree of maxillomandibular osteotomy and advancement.

Hochban[54] reported on a series of 21 consecutive patients treated for OSA with maxillomandibular osteotomy as the sole treatment in 20 of 21 patients. All 20 patients achieved a postoperative RDI of less than 10 (mean preoperative RDI, 44.9 ± 17.5; mean postoperative RDI, 3.5 ± 4.7).

Riley, Powell, and Guilleminault[98] reported that 306 patients who underwent maxillomandibular operations developed transient anesthesia of the cheek and chin area, which resolved in 87% of patients in 6 to 12 months. No patients experienced motor nerve deficits, postoperative bleeding, or major skeletal relapse. Waite and others[144] reported that of their 23 patients who underwent MMO, 12% developed cardiac arrhythmias, including cardiac arrest.

Hyoid expansion

Hyoid expansion is an experimental procedure in which the hyoid is separated into three pieces: one anterior and two lateral.[86] These segments are wired to an arch bar-like device, which holds the segments in an expanded manner, thus enlarging the hypopharyngeal lumen. Although effective as an experimental model, it has not been shown to be effective in patients with OSA.

Tracheotomy

Tracheotomy bypasses the upper airway obstruction and is known to reverse the obstructive components of OSA. Tracheotomy is indicated for those with this condition if the apnea is severe and if conservative therapy, including weight loss, removal of obstructive tissue, avoidance of sedatives, and nasal CPAP, has failed to change these symptoms dramatically. Generally, the indications for tracheotomy in patients with OSA are cor pulmonale, chronic alveolar hypoventilation, serious nocturnal arrhythmias, and disabling hypersomnolence if these symptoms have been unresponsive to attempted weight loss and avoidance of sedatives and alcohol and if the patient has not responded to or tolerated a trial of nasal CPAP.

The immediate improvement in symptoms after tracheot-

omy is dramatic. Its effectiveness in controlling cardiac arrhythmias and improving symptoms of pulmonary hypertension and oxygenation is well documented.[145] The disappearance of marked sinus arrhythmia and extreme sinus bradycardia and atrioventricular block after tracheotomy and their reappearance during sleep if the tracheostoma has been occluded indicate that these characteristic rhythm disorders are directly related to the airway occlusion during sleep. Tracheotomy also changes the sleep patterns in these patients. After tracheotomy, there is an almost immediate reversal of excessive daytime sleepiness and frequent sleep periods during the day.[147]

The marked improvement in the nocturnal sleep pattern is a result of a major reduction in the frequency of transient awakenings. There also is a decrease in the number of stage changes and the establishment of periods of sustained sleep, especially in stages 3 and 4. The tracheotomy reverses the frequency of transient awakenings. The tracheotomy reverses the fragmentary unsustained sleep stage organization that is associated with marked decreases in stage 3 and 4 sleep in patients with OSA. Oxygen saturation usually is improved after tracheotomy. The obstructive and mixed-type apneas essentially are eliminated by tracheotomy, and although nonobstructive apneas and hypopneas may persist and may even initially increase, usually after 3 or 4 weeks they will return to their normal pattern. It therefore is clear that tracheotomy is a effective treatment for the patient with severe OSA.

The decision regarding tracheotomy is made by a team of medical specialists and otolaryngologists. When life-threatening cardiac arrhythmias are identified in association with an OSA, tracheotomy should be performed. The other main indication of tracheotomy is severe hypoventilation with a marked decrease in arterial oxygen saturation. If the patient is severely obstructed and if the cardiac status is tenuous, tracheotomy may be performed, followed by appropriate medical, cardiac, and pulmonary therapy. After the patient has stabilized weeks later, he or she may be returned to the operating room for a uvulopalatopharyngoplasty. Some surgeons elect to perform a tracheotomy on patients undergoing uvulopalatopharyngoplasty to maintain a safe postoperative airway. Once the patient has satisfactorily healed over a few days, the tracheotomy tube may be removed quickly. Generally, if a tracheotomy is performed concomitantly with a uvulopalatopharyngoplasty, the tube is left in place for approximately 6 weeks, at which time a repeat sleep study is performed with the tracheostoma unplugged and plugged to determine the effectiveness of the uvulopalatopharyngoplasty. If there has been satisfactory improvement in the sleep study parameter with the tracheostoma closed, the tracheotomy tube is removed. If major cardiac problems persist or if there is major remaining daytime sleepiness and disturbed sleep patterns, the tracheotomy tube is left in place.[149]

The tracheotomy usually is performed during general and

endotracheal anesthesia. The induction of anesthesia may present problems because excessive tissue in the oropharynx may make it difficult for the anesthesiologist to intubate the patient. If the patient can be safely ventilated and intubated, routine induction of anesthesia with muscle relaxation is performed. However, if there is a question about the ability to ventilate the patient after muscle relaxation, the anesthesiologist may elect to perform intubation with the patient awake and during topical anesthesia. This may be performed by direct laryngoscopy through the oral approach, or the trachea may be intubated by using a fiberoptic direct scope that has been threaded down an endotracheal tube. This may be performed orally or transnasally. Tracheotomy may in some instances be performed during local anesthesia. Generally, this is not recommended because there usually is a large amount of excessive tissue in the surgical field. Tracheotomy in these patients requires a large amount of manual manipulation in the neck area. The time required for tracheotomies in these extremely obese patients with short necks typically is much longer than that for a routine, simple tracheotomy in a normal-weight or thin patient.

Several different types of tracheotomy techniques are available. The simple tracheotomy technique consists of a midline incision with dissection deep to the anterior wall of the trachea. A vertical incision is performed in the second or third tracheal ring, and a standard tracheotomy tube is placed. If the patient is not excessively obese, this technique may be satisfactory, although most of these patients are obese with thick necks, and this technique commonly leads to problems. The problems associated with the performance and care of the standard tracheotomy in obese patients may be dramatic. The surgical performance of the technique may be difficult because there are large amounts of fatty tissue that may interfere with exposure of the trachea. The trachea may be deep in the neck, and the proper fitting and maintenance of a standard tracheotomy tube in such a deep trachea may be difficult. In obese patients, granulation tissue commonly forms in the tracheostoma site (Fig. 81-19). This seems to be related to the large surface area of fatty tissue that is exposed.[26] This also may lead to granulation tissue within the trachea, may require repeated removal and treatments, and may, on occasion, even lead to obstruction of the airway. If the patient coughs out the tracheotomy tube during the early postoperative period, it may be difficult, if not impossible, to reinsert the tube quickly enough through the excessive amounts of tissue. To reduce these complications, many surgeons perform a modified tracheotomy that allows resection of large amounts of fatty tissue at the tracheostoma site and the creation of skin flaps that funnel down to the trachea (Fig. 81-20).[33] This permits easier and safer care of the tracheostoma site; it essentially connects the skin to the trachea wall and eliminates the exposure of the fatty tissue to the air.[80] The amount of granulation tissue is dramatically decreased, and there is greater ease in safely maintaining a tracheotomy tube in place. The actual incision

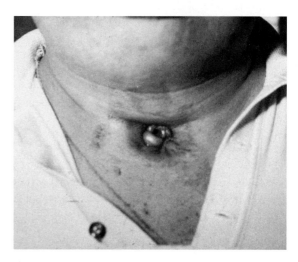

Fig. 81-19. Granulation tissue at tracheostoma site. (From Thawley SE: Surgical treatment of obstructive sleep apnea, *Med Clin North Am* 69:1337, 1985.)

into the trachea may be a simple vertical one or an inferior or superior flap of anterior tracheal wall may be rotated to the skin surface. Although this tracheotomy technique is better suited for permanent use, the procedure may be satisfactorily reversed with closure of the tracheostoma.

Although tracheotomy is an effective therapeutic method for patients with major OSA, the performance, postoperative care, and long-term follow-up evaluations require an active understanding of the potential problems. The major tracheal complications are granulation, tissue formation, bleeding, stoma narrowing, bronchitis, pneumonia, and psychological stigmata. Granulomas may form at the upper margin of the stoma site, as a result of chronic irritation and infection from the tube. The sharp edges of the tube rubbing against the anterior tracheal wall can aggravate the inflammation. The standard tracheotomy leaves fatty tissue that is easily inflamed and consequently tends to form granulation tissue, resulting in bleeding and local infection. When the skin flap technique is used, it keeps the stoma patent more easily and provides skin coverage of the fat, decreasing inflammation and granulation tissue formation. It also decreases the need for a long intratracheal prosthesis. Granulation tissue may be increased as a result of chronic bronchitis, which aggravates inflammation at the stoma site, although the development of tracheal granulation seems to be directly related to the type of tracheotomy performed and less to the chronic bronchial pulmonary disease.

There may be postoperative wound infections with bronchitis and occasional pneumonia. The complication rate is dramatically reduced by debridement of the excessive fatty tissue and the use of local skin flaps. Recurrent purulent bronchitis seems to occur more in patients who are predisposed to pulmonary infections because of associated chronic lung disease. Many of these patients continue to smoke. Bronchitis and pulmonary infections increase if patients fail

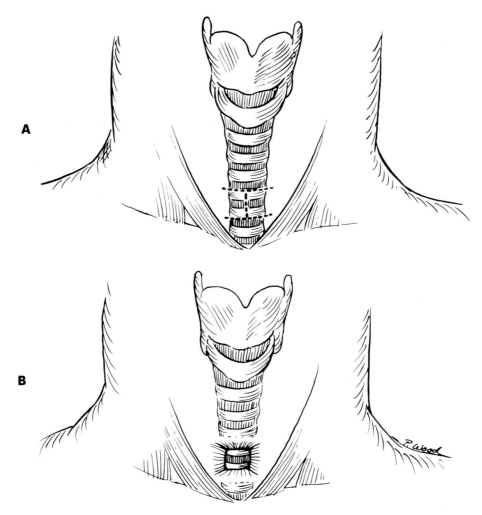

Fig. 81-20. A, Skin flaps overlying trachea. These are elevated, and fat in tracheostoma site is removed, allowing skin flaps to be beveled into tracheostoma area. **B,** Completed skin flap tracheotomy technique. Note skin directed to the tracheal level. This reduces amount of soft tissue exposed and decreases problems with granulation. (Modified from Thawley SE: Surgical treatment of obstructive sleep apnea, *Med Clin North Am* 69:1337, 1985.)

to use humidifiers at night, which results in inspissated bronchial secretions.

Psychosocial problems may develop after a tracheotomy. It is not unusual for patients to be depressed during the initial early postoperative period. This depression usually resolves with supportive care and through the patient's active understanding and management of the tracheostoma.

Although major depression and personality changes related to sleepiness respond to tracheotomy, the tracheotomy may produce transient adjustment reactions, spousal rejection, and increased dependency. Although tracheotomy in these patients produces more problems than the standard type of simple tracheotomy in other patients, these patients can be satisfactorily handled if their problems are anticipated and adequately treated. The results are improved through a thorough, perioperative teaching program aimed at educating the patient and the spouse and other family members regarding care of the tracheostoma.

OUTCOMES RESEARCH

Outcomes research is the scientific study of the results of diverse therapies that are used for a particular disease, condition, or illness.[30,133] The need to determine the outcomes of medical care is fundamental to the successful and cost-effective practice of medicine. The key features of outcomes research are the study of the effects of all major therapies on a condition, the expanded definition of outcome to include patient-based measures, and the central role of the patient in treatment selection.[89] The goals of this type of research are to document treatment effectiveness and create treatment guidelines. Treatment effectiveness implies the value or strength of a treatment as is used in the community during usual situations. Outcomes research also uses a broadened description of patient outcomes, which includes health status, quality of life, and satisfaction with care.

In 1992, the American Academy of Otolaryngology-Head and Neck Surgery Foundation, Inc. (AAO-HNSF) sponsored the Obstructive Sleep Apnea Treatment Outcomes Pilot Study (OSATOPS).[88] The main goals of OSATOPS were (1) to serve as a demonstration of multicenter treatment effectiveness and patient outcomes research project sponsored by the AAO-HNSF, (2) to validate the outcomes assessment methodology developed for this study, including the clinical severity index and OSA Patient-Oriented Severity Index (POSI), a disease-specific health-related quality of life index, and (3) to acquire pilot data to support a future, large-scale formal study of the effectiveness of common treatments for OSA.

There were 10 study centers in this project; 274 patients were screened, and 142 eventually were enrolled. Of those enrolled, 122 received some form of treatment: 71 (50%) received CPAP; 48 (34%) underwent surgery; and 3 (2%) altered diet and exercise. Outcomes were assessed 4 months after enrollment. The clinical severity index seemed to be able to classify patients accurately into three severity classes (mild, moderate, and severe) based on pretreatment factors. All patients were able to complete the obstructive sleep apnea patient-oriented severity index, and the responses seemed to describe well the patient's disease-specific health-related quality of life.

This project shows that the AAO-HNS can conduct multicenter treatment effectiveness studies. The various forms, instruments, and pilot data created and used for this project can serve as a solid foundation for future OSA treatment effectiveness studies.[88]

SUMMARY

Manifestations of SDB have been present in our society for many years. Snoring, restless sleep, and daytime drowsiness have been well recognized by the lay public, but until recently the understanding, evaluation, and treatment of these symptoms have largely eluded physicians. The prevalence of OSA in adults has been estimated to be around 4% for men and 2% for women. Sleep studies have shown the serious cardiopulmonary problems that may be associated with OSA.

Sleep apnea may present as a broad spectrum of symptoms that can range from snoring to life-threatening cardiac and pulmonary complications. Otolaryngologists are increasingly being asked to evaluate symptoms that may be related to sleep apnea. The public is becoming more educated concerning the importance of snoring, restless sleep, and daytime drowsiness. With the availability of more information, it has become obvious that sleep apnea has great importance to a range of cardiopulmonary and other medical problems.

The mainstay of treatment for patients with moderate-to-severe OSA is CPAP. Surgical therapy remains a viable alternative for treatment of SDB for patients who are unresponsive or unwilling to wear CPAP. There are many options available for surgical therapy, with the uvulopalatopharyngoplasty being the most widely used at the present time. However, active, basic, and clinical research is ongoing, and our concepts of pathophysiology and treatment continue to evolve.

REFERENCES

1. Afzelius LE and others: Sleep apnea syndrome—an alternative to tracheostomy, *Laryngoscope* 91:285, 1981.
2. American Academy of Neurology: Assessment: techniques associated with the diagnosis and management of sleep disorders, *Neurology* 42:269, 1992.
3. American Sleep Disorders Association: Practice parameters for the use of portable recording in the assessment of obstructive sleep apnea, *Sleep* 17:372, 1994.
4. American Sleep Disorders Association Report: Practice parameters for the use of laser-assisted uvulopalatoplasty, *Sleep* 17:744, 1994.
5. American Sleep Disorders Association Report: Practice parameters for the treatment of obstructive sleep apnea in adults: the efficacy of surgical modifications of the upper airway, *Sleep* 19:152, 1996.
6. American Thoracic Society: Sleep apnea, sleepiness, and driving risk, *Am J Respir Crit Care Med* 150:1463, 1994.
7. Anand V, Ferguson PW, Schoen LS: Obstructive sleep apnea: a comparison of continuous positive airway pressure and surgical treatment, *Otolaryngol Head Neck Surg* 105:382, 1991.
8. Baker TL: Introduction to sleep and sleep disorders, *Med Clin North Am* 69:1123, 1985.
9. Bearpark H and others: Snoring and sleep apnea: a population study in Australian men, *Am J Crit Care Med* 151:1459, 1995.
10. Blakley BW, Mahowald MW: Nasal resistance and sleep apnea, *Laryngoscope* 97:752, 1987.
11. Blakley BW and others: Sleep parameters after surgery for obstructive sleep apnea, *Otolaryngol Head Neck Surg* 95:23, 1986.
12. Block AJ, Wynne JW, Boysen PG: Sleep disordered breathing and nocturnal oxygen desaturation in post-menopausal women, *Am J Med* 69:75, 1980.
13. Block AJ and others: Sleep apnea hyponea and oxygen desaturation in normal subjects: a strong male predominance, *N Engl J Med* 300:513, 1979.
14. Bornstein SK: *Respiration during sleep: polysomnography.* In Guilleminault C, editor: *Sleep and waking disorders: indications and techniques,* Menlo Park, Calif, 1982, Addison-Wesley.
15. Borowiecki B and others: Fiberoptic study of pharyngeal airway during sleep in patients with hypersomnia obstructive sleep apnea syndrome, *Laryngoscope* 88:1310, 1978.
16. Boysen PG and others: Nocturnal pulmonary hypertension in patients with chronic obstructive pulmonary disease, *Chest* 76:536, 1979.
17. Bresnitz EA, Goldberg R, Kosinski RM: Epidemiology of obstructive sleep apnea, *Epidemiol Rev* 16:210, 1994.
18. Brownwell LG and others: Protriptyline in obstructive sleep apnea, *N Engl J Med* 307:1037, 1982.
19. Burstone CJ and others: Cephalometrics for orthognathic surgery, *J Oral Surg* 36:269, 1978.
20. Caldarelli DD, Cartwright R, Lilie JK: Severity of sleep apnea as a predictor of successful treatment by palatopharyngoplasty, *Laryngoscope* 96:945, 1986.
21. Carenfelt C: Laser uvulopalatoplasty in treatment of habitual snoring, *Ann Otol Rhinol Laryngol* 100:451, 1991.
22. Carskadon MA, Dement WC: *Normal human sleep: an overview.* In Kryger MH, Roth T, Dement WC, editors: *Principles and practice of sleep medicine,* Philadelphia, 1994, WB Saunders.

23. Cartwright RD, Samelson CF: The effects of non-surgical treatment for obstructive sleep apnea, *JAMA* 248:705, 1982.

24. Clark RW and others: Sleep apnea: treatment with protriptyline, *Neurology* 29:1287, 1979.

25. Clark RW and others: Adrenergic hyperactivity and cardiac abnormality in primary disorders of sleep, *Neurology* 30:113, 1980.

26. Conway WA and others: Adverse effects of tracheostomy for sleep apnea, *Arch Otolaryngol* 246:346, 1981.

27. Dierks E and others: Obstructive sleep apnea syndrome: correction by mandibular advancement, *South Med J* 83:390, 1990.

28. Eli SR and others: Demonstration of fixed upper airway obstruction, *Am J Radiol* 146:669, 1986.

29. Emirgil C, Sobol BJ: The effects of weight reduction on pulmonary function and the sensitivity of the respiratory center in obesity, *Am Rev Respir Dis* 108:831, 1973.

30. Epstein AM: The outcomes movement—will it get us where we want to go? *N Engl J Med* 323:266, 1990.

31. Esclamado RM and others: Perioperative complications and risk factors in the surgical treatment of obstructive sleep apnea syndrome, *Laryngoscope* 99:1125, 1989.

32. Fairbanks DNF: Uvulopalatopharyngoplasty complications and avoidance strategies, *Otolaryngol Head Neck Surg* 102:239, 1990.

33. Fee WE, Ward PH: Permanent tracheostomy: a new surgical technique, *Otol Rhinol Laryngol* 86:635, 1977.

34. Ferber R and others: Portable recording in the assessment of obstructive sleep apnea, *Sleep* 17:378, 1994.

34a. Flemons WW and others: The clinical prediction of sleep apnea, *Sleep* 16:S10, 1993.

35. Fujita S and others: Laser midline glossectomy as a treatment for obstructive sleep apnea, *Laryngoscope* 101:805, 1991.

36. Fujita A and others: Evaluation of the effectiveness of uvulopalatopharyngoplasty, *Laryngoscope* 95:70, 1985.

37. Fujita S and others: Surgical correction of anatomic abnormalities in obstructive sleep apnea syndrome: uvulopalatopharyngoplasty, *Otolaryngol Head Neck Surg* 89:923, 1981.

38. Gastaut H, Tassinari CA, Duron B: Etude polygraphique des manifestations épisodique (hyponique et respiratoires), diurnes et nocturne, du syndrome de Pickwick, *Rev Neurol (Paris)* 112:568, 1965.

39. Gislason T and others: Uvulopalatopharyngoplasty in the sleep apnea syndrome, *Arch Otolaryngol Head Neck Surg* 114:45, 1988.

40. Guilleminault C: *Clinical features and evaluation of obstructive sleep apnea.* In Kryger MH, Roth T, Dement WC, editors: *Principles and practice of sleep medicine,* Philadelphia, 1994, WB Saunders.

41. Guilleminault C, Stoohs R: Upper airway resistance syndrome, *Sleep Res* 20:250, 1991.

42. Guilleminault C, Partinen M, editor: *Obstructive sleep apnea syndrome: clinical research and treatment,* New York, 1990, Raven Press.

43. Guilleminault C, van den Hoed J, Mitler MM: *Clinical overview of the sleep apnea syndromes.* In Guilleminault C, van den Hoed J, Mitler MM, editors: *Sleep apnea syndromes,* New York, 1978, Alan R Liss.

44. Guilleminault C, Dement WC: *Sleep apnea syndromes and related sleep disorders.* In Williams RL, Karacan I, editors: *Sleep disorders: diagnosis and treatment,* New York, 1978, Wiley.

45. Gyulay S and others: A comparison of clinical assessment and home oximetry in the diagnosis of obstructive sleep apnea, *Am Rev Respir Dis* 147:50, 1993.

46. Kribbs NB and others: Objective measurement of patterns of nasal CPAP use by patients with obstructive sleep apnea syndrome, *Am Rev Respir Dis* 147:887, 1993.

47. Haponik EF: Computerized tomography in obstructive sleep apnea: correlation of airway size with physiology during sleep and wakefulness, *Am Rev Respir Dis* 127:221, 1983.

48. Harman EM, Block AJ: Why does weight loss improve the respiratory insufficiency of obesity, *Chest* 90:153, 1986.

49. Harman EM, Wynne JW, Block AJ: The effect of weight loss on sleep disordered breathing and oxygen desaturation in morbidly obese men, *Chest* 82:291, 1982.

50. Haavisto L, Suonpaa J: Complications of uvulopalatopharyngoplasty, *Clin Otolaryngol* 19:243, 1994.

51. He J and others: Mortality and apnea index in obstructive sleep apnea, *Chest* 94:9, 1988.

52. Herlihy JP, Whitlock WL, Dietrich RA: Sleep apnea syndrome after irradiation of the neck, *Arch Otolaryngol Head Neck Surg* 115:1467, 1989.

53. Hla KM and others: Sleep apnea and hypertension: a population-based study, *Ann Intern Med* 120:382, 1994.

54. Hochban W, Brandenburg U, Peter JH: Surgical treatment of obstructive sleep apnea by maxillomandibular advancement, *Sleep* 17:624, 1994.

54a. Hoffstein V, Szalai JP: Predictive value of clinical features in diagnosing obstructive sleep apnea, *Sleep* 16:118, 1993.

55. Ichioka M and others: A dental device for the treatment of obstructive sleep apnea: a preliminary study, *Otolaryngol Head Neck Surg* 104:555, 1991.

56. Ikematsu T: Study of snoring—fourth report: therapy, *J Jpn Otorhinolaryngol* 64:434, 1964.

57. Issa FG, Sullivan CE: Reversal of central sleep apnea using nasal CPAP, *Chest* 90:165, 1986.

58. Johns MW: A new method for measuring daytime sleepiness: the Eppworth Sleepiness Scale, *Sleep* 14:540, 1991.

59. Johnson NT, Chinn J: Uvulopalatopharyngoplasty and inferior sagittal mandibular osteotomy with genioglossus advancement for treatment of obstructive sleep apnea, *Chest* 105:278, 1994.

60. Kamami YV: Outpatient treatment of snoring with CO2 laser: laser-assisted UPPP, *J Otolaryngol* 23:391, 1994.

61. Kamami YV: Outpatient treatment of sleep apnea syndrome with CO2 laser: laser-assisted UPPP, *J Otolaryngol* 23:395, 1994.

62. Kaplan J, Staats BA: Obstructive sleep apnea syndrome, *Mayo Clin Proc* 65:1087, 1990.

63. Katsantonis GP, Friedman WH: A surgical treatment of snoring: a patient's perspective, *Laryngoscope* 100:138, 1990.

64. Katsantonis GP, Miyazake S, Walsh JK: Effects of uvulopalatopharyngoplasty on sleep architecture and patterns of obstructed breathing, *Laryngoscope* 100:1068, 1990.

65. Katsantonis GP, Walsh JR: Further evaluation of uvulopalatoplasty in the treatment of obstructive sleep apnea symptoms, *Otolaryngol Head Neck Surg* 93:244, 1985.

66. Katsantonis GP and others: Nasopharyngeal complications following uvulopalatoplasty, *Laryngoscope* 97:309, 1987.

67. Kravath RE, Pollack CP: Hypoventilation during sleep in children who have lymphoid obstruction treated by nasopharyngeal tube and T & A, *Pediatrics* 59:865, 1977.

67a. Kribbs NB and others: Objective measurement of patterns of nasal CPAP use by patients with obstructive sleep apnea, *Am Rev Respir Dis* 147:887, 1993.

68. Krol RC, Knuth SL, Bartlett D Jr: Selective reduction in genioglossal muscle activity by alcohol in normal human subjects, *Am Rev Respir Dis* 129:247, 1984.

69. Kryger MH, Roth T, Dement WC: *Principles and practice of sleep medicine,* ed 2, Philadelphia, 1994, WB Saunders.

70. Lenders H, Schaefer J, Pirsig W: Turbinate hypertrophy in habitual snorers and patients with obstructive sleep apnea: findings of acoustic rhinometry, *Laryngoscope* 101:614, 1991.

71. Lopata OE: Mass loading sleep apnea and the pathogenesis of obesity hypoventilation, *Am Rev Respir Dis* 126:640, 1982.

72. Lowe AA: Dental *appliances for the treatment of snoring and obstructive sleep apnea.* In Kryger MH, Roth T, Dement WC, editors: *Principles and practice of sleep medicine,* ed 2, Philadelphia, 1994, WB Saunders.

73. Lowe AA and others: Three dimensional CT reconstructions of tongue

and airway in adult subjects with obstructive sleep apnea, *Am J Orthod Dentofac Orthop* 90:364, 1986.

74. Lugaresi E and others: *Snoring: pathogenic, clinical, and therapeutic aspects.* In Kryger MH, Roth T, Dement WC, editors: *Principles and practice of sleep medicine,* ed 2, Philadelphia, 1994, WB Saunders.

75. Lyons HA, Huang CT: Therapeutic use of progesterone in alveolar hypoventilation associated with obesity, *Am J Med* 44:881, 1968.

76. Moran WB, Orr WC, Fixley MS: Nonhypersomnolent patients with obstructive sleep apnea, *Otolaryngol Head Neck Surg* 92:608, 1984.

77. Motta J, Guilleminault C: *Effects of oxygen administration in sleep induced apneas.* In Guilleminault C, van den Hoed J, Mitler MM, editors: *Sleep apnea syndromes,* New York, 1978, Alan R Liss.

78. Nocturnal Oxygen Therapy Trial Group: Continuous or nocturnal oxygen therapy in hypoxemic chronic obstructive lung disease, *Ann Intern Med* 93:391, 1980.

79. National Commission on Sleep Disorders Research: *Wake up America: a national sleep alert,* vol 2, Washington, DC, 1993, U.S. Government Printing Office.

80. O'Leary MJ, Farrell G: Myocutaneous fenestration in sleep apnea patients, *Laryngoscope* 96:356, 1986.

81. Orr WC: Utilization of polysomnography in the assessment of sleep disorders, *Med Clin North Am* 69:1153, 1985.

82. Orr WC, Imes NK, Martin RJ: Progesterone therapy in obese patients with sleep apnea, *Arch Intern Med* 83:476, 1975.

83. Orr WC, Males JL, Imes NK: Myxedema and obstructive sleep apnea, *Am J Med* 70:1061, 1981.

84. Panje WR, Holmes DK: Mandibulectomy without reconstruction can cause sleep apnea, *Laryngoscope* 94:1591, 1984.

85. Partinen M, Guilleminault C: Daytime sleepiness and vascular morbidity at seven-year follow-up in obstructive sleep apnea patients, *Chest* 97:27, 1990.

86. Patton TJ, Thawley SE: Expansion hyoidplasty, *Laryngoscope* 93:1387, 1983.

87. Pelausa EO, Tarshis LM: Surgery for snoring, *Laryngoscope* 99:1006, 1989.

88. Piccirillo JF and others: Obstructive sleep apnea: treatment outcomes pilot study, *Otolaryngol Head Neck* 1997.

89. Piccirillo JF: Outcomes research and otolaryngology, *Otolaryngol Head Neck Surg* 111:764, 1994.

90. Powell NB, Guilleminault C, Riley RW: *Surgical therapy for obstructive sleep apnea.* In Kryger MH, Roth T, Dement WC, editors: *Principles and practice of sleep medicine,* ed 2, Philadelphia, 1994, WB Saunders.

91. Powell N, Guilleminault C: Mandibular advancement and obstructive sleep apnea syndrome, *Bull Eur Physiopathol Respir* 19:604, 1983.

92. Powell NB and others: Obstructive sleep apnea, continuous positive airway pressure, and surgery, *Otolaryngol Head Neck Surg* 99:362, 1988.

93. US Department of Health and Human Services: *Polysomnography and sleep disorder centers,* Rockville, Md, May 1992, AHCPR Pub No. 92-0027, Agency for Health Care Policy and Research.

94. Puchalski R, Piccirillo JF, Spitznagel EA: Clinical and patient-based factors in predicting the respiratory distress index, *Laryngoscope* (submitted for publication).

95. Rajagorpal KR, Bennett LL: Overnight nasal CPAP improves hypersomnolence in sleep apnea, *Chest* 90:172, 1986.

96. Remmers JE and others: Pathogenesis of upper airway occlusion during sleep, *J Appl Physiol* 44:931, 1978.

97. Riley RW, Powell NB, Guilleminault C: Obstructive sleep apnea and the hyoid: a revised surgical procedure, *Otolaryngol Head Neck Surg* 111:717, 1994.

98. Riley RW, Powell NB, Guilleminault C: Obstructive sleep apnea syndrome: a review of 306 consecutively treated surgical patients, *Otolaryngol Head Neck Surg* 108:117, 1993.

99. Riley RW, Powell NB, Guilleminault C: Maxillofacial surgery and

nasal CPAP. A comparison of treatment for obstructive sleep apnea syndrome, *Chest* 98:1421, 1990.

100. Riley RW, Powell NB, Guilleminault C: Inferior mandibular osteotomy and hyoid myotomy suspension for obstructive sleep apnea: a review of 55 patients, *J Oral Maxillofac Surg* 47:159, 1989.

101. Riley RW, Powell NB: Maxillary, mandibular, and hyoid advancement: an alternative to tracheotomy in obstructive sleep apnea syndrome, *Otolaryngol Head Neck Surg* 94:584, 1986.

102. Riley RW, Powell NB, Guilleminault C: Inferior sagittal osteotomy of the mandible with hyoid myotomy and suspension—a new procedure for obstructive sleep apnea, *Otolaryngol Head Neck Surg* 94:589, 1986.

103. Riley RW, Powell NB, Guilleminault C: Maxillofacial surgery and obstructive sleep apnea: a review of 80 patients, *Otolaryngol Head Neck Surg* 101:353, 1989.

104. Riley RW and others: Cephalometric analyses and flow-volume loops in obstructive sleep apnea patients, *Sleep* 6:303, 1983.

105. Rodgers GK, Chan KH, Dahl RE: Antral choanal polyp presenting as obstructive sleep apnea syndrome, *Arch Otolaryngol Head Neck Surg* 117:914, 1991.

106. Rojewski TE, Schuller DE, Clark RW: Videoendoscopic determination of the mechanism of obstruction in obstructive sleep apnea, *Otolaryngol Head Neck Surg* 92:127, 1984.

107. Rundell OH, Jones RK: Polysomnography methods and interpretations, *Otolaryngol Clin North Am* 23:583, 1990.

108. Ryan CF and others: Upper airway measurements predict response to uvulopalatopharyngoplasty in obstructive sleep apnea, *Laryngoscope* 100:248, 1990.

109. Sanders MH and others: Adequacy of prescribing positive airway pressure therapy by mask for sleep apnea on the basis of a partial-night trial, *Am Rev Respir Dis* 147:1169, 1993.

110. Sanders MH, Gruendl CA, Rogers RM: Patient compliance with nasal CPAP therapy for sleep apnea, *Chest* 90:330, 1986.

111. Sanders MH and others: The detection of sleep apnea in the awake patients: the saw tooth sign, *JAMA* 245:2414, 1981.

112. Sauerland EK, Orr WC, Hairston LE: EMG patterns of oropharyngeal muscles during respiration in wakefulness and sleep, *Electromyogr Clin Neurophysiol* 21:307, 1981.

113. Schechtman KB, Piccirillo JF, Sher AE: Methodological and statistical problems in sleep apnea research: the literature on uvulopalatopharyngoplasty, *Sleep* 18:659, 1996.

114. Schmidt-Nowara W and others: Oral appliances for the treatment of snoring and obstructive sleep apnea: a review, *Sleep* 18:501, 1995.

115. Series F, St. Pierre S, Carrier G: Effects of surgical correction of nasal obstruction in the treatment of obstructive sleep apnea, *Am Rev Respir Dis* 146:1261, 1992.

116. Shepard JW and others: Evaluation of the upper airway in patients with obstructive sleep apnea, *Sleep* 14:361, 1991.

117. Shepard JW: Pathophysiology and medical therapy of sleep apnea, *Ear Nose Throat J* 63:24, 1984.

118. Shepard JW: Cardiopulmonary consequences of obstructive sleep apnea, *Mayo Clin Proc* 65:1250, 1990.

119. Shepard JW, Olsen KD: Uvulopalatopharyngoplasty for treatment of obstructive sleep apnea, *Mayo Clin Proc* 65:1260, 1990.

120. Shepard JW and others: Evaluation of the upper airway by computerized tomography in patients undergoing uvulopalatopharyngoplasty for obstructive sleep apnea. Paper presented at the meeting of the American College of Chest Physicians, Dallas, October, 1984.

121. Shepard JW and others: Evaluation of the upper airway by computerized tomography in patients undergoing uvulopalatopharyngoplasty for obstructive sleep apnea, *Am Rev Respir Dis* 140:711, 1989.

122. Sher AE, Schechtman KB, Piccirillo JF: The efficacy of surgical modifications of the upper airway in adults with obstructive sleep apnea syndrome, *Sleep* 19:156, 1996.

123. Sher AE: Obstructive sleep apnea syndrome: a complex disorder of the upper airway, *Otolaryngol Clin North Am* 23:593, 1990.

124. Sher AE and others: Predictive value of the Mueller maneuver in selection of patients with uvulopalatopharyngoplasty, *Laryngoscope* 95:1483, 1985.

125. Simmons FB, Guilleminault C, Miles LE: The palatopharyngoplasty operation for snoring and sleep apnea: an interim report, *Otolaryngol Head Neck Surg* 92:375, 1984.

126. Simmons FB, Guilleminault C, Silvestri R: Snoring, and some obstructive sleep apnea, can be cured by oropharyngeal surgery, *Arch Otolaryngol* 109:503, 1983.

127. Simmons FB, Hochman M: Severity of obstructive sleep apnea, *Otolaryngol Head Neck Surg* 103:625, 1990.

128. Skatrud J and others: Disordered breathing during sleep in hypothyroidism, *Am Rev Respir Dis* 124:325, 1981.

129. Smith PL and others: The effects of protriptyline in sleep disordered breathing, *Am Rev Respir Dis* 127:8, 1983.

130. Strobl KP, Redline S: Nasal CPAP therapy, upper airway muscle activation, and obstructive sleep apnea, *Am Rev Respir Dis* 134:555, 1986.

131. Strollo PJ Jr, Rogers RM: Obstructive sleep apnea, *N Engl J Med* 334:99, 1995.

132. Sullivan CE, Issa EG, Berthon-Jones M: Reversal of obstructive sleep apnea by continuous positive airway pressure applied through the nares, *Lancet* 1:862, 1982.

133. Sullivan LW: The need for medical treatment effectiveness research, *JAMA* 226:3264, 1991.

134. Suratt PM and others: Fluoroscopic and computed tomographic features of the pharyngeal airway in obstructive sleep apnea, *Am Rev Respir Dis* 127:487, 1983.

135. Sutton JR and others: Effect of acetazolamide on hypoxemia during sleep at high altitude, *N Engl J Med* 301:1329, 1979.

136. Taasan VC and others: Alcohol increases sleep apnea and oxygen desaturation in asymptomatic men, *Am J Med* 71:240, 1981.

137. Thawley SE: Surgical treatment of obstructive sleep apnea, *Med Clin North Am* 69:1337, 1985.

138. Thawley SE, Shepard JW: Understanding of the sleep apnea syndrome: causes and treatment, *VA Practitioner* 2:60, 1985.

139. Tilkian AG and others: Hemodynamics in sleep induced apnea: studies during wakefulness and sleep, *Ann Intern Med* 85:714, 1976.

140. Tilkian AG and others: Sleep-induced apnea syndrome, *Am J Med* 63:348, 1977.

141. Tusiewicz K and others: Mechanics of the rib cage and diaphragm during sleep, *J Appl Physiol* 43:146, 1977.

142. Vaughan RW, Cork RC, Hollander D: The effect of massive weight loss on arterial oxygenation and pulmonary function tests, *Anesthesiology* 54:325, 1981.

142a. Viner S, Szalai JP, Hoffstein V: Are history and physical examination a good screening test for sleep apnea? *Ann Intern Med* 115:356, 1991.

143. Wagner DR, Pollack CP, Weitzman ED: Nocturnal nasal airway pressure for sleep apnea, *N Engl J Med* 308:461, 1983.

144. Waite PD and others: Maxillomandibular advancement surgery in 23 patients with obstructive sleep apnea, *J Oral Maxillofac Surg* 47:1256, 1989.

145. Walsh JK, Katsantonis GP: Somnofluoroscopy as a predictor of UPP efficacy, *Sleep Res* 13:21, 1984.

146. Weider DJ, Sateia MJ, West RP: Nocturnal enuresis in children with upper airway obstruction, *Otolaryngol Head Neck Surg* 105:427, 1991.

147. Weitzman ED, Kahn E, Pollack CP: Quantitative analysis of sleep and sleep apnea before and after tracheostomy in patients with the hypersomnia–sleep apnea syndrome, *Sleep* 3:407, 1980.

148. Wetmore SJ, Scrima S, Hiller FC: Sleep apnea in epistaxis patients treated with nasal packs, *Otolaryngol Head Neck Surg* 98:596, 1988.

149. Wetmore SJ and others: Postoperative uvulopalatopharyngoplasty, *Laryngoscope* 96:738, 1986.

150. White DP and others: Central sleep apnea: improvement with acetazolamide therapy, *Arch Intern Med* 142:1816, 1982.

151. Wickwire NA, White RP, Proffit WR: The effect of mandibular osteotomy on tongue position, *J Oral Surg* 30:184, 1972.

152. Woodson BT, Fujita S: Clinical experience with lingualplasty as part of the treatment of severe obstructive sleep apnea, *Otolaryngol Head Neck Surg* 107:40, 1992.

153. Young T and others: The occurrence of sleep-disordered breathing among middle-aged adults, *N Engl J Med* 328:1230, 1993.

154. Zohar Y and others: Uvulopalatopharyngoplasty: evaluation of postoperative complications, sequelae, and results, *Laryngoscope* 101:775, 1991.

Chapter 82

Odontogenesis and Odontogenic Cysts and Tumors

Peter E. Larsen
Arden K. Hegtvedt

Cysts and tumors derived from the odontogenic tissues constitute an unusually diverse group of lesions. This diversity reflects the complex development of the dental structures because these lesions all originate through some alteration from the normal pattern of odontogenesis. Some lesions included in this category may in fact not represent neoplasia at all, but are only minor alterations in the normal process of tooth development. Lesions such as cysts also are tumors only in the broadest sense of the word and do not represent true neoplasms.

The purpose of this chapter is to review the process of odontogenesis with emphasis on the potential origin of cells that produce the most common odontogenic cysts and tumors. Diagnostic modalities will be discussed with emphasis on the practical approach to development of a differential diagnosis. Common odontogenic cysts and tumors will be presented, and treatment approaches to various odontogenic cysts and tumors outlined.

ODONTOGENESIS[18,27]

The primitive oral cavity, also called the *stomodeum*, is lined with ectoderm. At its deepest portion it contacts the blind superior aspect of the foregut, which is lined with endoderm. The union of these ectodermal and endodermal layers is called the *buccopharyngeal membrane*. At approximately the twenty seventh day of development, this membrane ruptures and the stomodeum becomes connected with the foregut. The primitive oral cavity is therefore an ectodermal lined structure beneath which lies the ectomesenchyme. The mesenchyme of the head is termed *ectomesenchyme* because of its ectodermal origin from neural crest cells. This is distinct from the mesenchyme of the rest of the body, which is of mesodermal origin.

Each tooth develops from a tooth bud that forms from the lining of the oral cavity. The tooth bud consists of three separate parts: (1) the enamel organ, which is derived from the oral ectoderm; (2) the dental papilla, which is derived from the ectomesenchyme; and (3) the dental sac, which also is derived from the ectomesenchyme. The portion of the developing tooth known as the *enamel organ* produces tooth enamel, whereas the dental papilla produces the tooth pulp and dentin; the dental sac is the precursor of the cementum and periodontal ligament. Tooth development has been broken down into stages primarily based on morphologic changes of the tooth bud. These stages include: (1) the dental lamina stage, (2) the bud stage, (3) the cap stage, and (4) the bell stage.

Dental lamina and bud stage

About 2 or 3 weeks after the rupture of the buccopharyngeal membrane, when the embryo is about 6 weeks old, the first sign of tooth development is seen. Along the oral ectoderm a ridge of basal cells begin proliferation at a more rapid rate than those cells adjacent to them. This leads to formation of a band of epithelium that runs along the crest of what will be the future dental arches. This band of proliferating epithelium is called the *dental lamina*.

At certain points along the dental lamina, each representing a location of the 10 mandibular and 10 maxillary deciduous teeth, an even more rapid cellular proliferation is seen.

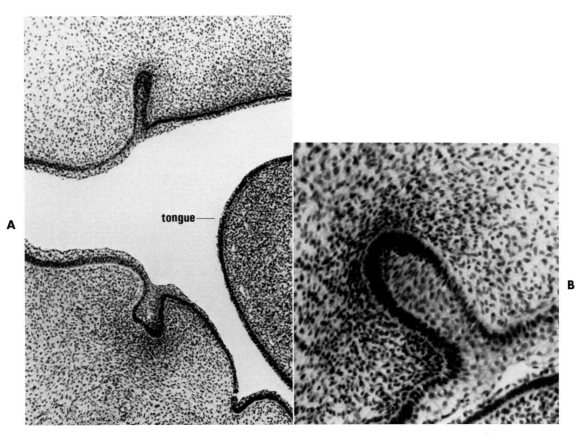

Fig. 82-1. Photomicrograph of a coronal section showing the bud stage of tooth development. **A,** Epithelial downgrowth along the dental lamina in the upper and lower jaws. **B,** A magnified view of the bud stage of development.

This further epithelial downgrowth and proliferation forms invaginations into the underlying ectomesenchymal tissue. These invaginations or buds represent the beginning of tooth development (Fig. 82-1).

Cap stage (proliferation)

As cellular proliferation continues, unequal growth occurs at various parts of the bud. A shallow depression occurs on the deep surface of the bud. Concomitant to this morphologic change in the developing bud, histologic differentiation occurs within the cells of the enamel organ. The single layer of the cuboidal cells lining the convexity of the enamel organ are known as the *outer enamel epithelium* and the more columnar cells along the concavity of the organ are called the *inner enamel epithelium.* As cells within the center of this epithelial enamel organ begin to separate because of an increase in intercellular fluid, they assume a more branched or reticular form. This area is now called the *stellate reticulum.* These changes within the enamel organ produce a figure reminiscent of a cap, hence the name given to this stage of development (Fig. 82-2).

While this differentiation is occuring within the enamel organ itself, changes within the associated ectomesenchyme

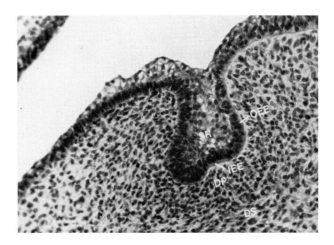

Fig. 82-2. Photomicrograph of a longitudinal section through a developing tooth showing the cap stage (proliferation) of development: *OEE,* outer enamel epithelium; *IEE,* inner enamel epithelium; *SR,* stellate reticulum; *DP,* dental papilla; *DS,* dental sac.

also occur. The portion of the ectomesenchyme that is partially surrounded by the proliferating inner enamel epithelium begins to condense, forming the dental papilla.

At the same time there is marginal condensation in the ectomesenchyme surrounding the enamel organ and the dental papilla. In this zone a denser and more fibrous layer gradually develops, forming the dental sac.

Bell stage (histodifferentiation and morphodifferentiation)

The differential growth of the epithelium into the underlying ectomesenchymal tissue continues, changing the form from a cap shape to a bell shape.

At this stage, the inner enamel epithelium consists of a single layer of columnar cells that further differentiates into tall columnar cells with oval nuclei that are polarized away from the basal lamina. These cells will become ameloblasts and be responsible for amelogenesis (enamel formation). These preameloblasts exert an organizing influence on the underlying ectomesenchymal cells of the dental papilla, causing them to begin differentiation into odontoblasts,

which will be responsible for forming the dentin of the developing tooth (Fig. 82-3).

By the time the primary tooth germ has reached the bell stage, other changes also are taking place. Lingual to the enamel organ of this primary tooth germ, the dental lamina is giving rise to the beginning of the enamel organ of the permanent tooth (Fig. 82-4). Concurrently, the dental lamina of the primary tooth begins to disintegrate. As the lamina breaks up, the cells that compose it either disappear or remain as small islands known as the *rest of Serres*.

Apposition

After differentiation of ameloblasts and odontoblasts is complete, apposition of the dental hard tissues begins. Dentinogenesis begins at approximately the fifth month *in utero*. Dentin formation begins as odontoblasts elaborate an eosinophilic material along the interface between the odontoblasts and ameloblasts. This material is predentin, which upon calcification forms dentin, the principal hard structure of the tooth. This dentin formation begins at the incisal region of the tooth and progresses toward the root.

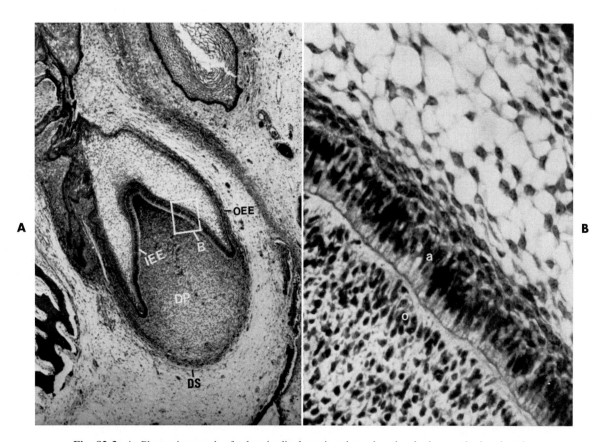

Fig. 82-3. A, Photomicrograph of a longitudinal section through a developing tooth showing the bell stage (histodifferentiation and morphodifferentiation) of development. The inner enamel epithelium has differentiated into columnar cells with polarized nuclei that will become ameloblasts *(a)*, and the ectomesenchymal cells within the dental papilla immediately adjacent to these developing ameloblasts are forming cuboidal cells that will become the odontoblasts *(o)*; IEE, inner enamel epithelium; OEE, outer enamel epithelium; DP, dental papilla; DS, dental sac. **B,** A magnified view of the developing ameloblasts and odontoblasts.

Amelogenesis or enamel formation begins immediately adjacent to the forming dentin and progresses toward the incisal edge. Similar to dentin formation, the first stage of enamel formation is the laying down of enamel as an organic material that subsequently undergoes calcification (Fig. 82-5). Normal amelogenesis relies on prior occurrence of normal dentinogenesis, hence the lack of enamel formation in odontogenic tumors such as ameloblastoma, where although normal-appearing ameloblasts are present, no odontoblasts or dentin formation is present to initiate enamel formation.

Root formation

After much of the crown formation has occurred, development of the root begins. The outer and inner enamel epithelia lie immediately adjacent to each other without an intervening stellate reticulum at the periphery of the developing tooth. These two layers together form Hertwig's epithelial root sheath, which grows into the surrounding connective tissue. Dentin formation continues toward the root of the tooth and is guided by this root sheath (Fig. 82-6). Root formation typically is complete 2 to 3 years after tooth eruption, at which time the root sheath breaks down and disappears with the exception of occasional epithelial remnants called the *rests of Malassez* (Fig. 82-7).

As the dentin grows downward into what will be the root of the tooth, the surrounding dental sac forms a thin calcified layer called *cementum* around the developing root; the dental sac also develops into connective tissue fibers that will become the periodontal ligament. On a radiograph of an unerupted and incompletely formed tooth, the dental sac is also called the *dental follicle*.

Eruption

As amelogenesis occurs, the layer of ameloblastic cells moves progressively closer to the outer enamel epithelium, squeezing the stellate reticulum in between. At the termination of crown development, the ameloblastic layer, the stellate reticulum, and the outer enamel epithelium will all essentially be fused and become known as the *reduced enamel*

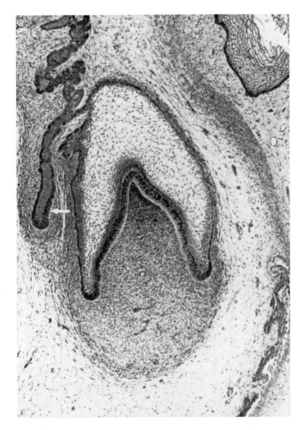

Fig. 82-4. Photomicrograph of a coronal section of developing permanent tooth lingual to the deciduous tooth *(arrow).*

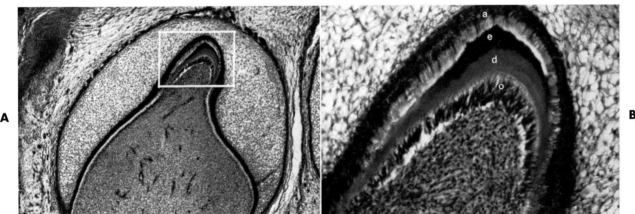

Fig. 82-5. A, Photomicrograph of a longitudinal section through a developing tooth during apposition of dentin and enamel. Apposition begins at the incisal tip and proceeds apically. **B,** Magnification of the area outlined showing the relationship of the ameloblasts *(a),* enamel *(e),* dentin *(d),* and odontoblasts *(o).*

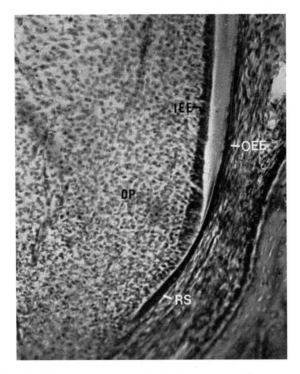

Fig. 82-6. Photomicrograph of a developing tooth. The outer enamel epithelium and inner enamel epithelium fuse and form the root sheath *(RS)*, which will determine the shape of the developing root. IEE, inner enamel epithelium; OEE, outer enamel epithelium; DP, dental papilla.

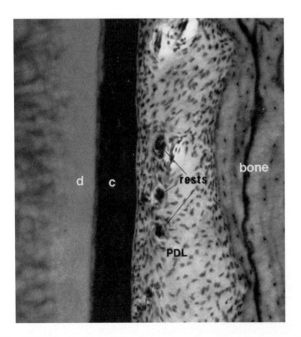

Fig. 82-7. Photomicrograph of a section along the root of a developed tooth. Note the relationship between the dentin *(d)* and cementum *(c)* forming the root and the adjacent periodontal ligament *(PDL)* and aveolar bone. Note the epithelial rests of Malassez within the periodontal ligament.

epithelium. This reduced enamel epithelium will remain around the developed crown until eruption of the tooth.

THE FORMATION OF ODONTOGENIC CYSTS AND TUMORS

The epithelium associated with odontogenic cysts and tumors is derived from one of the following sources (Fig. 82-8): (1) the reduced enamel epithelium of the tooth crown; (2) epithelial rests of Malassez, which are remnants of the Hertwig root sheath; (3) epithelial rests of Serres, which are remnants of the dental lamina; (4) the tooth germ itself, which includes the enamel organ, dental papilla, and dental sac. For example, an increased space between the crown of an unerupted tooth and the surrounding reduced enamel epithelium is frequently an early indication of cyst or tumor formation (Fig. 82-9).

In addition, some odontogenic tumors develop partially or entirely from cells of ectomesenchymal origin. The cellular origin for these lesions is either the dental papilla, the follicle, or the periodontal ligament.

CLASSIFICATION OF CYSTS AND TUMORS OF THE JAWS

Several systems have been devised for classifying cysts and tumors of the jaws. Some of these systems rely on morphologic differences between different lesions, either based on clinical or radiographic parameters, whereas others rely on histologic differences. Other systems categorize lesions totally on their etiology.[17,22] A modification of the World Health Organization (WHO) classification,[17] which divides cysts according to etiology is effective (Box 82-1). In this classification, the basic division is etiologic. A distinction is drawn between the autonomous development of the majority of cyst varieties and the inflammatory pathogenesis of the most common, the radicular cyst. This is preferable to classification based on histogenesis because opinions differ regarding the histology of several categories of cysts.

Unlike cysts, odontogenic tumors are most often classified according to their histogenesis. Tumors are either of epithelial, mesenchymal, or unknown origin. Tumors of epithelial origin are further classified into those that have a minimal inductive changes within the surrounding connective tissue. Lesions within this last group have in the past been called *mixed epithelial/mesenchymal tumors.*[21] This is incorrect because it is now believed that the neoplastic portion of the lesion is epithelial in nature and that this epithelium produces significant inductive changes within the connective tissue; this leads to the misconception that the connective tissue also is neoplastic. Box 82-2 outlines the classification of odontogenic tumors.

DIAGNOSIS

Clinical findings

The physical signs and symptoms of odontogenic cysts and tumors will depend to a certain extent on the dimensions of the lesion. A small lesion is unlikely to be diagnosed on a

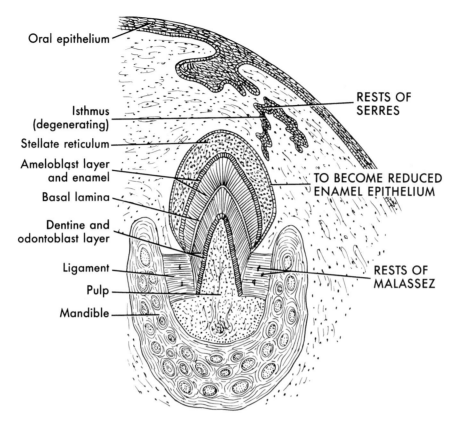

Fig. 82-8. Illustration showing the potential sources of odontogenic epithelium responsible for the formation of odontogenic cysts and tumors. Included are the rests of Serres, the rests of Malassez, and the reduced enamel epithelium.

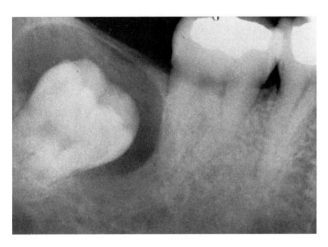

Fig. 82-9. Radiograph of an unerupted permanent tooth with increased space between the crown and reduced enamel epithelium that may be indicative of early cyst formation.

routine examination of the mouth because signs will not be demonstrable. Such lesions are only likely to be detected at an early stage as the result of routine radiographic examination. Exceptions are some early lesions that may present in conjunction with a devitalized tooth, which is detectable on clini-

cal examination. Some cystic lesions may become secondarily infected, leading to their diagnosis. Clinical absence of one or more teeth without the history of extraction also may be a clinical indicator of an undiagnosed odontogenic cyst or tumor because many of these lesions are associated with impacted or congenitally missing teeth (Fig. 82-10).

As the lesion grows, other indirect changes may occur. An enlarging lesion between two teeth can cause the crowns to converge and the roots to diverge (Fig. 82-11). Growth that is nearly undetectable visually may lead to difficulty with denture retention.

As the lesion enlarges even further, expansion of the bone may be seen directly. This is usually toward the buccal surface of the alveolar bone because this is the thinnes area and expansion occurs here most easily (Fig. 82-12). Clinically evident expansion is often a late finding, especially in lesions developing within the ramus or angle of the mandible or within the maxillary sinus. Lesions in these areas may become extremely large before expansion is observed clinically (Fig. 82-13).

Radiologic examination

Radiographic appearance of various odontogenic cysts and tumors varies considerably from lesion to lesion, with certain lesions having almost a pathognomonic appearance,

Box 82-1. Classification of jaw cysts

A. Developmental
   1. Odontongenic
      a. Follicular cyst
      b. Odontogenic keratocyst
      c. Eruption cyst
      d. Alveolar cyst of infants
      e. Gingival cyst of adults
      f. Developmental lateral periodontal cyst
   2. Nonodontogenic
      a. Nasopalatine duct cust
      b. Midpalatal cyst of infants
      c. Nasolabial cyst
      d. Globulomaxillary cyst, median mandibular cyst, and median alveolar cyst*
B. Inflammatory
      a. Radicular cyst
         1) Periapical cyst
         2) Inflammatory lateral periodontal cyst
C. Nonepithelial†
      a. Idiopathic bone cavity (traumatic, solitary, hemorrhagic bone cyst)
      b. Aneurysmal bone cyst
      c. Stafne's mandibular lingual cortical defect

* These cysts were previously regarded as developmental nonodontogenic cysts. This is no longer believed to be true, and this category is no longer used; it is of historical interest only.
† These lesions are often classified as cysts but do not have a distinct epithelial lining.

Box 82-2. Classification of odontogenic tumors

A. Benign epithelial odontogenic tumors
   1. Tumors producing minimal inductive change in the connective tissue
      a. Ameloblastoma
      b. Calcifying epithelial odontogenic tumor (Pindborg tumor)
      c. Odontogenic adenomatoid tumor (adenoameloblastoma, adenomatoidodontogenic tumor)
      d. Calcifying odontogenic cyst (Gorlin's cyst)
   2. Tumors producing extensive inductive change in the connective tissue
      a. Ameloblastic fibroma
      b. Ameloblastic fibroodontoma
      c. Ameloblastic odontoma (odontoameloblastoma)
      d. Odontoma
         1) Compound-composite odontoma
         2) Complex odontoma
B. Mesenchymal odontogenic tumors
   1. Odontogenic fibroma
   2. Odontogenic myxoma
   3. Cementoma
      a. Periapical cemental dysplasia
      b. Cementifying fibroma
      c. Benign cementoblastoma
   4. Dentinoma
C. Tumors of unknown origin
   1. Melanotic neuroectodermal tumor of infancy
D. Malignant odontogenic tumors
   1. Primary intraosseous carcinoma
   2. Ameloblastic fibrosarcoma
   3. Ameloblastic dentinosarcoma
   4. Ameloblastic odontosarcoma

whereas the only consistent thing about the appearance of other lesions is the total lack of any consistent radiographic presentation. The common lack of physical findings and the development of the majority of these lesions within the confines of bone makes the radiologic investigation and interpretation uniquely important. The radiographic appearance of various lesions will be discussed more completely as each individual lesion is described. There are some general principles that can be applied to the radiographic diagnosis of cysts and tumors of the jaws. This section will address these principles.

For a radiograph to provide useful information, it must be of good quality. Artifacts caused by inappropriate placement of film labels, patient jewelry, movement, or poor technique can mask the presence of a lesion.

Radiographs also are important in treatment planning for surgical removal of odontogenic lesions. Encroachment on vital structures, extent into soft tissue, size of the lesion, and requirements for reconstruction can all be evaluated. This will be more completely discussed in the section on treatment of cysts and tumors.

Various radiographic modalities are available for use in evaluating cysts and tumors of the jaws. Many lesions are detected on routine intraoral radiographs taken for screening purposes or for evaluation of other dental disease such as

caries. Because intraoral radiographs such as the periapical or bite-wing radiograph are most often used, this screening may be the first opportunity to evaluate an asymptomatic lesion. Intraoral radiographs have the advantage of providing excellent detail because the film-to-object distance is small and the film is placed intraorally immediately adjacent to the involved bone. This eliminates the overlying osseous structures often seen in routine extraoral head and neck radiographs. The major disadvantage is the lack of availability of these radiographs outside a dental office, their size limitations, and their inability to evaluate the areas that are not accessible to film placement; these are the ramus, condyle, and inferior border of the mandible Fig. 82-14 demonstrates how a subtle change on an intraoral radiograph can lead to diagnosis of a large intraosseous lesion. Perhaps the most useful intraoral radiograph, one for which there is no good extraoral substitute, is the occlusal radiograph. This is taken with a larger film that the standard periapical or bite-wing. For lesions in the anterior maxillary alveolus and palate, there is no adequate substitute (Fig. 82-15).

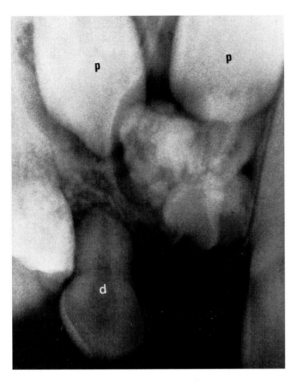

Fig. 82-10. An odontoma has formed leading to delayed eruption of the permanent tooth *(p)* and retention of the deciduous tooth *(d)*.

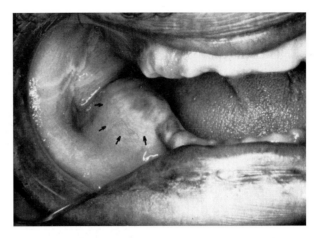

Fig. 82-12. Clinical photograph of buccal expansion resulting from growth of an odontogenic tumor in the body of the mandible *(arrows)*.

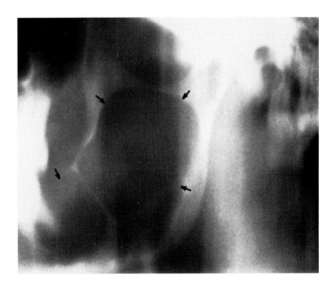

Fig. 82-13. Clinical expansion is difficult to detect in the ramus and angle region allowing large lesions to develop before detection. This radiograph shows a large odontogenic cyst in the ramus of the mandible that was not associated with any facial swelling *(arrows)*.

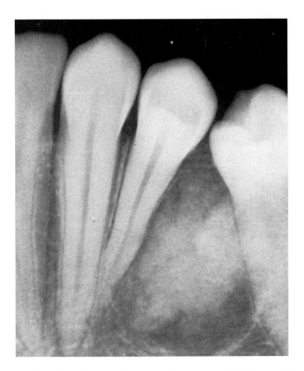

Fig. 82-11. An odontogenic tumor has caused clinically evident convergence of the crowns of adjacent teeth; the radiograph shows the resulting root of divergence.

Extraoral radiographs often are necessary for delineation of the entire lesion. They are useful in showing the extent of the lesion and its effect on adjacent structures. These radiographs also serve as a screening mechanism should multiple lesions be present. The panoramic radiograph is the most useful examination. It effectively shows the entire mandible including the ramus and condyle, the maxilla and maxillary sinuses, and the dentition. To reproduce this with other types of radiographs may require multiple views. The panoramic radiograph is actually a pantomogram. It makes use of the radiographic technique of tomography in which a collimated radiation source, and the film are rotated around the patient's head in opposite directions. This results in blur-

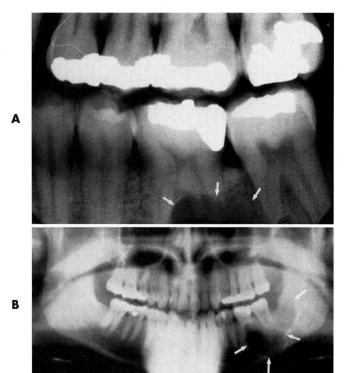

Fig. 82-14. A, A subtle change on this intraoral dental film *(arrows)* lead to the diagnosis of **B,** this large ameloblastoma.

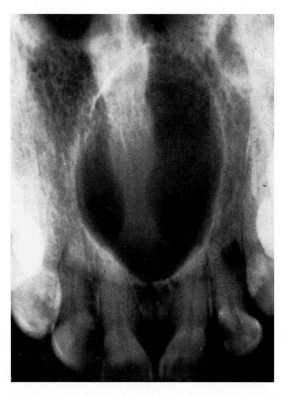

Fig. 82-15. Occlusal films are the only good method of evaluating lesions of the hard palate due to the bony overlap seen with other techniques. This is a nasopalatine duct cyst.

ring of structures on either side of a predetermined focal trough and has the advantage of eliminating much of the surrounding osseous interference that is seen with plain radiographs. However, this advantage also is a source of one of the major problems of the panoramic radiograph, which is that only structures within the focal trough are registered. This area of optimal focus is minimally adjustable and varies from machine to machine. It is possible that a lesion, even a rather large one, be incompletely visualized if it is outside the focal trough (Fig. 82-16). If a lesion is suspected on panoramic radiograph, an additional radiograph should be taken in the sagittal plane to help delineate any lateral and medial expansion that may be present. The panoramic radiograph also has the disadvantage of requiring the patient to remain still and in a sitting position for several seconds. This may not be possible in the debilitated, mentally retarded, or young patient.

Other extraoral films may be used to evaluate the lesion further or as a substitute when the panoramic radiograph is not possible. For mandibular lesions, the lateral oblique radiograph will allow the body, angle, ramus, and condyle

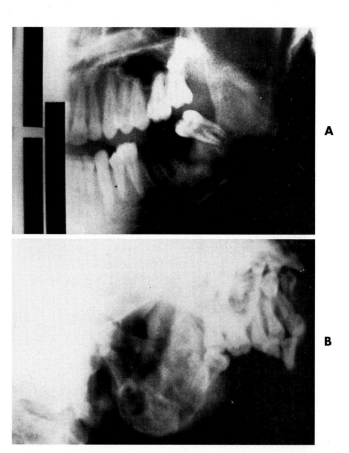

Fig. 82-16. A, Panoramic radiograph that appears essentially normal despite the large osseous lesion in the body of the mandible, which is shown on the lateral oblique film, **B,** This is caused when the object of importance is outside the focal trough.

to be seen. The parasymphysis and symphysis is often difficult to see because of overlying dentition and bone from the contralateral side. The teeth are also difficult to identify because teeth from the ipsilateral maxilla and the contralateral mandible and maxilla may overlie each other. For examination of maxillary cysts and tumors, the Waters view is very helpful as a screening tool. Maxillary lesions are difficult to delineate even on the best plain films; computed tomography (CT) may be necessary.

CT is not a cost-effective method of evaluating most routine odontogenic cysts and tumors. There are certain indications for the use of CT scans. For example, CT is helpful in defining the extent of very large lesions, especially if there is significant distortion of normal anatomy, which makes plain radiographs difficult to evaluate. CT can also be used to determine if the lesion is contained entirely within the involved bone, or if it has eroded through the cortex. Although malignant odontogenic tumors are extremely rare, some benign cysts and tumors behave aggressively and tend to have high recurrence rates, especially if they have perforated through cortical bone and into adjacent soft tissue; CT is extremely valuable in treatment planning for the removal of such lesions (Fig. 82-17).

Differential diagnosis

Once adequate clinical and radiographic examination is complete and before a biopsy has been performed, a differential diagnosis should be formulated. This should take into account information from both the clinical and radiologic examination, but because of the limited clinical findings associated with most odontogenic cysts and tumors, this is primarily a radiographic differential.

Much can be learned about the behavior of an odontogenic cyst or tumor by paying close attention to the radiograph. Benign, slow-growing lesions tend to cause tooth movement, blunting of the roots of teeth, displacement of vital structures such as nerves and vessels, and bony hard expansion with intact cortical bone. These lesions are usually well circumscribed by a radiopaque border (Fig. 82-18). Aggressive, fast-growing, or malignant lesions tend to resorb bone around the roots of teeth and not cause tooth movement. The teeth themselves are of such increased hardness in comparison to the surrounding bone that fast-growing lesions do not have time to cause resorption of the roots before the lesion is detected. Fast-growing and aggressive lesions also tend to resorb cortical bone and spread into soft tissue without significant cortical expansion. They also are poorly delineated radiographically without much cortical bone along the periphery of the lesion (Fig. 82-19).

From a radiographic approach, a simplified method of grouping these lesions is by some common radiographic findings. Each specific radiographic appearance may be associated with several different lesions, some of which are odontogenic in origin, some of which are not, but significant reduction in the number of different lesions that must be considered in a given differential is possible by grouping lesions according to their radiographic appearance. Other clinical findings such as age, sex, symptoms if any, and so

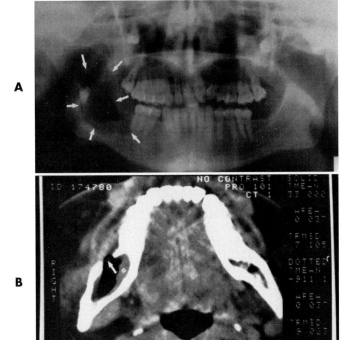

Fig. 82-17. A, The large cystic lesion in the right mandibular ramus is shown on this panoramic radiograph *(arrows).* **B,** Computed tomography allows visualization of the perforation of the lateral cortex by the lesion *(arrow).*

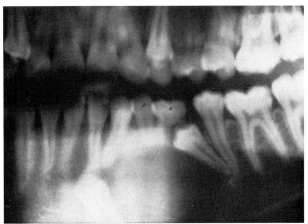

Fig. 82-18. Typical radiographic appearance of a benign lesion with blunting of tooth roots, displacement of teeth, a sclerotic, well-circumscribed border, and displacement of the inferior alveolar nerve.

on, can be used to further narrow the differential beyond what is possible radiographically. The classic radiographic presentations are radiolucent lesions, radiopaque lesions, and mixed radiopaque/radiolucent lesions. Within the purely radiolucent group, there are several subclassifications according to location and appearance of the lesion. In an attempt to facilitate the development of a differential diagnosis, the most common lesions occurring in the jaws have been categorized according to their radiographic appearance in Box 82-3. This list includes some nonodontogenic processes, which must also be considered in the differential.

Biopsy

Perhaps the simplest biopsy technique for intraosseous lesions of the jaws is aspiration. Although no tissue is obtained with aspiration, it is a biopsy in the broadest sense of the word. Aspiration can yield extremely valuable information about the nature of the lesion, yet it causes little patient discomfort. It may be done as a procedure itself or as a prelude to incisional or excisional biopsy. A radiolucent lesion that yields straw-colored fluid on aspiration is most likely to be a cystic lesion. If pus is aspirated, an inflammatory or infectious process should be considered. White keratin-containing fluid is indicative of an odontogenic keratocyst, whereas air may indicate a traumatic bone cavity. The inability to aspirate (vacuum within the syringe) is usually indicative of a solid process such as a neoplasm. Blood on aspiration could represent several lesions, the most important of which is the vascular malformation. The most common presentation of high-flow vascular lesions of the jaws is exsanguination or near-exsanguinating hemorrhage associated with a simple procedure such as biopsy of an innocuous asymptomatic radiolucency. For this reason, all radiolucent lesions should be aspirated before a biopsy is performed.

Whether to perform an incisional or excisional biopsy

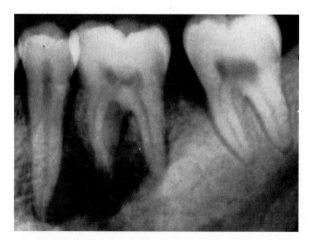

Fig. 82-19. Typical radiographic appearance of an aggressive lesion that has resorbed bone around teeth without displacement, has an ill-defined margin, and no sclerotic border.

Box 82-3. Radiographic presentation

I. Radiolucent Lesion of the Jaws
   A. Lesions at the apex of the tooth
      1. Dental granuloma
      2. Periapical cyst (inflammatory)
      3. Residual cyst
      4. Periapical (dental) abscess
      5. Cementoma (first stage)
      6. Odontogenic keratocyst
   B. Lesions in the midline of the maxilla
      1. Median palatine cyst
      2. Nasopalatine duct cyst (incisive canal)
   C. Lesion around the crown of an impacted tooth
      1. Follicular cyst
      2. Ameloblastoma
      3. Ameloblastic fibroma
      4. Odontogenic adenomatoid tumor
      5. Odontogenic myxoma
      6. Odontogenic keratocyst
   D. Soap-bubble-like radiolucencies
      1. Multilocular cyst
      2. Aneurysmal bone cyst
      3. Ameloblastoma
      4. Odontogenic myxoma
      5. Central giant-cell granuloma
      6. Odontogenic keratoycyst
   E. Lesions that destroy the cortical plate
      1. Metastatic tumor
      2. Primary malignant tumor
      3. Osteomyelitis
   F. Miscellaneous radiolucent lesions
      1. Lateral periodontal cyst
      2. Idiopathic bone marrow cavity
      3. Hematopoietic marrow
      4. Gingival cyst
      5. Hemangioma (central)
      6. Osteoporosis
      7. Stafne's bone cavity
II. Radiopaque Lesions of the Jaws
      1. Cementoma (third stage)
      2. Compound or complex odontoma
      3. Ossifying fibroma
      4. Osteoma
      5. Torus
      6. Root fragment or foreign body
      7. Focal sclerosing osteomyelitis
      8. Osteogenic sarcoma
      9. Chondrosarcoma
      10. Metastatic tumor
      11. Paget's disease
III. Mixed Radiolucent/Radiopaque Lesions of the Jaws
      1. Cementoma (second stage)
      2. Cystic odontoma
      3. Ossifying fibroma
      4. Adenomatoid odontogenic tumor
      5. Calcifying epithelial odontogenic tumor (Pindborg)
      6. Calcifying odontogenic cyst (Gorlin)
      7. Ameloblastic fibroodontoma
      8. Ameloblastic odontoma
      9. Osteogenic sarcoma
      10. Chondrosarcoma

initially is not always clear. Most odontogenic cysts and tumors are benign, and definitive treatment may be as simple as obtaining an excisional biopsy. However, there are some lesions that are more aggressive and require extensive curettage or marginal resection, and it is desirable to know this before the onset of surgery.

Indications for excisional biopsy include small, radiographically benign lesions that are readily accessible and can be removed without encroachment on adjacent structures. In cases where the access is more invasive than the surgical removal of the lesion itself, complete excision at the initial biopsy is preferred, even if the lesion is relatively large. This would include lesions in the mandibular condyle and lesions in young patients for whom a general anesthetic is required for any surgical intervention, even for incisional biopsy. Incisional biopsy is indicated in large lesions and in lesions suspected of aggressive behavior so that a definitive diagnosis can be made before treatment is instituted.

CLINICAL, RADIOGRAPHIC, AND HISTOLOGIC FEATURES OF COMMON ODONTOGENIC CYSTS

The more classic description of a cyst is that it is an epithelial-lined sac filled with fluid or semifluid material.[11] All odontogenic cysts fit this description, but certain nonepithelial cysts commonly included with odontogenic cysts do not. Because of this, a broader definition has been accepted. A cyst is a pathologic cavity having fluid, semifluid, or gaseous contents that are not created by the accumulation of pus; frequently, but not always, it is lined by epithelium.[12]

For the purpose of discussion and to simplify development of a differential diagnosis, this section will present a brief overview of each common cyst, its clinical and radiographic presentation, and recommended treatment. Because the histopathology of jaw cysts is confusing and the terminology is not always used consistently by general pathologists, these lesions are frequently misdiagnosed or incorrectly named, which can lead to improper treatment. Lesions that are frequently misdiagnosed will have special mention with regard to histopathology.

Lesions will be categorized according to the classification outlined previously. The more common inflammatory cysts will be described first, followed by the developmental odontogenic and nonodontogenic cysts, and lastly, the nonepithelial cysts.

Inflammatory cysts

Inflammatory cysts make up 85% of the cysts found in the jaws.[10] This high frequency is the result of the prevalence of dental disease, which frequently initiates the process. Inflammatory cysts result after bacterial invasion of the dental pulp leads to a chronic low-grade infection that results in a periapical granuloma around the root of the tooth. The normally quiescent epithelial cell rests of Malassez, which are within the periodontal ligament, are activated and proliferate to surround the granuloma, leading to cyst formation. These

cysts then grow by mechanisms that are not clearly defined to produce the inflammatory cyst associated with the root of the involved tooth, hence appropriately named *radicular cyst*. When the cyst is associated with the apex of the tooth root, it is called a *periapical cysts;* when it is along the side of the root, it is called a *lateral periodontal cyst.*

Periapical cyst

The periapical cyst is well recognized as the cystic lesion most likely encountered.

Clinical features. The majority of these lesions are asymptomatic. The associated tooth is nonvital and may have evidence of the source of the initial offending infection such as large unrestored decay, a large filling, or a history of pain in the tooth in the past.

Radiographic features. The radiographic presentation is fairly consistent. It is usually a radiolucent area of variable size attached to the root apex. The radiolucency is usually rounded or oval and surrounded by a radiopaque sclerotic bony periphery (Fig. 82-20).

Histology. The cyst is lined by stratified squamous epithelium. Pseudostratified ciliated columnar epithelium also may be seen in lesions occurring near the maxillary sinus. The thickness of the lining usually varies, and it seldom exhibits keratin formation.

Treatment. Treatment requires only that the source of infection be treated. This involves endodontic therapy (root canal) of the tooth to remove the necrotic pulpal tissue or extraction of the tooth. The lesion will generally resolve after this but should be followed radiographically and enucleated if it enlarges or fails to resolve.

Lateral inflammatory periodontal cyst

The lateral inflammatory periodontal cyst is less common than the periapical cyst. When the radicular cyst forms around an opening between the pulp and the periodontal

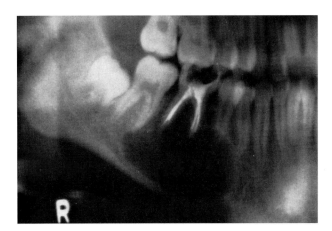

Fig. 82-20. Radiographic appearance of an inflammatory periapical cyst that is secondary to decay with failed root canal therapy in the associated tooth.

ligament that is along the lateral aspect of the tooth instead of at the apex, a lateral inflammatory periodontal cyst is produced.

Clinical features. These lesions are clinically asymptomatic except for the associated nonvital tooth.

Radiographic features. These lesions usually are small, well-circumscribed radiolucencies associated with the lateral aspect of the tooth root. There may be signs of previous tooth injury such as dental decay or large restoration of the tooth.

Treatment. Treatment is the same as for periapical cysts.

Developmental odontogenic cysts

Developmental odontogenic cysts account for 10% of all cysts of the jaws. The odontogenic keratocyst and the follicular cyst account for 8%, whereas all other developmental odontogenic cysts account for the other 2%.[29] Emphasis will be placed on the two most common lesions in this group.

Follicular cyst

This cyst also has been called a *dentigerous cyst* because of its association with the crown of unerupted teeth, but as other types of cysts also can be found around the crowns of unerupted teeth, the term *follicular cyst* is more correct because of the suspected development of the lesion from the follicle of the tooth. This cyst is most frequently identified in the mandible and is associated with the completed crown of an unerupted or impacted tooth. The cyst is thought to originate from accumulation of fluid between the reduced enamel epithelium and the completed tooth crown (see Fig. 82-9). Its incidence is the same in both sexes and is most common in childhood and adolescence. The growth rate may be rapid, with lesions growing up to 5 cm in diameter in 3 to 4 years.

Clinical features. Follicular cysts may get large before they are diagnosed, and facial swelling may be the first clinical sign. They are always associated with an unerupted or impacted tooth, most commonly the mandibular or maxillary third molar or maxillary canine.

Radiographic features. The follicular cyst appears as a radiolucent area within the jaw and is in some way associated with an unerupted tooth crown. It is usually a well-circumscribed lesion that is unilocular and has a sclerotic bony border. There may be significant expansion of the cortical plate and displacement of tooth roots or the inferior alveolar canal. The cyst may cause displacement of the associated tooth, sometimes for a large distance (Fig. 82-21).

Histology. The follicular cyst typically has a thin connective tissue wall that is lined by a thin layer of stratified squamous epithelium within the lumen (Fig. 82-22). Hyaline bodies frequently are found within the epithelial lining, as well as clefts from cholesterol crystals. Some cysts also may have mucous cells within the lining, which is of importance when considering the possibility that other lesions may develop within the wall or lumen of a follicular cyst. The lesions that may develop within the cyst arise from the actual

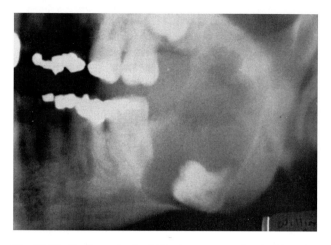

Fig. 82-21. Radiograph of a follicular cyst associated with an impacted third molar tooth. The lesion is large and has caused significant displacement of the associated tooth.

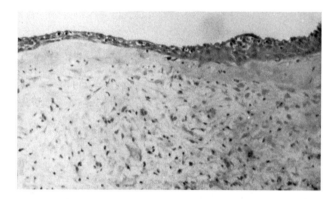

Fig. 82-22. Photomicrograph of the lining of a follicular cyst. Note the difference between this appearance and that of the odontogenic keratocyst (see Fig. 82-23).

epithelial lining or from rests of odontogenic epithelium that are in the connective tissue around the cyst. Odontogenic tumors such as the ameloblastoma frequently arise from the lining of the follicular cyst. Less common but of importance is the occurrence of epidermoid carcinoma arising from the lining of a follicular cyst or of mucoepidermoid carcinoma arising from the mucous glands within the wall of the cyst. This is the suspected origin of most intraosseous mucoepidermoid carcinomas.

Treatment. Treatment depends on the size of the lesion, but enucleation and curettage is adequate. For large lesions, decompression to allow some decrease in size is possible but the lesion should ultimately be treated with enucleation and curettage to allow histologic evaluation of the entire lesion and to prevent recurrence.

Odontogenic keratocyst

The odontogenic keratocyst is so named because of its characteristic histologic appearance. Clinically and radiographically it may appear as a follicular cyst associated with the crown of an unerupted tooth. It also may appear associated with the root of a tooth as a radicular cyst or by itself. When it occurs by itself, it is frequently called a *primordial cyst,* which is a cyst that arises where there is no apparent tooth formation associated. Virtually all primordial cysts have the histologic appearance of an odontogenic keratocyst. The odontogenic keratocyst is thought to develop from the remnants of the dental lamina, which are the rests of Seres.[9,16]

Clinical features. The odontogenic keratocyst may occur in many clinical situations. It may appear at any age but is rare in those less than 10 years of age. The peak incidence is in the second and third decades, and there is a predilection for males of 1.8 : 1. Anatomically the mandible is affected more frequently than the maxilla with 75% of the lesions occurring there. The third molar and ramus areas are the most frequently involved, with the first and second molar areas following. No clinical presentation is specific. The patient may be asymptomatic until gradual expansion is noted or until a secondary infection occurs.

Radiographic features. The odontogenic keratocyst may be identified in a variety of anatomic locations. The majority of the lesions are present in the third molar and ramus area of the mandible. The cyst itself may have several radiologic variations. Approximately 50% of these cysts have a unilocular appearance, but a multiocular appearance can occur. As already mentioned, the diagnosis of odontogenic keratocyst is a histologic one, and the cyst may have several radiographic appearances such as of a follicular or radicular cyst. The lesion is slow growing and usually will be well circumscribed with a sclerotic border. Teeth may be displaced, and cortical perforation may be more common than in other cystic lesions.

Histology. Specific histologic criteria exist for diagnosis of a keratocyst (Fig. 82-23). These include: (1) a thin, stratified squamous epithelium that is a uniform 6 to 8 cells thick, without rete ridge formation; (2) prominent columnar or cuboidal basal cell layer with dense nuclear staining; (3) a corrugated surface layer of parakeratin or orthokeratin; and (4) a thin, connective tissue wall. The lumenal material may vary from a straw-colored clear substance to a creamy white keratin-filled material. The importance of the histologic diagnosis is that an untrained pathologist may mistake the odontogenic keratocyst for a simple follicular cyst. The recurrence rate for these lesions is much higher, and this misdiagnosis may lead to improper treatment.

Treatment. As mentioned previously, distinguishing the odontogenic keratocyst from other odontogenic cysts is important because of its higher recurrence rate. Recurrence rates from 10% to 60% have been reported. The large difference in rate of recurrence may be related to inconsistencies in reporting of the data and inadequate follow-up because these lesions can take many years to recur. In a recent review of 426 patients, a composite recurrence rate of 34% was seen.[32] This is consistent with other well-documented reports

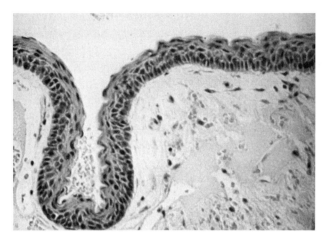

Fig. 82-23. Photomicrograph of an odontogenic keratocyst. Note the uniformly thin epithelial layer 6 to 8 cells thick with a corrugated surface layer of perakeratin. The basal cells are prominent and cuboidal and the underlying connective tissue is thin.

citing recurrence rates of 33%[19] and 44%,[28] respectively. The high incidence of recurrence is possibly due to several factors: (1) some lesions are multilocular, making complete removal difficult; (2) the cyst lining is thin and friable, which makes it easy to leave fragments behind during enucleation; (3) odontogenic keratocysts have been shown to have a higher mitotic rate than other cysts, which may make any residual epithelium more likely to proliferate and lead to recurrence; (4) the cyst itself may have areas of epithelial budding that are left behind during enucleation; (5) as these lesions tend to perforate cortical bone more frequently, cystic epithelium may be located in the soft tissue from where it is more difficult to completely remove it; and (6) the lesion is often clinically mistaken for more benign cysts and treated less aggressively, only to have the diagnosis of keratocyst rendered after treatment is complete.[29]

Treatment consists of enucleation and curettage. If the lesion is large, decompression with subsequent enucleation is advantageous.[31] In the case of the odontogenic keratocyst, this is particularly useful because even after a short period of exposure to the oral cavity by temporary decompression, the lining epithelium of the cyst cavity undergoes a thickening and the fibrous connective tissue thickens as well. This makes removal easier and decreases the chance of leaving remnants of epithelium behind. It has been shown that if the cystic lining can be removed in one piece, the incidence of recurrence is small; however, if the lining is removed in fragments, the incidence of recurrence is greater than 50%.[4] If a wedge of tissue is removed from the mucosa overlying the cyst, the potential source of other lesions may be removed.[26] Once the lesion has been enucleated, aggressive curettage of the bony walls with rotary instruments is recommended. Others have used chemical or cryotherapy modalities to further remover any remaining epithelium, but data proving that this is helpful is inadequate. If the lesion recurs, especially if it is located in the posterior mandible or maxilla, more aggressive treatment, such as marginal resection, may be indicated.

Special considerations. If multiple keratocysts are found, suspicion should be high for basal cell nevus syndrome (Gorlin's syndrome).[6,7] Patients with this syndrome also exhibit skeletal anomalies such as calcified falx, bifid ribs, fused vertebrae, and scoliosis. They also have soft-tissue aberrations such as multiple basal cell carcinomas, even in young patients and in non–sun-exposed areas; palmar pitting; and epidermoid cysts. Patients have a characteristic facies of frontal and temporoparietal bossing of the skull, well-developed supraorbital ridges, and ocular hypertelorism.

The remaining developmental odontogenic cysts only account for 2% of all jaw cysts, making their clinical significance relatively low. Some of them can present an unusual clinical picture, and they deserve some review.

Eruption cyst

The eruption cyst is generally recognized as the soft-tissue analogue of the follicular cyst. It is entirely within the soft tissue and does not usually produce any radiographic change. The cyst will generally undergo spontaneous rupture and resolution without any treatment. The clinical appearance is that of a smooth, tense, dark blue or purple swelling over the crown of an erupting tooth (Fig. 82-24). The lesion may cause some alarm for the parent and also may be symptomatically painful. If symptomatic, a portion of the sac can be excised leading to resolution of the symptoms.

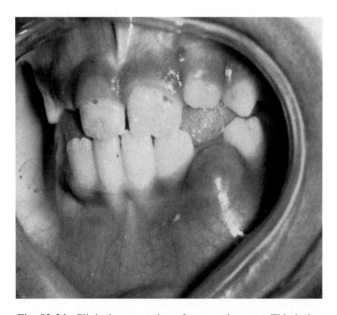

Fig. 82-24. Clinical presentation of an eruption cyst. This lesion may be confused with lesions that need biopsy or surgical removal. Treatment is observation.

Alveolar cyst of infants

These small cysts also are known as *dental lamina cysts of the newborn*. The correct term is *alveolar cyst of infants,* and they are small discrete white swellings located on the crest of the alveolus in newborns. These small soft-tissue cystic lesions arise from the dental lamina. They are asymptomatic, require no treatment, and will resolve spontaneously.

Gingival cyst of adults

The gingival cyst (called the *gingival cyst of adults* to distinguish it from the alveolar cyst of infants) is an uncommon soft-tissue lesion. The term is used to identify a cyst that occurs in either the attached or unattached gingival tissue. It is believed to originate in the dental lamina. It occurs at any age but is much more common in patients over the age of 40. It occurs most commonly in the cuspid-bicuspid region of the mandible. The cyst is typically asymptomatic and presents as a localized swelling in the involved area. There is usually no radiographic evidence and no tendency for recurrence after excisional biopsy, which is the treatment of choice.

Developmental lateral periodontal cyst

This is the developmental counterpart of the inflammatory periodontal cyst. The cyst develops from epithelial rests of Malassez, but pulpal necrosis of the tooth is not the initiating factor. These lesions occur primarily in adults and local excision is the treatment of choice. Recurrence is rare.

Developmental nonodontogenic cyst

The remaining 5% of cysts within the jaws are made up of nondontogenic cysts. Developmental nonodontogenic cysts within the jaws must arise from epithelium not associated with tooth development. In the past, several entities were described as fissural cysts because they were suspected to have arisen from tissue entrapped during fusion across various fissures during facial development. It has now been clearly shown that the only true fissural cyst is the midpalatal cyst of infants. Other so-called fissural cysts such as the globulomaxillary cyst, the median alveolar cyst, and the median mandibular cyst are most likely to be developmental or inflammatory odontogenic cysts.[17,22,33] The other two lesions within this category are the nasopalatine duct cyst, which arises from the cystic degeneration of the vestigule bilateral oronasal ducts, and the nasolabial cyst, which is a soft-tissue cyst arising from dystopic rests of the nasolacrimal ducts.

Nasopalatine duct cyst

The nasopalatine duct cyst, also known as the *incisive canal cyst* is formed from cystic degeneration of the oronasal ducts that connect the nasal cavity to the oral cavity during development. It is the most common nonodontogenic developmental cyst. The nasopalatine duct cyst is usually asymptomatic and is discovered on routine radiographic investigation. It also may become secondarily infected leading to rapid enlargement and pain. The cyst appears as a round to ovoid or heart-shaped radiolucency lying between the maxillary central incisors (see Fig. 82-15). It may be difficult to distinguish a small lesion from the nasopalatine duct itself. The nasopalatine duct cyst is lined by stratified squamous epithelium, pseudostratified ciliated columnar epithelium, cuboidal epithelium, or a combination. The cyst has a connective tissue wall that may have mucous glands, nerves, and blood vessels within it. Small cysts may just be observed with regular radiographic examination, whereas larger lesions or those that become secondarily infected should be treated with enucleation and curettage.

Midpalatal cyst of infants

The midpalatal cyst of infants arises from epithelium entrapped along the line of fusion of the palatal processes of the maxilla. The reason for induction of this epithelium to cyst formation is unknown. It is located at the midline of the hard palate of the maxilla. It is usually asymptomatic unless secondarily infected. It may produce a midpalatal swelling. An intraoral occlusal radiograph will often show the lesion, which is a well-circumscribed radiolucency with a sclerotic border, located in the midline of the hard palate. The histology shows stratified squamous or pseudostratified columnar epithelium. Treatment is access through a full-thickness palatal flap and enucleation and curettage. Recurrence is low.

Nasolabial cyst

The nasolabial cyst is a soft-tissue lesion developing within the labial vestibule just below the attachment of the nasal ala in the maxilla. It has been identified incorrectly as a fissural cyst in the past and does not originate from fissural epithelium but from remnants of the nasolacrimal ducts.[17] The clinical presentation is one of upper-lip swelling or of swelling within the floor of the nose. Nearly 75% of these lesions occur in women. The cyst rarely produces a radiographic appearance. Histologically, it is a true cyst with an epithelial lining with stratified squamous, or cuboidal, or respiratory epithelium. The cyst should be treated with local excision from an intraoral approach.

Nonepithelial cysts

The nonepithelial cysts are a group of unrelated lesions that typically have been termed cysts although they do not have an epithelial lining. These lesions must be included in any discussion of cysts of the jaws because they must be considered in the differential diagnosis. They are best included here because they do not fall into the group of odontogenic tumors or benign diseases of bone.

Idiopathic bone cavity

The idiopathic bone cavity is also known as *solitary bone cyst, hemorrhagic cyst, extravasation cyst,* and *simple bone cyst.* The lesion is not a true cyst and its etiology is unclear, so names that imply an etiology of true cyst formation should be avoided. Of the several theories regarding the development of this cavity, trauma that initiates an intramedullary hemorrhage with subsequent degeneration of the clot without bony filling, leading to an empty bone cavity, is the favored explanation. The idiopathic bone cavity occurs most frequently in the second decade of life and is most often identified in the region of the posterior body and ascending ramus of the mandible. The patient is usually asymptomatic, and the defect is discovered on routine radiographic investigation (Fig. 82-25). The idiopathic bone cavity is usually a radiolucent lesion of variable size. It may become very large and surround the mandibular posterior teeth. This is different from other lesions that tend to push the teeth roots apart. The lesion also may extend to the inferior border but does not usually displace the inferior alveolar nerve, which also is unusual because other lesions tend to displace the nerve. Histologically, the lesion shows bony walls without a lining. It is fluid- or air-filled. Treatment requires biopsy to rule out other lesions, but the process of opening the lesion and causing hemorrhage within the cavity is usually enough to lead to resolution of the lesion.

Stafne's mandibular lingual cortical defect

This entity also is known by several other terms including *lingual mandibular bone cavity, static bone cavity,* and *lingual salivary gland defect.* This is an asymptomatic lesion. It usually occurs in adults over the age of 25. Radiographically, the lesion is a solitary radiolucency below the inferior alveolar canal near the angle region of the mandible (Fig. 82-26). The lesion usually is oval and exhibits no growth over long periods of time. The periphery is smooth and symmetric. The lesion is benign, has no growth potential, and a

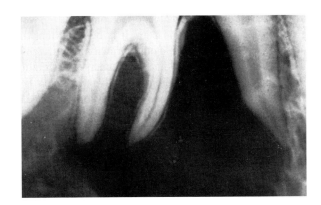

Fig. 82-25. Radiograph of an idiopathic bone cavity. This is not a true cyst. It differs in appearance from most odontogenic cysts in that it grows around and between the roots of associated teeth, giving it a scalloped appearance.

2. Plexiform. In this form the epithelial component is arranged in strands, bounded by strands of columnar cells between which may be found stellate reticulum-like cells. Occasionally, double rows of columnar cells are present. The stellate reticulum-like component is less prominent in this histologic pattern. Cystic degeneration is often present. The supporting stroma is usually loose and vascular (Fig. 82-30). Follicular and plexiform types frequently exist within the same tumor.

3. Basal cell. In this infrequently occurring variant, the cells are more cuboidal and may be arranged in sheets. This form bears resemblance to basal cell carcinoma of the skin.

4. Acanthomatous. The stellate reticulum-like cells undergo squamous metaplasia and sometimes produce keratin in this form. This type is usually present within the follicular ameloblastoma.

5. Granular cell. The stellate reticulum-like cells and frequently the peripheral layer undergo cytoplasmic transformation and take on a granular, eosinophilic appearance. The granules represent lysosomal aggregates. This form appears to be an aggressive lesion with numerous recurrences and reports of metastasis.

6. Desmoplastic. This form generally occurs in the anterior mandible and bears resemblance to fibroosseous disease. There is an abundant hyalinized stroma with distorted epithelial islands.

Treatment and prognosis. Unlike the unicystic ameloblastoma, the recurrence rate for solid ameloblastoma is more than 55% if treated with only enucleation and curettage, therefore, it is recommended that treatment include resection with 1-cm margins. If the lesion has perforated bone, the periosteum or overlying mucosa is sacrificed. If the lesion has extended beyond the confines of periosteum, surgical margins should be assessed using frozen sections. Care should be taken to avoid entering the tumor mass during resection, and rotary burrs should not be used for curettage because neoplastic cells may be seeded to other areas.[15]

Calcifying epithelial odontogenic tumor (Pindborg tumor)

Clinical features. This tumor occurs in patients over a broad age distribution with most cases occurring in middle age. Lesions occur twice as frequently in the mandible as

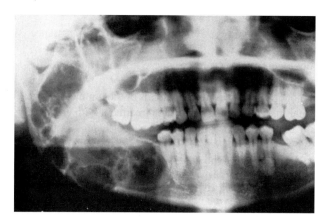

Fig. 82-28. Radiograph of a central ameloblastoma displaying multilocularity. Ameloblastomas may have either a unilocular or multilocular appearance.

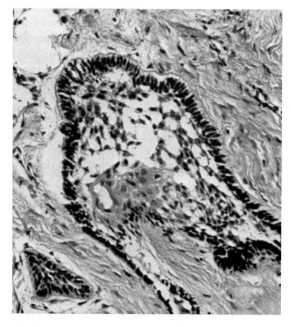

Fig. 82-29. Photomicrograph of a follicular ameloblastoma. Note the epithelial nests and islands and polarized nuclei.

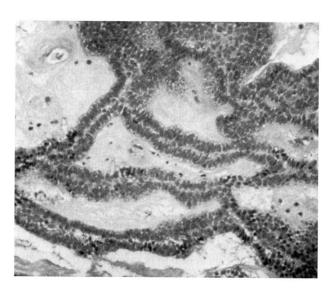

Fig. 82-30. Photomicrograph of a plexiform ameloblastoma. Histologic examination of this lesion reveals epithelial trabeculae in an interlacing pattern as well as nuclear polarization.

the maxilla, with the premolar-molar area most often affected. Most cases present as an asymptomatic swelling. Although reported, extraosseous cases are rare. Usually the tumor occurs at an intraosseous site, and it is associated with an impacted tooth in approximately one half of the patients.

Radiographic features. This lesion may appear as either a diffuse or well-circumscribed unilocular radiolucency. In some cases there will be a mixed pattern of radiolucency and radiopacity. Scattered flecks of calcification are sometimes seen within a radiolucent field.

Histology. Polyhedral epithelial cells arranged in sheets or small islands are seen. These cells have distinct borders and a granular eosinophilic cytoplasm. In some regions a homogeneous eosinophilic material that stains positive for amyloid may be present. Calcification, often in the form of concentric Liesegang rings may be produced within the amyloid-like material (Fig. 82-31). Intercellular bridges are frequently prominent. The nuclei are often pleomorphic with multinucleated forms being relatively common, but mitotic figures are rare. The morphologic variability that is sometimes present may mimic adenocarcinoma or other malignancies.

A clear-cell variant that exhibits a vacuolated cytoplasm is seen occasionally. This cell types may easily be confused with mucoepidermoid carcinoma or metastatic malignancy.

Treatment. This tumor is slow growing and locally invasive. However, because it has certain features in common with ameloblastoma some surgeons choose to treat it in the same fashion. There have been relatively few cases reported that have been followed up in the long term. Controversy exists as to whether to treat this lesion as aggressively as ameloblastoma; however, current therapy consists of either resection with a 1-cm margin or surgical excision with peripheral resection. The peripheral form of the lesion may be treated by local excision.

Odontogenic adenomatoid tumor (adenomatoid odontogenic tumor, adenoameloblastoma)

It is speculated that this lesion arises because of a late disturbance in odontogenesis. Some investigators consider it to be a benign neoplasm, whereas others believe it is a hamartoma or an odontogenic cyst. As the name implies, the structure contains duct-like elements.

Clinical features. Patients are typically aged less than 20 years old, and approximately two out of three lesions occur in females. About two thirds of these tumors are found in the anterior maxilla, usually associated with an impacted tooth, most frequently the maxillary canine. This tumor generally presents as a painless swelling. In rare instances, it has been reported as an extraosseous lesion.

Radiographic features. The lesion generally presents as a unilocular radiolucency that resembles a dentigerous cyst, but it extends further apically than the cementoenamel junction and may contain focal radiopacities. Although separation of roots and displacement of teeth is a frequent finding, root resorption is rare (Fig. 82-32).

Histology. This tumor is encapsulated and often appears contained within a cystic structure. It is composed of colum-

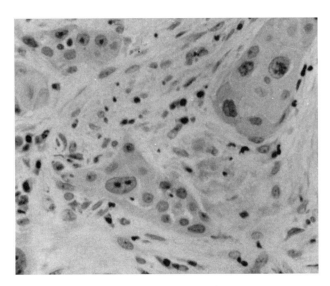

Fig. 82-31. Photomicrograph of a calcifying epithelial odontogenic tumor. Islands of polyhedral epithelial cells are present. Note the granular appearance of the cytoplasm. The epithelium may be pleiomorphic and appear malignant even though the lesion is benign.

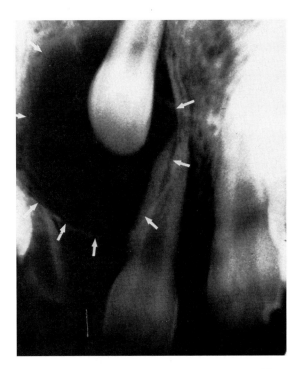

Fig. 82-32. Radiograph of an odontogenic adenomatoid tumor. The unilocular radiolucent appearance with displacement of adjacent teeth is characteristic of many of the benign odontogenic tumors.

nar or cuboidal epithelial cells in a duct-like arrangement. The ducts may contain an eosinophilic coagulum, and calcifications may be present. There is a sparse connective tissue stroma. In other areas the epithelial cells are spindle-shaped or polyhedral and are arranged in nests, whorls, or cords. The tumor is structurally similar to the enamel organ (Fig. 82-33).

Treatment. Because the lesion is encapsulated and noninvasive, the treatment of choice is enucleation. Recurrence is extremely rare.

Calcifying odontogenic cyst (Gorlin's cyst: keratinizing and calcifying odontogenic cyst)

Although this lesion is called a cyst, it is now considered by most investigators to be an odontogenic tumor. This remains an area of debate because the lesion frequently contains both tumor and cystic elements.

Clinical features. Most lesions are found in the mandible and occur over a wide age range. There generally is no associated pain, and the lesion can occur extraosseously.

Radiographic features. A well-circumscribed radiolucency is present in the central intrabony lesion. Calcified radiopaque material is usually present within the radiolucency (Fig. 82-34). The tumor is usually small, but can become large, occupying much of the jaw.

Histology. The lesion may be cystic or may appear solid. A squamous, cuboidal, or columnar epithelial lining is present, within which is contained pale eosinophilic cells and "ghost" cells, which may keratinize and calcify. The eosinophilic cells and "ghost" cells may penetrate the surrounding connective tissue to stimulate a giant-cell reaction and dystrophic calcification. Stellate reticulum-like formations

as well as sheets and duct-like configurations of epithelial cells may be seen. On occasion, melanin may be found.

Praetorius and others[20] have classified the calcifying odontogenic cyst as:

Type I (Cystic)
A. Simple unicystic
   Thin epithelial lining. Focal areas of stellate reticulum and "ghost" cells. Scant dysplastic dentin.
B. Odontoma type
   Same as previous, but also contains calcified tissue in its wall.
C. Ameloblastomatous type
   Contains ameloblastoma-like proliferations in cyst capsule and lumen.
Type II (Neoplastic)
   Ameloblastoma-like odontogenic epithelium invading connective tissue is characteristic. Ghost cells and dentinoid are present.

Treatment. All type I lesions are treated by enucleation and curettage. Extraosseous lesions are treated by local excision. Type II lesions are rare and present an invasive and infiltrative behavior. Treatment should consist of marginal or *en bloc* resection, depending on the size of the lesion.

Ameloblastic fibroma

This is an uncommon neoplasm arising from simultaneous proliferation of both epithelial and mesenchymal tissue without formation of calcified tissue.

Clinical features. This lesion most commonly arises in the molar region of the mandible. Forty percent of the pa-

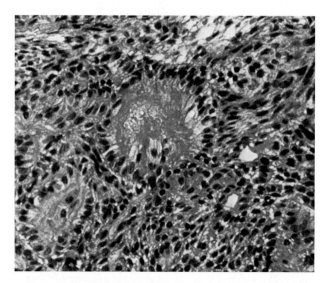

Fig. 82-33. Photomicrograph of an odontogenic adenomatoid tumor. Note the duct-like arrangement of cuboidal cells with an amorphous coagulum within the center of the duct. Calcifications may be present.

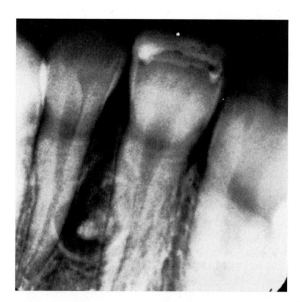

Fig. 82-34. Radiograph of a calcifying odontogenic cyst. Note the presence of densely radiopaque material within the radiolucency.

tients are under the age of 10, with a mean age at diagnosis of 14.6 years.[24] It is a slow-growing lesion that does not tend to infiltrate and rarely causes pain.

Radiographic features. The appearance of ameloblastic fibroma is very similar to that of ameloblastoma. It is of variable size, is usually unilocular but may be multilocular, and has a smooth outline. It is frequently associated with unerupted teeth.

Histology. Scattered islands of columnar or cuboidal epithelial cells are arranged in nests, cords, and strands similar to primitive odontogenic epithelium. Occasionally, stellate reticulum-like tissue is present. The surrounding connective tissue resembles dental papilla.

Treatment. Treatment of this lesion consists of enucleation and curettage. There is little tendency for recurrence. However, patients should continue to be followed on an annual basis because causes of ameloblastic fibrosarcoma have originated from recurrent ameloblastic fibroma.[13]

Ameloblastic fibroodontoma

This lesion represents an immature form of complex odontoma and therefore represents a hamartoma rather than a neoplastic process.

Clinical features. Most patients are aged less than 15 and male. The maxilla and mandible are affected with equal frequency. The lesion is most often associated with an impacted tooth in the molar region. The most common complaints are swelling and failure of tooth eruption.

Radiographic features. This is a well-circumscribed expansile radiolucency containing a single or multiple radiopaque masses. The lesion's size is extremely variable.

Histology. The microscopic picture is a combination of that found in ameloblastic fibroma and composite odontoma.

Treatment. This lesion is treated by enucleation and curettage because it has little tendency for recurrence.

Ameloblastic odontoma (odontoameloblastoma)

This is an extremely rare lesion that consists of ameloblastoma and composite odontoma. It is unusual in that it consists of a relatively undifferentiated neoplastic tissue associated with a highly differentiated tissue. Recurrence may occur with inadequate removal.

Clinical features. This lesion tends to occur at any age but is more frequent in children. It is more often found in the mandible than the maxilla. Presenting symptoms include mild pain and delayed eruption of teeth.

Radiographic features. Central destruction of bone with expansion of the cortical plates is common. Many small radiopaque masses are present within the lesion.

Histology. There is a great variety of cells in a complex distribution. There are many structures resembling normal or atypical tooth germ. Sheets of typical ameloblastoma are present.

Treatment. Management of this lesion is controversial because there are so few cases. The general behavior is the same as for ameloblastoma, so marginal or *en bloc* resection is suggested, depending on the size of the lesion.

Odontoma

Odontoma is a hamartoma derived from functional ameloblasts and odontoblasts and forms enamel and dentin in an abnormal pattern. It is frequently called *composite* because it contains more than one type of tissue. If the enamel and dentin form structures that bear resemblance to normal teeth, it is called a *compound composite odontoma*. If the dental hard tissues form a more disorganized mass, it is termed *complex composite odontoma*. The compound type is more common.

Clinical features. Odontomas are found in patients of all ages and in all locations within the jaws. These lesions are frequently associated with dentigerous cysts.

Radiographic features. This lesion appears as an irregular radiopaque mass surrounded by a thin radiolucent region. It is often located between tooth roots. Frequently, odontomas are associated with unerupted teeth. Compound composite odontomas may have the appearance of a mass of tooth-like structures (Fig. 82-35).

Histology. The microscopic appearance is that of enamel, dentin, pulp, and connective tissue, similar to a dental follicle (Fig. 82-36). ''Ghost'' cells also may appear in this lesion (as seen in the calcifying odontogenic cyst). This

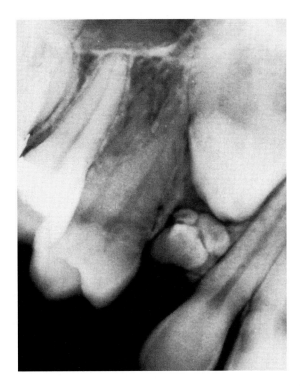

Fig. 82-35. Radiograph of a compound composite odontoma. Multiple tooth-like structures are present near the crest of the anterior maxillary aveolar bone in association with an impacted canine tooth.

lesion should not be confused with ameloblastic fibro-odontoma.

Treatment. Because there is no tendency for recurrence, odontomas are treated by simple enucleation.

Mesenchymal odontogenic tumors

Odontogenic fibroma

This is a rare lesion composed of connective tissue and odontogenic islands and resembles a dental follicle. It appears to arise from periodontal ligament, dental papilla, or dental follicle. It occurs around the crown of unerupted teeth and appears much like a follicular cyst.

Clinical features. This tumor occurs most frequently in the mandibles of children, adolescents, and young adults. It exhibits slow, expansile growth and rarely produces pain.

Radiographic features. A unilocular or multilocular radiolucency with smooth borders is common.

Histology. The lesion contains collagen fibers and fibroblasts with occasional osteoid, dysplastic dentin, or cemental tissue. Its appearance must be distinguished from the Antony B type configuration found in neurofibromas.

Treatment. Enucleation is the treatment of choice because recurrence has not been reported.

Odontogenic myxoma

This tumor also has a mesenchymal origin, arising from periodontal ligament, dental follicle, or dental papilla.

Clinical features. It occurs most often in the second and third decades and slightly more frequently in the mandible than the maxilla. It is often associated with missing or impacted teeth. This is a slow-growing, expansile lesion.

Radiographic features. A multilocular radiolucency is often present although it may present as a mottled unilocular radiolucency. Displacement of teeth is common, but root resorption is rare. The lesion tends to erode through cortical bone and frequently involves the maxillary sinus if it occurs in the upper jaw.

Histology. There are few cells present in this tumor, but there is a prominent mucoid intercellular substance. The cells are stellate or spindle-shaped with long fibrils. Occasional nests of odontogenic eipthelium or collagen fibers may be seen. Hyaluronic acid and chondroitin sulfate are produced by this lesion (Fig. 82-37).

Treatment. Although this tumor is benign, it behaves rather aggressively. Because of its invasive nature, this lesion is frequently large by the time it is diagnosed. The treatment of choice is either marginal or *en bloc* resection with 1-cm margins. It is not responsive to radiotherapy.

Cementoma

Cementoma is the broad classification for lesions that have in common the production of cementum. All cementomas are benign; however, treatment will vary depending on the specific type.

Periapical cementoosseous dysplasia

This lesion appears to arise from the periodontal ligament and contains various amounts of fibrous tissue, cementum, and bone. Although it occurs frequently, its etiology has not been fully explained.

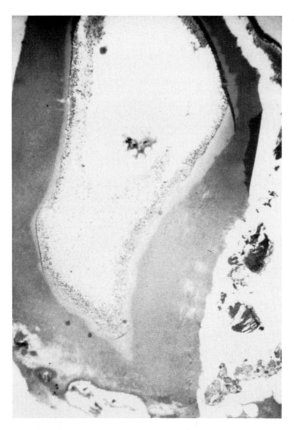

Fig. 82-36. Photomicrograph of a compound composite odontoma. The appearance is that of mature enamel, dentin, and cementum within connective tissue.

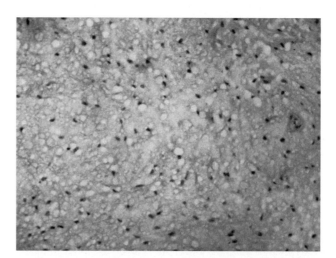

Fig. 82-37. Photomicrograph of an odontogenic myxoma. The lesion is sparsely cellular with large quantities of mucoid intercellular substance.

Clinical features. Patients are predominantly black women over the age of 20. In most cases, multiple lesions are present that are asymptomatic and usually involve the mandibular incisor root apices.

Radiographic features. This lesion passes through three stages in its maturation. The osteolytic stage occurs first and is characterized by localized dental periapical radiolucencies similar in appearance to those that occur with a dental abscess. The next period is termed the *cementoblastic stage.* During this time cementoblasts become more active and produce spicules of cementum, which produce a mixed radiolucent/radiopaque appearance. The final or mature stage consists of an abnormally large amount of calcification that appears as a dense periapical radiopacity surrounded by a thin radiolucent border (Fig. 82-38).

Histologic description. This lesion contains varying amounts of fibrous connective tissue, cementoblasts, and cemental tissue depending on the stage of the lesion.

Treatment. Periodic radiographic observation is appropriate. The teeth are vital and should not be treated by extraction or endodontic therapy. Electrical, thermal, and mechanical stimulation of the teeth can aid the clinician who is attempting to rule out dental infection during the osteolytic or cementoblastic stages.

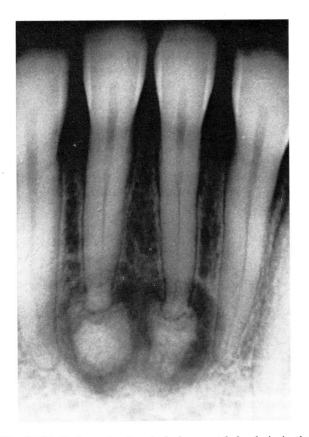

Fig. 82-38. Radiograph of periapical cemental dysplasia in the cementoblastic stage. A mixed radiolucent/radiopaque appearance is present.

Cementifying fibroma or cementoossifying fibroma

This lesion closely resembles the ossifying fibroma and it probably arises from the same progenitor cell.

Clinical features. It occurs most often in young and middle-aged adults, more frequently in the mandible, and there is a marked female predilection. This is a slow-growing expansile tumor that can displace teeth and produce swelling, but rarely causes pain.

Radiographic features. The radiographic appearance of this lesion changes depending on its state of maturation. Independent of the stage of development, the lesion will always appear well circumscribed. Initially it will appear as a radiolucency and will later pass through a stage in which flecks of calcification are present. Finally it will become densely radiopaque. This tumor exhibits a centrifugal growth pattern, such that the lesion is always found to be round.

Histology. Collagen fibers and fibroblasts or cementoblasts as well as small masses of calcified tissue are present. The name of the lesion depends on the type(s) of calcified tissue present.

Treatment. This lesion is benign, noninvasive, and has demonstrated no propensity for recurrence. It is best treated by simple enucleation.

Benign cementoblastoma (true cementoma)

This relatively uncommon lesion probably represents a benign neoplasm of cementoblasts that produces a large mass of cemental tissue at the tooth root.

Clinical features. Patients are usually aged less than 25 years, but the age range extends into the eighth decade. The mandible is more often affected than the maxilla, with the mandibular permanent first molar being the most frequent site of involvement. The involved tooth is vital and usually pain-free. The slow growth of this lesion may result in cortical expansion.

Radiographic features. A well-circumscribed dense radiopacity is attached to the tooth root and is often surrounded by a narrow radiolucent line. The affected root is frequently obscured by the mass secondary to root resorption and fusion of the tumor to the tooth.

Histology. Sheets of cementum-like tissue surrounded by cementoblasts are a prominent feature. Reversal lines are sometimes present, as are cementoblasts. Fibrovascular tissue is present to a varying degree. The periodontal ligament is obliterated, and the tooth may show resorption. A soft-tissue capsule may be seen at the periphery with cemental trabeculae positioned at right angles. The lesion may resemble a benign osteoblastoma, osteoid osteoma, or osteosarcoma.

Treatment. Removal of the affected tooth is indicated. The dental extraction can usually be performed easily because there is cortical thinning as a result of expansion of the lesion. This tumor must be distinguished from hypercementosis or chronic sclerosing osteomyelitis. Benign cementoblastomas do not recur after treatment.

Dentinoma

This is an extremely rare tumor composed of connective tissue, odontogenic epithelium, and abnormal dentin.

Clinical features. This lesion occurs in the mandibular molar region in young adults. It is often associated with an impacted tooth; however, extraosseous cases can occur. Pain, swelling, and mucosal perforation have been reported.

Radiographic features. The radiographic picture may be extremely variable. It may appear as a radiolucency, a radiolucency with small radiopaque flecks, or a solitary radiopaque mass.

Histology. The connective tissue stroma resembles dental papilla. Masses of irregular dentin with demonstrable dentinal tubules are present. Undifferentiated odontogenic epithelium is present and enamel is absent. If enamel were present the lesion would be called a *complex composite odontoma.*

Treatment. This lesion is treated by enucleation and curettage.

Tumors of unknown origin

Melanotic neuroectodermal tumor of infancy

This appears to be a tumor of neural crest origin. High urinary excretion of vanillylmandelic acid is consistent with other neural crest tumors.

Clinical features. This lesion usually arises in the anterior maxillary region in children aged less than 6 months. The lesion is not present at birth. The tumor is benign and has exhibited little tendency to recur; however, it does grow rapidly. It has a darkly pigmented appearance and does not ulcerate (Fig. 82-39).

Radiographic features. It presents as a ragged radiolucent lesion that resembles a malignancy. The primary central incisor is carried with the lesion when it occurs in the anterior maxilla.

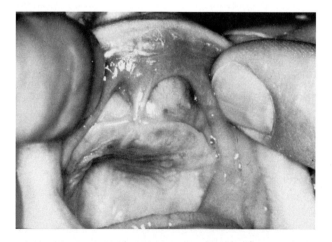

Fig. 82-39. Clinical photograph of a melanotic neuroectodermal tumor of infancy. There is an anterior maxillary swelling that extends from the labial vestibule to the palate.

Histology. The tumor is nonencapsulated and infiltrative. Cuboidal cells, many with melanin pigmentation, form alveoli that contain neuroblast-like cells. These cells have prominent round nuclei with little cytoplasm. The stroma consists of vascular and fibrous tissue.

Treatment. This lesion is treated by local excision with curettage. It may be confused with a neuroblastoma or congenital epulis of the newborn.

Malignant odontogenic tumors

Primary intraosseous carcinoma

This is an extremely rare tumor. The diagnosis is often made after metastasis has occurred. Primary intraosseous carcinomas may be of three different types:[3]

1. Arising from an odontogenic cyst
2. Developing from an ameloblastoma
   Well differentiated (malignant ameloblastoma)
   Poorly differentiated (ameloblastic carcinoma)
3. Arising from odontogenic epithelium

Clinical features. Aggressive local invasion with destruction of adjacent tissues is the major feature. Regional and distant metastasis will occur.

Radiographic features. The lesion will present as a radiolucency with poorly defined margins. Destruction of bone and tooth root structure may occur.

Histology. This highly depends on the tissue from which the tumor arises. However, invasiveness, cellular pleomorphism, atypical mitotic figures, and large hyperchromatic nuclei will be present.

Treatment. Resection of the tumor with 1-cm margins and frozen sections is generally indicated. Radiotherapy is usually recommended. Treatment of metastases may involve surgical removal, radiation, or chemotherapy.

Ameloblastic fibrosarcoma (ameloblastic sarcoma)

This is a rare tumor and is the malignant counterpart of the ameloblastic fibroma.

Clinical features. It occurs more frequently in young adults and is more common in the mandible than in the maxilla. The tumor is generally painful, exhibits rapid growth, and destroys bone. Teeth may become loose and there may be ulceration of the overlying mucosa with associated bleeding.

Radiographic features. The borders of the lesion are poorly defined, and local bone destruction is present.

Histology. Most cases have occurred through malignant transformation of a preexisting ameloblastic fibroma. The odontogenic epithelium does not undergo malignant conversion. However, the mesenchymal portion displays increased cellularity, cellular pleomorphism, hyperchromatic nuclei, and atypical mitotic figures.

Treatment. Wide surgical resection is indicated. The recurrence rate is high. Radiotherapy is not recommended because it has not proven to be effective in management of this tumor.

Ameloblastic dentinosarcoma

This lesion is identical to the ameloblastic fibrosarcoma except that it contains dysplastic dentin but no enamel.

Treatment. Wide surgical resection is necessary as recurrences are frequent. The lesion is poorly responsive to radiation.

Ameloblastic odontosarcoma

This tumor is similar to the ameloblastic fibrosarcoma and ameloblastic dentinosarcoma except that it contains both dysplastic enamel and dentin.

Treatment. Wide surgical resection is necessary because recurrences are frequent. The lesion is poorly responsive to radiation.

SURGICAL MANAGEMENT OF ODONTOGENIC CYSTS AND TUMORS

Surgical goals

The vast majority of odontogenic lesions are benign, and most are only minimally aggressive. This makes it crucial to define carefully the ultimate goal of surgery. Unlike malignant lesions where the primary goal is preservation of life, with other factors being of secondary importance, the treatment of odontogenic cysts and tumors must not be accomplished at the expense of function or esthetics.

The goals of management of benign odontogenic cysts and tumors are:[2] (1) remove all abnormal tissue; (2) conserve healthy bone and dental structures; (3) preserve adjacent structures such as the inferior alveolar nerve; (4) restore the surgical defect to its presurgical state of anatomic form and function; and (5) prevent recurrence of the lesion.

Principles in surgical management

Cysts and tumors of the jaws are treated in a variety of ways depending on several factors (Fig. 82-40). Virtually all cysts are treated with either enucleation or enucleation and curettage. Occasionally, decompression or marsupialization can be done first to allow the lesion to decrease in size before it is removed definitively. Odontogenic tumors are treated by enucleation with or without curettage, by marginal or partyal resection, and occasionally by composite resection (Box 82-4).

A definition of terms is necessary before proceeding. Enucleation of a lesion involves local removal of the lesion by instrumentation in direct contact with the lesion (Fig. 82-41). If curettage also is used, 1 to 2 mm of the bony wall is removed after the lesion is enucleated (Fig. 82-42). This is accomplished with aggressive curettage by hand or by the use of rotary instrumentation. Resection involves incision or osteotomy through uninvolved tissue adjacent to the lesion without disruption of the lesion. Marginal resection does not

---

Box 82-4. Surgical modalities for treatment of odontogenic cysts and tumors

Enucleation and curettage
  Odontogenic cysts:
    Virtually all unless recurrent
  Odontogenic tumors:
    Odontoma
    Ameloblastic fibroma
    Ameloblastic fibroodontoma
    Adenomatoid odontogenic tumor
    Calcifying odontogenic cyst
    Cementoblastoma
    Central cementifying fibroma
    Unicystic ameloblastoma (except mural type)
Marginal or partial resection
  Odontogenic cysts:
    Recurrent odontogenic keratocyst
  Odontogenic tumors:
    Ameloblastoma (solid and mural type unicystic)
    Calcifying epithelial odontogenic tumor (Pindborg tumor)
    Odontogenic myxoma
    Ameloblastic odontoma
    Squamous odontogenic tumor
Composite resection*
  Odontogenic tumors:
    Malignant ameloblastoma
    Ameloblastic fibrosarcoma
    Ameloblastic odontosarcoma
    Primary intraosseous carcinoma

* These lesions are malignancies and may be treated variably and with additional modalities such as radiation or chemotherapy.

---

produce a continuity defect of the involved bone, for example, leaving a portion of the inferior border of the mandible intact (Fig. 82-43). Partial resection removes a full-thickness portion of the involved bone. In the maxilla this may not differ much from a marginal resection; however, in the mandible, it produces a continuity defect (Fig. 82-44). Composite resection involves removal of tumor, adjacent bone, soft tissue, and contiguous lymph node channels. The only odontogenic lesions treated with composite resection are malignant neoplasms.

The decision as to which method of treatment to use for the management of a given odontogenic lesion is based primarily on the histologic diagnosis because it provides the most information about the lesion's aggressiveness and its potential for recurrence. Other factors may play a role in helping to decide between a more or less aggressive therapy. These factors include the anatomic location of the lesion, its proximity to adjacent vital structures, the size of the lesion, its spread to adjacent soft tissue, the duration of the lesion, and the plans for reconstruction.

Lesions in the mandible are more readily diagnosed, are

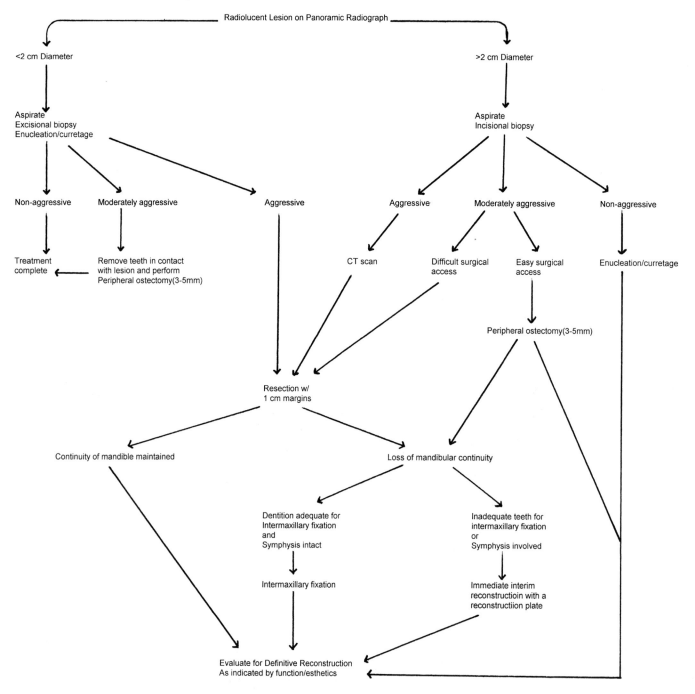

Fig. 82-40. Management of an odontogenic lesion of the mandible.

usually smaller at the time of diagnosis, and are more easily followed for recurrence than their counterparts in the maxilla. Lesions in the anterior of either the maxilla or mandible are easier to diagnose, treat, and follow than their counterparts in the posterior of each respective jaw. Because of

this, a more aggressive approach is often recommended for lesions in the posterior maxilla than for those in the anterior mandible.

Proximity of adjacent vital structures should not deter adequate removal of a lesion. It may be possible to decom-

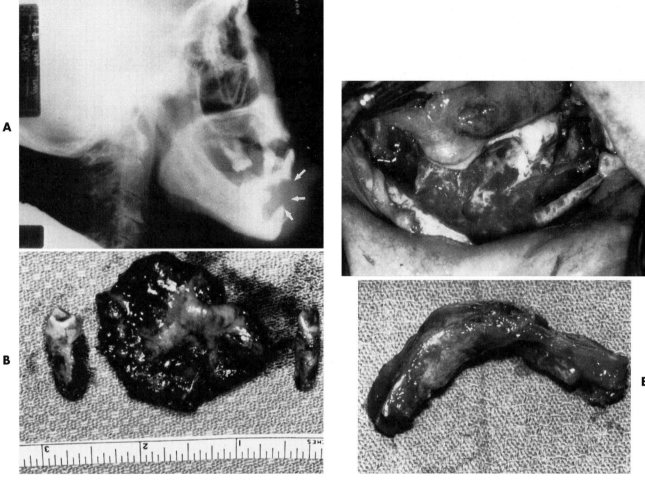

Fig. 82-41. Enucleation of a cyst. **A,** Radiograph showing large cystic lesion in the anterior mandible. **B,** The specimen and involved teeth after enucleation.

Fig. 82-42. Bony cavity in anterior mandible after removal of odontogenic myxoma. **A,** Note the multilocular nature of osseous resorption; **B,** the specimen immediately after removal.

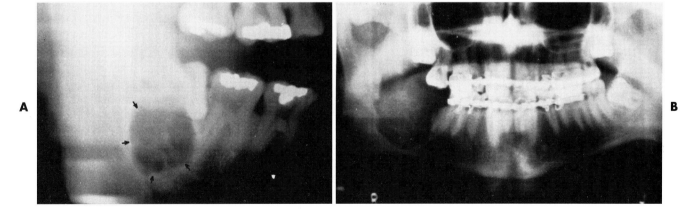

Fig. 82-43. Odontogenic myxoma of the mandibular angle associated with a developing mandibular third molar. **A,** Preoperative radiographic appearance. The lesion was treated with marginal resection from an extraoral approach with immediate reconstruction using a cancellous bone graft from the ilium and a sural nerve graft of the inferior alveolar nerve. **B,** Postoperative radiographic appearance.

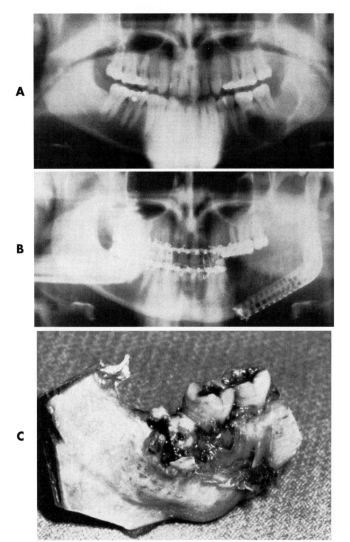

Fig. 82-44. Ameloblastoma of the angle and body of the mandible. **A,** Preoperative radiographic appearance. The lesion was treated with partial resection from an extraoral approach. **B,** Specimen with cortical perforation of the lesion. **C,** The defect was immediately reconstructed with a cancellous bone graft from the ilium and a titanium mesh tray.

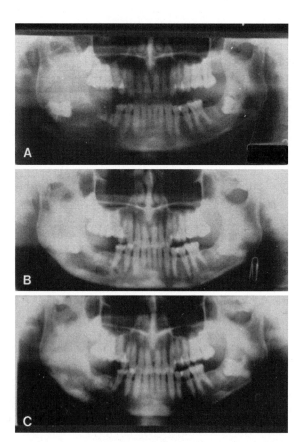

Fig. 82-45. Sequential panoramic radiographs of a large follicular cyst in the right mandibular body. **A,** Initial appearance of the lesion, which is large. Enucleation at this time would have involved the inferior alveolar nerve and threatened pathologic fracture. The lesion was decompressed and allowed to remain open to the oral cavity. **B,** Appearance 6 months after decompression. Note decrease in size of the lesion, which allowed enucleation and removal of the involved tooth without injury to associated structures. **C,** Six months after enucleation. With remodeling and bony fill, the lesion has all but resolved.

press a cyst to allow some bony fill before enucleation in an attempt to preserve adjacent teeth and nerves (Fig. 82-45). This decompression should be distinguished from marsupialization where no follow-up enucleation is accomplished. Marsupialization as treatment alone is not recommended because it requires a compliant patient, does not allow histopathologic diagnosis of the entire lesion, and may leave remnants of tissue behind, leading to recurrence. This type of treatment is not applicable for odontogenic tumors.

Extremely large lesions may require more aggressive treatment than smaller lesions of the same histologic type. Large lesions are more difficult to remove completely with enucleation alone. They may be large because they are more aggressive in behavior or because diagnosis was delayed because of poor patient reliability or difficulty in detection. Whichever the case, a more aggressive approach may be indicated to prevent recurrence.

Virtually all odontogenic cysts and tumors originate within bone. Aggressive lesions such as ameloblastomas and odontogenic keratocysts may perforate the cortical plate that usually surrounds the intraosseous lesion, enabling communication with the adjacent soft tissue. This is associated with increased difficulty in total removal (see Fig. 82-44, *B*). Although these lesions do not usually spread within the soft tissue and tend to remain encapsulated by the periosteum, the likelihood of removing the lesion incompletely is greater.

Several odontogenic tumors exhibit very slow growth, eventually reaching a static point in size. These lesions should be treated less aggressively than lesions that have exhibited rapid enlargement. Regardless of the treatment used, the attention to restoration of esthetics, and function should be considered before treatment is begun. Preservation of a portion of the condyle and ramus can greatly improve reconstruction, as can maintenance of the mandible's continuity and range of motion during the interval between tumor removal and reconstruction.

SUMMARY

The normal development of teeth and associated structures of the jaws have been reviewed. Odonogentic epithelium that is trapped within the developing hard and soft tissue of the head and neck can degenerate and develop into a variety of odonogenic cysts and tumors. These lesions are generally benign, but some may behave in an aggressive manner. Malignant variants exist but are extremely rare. Key features to remember are that the clinical and radiographic appearance of these lesions are similar, and histopathologic diagnosis is key to development of a proper treatment plan. Subtle variations between the histologic presentation of many of these lesions may cause them to be confused with each other. The assistance of an oral and maxillofacial pathologist in making the proper diagnosis is frequently helpful.

Odontogenic lesions are managed surgically with enucleation, enucleation and curettage, or resection, depending on their extent and histopathologic behavior. Reconstruction of not only the lost osseous structure but associated dentition is critical for the rehabilitation of these patients.

REFERENCES

1. Browne RM: The odontogenic keratocyst—clinical aspects, *Br Dent J* 128:225, 1970.
2. Cherrick HM: *Odontogenic tumors of the jaws.* In Laskin DM, editor: *Oral and maxillofacial surgery,* vol 2, St Louis, 1985, Mosby.
3. Elzay RP: Primary intraosseous carcinoma of the jaws: review and update of odontogenic carcinomas, *Oral Surg* 54:299, 1982.
4. Forsell K: The primordial cyst: a clinical and radiographic study, *Proc Finn Dent Soc* 76:129, 1980.
5. Gold L: Biologic behavior of the ameloblastoma, *Oral Maxillofac Surg Clin North Am* 3:21, 1991.
6. Gorlin RJ: Nevoid basal-cell carcinoma syndrome, *Medicine* 66:98, 1987.
7. Gorlin RJ, Goltz RW: Multiple nevoid basal-cell epithelioma, jaw cysts and bifid rib, *N Engl J Med* 262:908, 1960.
8. Greer RO, Hammond WS: Extraosseous ameloblastoma: light microscopic and ultrastructural observations, *J Oral Surg* 36:553, 1978.
9. Harris M: A review of recent experimental work on the dental cyst, *Proc R Soc Med* 67:1259, 1974.
10. Kay LW, Laskin DM: *Cysts of the jaws and oral and facial soft tissues.* In Laskin DM, editor: *Oral and maxillofacial surgery;* vol 2, St Louis, 1985, Mosby.
11. Killey HC, Kay LW: *Benign cystic lesions of the jaws, their diagnosis and treatment,* ed 3, London, 1966, Churchill Livingstone.
12. Kramer IRH: Changing views on oral disease, *Proc R Soc Med* 67: 271, 1974.
13. Leider AS, Nelson JF, Trodahl JN: Ameloblastic fibrosarcoma of the jaws, *Oral Surg* 33:559, 1972.
14. Livingstone A: Observations of the development of the dental cyst, *Dent Rec* 47:531, 1927.
15. MacIntosh RB: Aggressive surgical management of the ameloblastoma, *Oral Maxillofac Surg Clin North Am* 3:73, 1991.
16. Main DMG: Epithelial jaw cysts: a clinicopathological reappraisal, *Br J Oral Surg* 8:114, 1970.
17. Main DMG: Epithelial jaw cysts: 10 years of the WHO classification, *J Oral Pathol* 14:1, 1985.
18. Melfi RC: *Permar's oral embryology and microscopic anatomy,* ed 8, Philadelphia, 1988, Lea & Febiger.
19. Pindborg JJ, Hansen J: Studies on odontogenic cyst epithelium, *Acta Pathol Microbiol Scand* 58:283, 1963.
20. Praetorius F and others: Calcifying odontogenic cyst: range, variations, and neoplastic potential, *Acta Odontol Scand* 39:227, 1981.
21. Shafer WG, Hine JK, Levy BM: *A textbook of oral pathology,* ed 4, Philadelphia, 1984, WB Saunders.
22. Shear M: Cysts of the jaws: recent advances, *J Oral Pathol* 14:43, 1985.
23. Simpson HE: Basal cell carcinoma and peripheral ameloblastoma, *Oral Surg* 38:233, 1974.
24. Small IA, Waldron CA: Ameloblastomas of the jaws, *Oral Surg* 8: 281, 1955.
25. Stanley HR, Diehl DL: Ameloblastoma potential of follicular cysts, *Oral Surg* 20:260, 1965.
26. Stoelinga PJW, Peters JH: A note on the origin of keratocysts of the jaws. *Int J Oral Surg* 2:37, 1973.
27. Ten Cate AR: *Oral histology: development, structure and function,* ed 3, St Louis, 1989, Mosby.
28. Toller PA: New concepts of odontogenic cysts, *Oral Surg* 1:3, 1972.
29. Trimble DL: *Odontogenesis and jaw cysts.* In Cummings CW and others, editors: *Otolaryngology—head and neck surgery,* St Louis, 1986, Mosby.
30. Waldron CA: *Odontogenic cysts and tumors.* In Neville and others, editors: *Oral and maxillofacial pathology,* Philadelphia, 1991, WB Saunders.
31. Waldron CW: Cystic tumors of the jaws: conservative and two-stage operative procedures to prevent deformity and the loss of useful teeth, *Am J Orthod* 27:313, 1941.
32. Williams TP: Surgical treatment of odontogenic keratocysts, *Oral Maxillofac Clin North Am* 3:137, 1991.
33. Wysocki GP: The differential diagnosis of globulomaxillary radiolucencies, *Oral Surg* 51:281, 1981.

Chapter 83

Temporomandibular Joint Disorders

Daniel M. Laskin

It has been estimated that as many as 10 million people in the United States suffer from disorders of the temporomandibular joint (TMJ), and such disorders constitute a major health problem. Because many of these patients complain about facial pain, earache, and headache, they are frequently seen by the otolaryngologist. Therefore it is important for the otolaryngologist to be familiar with the diagnosis and treatment of these various conditions.

The term, *temporomandibular disorders* (TMD), is an "umbrella" term actually encompassing two groups of patients: those with true abnormality of the TMJ and those with primary involvement of the masticatory muscles (myofascial pain-dysfunction [MPD] syndrome). Much of the difficulty encountered in the treatment of TMDs relates to the failure to distinguish between these two groups because of the similarity of the signs and symptoms with which they present. Adding further to the confusion is the fact that there also are a variety of other conditions unrelated to the TMJ occurring in the same region that can produce similar signs and symptoms; these also should be considered in the differential diagnosis. The emphasis in this chapter is on the diagnosis of TMDs, with a subsequent discussion of what is known about the etiology of the various conditions forming the basis for a rational approach to therapy.

ANATOMY

To understand some of the clinical problems that can originate in the TMJ, it is first necessary to understand something about the anatomy of this unique structure. The TMJ consists of the movable condyloid process and its articulating counterpart, the articular eminence, which forms the an-

terior aspect of the glenoid fossa. The articulating surfaces are lined with fibrous connective tissue beneath which, on the condyle, is a layer of hyaline cartilage. This relatively unprotected cartilage layer is an important growth site for the mandible, and damage to it can have major effects, not only on mandibular growth and morphology but also ultimately on growth of the maxilla and midface. Thus, whenever there is any abnormality involving the TMJ in a growing child, there is need for concern about the primary condition and its possible secondary effects on facial growth.

The TMJ also differs from most other joints in the body because it has a disc interposed between the articulating components. This disc adds stability to the joint by compensating for the incongruity between the articulating surfaces. It also serves as a shock absorber and contributes to the ability of the condyle to undergo rotational and translatory movements. Certain conditions can lead to displacement of the intraarticular disc (internal derangement), and this can result in abnormal sounds and altered function.

Another difference between the TMJ and other joints in the body is the influence of the teeth on the relationship of the articulating components. When the teeth are not in occlusion, this relationship is determined by the morphology of the bones and the muscles and ligaments that cross the joint (just as in any other joint). When the teeth come into contact, they determine the final position of the condyle. This factor has clinical implications that have to be considered in the treatment of many conditions involving the TMJ.

The final difference between the TMJ and other joints in the body relates to the functional relationship between the two joints. The mandible is the only bone in the body hinged on both ends that is not capable of independent movement at one end. This also has clinical implications because any dysfunctional movement on one side will result in altered movement on the contralateral side. Thus, a unilateral condition ultimately can lead to pain and dysfunction in the opposite joint even though the underlying problem does not affect it primarily. This phenomenon has to be considered whenever a patient presents with bilateral TMJ symptoms.

DISEASES AND DISORDERS

The TMJ is susceptible to the same conditions that affect other joints in the body such as congenital and developmental anomalies, traumatic injuries, dislocations, ankylosis, various forms of arthritis, and occasional neoplastic diseases (Table 83-1). There also may be internal derangements of the intraarticular disc. Although many of these conditions are treated in the same manner as when they occur in other joints, the previously described anatomic and functional differences of the TMJ often require some variations of therapy.

Congenital and developmental anomalies

Because the condyle has an important role in mandibular growth, congenital absence of the condyle (condylar agenesis, otomandibular dysostosis, hemifacial microsomia), con-

dylar hypoplasia, or condylar hypoplasia can produce severe facial deformity. It is important to distinguish between these conditions because of the variations in their treatment.

Condylar agenesis

With condylar agenesis, the coronoid process, the ramus, and parts of the mandibular body also may be absent, and there can be associated abnormalities of the internal and external ear, the temporal bone, the parotid gland, the muscles of mastication, and the facial nerve. Radiographs of the mandible and TMJ show the degree of bony involvement and help distinguish this condition from others that produce similar facial deformities but are not associated with such severe structural loss.

Early treatment of condylar agenesis is indicated to limit the degree of deformity. The objectives are to reestablish normal ramal height and to restore the missing growth site so that further mandibular deformation is prevented. When a large portion of the condyle and ramus is absent, this is best accomplished by reconstruction of the TMJ with a costochondral graft.[4,15] However, in patients with less severe deformities, distraction osteogenesis may be used to help correct the problem.[11,16] Orthodontic therapy, orthognathic surgery, otoplasty, and soft- and hard-tissue grafts for facial

Table 83-1. Differential diagnosis of temporomandibular joint disease

Disorder	Pain	Limitation	Diagnostic features
Agenesis	No	Yes	Congenital; usually unilateral; mandible deviates to affected side; unaffected side long and flat; severe malocclusion; often ear abnormalities; radiograph shows condylar deficiency
Condylar hypoplasia	No	No	Congenital or acquired; affected side has short mandibular body and ramus, fullness of face, deviation of chin; body of mandible elongated and face flat on unaffected side; malocclusion; radiograph shows condylar deformity, antegonial notching
Condylar hyperplasia	No	No	Facial asymmetry with deviation of chin to unaffected side; cross-bite malocclusion; prognathic appearance; lower border of mandible often convex on affected side; radiograph shows symmetric enlargement of condyle
Neoplasia	Possible	Yes	Mandible may deviate to affected side; radiographs show enlarged, irregularly shaped condyle or bone destruction depending on type of tumor; unilateral condition
Infectious arthritis	Yes	No	Signs of infection; may be part of systemic disease; radiographs may be negative early, later can show bone destruction; fluctuance may be present; plus may be obtained on aspiration; usually unilateral
Rheumatoid arthritis	Yes	Yes	Signs of inflammation; findings in other joints (hands, wrists, feet, elbows, ankles); positive laboratory tests; retarded mandibular growth in children; anterior open bite in adults; radiograph shows bone destruction; usually bilateral
Traumatic arthritis	Yes	Yes	History of trauma; radiograph negative except for possible widening of joint space; local tenderness; usually unilateral
Degenerative arthritis	Yes	Yes	Unilateral joint tenderness; often crepitus; temporomandibular joint may be only joint involved; radiograph may be negative or show condylar flattening, lipping, spurring, or erosion
Ankylosis	No	Yes	Usually unilateral but can be bilateral; may be history of trauma; young patient may show retarded mandibular growth; radiographs show loss of normal joint architecture
Internal disc derangement	Yes	Yes	Pain exacerbated by function; clicking on opening, or opening limited to under 25 mm with no click; positive arthrographic or magnetic resonance imaging findings; may be history of trauma; usually unilateral

From Laskin DM, Block S: Diagnosis and treatment of myofascial pain dysfunction (MPD) syndrome, *J Prosthet Dent* 56:75, 1986.

augmentation often are necessary to complete the reconstructive process.

Condylar hypoplasia

Hypoplasia of the mandibular condyle may be congenital, but it usually results from trauma, infection, or irradiation during the postnatal growth period. The decreased condylar growth produces a facial deformity characterized by shortness of the mandibular body, fullness of the face, and deviation of the chin to the affected side. On the contralateral side, the body of the mandible is elongated, and the face appears flattened. The degree of mandibular and facial deformity relates to the severity of the hypoplasia and the age at which it occurred. The diagnosis is based on the history of progressive facial deformity during the growth period, radiographic evidence of condylar deformity and antegonial notching, and a frequent history of trauma.

If the condition is recognized during the growth period, replacement of the condyle with a costochondral graft may be indicated.[10,13] However, recent reports have suggested that distraction osteogenesis may offer another alternative.[11,16] In adults, either shortening of the normal side of lengthening of the abnormal side by orthognathic surgery is aesthetically and functionally corrective. Previous orthodontic therapy often is necessary to establish a normal occlusion.

Condylar hyperplasia

Condylar hyperplasia is a disturbance of unknown etiology characterized by a slowly progressing, unilateral overgrowth of the mandible, resulting in facial asymmetry, malocclusion, and deviation of the chin to the unaffected side. In contrast with condylar hypoplasia, which produces changes in facial symmetry during normal mandibular growth, this condition usually first becomes apparent in those in the second decade of life when one condyle continues to grow, whereas the other side is no longer active. On radiographic examination, the condyle may have a normal shape, but the mandibular neck is elongated or the entire condyloid process may be symmetrically enlarged. This is in contradistinction to osteoma or osteochondroma of the condyle, which can sometimes produce a similar facial deformity, but which produce condylar asymmetry.

Treatment of condylar hyperplasia depends on whether the condyle is still growing,[2] which can be determined by the use of scintigraphy. If growth is still occurring, condylectomy is the treatment of choice. If growth has ceased, the condition is corrected by orthognathic surgery, usually preceded by orthodontic alignment of the teeth.

Traumatic injuries

The condyloid process is one of the most frequent sites of fracture after trauma to the mandible. The diagnosis generally is based on the physical and radiographic findings. There usually is preauricular pain and tenderness and difficulty in opening the mouth. When there is a unilateral frac-

ture, the jaw will deviate to the affected side on attempted mouth opening. In patients with bilateral fractures, there is no deviation, but there frequently is an anterior open bite.

Intracapsular condylar fractures are treated by short periods of maxillomandibular fixation. In adults, fractures of the condyloid process are also treated by maxillomandibular fixation unless the malposed segment interferes with jaw function, there are no occluding teeth on the involved side, or if the condyloid processes are fractured bilaterally and grossly displaced. In the latter instances, open reduction should be done.[19] Other conditions that may necessitate open reduction are a lack of adequate teeth for maxillomandibular fixation and the presence of associated fractures in the mandible or the maxilla and midface. In children, closed reduction and fixation also is the method of choice, except that a fractured, severely displaced, condyloid process may require surgical repositioning to avoid a possible growth deformity occurring subsequently.[8]

Dislocation

When the jaw is dislocated, the mandible is fixed in an open position with only the most posterior teeth contacting. Three forms of dislocation can be distinguished based on the frequency of the condition: the single, acute episode; chronic recurrent dislocation; and chronic persistent dislocation. Only the last two conditions may require surgical treatment; acute dislocation is treated by manual reduction supplemented by the use of local anesthesia, intravenous sedation, or general anesthesia.

Chronic recurrent dislocation can be treated by injection of a sclerosing agent into the TMJ capsule and ligament to produce scarring of the stretched tissues,[17] or the same effect can be accomplished by capsulorrhaphy. If the factors leading to the capsular laxity, such as frequent epileptic seizures or dyskinetic jaw movements, are uncontrollable, the patient may require lateral pterygoid myotomy.[6]

Some cases of chronic persistent dislocation can be reduced manually with the aid of traction wires placed through the bone at the angles of the mandible. When this fails, temporal myotomy performed through a vertical incision over the anterior border of the coronoid process generally is effectual.[6] As a last resort, direct manipulation of the condyles through preauricular incisions or condylectomy can be done.

Ankylosis

The most common causes of TMJ ankylosis are traumatic injuries and rheumatoid arthritis, although it also may result from congenital abnormalities, infection, or neoplasia. It is important to distinguish between true ankylosis, which involves the joint, and false ankylosis, which involves extraarticular conditions such as enlargement of the coronoid process, depressed fractures of the zygomatic arch, or scarring from surgery or irradiation. Radiographic examination of the TMJs and a careful clinical history generally are sufficient to establish the diagnosis of true ankylosis. The radiographs usually show condylar deformity and either a narrowing or irregularity of the joint space or obliteration of the normal bony morphology.

There are three basic principles involved in the surgical treatment of ankylosis.[8] First, the new joint should be established at the highest possible point on the ramus to maintain maximum ramal height and to minimize postoperative shift of the mandible; second, an interpositional material should be placed to avoid fusion of the parts; and third, it is important to initiate long-term physical therapy postsurgically. In the growing child, consideration should not only be given to maintenance of ramal height but also to replacement of the condylar growth site. A costochondral graft serves this purpose and provides an excellent interpositional material.[14]

Arthritis

Arthritis is the most frequent abnormal condition affecting the TMJ. All of the various types that occur in other joints can occur in this region, but infectious, traumatic, rheumatoid, and degenerative are the most common.

Infectious arthritis

Infectious arthritis condition is rare in the TMJ. It may be associated with a systemic disease such as gonorrhea, syphilis, or tuberculosis, may develop as an extension of a local infection, or occasionally may result from blood-borne organisms. Clinically, there are local signs of inflammation and limited jaw movement. There also may be signs and symptoms of the associated systemic disease. The results of radiographs are negative initially, but later may show extensive bone destruction. Treatment includes antibiotics, proper hydration, control of pain, and restriction of jaw movement. Suppurative infections may require aspiration, incision and drainage, or sequestrectomy.

Traumatic arthritis

Acute trauma to the mandible that does not cause a fracture still can produce injury to the TMJ. When this occurs in a child, it is important to warn the parents about the possibility of future retardation of mandibular growth.

Traumatic arthritis is characterized by TMJ pain and tenderness and limitation of jaw movement. The radiograph may be negative or show widening of the joint space caused by intraarticular edema or hemorrhage. Treatment consists of nonsteroidal antiinflammatory drugs (NSAIDs), application of heat, soft diet, and restriction of jaw movement.

Rheumatoid arthritis

Although the earliest symptoms of rheumatoid arthritis occasionally may occur in the TMJ, generally other joints are involved first. When the TMJ is involved, there usually is bilateral pain, tenderness and swelling, and limitation of jaw motion. In the early stages, there may be no radiographic changes, but with progression of the disease, the articular surface of the condyle is destroyed and the joint space is obliterated; as a result, an anterior open bite can occur. In children, such destruction also can cause mandibular growth retardation and facial deformity. In all patients, there is a possibility of ankylosis.

Treatment of rheumatoid arthritis in the TMJ is similar to that in other joints.[18] Antiinflammatory drugs are used during the acute phases, and mild jaw exercises are used to prevent excessive loss of motion when the acute symptoms subside. In patients with severe cases, drugs such as hydroxychloroquine, gold, and penicillamine also are used to control the pain and inflammation. Surgery may be necessary if ankylosis develops.

Degenerative arthritis

Primary degenerative arthritis is seen in older persons and is associated with normal aging. Its onset is insidious; the symptoms generally are mild, and patients rarely complain about the condition. Secondary degenerative arthritis, which usually is caused by trauma or the chronic clenching associated with MPD syndrome, occurs in younger patients and produces more severe symptoms of pain, joint tenderness, clicking or crepitation, and limitation of jaw movement. The condition usually is unilateral. The radiograph frequently will show flattening, lipping, osteophyte formation, or erosion of the articular surface of the condyle.

Treatment of degenerative joint disease includes administration of NSAIDs, a soft diet, limited jaw movement, and use of a bite appliance if the patient has a chronic clenching or grinding habit. When nonsurgical management for 3 to 6 months fails to relieve the symptoms, and when there is radiographic evidence of bony change on the articular surface of the condyle, surgical intervention may be indicated. This should involve removal of only the minimal amount of bone necessary to produce a smooth articular surface. Unnecessary removal of the entire cortical plate, as occurs with the so-called condylar shave or condylotomy, can lead to continued resorptive changes in some instances and should be avoided if possible.

Neoplasms

Primary neoplasms originating in the TMJ are uncommon. Chondroma, osteochondroma, and osteoma are the most common benign tumors. There also have been isolated cases of myxoma, fibrous dysplasia, giant cell reparative granuloma, synovialoma, chondroblastoma, osteoblastoma, and synovial hemangioma reported. Malignant tumors are even more uncommon, with infrequent reports of fibrosarcoma, chondrosarcoma, and multiple myeloma. The TMJ also can be invaded by neoplasms from the cheek or parotid gland, and metastasis to the condyle from distant neoplasms also has been noted on occasion.

Tumors of the TMJ cause pain, limited jaw movement, and difficulty in occluding the teeth. Depending on the nature of the condition, the radiographs may show bony deformation, apposition, or resorption. Biopsy is necessary to establish a definitive diagnosis.

Surgery is the treatment of choice for primary neoplasms, whether they are benign or malignant. Most of the malignant neoplasms are not radiosensitive, and therefore radiotherapy seldom is used.

Internal derangements

Internal derangements of the TMJ take three forms: anterior disc displacement with reduction on opening the mouth, which is characterized by clicking or popping sounds (Fig. 83-1); anterior disc displacement without reduction on attempted mouth opening, which is characterized by locking (Fig. 83-2); and disc adhesion to the articular eminence, which also is characterized by limitation of mouth opening resulting from inability of the condyle to translate (Fig. 83-3). As a result of an internal derangement, the patient also may develop a perforation in the disc or, more commonly, at the junction between the disc and the retrodiscal tissue.

Internal derangements may be caused by trauma, the lateral pterygoid spasm that frequently accompanies MPD syndrome, or the alterations in the frictional properties of the joint and the resultant degenerative changes that are pro-

duced by chronic clenching. In addition to the sounds produced and the difficulties with jaw movement, the most common symptom caused by an internal derangement is pain. The diagnosis generally is made based on the history and physical examination and is confirmed by visualization of disc position by magnetic resonance imaging (MRI).

A patient with a painless click and no jaw dysfunction

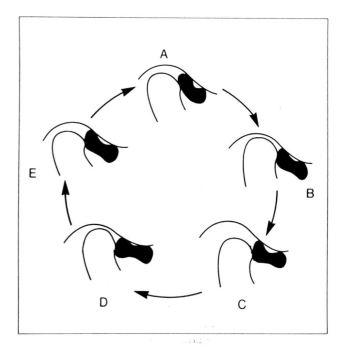

Fig. 83-2. Anterior displacement of the intraarticular disc without reduction on attempted mouth opening. The displaced disc acts as a barrier and prevents full translation of the condyle. (Modified with permission from McCarty W: *Diagnosis and treatment of internal derangements of the articular disc, articular disc and mandibular condyle.* In Solberg WK, Clark GT, editors: *Temporomandibular joint problems: biologic diagnosis and treatment,* Chicago, 1980, Quintessence.)

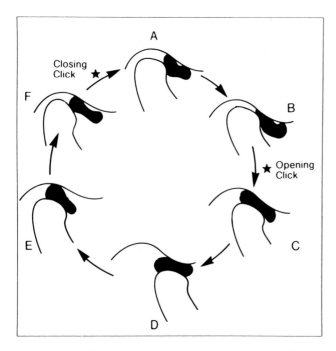

Fig. 83-1. Anterior displacement of the intraarticular disc with reduction on opening of the mouth. A clicking or popping sound occurs as the disc returns to its normal position in relation to the condyle. During closure, the disc again become anteriorly displaced, sometimes accompanied by a second sound (reciprocal click). (Modified with permission from McCarty W: *Diagnosis and treatment of internal derangements of the articular disc and mandibular condyle.* In Solberg WK, Clark GT, editors: *Temporomandibular joint problems: biologic diagnosis and treatment,* Chicago, 1980, Quintessence.)

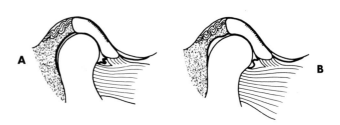

Fig. 83-3. Adhesion of the intraarticular disc causing limitation of mouth opening. **A,** The disc is adherent to the articular eminence in a normal position when the mouth is closed. **B,** During mouth opening, the disc does not move and this limits condylar translation. Because the condyle only rotates, opening is limited to 25 to 30 mm. (Reprinted with permission from Kaplan AS, Assael LA: *Temporomandibular disorders: diagnosis and treatment,* Philadelphia, 1991, WB Saunders.)

requires no treatment. For those who have associated pain, treatment consists of NSAIDs, a bite-opening appliance, and a muscle relaxant when there is lateral pterygoid spasm. For patients with persistent pain and clicking unresponsive to such modalities, the disc can be repositioned by open surgery (discoplasty) or arthroscopically.

In patients with anterior disc displacement without reduction (locking), surgical correction is urgent because if untreated for a long period, degenerative changes in the disc and condyle can occur, complicating the treatment. When open surgery is used, repositioning of the disc should be attempted first, although if the disc is extremely deformed and cannot be repositioned or if there is a large, nonreparable perforation in the disc or retrodiscal tissue, it should be removed and replaced with an auricular cartilage or dermal graft. Currently, there are no acceptable alloplastic substitutes for the disc.

Arthroscopic lysis of adhesions and joint lavage also is used to treat anteriorly displaced, nonreducing discs. Although this procedure does not restore the disc to its normal position,[1] it does restore disc mobility, and this reduces the pain and improves function in most patients.[3] The good results obtained with arthroscopic lysis and lavage have led to the use of arthrocentesis as an even less invasive form of treatment. This involves establishing inlet and outlet portals in the upper joint space with hypodermic needles, irrigation with lactated Ringer's solution, and lysis of adhesions by hydraulic distention and manual manipulation of the joint. The results of arthrocentesis parallel those achieved with arthroscopic lysis and lavage.[12]

Patients who have locking as a result of adhesion of the disc to the articular eminence are not candidates for open surgery because the disc is in a relatively normal position. Such patients can be treated successfully with either arthroscopic lysis and lavage or by arthrocentesis, which restore normal disc mobility.

MYOFASCIAL PAIN-DYSFUNCTION SYNDROME

MPD syndrome is a psychophysiologic disease that primarily involves the muscles of mastication.[5] The condition is characterized by poorly localized, dull, aching, radiating pain that may become acute during use of the jaw and by mandibular dysfunction that usually involves a limitation of opening. The condition generally involves only one side of the face, and on examination, tenderness usually can be elicited in one or more of the muscles of mastication or their tendinous attachments. Although headache frequently is mentioned as a symptom, the only type of headache that may be directly or indirectly part of the syndrome is muscle spasm or tension-type headache, with other types being coincidental findings. The same is true for such complaints as decreased hearing, tinnitus, burning tongue, and neuralgic pains. However, when there is lateral pterygoid spasm, the patient may complain of earache and deep pain behind the eye. Although MPD syndrome starts as a functional disorder,

it ultimately can lead to organic changes in the TMJ and the masticatory muscles and even may cause alterations in the dentition.

MPD syndrome is believed to be a stress-related disorder. It is hypothesized that centrally induced increases in muscle tension, frequently combined with the presence of parafunctional habits such as clenching or grinding of the teeth, result in the muscle fatigue and spasm that produce the pain and dysfunction. Similar symptoms occasionally also can result from muscular overextension, muscle overcontraction, or trauma (Fig. 83-4).

Women are affected by MPD syndrome more frequently than men, with the ratio in various reports ranging from 3 : 1 to 5 : 1. Although the condition can occur in children, the greatest incidence appears to be in the 20- to 40-year age group.

Differential diagnosis

Because the cardinal signs and symptoms of MPD syndrome are similar to those produced by such organic problems involving the TMJ as degenerative joint disease and internal disc derangement and by a variety of nonarticular conditions (Tables 83-2 and 83-3), the diagnosis of this syndrome can be difficult, requiring a careful history and a thorough clinical evaluation to rule out other conditions. Periapical radiographs of the teeth and screening radiographs (transcranial, transpharyngeal, or panoramic) of the TMJs may be helpful. If the screening views of the TMJs show some abnormality, tomographic views or computed tomography (CT) scans usually are advisable. MRI also can be useful in determining the position of the disc when an internal derangement of the TMJ is being considered. Depending on the suspected condition, other radiographic views of the head and neck and scintigraphy may be needed to establish a final diagnosis. In addition, certain laboratory tests may be helpful in some patients. These tests include a complete blood cell count if an infection is suspected; serum calcium, phosphorous, and alkaline phosphatase measurements for possible bone disease; serum uric acid determination for gout; serum creatinine and creatine phosphokinase levels as indicators of muscle disease; and erythrocyte sedimentation rate, rheumatoid factor, latex fixation, and antinuclear antibody tests for suspected rheumatoid arthritis. Electromyography can be used to evaluate muscle function. Psychologic evaluation and psychometric testing are good research tools, but they have little diagnostic value other than to determine the presence of any associated abnormal behavioral characteristics.

Treatment

The treatment of MPD syndrome is divided into four stages (Fig. 83-5).[9] Once a definitive diagnosis is made, stage I therapy is started. This initially involves providing the patient with some understanding of the problem. Because patients often have difficulty accepting a psychophysiologic

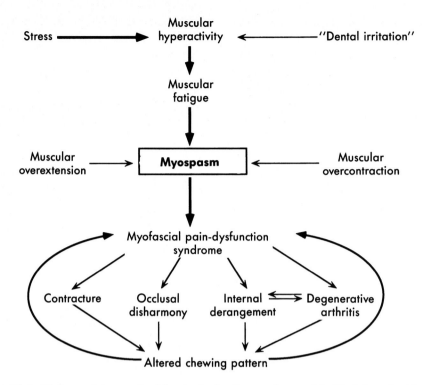

Fig. 83-4. Etiology of the myofascial pain-dysfunction syndrome. (Modified from Laskin DM: Etiology of the pain-dysfunction syndrome, *J Am Dent Assoc* 79:147, 1969.)

Table 83-2. Differential diagnosis of nonarticular conditions mimicking pain of myofascial pain dysfunction syndrome

Disorder	Limitation	Muscle tenderness	Diagnostic features
Pulpitis	No	No	Mild to severe ache or throbbing; intermittent or constant; aggravated by thermal changes; eliminated by dental anesthesia; positive radiograph findings
Pericoronitis	Yes	Possible	Persistent mild to severe ache; difficulty swallowing; possible fever; local inflammation; relieved with dental anesthesia
Otitis media	No	No	Moderate to severe earache; pain constant; fever; usually history of upper respiratory infection; no relief with dental anesthesia
Parotitis	Yes	No	Constant aching pain, worse when eating; pressure feeling; absent salivary flow; ear lobe elevated; ductal suppuration
Sinusitis	No	No	Constant aching or throbbing; worse when change head position; nasal discharge; often molar pain not relieved by dental anesthesia
Trigeminal neuralgia	No	No	Sharp stabbing pain of short duration; trigger zone; pain follows nerve pathway; older age group; often relieved by dental anesthesia
Atypical (vascular) neuralgia	No	No	Diffuse throbbing or burning pain of long duration; often associated autonomic symptoms; no relief with dental anesthesia
Temporal arteritis	No	No	Constant throbbing preauricular pain; artery prominent and tender; low grade fever; may have visual problems; elevated sedimentation rate
Trotter's syndrome (nasopharyngeal carcinoma)	Yes	No	Aching pain in ear, side of face, lower jaw; deafness; nasal obstruction; cervical lymphadenopathy
Eagle's syndrome (elongated styloid process)	No	No	Mild to sharp stabbing pain in ear, throat, retromandible; provoked by swallowing, turning head, carotid compression; usually posttonsillectomy; styloid process longer than 2.5 cm

From Laskin DM, Block S: Diagnosis and treatment of myofascial pain dysfunction (MPD) syndrome, *J Prosthet Dent* 56:75, 1986.

Table 83-3. Differential diagnosis of nonarticular conditions producing limitation of mandibular movement

Disorder	Pain	Muscle tenderness	Diagnostic features
Odontogenic infection	Yes	Yes	Fever; swelling; positive radiographic findings; tooth tender to percussion; pain relieved and movement improved with dental anesthesia
Nonodontogenic infection	Yes	Yes	Fever; swelling; negative dental findings on radiograph; dental anesthesia may not relieve pain or improve jaw movement
Myositis	Yes	Yes	Sudden onset; movement associated with pain; areas of muscle tenderness; usually no fever
Myositis ossificans	No	No	Palpable nodules seen as radiopaque areas on radiograph; involvement of nonmasticatory muscles
Neoplasia	Possible	Possible	Palpable mass; regional nodes may be enlarged; may have paresthesia; radiograph may show bone involvement
Scleroderma	No	No	Skin hard and atrophic; mask-like faces; paresthesias; arthritic joint pain; widening of periodontal ligament
Hysteria	No	No	Sudden onset after psychological trauma; no physical findings; jaw opens easily during general anesthesia
Tetanus	Yes	No	Recent wound; stiffness of neck; difficulty swallowing; spasm of facial muscles; headache
Extrapyramidal reaction	No	No	Patient on antipsychotic drug or phenothiazine tranquilizer; hypertonic movement; lip smacking; spontaneous chewing motions
Depressed zygomatic arch	Possible	No	History of trauma; facial depression; positive radiographic findings
Osteochondroma coronoid process	No	No	Gradual limitation; jaw may deviate to unaffected side; possible clicking sound on jaw movement; positive radiographic findings

From Laskin DM, Block S: Diagnosis and treatment of myofascial pain dysfunction (MPD) syndrome, *J Prosthet Dent* 56:75, 1986.

explanation for their condition, the discussion should deal with the issue of muscle fatigue and spasm as the cause of the pain and dysfunction, delaying consideration of the role of stress and psychologic factors until the symptoms have improved and until the patient's confidence has been gained. Relating the symptoms to the specific masticatory muscles from which they originate helps the patient understand the reason for the type and location of the pain; for example, headache from the temporalis muscle, jaw ache from the masseter muscle, discomfort when swallowing and stuffiness in the ear from the medial pterygoid muscle, and earache and pain behind the eye from the lateral pterygoid muscle.

In addition to the initial explanation, the patient is counseled regarding home therapy. Counseling includes recommendations about avoidance of clenching and grinding of the teeth; eating a soft, nonchewy diet; use of moist heat on, and massage of, the masticatory muscles; and limitation of jaw motion. Because the patient has muscle spasm and pain, a muscle relaxant and a NSAID are prescribed. Diazepam and ibuprofen are commonly used.

About 50% of the patients will have a resolution of their symptoms within 2 to 4 weeks with stage I therapy. For those whose symptoms persist, stage II therapy is initiated. Home therapy and medications are continued, but at this point, a bite appliance is made for the patient. Although numerous types have been used, the Hawley-type maxillary appliance probably is most effective because it prevents con-

tact of the posterior teeth and thereby also prevents most forms of parafunctional activity. Generally, the appliance is worn at night, but it can be worn for 5 to 6 hours during the day if necessary. It should not be worn continuously because the posterior teeth may supraerupt in some patients.

With stage II therapy, another 20% to 25% of patients will become free of symptoms in 2 to 4 weeks. The medications are stopped first and wearing the bite appliance is discontinued next. If the patient has a return of symptoms when the appliance is not worn at night, its use can be continued indefinitely.

Patients who do not respond to the use of a bite appliance are entered into stage III of treatment for 4 to 6 weeks. In this phase, either physical therapy (ultrasound, electrogalvanic stimulation) or relaxation therapy electromyographic (biofeedback, conditioned relaxation) are added to the regimen. There is no evidence to show that one form of treatment is better than the other, and either can be used first. If one is not successful, the other then can be tried. Stage III therapy usually helps another 10% to 15% of patients.

If all of the previous approaches fail and if there is no question about the correctness of the diagnosis, psychologic counseling is recommended. This involves helping patients identify possible stresses in their life and learning to cope with such situations. If there is doubt about the diagnosis, the patient should first be referred for appropriate dental and neurologic consultation and evaluation. Another alternative is to refer patients with recalcitrant MPD syndrome to a TMJ

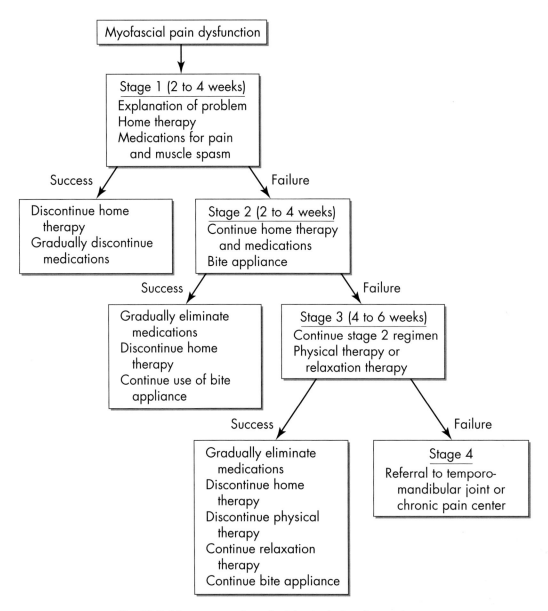

Fig. 83-5. Management of myofascial pain dysfunction syndrome.

center or pain clinic because such patients generally require a multidisciplinary approach for successful treatment.

SUMMARY

The successful treatment of patients with TMDs depends on establishing an accurate diagnosis and using proper therapy based on an understanding of the etiology of the condition being managed. Of particular importance is separating those patients with MPD syndrome, who constitute the major group encountered and who are not surgical candidates, from those with TMJ abnormality, who frequently require surgical treatment. Even in the latter group, many of the commonly encountered conditions, such as arthritis and internal disc derangements, often respond to nonsurgical therapy, and this type of treatment should be given a fair trial before more aggressive treatment is considered.

REFERENCES

1. Gabler MJ and others: Effect of arthroscopic temporomandibular joint surgery on articular disc position, *J Craniomand Disord Facial Oral Pain* 3:191, 1989.
2. Hampf G, Tasanen A, Nordling S: Surgery in mandibular condylar hyperplasias, *J Max Fac Surg* 13:74, 1985.
3. Indresano AT: Arthroscopic surgery of the temporomandibular joint: report of 64 patients with long-term follow-up, *J Oral Maxillofac Surg* 47:439, 1989.
4. Kaban LB, Moses MH, Mulliken JB: Surgical correction of hemifacial microsomia in the growing child, *Plast Reconstr Surg* 82:9, 1988.
5. Laskin DM: Etiology of the pain-dysfunction syndrome, *JADA* 59:147, 1969.

6. Laskin DM: *Myotomy for the management of recurrent and protracted mandibular dislocation.* In Kay L, editor: *Oral surgery,* Copenhagen, 1972, Munksgaard.

7. Reference deleted in pages.

8. Laskin DM: *Surgical management of diseases of the temporomandibular joint.* In Hayward JR, editor: *Oral surgery,* Springfield, Ill, 1976, Charles C Thomas.

9. Laskin DM, Block S: Diagnosis and treatment of myofascial pain-dysfunction (MPD) syndrome, *J Prosthet Dent* 56:75, 1986.

10. Lindqvist and others: Adaptation of autogenous costochondral grafts used for temporomandibular joint reconstruction: a long-term clinical and radiographic follow-up, *J Oral Maxillofac Surg* 48:465, 1988.

11. McCarthy JG and others: Lengthening of the mandible by gradual distraction, *Plast Reconstr Surg* 89:1, 1992.

12. Nitzan DW: *Arthrocentesis for management of severe closed lock of the temporomandibular joint.* In Laskin DM, editor: *Current controversies in surgery for internal derangements of the temporomandibular joint,* Philadelphia, 1944, WB Saunders.

13. Obeid G, Guttenberg SA, Cannole PW: Costochondral grafting in condylar replacement and mandibular reconstruction, *J Oral Maxillofac Surg* 48:177, 1988.

14. Politis C, Fossion E, Bossuyt M: The use of costochondral grafts in arthroplasty of the temporomandibular joint, *J Cranio Max Fac Surg* 15:345, 1987.

15. Poswillo DE: Biological reconstruction of the mandibular condyle, *Br J Oral Maxillofac Surg* 25:149, 1987.

16. Rachmiel A, Levy M, Laufer D: Lengthening of the mandible by distraction osteogenesis: report of cases, *J Oral Maxillofac Surg* 53:838, 1995.

17. Schultz LW: Twenty years' experience in treating hypermobility of the temporomandibular joints, *Am J Surg* 92:925, 1956.

18. Zide MF, Carlton D, Kent JH: Rheumatoid arthritis and related arthropathies: systemic findings, medical therapy, and peripheral joint surgery, *Oral Surg* 61:119, 1986.

19. Zide MF, Kent JH: Indications for open reduction of mandibular condyle fractures, *J Oral Maxillofac Surg* 41:89, 1983.

Chapter 84

Cosmetic and Functional Prosthetic Rehabilitation of Acquired Defects

Alan B. Carr

The otolaryngologist is routinely faced with the need to prescribe reconstructive treatment for acquired defects of the head and neck region. Whether the defect has been acquired through disease and its removal or as a result of trauma, the surgeon should have an understanding of the benefits and risks associated with the various surgical and prosthetic options available to their patients. It is the intent of this chapter to provide information regarding the unique challenges this population of patients presents for prosthetic management of common acquired defects to guide decision-making regarding the combined surgical–prosthetic treatment of these patients. Although the major emphasis will be for acquired defects resulting from treatment of head and neck cancer, the principles presented are largely applicable to traumatic defects as well.

SOCIAL IMPACT OF HEAD AND NECK CANCER

Although the incidence of head and neck cancer is not as high as cancers in other regions of the body, its importance in the head and neck region relates to the heightened functional impairment and psychosocial impact that result from such diseases and their treatment. The complex functional arrangement of the human aerodigestive and specialized sensory systems provide the basic functions of respiration and feeding; the learned behaviors of mastication and speech; the special sensory functions included in the head and neck region (vision, hearing, taste, balance, smell); the specialized senses, coordinated in function, sensate, moist and mobile local mucosal environment of this region; and the psychosocial importance associated with the facial–oral–laryngeal structures, which all make surgical management in this region a complex undertaking.

MULTIDISCIPLINARY CARE

For the provider of care and the patient, the diversity of the local region often presents multifaceted problems associated with the management of cancer in the region, and consequently the best management is through the coordinated efforts of a multidisciplinary team. Because of the complexity of the functional deficits associated with removal of some head and neck tumors (and the required adjacent tissue), surgical management may not be adequate as a sole reconstructive procedure. For tumors that involve regions of anatomy that participate in different but coordinated functions or for defects that involve large areas, surgical replacement of useful anatomy using the best available methods often is less than ideal and less predictable than prosthetic management. The challenge for the surgeon is to recognize the surgical reconstructive limits for complex defects, understand when prostheses provide a better functional and cosmetic result compared with the surgical options, understand when prostheses are required in coordination with surgical reconstruction, and to design and provide a surgical site as required for optimum prosthetic usefulness.

The surgeon who provides head and neck cancer management services needs the support of a dental colleague to maximize this service. Many well-meaning general dentists have helped in these challenging endeavors, although the interaction too often has been less than ideal because of the limited training and expertise of the dentist. This has unfortunately often placed the surgeon in a position to offer more surgery when adequate prosthetic support is not available. Maxillofacial prosthetics, a subdiscipline of the specialty prosthodontics, is the branch of dentistry that provides prostheses to treat or restore tissues of the stomatognathic system and associated facial structures that have been affected by disease, injury, surgery, or congenital defect, providing restoration of all possible functions and esthetics. The maxillofacial prosthodontist is a vital resource to the total head and neck patient management service and is best qualified to provide the prosthetic support to the surgeon. Given the requirement of coordinated surgical–prosthetic management, the patient with an acquired defect is best served by the coordinated efforts of the surgeon and maxillofacial prosthodontist. Consequently, to facilitate the coordination of treatment for patients with acquired defects, the following aspects related to prosthetic care in these patients will be discussed:

1. The degree to which prosthetic reconstructions can approach presurgical functional measures;
2. The timing of prosthetic care with examples of prostheses for the most common head and neck surgical defects, and the surgical outcomes that improve prosthetic success for different regions;
3. The prosthetic management of extraoral defects with descriptions of favorable surgical outcomes; and
4. The use of implants for the patient with acquired defects.

INTRAORAL MAXILLOFACIAL PROSTHETIC FUNCTION COMPARED TO PRESURGICAL STATE

In this region of the body, which is vital to the normal social interaction of the patient, it is important that the patient's understanding of the impairment associated with the surgical resection and the degree to which the surgical or prosthetic reconstructions will provide restoration be as clear as possible. This is not easily accomplished because (1) it often is difficult to precisely describe the anatomic involvement of the disease presurgically (and the degree of impairment associated with the treatment), and (2) the subject of cancer is such a psychologic burden to most patients that it makes the patient–provider interaction difficult. However, to help develop an understanding of realistic maxillofacial prosthetic expectations of restoration, it is helpful to have an appreciation of the functional capacity of conventional dental prosthetic management against a background of normative dentate function.

Functional normal

Because patients present with varying presurgical intraoral conditions, their basis for comparison is from their unique oral–dental experience. A knowledge of the variation of objective and subjective measures of oral function helps in the development of realistic goals and expectations for the patient with an acquired defect. Functional impairment after surgery most often relates to mastication, swallowing, and speech, whereas cosmetic impairment resulting from intraoral defects most often is characterized by disfigurement of the lower third of the face.

Mastication

Although functionally considered a separate act, mastication as part of the feeding continuum precedes the activity of deglutition and is not an end to itself. The interaction of the two distinct but coordinated aspects of feeding suggests some judgment of mastication termination or completeness precedes the initiation of deglutition. Although the mastication–deglutition sequence is obvious, the interaction of the two functions is not widely understood and underlies some of the subtle but important functional deficits inherent in the head and neck cancer patient after surgery.

Mastication involves two discrete but well-synchronized activities: subdivision of food by applied force, and manipulation by the tongue and cheeks to sort out coarse particles and bring them to the occlusal surfaces of teeth for further breakdown.[23] The initial subdivision or comminution phase involves the processes of (1) selection, which is the chance that a particle is placed between the teeth in position to be broken, and (2) breakage, which is the degree of fragmentation of a particle once selected.[33] The size, shape, and texture of the food particles provide the sensory input that influences the configuration and area of each chewing stroke. The larger particles are selectively reduced more rapidly than fine particles in efficient mastication.[57] The process of mastication therefore is greatly influenced by factors that impact the physical ability to reduce food and to monitor the reduction process by neurosensory means.

Food reduction. An index of food reduction is described as *masticatory efficiency*, which is the ability to reduce food to a certain size in a given time frame.[4] It has been shown that there is a strong correlation between masticatory efficiency and the number of occluding teeth in dentate patients, which would suggest variability of particle selection related to contacting teeth.[16] The reliability of this process is shown in duplication of masticatory efficiency tests in the same patient over time when no change in the number of contacting teeth has been made.[57] This reliability of masticatory efficiency is not seen across populations of patients with an identical number of occluding teeth. Performance measures reveal a great deal of functional variability in patients with similar numbers of contacting teeth, and an even greater variability is seen within populations with greater loss of teeth (increasing degrees of edentulousness).

Occlusal contact area is highly correlated with masticatory performance.[57] Therefore the loss of molar teeth, which because of an increased size provide more opportunity for contacting surfaces, would be expected to be impact measures of performance greater. This has been shown in patients with missing molars who required a greater number of chewing strokes and a greater mean particle size before swallowing.[44] The point at which a person is prepared to swallow the food bolus is another measure of performance and is described as the *swallowing threshold*. Superior masticatory ability that is highly correlated with occlusal contact area also achieves greater food reduction at the swallowing threshold. Conversely, a decreased ability to chew is reflected in larger particles at the swallowing threshold.

Prosthetic replacement of teeth reveals that functional restoration often is less than the complete natural dentition state. Functional measures are closest to the natural state when replacements are fixed partial dentures rigidly supported by teeth or implants, intermediate in function when replacements are removable and supported by teeth, lower in function when replacements are removable and supported by teeth and edentulous ridges, and lowest in function when replacements are removable and supported on edentulous ridges alone.[4,13,34]

Subjective measures of oral function provide information as to the level of concordance between the patient's objective measures of oral function and his or her perception. It has been shown that subjective measures of masticatory ability often are overrated compared with functional tests and that for complete denture wearers, the subjective criteria may be preferred in monitoring care.[3] The literature also suggests that removable partial dentures frequently are described by patients as adding little benefit over no prostheses,[31,44] although this most likely is related to the lack of maintenance of the occluding tooth relationships[30,52] and indicates the limitations of this form of dental prosthesis for patient populations that may be unreliable in maintaining follow-up visits.

Monitoring of food reduction. Food reduction also is influenced by the ability to monitor the process that is required to determine the point at which swallow is initiated. As mentioned previously, the size, shape, and texture of food is monitored during mastication to allow modification in mandibular movement for efficient food reduction. This has been shown in dentate patients who were given food particles of varying size and concentration suspended in yogurt and who revealed that increased concentrations and particle size required more time to prepare for swallowing (i.e., greater swallowing threshold).[47] These findings suggest that the oral mucosa has a critical role in detecting characteristics necessary for efficient mastication.

If afferent sensory input is necessary for efficient mastication, might this help explain why complete denture patients (with so much mucosa covered by the prostheses) exhibit much lower scores of oral function? Could an understanding of the underlying reasons for this reduced functional capacity have any bearing on maxillofacial deficits after head and neck surgery? One study addressed this reduced sensory input related to masticatory efficiency hypothesis by anesthetizing the oral mucosa of dentate patients and measuring masticatory efficiency.[22] They found a profound effect on masticatory efficiency with unilateral anesthesia. In this study, patients who normally required approximately 20 chewing strokes to prepare food for swallowing required approximately 40 chewing strokes for the same task after unilateral anesthesia. These dentate patients, who normally were more selective of coarse particles for more rapid reduction characteristic of efficient mastication, had more random reduction of food particles as seen in complete denture patients. This finding of an increased number of chewing strokes as a compensatory reaction in mastication is common to complete denture patients,[13,34] and as with the measure of bite force, is variable among patients for satisfactory and unsatisfactory prostheses.[4,13] The relationship between decrease in sensation and functional performance may help partly explain the functional scores of patients after intraoral resections and reconstructions and is the underlying reason for the increased interest in sensate flaps for oral reconstructions.[15]

Swallowing

The act of swallowing, or deglutition, is a complex functional task involving the oral cavity, pharynx, and esophagus, where the transition from the oral cavity phase to the pharyngeal phase is initiated by the patient. The previous discussion involving the judgment by the patient as to the preparedness of the reduced food for swallowing gives an indication of the varying degree of reduction or masticatory efficiency based on the number of contacting teeth. At this stage, the decision to swallow has been made, and the major controlling factors for normal deglutition are the structural integrity of the component parts and their coordinated neuromuscular activity. Although surgical management can impact all phases of the swallowing mechanism, prosthetic management is chiefly concerned with components in the oral and pharyngeal phase related to structural integrity: the tongue, the hard palate, and the soft palate–pharyngeal functional unit commonly referred to as the *palatopharyngeal complex*. Objective measures of normal swallowing, as determined from videofluoroscopic studies, provide an understanding of the timing and coordination of tongue loading and pulsion, nasopharyngeal closure, pharyngeal clearance, airway protection, and upper esophageal opening.[20] Prosthetic management only directly affects the first three mentioned measures.

The tongue exhibits a highly complex capacity for motion because of its arrangement of muscles with external attachments, allowing for a range of movement about the oral cavity, and internal or intrinsic attachments, allowing for task-specific shape modifications. Studies of the surface motion of the tongue during swallowing reveal perimeter contact with the alveolar ridge and a central groove, which exhibits centripetal and centrifugal motion.[21] Such motion combined with the pharyngeal walls creates an oropharyngeal chamber that expels its contents into the hypopharynx. The tongue is capable of modulation of its propulsive force based on bolus viscosity and volume. The modulation capacity of the anterior two thirds of the tongue exceeds that of the posterior base of the tongue.[46] Consequently, the tongue functions in swallowing include bolus containment, volume accommodation, and the major contributor of bolus propulsion.

Palatopharyngeal closure for the purpose of separating the oral and pharyngeal cavities from the nasal cavities is required for speech, swallowing, and forced, sustained inhalation and exhalation. Separation during swallowing, which is necessary to prevent reflux of food and liquid into the nose, only appears to be similar to closure during speech. Swallowing closure is more forceful or ballistic in the action, includes more regional muscular recruitment,[49] and the reflex control for swallowing has been stated to be different from that for speech.[53] Therefore, diagnostic measures of closure for swallowing function are not necessarily transferable to the function of speech.

Because closure includes portions of the palate and pharynx, it frequently is referred to as *palatopharyngeal closure*. When the food bolus is propelled into the pharynx, stimulation of the surrounding mucosa of the tonsillar pillars initiates involuntary pharyngeal contractions beginning with palatal elevation in coordination with pharyngeal wall movement, hyoid bone elevation, and epiglottis closure of the airway with opening of the pharyngoesophageal sphincter. These events in humans have been described as being impressively constant.[53] The components of major interest for prosthodontic impact are the soft palate and pharyngeal wall movement.

The position and movement of the soft palate varies with age, and at closure, it is characteristically above the level of the palatal plane in adults.[1] The pattern of movement also varies between men and women, with men showing a longer portion of palate in contact, less length, and a higher point of contact with the posterior pharyngeal wall.[41] Pharyngeal wall movement is less predictable from the posterior wall than from the lateral walls and the soft palate. Posterior wall movement has been shown in patients in whom compensatory movement may provide a functional benefit because of long-term structural inadequacy (i.e., cleft palate). Lateral pharyngeal wall movement contributes significantly to palatopharyngeal closure for swallowing and speech. The level of movement is greatest at the region of the hard palatal plane, making transoral inspection of this movement difficult. The character of movement is sphincteric in nature, not always bilaterally similar, in contact with the soft palate for about 1 cm,[18] and in contact at the midline for varying lengths, depending on whether the swallow was a reflex or dry swallow.[53] The musculature responsible for this pharyngeal wall movement has been debated, but current research supports the bilateral superior constrictor, levator palati, and possibly the salpingopharyngeus muscles.

Unlike the learned and voluntary function of mastication, once initiated, swallowing is largely a reflex phenomenon. The integrated phases of swallowing proceed in a preordained manner and can run their full course without benefit of, or modification by, afferent support.[10] Consequently, for patients with acquired defects that impact swallowing, prosthetic management can only serve a mechanical role that addresses loss of structural integrity. The altered functional capacity of the reconstructed environment will be the overriding factor in swallow rehabilitation.

Speech

Speech is a learned function that uses the structural anatomy intended for the more basic functions of respiration and deglutition. For successful speech, multiple component systems are required and include respiration, phonation, resonation, articulation, neurologic integration, and the ability to hear sounds. The usefulness of speech lies in the ability to communicate, therefore the most useful objective measure of speech is a measure of speech intelligibility.

Surgical management of head and neck tumors can result in acquired speech disorders, including impaired articulation, decreased speech intelligibility, altered oral and nasal resonance, impaired voice quality, changed speech rates and prosody, and decreased global speech proficiency.[37] Surgical reconstructions for tongue, floor of mouth, and mandible tumors also can alter speech through an effect on the mobility of the tongue, mandible, and lips. Reconstruction of pharyngeal areas with tissue that does not allow dynamic movement and is bulkier than the original tissue also may alter the resonance quality of speech. Prosthodontic management mainly addresses the resonation and articulation deficits created by the tumor management.

The acquired defects that most frequently impact speech are caused by resections of the tongue, floor of mouth, retromolar trigone, mandible, and the hard and soft palates. Defects that create communication between separate cavities (maxillary or soft palate defects) or defects that are large and dramatically increase the size of a cavity can alter speech resonance. Resonant quality to speech is derived from the airway chambers above the level of the larynx and include the pharynx at all levels, the nasal cavities, and the oral cavity. For the mucosal-lined pharyngeal chamber, changes in the static dimensions or the opportunity for dynamic movement that influences resonance will not be improved with the use of a prosthesis.

The soft palate serves to couple and uncouple the oral and nasal cavities for selective production of consonant phonemes. This valve-like function has the purpose of helping to direct the airstream selectively for oral and nasal consonant production, and as such, the soft palate controls the use of the different resonant chambers of the upper airway. The soft palate also is important to the articulatory function of speech by virtue of its control of the airway for creation of the oral articulatory valves. Altered function of the soft palate consequently impacts articulation and resonation components. One study has shown that when resections are limited to the anterior portion of the soft palate, prosthetic treatment has sufficed (and surgical reconstruction is not indicated), whereas more total resections to the posterior pharyngeal wall were equally successful with surgery and prosthetics.[55] The challenge for prosthetic management is to determine the altered soft palatal or surrounding pharyngeal wall movement and the associated palatopharyngeal incompetency and to place a static palatal component of a prosthesis within this region to artificially redirect the airstream for optimum articulation. Successful management of soft palatal defects with such speech aid prostheses is best determined through coordinated speech intelligibility testing by a speech pathologist.

Surgical management of tumors involving the tongue impact the articulatory function of this highly specialized organ. The extrinsic muscles chiefly provide a stable postural background from which the intrinsic muscles control fine, discrete movements, as are those associated with speech. It has been shown that the articulatory movements of the tongue apex are more active in consonant production, and the body of the tongue is active in consonant and vowel production.[45] A comparison of speech function in a group of 11 patients who had resection of greater than 1-cm tumors of the tongue base, tonsillar pillar, and mandible (with primary closure) with another group of patients who had anterior tongue resections revealed that speech performance was better in the group with tongue base resection.[32] The maintenance of anterior tongue mobility was an important finding and suggests efforts to minimize the surgical impact on tongue mobility after surgery are warranted.

For useful production of consonants in speech, the tongue must be able to contact variable regions of the maxilla, teeth, and possibly the lips. Surgical defects that result in hindered movement can be compensated for by artificial lowering of the maxilla and palate to the altered functional level of the tongue to attempt to improve consonant production. For those with total glossectomy defects, prostheses can be provided to statically fill the space in the floor of the mouth to facilitate deglutition and speech. The success of such prostheses for both functions largely depends on the mobility of the mandible and whether the base of tongue was preserved. It is common that each function will require different static forms for optimum results.

Cosmetic impact of intraoral acquired defects

Surgical management of intraoral or perioral tumors that requires removal of portions of the facial skeleton can cause disfigurement of the face. The most common disfiguring procedure involves resection of the mandible with either no reconstruction or reconstruction resulting in altered contours of the lower third of the face. The past decade has seen increased attention directed toward the cosmetic impact of resective surgery of the head and neck region, and this has resulted in the established current minimal reconstructive option for mandibular resections as the prosthetic plate.[7]

Other forms of cosmetic defects that are not classified as deformities include drooling, oral incompetence, facial paralysis, and unintelligible speech. Drooling and oral incompetence are associated with similar deficits and are closely related to impaired mandibular lip sensation or posture, a decreased labial and lingual sulcus reflection that does not encourage posterior flow of saliva and liquids in the diet, and a decreased ability to approximate and seal the lips during swallowing. These deficits typically are not managed with prostheses. Unilateral facial paralysis, which results in an inferior positioning of the oral commissure, has been treated with the use of a lip-supportive prosthesis that simply attempts to place the commissure in a bilaterally appropriate position.[29] Such a prosthesis does not address the paralysis affect on the lower eyelid or cheek, is not able to mimic the dynamic movement of a normal commissure, and requires considerable patient accommodation. The social impact of speech carries a cosmetic characteristic that needs to be appreciated in its restoration.

Prosthetic physiology

Tooth loss has been successfully treated with various dental prostheses to provide cosmetic and functional restoration. The nature of the tooth loss (the number and location of teeth and associated structures) determines the types of prostheses to be considered for this restoration and includes fixed or removable partial dentures, removable complete dentures, and maxillofacial prostheses. The most important consideration for prosthetic treatment where artificial replacements are placed within an environment subjected to functional loads associated with mastication, deglutition, speech, and other related oromandibular movements is the ability to resist the anticipated loads. For prostheses that are removable, the additional requirement of being retained in place while not in function is obvious, especially for the dislodging effect of gravity on maxillary prostheses.

Normal resistance to functional loads is achieved by the highly sophisticated periodontal attachment of the natural dentition, which provides support and stability to teeth. When the dentition is partially depleted and replaced by prostheses that are tooth-supported, the support and stability of the replacement teeth remain to be provided by the natural attachment supporting the prosthesis. When tooth loss includes several posterior teeth, replacements are placed over the residual edentulous ridge, and the prosthesis receives support and stability from teeth and mucosa. When all the teeth are lost, the support and stability are totally provided by the mucosa covering the residual edentulous ridges. Finally, when surgical removal of tumors results in tooth and supporting structure loss, the support and stability are provided by combinations of remaining teeth or residual ridges and suitable areas within the surgical defect. For partial and complete tissue-supported prostheses, the mechanism of functional load support, as provided by the mucosa, is unsuited to the task from a biologic standpoint. Given this understanding, when a maxillofacial prosthesis is required to use tissue within a surgical defect for support and stability, it is obvious that this defect environment is even less suited to the task.

Maxillofacial prosthetics is largely a removable prosthetic discipline, with the exception of dental implant-retained prostheses for some applications. Removable prostheses generally can be categorized into prostheses prescribed for completely edentulous patients and prostheses prescribed for patients with some teeth remaining. The typical goal of treatment for each category of patient is a well-supported, stable, retentive prosthesis that is acceptable in appearance and exhibits minimal movement under function, thereby preserving the maximum amount of supporting tissue over time. A conceptual strategy for achieving this goal includes maximum coverage of the edentulous ridge within the movement capacity of the muscular attachments, maximum engagement of the remaining teeth to help control retention and movement under function, and placement of artificial teeth to facilitate maintenance of this prescribed tooth–tissue contact during normal functional contacts. Maintaining these basic concepts within an otherwise normal anatomic environment (relative to food control and deglutition) has provided reasonable success for patients requiring replacement of missing teeth.

Measures of function related to mastication and deglutition reveal that, in general, conventional removable prostheses more closely approach the normal dentate state when more natural teeth remain, the prosthetic teeth replace lost functional tooth contacts, and edentulous ridge quality and contour are optimum. As the size of the edentulous component of the prostheses increases, more demand is placed on the adjacent oral structures to control the removable prosthesis. The fact that control of such prostheses is a skilled performance acquired by some patients suggests that oral structures adjacent to the prostheses are important for successful performance.[5] This is crucial to an understanding of the impact postsurgical defect characteristics and soft-tissue reconstruction have on maxillofacial prosthesis management. This is because of the major contribution of the cheek and tongue under the control of the patient for controlling large removable prostheses and because of the potential that after surgery such control may be dramatically hindered. It also is critical to note that the measures of oral competence and mastication, specifically as they relate to food manipulation (bolus preparation and swallow), are related to soft-tissue reconstruction goals difficult to obtain with large flaps.

The patient who is most negatively impacted by surgical intervention is the patient who has been functioning with sufficient natural teeth and who, after a large surgery that has removed most of the functioning teeth, is required to function with a removable prosthesis that replaces one half or more of the dentition. These patients have the most favorable presurgical functional condition, natural teeth, and a severely compromised postsurgical state. They often are most discouraged by the prosthetic result. Consequently, for the patient who presurgically has sufficient teeth (or prosthetic replacements totally supported by teeth) to function normally, the functional baseline for comparison of the postsurgical maxillofacial prostheses is the most optimum for comparison. Existing measures of removable prosthesis function suggest a restoration of function that is less than ideal and is best in an environment that enables patient manipulation of prostheses with tongue, cheeks, and lips.

TIMING OF DENTAL AND MAXILLOFACIAL PROSTHETIC CARE

A conceptual model for the timing of dental and oral care that best emphasizes the initial more important surgical requirements and then the later more important prosthetic ones is helpful for the coordination of care. Such a strategy considers preoperative, intraoperative, interim, and definitive care.

Pre- and intraoperative care

The planning of prosthetic treatment for acquired oral defects should begin before surgery. For the patient undergoing head and neck surgery, consideration should be given to dental needs that will improve the immediate postoperative course (Table 84-1). Consequently, the prosthodontist who will help with management of the patient's care should see the patient before surgery. The dental objectives of the pre- and intraoperative care stage are to remove potential dental postoperative complications, to plan for the subsequent prosthetic treatment, and to make recommendations for surgical site preparation to improve structural integrity. A major benefit of such a preoperative consultation is the opportunity to discuss the functional deficits associated with the anticipated surgical procedure and how the stages of prosthetic management will address them.

The immediate postoperative period will be challenging

Table 84-1. Presurgical oral considerations

- Patient consultation to discuss anticipated postsurgical impairment and manner of prosthesis management
- Determine potential for dental complications and prescribe the required treatment
- Plan subsequent prosthetic treatment from records (dental casts and radiographs)
- Make recommendations for surgical site preparation to optimize prosthetic management

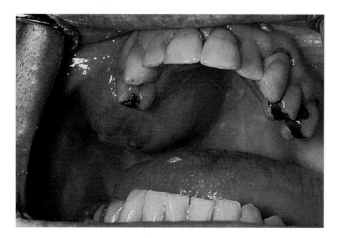

Fig. 84-1. Presurgical evaluation of this maxillary tumor and dentition will guide decision-making that can improve the interim treatment of the patient. Anticipating a large resection, the preservation of questionable teeth during the interim phase is warranted to improve the function of the interim prosthesis. Presurgical management should include débridement and caries control, along with obtaining dental records.

to the patient. If preexisting dental disease is severe enough to potentially create symptoms during the immediate postoperative period, treatment should be provided to remove such a complication (Fig. 84-1). Large carious lesions that could create pain can be temporarily restored or treated endodontically, if they offer some advantage to postoperative prosthetic function. Teeth exhibiting acute periodontal disease (such as acute necrotizing ulcerative gingivitis) should be treated, as should any periodontal condition that could potentially cause postoperative pain as a result of excessive mobility. Any tooth that is deemed nonrestorable because of advanced caries or periodontal disease and that is not critical for temporary use during the interim care period after temporary treatment should be removed at the time of resective surgery. Teeth that may appear to have a limited long term-prognosis may dramatically enhance prosthetic service during the initial postsurgical period and should be maintained until definitive care is initiated.

Impressions are made of the maxillary and mandibular arches to provide a record of existing conditions and occlusion, to allow fabrication of immediate or interim prostheses, and to assess the need for immediate and delayed modification of the teeth or adjacent structures to optimize prosthetic care. It is important at this stage to begin planning for the definitive prosthesis because the greatest impact on the success of the maxillofacial prosthesis stems from the integrity of the surrounding structures.[9]

Interim care

The major emphasis during this stage of care is the surgical (and adjunctive) management needs of the patient. In today's environment of appropriately aggressive mandibular surgical reconstruction, mandibular discontinuity defects seldom are a surgical outcome; consequently, interim care for mandibular defects is not indicated, and the discussion will be directed toward the maxillary defect.

The maxillary defect allows oronasal communication that creates physiologic deficiencies in mastication, deglutition, and speech. Such defects have a negative impact on the psychologic disposition of patients, especially if the defect also affects cosmetic appearance. The major deficiencies directly addressed by prosthetic management at this time are deglutition and speech. The patients are counseled that chewing on the defect side is not allowed because of the effect on prosthesis movement. The objective of this prosthesis is to separate the oral and nasal cavities by obturating the communication. Such obturator prostheses are most commonly referring to obturation of a hard palatal defect but conceptually can be considered the same for soft palatal defects at this stage of management because both attempt to artificially block the free transfer of speech sounds and food and liquids between the oral and nasal cavities. The advantages of having the ability to take nourishment by mouth without nasal reflux (allowing for nasogastric tube removal) and to communicate with family members is a major component of early prosthetic management. How immediate such care should be provided depends on a number of factors.

A prosthesis could be provided at surgery. Such a prosthesis is placed at the time of surgical access closure and serves to control the surgical dressing and split-thickness skin graft during the immediate postsurgical period. Such prostheses are best stabilized by appropriate wiring to remaining teeth or alveolar bone, or suspended from superior skeletal structures. For some patients who have teeth remaining, such an immediate surgical prostheses could be retained by wires in the prosthesis that engage undercuts on the teeth and would be removable, although the ability to control the surgical dressing may be less predictable with such an approach. Immediate placement of a prosthesis has been suggested to improve patient acceptance of the surgical defect, although no measure of this psychologic impact has been shown and offers greater assurance of adequate nourishment by mouth potentially precluding the use of a nasogastric tube.

It may be preferable to stabilize the surgical dressing by suturing a sponge bolster to place providing stabilization to the split-thickness skin graft. After the primary healing stage, the sponge and packing (or the immediate prosthesis if used) are removed by the surgeon, and an interim obturator prosthesis can be placed. For the patient who has been provided with bolster obturation, the presurgical prosthodontic evaluation is important to ensure the patient is prepared for the transition from bolster to prosthesis and to ensure plans for the prosthesis are made, especially if an interim prosthesis is to be fabricated from a presurgical impression.

For edentulous patients with acceptable maxillary complete dentures, the existing prosthesis can be modified to

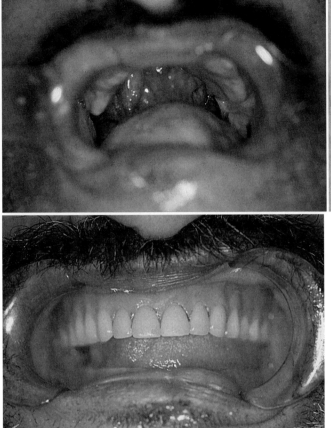

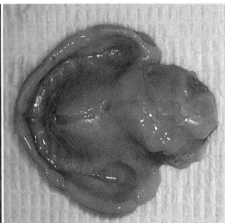

Fig. 84-2. Immediate modification of an existing complete denture to obturate a combined hard and soft palatal defect. The benefit of this temporary modification is immediate improvement of speech and swallowing, which help improve the patient's ability to cope with the postsurgical defect.

adequately obturate the defect and can serve satisfactorily during the healing stage (Fig. 84-2). An advantage to the use of an existing prosthesis is that accommodation is less challenging to the patient because of the use of a prosthesis with contours normal to the presurgical state. When an edentulous patient has no prosthesis or if the existing prosthesis is unacceptable, it may be necessary to make an impression after surgical pack removal to fabricate an interim obturator prosthesis. For patients with teeth, an interim prosthesis is made from the preoperative cast, which has been altered with input from the surgeon regarding the location of remaining teeth and uses retaining clasps to stabilize the prosthesis (Fig. 84-3). Subsequent addition of a resilient lining material to the prosthesis portion that covers the defect provides for obturation to the level of toleration of the surgical wound. As the defect margins and lining tissue mature, more aggressive filling of the defect improves the opportunity for maximum seal and benefit.

When surgical defects become large, as in a near total maxillectomy defect, prosthesis support, stability, and retention is not likely to be satisfactory unless extension into the defect can be accomplished (Fig. 84-4). When teeth remain, this defect size impact is somewhat lessened, but when the remaining teeth are few or located in a straight line, the mechanical advantage for prosthesis stability is less. The ability of the defect tissues to offer the needed mechanical characteristics to the interim prosthesis is unpredictable at best. It is this patient that benefits the most from the surgeon who understands the prosthetic benefits to various surgical defect conditions that provide for the most advantageous structural integrity.

Potential complications

The duration for the interim phase of prosthetic management can be a period of 3 or more months. The primary objective is to allow the patient to pass from an active surgical (and adjunctive treatment) phase to an observational phase of management with minimal complications. During the transition, the patient recovers from the systemic effects of the treatment, deals with the psychologic impact of the defect using his or her own coping strategy, and becomes more aware of the functional deficits associated with the surgical defect(s). Minimizing potential complications during the transition, which includes preparing the patient for those anticipated to occur, facilitates the process for the patient and family. Common interim prosthetic complications relate to tissue trauma and the associated discomfort, inadequate retention (looseness) of the maxillary prosthesis, in-

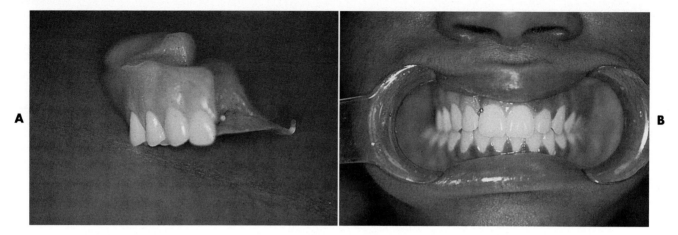

Fig. 84-3. A, An interim obturator prosthesis made of acrylic resin and wire clasps. Teeth have been included on the prosthesis for cosmetic reason only. **B,** This photograph was taken 5 weeks after a right partial maxillectomy procedure.

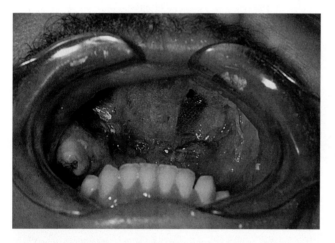

Fig. 84-4. A maxillary defect after a motor vehicle accident; only one remaining molar is available for prosthetic use in providing support, stability, and retention. The need to engage the defect for prosthetic management is apparent.

Table 84-2. Interim prosthetic treatment

Mandibular defects	Not usually indicated
Maxillary defects	
Goals	Obturate surgical defect
	Improve speech and deglutition
Instructions	Head level when swallowing
	Cannot chew on defect side
	Looseness, leakage, or discomfort require a check-up
Complications	Loss of seal, which creates nasal speech and leakage of food and liquids
	Lack of retention or looseness
	Unable to place prosthesis because contracture of lateral scar band
	Discomfort because of mucositis (radiotherapy or chemotherapy), prosthesis pressure, overly aggressive defect cleaning

complete obturation with leakage of air, food, and liquid around the obturator portion of the prosthesis, and the tissue effects of chemotherapy and radiotherapy (Table 84-2).

Discomfort related to the use of interim prostheses can be a result of surgical wound healing dynamics, defect conditions, mucosal effects of adjunctive treatment, or prosthetic fit. Common areas of surgical wound pain include junctions of oral and lip or cheek mucosa, especially at the anterior alveolar region for maxillectomy patients (Fig. 84-5). The lateral scar band produced when the skin graft heals to the oral mucosa also can be the site of discomfort in some patients. When a split-thickness skin graft is not placed, discomfort caused by prosthesis fit within the defect can be a consistent and long-term problem. The hard palate surgical margin when not covered with surgically reflected oral mucosa most often will be covered by nasal epithelium, which

also is prone to discomfort. Alveolar bone cuts that have not been rounded will perforate the oral mucosa and be painful whether a prosthesis is worn or not. This is most frequently a finding for mandibular resection superior alveolar margins when the reconstruction has restored the lower and labial contour to the mandible, but the intraoral mucosa at the superior surface is under tension because of a difference in height (Fig. 84-6).

The prosthesis can create discomfort from excessive static pressure from the internal surfaces or from overextension into the vestibular tissues. The prosthesis also can create discomfort as a result of functional movement associated with swallowing and speech. As discussed previously, prosthesis movement depends on the quality of the supporting structures. Teeth offer the best support, followed by firm edentulous ridges, and lastly the surgical defect structures. The tongue, opposing dentition, and cheeks and lips place

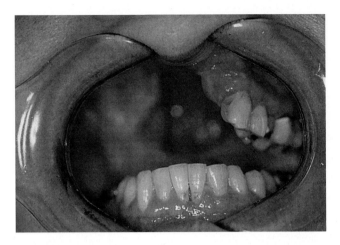

Fig. 84-5. The anterior maxillary resection region often is a source of discomfort for maxillectomy patients. The attachment of sensitive lip or cheek lining mucosa and the split-thickness skin graft to the alveolus, especially in this region of excessive prosthetic movement, creates a combination prone to discomfort.

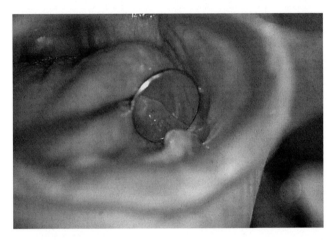

Fig. 84-6. Exposed alveolar bone at the anterior resection region of a mandibular left segmental resection. This condition hinders prosthesis use, and for patients treated with radiotherapy requires careful monitoring.

force on the prosthesis that should be resisted over a large area to prevent movement. Because the defect is least likely to be able to resist movement, the relative size and structural integrity of the defect compared with the remaining teeth or edentulous ridge determines the potential prosthesis movement and most impacts the discomfort related with such movement.

When teeth are available (and especially if located close to and far away from the defect), retention is enhanced by engaging them with prosthetic clasps for retention. Tooth-clasp retention is the most efficient means for effectively resisting dislodgement. The clasps will require periodic adjustment to maintain their effectiveness as the movement of the prosthesis flexes the clasps beyond their elastic recovery

capacity. For edentulous patients, because the surgical defect allows communication between cavities, the fitting surface of the prosthesis can no longer create a closed environment to develop a seal for resisting dislodgement. Consequently, during the interim phase when complete engagement of the defect is not possible because of tissue sensitivity, the careful use of denture adhesives is required to facilitate retention. The patient should be instructed that adhesives can alter the prosthesis fit and can disrupt the close adaptation of the prosthesis to the remaining tissues. Used adhesive should be removed before reapplying new adhesive to maintain fit and hygiene. The inability to completely place the prosthesis, which for maxillectomy patients can be because of contracture of the scar band, also can affect retention. When the maxillary resection leaves the cheek unsupported by bone, the prosthesis provides the necessary support for wound maturation. If the patient removes the interim obturator prosthesis for a period sufficient to allow contraction, the prosthesis will be more difficult to place. Once placed, the scar band will relax, and subsequent removal and placement will be more easily accomplished. The discomfort associated with this phenomenon is mostly a result of patient anxiety and can be effectively addressed by reassuring the patient that this is an easily handled complication.

During the immediate postoperative healing stage, the surgical defect will undergo a change in dimension that impacts the prosthesis fit and seal. If space is created with the change, speech will be altered (increase in nasality), and nasal reflux with swallowing will occur. The interim prosthesis is made of easily adjustable material to allow accommodation for such changes. The most common manner of adjustment is through the use of temporary resilient denture lining materials, which mold to the tissues directly and reduce the mechanical effects of movement by their viscoelastic nature. Leakage can occur easily when swallowing unless the patient follows certain instructions. Because the prosthesis cannot offer a water-tight seal that matches the presurgical state, patients will be instructed not to swallow large quantities at one time and to hold their head horizontal when swallowing. When the head posture is forward, as in taking soup from a spoon, leakage easily occurs around the obturator component of a prosthesis. Another difficult condition that presents difficulty in controlling leakage on swallowing is the midline soft palatal resection. The functional movement of the remaining soft palate often is difficult to fit a prosthesis to and to provide an adequate seal during the interim prosthesis stage (Fig. 84-7).

When combination treatment is prescribed for the patient, it is commonly provided during the postsurgical phase when the patient is using an interim prosthesis. The major intraoral complication associated with radiotherapy and chemotherapy that impacts interim prosthetic service is mucositis. A careful balance between comfort and adequate fit for speech and swallowing needs should be determined with input from the patient. If prosthesis adjustment can offer relief to ensure

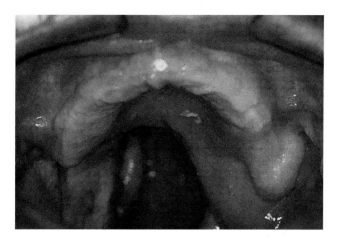

Fig. 84-7. A maxillary combination hard and soft palatal defect. The remaining edentulous ridge provides a good prosthetic foundation, although the soft palatal resection and unpredictable movement of the residual soft palate can make optimum speech improvement difficult to achieve with a prosthesis.

completion of treatment and if the patient understands the impact adjustment may have on speech and swallowing, then it should be accomplished.

The long-term effects of radiotherapy, especially radiation-induced xerostomia and capillary bed changes (obliterative endarteritis) within the mandible, present a potentially serious threat to any remaining dentition and to the development of osteoradionecrosis. During the interim prosthesis stage, the patient will begin to notice the xerostomic effects, which include development of thick, ropy saliva that makes swallowing more difficult and an increase in discomfort associated with removable prostheses.

Defect and oral hygiene

After surgical pack removal, the defect site will mature with time and with exposure to the external environment. Initial loss of incompletely consolidated skin graft, mucous secretions mixed with blood, and residual food debris within the cavity are common oral findings for the patient with a maxillary defect. These cause concern for patients who are unprepared and unfamiliar with these new oral findings. As they become more familiar with the surgical defect, the patients should be encouraged to clean the defect of food debris and mucous secretions routinely. Defect hygiene will allow more timely healing and will improve the ability to adequately fit a prosthesis. Common defect hygiene practices are either lavage procedures, which include rinsing of the defect during normal showering, rinsing of the defect using a bulb syringe or a modified oral irrigating device (modified to provide a multiple orifice "shower" effect), or manual cleaning procedures such as the use of a sponge-handled cleaning aid. Frequently, dried mucous secretions are difficult to remove and require adequate hydration before mechanical removal.

After surgical pack removal, the patient may be reluctant to begin oral hygiene practices because of oral discomfort. As the patient uses the interim prosthesis, which requires daily removal and cleaning at a minimum, he or she will realize the need for and benefit from normal oral hygiene practices because of improved prosthesis fit and tolerance. When teeth are remaining, it is important to the success of long-term prosthetic care to maintain a high level of oral hygiene. This is more critical for patients who exhibit xerostomia and have an increased risk of caries. For these patients, a daily application of fluoride in custom-formed carriers is prescribed along with frequent professional cleanings. The successful use of maxillofacial prostheses is enhanced greatly by the support provided by natural teeth. Consequently, during the interim prosthetic period, periodontal management procedures are begun in anticipation of the definitive treatment to allow a smooth transition from the interim to definitive prosthetic stages.

Definitive care

Definitive prosthetic management can be initiated when the surgical and adjunctive treatment phases have been completed for an amount of time so that the defect tissue has matured sufficiently to tolerate more aggressive prosthetic manipulation and obturation. This phase can be considered a transition for the patient–physician relationship, wherein the primary surgical emphasis shifts from active treatment to observation. The primary emphasis from the patient's standpoint shifts to the prosthetic management. However, for some patients, more definitive prostheses are delayed because of general health concerns or questionable tumor prognosis or control, or when the patient has failed to reach a level of oral or defect hygiene that warrants more sophisticated treatment. Although this phase of management may be considered elective, without definitive prostheses, patients are not afforded the opportunity for complete rehabilitation. It is the extended use of temporary prostheses beyond their serviceable lifespan that has given a poor impression of prosthetic service to many surgeons and patients. Every opportunity should be provided to the patient for the most complete rehabilitation possible, which requires consideration of more definitive prostheses.

The inability of prostheses to mimic their natural counterparts results in less-than-ideal functional measures. Factors related to the structural integrity of the surgical defect and associated reconstructions as they impact this already compromised functional capacity are important considerations. As stated previously, the fact that control of removable maxillofacial prostheses requires the skilled performance of patients suggests that oral and defect structures adjacent to the prostheses are important for successful performance.[5] This is crucial to the understanding of the impact postsurgical defect characteristics and soft-tissue reconstruction have on maxillofacial prosthesis management. The reason for this is twofold: (1) the opportunity for maximum prosthetic benefit requires consideration of surgical site characteristics that are

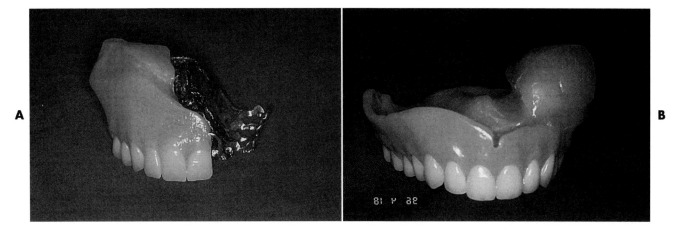

Fig. 84-8. Examples of obturator prostheses for **A**, a patient with teeth in whom the support, stability, and retention are dramatically improved through clasp engagement of all the remaining teeth, and **B**, a completely edentulous patient in whom maximum extension into the defect is required to optimize performance.

separate from classic tumor control approaches, and (2) the ability of the patient to biomechanically control large removable prostheses after surgery may be significantly hindered by surgical closure or reconstruction options. Surgical outcomes that can improve prosthetic function without adversely affecting tumor control should be considered and will be described for the more common surgical defects and associated prostheses.

Maxillary defects

Surgical outcomes that impact prosthetic success can be considered as either those that impact the amount of maxillary structures removed or those that impact the structural integrity and quality of the defect. For surgical defects of the hard or soft palate, the primary prosthetic objectives are restoration of the physical separation of the oral sinus, and nasal cavities in a manner that restores mastication, deglutition, speech, and facial contour to as near normal as possible. The typical prostheses that are used to achieve these objectives include the obturator prosthesis (Fig. 84-8), typically referring to prostheses that obturate defects within the bony palate, and the speech aid prosthesis (Fig. 84-9), which typically refers to prostheses that restore palatopharyngeal function for defects of the soft palate.

Current preoperative diagnostic procedures have improved the ability to discern the location and regional bone involvement of tumors of the maxilla and associated paranasal sinuses. Relative to prosthetically important surgical modifications, if it can be determined that tumor control does not require a classic radical maxillectomy approach or that the inferior sinus floor, hard palate, and alveolus are uninvolved, preservation of as much hard palate, alveolar bone, and teeth as possible should be considered. Tooth preservation has the greatest impact on success because of the stabilizing effect on prosthetic movement. When teeth can be

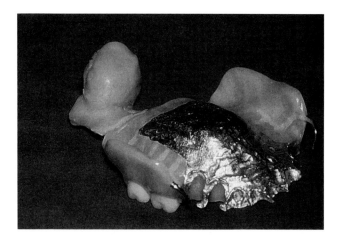

Fig. 84-9. A speech aid prosthesis that attempts to position an extension of the prosthesis into the region of maximum palatopharyngeal movement to obturate the remaining space in a manner that facilitates speech intelligibility.

retained in the premaxilla, for more posterior tumors, or in the posterior molar region, for more anterior tumors, control of prosthesis movement is more easily accomplished, and prosthetic success can be considerably improved (Fig. 84-10). Because the classic midline maxillectomy defect is dramatically more debilitating for the average patient than a defect wherein preservation of the premaxillary component was accomplished, inclusion of the anterior premaxillary component should be decision based on tumor control alone, rather than on surgical convenience.

For resections in patients with teeth, the tooth adjacent to the defect is subjected to the most force from prosthesis movement. When planning the surgical alveolar ostectomy cut, the resection should be made through the extraction site of the adjacent tooth to provide the most favorable prognosis

segments of the mandible should be based on tumor control and patient survival and not on access. Surgical outcomes of mandibular osteotomy that may impact prosthetic management relate to the fixation placement. For edentulous patients who will need mucosal-supported complete dentures, the internal rigid fixation should be placed below the level of the anterior labial vestibule extension of the prosthesis, which can be accomplished by using the mental foramen as a guide and by placing the fixation just below a line joining the bilateral foramina.

A recognition of the pattern of tumor invasion and spread within the mandible has led to a better understanding of appropriate application of another mandible preservation procedure, the rim resection.[40,43] For the mandibular rim resection, the optimum surgical outcome for prosthetic use would be a soft-tissue reconstruction that provides a firm, thin attachment to the remaining bone, which exhibits a smooth, inverted U-shaped surface contour. This surgical result offers the best opportunity for prosthetic options, including removable prostheses or an implant-supported prosthesis. If an implant-supported prosthesis is planned, the prognosis is improved if the remaining bone allows placement of multiple implants 1 cm or longer in length. Because these preservation procedures maintain the original maxillomandibular relations, the opportunity to replace the missing dentition in an anatomically useful position is afforded. The difficulty in maintaining these relations and in providing the reconstruction of the adjacent soft tissues in a manner that allows separate but coordinated function of all components is the challenge when mandibular segmental resection is necessary for tumor control.

Mandibular resection. When tumors are primary to the mandible, such as an ameloblastoma, or involve the mandible from adjacent regions, surgical resection of segments of the mandible is required for tumor control. It may be difficult to always predict the functional deficit and the exact plan of reconstruction because the surgeon determines the extent of the resection based on a combination of presurgical and surgical findings. However, the common anatomically based mandibular resections include the lateral mandibular resection, the anterior mandibular resection, and the hemimandibular resection. From the standpoint of the surviving mandibular resection patient, the most important decision regarding patient treatment is the decision to maintain mandibular continuity that allows maintenance of position for adjacent intraoral and extraoral soft tissue.

Reconstruction decisions. No reconstruction is no longer a planned option. Surgical evolution of procedures that maintain continuity to the mandible have dramatically improved the opportunity for functional restoration of mastication, deglutition, and speech. The debilitating effects of the discontinuity defect included a major cosmetic deformity to the lower third of the face, decreased masticatory function as a result of unilateral closure, and a compromised coordination of tongue and teeth, altered speech ability, and im-

paired deglutition. Given an appreciation of the decreased performance seen with conventional mucosal-borne denture prostheses, it should be obvious that masticatory rehabilitation for the resection patient without mandibular continuity is unpredictable at best and never achieved for most patients. Even for patients with remaining teeth, the altered mandibular position presents a major functional and cosmetic handicap. From a prosthetic rehabilitation standpoint, one of the most significantly handicapped postsurgical head and neck conditions is the discontinuous mandible. Consequently, such a postsurgical condition should be the rare exception (typically a result of reconstruction plate failure) and should not be the planned surgical outcome.

Reconstruction plates. The cosmetic deformity associated with mandibular resection is improved through the use of reconstruction plates to maintain the presurgical contour to the lower jaw.[7] This form of mandibular contour and position maintenance should be considered the minimal standard of care for mandibular resection patients from a functional standpoint. Use of reconstruction plates can maintain cosmetic appearance and preserve the bilateral nature of mandibular movement. However, the use of reconstruction plates alone precludes replacement of teeth in the region of resection. Prosthetic replacement of teeth cannot be provided for regions superior to the reconstruction bar because of the potential for mucosal perforation and exposure of the bar from functional loading of the soft tissue. From a masticatory function standpoint, this may not be a significant negative impact for some patients because of the maintenance of sufficient numbers of occlusal contacts postsurgically.

Plate and soft-tissue reconstruction versus more aggressive techniques. Although it is clear to the surgeon that the real challenges for those with head and neck cancer are control of local, neck, and metastatic disease, the surviving patients (and the resection patients with benign disease) should have every reasonable opportunity for complete rehabilitation. Regarding the management target referred to as rehabilitation, there appears to be some confusion in the literature as to what constitutes a functional rehabilitation. It is possible that the terminology has not kept pace with the evolution of surgical reconstructive techniques that now allow a broad range of functional outcomes to be considered in a true functional rehabilitation.[51] The argument that bigger operations, referring to more aggressive reconstructions, have not shown a statistically significant change in survival rates is true,[24] but the outcome of interest regarding decisions of reconstruction is not a positive effect on survival but is a positive effect on quality of survival. As has been stated previously, if surgical reconstruction is to be best applied to each patient, a complete understanding of the defects involved is needed, the magnitude of the disability associated with the ablative surgery (from the standpoint of the patient) should be identified, and the rehabilitative efforts should be measured.[50] An important measure that will help this area of healthcare evolve is the measure of cost-effectiveness, and the challenge is to develop reliable and valid means for measuring the functional and psychosocial outcomes of various treatment options for mandibular resection management.

The identification of the surgical result as being disabling is an important point to address regarding patient decisions for reconstruction. The magnitude of the disability is a patient-specific, patient-perceived disability that is determined against the patient's recollection of the presurgical condition. Consequently, the patient has a role in the process of reconstruction outcome assessment that is the truest measure of its success, and therefore he or she should be a part of planning for maximum patient benefit. In the reconstruction decision-making process, there may be a lack of concordance between the patient and surgeon regarding expectations and outcomes.[25] Such a problem is common in healthcare and is critical to understand for outcome measures that have a strong psychosocial component. In this region of the body, which is vital to social interaction, it is important that the patient's understanding of the impairment and subsequent disability associated with the surgical resection and surgical or prosthetic reconstructions be as clear as possible. This is not easily accomplished because it often is not only difficult to precisely describe the anatomic involvement of the disease presurgically (and the degree of disability associated with the treatment), but the subject of cancer is such a psychologic burden to most patients that it makes the patient–provider interaction difficult. Nevertheless, it has been shown that long-term survivors (between 2 and 6 years) of composite head and neck resections still experience severe psychosocial distress[8] and that presurgical counseling regarding treatment and its sequelae has a positive effect on psychosocial outcome.[12] Discussing patient expectations and goals is a critical step for clinical decisions wherein preferences play a role,[17] although an added benefit to this type of patient–provider interaction is the opportunity to educate patients when their expectations are unrealistic.[8] The surgeon and maxillofacial prosthodontist team, after developing protocols for management of common reconstruction options, can share in the patient education needs as they arise.

Mandibular reconstruction with replacement of bone. The evolution of head and neck reconstructive surgery has been dramatic over the past three decades. The vascularized tissue options of the forehead and deltopectoral regions gave way to the more popular pedicled myocutaneous flaps from the 1960s to the 1970s. By the 1980s, numerous osteomyocutaneous free-flap donor sites were identified and were used for mandibular reconstruction. At this time particulate cancellous bone marrow in formed allogeneic frames was also used for mandibular reconstruction. Equally important to the functional outcome of mastication was the development of the science and clinical application of the osseointegration phenomenon in the area of dental implants.

Immediate versus delayed reconstruction. Because the minimal reconstructive effort for any mandibular seg-

mental resection should include immediate stabilization with maximum tongue mobility, which facilitates secondary reconstructive efforts by reducing the negative outcomes of fibrosis and contracture seen when no stabilization is provided,[36] the decision whether to reconstruct immediately or at a delayed time is one made regarding the immediate or delayed use of bone. It may be important when making this decision to consider the functional requirement of dental prostheses given the extent of the surgery and the remaining teeth. For some patients, the option of no prosthesis is the most favorable option. If a lateral resection leaves sufficient numbers of teeth for functional benefit, the patient may be better served by providing no additional intervention, especially if a serious medical risk exists. The number of teeth required for functional benefit will vary for each patient, although the patient with a full complement of teeth on the nonresected side of the mandible and with an optimally preserved occlusion through the ipsilateral canine or premolar region may be a candidate for no prosthetic consideration. For the patient with a conservative lateral resection, the ability to function with a mandibular removable resection prosthesis is variable (especially for edentulous patients) (Fig. 84-13). For these patients, strong consideration for bone reconstruction and possibly secondary preprosthetic surgery of the reconstructed region should be given. In this patient, maximum functional benefit will be achieved through the use of endosseous implants for complete support (totally implant-supported) or assisted support (implant-tissue supported) of the prostheses (Fig. 84-14).

When the decision is made to proceed with a reconstruction that provides the best chance for dental reconstruction after mandibular resection, the use of bone as a component of the reconstruction is necessary. As stated previously, the most important effect on reconstructive outcomes stems from the soft-tissue defect size and the degree to which the replacement soft tissue can match the presurgical functional characteristics. A patient can receive a stable bone replacement and be provided with a well-supported, stable, and retentive prosthesis for a mandible that exhibits adequate functional movement capability, and the cheek and tongue cannot manipulate food or liquids in a coordinated fashion for mastication. Given this understanding, the following discussion of mandibular bone reconstruction stresses the need for an adequate functional soft-tissue environment, which is highlighted by the characteristics of preserved or restored sensation, sufficient tongue mobility, and the opportunity for oral competence.

The literature provides numerous descriptions of the surgical options for mandibular hard- and soft-tissue reconstruction.[24,26,28,35,38] A healthy concern exists regarding the cost–benefit of such procedures.[36,50,54] Options for mandibular replacements include particulate cancellous bone marrow in an allogeneic frame shaped to the contour of the replaced anatomy,[38] nonvascularized free bone grafts, pedi-

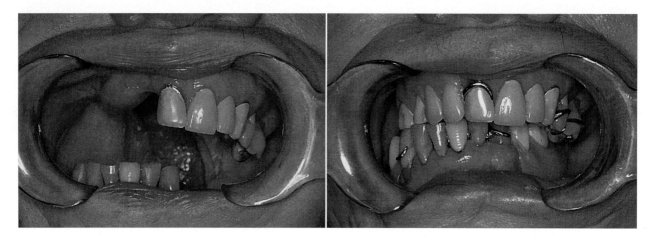

Fig. 84-13. A patient with right maxillary and mandibular defects. The mandibular discontinuity defect is illustrated by the right deviated dental midline. The mandibular resection prosthesis attempts to restore occlusion in a manner that accommodates the altered closure pattern of the residual hemimandible. With adequate soft-tissue reconstruction, functional improvement is minimal for such prostheses and less for edentulous resection prostheses when implants are not used.

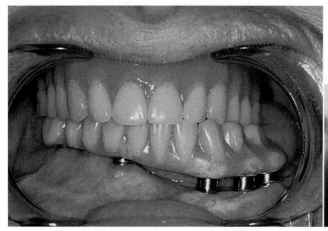

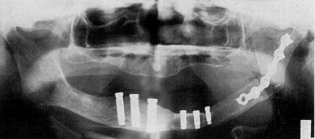

Fig. 84-14. A patient who has received a left mandibular resection with immediate free graft transfer using a fibula, stabilized with a reconstruction plate. The radiograph was taken after the patient received a full course of radiotherapy, hyperbaric oxygen therapy, partial plate removal that was required for the split-thickness skin graft vestibuloplasty, and dental implant placement. The functional stability of the mandibular prosthesis is excellent, and because of the adequate mobility of the tongue, masticatory performance is good.

cled osteocutaneous flaps, and free revascularized bone and composite grafts.[26] Of these options, particulate cancellous bone marrow with allogeneic frames and free revascularized bone and composite grafts are most commonly used. The proponents of each technique make decisions based on issues of reconstruction timing needs, morbidity associated with the donor site, and potential for perioperative and postoperative complications. Regarding complications, an important adjunctive therapy in the postradiation patient is hyperbaric oxygen, especially to improve the healing dynamics associated with the soft-tissue environment, the graft bone, and dental implants. The important surgical outcomes that im-

pact prosthetic care after successful transfer, stabilization, and union relate to the replacement bone size, shape, position, and type of prosthesis planned. The ideal prosthetic characteristics of the replacement mandible are shown in Table 84-3. Regardless of the type of prosthesis to be used, the appropriate placement of the bone relative to the opposing arch is vital to the intended functional use. If a removable prosthesis is expected to cover the bone reconstruction, the contour of the developed ridge should provide a surface covered with firm thin soft tissue and a rounded superior contour with buccal and lingual slopes approaching parallel to each other and with sufficient vestibular depth to provide horizon-

Table 84-3. Ideal dental prosthetic characteristics of a mandibular reconstruction

Spatial relationship to	
Remaining mandible	Should be continuous at superior and inferior borders with the proximal/distal segments of resident mandible
Facial contour	Should restore presurgical external contour to the lower third of the face
Maxillary teeth—horizontal concern	Should be positioned beneath the opposing teeth to allow functional placement of the replacement teeth
Maxillary teeth—vertical concern	Should provide a minimum of 1-cm spacing between the soft tissue covering the bone and the opposing occlusion (not the opposing ridge)
Size and shape	
Intraoral form	Should exhibit a rounded superior surface with nearly parallel buccal and lingual surfaces at least 1 cm in height from vestibule
Bulk	Should provide a minimum bulk for implants of 1 cm in width and 1.5 cm in height
Soft-tissue relationships	
Separate movement	Should provide a 1-cm vestibular depth and distensibility that allows independent movement of the cheek and tongue relative to the mandible
Ridge covering	Should provide soft tissue covering the bone that is firm (bound to the bone) and approximately 0.3 cm thick

tal stability. Such a ridge condition is the surgical analog of a minimally resorbed edentulous ridge, and with adequate cheek and tongue movement, it should provide a reasonable prognosis for prosthetic success, provided sufficient numbers of teeth remain on the nonresected side. For the optimum chance of prosthetic function, dental implants should be considered, and with sufficient bulk of bone and the same characteristics listed for the removable prosthesis, the prognosis for success is optimum. To reiterate, the major determining factor for improved function will be the quality of the soft-tissue reconstruction.

Complications

The major complications seen in patients with mandibular reconstructions relates to the bulk of the soft-tissue component and lack of mobility of the tongue. When these factors are controlled for, complications are mostly a result of bone placement and size. The common use of free flaps, including bone from other regions of the body that do not possess the native mandible shape, presents a major degree of technical difficulty associated with the procedure. The fibula, which is a popular choice for mandibular replacement, presents some challenges in meeting the ideal requirements as listed in Table 84-3.[27] Because of the straight nature of the bone, it is easy to err in the horizontal and vertical positioning, especially for reconstructions that span to the midline. Lingual positioning requires prosthetic placement at a position that may be functionally unstable with time (Fig. 84-15). Such a location requires implant positions that create a mechanical cantilever that can be detrimental to the long-term success of the implant-supported prosthesis. Posteriorly, the inability to recreate the natural ascending curve of the mandible can restrict placement of teeth and preclude restoring complete occlusion on the resected side. It is common to have a mismatch in height at the anterior junction of the graft with the resident mandible (Fig. 84-16). For implant-

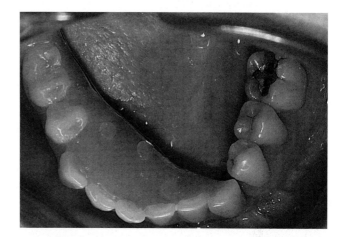

Fig. 84-15. Implant placement is dictated by the location of the bone graft. Horizontal discrepancies in implant-bone location relative to the necessary functional tooth position can cause high-torque stress to develop in the implant supporting bone. Also, the mobility of the tongue should be optimum to have the opportunity to place food over such a span of prosthesis.

supported prostheses, this area can present major challenges to adequate hygiene of the implants and with time can compromise implant health. For removable prostheses, this can become a source of irritation if fulcruming occurs with movement. The concern regarding the size of the fibula is that implant length seems to be a factor in predicting success. When implant failure is correlated with length, increasing length, especially greater than 1 cm, predicts a dramatic improvement in survival. There may be a tendency to place dental implants primarily at the time of immediate reconstruction. When radiotherapy is planned after surgery, implant placement delay after a course of hyperbaric oxygen improves the chance for implant survival and reduces the chance for developing osteoradionecrosis of the resident mandible (see Fig. 84-14). Additionally, the maxillofacial prosthodontist will be able to provide the most useful input regarding the placement of implants after a survey of the relationships provided by the bone reconstruction. Although immediate placement can be accomplished, it often has resulted in dental implant positions that are not useful for prosthetic support.[48]

PROSTHETIC MANAGEMENT OF EXTRAORAL ACQUIRED DEFECTS

An acquired facial defect, which can result from traumatic injury or surgical management of disease, often is a major burden to a patient functionally and cosmetically because of the tremendous social disability associated with such conditions. The loss of external facial features, such as the nose or ear, present largely cosmetic defects, whereas the loss of an eye presents a cosmetic defect and functional impairment. Surgical and prosthetic management of these acquired defects address mainly the cosmetic deficit.

The decision to reconstruct facial defects surgically or prosthetically often is difficult. Both management procedures have limitations that are general to patients with cosmetic defects and specific to the site involved. In general, surgical limitations are related to the need to monitor the local site if the defect is of oncologic origin, the frequently compromised local tissue quality and color, the multistage requirement for reconstruction (especially for large defects), and the unpredictable maintenance of form often seen. The prosthetic limitations relate to (1) material deficiencies that require frequent intervention, (2) problems of retention and unpredictable placement when implants cannot be used, (3) prosthetic–tissue margin visibility (especially for midface prostheses), (4) and lack of acceptance of an artificial body part by some patients. Generally, prostheses are indicated when surgical intervention is to be delayed or is contraindi-

cated, as is the case for postsurgical cancer patients. For these patients, it is inadvisable to immediately surgically reconstruct a defect that requires monitoring; frequently, the use of radiotherapy complicates wound healing dynamics and predictability, and for larger defects, the benefits do not outweigh the multistage approach often required.

Because the major objective of the management is cosmetic, the emphasis is to achieve a natural-looking prosthetic replacement of the previous facial part and to place it on or around the postsurgical wound. The retention of the prostheses historically has been provided by mechanically engaging anatomic undercuts, the use of eyeglass frames or straps, or more commonly, the use of skin adhesives. Adhesives are the predominant means of providing retention for extraoral prostheses, although concern exists because of the deleterious effect of adhesives and their clean solvents on the prosthetic material and skin. This skin effect is more pronounced for patients who have had radiotherapy to the region. The manner of retention is evolving from adhesive use to a craniofacial implant-based mechanical retention procedure. The application of craniofacial implants has improved the quality of service available to these patients by the impact on accurate positioning, increased confidence in the retention of these prostheses, the ability to provide thinner, less visible prosthetic margins and the reduction of adhesive-induced skin and material complications.

The psychosocial aspect of patient care involving facial defects includes knowledge of patient coping skills, patient expectation development (especially given the material limitations), and the patient's perceived ability to physically manipulate the prosthesis. These issues can be as important to a successful result as the natural appearance of the prosthesis. Given this understanding and because the resulting surgical environment can impact the cosmetic result, the following discussion will focus on the surgical outcomes that may im-

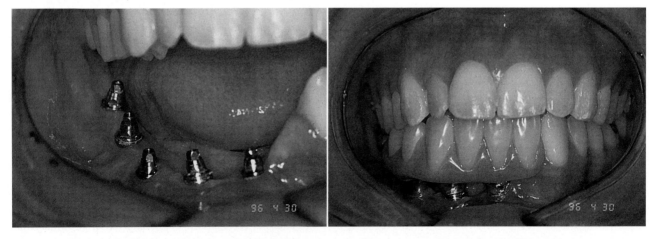

Fig. 84-16. Good horizontal positioning of implants in a fibula graft, although the step in height at the anterior and the lack of interocclusal space posteriorly caused prosthetic complications with hygiene and discomfort.

pact prosthetic management of nasal, orbital, and auricular defects (Table 84-4).

Nasal defects

When a prosthesis is planned for a nasal defect, partial rhinectomy procedures can seriously complicate the result. A total rhinectomy is ideal (Fig. 84-17).

When the surgical procedure emphasizes preservation, as (e.g., when the nasal bones or alae are not resected, the prosthesis must cover the remaining anatomy, resulting in an oversized, unacceptable prosthesis. Attempts to cover these regions with thin portions of the prosthetic material often

Table 84-4. Ideal extraoral defect characteristics for prosthetic use

Nasal
    Total rhinectomy, which includes nasal bones
    No distortion of lateral anatomy (i.e., nasolabial folds)
    Undisturbed maxillary lip
    Firm inferior base with split-thickness skin graft (STSG)
Orbital
    Sufficient depth for prosthetic components
    STSG lining interior surface
    No marginal tissue distortion
    Eyebrow preservation
    Rounded orbital margin
Auricular
    Firm, thin base with STSG
    Contour irregularities to aid placement
    Anterior–inferior margin free of condyle
    Maintenance of tragus and patent external auditory meatus

result in easily distorted and torn margins. The base of the defect can be lined with a split-thickness skin graft, which allows for an adequate supporting tissue and can help prevent lip distortion from wound contracture. Similarly, the lateral nasolabial folds should be undistorted to allow for a more normal appearance and to facilitate camouflaging the prosthesis margins. When the decision is made to include implants for the nasal defect, the preferred site is the anterior floor of the nose and maxilla region, where the greatest bulk of bone exists within the defect. Implant placement should result in the percutaneous (when a skin graft is used) portion penetrating into the bulk of the anticipated prosthesis.

Orbital defect

The most common acquired defect involving the orbit is the exenteration defect, resulting from tumor removal. If confined to the orbit, the prosthesis is more easily disguised than if the surgical margins extend beyond the orbit into adjacent facial regions, which often exhibit more displaceable soft tissue that move with function (especially under the influence of the muscles of facial expression). Movement at a junction of the skin and prosthesis easily can dislodge an adhesive-retained prosthesis.

As with the nasal defect, the orbital region is highly exposed to the casual observer, and any surgical boundaries that are distorted limit the effectiveness of the prosthesis. The ideal defect has been lined with a split-thickness skin graft, has sufficient depth to allow placement of the required prosthetic components, exhibits minimal or no orbital margin tissue distortion, preserves the eyebrow position, and provides a rounded orbital margin entry to the depth of the defect (Fig. 84-18).

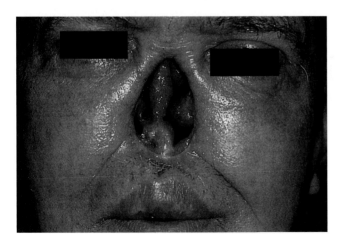

Fig. 84-17. A total rhinectomy defect that illustrates distorted lateral margins, a full left cheek, and a distorted maxillary lip. Because these presenting conditions impact the overall cosmetic appearance of the nasal prosthesis, the patient should recognize the limitations of the prosthesis to correct for undesirable surgical outcomes.

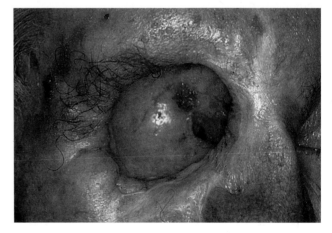

Fig. 84-18. An orbital defect that is confined to the bony orbit, leaving the orbital margin relatively intact. The defect is lined with a split-thickness skin graft, has rounded and slightly displaceable orbital margins that facilitate retention, and a firm inferior margin providing a good supportive base. The eyebrow is distorted into the defect, and the lateral and inferior margins are somewhat irregular, although the opportunity to provide a camouflaged prosthesis with adequate retention is good.

The inferior margin, as with the nasal defect, should ideally have a firm, broad supportive base. The split-thickness skin graft provides an interior surface, which is an ideal, nonsensitive bearing surface that is easily cleaned. The graft also may facilitate the development of rounded contours to the superior and lateral walls of the orbital rim, which allows for ease of prosthesis placement and removal. When the surgical wound is allowed to heal secondarily, the resulting surface is more sensitive, less easily maintained by the patient, and does not provide an ideal internal configuration for retention. The interior anatomic retention of a well-healed orbital defect is less likely to need the assistance of implant retention. The eyebrow should be maintained, if possible, to allow the superior margin placement of the prosthesis to be hidden inferior to the brow line. However, the preservation of the eyelids limits the access to the defect and the opportunity for a successful prosthesis.

When the defect extends beyond the normal orbital margins, the need for implant assistance increases. Craniofacial implant placement in the orbital region is most successful when the lateral and superior rims are used. Because placement angulation is difficult in this region, care should be exercised to ensure that the retentive components of the prosthesis and implants are within the bulk of the prosthesis and are not protruding from the defect.

Auricular defect

The advantage of an auricular defect compared with the previous defects relates to the lateral face position and the opportunity to use hair to disguise the superior and posterior margins. When a prosthesis is indicated, the entire ear should be removed except for the tragus, which helps to hide a portion of the anterior margin and provides a landmark for repeated placement. If previous reconstructions have been attempted, remaining tissue remnants also should be removed because they can require distorted contours to the prosthesis.

The ideal auricular defect has a firm, thin base (Fig. 84-19). This region has the most successful performance record for the use of craniofacial implants, more successful than either the orbit or the nasal region.

IMPLANT USE FOR ACQUIRED DEFECTS

As described previously, the common use of intraoral mucosal tissues for support of removable dental prostheses often has resulted in limited restoration of function when compared with the fully dentate mouth. When bone-anchored implants have been substituted for this mucosal support, the performance measures describe a more completely restored condition.

Additionally, part of the success of bone-anchored prostheses is related to the reduced progression of the residual ridge resorption commonly seen in populations of remov-

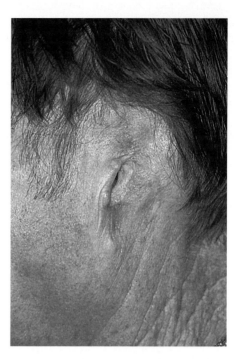

Fig. 84-19. An auricular defect that exhibits a firm and thin soft-tissue foundation, a slight irregular contour superior and posterior to the external auditory meatus, preservation of the tragus, and the opportunity to camouflage the margins with the hair and eyeglass frames.

able prosthesis-wearing patients. For patients requiring conventional prosthetic replacement of teeth, those with the most depleted dentitions benefit the most from the use of implants. For patients with acquired defects of the oral cavity, an even greater advantage for implant use lies in the ability to provide retention and support to prostheses that are dramatically compromised because of a qualitatively and quantitatively decreased supportive foundation. It is the patient with an acquired defect who benefits the most from the use of dental implants because the improvement in prosthetic support frees the adjacent tissues, which frequently are reconstructed structures, from the function of removable prosthesis movement control.

Implant use in the nonradiated mandible and maxilla to support typical maxillofacial prostheses has revealed cumulative success rates similar to those for conventional implants—approximately 75% for the maxilla and 90% for the mandible whether placed in nonvascular or revascularized free bone grafts.[2] Similarly, the success rates for extraoral implants reveal some location-specific effect, with the temporal region having the highest success (95%), followed by the base of the nose and maxilla (90%), and the frontal bone of the orbital rim (77%). Although reports continue to accumulate and exact success rates vary between reports, in general the opportunity to provide a management procedure that, at worst, has an 8 in 10 chance of success is a favorable risk for the benefit derived.

When the patient has been exposed to adjunctive radiotherapy, the recipient bone offers decreased healing potential because of the normal tissue damage and sublethal cellular damage, which leads to progressive obliterative endarteritis with resultant tissue ischemia and fibrosis. This is reflected in a higher implant failure rate as a result of the reduced capacity of the bone to primarily heal and remodel under functional loads. This finding has been reported for intraoral and extraoral maxillofacial implant use.[11] It also has been reported that the use of hyperbaric oxygen (HBO) treatment, as originally provided for osteoradionecrosis patients, provides a protective effect against this decreased success rate for radiated bone.[38] A course of HBO management is described as being indicated for patients who require reconstructions within tissue that has received a dose of radiation greater than 5000 cGy because this is the only means of developing capillary angiogenesis and fibroplasia within radiated tissue.[42] The use of HBO reduces the incidence of complications associated with implant use, which include implant loss and soft-tissue inflammatory reactions. The timing of implant placement relative to the primary surgical–radiation combination protocols is continuing to be investigated. Because bone exhibits a delayed response to radiation damage of 2 to 3 months, current reports suggest to either take advantage of this window of time for implant placement or to delay placement until approximately 1 year or more after treatment.

SUMMARY

This chapter attempts to describe the functional and cosmetic aspects of maxillofacial prosthetic management of acquired defects in light of the realistic function provided by removable prostheses. The goal is to facilitate the decision-making for combined surgical and prosthetic treatment of patients with acquired defects of the head and neck.

The functional impairment associated with common surgical procedures is discussed, and an attempt is made to describe prosthesis goals and limitations and to provide an understanding of the expectations of prosthetic reconstruction. Also, the timing of prosthetic management and the types of common prostheses associated with the stages of prosthetic management are discussed. For extraoral defects, the ideal surgical site preparation for nasal, orbital, and auricular defects is described, and the use of bone-anchored implants for maxillofacial applications is discussed.

REFERENCES

1. Aram A, Subtelny JD: Velopharyngeal function and cleft palate prostheses, *J Prosthet Dent* 9:149, 1959.
2. Beumer J, Roumanas E, Nishimura R: Advances in osseointegrated implants for dental and facial rehabilitation following major head and neck surgery, *Semin Surg Oncol* 11:200, 1995.
3. Boretti G, Bickel M, Geering AH: A review of masticatory ability and efficiency, *J Prosthet Dent* 74:400, 1995.
4. Carlsson GE: Masticatory efficiency: the effect of age, the loss of teeth and prosthetic rehabilitation, *Int Dent J* 34:93, 1984.
5. Culver PAJ, Watt L: Denture movements and control, *Br Dent J* 135:111, 1973.
6. Curtis T, Beumer J: *Restoration of acquired hard palate defects: etiology, disability and rehabilitation.* In Beumer J, Curtis T, Firtell D, editors: *Maxillofacial rehabilitation,* St Louis, 1979, Mosby.
7. Davidson MJ, Gullane PJ: Prosthetic plate mandibular reconstruction, *Otolaryngol Clin North Am* 24:1419, 1991.
8. de Boer MF and others: Rehabilitation outcomes of long-term survivors treated for head and neck cancer, *Rehabil Head Neck Cancer* Nov/Dec: 503, 1995.
9. Desjardins RP: Early rehabilitative management of the maxillectomy patient, *J Prosthet Dent* 38:311, 1977.
10. Doty RW: *Neural organization of deglutition.* In *Handbook of physiology,* IV, 1968.
11. Granstrom G and others: *Bone-anchored rehabilitation of irradiated head and neck cancer patients,* First International Congress on Maxillofacial Prosthetics, Memorial Sloan-Kettering Cancer Center, April, 1994, New York, MSK Publishers.
12. Greenfield S, Kaplan S, Ware JE: Expanding patient involvement in care. Effects on patient outcomes, *Ann Intern Med* 102:520, 1985.
13. Hans S, Gunne J: Masticatory efficiency and dental state: a comparison between two methods, *Acta Odont Scand* 43:139, 1985.
14. Haribhakti VV, Kavarana NM, Tibbrewala AN: Oral cavity reconstruction: an objective assessment of function, *Head Neck* Mar/Apr:119, 1993.
15. Hayden RE: Free flap transfer for restoration of sensation and lubrication to the reconstructed oral cavity and pharynx, *Otolaryngol Clin North Am* 27:1185, 1994.
16. Helkimo M, Carlsson GE, Helkimo MI: Chewing efficiency and state of the dentition, *Acta Odont Scand* 36:33, 1978.
17. Hornberger JC, Habraken H, Bloch DA: Minimum data needed on patient preferences for accurate, efficient medical decision making, *Med Care* 33:297, 1995.
18. Isshiki N, Honjow I, Morimoto M: Cineradiographic analysis of movement of the lateral pharyngeal wall, *Plast Reconstr Surg* 44:357, 1969.
19. Jacob RF, Bowman J, Perez D: *Postsurgical palatal augmentation prostheses for improved speech and swallowing.* First International Congress on Maxillofacial Prosthetics, April 1994, Memorial Sloan Kettering Cancer Center, New York, MSG Publisher.
20. Kahrilas PJ: Current investigation of swallowing disorders, *Baillieres Clin Gastroenterol* 8:651, 1994.
21. Kahrilas PJ and others: Deglutitive tongue action: volume accommodation and bolus propulsion, *Gastroenterology* 104:152, 1993.
22. Kapur KK, Garett NR, Fisher E: Effects of anesthesia of human oral structures on masticatory performance and food particle size distribution, *Arch Oral Biol* 35:397, 1990.
23. Kawamura Y: Recent concepts of the physiology of mastication, *Adv Oral Biol* 1:77, 1964.
24. Komisar A: The functional result of mandibular reconstruction, *Laryngoscope* 100:364, 1990.
25. Kravitz RL: Patients' expectations for medical care: an expanded formulation based on review of the literature, *Med Care Res Rev* 53:3, 1996.
26. Kuriloof DB, Sullivan MJ: Mandibular reconstruction using vascularized bone grafts, *Otolaryngol Clin North Am* 24:1391, 1991.
27. Larsen, PE: Discussion for evaluation of osseointegration of endosseous implants in radiated, vascularized fibula flaps to the mandible, *J Oral Maxillofac Surg* 53:644, 1995.
28. Larson DL, Sanger JR: Management of the mandible in oral cancer, *Semin Surg Oncol* 11:190, 1995.
29. Lazzari JB: Intraoral splint for support of the lip in Bell's palsy, *J Prosthet Dent* 5:579, 1955.

30. Leake JL, Hawkins R, Locker D: Social and functional impact of reduced posterior dental units in older adults, *J Oral Rehabil* 21:1, 1994.

31. Liedberg B, Spiechowicz E, Owall B: Mastication with and without removable partial dentures: an intraindividual study, *Dysphagia* 10:107, 1995.

32. Logemann JA and others: Speech and swallowing function after tonsil/base of tongue resection with primary closure, *J Speech Hearing Res* 36:918, 1993.

33. Lucas W, Luke H: The processes of selection and breakage in mastication, *Arch Oral Biol* 28:813, 1983.

34. Manly RS, Vinton P: A survey of the chewing ability of denture wearers, *J Dent Res* 30:314, 1951.

35. Markowitz BL, Calcaterra TC: Preoperative assessment and surgical planning for patients undergoing immediate reconstruction of oromandibular defects, *Clin Plast Surg* 21:9, 1994.

36. Martin PJ, O'Leary MJ, Hayden RE: Free tissue transfer in oromandibular reconstruction, *Otolaryngol Clin North Am* 27:1141, 1994.

37. Mathog RH and others: Rehabilitation of head and neck cancer patients: consensus on recommendations from the international conference on rehabilitation of the head and neck cancer patient—speech production, *Head Neck* Jan/Feb:1, 1991.

38. Marx RE: Mandibular reconstruction, *J Oral Maxillfac Surg* 51:466, 1993.

39. McConnel FMS, Teichgraeber JF, Adler RK: A comparison of three methods of oral reconstruction, *Arch Otolaryngol Head Neck Surg* 113:496, 1987.

40. McGregor AD, MacDonald DG: Patterns of spread of squamous cell carcinoma within the mandible, *Head Neck Surg* 11:457, 1989.

41. McKerns D, Bzoch KR: Variations in velopharyngeal valving: the factor of sex, *Cleft Palate J* 7:652, 1970.

42. Myers RAM, Marx RE: Use of hyperbaric oxygen in postradiation head and neck surgery, *NCI Monographs* 9:151, 1990.

43. O'Brien CJ and others: Invasion of the mandible by squamous carcinomas of the oral cavity and oral pharynx, *Head Neck Surg* 8:247, 1986.

44. Oosterhaven SP and others: Social and psychological implications of missing teeth for chewing ability, *Comm Dent Oral Epid* 16:79, 1988.

45. Perkell JS: *Physiology of speech production, Research monograph No. 53*, Cambridge, Mass, 1969, MIT Press.

46. Pouderoux P, Kahrilas PJ: Deglutitive tongue force modulation by volition, volume, and viscosity in humans, *Gastroenterology* 108:1418, 1995.

47. Prinz JF, Lucas PW: Swallow thresholds in human mastication, *Arch Oral Biol* 40:401, 1995.

48. Roumanas ED and others: *Reconstruction of mandible defects: conventional prosthodontics vs use of implants.* In First International Congress on Maxillofacial Prosthetics, Memorial Sloan-Kettering Cancer Center, April 1994, New York, MSG Publishers.

49. Shprintzen RJ and others: A three dimensional cinefluoroscopic analysis of velopharyngeal closure during speech and nonspeech activities, *Cleft Palate J* 11:412, 1974.

50. Shusterman M: The proof of the pudding is in the eating, or the functional evaluation of surgical reconstruction, *Head Neck Surg* 2:203, 1989.

51. Urken ML and others: Functional evaluation following microvascular oromandibular reconstruction of the oral cancer patient: a comparative study of reconstructed and nonreconstructed patients, *Laryngoscope* 101:935, 1991.

52. van Waas M and others: Relationship between wearing a removable partial denture and satisfaction in the elderly, *Comm Dent Oral Epid* 22:315, 1994.

53. Weinberg B: Deglutition: *a review of selected topics.* In *Speech and the dentofacial complex: The state of the art.* ASHA Reports 5, NIDR/NIH publication 69-2228, October 1970.

54. Weymuller EA and others: Cost-benefit management decisions for carcinoma of the retromolar trigone, *Head Neck* Sep/Oct:419, 1995.

55. Yoshida H and others: A comparison of surgery and prosthetic treatment for speech disorders attributable to surgically acquired soft palatal defects, *J Oral Maxillfac Surg* 51:361, 1993.

56. Yousif NJ and others: Soft-tissue reconstruction of the oral cavity, *Clin Plast Surg* 21:15, 1994.

57. Yurkstas AA: The masticatory act, *J Prosthet Dent* 15:248, 1965.

Chapter 85

Oral Cavity and Oropharyngeal Reconstruction

William R. Panje
Michael R. Morris

Reconstructive head and neck surgery is an art dictated by the extent of a surgeon's knowledge, perception, and vision. The efforts of earlier pioneers, despite being restricted by the quality and number of reconstructive options, showed remarkable ingenuity and understanding of wound healing. Their experiences engendered the sound surgical principles and management guidelines that are the cornerstones of head and neck reconstruction today.

The foremost principle is that total tumor removal cannot be compromised. A preconceived notion about how to reconstruct or a limited experience in reconstruction will influence an operator's aggressiveness and thoroughness in ablating a large cancer. This indiscretion may then adversely affect a patient's survival and quality-of-life.

Head and neck surgical defects can be physically mutilating and functionally assaulting to breathing, eating, speaking, smelling, tasting, hearing, and seeing. The surgeon is faced with restoring a patient's esthetic integrity and recreating the essence of day-to-day living.[11] Only after the final surgical defect is created can reconstructive planning and design be finalized. The multitude of techniques developed over the past 20 years allows for an individualized and refined approach to reconstruction.

The second major lesson is that all patients with major resections in the oral cavity and oropharynx will have some degree of dysphagia and aspiration. Most patients can overcome the loss of up to 50% of any single region without debilitating morbidity. Larger resections can encompass adjoining regions, which may lead to serious disability. The finest, state of the art reconstruction cannot recreate the complex neuromuscular interactions necessary for a normal swallow. Rehabilitation and patient training are of paramount importance to the ultimate success of the reconstructive effort.

The art of head and neck reconstruction, therefore, begins with synthesizing all the pertinent preoperative factors: the patient, the tumor, the defect, the surgeon, and the hospital. A workable plan is developed and instituted. Intense rehabilitation and support then is provided to the patient to maximize his or her physical integrity, self-esteem, and quality-of-life.

PREOPERATIVE CONSIDERATIONS

Patient factors

The general health and mental stamina of a patient influence a surgeon's choice for reconstruction. A vibrant 70-year-old probably will have several more productive years and should be treated as such. A 50-year-old with significant heart disease has increased perioperative risk with longer anesthesia times, which should limit options. Diabetes, peripheral vascular disease, and malnutrition adversely affect wound healing and decrease the reliability of musculocutaneous and free-flap survival. A patient with poor self-esteem will not tolerate a cosmetic or functional deformity and will resist rehabilitation. Delaying an elaborate reconstruction on such patients may prove beneficial to their motivation. Limited mental faculties also will severely hinder postoperative rehabilitation and make aspiration a major concern.

Patients who are fortunate enough to have a supportive family tend to accept their disability and rehabilitate better.

A surgeon should involve the family in preoperative discussions whenever a major reconstruction is contemplated.

Last and most important is the assessment of the patient's rehabilitative potential. For example, can he or she expect to return to work, resume his or her hobbies, or fulfill a life-long ambition? A surgeon must understand precisely the donor morbidity associated with each of the reconstructive options chosen. For example, golfing, tennis, and swimming involve different actions of the trunk and shoulder girdle. If a patient has a strong desire to maintain or pursue a skill or hobby, every effort should be made to preserve the necessary muscle function. On the other hand, a public figure or model may desire a more cosmetic but functionally inferior option.

Tumor factors

The size and location of the primary tumor greatly influences any need for elaborate reconstruction. The presence of significant neck or distant metastasis significantly reduces long-term survival, and simpler, more functional reconstructions are appropriate. Tumor recurrences, especially in previously irradiated areas, generally require a more aggressive resection. Previous exposure to radiotherapy will negate the jaw periosteum as a reliable oncologic barrier[24] and will make frozen sections unreliable. This often will cause a surgeon to delay a reconstruction. Lastly, the biologic behavior of the tumor will dictate the need for combination therapy. When postoperative radiotherapy is necessary, it should be instituted within 4 to 6 weeks for maximum effect. The reconstructive plan should allow for this so that prognosis is not adversely affected.

Defect factors

Specific defects will be dealt with later in this chapter, although several general factors should be considered. When vital structures such as the carotid artery or brain parenchyma are exposed, it is imperative that the reconstruction provide adequate protection. The condition of the remaining oral cavity and oropharyngeal tissue is a key factor. A densely irradiated or scarred recipient bed generally requires vascularized tissue for closure. A control fistula or even a delayed reconstruction sometimes is necessary. Exposed bone, especially mandible, should be covered if radiation is planned.

A systematic analysis of what regions have been removed or affected by the ablation will help delineate the extent of the dysphagia expected. Surgery or irradiation involving the pterygoids will promote scarring and trismus, which may be severe enough to interfere with prosthesis or denture insertion or even oral intake. Consideration for coronoidectomy and subperiosteal detachment of the medial pterygoid, temporalis, and masseter sometimes is appropriate. Oral competence is the next requisite in an orderly swallow. Any lip reconstruction should be done with local tissue of the face, maintaining muscular integrity if possible. An incompetent lip or one lacking bony support should be suspended.

Bolus preparation and transport are the next considerations. The action of the tongue against the hard palate is crucial. In general, the tongue and floor of mouth are reconstructed as separate structures with care to maintain a lingual vestibule and restore sufficient height to the floor of mouth. Tongue mobility, not necessarily bulk, should be a primary goal of any reconstructive technique.

The oropharyngeal complex begins the involuntary portion of swallowing. The tongue base moves posteriorly, and the hyoid moves anteriorly and superiorly as a result of submental muscular activity.[21,38] This leads to laryngeal movement forward and up under the base of the tongue. The velopharynx will concomitantly seal off to prevent reflux. When a radical resection interferes with this sequential reflex, significant dysphagia will result. Laryngeal suspension from the anterior jaw sometimes can help postoperative deglutition and should be a consideration.[9] When soft palate competence is lost, velopharyngeal narrowing through a palatal or pharyngeal flap will help reduce nasal regurgitation.

The last part of the swallowing act is cricopharyngeal or upper esophageal sphincter (UES) relaxation. This relaxation occurs in conjunction with laryngeal elevation, which moves the cricoid anteriorly and superiorly, pulling the cricopharyngeal region open maximally.[21,38] The vocal cords and arytenoids approximate as soon as fluid contacts the anterior mouth. The arytenoids then contact the base of the epiglottis during the pharyngeal swallow, providing maximum airway protection while the bolus passes. The cords then open just after the UES closes. This whole action takes place in just over 2 seconds.[38] The surgeon should understand that if bolus transport or oropharyngeal contraction is hindered, the UES relaxation and cricopharyngeal opening will not be synchronized, which causes pharyngeal pooling and aspiration. Any compromise of laryngeal function as a result of the ablation increases the risk of aspiration substantially. A cricopharyngeal myotomy often is an essential part of the reconstructive effort if swallowing rehabilitation is to be successful.

Surgeon factors

The surgeon ultimately chooses the reconstructive option to be applied based on a careful analysis of the points already discussed. His or her choice will be influenced by his or her level of training, experience, perception, and basic understanding of the art. Any surgeon involved with this type of reconstruction should have a keen understanding of the expected morbidity and the resources to provide a contemporary rehabilitation. The reconstruction often can be more technically demanding and take longer to perform than the ablation. It often can tax the stamina and capabilities of a surgeon attempting a primary repair. An elaborate reconstruction always can be delayed so that it can be approached with the necessary enthusiasm. Many centers have instituted a team approach, splitting the tasks of resection and reconstruction, although such an approach also divides the responsibility for patient care and has the potential for alienating a patient and his or her family. Remember that the most important "team" is the partnership between surgeon and patient.

Hospital factors

The success or failure of any reconstruction rarely is based simply on whether the defect heals but rather on how well the patient ultimately can get on with his or her day-to-day living. Success requires the availability and input of several other departments, including radiotherapy, oncology, dentistry, speech and swallowing, nursing, prosthodontics, and social work. The surgeon should orchestrate the efforts of all these specialties, and the surgeon ultimately is responsible if complications or problems occur.

SPECIFIC SITUATIONS

Reconstruction of small defects of the tongue and floor of mouth

Laser (KTP, CO$_2$) excision is the preferred method for T$_1$ and T$_2$ cancers of the tongue and floor of mouth. Because it causes limited thermal injury to adjacent tissues reducing postoperative edema and pain, the laser can play a key role in limiting reconstructive needs. Wounds can be left to granulate, with little worry about slough, infection, pain, or significant scar formation with secondary contracture.[33] Wounds produced by the cold knife or diathermy should be closed primarily if no significant reduction of oral function will result or covered with a split-thickness skin graft (STSG).

If the cancer encroaches on Wharton's duct, the entire submandibular system should be removed in continuity with the floor of mouth through a pull-through approach. The ablation or reconstruction occasionally can compromise the patency of Wharton's duct, necessitating a formal ductoplasty. Rehabilitation generally is limited to the immediate postoperative period. With open laser wounds, a clear liquid diet usually is initiated on the first postoperative day if tolerated. The diet is advanced to soft foods as tolerated, and yogurt, 1 cup per day, is added. Proper mouth care is critical and includes brisk rinsing with a half-strength peroxide solution after any oral intake. Patients with skin grafts should take nothing by mouth until the bolster is removed after 8 to 10 days.

Split-thickness skin graft technique

A dermatome can be used to harvest a 0.012-inch (0.46 to 0.51 mm) graft from the anterolateral thigh. Alternative donor sites include the postauricular, cervical, supraclavicular, or triceps skin. A full-thickness skin graft usually is harvested from these alternative sites, and the donor defect is closed primarily. The full-thickness skin then can be converted to a STSG, which is sutured into the defect at its peripheral margin and centrally. Multiple pie-crust incisions

are placed in the graft after it is secured. A bolster of sponge or rolled adaptic also is used to fix the graft when reconstructing a high-motion area or one that is subject to excessive trauma. The intraoral bolster also is important in creating a new paralingual sulcus (Fig. 85-1).

Reconstruction of through-and-through defects of the tongue and floor of mouth with or without marginal mandibulectomy

A marginal mandibulectomy generally is included in a floor of mouth resection to provide a more adequate excision margin. Whenever a submandibular or more formal neck dissection is done in conjunction with the primary tumor, a pull-through (in-continuity) approach provides an oncologically sound resection.[7] Soft-tissue replacement is all that is required because mandibular continuity is maintained. The key to reconstructing the through-and-through oral cavity defect is to reestablish the muscular support for the floor of mouth. The extent of the defect will dictate the appropriate options.

Primary closure of the myelohyoid defect can be done on patients with small defects with excellent preservation of function. Another method is to detach the hyoglossus muscle from the hyoid and attach it to the mandibular periosteum or myelohyoid remnant.[7] This method requires removal of

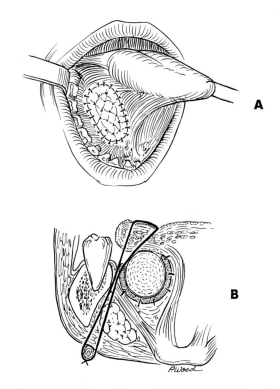

Fig. 85-1. Split-thickness skin graft (STSG). **A,** STSG applied to cover the floor of mouth defect. Note the quilting sutures for better contact and fixation. **B,** Cross-section showing placement of bolster with through-and-through fixation sutures to recreate a paralingual sulcus.

the digastric muscle but provides excellent rehabilitation. Larger defects can be managed easily by rotating in a superiorly based sternocleidomastoid muscle flap.[16,22,41] The intraoral reconstruction generally is done with a bolstered STSG as previously described. Great care is taken to recreate an adequate paralingual sulcus to avoid tethering the tongue. The exposed bone is covered with a buccoalveolar mucosal advancement flap. When covering the exposed bone is problematic, other methods can be applied. The myelohyoid can be rotated superiorly on its periosteal attachments to cover the bone. Larger defects can be covered with a temporoparietal fascial flap tunneled intraorally.[3,17] Lastly, a posteriorly based tongue flap has limited usefulness for this situation.[19] Musculocutaneous flaps tend to be too bulky to be a wise choice in this situation. The one exception would be the platysma musculocutaneous flap, which can be useful in oral cavity reconstruction.[10,13] Neck incisions should be appropriately designed, and great care should be taken to avoid compromising the blood supply during submandibular triangle dissection, which greatly limits its unplanned use. Many authors advocate a free radial forearm flap for these defects.[26,40,44] The flap has an excellent success rate (90%) and holds up well to postoperative radiation. It can be harvested with cutaneous nerves that after microneural anastamosis with the lingual nerve will create a sensate reconstruction. Use of this flap requires microvascular expertise, increased operative time, and possibly a two-team approach. There generally is limited donor site morbidity, although some significant and unacceptable complications have occurred.[6,39] These advantages and drawbacks should be considered in light of the excellent availability of local and regional tissue to rebuild these relatively minor defects.

Superiorly based sternocleidomastoid flap technique[16,22,41]

The sternocleidomastoid muscle receives its dominant blood supply from a branch of the occipital artery and a regular and necessary contribution of blood from a branch of the superior thyroid artery. The inferior supply from the thyrocervical trunk is of lesser importance, making a superiorly based flap the most reliable. The arc of use of a superiorly based sternocleidomastoid flap is ideal for oral cavity and oropharyngeal reconstruction. The muscle is released from its sternal and clavicular attachments and is dissected superiorly. Dissection never proceeds any higher than is necessary to provide the arc needed for the reconstruction. The spinal accessory nerve may restrict the forward rotation of the muscle, and the superior thyroid artery should be preserved if at all possible. Once the muscle is rotated into the surgical defect, it is tacked down in the neck and intraorally. The mucosal edges of the defect are sutured to the muscle so that a "vest-over-pants" type of overlapping is created. The wound then can be left to granulate or a STSG can be applied intraorally as previously described. Adequate drainage and a pressure dressing are essential for successful healing.

An alternative method is to develop a sternocleidomastoid musculocutaneous flap. The amount of cervical skin that can be transferred is limited to the width of the muscle and can be extended below the clavicle for 1 to 2 cm. In previously irradiated patients, island-type cutaneous pedicles are discouraged because of their poor reliability. Skin over the entire muscle is left intact, and the muscle is mobilized as described, carefully preserving the superior thyroid artery supply. The skin covering that portion of the muscle tunneled through the neck then is deepithelialized. The donor site is closed primarily (Fig. 85-2).

Temporoparietal fascial flap technique[3,17]

The temporoparietal fascia is a 2- to 4-mm thick connective tissue that is the lateral extension of the galeal layer of the scalp. It joins the epicranius muscle anteriorly and posteriorly, the tendinous galea superiorly, and blends with the superficial musculoaponeurotic system inferiorly. There is a vascular plexus composed of branches from the occipital and superficial temporal arteries that supply the fascia in an axial pattern. This tissue is vascular, thin, and pliable, making it ideal for intraoral reconstruction.

Flap dissection begins with a careful mapping of the superficial temporal artery and its branches. A curvilinear scalp incision is placed over the lateral scalp, and dissection begins inferiorly. Bipolar cautery is essential in maintaining hemostasis because numerous perforating vessels will be encountered. The edges of the flap are incised down to the deep temporal fascia, and the flap is quickly elevated off of it. The vascular pedicle can be carefully narrowed at the zygoma and traced 2 to 6 cm caudally if needed. The donor area then can be closed primarily over a suction drain. The temporoparietal fascial flap (TFF) is delivered into the oral cavity and oropharynx and is used to bridge the surgical defect (Fig. 85-3). A STSG can be applied intraorally, or the tissue can be left exposed to granulate. This flap can easily reach the anterior floor of mouth, posterior cranial fossa, and into the neck for carotid coverage.

Platysmal flap technique[10,13]

The submental branch of the facial artery is the major arterial supply to this flap. It has a fairly protected position under the mandible with numerous anastomoses with the ipsilateral and contralateral labial arteries, the superior thyroid artery, and the superior labial artery. Ligation of the facial artery distal to the submental artery branching (e.g., where it courses over the mandible) does not compromise the flap. The platysma muscle can even be incised superior to this take-off to improve mobility and axis of use if needed. An added advantage to this flap is its innervation by the facial nerve. This motor innervation can be preserved and used advantageously in rehabilitating an incompetent lip. The flap also has the capacity for sensory nerve reanastomosis, providing sensation to the reconstructed area.

The platysmal flap should be designed and raised before

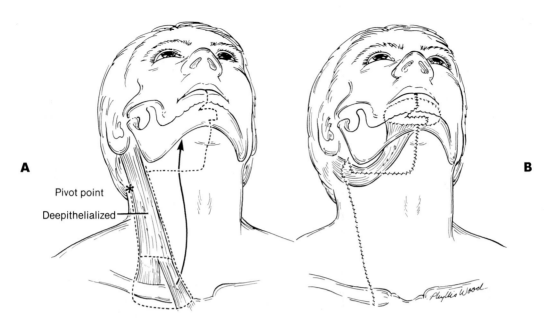

Fig. 85-2. Sternocleidomastoid flap. **A,** Superiorly based sternocleidomastoid musculocutaneous flap. Note the posterior pivot point. Only dissect to the degree necessary to adequately reconstruct the defect. **B,** Flap rotated into floor of mouth defect and primary closure of donor site.

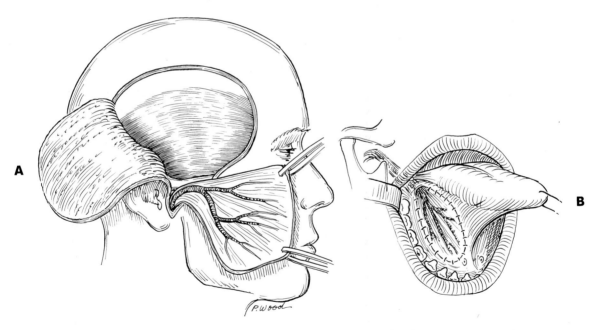

Fig. 85-3. Temporoparietal fascial flap. **A,** Temporoparietal fascial flap incised and rotated inferiorly. Note that the pedicle is dissected below the zygoma. **B,** The flap is tunneled into the oropharynx and oral cavity and used to close the surgical defect. A skin graft can be applied intraorally.

any neck surgery is performed. The cutaneous paddle is designed as an ellipse up to 6 to 7 cm × 10 to 12 cm as dictated by the defect. A minimum of a 5-cm ellipse is required to ensure an adequate number of perforators are included. The inferior aspect of the cutaneous paddle coincides with the inferior segment of the neck incision, which is carried

through skin and platysma and continued superiorly to the mastoid tip. The incision along the superior edge of the skin paddle is carried down to platysma only. The musculocutaneous flap then is elevated in the subplatysmal plane commonly used in neck surgery. If a cutaneous branch from the superior thyroid artery is encountered, it should be preserved

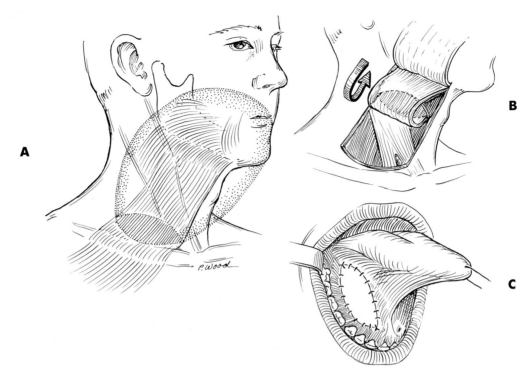

Fig. 85-4. Platysma flap. **A,** Platysma musculocutaneous flap after incising cutaneous island. **B,** Flap is elevated and rotated 270° inward medial to the mandible into the floor of mouth defect. **C,** Flap in place after reconstructing the oral defect.

if possible. Once mobilized, the flap is turned 180° through the defect into the oral cavity (Fig. 85-4).

Radial forearm flap technique[6,26,39,40,44]

The radial forearm flap is a ready source of thin, pliable, relatively hairless skin ideally suited for intraoral reconstruction. The radial artery provides the arterial supply for the flap. It travels within the lateral intermuscular septum of the forearm and gives off multiple branches to the forearm muscles, the volar skin, and the periosteum of the radius. The venous drainage for the flap can be through either a venae comitantes or a cutaneous vein (usually the cephalic). The medial and lateral cutaneous nerves can be harvested with the radial forearm flap permitting a reinnervation of the tissue at the recipient site. A segment of radius comprising 40% of its circumference and up to about 12 cm of its length can be included with the radial forearm flap, which allows this flap to reconstruct composite defects of the jaw with relative ease.

Preoperative assessment should include an Allen test to verify adequate collateral hand perfusion by the ulnar artery. The radial artery is located by palpation or a Doppler ultrasound examination, and the flap is designed as dictated by the reconstructive situation. A tourniquet is applied to the upper arm to reduce operative blood loss and oozing. The distal skin and underlying fascial septum are incised, and

the radial artery is located and ligated. The flap then is raised in a distal-to-proximal direction.

The vascular pedicle is isolated proximal to the cutaneous paddle and can be developed for several centimeters if desired, which allows great flexibility for reanastomosis at the recipient site (Fig. 85-5).

Adapting the radial forearm flap to the surgical reconstruction generally is easy. The workability of the tissue allows it to readily conform to the defect.

The donor site can be covered with a STSG or closed primarily. The morbidity of the radial forearm flap usually is minor and well accepted by the patient. If a STSG is used, there often is a problem with skin breakdown over the exposed forearm tendons, which can be minimized by covering all tendons with muscle before applying the graft and never using a meshed STSG. An ulnar transposition flap often can permit primary closure and avoid the problem of delayed healing. A minor loss of sensation centered over the snuffbox is common, and painful neuromas of the radial nerve develop infrequently. A significant loss of hand function can occur postoperatively, although this is rare. It can consist of either stiffness or actual contracture and is a result of inadequate collateral perfusion from the ulnar artery after radial artery sacrifice. Some surgeons advocate reestablishing the radial artery with an interposition graft after harvesting the radial forearm flap, although this has proven to be

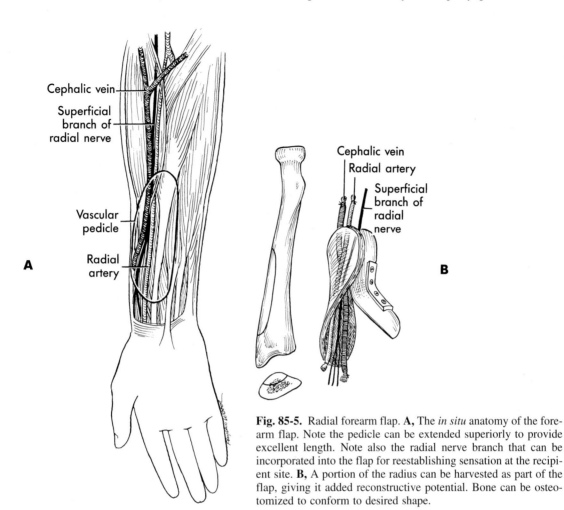

Fig. 85-5. Radial forearm flap. **A,** The *in situ* anatomy of the forearm flap. Note the pedicle can be extended superiorly to provide excellent length. Note also the radial nerve branch that can be incorporated into the flap for reestablishing sensation at the recipient site. **B,** A portion of the radius can be harvested as part of the flap, giving it added reconstructive potential. Bone can be osteotomized to conform to desired shape.

unreliable and is not routinely recommended. This reconstructive technique is widely applied and has become popular with head and neck surgeons, although there are several other excellent techniques available that do not require microvascular expertise and do not entail the risk of rendering a hand nonfunctional.

Reconstruction of defects in the oropharynx and base of tongue with an intact mandibular arch

Small defects (up to 3 to 4 cm) as a result of transoral laser resection of oropharyngeal, tongue base, retromolar trigone, or palatal tumors can be left to granulate. Postoperative care is as described for oral cavity defects.

A STSG or dermal graft is a rapid and useful technique for reconstructing smaller defects of the oropharynx and retromolar trigone. Partial graft loss is common and may result in scarring and eventual tethering of the tongue.

Larger defects, especially those with exposed mandible, require a vascularized flap for adequate reconstruction. The temporalis musculofascial flap[20,37] or TFF[3,17] are excellent, readily available alternatives. Other less useful local flaps include a laterally or posteriorly based tongue flap,[12,19] a masseter crossover flap,[42] and a hard palatal mucosal flap.[15] The extent and nature of the defect to be closed will determine the applicability of these secondary options.

Regional musculocutaneous flaps generally have too much bulk for these defects. A pectoralis major musculofascial flap avoids the problem of bulkiness and provides ample tissue to reconstruct large oropharyngeal defects.[25] One potential misuse of this method is to apply it to defects that include a major portion of the tongue base. As previously stressed, the tongue should be reconstructed separately from the floor of the mouth or oropharynx if at all possible to maximize postoperative function. Regional flaps whose pedicles are buried subcutaneously will contract and atrophy substantially over time, which can easily lead to significant tethering of the tongue. A secondary procedure to release the tongue from the pedicle then is needed to limit the patient's dysphagia. Large defects limited to the base of the tongue can be closed with a set back tongue flap.[28] This method maintains maximum tongue mobility and posterior bulk and generally leaves the patient with excellent function.

Several different free flaps have been used successfully to reconstruct these defects. The radial forearm flap is perhaps the most popular, but cutaneous flaps from the groin,[34] dorsum of the foot,[1] and mucosal flaps[36] (primarily split-jejunum) have been used. The same drawbacks discussed previously apply to this situation. The need for increased operative time and microvascular expertise plus an ample supply of excellent locally available tissue limits the widespread application of free flaps to this reconstructive situation.

Temporalis flap technique[20,37]

The temporalis muscle receives its blood supply from the internal maxillary artery through the anterior and posterior deep temporal arteries. These vessels arborize within the temporalis in such a way that the muscle can be split coronally into anterior and posterior segments or sagittally into medial and lateral halves. The deep temporal fascia, which frequently is harvested with the temporalis muscle, has a separate axial supply originating from the superficial temporal artery—the middle temporal artery.

The coronoid process is identified transorally, and the temporalis insertion is elevated off of the medial surface, taking care to preserve the vascular supply to the muscle. The coronoid process then is transected at its base. A curvilinear incision is placed in the temporal scalp and carried down through the superficial temporal fascia to expose the deep fascia. Scalp flaps are reflected anteriorly and posteriorly,

exposing the full extent of the muscle. The fascial attachments to the zygomatic arch are incised, and the bony arch is removed. Exposure for the anterior osteotomy sometimes can require a second incision, especially if replacement of the arch is planned. The musculofascial flap is lifted off of the temporal squama distally to proximally. Once adequate mobilization has been accomplished, a tunnel is developed bluntly into the oral cavity. The flap then is delivered through the tunnel for use in the reconstruction. The mucosal edges of the defect are sewn to the deep temporal fascia so that there is a ''vest-over-pants'' overlap (Fig. 85-6).

This muscle is locally available, fairly thin, and supple, making it useful in intraoral and oropharyngeal reconstruction. The ability to split the muscle sagittally or coronally allows the operator a degree of dimensional flexibility. Functional donor morbidity is minor, and the cosmetic appearance of the defect can be improved with the intraoperative implantation of Instat collagen or Gore-Tex. The zygomatic arch can be replaced after rotating the flap intraorally, but this often is unnecessary. The bulk of the muscle turned on itself will adequately recreate the arch contour. If the arch is to be replaced, it can be wired or plated at the conclusion of the case. Paralysis of the temporal branch of the facial nerve occurs in as many as 20% of patients with the temporalis flap technique. The nerve function probably is lost as a result of stretch injury, so surgical technique should be refined.

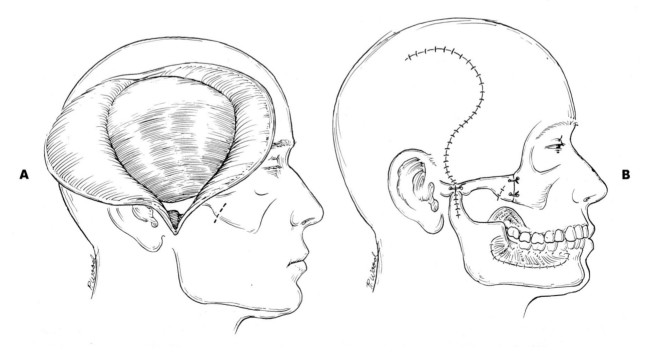

Fig. 85-6. Temporalis flap. **A,** The temporalis muscle and overlying deep temporal fascia are exposed. A second incision at the medial extent of the zygoma can be placed to facilitate removal. **B,** The flap is lifted and turned into the oropharyngeal defect. The zygoma can be replaced if deemed necessary.

Laterally based tongue flap technique[12,19]

The tongue offers an excellent source of tissue for reconstructing defects of the posterior oral cavity and oropharynx. Advantages of this flap include local accessibility, well-vascularized and reliable tissue, no separate donor site defect, and limited operative time for reconstruction. The major disadvantage is the unavoidable reduction of tongue function. This morbidity is relatively minor if only one half of the tongue is used. The laterally based tongue flap can survive when the ipsilateral lingual artery has been ligated if it is carefully dissected. Previous irradiation does not seem to influence the reliability or usefulness of this flap.

The laterally based tongue flap is pedicled on the remaining floor of mouth. A midline mucosal cut is made from the tongue base to the tongue tip. This incision is carried into the tongue musculature for 1 to 2 mm. The myomucosal flap then is dissected laterally, unrolling the mobile tongue. The flap then can be rotated into the surgical defect for primary closure. The remaining anterior hemitongue is closed by approximating the dorsal and ventral surfaces. This narrowed mobile tongue will hypertrophy over time, minimizing any functional morbidity (Fig. 85-7).

Hard palate mucosal flap technique[15]

The mucoperiosteum of the hard palate can be pedicled on a single greater palatine artery, which can be up to 24 cm² of locally available, thin, well-vascularized tissue. The arc of use is somewhat limited, but defects of the buccal mucosa, retromolar trigone, tonsillar region, or soft palate can be easily covered. The tissue is not very pliable and does not tolerate tension. Previous irradiation to the oral cavity should be considered a relative contraindication to the use

of this flap because the denuded palatal bone is predisposed to develop osteitis.

An incision is placed approximately 1 cm medial to the maxillary alveolus circumferentially around the hard palate. The greater palatine artery is protected within a 1-cm pedicle at the flap's base. The flap then is rotated into the surgical defect. The vascular pedicle can be skeletonized further to increase the arc of use, but this increases the risk for vessel torsion and subsequent total flap loss. The donor defect is left to granulate. A palatal prosthesis can be placed to cover the denuded bone until healing has progressed (Fig. 85-8).

Reconstruction of defects in the buccal area

As in other sites, smaller wounds can be left to granulate or are closed primarily. STSGs or mucosal grafts are easily applied to this area. Bolstering seldom is necessary for the success of these grafts, provided they are peripherally fixed and quilted appropriately. More extensive tissue loss generally requires replacement of adequate bulk to prevent dimpling of the cheek or restriction of mouth opening subsequent to wound contracture. The temporalis muscle flap[20,37] or TFF[3,17] offer the same advantages described for oropharyngeal defects. The internal surface of the flap can be easily skin-grafted, providing an excellent reconstruction of the area.

Through-and-through defects provide more of a surgical challenge because internal and external coverage is required. The lateral scalp flaps already discussed can be skin-grafted on both surfaces, although this would be a cosmetically inferior option. Combining a cervical rotation flap[35,46] externally with a lateral scalp flap internally would be a good option.

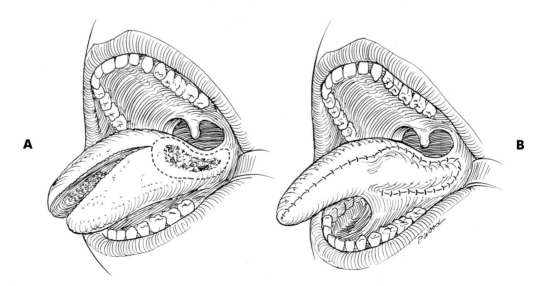

Fig. 85-7. Tongue flap. **A,** A midline incision is made through the mobile tongue. The tongue then is unfurled, developing a laterally based myomucosal flap. **B,** The flap covering the oropharyngeal defect. The remainder of the tongue is closed on itself.

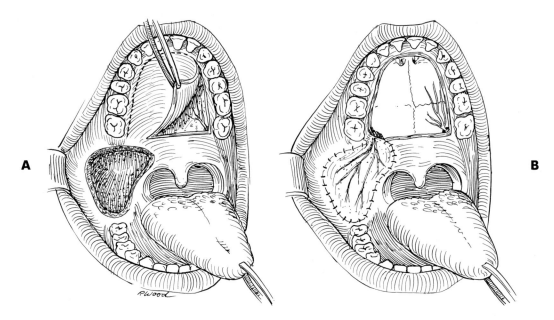

Fig. 85-8. Palatal flap. **A,** The palatal mucoperiosteal flap is developed with care to preserve one greater palatine pedicle. **B,** Flap rotation into place to cover the oropharyngeal defect.

Musculocutaneous flaps such as the pectoralis major,[4,25] latissimus,[23] or trapezius[27] have some applicability to large through-and-through buccal defects. Separate skin islands can be made and the muscle turned on itself to provide an internal lining and external coverage. An alternative would be to skin-graft the internal surface of the muscle and to use the cutaneous portion of the flap externally. Any of the cutaneous or musculocutaneous free flaps can be applied to this situation. The free scapular flap[8,14] deserves special mention because the vascular anatomy allows the dissection of two separate cutaneous paddles, which allows the surgeon a three-dimensional flexibility that is ideally suited for through-and-through defects.

Cervical rotation advancement flap technique[35,46]

The cervical rotation advancement flap is a cosmetically excellent option for reconstructing the external aspect of a through-and-through buccal defect. The internal lining can be reestablished with a temporalis muscle STSG covered flap. This combination provides excellent bulk and cosmesis. An alternative would be to apply a STSG to the undersurface of the cervical rotation advancement flap.

Flap design is influenced by the size of the buccal defect, but it generally involves an incision running from the posterior aspect of the facial defect to the ear. The incision then curves under the lobule of the ear onto the neck about 1 to 2 cm behind the anterior border of the trapezius. The incision can be continued onto the chest wall when maximum rotation is needed. This incision affords exposure to allow radical neck dissection if necessary. A subplatysmal plane is developed, and the flap is lifted just enough to provide a tension-free closure. The neck incision usually can be closed primarily (Fig. 85-9).

Latissimus dorsi musculocutaneous flap technique[23]

The latissimus dorsi musculocutaneous flap can be harvested as a free flap or transferred transaxillary into the head and neck for reconstructive uses. The dominant blood supply to the flap is through the thoracodorsal artery, which is a branch of the circumflex scapular artery. The vascular pedicle enters the latissimus on its medial surface about 8 to 10 cm distal to its humeral insertion. The artery usually bifurcates after entering the muscle, sending a dominant branch parallel and about 2 cm posterior to the free lateral border of the muscle. The upper branch courses transversely parallel and about 3.5 cm inferior to the upper border of the muscle. Numerous perforating vessels originate from these musculocutaneous arteries to supply the subdermal plexus of the overlying skin. The density of perforating vessels is greater in the proximal two thirds of the muscle, making this skin more reliable to transfer with the flap. The latissimus dorsi musculocutaneous flap has a potential of 40 × 25 cm of tissue available for transfer if needed. The arc of use is substantial, reaching to the vertex of the skull if necessary. The thoracodorsal nerve travels with the vascular bundle, giving the flap the ability to be reinnervated at the recipient site.

The patient should be in the lateral position to use this flap, which necessitates preoperative planning and coordination. Preoperative marking of the anterior border of the latissimus facilitates easy intraoperative location. The ipsilateral arm should be sterilely draped and mobile and is supported on a Mayo stand during flap dissection. Flap design is dic-

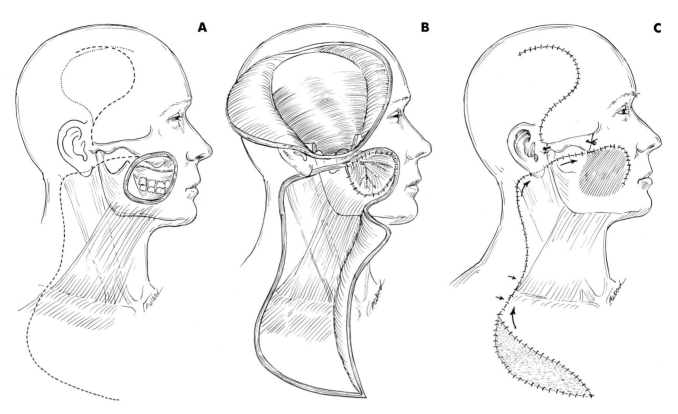

Fig. 85-9. Buccal defect. **A,** A patient with a through-and-through buccal defect with incisions diagrammed for a cervical rotation advancement flap. **B,** Temporalis muscle flap rotated into buccal defect and cervical flap lifted. **C,** External closure completed. Note that the intraoral surface can be covered with a skin graft.

tated by the defect to be reconstructed, but it should be remembered the cutaneous perfusion over the distal one third of the muscle can be tenuous. A Doppler ultrasound examination can be used to locate perforators and to allow flap design to be modified accordingly. The dissection begins with an incision through skin and subcutaneous tissue along the previously marked anterior border of the muscle. The plane between the latissimus and serratus is bluntly developed, and the vascular pedicle is located by Doppler examination and palpation. The cutaneous island is incised down to the muscle circumferentially. The inferior and medial muscular incisions are made as distal from the edge of the cutaneous island as possible. Dissection proceeds posteromedially toward the axilla. The neurovascular pedicle exits from the muscle well before it inserts onto the humerus, so great care should be taken when dissection approaches this area. To isolate the thoracodorsal pedicle, the branches to the serratus should be ligated. The pedicle can be traced proximally to the circumflex scapular artery. The tendonous insertion then is separated from the humerus, totally isolating the vascular pedicle. A plane is developed transaxillary superficial to the pectoralis minor muscle. The pectoralis major muscle is separated from the clavicle far enough to allow

the flap to be passed unrestricted into the neck (Fig. 85-10). If the lifted flap cannot reach the surgical defect, the pedicle can be exteriorized or the pedicle can be separated and the tissue transferred as a free flap. The donor site usually can be closed primarily, or an STSG can be applied. The patient's arm is placed in a shoulder immobilizer for 4 or 5 days, after which physical therapy is instituted.

When an internal and external lining is required, there are a few options available to the surgeon. The undersurface of the muscle can obviously be skin-grafted as has been previously described for other flaps. A second option would be to remove a strip of skin from the center of the cutaneous island to create two islands. This procedure would have to be planned according to the distribution of the perforators. Another alternative would be to develop two separate musculocutaneous segments supplied by either branch of the thoracodorsal. Incorporation of the flap into the defect should use the vest-over-pants overlap. This is possible by harvesting muscle distal to the cutaneous island.

Scapular free flap technique[8,14]

The scapular free flap is based on branches from the circumflex scapular artery. This artery originates from the subscapular artery, which is a major branch of the axillary ar-

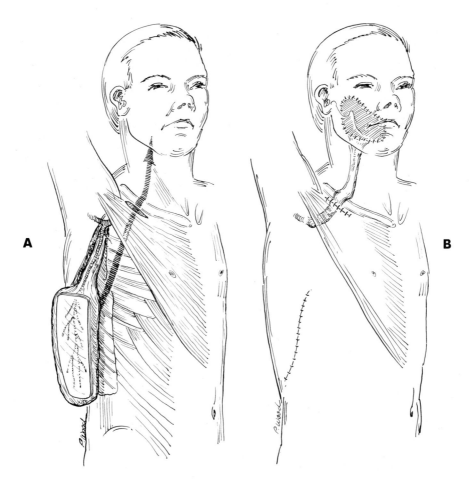

Fig. 85-10. Latissimus dorsi flap. **A,** The latissimus dorsi musculocutaneous flap lifted, and its insertion to humerus is severed above the vascular pedicle. A plane is developed over the pectoralis minor. **B,** The flap is delivered into the neck and face through the axilla through an incision between the clavicle and the pectoralis major.

tery. The circumflex scapular artery can be located externally within the triangular space bounded by the teres minor above, teres major below, and the long head of the triceps laterally. The circumflex scapular artery traverses this space and divides into a transverse and descending branch. This system supplies the skin from the posterior axillary fold to the midline and from the scapular spine to its tip. The nutrient arteries form a rich fascial plexus that sends vertical branches into the subdermal plexus of the skin, allowing peripheral debulking of excess fat and subcutaneous tissue with this flap. Two separate cutaneous flaps can be developed on the circumflex scapular artery, allowing great flexibility to the surgeon.

The patient should be rotated enough to allow access to the midline of the back. Tissue requirements are diagrammed on the patient and incorporated within an ellipse. The elliptical defect can be closed primarily if it is less than 10 to 12 cm. If only one paddle is required, the transverse branch is the preferred pedicle. The skin and subcutaneous tissue is incised, and dissection is started in a medial-to-lateral direc-

tion in the avascular plane of loose areolar tissue superficial to the fascia of the infraspinatus muscle. Dissection proceeds medially until the triangular space is reached where the circumflex scapular artery is easily located by palpation or Doppler examination. Pedicle dissection can proceed proximally to the subscapular or axillary artery as needed, creating a length of up to 10 cm. The CSA usually is between 2 to 3 cm, which makes microvascular anastomosis relatively easy (Fig. 85-11).

Reconstruction of defects of the hard palate

Hard palate mucosal defects can be closed with STSG or mucosal graft or left to granulate. Small through-and-through palatal defects can be closed with palatal rotation flaps. When surgical reconstruction has been delayed and palatal edges have healed, nasal mucosa can be back-dissected and turned into the defect. This tissue will provide a first layer of closure that can be covered with a palatal rotation flap. Larger through-and-through defects are best managed with prosthetics. Prosthetics allow for rapid rehabilita-

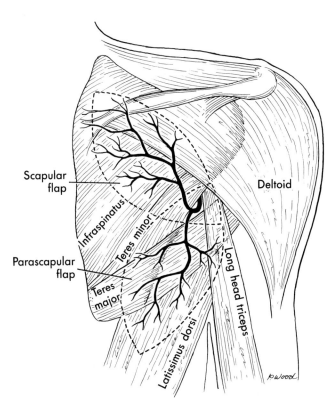

Fig. 85-11. Scapular flap. The scapular area provides an excellent source of cutaneous and osseous tissue. The latissimus dorsi can be lifted in conjunction with this tissue, which greatly expands its reconstructive potential.

tion and careful monitoring for tumor recurrence. The hard palate serves only a passive function in deglutition and speech, so obturation is a physiologically suitable alternative. The surgeon should always underestimate the amount of palate and the number of teeth to be removed, which will allow construction of a temporary obturator that is sure to fit the eventual defect. The surgeon should attempt to retain as much anterior palate and bone lateral to the midline of the defect side as possible to provide ledges for stabilizing a prosthesis. A dental prosthesis is not suitable for a mentally retarded or senile person or for anyone not competent to manage it. These patients often will require flap reconstruction of their palates. The radial forearm flap and temporalis flap have been used with success in these situations.

Total palatectomy defects present unique and complex reconstructive problems. Attempts to replace bone usually is fraught with difficulty. In general, the upper lip should be reconstructed with adjacent soft tissues, and the palate and nose should be replaced with a prosthesis. Special fixation techniques are required to provide adequate support for these large prostheses. Osseointegration[2] of the remaining maxilla and skull base will provide many sites for prosthesis support, but the process takes many operations and several months to complete. Another much simpler technique[30] is the placement of a stainless steel Steinmann's pin between the zygo-

matic arches. A small metal tray containing rare earth magnets then is attached to the pin. Counter-attaching magnets are placed within the prosthesis to provide a firm fixation point.

Reconstruction of composite defects of the lateral jaw oropharynx

When the oncologic ablation requires the removal of a segment of the jaw, the surgeon is faced with a more difficult reconstructive decision. He or she must decide if rebuilding a jaw is in the best interests of the patient. Several excellent sources of vascularized bone grafts have been discovered over the past several years and have added to the options available to the surgeon. These flaps provide excellent restoration of contour and an improved cosmetic result, although one should remember that functional rehabilitation generally is of greater concern to the patient. The benefits gained by reconstructing the jaw should be established before surgery. The patient should understand that the added surgical time, expense, risk for failure, and need for reoperation inherent in jaw restoration actually may be detrimental to his or her postoperative function. Reconstruction of the ramus and bony defect common with lateral composite resections leads to increased trismus and limited mandibular motion postoperatively.[18] This can have a direct impact on the patient's quality of life by reducing his or her chances for adequate oral function. Advocates of immediate jaw reconstruction cite mandibular drift as a major postoperative concern, although this worry seems unfounded. Drift is minimal as long as the soft-tissue defect is adequately replaced and isometric exercises are instituted in immediately after surgery. These exercises include having the patient practice bringing his or her remaining dentition into occlusion. External pressure on the jaw often is required to align it properly. Internal maxillary fixation is another method for maintaining occlusion and is recommended whenever the soft-tissue defect is not replaced with adequate bulk. The surgeon will find that these "unreconstructed" people will open their jaw along a deviated plane of motion but generally will have good function. They also will have an acceptable cosmetic appearance. With the understanding that the functional rehabilitation of this lateral defect depends most on the soft-tissue reconstruction, a few specific techniques will be discussed. Specific methods for reconstructing the jaw defect are discussed elsewhere in the book and will be mentioned in the next section.

Pectoralis major musculocutaneous flap technique[4,25]

The pectoralis major musculocutaneous flap certainly is a workhorse and the most familiar musculocutaneous flap for reconstructive surgeons. The muscle receives a dominant blood supply from the thoracoacromial artery, which originates from the axillary artery under the superior edge of the pectoralis minor muscle. The lateral thoracic artery is a second arterial supply to the pectoral muscle. These arteries travel in the clavipectoral fascia, allowing a safe and bloodless plane of dissection between the pectoralis major and pectoralis minor muscles.

The flap has limitations in application. Too much bulk and hair-bearing skin can be a problem in reconstruction of the tongue and the floor of the mouth. This is not a problem when a lateral composite defect is reconstructed. The bulk provides excellent contour for the patient and ample tissue to avoid excessive mandibular drift. Postoperative radiotherapy will deter any hair growth.

An island musculocutaneous flap, a musculofascial, or simply a muscular flap can be developed. If a pectoralis major musculocutaneous flap is needed, the skin requirements carefully are diagrammed on the patient's chest, and the arc of flap use is simulated with a sponge. It is most desirable to place the entire cutaneous paddle over the muscle, although random skin over the sternum, xyphoid, or rectus is sometimes needed to reach the surgical defect. The cutaneous paddle is circumferentially incised down to the pectoral fascia with care to bevel the cuts outward from the skin edges. Tacking sutures are placed to reduce the shearing of skin and subcutaneous tissue over muscle. The chest incision is continued from the superior aspect of the cutaneous paddle superiorly and laterally to create (and preserve for future use) a deltopectoral flap. The remaining chest skin is rapidly dissected off the pectoralis major, exposing its free lateral border and clavicular insertion. Care is taken not to dissect the chest skin too close to the sternum; the integrity

of the internal mammary perforators should be preserved. The avascular plane between the pectoralis major and minor muscles is bluntly developed, allowing palpation and even visualization of the vascular pedicle. The inferior and medial margin of the muscle is separated, obtaining as much muscle beyond the cutaneous paddle as possible. The vascular pedicle then is developed by incising the muscle medially and laterally. Care is taken to avoid skeletonizing the pedicle, and dissection is continued until enough of an arc is developed to rotate the tissue into the defect without excessive tension (Fig. 85-12). The clavicular fibers of the pectoralis major are preserved if possible to lessen donor morbidity to the patient. The vascular pedicle is turned over the clavicle, and the cutaneous paddle is used for the mucosal closure. The donor site usually can be closed primarily with undermining.

Gastroomental free flap technique[31]

The gastroomental free flap replaces the resected mucosa with antral mucosa, giving it a distinct advantage over alternative methods. This mucosa is soft, pliable, and moist, allowing easy molding to complex defects. By providing a secreting mucosal surface, deglutition and xerostomia are improved postoperatively. Previous gastric surgery may negate the use of the gastroomental free flap. Preoperative planning should include an upper gastrointestinal series and consultation with a general surgeon.

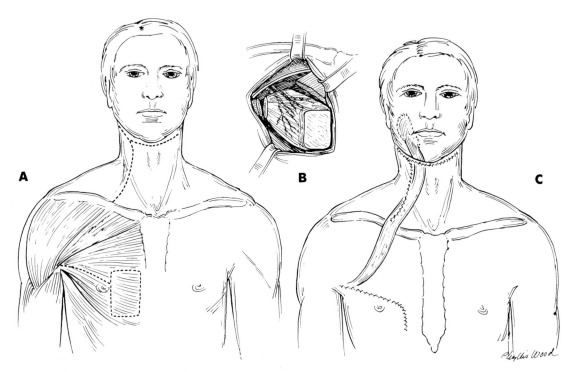

Fig. 85-12. Pectoralis major flap. **A,** The cutaneous island is incised down to the pectoralis major muscle. An incision is carried laterally from this island along the anterior axillary line. **B,** The medial and lateral muscle cuts are made, freeing up the pedicle and allowing the necessary arc for reconstruction in the head and neck. **C,** The flap in place and the donor area is closed primarily.

The harvesting of a gastroomental free flap can proceed simultaneously with the cancer excision. An upper abdominal incision is made, and the peritoneum is entered. A GIAR stapler is used to remove a portion of the greater curvature mucosa and simultaneously close the stomach. Up to 144 cm² of non–acid-secreting mucosa can be harvested without interfering with normal gastric function. A variable amount of omentum can be included with the gastric mucosa, depending on the vessel arcades and the gastroepiploic pedicle. A pedicle of up to 10 to 12 cm usually can be developed (Fig. 85-13). A feeding jejunostomy is placed before closing the abdomen. After microvascular anastomosis in the neck, the gastric patch easily reconstructs the internal defect. The major problem encountered with the use of gastric mucosa is the occasional production of excessive mucus, which can be severe enough to cause major aspiration. For this reason, tracheostomy is recommended in all patients undergoing this procedure.

Controlled fistula technique

Some wounds or reconstructive situations require the creation of a controlled fistula for safety. A MacFee type of neck incision is ideal for developing a fistula. The upper horizontal incision should be placed at least 3 to 4 cm from the jaw, which creates an upper cervical–facial flap that can be turned under the lower border of the jaw and approximated to the alveolar, buccal, or lateral floor of mouth mucosa. If secondary reconstruction is planned within 7 to 10 days, the wound is simply packed with bacitracin-coated adaptic. The central cervical flap provides coverage for the carotid system. If a regional flap is needed, it can be attached to the medial aspect of the oral defect and brought externally to cover the cervical skin defect (Fig. 85-14). When fistula closure is possible, the turn-in flap is released. The regional flap then is incised where it had been previously attached to the cervical skin. This edge then is brought into the oral cavity and attached to the lateral floor of mouth, alveolar ridge, or buccal mucosa. The cervical skin flaps then are closed in their normal anatomic position.

Reconstruction of composite defects of the anterior jaw and floor of mouth

Composite resection of the anterior floor of mouth and jaw produces devastating functional and cosmetic morbidity for a patient. There are instances when not attempting to reconstruct the jaw is the appropriate option even for these defects. Severely debilitated or elderly patients will not tolerate the extended operating time or degree of postoperative rehabilitation necessary. If tongue function is dramatically compromised, any hope of pleasurable oral intake is remote, and gastrostomy feeding will be necessary. The lower lip can be suspended from the zygomas to provide oral competence, making jaw restoration solely a cosmetic concern. The cosmetic impact of an "Andy Gump" appearance can be socially crippling for a patient. In general, adequate rehabilitation after this type of ablation will require a continuous jaw arch to support the lower lip and prevent oral incompetence. By replacing the lost bone, the patient also has the potential for dental rehabilitation with osseointegration.

The decision of whether to reconstruct the jaw primarily or in a second operation depends in large part on the resources available to a surgeon. The failure rate of bone grafts in primary reconstruction is too great to recommend their routine use. Vascularized autologous bone can tolerate limited exposure to oral contamination without becoming irreversibly infected. As long as the vascularized bone is well stabilized and protected from the oral cavity by adequate soft tissue, there is an acceptable success rate with primary reconstruction. It is unreasonable for a surgeon to perform a large anterior composite resection and then undertake a complicated reconstruction that includes a vascularized bone flap. This superhuman effort will surely produce compromises that not only risk complication and failure, but can reduce the quality of postoperative function for the patient. This is one circumstance where a surgical team approach probably is the best option. While one group of surgeons remove the cancer, another group harvests the tissue for re-

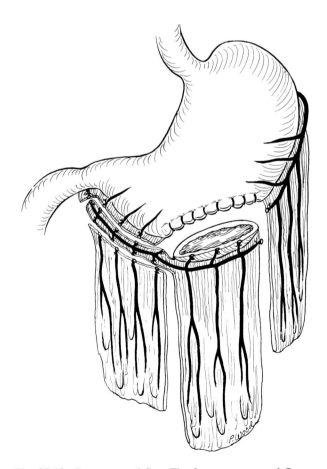

Fig. 85-13. Gastroomental flap. The free gastroomental flap can provide a large amount of omentum, and gastric mucosa is ideally suited to resurface the oral cavity and oropharynx.

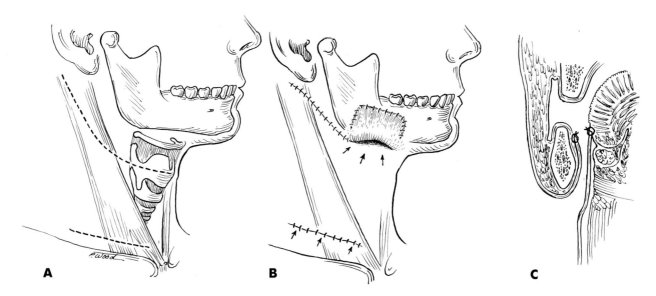

Fig. 85-14. Fistula. **A,** Placing the upper horizontal incision 3 to 4 cm from the edge of the jaw allows the development of a turn-in flap for a controlled fistula. **B** and **C,** Upper cervical flap turned into the oral cavity and sutured to the alveolar and buccal mucosa. The central cervical flap covers the great vessels.

construction, which maximizes the efficient use of time and best serves the patient.

Another option is to reconstruct the defect at a second operation. Surgical margins often are in question when resecting large tumor recurrences, especially in an irradiated failure. Frozen sections notoriously are inaccurate in these patients, and often it is in the patient's best interest to delay elaborate reconstruction until margins are cleared by permanent microscopic review. The surgical defect can be packed for the 2 to 3 days necessary for confirmation of margins. Additional tissue can be resected if needed, or the wound can be freshened and the reconstruction performed, which allows the single operator to be well rested and well prepared for the best reconstruction possible.

The last approach is to reconstruct the soft-tissue defect and to use a metal plate to span the mandibular defect to stabilize the remaining jaw segments. The final mandibular reconstruction then can be delayed for several weeks to months after radiotherapy and rehabilitation. By delaying the reconstruction, the surgeon can rebuild the jaw without entering the oral cavity. Bone grafts are more successful in these patients and are an acceptable alternative to vascularized bone. A full-thickness calvarial bone graft is preferred if appropriate for the defect.

Mandibular reconstruction bar technique

Maximizing success with mandibular plating requires a systematic approach and attention to detail. A minimum of three-screw fixation is required on each fragment plated. If possible, plates always are adjusted, and preliminary marking holes are drilled before any jaw is resected. Titanium or

vitallium (cobalt–chromium alloy) is the preferred plating material. Drilling is done at extremely slow speeds (25 to 50 rpm) under copious cool saline irrigation. Anterior defects always are underprojected when using plates. This can be accomplished simply by applying the bar to the lingual surface of the remaining jaw. When plates are to be left for long periods of time, all screw holes are manually tapped. The hollow screw reconstruction plate system also should be considered for this situation.[45]

Trapezius osteomusculocutaneous flap technique[27,29]

The trapezius osteomusculocutaneous flap can provide up to 12 × 2.5 cm of vascularized bone for mandibular reconstruction. The posteromedial scapular spine is the bone portion of the flap, and it is combined with either a superiorly based or island-type trapezius flap.

The anterior incision for the superiorly based flap follows the anterior border of the trapezius muscle. The posterior incision is roughly parallel to this traveling to the midline at about C5 or C6. The incision crosses the midline and turns cephalad only enough to allow the necessary arc to reach the surgical defect. The superiorly based flap can be successfully used even when previous neck surgery has sacrificed the transverse cervical or occipital vessels. The paraspinous perforators are the key supply to the flap. The caudal incision is placed below the scapular spine. The muscular attachments to the scapular spine are carefully preserved. The bone cuts are made with care to preserve the integrity of the acromion. The remaining attachments of the trapezius to the clavicle and acromion are separated, and the flap is rotated superiorly. The transverse cervical vessels are divided if necessary. The muscle pedicle can be externalized to improve the arc of use. The scapular spine should be rigidly fixed into the jaw defect, which is accomplished with metal plating or by transcutaneous suspension wires connected to an external acrylic bar.

The island flap is based on the transverse cervical vessels. The integrity of these vessels should be verified before the flap is dissected. The transverse cervical vein usually dictates the arc of use of this flap. Once the vessels have been isolated and clearly identified, the flap can be designed. The cutaneous paddle usually is centered over the acromion, and up to 40% of the skin can be over the deltoid. The distal skin is lifted superiorly to the spine. The bone is harvested for the superiorly based flap. The anterior, superior, and posterior skin incisions are made down to the trapezius fascia. Blunt dissection under the vascular pedicle provides the necessary undermining. The posterior and superior muscle cuts are made, and the flap is rotated superiorly (Fig. 85-15).

Sacrificing the function of the trapezius muscle solely for reconstructive purposes is not recommended because the resultant shoulder morbidity is too great. The flap is ideal for those situations wherein the spinal accessory nerve is sacrificed as part of a radical neck dissection. It is noteworthy that these flaps can be dissected without having to cut the spinal accessory nerve, although the arc of use will be restricted without its sacrifice. Donor defects can be closed primarily, or an STSG can be applied.

Internal oblique–iliac crest osteomusculocutaneous flap technique[43]

Including the internal oblique muscle with an iliac bone flap based on the deep circumflex vessels has solved some of the problems previously associated with this donor tissue. The skin paddle and muscle cuffs that comprised the original flap often were inadequate to restore the soft-tissue portion of the defect and were unmaneuverable. The internal oblique, which is thin and well vascularized, is ideal for covering the intraoral surface of the bone and provides an excellent bed for an STSG. Deep labial and lingual sulci can be created with the STSG, providing maximum tongue mobility and best intraoral contour for denture support. The iliac crest has the largest supply of bone adequate for mandibular reconstruction of any donor area. It is of such quality that immediate osseointegration for total dental rehabilitation is possible. The separate donor areas allows for a two-team approach to the operation. Without this team approach, combined ablation and reconstruction with this flap would take an unacceptably long time to perform. Flap dissection is an involved procedure and is in an area unfamiliar to most head and neck surgeons. Donor morbidity associated with this flap is minimal and well tolerated by patients.

Scapular osteocutaneous flap technique[5]

The lateral border of the scapula provides another source for a vascularized bone flap. A segment of bone 1.5 × 3 cm thick and up to 14 cm long can be pedicled on the circumflex scapular vessels. A portion of the inferior tip and medial border of the scapula can be included and has an ideal shape for the mandibular angle. The free scapular flap can be developed at the same time, providing two separate cutaneous paddles. These cutaneous paddles, which can be positioned virtually independent of the bone, allow great reconstructive versatility. The two-team approach can be applied with this flap and allows the patient to be positioned properly. Donor site morbidity has been relatively minor.

The major drawback with this donor bone is its thinness (only 1.5 cm) as an alveolar surface, which limits the potential total dental rehabilitation obtainable with osseointegration. It is noteworthy that the latissimus dorsi musculocutaneous flap can be included on the same vascular pedicle as the scapular osteocutaneous flap, providing the reconstructive surgeon with a tremendous amount of tissue capable of rebuilding virtually any defect imaginable.

Radial forearm–radius flap technique[6,26,39,44]

A portion of the radius can be incorporated into the radial forearm flap to provide another source of vascularized bone. Flap dissection is relatively straightforward and can be completed quickly, which explains the popularity of the radial forearm–radius flap. The amount of donor bone is limited, and there is potential for significant morbidity if certain principles are not adhered to. The drawbacks are discussed in the radial forearm flap section, and the fact that the radius is not the best bone available for jaw reconstruction limits the applicability of the radial forearm–radius flap.

Reconstruction of oropharyngocutaneous fistula

Fistulas can occur immediately after surgery as a result of infection and poor wound healing. They generally can be managed conservatively by opening the neck to provide salivary egress and starting local wound care. Often patients cannot afford the extended period of secondary healing because they need to start radiotherapy or because of family or work needs, and surgical intervention is needed.

Another situation wherein a surgical reconstruction may be needed is a chronic fistula that has not responded to conservative treatment and is causing the patient major morbidity. Many patients have been irradiated or suffer a medical condition that adversely affects wound healing, such as diabetes or hypothyroidism.

Many separate factors influence the surgical management of a salivary fistula. Previous irradiation, general medical status of the patient, size of the dehiscence, exposure of vital structures, type of neck flaps used, and type of reconstruction previously performed are but a few of the more important factors. In general, the surgeon should strive for a three-layer closure, consisting of internal mucosa, intervening well-vascularized tissue, and skin. There should be a vest-over-pants type of overlap between the intervening tissue

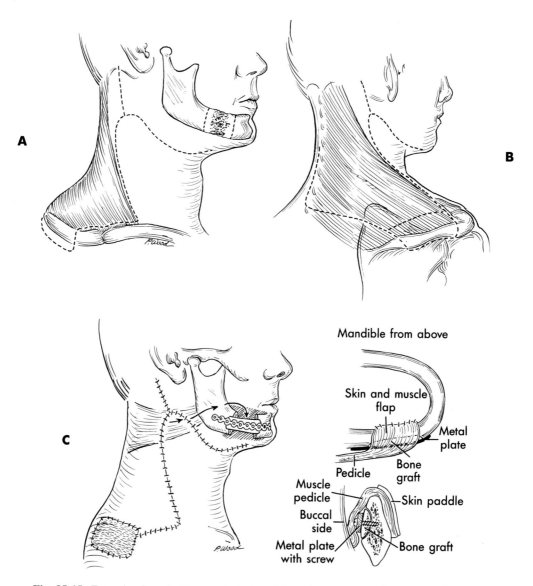

Fig. 85-15. Trapezius flap. **A,** The superiorly based trapezius osteomusculocutaneous flap can be easily developed with a Conley-type neck incision. **B,** The posterior incision runs roughly parallel to the anterior border of the trapezius to about C6 where it turns superiorly only enough to allow the necessary arc for reconstruction. **C,** The spine is plated to the remaining jaw, and the donor site is closed primarily or with a skin graft.

and the mucosal closure. In the acute situation, a muscle or musculocutaneous flap usually is necessary. The sternocleidomastoid,[16,22,41] pectoralis major,[4,25] latissimus,[23] or superiorly based trapezius flap[27] have been extremely useful. With a chronic fistula, local turn-in flaps can provide the internal closure. A muscle flap provides the intervening tissue, and an STSG provides the skin closure.

Free flaps are useful alternatives to local and regional muscle flaps, although suitable recipient vessels for reanastomosis can be hard to find. The omental free flap[32] is perhaps the best at healing virtually any chronic defect the head and neck surgeon will face.

Omental free flap technique[32]

The omentum is the body's best reparative tissue. It will conform to any defect almost like a liquid. Its abundant vascularity is unsurpassed and facilitates the rapid healing of difficult surgical wounds, even osteoradionecrosis. The rich lymphatic network within the omentum may provide conduits to improve the lymphedema commonly found in postsurgery and in radiotherapy patients. An upper abdominal incision and dissection as described for the gastroomental flap are used. Work on the recipient site can proceed while the free omental flap is being harvested. The recipient site is thoroughly debrided, and the mucosal and skin edges are back-dissected by 1 to 2 cm. The omentum then is tucked into the defect so that there is good vest-over-pants overlap. The internal and external surfaces of the omentum do not need any coverage because any exposed portion epithelializes rapidly. If an STSG is applied, it develops into a supple surface with minimal contraction. The surgeon should remember that the omentum is an option whenever there is a difficult reconstructive situation in a poor recipient bed.

REFERENCES

1. Acland RD, Flynn MB: Immediate reconstruction of oral cavity and oropharyngeal defects using microvascular free flaps, *Am J Surg* 136: 419, 1978.
2. Albrektsson T and others: Present clinical applications of osseointegrated percutaneous implants, *Plast Reconstr Surg* 79:721, 1987.
3. Antonyshyn O, Gross JS, Birt BD: Versatility of temporal muscle and fascial flaps, *Br J Plast Surg* 41:118, 1988.
4. Ariyan S: The pectoralis major myocutaneous flap, *Plast Reconstr Surg* 63:73, 1979.
5. Baker SR, Sulivan MJ: Osteocutaneous free scapular flap for one-stage mandibular reconstruction, *Arch Otolaryngol* 114:267, 1988.
6. Bardsley AF and others: Reducing morbidity in the radial forearm flap donor site, *Plast Reconstr Surg* 86:287, 1990.
7. Barton RT, Ucmakli A: Treatment of squamous cell carcinoma of the floor of the mouth, *Surg Gynecol Obstet* 145:21, 1977.
8. Barwick WJ, Goodkind KDJ, Scrafin D: The free scapular flap, *Plast Reconstr Surg* 69:779, 1982.
9. Calcaterra T: Laryngeal suspension after supraglottic laryngectomy, *Arch Otolaryngol* 102:716, 1976.
10. Coleman JJ, Nahai F, Mathes SJ: Platysmal musculocutaneous flap: clinical and anatomic considerations in head and neck reconstruction, *Am J Surg* 144:477, 1982.
11. Conley JJ: *Regional flaps of the head and neck*, Philadelphia, 1976, WB Saunders.
12. DeSanto LW, Whicker JH, Devine KD: Mandibular osteotomy and lingual flaps, *Arch Otolaryngol* 101:652, 1975.
13. Futrell JW and others: Platysma myocutaneous flap for intraoral reconstruction, *Am J Surg* 136:504, 1978.
14. Granick MS, Newton D, Hanna DC: Scapular free flap for repair of massive lower facial composite defects, *Head Neck Surg* 8:436, 1986.
15. Gullane PJ, Arena A: Palatal island flap for reconstruction of oral defects, *Arch Otolaryngol* 103:598, 1977.
16. Haymaker RC: *Oral cavity and oropharyngeal reconstruction*. In Cummings CW and others, editors: *Otolaryngology—head and neck surgery*, St Louis, 1986, Mosby.
17. Horowitz JH and others: Galeal-pericranial flaps in head and neck reconstruction, *Am J Surg* 148:489, 1984.
18. Komisar A: The functional result of mandibular reconstruction, *Laryngoscope* 100:364, 1990.
19. Komisar A, Lawson W: A compendium of intraoral flaps, *Head Neck Surg* 8:91, 1985.
20. Koranda FC, McMahon MF: The temporalis muscle flap for intraoral reconstruction: technical modifications, *Otolaryngol Head Neck Surg* 98:315, 1988.
21. Logemann JA: *Normal swallowing and the effects of oral cancer on normal deglutition*. In *Head and neck cancer*, vol 2, Toronto, 1990, Mosby.
22. Marx RE, McDonald DK: The sternocleidomastoid muscle as a muscu-

lar or myocutaneous flap for oral and facial reconstruction, *J Oral Maxillofac Surg* 43:155, 1985.
23. Maves MD, Panje WR, Shagets FW: Extended latissimus dorsi myocutaneous flap reconstruction of major head and neck defects, *Otolaryngol Head Neck Surg* 92:551, 1984.
24. McGregor AD, MacDonald DG: Routes of entry of squamous cell carcinoma to the mandible, *Head Neck Surg* 10:294, 1988.
25. Moloy PJ: Reconstruction of intermediate-sized mucosal defects with the pectoralis major myofascial flap, *J Otolaryngol* 18:32, 1989.
26. Muldowney JB and others: Oral cavity reconstruction using the free radial forearm flap, *Arch Otolaryngol Head Neck Surg* 113:1219, 1987.
27. Netterville JL, Panje WR, Maves MD: The trapezius myocutaneous flap, *Arch Otolaryngol* 113:271, 1987.
28. Panje WR: *Immediate reconstruction of the oral cavity*. In *Comprehensive management of head and neck tumors*, Philadelphia, 1987, WB Saunders.
29. Panje WR, Cutting C: Trapezius osteomyocutaneous island flap for reconstruction of the anterior floor of mouth and the mandible, *Head Neck Surg* 3:66, 1980.
30. Panje WR, Lavelle WH: *Combined external musculocutaneous flap and internal prosthesis for reconstruction of the total midfacial defect*. In *Plastic reconstructive surgery of the head and neck: proceedings of the fourth international symposium*, St Louis, 1984, Mosby.
31. Panje WR, Little AG, Moran WJ: Immediate free gastro-omental flap reconstruction of the mouth and throat, *Ann Otol Rhinol Laryngol* 96: 15, 1987.
32. Panje WR, Pitcock JK, Vargish T: Free omental flap reconstruction of complicated head and neck wounds, *Otolaryngol Head Neck Surg* 100: 588, 1989a.
33. Panje WR, Scher N, Karnell M: Transoral carbon dioxide laser ablation for cancer, tumors, and other diseases, *Arch Otolaryngol* 115:681, 1989.
34. Panje WR and others: Reconstruction of intraoral defects with the free groin flap, *Arch Otolaryngol* 103:78, 1977.
35. Patterson HC and others: The cheek-neck flap for closure of temporozygomatic cheek wounds, *Arch Otolaryngol* 110:388, 1984.
36. Reuther JF, Steinau HU, Wagner R: Reconstruction of large defects in the oropharynx with a revascularized intestinal graft: an experimental and clinical report, *Plast Reconstr Surg* 73:345, 1984.
37. Shagets FW, Panje WR, Shore JW: Use of temporalis muscle in complicated defects of the head and face, *Arch Otolaryngol Head Neck Surg* 112:60, 1986.
38. Shaker R and others: Coordination of deglutitive glottic closure with oropharyngeal swallowing, *Gastroenterology* 98:1478, 1990.
39. Swanson E and others: The radial forearm flap: reconstructive applications and donor-site defects in 35 consecutive patients, *Plast Reconstr Surg* 85:258, 1990.
40. Takato KT and others: Oral and pharyngeal reconstruction using the free forearm flap, *Arch Otolaryngol Head Neck Surg* 113:873, 1987.
41. Tiwari R: Experiences with the sternocleidomastoid muscle and myocutaneous flaps, *J Laryngol Otol* 104:315, 1990.
42. Tiwari RM, Snow GB: Role of masseter crossover flap in oropharyngeal reconstruction, *J Laryngol Otol* 103:298, 1989.
43. Urken ML and others: The internal oblique-iliac crest osseomyocutaneous free flap in oromandibular reconstruction, *Arch Otolaryngol Head Neck Surg* 118:339, 1989.
44. Urken ML and others: The neurofasciocutaneous radial forearm flap in head and neck reconstruction: a preliminary report, *Laryngoscope* 100:161, 1990.
45. Vuillemin T, Raven J, Sutter F: Mandibular reconstruction with the titanium hollow screw reconstruction plate (THORP) system: evaluation of 62 cases, *Plast Reconstr Surg* 82:804, 1988.
46. Wallis A, Donald P: Lateral face reconstruction with the medial-based cervicopectoral flap, *Arch Otolaryngol Head Neck Surg* 114:729, 1988.

Chapter 86

Oromandibular Reconstruction

Mark L. Urken
Daniel Buchbinder

The causes of segmental mandibular defects are varied, ranging from congenital to acquired. By far, the most common causes are postoncologic surgery, severe avulsive trauma and inflammatory diseases such as osteomyelitis or osteoradionecrosis. All of these etiologies result in a spectrum of aesthetic deformities and functional disability that vary with the size and location of the segmental defect. Loss of a small segment of the posterior body or ramus seldom leads to a cosmetic or functional disturbance. Rather, the mandible shifts to the affected side, resulting in malocclusion, but the patient is generally able to function adequately. As the defect becomes more extensive to include a significant portion of the body or the anterior arch, the resultant deformity can become crippling. Loss of the structural support for the tongue and laryngeal suspension will not only lead to problems of mastication and deglutition, but prolapse of the tongue also may compromise the airway, requiring a permanent tracheostomy. Clearly these types of defects must be reconstructed if the patient is to rehabilitated.

METHODS OF RECONSTRUCTION

Many surgical procedures have been advocated for mandibular reconstruction. The most common involves the use of autogenous bone grafting. However, allogeneic bone and, to a lesser extent, xenogeneic bone have been used in combination with autogenous bone with some degree of success. Prosthetic devices, pedicled bone flaps, and, more recently, free vascularized bone-containing flaps also have been used, each having its own indications, limitations, and complications. An overview of each of these techniques is presented here.

Bone grafting in mandibular reconstruction

Several types of bone grafts have been used for mandibular reconstruction, including autogenous, homologous, and xenogeneic grafts. These grafts differ in their potential to cause host–graft immunologic response and in their osteoconductive/osteoinductive properties.

Autogenous bone grafts

Autogenous bone grafts, or autografts, are procured from the affected patient, usually from another body site. Autogenous grafting is the procedure of choice for mandibular reconstruction because it provides viable and immunocompatible osteoblastic cells as well as pluripotential mesenchymal cells that can differentiate into osteoblastic cells in the presence of bone morphogenic proteins. Autogenous bone graft sources used in mandibular reconstruction include the calvarium, rib, ilium, tibia, fibula, scapula, humerus, radius, and metatarsus.

Three forms of autogenous bone grafts can be harvested: cancellous, cortical, and corticocancellous. The form of graft to be used depends on the type of defect to be reconstructed.

Cancellous bone grafts consist of medullary bone and bone marrow. This type of graft contains the highest percentage of viable transplanted cells. Furthermore, because of its particulate structure and large surface area, cancellous bone becomes revascularized more rapidly, resulting in a higher percentage of cells surviving the transplantation procedure.

Cortical grafts, conversely, are lamellar bone struts. The predominant cell type transferred in this type of graft is the osteocyte. Osteocytes rarely survive transplantation because of the relatively long amount of time needed for revascularization of this type of graft.

Corticocancellous grafts consist of a piece of cortical bone with its underlying cancellous portion. The advantage of this type of graft is that it provides not only viable osteoblastic cells but also the structural integrity necessary to bridge discontinuity defects. A drawback to large corticocancellous bone blocks is the slow revascularization of the cortical portion of the graft, sometimes resulting in decreased survival of the cancellous portion as well.

Homologous bone grafts

Homologous, or allogeneic, bone grafts are obtained from individuals within the same species. Obviously, because they are genetically dissimilar to the host, these grafts are a potential source of antigens. Their antigenicity is usually reduced by a process such as lyophilization. Unlike autogenous bone, allogeneic grafts do not provide viable cells. The cells garnered from allogeneic grafts are believed to contain osteoinductive elements that will ''turn on'' the host's pluripotential cells to differentiate into the osteoprogenitor cells. This type of graft material is often used as a bioresorbable crib or as an expander of antogenous bone graft when additional bone is difficult to obtain.

The most popular graft used in secondary mandibular reconstruction is a combination graft consisting of an allogeneic crib (usually a freeze-dried iliac bone or mandible) that is hollowed out and filled with autogenous corticocancellous bone chips.[23] The bone chips provide a sufficient amount of viable material for phase-I bone healing while the crib acts as a biodegradable tray that is replaced by host bone during the remodeling phase of bone healing.

Xenogeneic bone grafts

Xenogeneic grafts, which were popular in the 1950s and 1960s, are transferred across species. Bovine bone has been used extensively in reconstructive surgery. Because of its high antigenic potential, this type of bone graft material is no longer widely used today except in limited periodontal applications.

Graft healing

Bone graft healing is unique. New bone is formed during the healing phase as opposed to scar, which would normally result in other types of connective tissue repair. Graft healing is termed *incorporation*. The quality and vascularity of the recipient bed, into which the graft is placed, plays a significant role in successful incorporation. The bed provides the cellular elements that are transformed into osteoblasts mediated by inductive factors contained within the bone graft. The bed also supplies the vessels that provide the nutrients needed to ensure survival of the transplanted osteoblasts contained within the compressed cancellous moiety of the bone graft.

Radiotherapy greatly affects the quality of the soft tissues. Radiation injury usually causes hypocellularity, hypovascularity, and hypoxia of the recipient bed, creating an environment that is inadequate for graft incorporation. Under these circumstances adjunctive hyperbaric oxygen therapy has been used preoperatively to improve the quality of the recipient bed. Hyperbaric oxygen creates a marked oxygen tension gradient between the hypoxic radiated bed and the surrounding normal tissues. This leads to osteoangiogenesis and invasion of the hypoxic area by blood vessels and fibroblasts, which in turn improves the vascular and cellular components of the site, providing the elements required to support the incorporation of a free bone graft. When hyperbaric oxygen is not available, the quality of the soft tissues can be improved by the transfer of well-vascularized soft tissue such as pedicled myocutaneous flaps or, alternatively, the microvascular transfer of bone-containing flaps that have their own blood supply and do not rely on the recipient bed for revascularization.

Two-phase theory of bone graft incorporation

Barth in 1893[3] and Axhausen in 1907[2] studied serial histologic specimens to better define the process of graft incorporation. They concluded that the vascularity of the recipient bed was critical in providing vessels that eventually invaded the inert graft and replaced it with living host bone. This concept, initially termed *death and resurrection*, became known as *creeping substitution* and remained unchallenged until the introduction of the two-phase theory of osteogenesis.

The first phase of osteogenesis consists of new osteoid formation from cells that survive and proliferate following transplantation. This usually begins soon after the transplantation and can last up to 4 weeks. The amount of bone that is formed during this phase is proportional to the number of bone cells that survive the transplantation procedure. It is therefore important to provide the greatest number of cells per given volume to ensure adequate bone formation. Phase I bone determines the volume of the bone graft. The second phase of bone formation contributes little to the new bone mass. Phase II usually begins approximately 2 weeks after transplantation and lasts indefinitely, as long as the bone-remodeling process continues. This phase is marked by a period of intensive angiogenesis and fibrogenesis, followed by host bone formation. Fibroblasts and mesenchymal bone cells are induced by a substance present within bone that promotes their differentiation into osteoblasts that lay down new bone. Urist[39] proposed that this inductive substance that ''turned on'' the host mesenchymal cells was a protein aggregate of low molecular weight present in the bone matrix. This substance, which later became known as *bone morphogenic protein*, is acid insoluble but can easily be destroyed by heat in excess of 80°, gamma irradiation, and proteolytic enzymes.

Other factors responsible for the differentiation of mesenchymal cells into chondrocytes and ultimately bone also have been described. For example, two cartilage-inducing factors have been isolated and characterized. However, experimental studies have shown that the cartilage-inducing factors alone were insufficient to cause endochondral bone formation when placed in ectopic, subcutaneous sites. Endochondral bone formation did occur when the cartilage-inducing factors were mixed with yet another bone protein, termed *osteoinductive factor*. It then became evident that these two factors must work in tandem to produce heterotopic bone formation. The best source of inductive substances is autogenous bone and demineralized allogeneic bone. The action of bone morphogenetic protein was found to be somewhat suppressed in nondecalcified allogeneic struts. Senn[30] and Narang and Wells[22] confirmed that demineralized allogeneic grafts outperformed similar nondemineralized grafts in terms of earlier calcification and ultimate incorporation to the host bone.

Donor site selection

In a thorough review of the literature, Ivy[12] reported that the first attempts at mandibular reconstruction with autogenous bone were accomplished using long bones such as the femur and tibia. Other sites that have been advocated include the ribs, cortical strips of iliac bone, and the fourth metatarsal (used in condylar head replacement).

Major advances in grafting techniques for mandibular reconstruction followed World Wars I and II, which resulted in significant numbers of patients with traumatic mandibular defects. Lindenman[14] reported clearly better results with iliac bone grafts in 160 patients than with tibial grafts, which were reported in his previous series. Waldron and Risdon reported similar results with use of the iliac bone.[27,47] Chubb,[6] Billington and Round,[5] Ivy,[12] and others reported similar findings. By the end of the World War II it had become apparent that a bone graft with a high percentage of cancellous bone was superior to one with cortical bone, as demonstrated by the increased rate of healing and graft incorporation and the higher rates of resistance to infection.[21] The iliac bone, rib, and calcarium are the donor sites of choice today for free bone grafts to the craniomaxillofacial region.

Iliac bone. The ilium is an excellent donor site because of its ability to harvest cancellous bone, cortical strips, and corticocancellous blocks that can be ''ground'' down using a bone mill to provide corticocancellous bone chips. These in turn can be condensed into bone defects or packed in alloplastic or allogeneic bone cribs. Harvesting bone from the ilium can be performed through an anterior or a posterior approach (Fig. 86-1). The major difference between the two approaches is the amount of cancellous bone that can be harvested. Finally, when a small amount of bone is needed, a bone trephine can be passed through a small skin incision to harvest cancellous bone from the anterior iliac crest region. With the use of an open technique, approximately 50 ml of cancellous bone can be harvested from the anterior ilium.

Both the lateral and medial approaches to the anterior

ilium have been described. It is generally believed that the anteromedial approach minimizes postoperative gait disturbance because the attachment of the lateral thigh and gluteal muscles is maintained. These muscles are active in walking, and detaching their bone insertion leads to a transient gait disturbance secondary to surgical pain and guarding. Marx and Morales[17] reported that 42% of patients undergoing bone harvest from the anterior ilium through a lateral approach exhibited a gait disturbance on the tenth postoperative day. At 8 weeks, 10% of those patients continued to have some gait disturbance. Only 6% of patients who underwent bone harvest from the posterior hip had similar gait problems in the immediate postoperative period.

Fortunately, long-term disturbances are relatively rare. A gluteal gait may develop in a small number of patients usually as a result of weakness of the gluteal musculature or tensor fascia lata. When this occurs, the patient is unable to lock the knee in extension and a limp results. When a larger amount of cancellous bone is needed, the posterior ilium is the donor site of choice. Twice as much cancellous bone can usually be harvested from the posterior ilium as from the anterior ilium.

Donor site complications are not limited to gait distur-

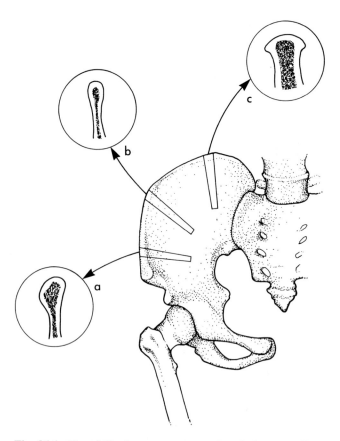

Fig. 86-1. Use of iliac bone as a source of cortical or cancellous bone. Note the amount of cancellous bone available in the anterior ilium (*a* and *b*) versus the amount available in the posterior ilium (*c*).

bances. Injury to the abdominal contents can be caused by inadvertent perforation of the peritoneal cavity by a surgical instrument. It is for this reason that a medial approach to the ilium is preferred by the majority of surgeons. The peritoneal contents and iliac muscle are retracted medially and protected by a Deaver retractor. Paralytic or mechanical ileus is a more common complication of this type of surgery. A mechanical ileus may result from the lateral approach, probably as a result of hematoma formation when the medial cortex is violated and the iliac muscle is injured.

Other complications of lilac bone harvesting include sensory disturbances from injury to the lateral femoral cutaneous nerve or branches of the subcostal and iliohypogastric nerves. The latter run across the iliac crest in the area of the tubercle and can easily be damaged during surgery. Abdominal hernias, although rare, have been associated with bicortical block harvest.

Rib. The rib remains a popular source of bone-grafting material. It is most often used in conjunction with its costochondral junction for condylar replacement. This is especially useful in growing patients, in whom transfer of the growth center may assist in development of the mandible. Corticocancellous split rib grafts have been used as an autogenous onlay grafting material in craniomaxillofacial surgery, as struts spanning advancement defects in maxillofacial osteotomies, and as biodegradable autogenous cribs when used in combination with corticocanellous bone chips.

The fifth, six, or seventh rib is usually harvested (Fig. 86-2). When more than one rib is needed, alternate ribs can be harvested safely without the risk of producing a flail chest.

In children, closure of the periosteum following the rib harvest often leads to complete regeneration of the rib within a year. The advantage of this technique is that it allows for a renewable source of grafting material when multiple, staged procedures are planned.

The development of a pneumothorax is perhaps the most serious complication that has been described following rib harvesting. This is especially true when the costochondral junction also is harvested. The periosteum overlying the costochondral junction is preserved on the superior, anterior, and inferior surfaces, leaving the periosteum on the deep surface to avoid pleural tears. Inadvertent tears of the parietal pleura require placement of a chest tube to ensure reexpansion of the affected lung. Atelectasis, congestion, and even pneumonia are some of the other common pulmonary problems associated with hypoventilation secondary to guarding incisional pain. The use of long-acting nerve blocks reduces the chances for developing such pulmonary complications.

Alloplastic implants

A variety of alloplastic implants have been used in mandibular reconstruction. The use of prosthetic devices can be divided into three major categories. The first category is composed of implants that are used as temporary spacers when a more definitive bony reconstructive procedure is planned in the future. The second category consists of patients who are not considered good candidates for a more extensive bone-grafting procedure or for whom the nature of the defect does not warrant a more elaborate reconstructive procedure and the implant is used as a permanent gap-bridg-

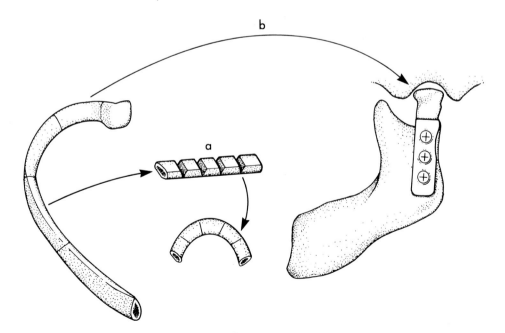

Fig. 86-2. Rib grafting in mandibular reconstruction. *a,* Rib contouring can be achieved through "Kurfing." *b,* The rib and costochondral junction are used to reconstruct the temporomandibular joint.

ing appliance. In the third group the implants are used as internal devices for fixation of a bone graft (Fig. 86-3).

Kirshner wires and Steinmann pins are perhaps the simplest forms of implants used as spacers in mandibular reconstruction. They are threaded into the medullary portion of the proximal and distal stumps to maintain their preoperative special relationship. Unfortunately, adequate long-term fixation is difficult to achieve, and these implants tend to loosen, causing their displacement, internal or external extrusion, and infection of the overlying soft tissues. Although several attempts have been made to increase implant stability by grooving the bone, contouring the appliance, and even adding retention bolts on either end of the appliance, results have been similarly disappointing. If is for these reasons that this method of reconstruction has been abandoned.

Metallic and polyurethane-coated Dacron mesh cribs also are used to bridge continuity defects of the mandible. These performed devices are trimmed and contoured *in situ* to the exact dimensions of the defect and fixed to the remaining mandible using wires, sutures, and bone screws. While a metallic tray is rigid enough to allow for immediate mandibular function, its long-term retention often leads to complications such as implant fracture. In addition, when these ribs are used in conjunction with a bone graft, there is often resorption of the graft, demonstrated by a radiographic "empty crib" appearance. This complication is most likely due to two phenomena: (1) poor revascularization and incorporation of the graft and (2) the stress-shielding effects of the crib on the graft.

The most popular prosthetic device currently being used in mandibular reconstruction is the transosteal bone plate with retention screws. Plating systems have been used routinely in orthopedic surgery for the treatment of long bone injuries. Over the past few years, the authors have witnessed an explosion in the number of plating systems specifically designed for maxillofacial reconstruction. These plating systems differ from their orthopedic counterparts in that they take into account the unique biomechanical requirements of the mandible. Mandibular reconstruction plates should be easy to contour during surgery yet rigid enough to withstand immediate masticatory loading, and they should not interfere with the delivery of radiotherapy.

Stainless steel, Vitallium, and titanium are the metals used most commonly in the fabrication of mandibular reconstruction plates. Titanium is generally considered the most biocompatible of the three. However, the low modulus of elasticity of titanium makes this type of implant more fragile and difficult to contour. This is a critical factor because one of the most important aspects in the use of these plates is their ease of adaptation. Certain basic principles must be followed to ensure a successful result. The plate must be contoured to fit passively over the outer aspect of the mandible, approximating the posterior and interior borders in the ramus and body areas, respectively. If the plate is to be used in the symphyseal area, it should be undercontoured to avoid overprojection in the area of the bony pogonion. The contoured plate is then fixed to the underlying bone using a minimum of four pretapped screws in the most proximal and distal holes. Pretapped screws are better suited for use in bone whose thickness exceeds 4 mm.[25] Tapping the bone leads to a significant reduction in the insertion torque forces when compared with self-tapping screws.[25] Following contour and fixation, the plate is removed and the bony resection completed. In cases in which the extent of the tumor completely distorts the normal mandibular anatomy or a total disarticulation of the condyle is expected, prebending of the plate before bony resection is an impossible task.

Other methods employed to maintain mandibular relationships include the use of temporary external pin fixators, maxillomandibular fixation, gunning-type splints, and skeletal fixation. When a prosthetic condyle is to be used, preservation of the cartilaginous temporomandibular joint disk or placement of a muscle flap (temporalis) to relieve the glenoid fossa is often necessary.

One of the major controversies resulting from the use of these metal implants has been their effect on the delivery of therapeutic radiation to the area. A number of studies have demonstrated that buried metallic bone plates cause a small increase in radiation at the entrance side and a decrease in radiation at the exit or deep aspect of the implant.[10,28,34] Slight variations were noted with different metals. The shape and size of the implant also were found to be significant. Current clinical opinion suggests that the use of these plates in a field that will be radiated does not have a serious effect on dosimetry. The radiation oncologist should be aware of the presence of the buried hardware so that it can be accounted for when calculating the dose and planning the portals.

A final issue that remains unclear is the necessity for removal of the hardware, when plates can be used to fix a bone graft, and the timing of this procedure. In general, removal of a reconstruction plate in an asymptomatic patient should be performed 6 to 8 months following the bone-grafting procedure. This will ensure that enough time has elapsed

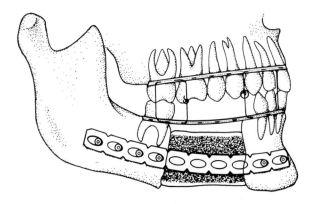

Fig. 86-3. Transosteal bone plate and screws used for fixation of a bone graft to the mandible.

to allow for complete integration of the bone graft. Perhaps the main reason for hardware removal is the prevention of the long-term effects of stress shielding.[13] Other benefits include improvement in lower facial contour and facilitation of preprosthetic surgery, such as a vestibular depth extension (vestibuloplasty) procedure.

PRIMARY VERSUS SECONDARY MANDIBULAR RECONSTRUCTION

There are many issues regarding the timing of mandibular reconstruction, some of which are based on technical considerations whereas others are philosophic. In the past, delayed reconstruction was considered the standard. Avoiding graft contamination by saliva resulted in a superior success rate with little or no infection or extrusion of the graft. However, a number of successful series of primary mandibular reconstruction using free bone grafts have been reported. Obwegesser and Sailer[23] reported a 70% success rate in cases in which an immediate bone graft was used through a transoral route. Strelzow[33] also reported good result in his series, with only two failures in 11 patients.

The major technical considerations are related to the use of vascularized versus nonvascularized bone. The exposure of a nonvascularized bone segment to oral contamination is fraught with high complication and failure rates. This fact alone has led the majority of reconstructive surgeons to adopt a policy of delayed reconstruction. Some clinicians also maintain the philosophy that the recurrence rate of oral cavity cancer is sufficiently high to impose a mandatory disease-free interval before undertaking a complex mandibular reconstruction.

This philosophy has been challenged as newer techniques using vascularized bone have led to high success rates (approaching 96%) despite exposure to oral flora and a previously irradiated site.[40] The predictable nature of this method of reconstruction allows it to be performed in the primary setting. This alternative approach is based on the philosophy that patients should not be forced to live with the aesthetics and functional deficits that follow ablative surgery. Rather, they should be restored to as near normal a lifestyle as possible for the duration of their lives.

The goals of primary oromandibular reconstruction are to reliably, safely, and quickly restore lower facial contour, occlusal relationships, functional lower dentition, and, most important, deglutition and mastication. In addition, through primary reconstruction, the surgeon avoids the major problems incurred in the secondary setting related to drift of the remaining mandibular segment, soft-tissue contracture, and risk of facial nerve injury when the ramus and condyle are reconstructed in a previously operated scarred and irradiated bed.

In most cases of secondary mandibular reconstruction, the soft-tissue coverage has been established and the surgeon is only concerned with restoring the bony mandibular archi-

tecture. Alternatively, primary mandibular reconstruction allows for the soft-tissue lining be restored at the same time as the bone. The remainder of this chapter addresses the techniques that are available for primary reconstruction.

TECHNIQUES OF RECONSTRUCTION

Classification of oromandibular defects

The recognition that the majority of mandibular discontinuity defects are problems of both the bone and the surrounding soft tissue makes the restoration of such defects more appropriately termed *oromandibular reconstruction*. Establishment of an accepted classification scheme to describe these defects is critical for a variety of reasons. Detailed definition of a patient's defect provides a framework for the surgeon to select the best method for reconstruction and permits critical evaluation of the functional and aesthetic outcome of the procedure so that different methods can be compared effectively. In addition, it allows the surgeon to predict the outcome for an individual patient with a particular defect. Finally, classification of a defect into its component parts forces the surgeon to approach each missing part in a more selective fashion in order to achieve optimum restoration of form and function.

Bone defects

The mandible can be divided into different parts based on a variety of schemes. The scheme we devised is based on functional considerations related to detachment of different muscle groups and on the degree of difficulty of achieving a successful esthetic outcome (Table 86-1). This classification is illustrated in Figure 86-4. The condyle is an important component that is difficult to reconstruct. The number of options in condylar replacement reflects the fact that no single technique is universally successful. The alternatives for reconstruction of the condyle include vascularized bone, costochondral grafts, and alloplastic condyles. Resection of the ramus of the mandible causes disruption of the masticator muscle sling. The division between defects of the ramus (R) and defects of the body (B) in the classification scheme is somewhat arbitrary. However, a defect of the ramus indicates a near-complete detachment of the muscles of mastica-

Table 86-1. Classification of bone defects

Defect	Abbreviation
Condyle	C
Ramus	R
Body	B
Symphysis	
Total	S
Hemi	S^H
Palate	P

tion. Body defects extend to the mental foramen. Defects of the symphysis are divided into total (S) and partial (S^H) defects based on the degree of disruption of the suprahyoid and tongue muscle attachments and the difficulty of restoring the contour of the mandibular arch.

Palatal defects are included in the scheme for bone for a very important functional reason. Defects of the hard and/or soft palate that require placement of an obturator interfere with the sensory feedback from a large mucosal surface. Loss of this sensation imposes a significant deficit in the oral cavity that is already partially anesthetized as a result of an ablative procedure and the introduction of foreign denervated tissue.

Soft-tissue defects

Classification of soft-tissue defects of the oral cavity is more challenging than that of bone defects because of the intricate three-dimensional geometry and the markedly different qualities of the soft tissue in different regions of the oral cavity. Classification becomes even more complex when consideration is given to the functional aspects related to the loss of motor activity of the tongue, the soft palate, or the muscles of facial expression.

In 1991 the authors introduced a detailed system for classifying soft-tissue defects (Table 86-2). The oral cavity and oropharynx were divided into different mucosal and myomucosal regions. The soft palate (SP) was divided into hemi (SP^H) and total (SP^T) defects (Fig. 86-6). The pharynx (PH) was subdivided into lateral (PH^L) and posterior (PH^P) pha-

Table 86-2. Classification of soft-tissue defects

Defect	Abbreviation
Mucosa	M
Labial	L
Buccal	B
Soft palate	SP
Hemi	SP^H
Total	SP^T
Floor of mouth	FOM
Anterior	FOM^A
Lateral	FOM^L
Pharynx	PH
Lateral	PH^L
Posterior	PH^P

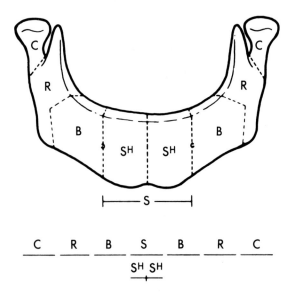

Fig. 86-4. Classification of mandibular defects. *P* indicates defects of the hard or soft palate that require an obturator. (From Urken ML and others: Oromandibular reconstruction using microvascular composite free flaps: report of 71 cases and a new classification scheme for bony, soft tissue and neurologic defects, *Arch Otolaryngol Head Neck Surg* 117:733, 1991.)

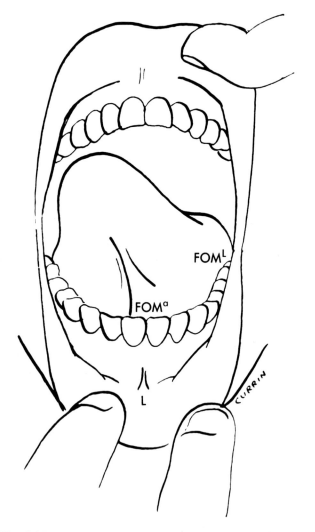

Fig. 86-5. Classification of mucosal defects of the oral cavity. (From Urken ML and others: Oromandibular reconstruction using microvascular composite free flaps: report of 71 cases and a new classification scheme for bony, soft tissue and neurologic defects, *Arch Otolaryngol Head Neck Surg* 117:733, 1991.)

ryngeal defects based on the requirements for soft-tissue augmentation to restore function and prevent pharyngeal stenosis. Defects of the labial (L) and buccal (B) mucosa were classified according to the need to place a flap or skin graft in order to restore normal sulcular anatomy. The same is true of floor of mouth defects (FOMs), which are divided into anterior (FOM^A) and lateral (FOM^L) defects (Fig. 86-5). In addition to restoration of sulcular anatomy, the effect on tongue mobility is assessed to determine the need for additional tissue to prevent ankylosis.

Tongue function is the most important determining factor in the overall success of oral rehabilitation. It is particularly difficult to classify tongue defects. However, because of the propensity of neoplasms to involve the lateral border, the tongue is longitudinally divided into quarters in addition to being divided into the mobile tongue (T^m) and the tongue base (T^b) (Fig. 86-7). Total glossectomy defects were designated *TG*, and resections that left a nonfunctional residual tongue were classified as *T$^m_{NF}$* or *T$^b_{NF}$* (Table 86-3).

Both traumatic and ablative defects may involve the skin of the face and neck. Classification of these deficits is outlined in Table 86-4. The division between the mentum (C^m)

and the cheek (C^{ch}) is based on a vertical line extending through the lateral oral commissures (Fig. 86-8). Perhaps one of the most challenging aspects of soft-tissue reconstruction is the restoration of aesthetically pleasing and functionally competent upper and lower lips.

Table 86-3. Classification of myomucosal defects of the tongue

Defect	Abbreviation
Mobile	T^M
One quarter	T$^M_{1/4}$
One half	T$^M_{1/2}$
Three quarters	T$^M_{3/4}$
Nonfunctional	T$^M_{NF}$
Base	T^B
One quarter	T$^B_{1/4}$
One half	T$^B_{1/2}$
Three quarters	T$^B_{3/4}$
Nonfunctional	T$^M_{NF}$

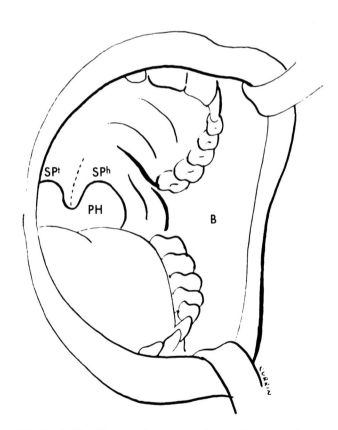

Fig. 86-6. Classification of mucosal defects of the oral cavity and oropharynx. (From Urken ML and others: Oromandibular reconstruction using microvascular composite free flaps: report of 71 cases and a new classification scheme for bony, soft tissue and neurologic defects, *Arch Otolaryngol Head Neck Surg* 117:733, 1991.)

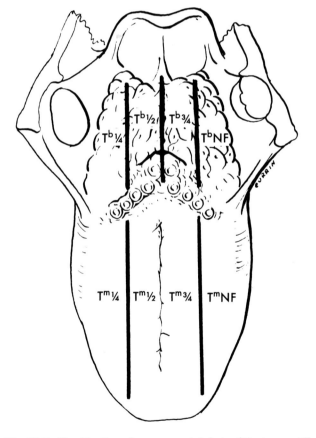

Fig. 86-7. Classification of myomucosal defects of the tongue, *T^m* and *T^b* refer to mobile tongue and tongue base, respectively. (From Urken ML and others: Oromandibular reconstruction using microvascular composite free flaps: report of 71 cases and a new classification scheme for bony, soft tissue and neurologic defects, *Arch Otolaryngol Head Neck Surg* 117:733, 1991.)

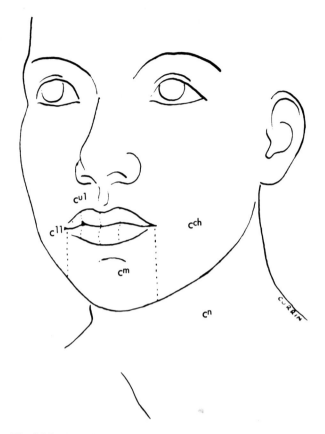

Fig. 86-8. Classification of cutaneous and lip defects. (From Urken ML and others: Oromandibular reconstruction using microvascular composite free flaps: report of 71 cases and a new classification scheme for bony, soft tissue and neurologic defects, *Arch Otolaryngol Head Neck Surg* 117:733, 1991.)

Table 86-4. Classification of cutaneous defects

Defects	Abbreviation
Cheek	C^{CH}
Neck	C^{N}
Mentum	C^{M}
Lips	C^{L}
Upper	$C^{UL}_{1/4}$, $C^{UL}_{1/2}$, $C^{UL}_{3/4}$, C^{UL}_{total}
Lower	$C^{LL}_{1/4}$, $C^{LL}_{1/2}$, $C^{LL}_{3/4}$, C^{LL}_{total}

Neurologic defects

A critical assessment of functional and aesthetic deficits following ablative oral cavity surgery demands that neurologic defects be included in a classification scheme (Table 86-4). The nerves most often involved in an ablative procedure include the lingual (N^{L}), hypoglossal (N^{H}), facial (N^{F}), and inferior alveolar (N^{IA}). When the neurologic problem is bilateral, the subscript B is used. Therefore, a bilateral inferior alveolar nerve defect is denoted as N^{IA}_{B} (Table 86-5).

Table 86-5. Classification of neurologic defects

Defect	Abbreviation
Hypoglossal	N^{H}
Lingual	N^{L}
Facial	N^{F}
Inferior alveolar	N^{IA}
Bilateral	N_{B}

Vascularized bone in mandibular reconstruction

The advantages of using vascularized bone in mandibular reconstruction were outlined through a series of experimental studies performed in an animal model in the early 1970s.[18] Through the transfer of rib with its blood supply as an onlay graft or to bridge a segmental defect, it was found that vascularized bone resists infection and extrusion, has an osteogenic rate comparable to that of other bone in the skeleton, and heals to the surrounding bone in a fashion similar to the healing of fractures. Additional studies demonstrated that vascularized bone behaved in a comparable fashion whether it was placed in an irradiated or nonirradiated bed and was superior to nonvascularized bone.[24] The ability of vascularized bone to contribute both a blood supply and an osteogenic potential at the graft–mandible interface was particularly appealing.

A flurry of activity in the 1970s and early 1980s centered around the transfer of vascularized bone to the oral cavity through a variety of mechanisms. Staged procedures were devised whereby bone grafts were wrapped in regional cutaneous flaps and subsequently transferred as a composite flap once the bone had become vascularized.[7,32] Finally, as more and more muscle and musculocutaneous pedicle flaps were used for soft-tissue reconstruction, associated bone segments were transferred as composite flaps. The pectoralis major muscle flap was used to carry rib and sternum. Rib also was transferred with the latissimus dorsi muscle. The trapezius muscle flap was popularized as a composite flap with the scapular spine. The sternocleidomastoid muscle was used to carry a segment of clavicle, and the temporalis was a carrier for the outer table of the calvarium. None of the regional flaps achieved lasting popularity as a composite flap for the following reasons: (1) difficulty in harvesting, (2) tenuous blood supply to the bone, (3) poor bone stock, and (4) limited maneuverability of the soft-tissue component relative to the bone in order to allow accurate reconstruction of the intricate three-dimensional soft-tissue anatomy of the oral cavity.

During the time that much attention was being focused on regional flaps for head and neck reconstruction, developments were slowly being made in the microvascular transfer of a variety of vascularized bone flaps. The first reported vascularized bone–containing free flap (VBCFF) was used by McKee in 1970 to reconstruct the mandible.[19] It was not until 1978 that the first large series of mandibular reconstructions using VBCFFs was published.[9,20] Eight different donor sites have been reported in the literature for harvesting VBCFFs to be used in oromandibular reconstruction: ilium, scapula, radius, fibula, rib, humerus, metatarsus, and ulna.

Before discussing these donor sites and their relative use, it is important to separate the bone and soft-tissue components of the composite flaps to discuss the ideal qualities of each. The most desirable qualities for bone used in reconstruction of the mandible include the following: (1) it is of adequate length to restore a segmental defect of nearly any length; (2) it has a natural shape or easy contourability to conform to and restore the shape of the missing mandibular segment; (3) it is well vascularized; (4) it has a vascular anatomy that is readily preserved while contouring the graft; (5) it is of sufficient height and width for reliable placement of endosteal dental implants for prosthetic rehabilitation; and (6) there are no significant functional or esthetic deficits at the donor site following harvest. Any composite flap should have a consistent vascular anatomy with a pedicle that is long enough and of sufficient diameter to permit easy revascularization through anastomoses to recipient vessels in the neck. In an effort to shorten the total operative time, it also is beneficial to select a donor site that permits harvest of the flap by a second team of surgeons at the same time that the oncologic surgical procedure is performed and the recipient site is being prepared.

The soft-tissue component of the VBCFF is of equal or greater importance than the bone component in achieving the optimum functional result. Management of the tongue following floor of mouth resection or partial glossectomy is critical. There is currently no way to restore functional tongue musculature following ablation. However, one of the major goals in soft tissue reconstruction is to ensure that the remaining tongue mobility is preserved. This is achieved through the use of a pliable and redundant segment of tissue. A split-thickness skin graft or a thin sensate cutaneous flap is ideal for that purpose. When the resection is limited to the floor of the mouth and the lateral aspect of the tongue, the former technique is quite adequate.[43] When a significant portion of the tongue has been removed, a thin, cutaneous flap (e.g., the radial forearm free flap) can be fashioned to restore the volume, shape, and sensation while preserving overall tongue mobility. Therefore, the ideal qualities of the soft-tissue component of a VBCFF are as follows: (1) it is abundant; (2) it is well vascularized; (3) it is thin and pliable; (4) it has adequate mobility relative to the bone to permit easy reconstruction of the three-dimensional oral cavity and oropharyngeal anatomy; (5) it is sensate; (6) it is lubricated; and (7) there is minimal donor site morbidity. No single VBCFF currently provides all of these soft-tissue qualities.

Rib

The rib was the first vascularized bone to be used in mandibular reconstruction. It has been transferred to the oral cavity through a variety of techniques.[29] The direct blood supply to the rib may be based anteriorly on a branch of the internal mammary artery or posteriorly or posterolaterally on the posterior intercostal vessels. The approaches provide a VBCFF composed of skin and a segment of rib. Alternatively, vascularized rib has been transferred with the petoralis major, serratus anterior, or latissimus dorsi muscle as the carrier. The primary drawback to the use of the rib is its poor bone stock except for condylar reconstruction, regardless of the vehicle for maintaining its nutrient blood supply. Osteocutaneous flaps are limited because of the tenuous blood supply to the skin from an anterior approach and the risky dissection via a posterior approach. The rib has been relegated to a flap of historical interest in light of the alternatives now available for oromandibular reconstruction.

Metatarsus

The metatarsus was the next reported VBCFF in mandibular reconstruction.[4] This osteocutaneous flap based on the first dorsal metatarsal artery transfers a segment of thin, sensate skin with the second metatarsal. Use of this flap for small segmental defects is advantageous because of the quality of the skin; it is the thinnest sensate flap available in the body. However, the bone volume is limited, and the skin-grafted donor site on the dorsum of the foot is prone to breakdown from direct trauma. For these reasons, this donor site is not often used at this time.

Ilium

The length, natural curvature, and volume of bone that can be harvested from the ilium have made this a valuable source of VBCFFs for oromandibular reconstruction. The iliac crest is the only vascularized bone that has been used extensively with simultaneous or delayed endosteal dental implant placement, permitting functional dental restoration. This iliac crest and the overlying skin were initially transferred based on the superficial circumflex iliac artery. However, this vascular pedicle provided a tenuous supply to the bone and a variable anatomy that made it a difficult flap to harvest. Taylor, Townsend, and Corlett[36,37] introduced the use of this donor site based on the deep circumflex iliac artery, which provided a more favorable and more consistent vascular pedicle as well as a hardier blood supply to the bone through both the periosteal and direct endosteal feeders.

The introduction of the osteocutaneous iliac crest flap, based on the deep circumflex iliac artery, was one of the major landmarks in free-flap reconstruction of the oral cavity. Although it provided vascularized bone of excellent quality, the associated skin paddle was not ideal for relining the oral cavity. The skin and subcutaneous tissue were often too thick for accurate restoration of the three-dimensional anatomy. In addition, the blood supply to the skin may be tenuous. It is derived from fine musculocutaneous perforators that run in an array along the inner aspect of the iliac crest, coursing through the transversus abdominis muscle and internal and external oblique layers of the abdominal wall. That blood supply to the skin may be easily compromised when the skin is manipulated relative to the bone.

A second soft-tissue flap was added to the osteocutaneous flap by Ramasastry, Granick, and Futrell,[26] who described the combination of the internal oblique muscle vascularized through the ascending branch of the deep circumflex iliac artery. When first introduced in 1984, this osteomyocutaneous flap was used for reconstruction of the extremities.[26] The attractive feature of this composite flap was that it provided a broad sheet of internal oblique muscle that had an axial-pattern blood supply, improving both its reliability and its maneuverability relative to the bone (Fig. 86-8). The denervated muscle undergoes atrophy that leaves a thin, fixed, soft tissue coverage over the bone. The authors introduced this flap in 1989 for oromandibular reconstruction. In an effort to restore sulcular anatomy and maintain maximal tongue mobility, a redundant split-thickness skin graft is placed over the muscle (Fig. 86-9).[42,43]

The skin paddle is used as an external monitor or to resurface cutaneous defects when reconstructing composite defects involving mucosa, bone, and skin. When used solely as a monitor, it is subsequently removed to provide a more pleasing contour to the neck. The subcutaneous tissue in the flap can be maintained to augment radical neck deformities.

One of the limitations of this flap is related to the donor site, where a meticulous closure is required to prevent a postoperative hernia. In addition, the skin overlying the iliac crest is a poor color match for the face and cannot reliably be placed above the level of the oral commissure without

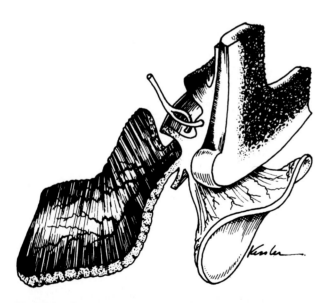

Fig. 86-9. Iliac crest–internal oblique muscle osteomyocutaneous flap. The three major components of this composite flap are supplied by the deep circumflex iliac artery and vein. (From Urken ML and others: The internal oblique-iliac osseomyocutaneous microvascular free flap in head and neck reconstruction, *J Reconstr Microsurg* 5:203, 1989.)

risking compromise of the skin's vascularity. For massive through-and-through defects that require resurfacing of large portions of the cheek integument, we prefer to combine the iliac crest–internal oblique muscle flap with a regional myocutaneous or cervicofacial advancement flap. Alternatively, the scapular system of flaps provides an abundance of skin with extensive mobility relative to the bone.[45]

Scapula

The lateral border of the scapula was introduced as a vascularized bone–containing free flap by Teot and others in 1981.[38] Based on the subscapular artery and vein, a large number and variety of soft-tissue components can be harvested, including the scapular cutaneous flap, parascapular cutaneous flap, latissimus dorsi myocutaneous flap, and serratus anterior flap. The large surface area and tremendous flexibility afforded by each of these soft-tissue components, supplied through a separate vascular leash, make this the most versatile donor site for VBCFFs. However, there are three major drawbacks to this composite flap: (1) the bone of the lateral scapular border is quite thin and does not readily accept endosteal dental implants; (2) the harvesting cannot be done simultaneously with the ablative procedure, necessitating a sequential approach; and (3) the cutaneous flaps have not been reported as sensate flaps.

Radius

The radial forearm flap has been a workhorse cutaneous free flap for head and neck reconstruction for over a decade. It offers a thin, well-vascularized supply of skin with an easily identifiable sensory supply. The radial artery and cephalic vein are long, large-diameter vessels that can be reliably revascularized to recipient vessels in the neck. A segment of the radius measuring 10 cm in length and no greater than 40% of the circumference can be transferred. Despite the favorable pedicle and soft-tissue component of this VBCFF, it usefulness for oromandibular reconstruction is limited by the small stock of bone that can be transferred. In addition, there is a high rate of donor site fractures that can lead to significant functional problems in the hand.[40]

Ulna

The ulnar composite flap, which is quite similar to that of the radius, is a fasciocutaneous flap supplied by the ulnar artery. This VBCFF has both a favorable vascular pedicle and an excellent cutaneous component for oral lining. However, the stock of bone also is limited to 40% of the circumference of the ulna. The reported experience with this VBCFF is quite small, in large part because of a reluctance to interrupt the dominant blood supply to the hand.[15]

Humerus

The lateral arm flap is the third sensate, fasciocutaneous composite flap that can be harvested from the arm. This flap is based on the posterior radial collateral artery, which is a terminal branch of the profunda branchii artery. In most cases, an oval flap of skin 6 to 7 cm wide can be harvested and still achieve primary closure. A segment of the humerus, measuring 10 cm in length and approximately 20% of the circumference, can be harvested safely. The posterior cutaneous nerve supplies sensation to the skin paddle. As with the ulna, there is limited experience with this VBCFF for oromandibular reconstruction.[16] Although the donor site is better camouflaged than the two forearm flaps and the sensate skin paddle and vascular pedicle are quite favorable, the bone stock is limited for functional dental restoration using osseointegrated implants.

Fibula

The vascularized fibular flap provides the longest expendable segment of bone that is available for transfer. Frequently used for bridging long bone defects in orthopedic surgery, it has been modified and used for oromandibular reconstruction.[11] The peroneal artery supplies up to 25 cm of bone as well as a segment of skin along the lateral aspect of the lower leg. The tenuous vascularity to the skin running through the septocutaneous perforators may be enhanced by harvesting a segment of soleus to capture additional musculocutaneous perforators. The straight segment of fibula must be contoured through numerous osteotomies and ostectomies to simulate the shape of the mandible. The bone stock of the fibula is more favorable than that of any other VBCFF, except for the ilium. The length of bone that can be harvested from this donor site makes it the flap of choice for near-total mandibular deformities. The reliability of the skin is questionable and both the surgeon and the patient should be prepared for the possible need for a second soft-tissue flap, either free or pedicled, when reconstructing composite defects with a fibular osteocutaneous flap.

The authors' philosophy in using dental implants is to place the longest possible implant into the VBCFF. The rate of marginal bone loss in vascularized bone graft is unknown at this time. Longitudinal studies using serial panoramic views over a 5-year period are needed to answer this question. If marginal bone loss is no greater than in the edentulous mandible, we will then be able to determine the minimum bone requirements for functional dental restoration.

COMBINED FREE FLAPS

As we strive to fine-tune the soft-tissue reconstruction the oral cavity to optimize functional results, a number of points should be emphasized. Restoration of function does not necessarily follow the restoration of form in the oral cavity. The reconstruction of the tongue as a separate unit assists in preventing tethering of this vital organ. Therefore it is helpful to try to separate the mobile tongue from the floor of the mouth and the soft tissue overlying the alveolar ridge. This can be achieved through the use of a redundant skin graft when there has been a limited glossectomy. However, when faced with a significant loss of tongue volume

and a disturbance in tongue form, the authors prefer to reconstruct these defects using a separate sensate cutaneous free flap. In so doing, the shape and volume of the tongue can be restored and the mobility maintained. To this end, we have resorted to the use of a separate single radial forearm free flap to reconstruct the tongue and an iliac crest osteomyocutaneous flap to reconstruct the mandible and the neoridge.[41] The restoration of sensation to the mobile tongue is a critical factor in achieving functional mastication. Proprioceptive feedback is needed to manipulate the food bolus between the occlusal surfaces as well as to prevent food trapping in the floor of the mouth. Sensation in the tongue base is probably even more critical in providing a warning system for the larynx to prevent aspiration following significant tongue base resection. Although the early results with this method of reconstruction are quite optimistic, its true efficacy must be delineated through more critical functional analyses.

ADJUNCTIVE TECHNIQUES

A number of additional measures are helpful in select cases of oromandibular reconstruction. Lower lip anesthesia following inferior alveolar nerve resection predisposes to the problem of drooling.[46] This is particularly debilitating in individuals requiring total lower-lip anesthesia. This problem can be partially overcome by the use of nerve grafts to bridge the gap between the stumps of the inferior alveolar and mental nerves once frozen sections confirm the absence of neural spread of the disease. The recovery of lip sensation has been valuable in postoperative oral rehabilitation.[44]

Limited ability to open the mouth as a result of fibrosis of the muscles of mastication following surgery and radiotherapy may cause a significant handicap in dental rehabilitation and overall oral function. This may be addressed through physical therapy, brisement force with the patient under anesthesia, and, finally, coronoidectomies when there is evidence of temporalis fibrosis or in secondary mandibular reconstruction cases in which the proximal segment is scarred.

Finally, in the authors' efforts to restore sulcular anatomy at the time of the initial reconstructive procedure, the final result may require intraoral revision through debulking of cutaneous flaps or the interposition of skin or dermal grafts as a vestibuloplasty. The primary indications for doing these procedures is to relieve ankyloglossia, reduce the soft-tissue height over the neomandible for prosthetic rehabilitation, or restore the anterior gingivolabial sulcus, which is most important for oral continence.

DENTAL REHABILITATION

One of the main goals of mandibular reconstruction is rehabilitation of the patient's masticatory function. Restoration of bony continuity without intraoral reconstruction of the denture-bearing surface cannot be considered a successful result. Surgical scarring and the inability to replace the intraoral tissues with a thin, well-vascularized, adherent surface over the neomandible have frustrated surgeons and prosthodontists in their attempts to achieve functional dental rehabilitation. Use of the internal oblique muscle as part of the osteomyocutaneous iliac crest tripartite flap has resulted in restoration of an adequate denture-bearing area. The high success rate of the root form of endosteal implants led to their widespread use in edentulous patients. Their use in mandibular reconstruction resulted in the ability to offer the patient a fixed, stable dental prosthesis. Patients undergoing this type of dental reconstruction are able to function according to objective criteria at levels equal to those of noncancer patients with similar appliances.[44]

Three types of dental appliance can be used in restoration of the occlusal aspect of the masticatory apparatus. The tissue-borne removable denture is the simplest prosthesis. Its stability and retention depend on the presence of a broad denture-bearing area with adequate sulcular extensions. This tissue-borne denture can be either complete or partial. With the latter, the remaining teeth are used to anchor the prosthesis. It is in this select group of mandibular reconstruction patients with residual lower dentition that a partial tissue-borne prosthesis may be used with a fair degree of success (Figs. 86-10 and 86-11). A relative contraindication to the use of a tissue-borne prosthesis is a history of radiotherapy. Xerostomia, which is often a result of radiation injury, creates problems with retention of the denture. Furthermore, these patients become more prone to osteoradionecrosis through repeated traumatic ulcerations caused by the acrylic base of the denture.[8] The use of endosteal osseointegrated implants allows for partial or total unloading of the oral mucosa.

The concept of osseointegration for dental rehabilitation was first described by Adell and others.[1] In a generic sense, osseointegration refers to direct contact of organized living bone to the implant surface without an intervening connective tissue interface. This process results in functional anchorage of the implant to the surrounding bone analogous to that of the tooth root (Fig. 86-12). A variety of materials have been used to make the implants, including vitreous carbon, crystal sapphire, and aluminum ceramic. Titanium screw/plasma-sprayed implants seem to offer the best anchorage. These implants allow for an increased surface area of contact with the surrounding bone and for transmission of the axial load to the surrounding bone through compression along the inclined surface of the screw threads.[31]

After initial placement of the implants using a meticulous surgical technique that protects the bone from the surgical trauma, the fixture is covered by the gingiva and left to heal for 4 to 6 months. Following this period the second-stage

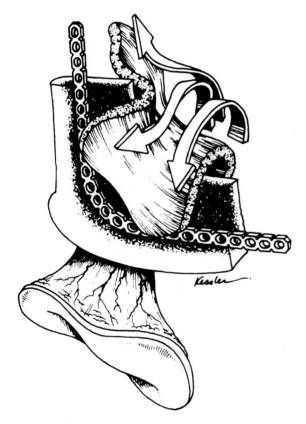

Fig. 86-10. Transposition of the internal oblique muscle over the neomandible allows resurfacing with pliable, well-vascularized tissue that undergoes progressive atrophy as a result of denervation. A split-thickness skin graft placed over the muscle with bolsters permits reestablishment of the sulci at the time of primary reconstruction. In addition, skin graft placed against the cut portion of the tongue or floor of the mouth maintains maximum mobility of tongue. (From Urken ML and others: The internal oblique-iliac osseomyocutaneous microvascular free flap in head and neck reconstruction, *J Reconstr Microsurg* 5:203, 1989.)

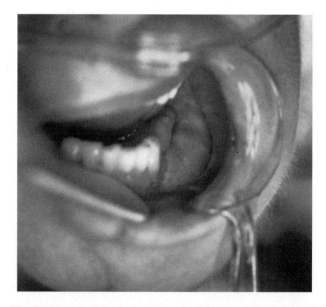

Fig. 86-11. Intraoral view at 6 months following left hemimandibular reconstruction with an internal oblique–iliac crest osteomyocutaneous flap.

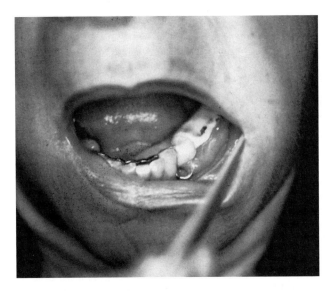

Fig. 86-12. Dental rehabilitation of this one-quadrant defect with a tissue-borne prosthesis is facilitated by sulcular extensions created by redundant skin graft placed over the internal oblique muscle. Denture retention is achieved through the surface area obtained from restoration of the sulcular anatomy and clasps to the residual dentition.

surgical procedure is performed, which involves placement of a transmucosal titanium cuff fastened to the fixture through an internal retention screw. Fabrication of the dental prosthesis can then be carried out. The soft-tissue requirements for implant-borne dentures are much less stringent because prosthetic retention is achieved primarily through the fixtures. Deep sulci are therefore not critical.

When implant-assisted prostheses are used, the load is usually shared by two or more implants placed in the symphyseal area and the oral mucosa. A number of denture connectors can be used, including magnets, ball-and-socket connectors and clip bar–type attachments. The purpose of these implants is to assist in the primary retention of the prosthesis and to help stabilize it functionally against lateral displacement forces. The use of implant-assisted prostheses is popular because they are more cost-effective than implant-borne prostheses (Figs. 86-13 through 86-16).

Fixed implant-borne dentures are the most stable form of dental restoration. These dentures are fully supported by five

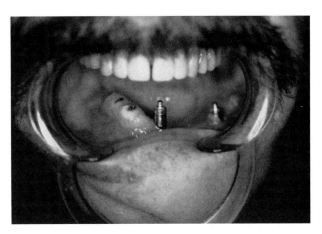

Fig. 86-14. Intraoral view at 4 months following reconstruction with an iliac crest free flap in which osseointegrated implants were placed primarily. Implants were activated and loaded to support an implant-assisted lower denture.

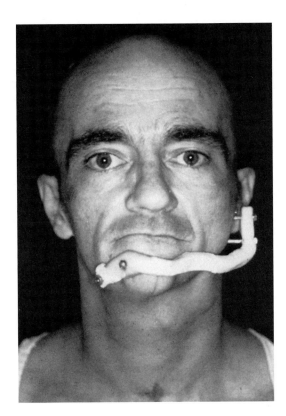

Fig. 86-13. Preoperative appearance of a 52-year-old man following left composite resection and postoperative radiotherapy.

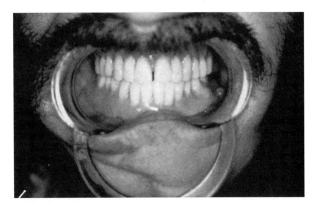

Fig. 86-15. Dental rehabilitation with a functional prosthesis with retention and stability achieved through the two implants.

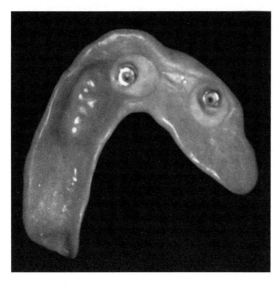

Fig. 86-16. A removable prosthesis attaches to dental implants through a ball-and-socket connection.

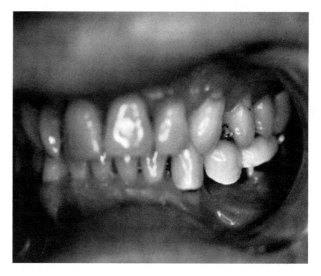

Fig. 86-18. Intraoral view at 5 months following surgery reveals one-quadrant restoration with an implant-borne fixed lower denture.

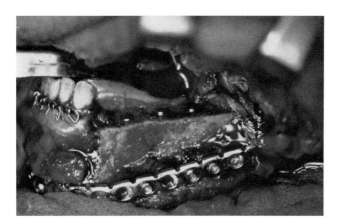

Fig. 86-17. Primary left hemimandibular reconstruction with an iliac crest free flap. Three dental implants were placed primarily into a vascularized bone graft.

to six fixtures, which are attached to the transepithelial connector implants by small fixation screws. These dentures can be removed by the prosthodontist for routine maintenance. The fixed implant-borne denture does not come into contact with the underlying mucosa. It is therefore ideally suited for the irradiated patient at high risk for developing osteoradionecrosis in their native mandible (Figs. 86-17 and 86-18).

CONCLUSION

Tremendous advances have been made in the reconstruction and rehabilitation of patients with oral cavity cancer. However, persistent problems continue to thwart our efforts to restore these patients to their predisease state. Radiation-induced fibrosis of the muscles of mastication and radiation-induced xerostomia are difficult problems to overcome. The loss of tongue musculature is perhaps the most debilitating and seemingly the most insurmountable problem. Functional reconstruction following significant glossectomy is one of the great challenges in oromandibular reconstruction today.

REFERENCES

1. Adell R and others: A 15-year study of osseointegrated implants in the treatment of the edentulous jaw, *Int J Oral Surg* 10:387, 1981.
2. Axhausen G: Histologische untersuch Ungen uber Knochen Transplantation am Menschen, *Dsch Ztshr Chir* 91:388, 1907.
3. Barth A: Ueber Histologishe befunde nach Knochen Implantationen, *Arch Klin Chir* 46:409, 1893.
4. Bell M, Barron P: A new method of oral reconstruction using a free composite free foot flap, *Ann Plast Surg* 5:281, 1980.
5. Billington W, Round H: Bone grafting of mandible with report of 7 cases, *Br J Surg* 497:13, 1926.
6. Chubb G: Bone grafting of the fractured mandible with an account of 60 cases, *Lancet* 9:2, 1920.
7. Conley J: Use of composite flaps containing bone for major repairs in the head and neck, *Plast Reconstr Surg* 49:522, 1971.
8. Daly TE, Drane JB, MacComb WS: Management of problems of the teeth and jaw in patients undergoing irradiation, *Am J Surg* 124:539, 1972.
9. Daniel R: Mandibular reconstruction with free tissue transfers, *Ann Plast Surg* 1:346, 1978.
10. Dutreix J, Bernand M: Dosimetry at interfaces for high energy x and gamma rays, *Br J Radiol* 39:205, 1966.
11. Hidalgo D: Fibula free flap: a new method of mandible reconstruction, *Plast Reconstr Surg* 84:71, 1989.
12. Ivy RH: Bone grafting for restoration of defects of the mandible: a collective review, *Plast Reconstr Surg* 7:333, 1951.
13. Kennady MC and others: Stress shielding effect of rigid internal fixation plates on mandibular bone grafts, *Int J Oral Maxillofac Surg* 18:207, 1989.
14. Lindenman A (cited in Dolomore WH): *Br Dent J* 38:201, 1917.
15. Lovie MJ, Duncan GM, Glasson DW: The ulnar artery forearm free flap, *Br J Plast Surg* 37:486, 1984.
16. Martin D and others: The osteocutaneous outer arm flap: a new concept

in microsurgical mandibular reconstructions, *Rev Stomatol Chir Maxillofac* 89:281, 1988.

17. Marx RE, Morales MJ: Morbidity from bone harvest in major jaw reconstruction: a randomized trial comparing the lateral anterior approach and posterior approaches to the ilium, *J Oral Maxillofac Surg* 48:196, 1988.

18. McCullough D, Fredrickson J: Neovascularized rib grafts to reconstruct mandibular defects, *Can J Otolaryngol* 2:96, 1973.

19. McKee D: Microvascular rib transposition for reconstruction of the mandible. Paper presented at the annual meeting of the American Society of Plastic and Reconstructive Surgeons, Toronto, Ontario, Canada, 1971.

20. McKee D: Microvascular bone transplantation, *Clin Plast Surg* 5:283, 1978.

21. Mowlen R: Bone grafting, *Br J Plast Surg* 16:293, 1963.

22. Narang R, Wells H: Experimental osteogenesis in periapical areas with decalcified allogenic bone matrix, *Oral Surg* 35:136, 1973.

23. Obwegesser HL, Sailer HF: Experience with intraoral resection and immediate reconstruction in cases of radio-osteomyelitis of the mandible, *J Maxillofac Surg* 6:257, 1978.

24. Ostrup L, Fredrickson J: Reconstruction of mandibular defects after radiation using a free living bone graft transferred by microvascular anastamoses: an experimental study, *Plast Reconstr Surg* 55:563, 1975.

25. Phillips J, Rahn B: Comparison of compression and torque measurements of self-tapping and pre-tapped screws, *Plast Reconstr Surg* 83:447, 1989.

26. Ramasastry SS, Granick MS, Futrell JW: Clinical anatomy of the internal oblique muscle, *J Reconstr Microsurg* 2:117, 1986.

27. Ridson F: Treatment of nonunion of fractures of the mandible with free autogenous bone grafts, *JAMA* 207:70, 1922.

28. Schwartz HC and others: Interface radiation dosimetry in mandibular reconstruction, *Arch Otolaryngol Head Neck Surg* 105:293, 1979.

29. Serafin D and others: Vascularized rib periosteal and osteocutaneous reconstruction of the maxilla and mandible: an assessment, *Plast Reconstr Surg* 66:718, 1980.

30. Senn N: On the healing of aseptic bone cavities by implantation of antiseptic decalcified bone, *Am J Med Sci* 98:219, 1989.

31. Skajak R: Biomechanical consideration in osseointegrated prostheses, *J Prosthet Dent* 49:843, 1983.

32. Snyder C and others: Mandibulofacial restoration with live osteocutaneous flaps, *Plast Reconstr Surg* 45:14, 1970.

33. Strelzow VV: Mandibular reconstruction using implantable stabilization plates, *Arch Otolaryngol Head Neck Surg* 109:333, 1983.

34. Tacher M and others: Perturbation of cobalt radiation doses by metal objects implanted during oral and maxillofacial surgery, *J Oral Maxillofac Surg* 42:108, 1984.

35. Reference deleted in pages.

36. Taylor GI, Townsend P, Corlett R: Superiority of the deep circumflex iliac vessels as the supply for clinical work, *Plast Reconstr Surg* 64:745, 1979.

37. Taylor GI, Townsend P, Corlett R: Superiority of the deep circumflex iliac vessels as the supply for free groin flaps: experimental work, *Plast Reconstr Surg* 64:595, 1979.

38. Teot L and others: The scapular crest pedicled bone graft, *Int J Microsurg* 3:257, 1981.

39. Urist MR: The substratum of bone morphogenesis, *Dev Biol* 4(suppl):125, 1970.

40. Urken ML: Composite free flaps in oromandibular reconstruction: review of the literature, *Arch Otolaryngol Head Neck Surg* 117:724, 1991.

41. Urken ML, Weinberg H, Vickery C: The combined sensate radial forearm and iliac crest free flaps for reconstruction of significant glossectomy-mandibulectomy defects. Paper presented at the annual meeting of the American Society for Head and Neck Surgery, Kona, Hawaii, May 7, 1991 (accepted by *Laryngoscope* for publication).

42. Urken ML and others: The internal oblique-iliac crest osseomyocutaneous free flap in oromandibular reconstruction: report of 20 cases, *Arch Otolaryngol Head Neck Surg* 115:339, 1989.

43. Urken ML and others: The internal oblique-iliac crest osseomyocutaneous microvascular free flap in head and neck reconstruction, *J Reconstr Microsurg* 5:203, 1989.

44. Urken ML and others: Functional evaluation following microvascular oromandibular reconstruction of the oral cancer patient: a comparative study of reconstructed and nonreconstructed patients, *Laryngoscope* 101:935, 1991.

45. Urken ML and others: The internal oblique-iliac crest free flap in composite defects of the oral cavity involving bone, skin, and mucosa, *Laryngoscope* 101:257, 1991.

46. Urken ML and others: Oromandibular reconstruction using microvascular composite free flaps: report of 71 cases and a new classification scheme for bony, soft tissue and neurologic defects, *Arch Otolaryngol Head Neck Surg* 117:733, 1991.

47. Waldron CW, Risdon F: Mandibular bone graft, *Proc R Soc Med* 12:11, 1919.

Index

Note: Page numbers set in italic indicate figures; those followed by *t* indicate tables; those preceded by *P* indicate material found in the Pediatric volume.